Patient Drug Facts

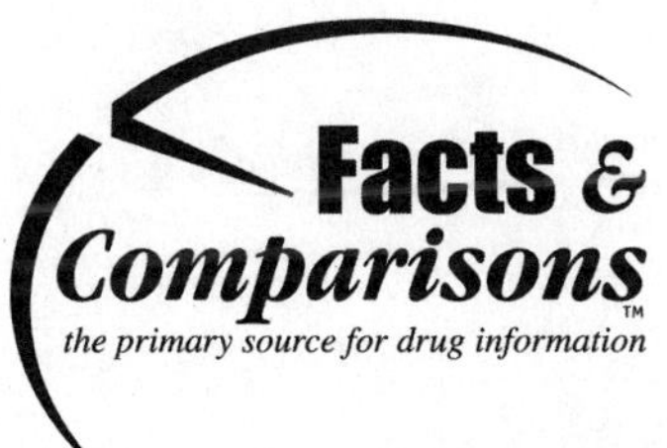

Patient Drug Facts

Publisher and CEO	Kenneth H. Killion
Senior Managing Editor	Teri H. Burnham
Managing Editor	Angela J. Schwalm
Senior Editor	Kimberly A. Faulhaber
Assistant Editors	Rachel E. Jackson Nicholas R. Weber
Quality Control Editor	Susan H. Sunderman
SGML Specialist	Linda M. Jones
Composition Specialist	Jennifer M. Reed
Director, Sales and Marketing	Robert E. Brown
Manufacturing Services Manager	Susan L. Polcyn
Consulting Editors	
Associate Editor	Timothy R. Covington, PharmD, MS Anthony and Marianne Bruno Professor of Pharmacy Director, Managed Care Institute School of Pharmacy, Samford University Birmingham, Alabama
Assistant Editors	Lawrence R. Borgsdorf, PharmD, FCSHP Pharmacist Specialist-Ambulatory Care Kaiser Permanente Bakersfield, California Richard M. Oksas, PharmD, MPH Family Practice Pharmacist Natividad Medical Center Salinas, California Karen J. Tietze, PharmD Professor of Clinical Pharmacy Philadelphia College of Pharmacy University of the Sciences in Philadelphia Philadelphia, Pennsylvania

Patient Drug Facts

Patient Drug Facts, First Edition, 2003

Adapted from *Professional's Guide to Patient Drug Facts* loose-leaf drug information service through the July 2002 update. Previous copyrights 1989-2002 by Facts and Comparisons.

ISBN 1-57439-160-7

Printed in the United States of America

Indexing by Coughlin Indexing Services, Inc., in Annapolis, Maryland.

The information contained in *Patient Drug Facts* is available for licensing as source data. For more information on data licensing, please call 1-800-223-0554.

Published by
Facts and Comparisons®
A **Wolters Kluwer** Company
111 West Port Plaza, Suite 300
St. Louis, Missouri 63146-3098
www.drugfacts.com
314-216-2100/800-223-0554

Facts and Comparisons Editorial Advisory Panel

Table of Contents

Preface ix

Introduction xi

Guidelines For Use xiii

Chapters (A detailed table of contents appears at the beginning of each chapter.)

1. Nutritionals 1
2. Blood Modifiers 69
3. Hormones 137
4. Cardiovasculars 311
5. Respiratories 453
6. Central Nervous System Agents 573
7. Gastrointestinals 915
8. Anti-Infectives 1029
9. Vaccines 1247
10. Ophthalmics and Otics 1307
11. Topicals 1403
12. Antineoplastics 1535
13. Miscellaneous Agents 1631
14. Home Testing Kits 1747

Appendices

The Home Medicine Cabinet A-3

Oral Dosage Forms That Should Not Be Crushed or Chewed A-7

International System of Units A-17

Normal Laboratory Values A-19

FDA Pregnancy Categories A-29

Poison Center Hotline A-31

Drug Names That Look Alike and Sound Alike A-33

Index I-1

Preface

The contemporary health care landscape is changing rapidly. The focus on quality of care and improved health outcomes is growing in intensity. Payers of health care goods and services are experiencing sticker shock, and they expect more value for each dollar spent on health care. Thus, managed care and managed cost are increasingly pervasive elements on one's professional life.

Drugs are the "best buy" in American health care. The total annual expenditure for drug therapy represents 7% to 10% of the total health care expenditure; however, 85% to 90% of patients with acute or chronic diseases get well or better because of drug therapy. The return-on-investment with regard to drug therapy is profound and irrefutable.

Drugs are truly two-edged swords. They have the potential to not only do great good but also great harm if used inappropriately. Providers of health care are being increasingly challenged to do the following:

- Promote safe, appropriate, effective, and economical drug use.
- Assist in producing optimal therapeutic outcomes by fostering precision in drug therapy management.
- Foster the evolution and delivery of highly cognitive, interactive, problem-based, outcome-oriented pharmaceutical care that maximizes the benefit of drug therapy while operating to prevent, identify, and resolve drug-related problems and therapeutic misadventures.

Optimal pharmacotherapy is central to the quest for disease management quality. System failures in drug therapy management are abundant, and there is much room for improvement.

Selected evidence of system failures in drug therapy management is included below:

- Approximately 30% to 50% of the 1.8 to 2 billion prescriptions dispensed annually are not taken properly by the patient.
- Approximately 7% to 8% of diagnosed patients never get their prescription(s) filled, the ultimate noncompliance error.
- The annual *direct* cost of therapeutic noncompliance and drug-induced morbidity and mortality is estimated to be $50 to $80 billion. The *indirect* cost (eg, lost productivity, lost wages) is estimated to be an additional $50 billion per year.[1,2]
- The economic consequences of managing the complications of inappropriate or mismanaged drug therapy exceeds the annual cost of all diabetes care ($45.2 billion in 1994) and approaches the cost of managing all cardiovascular disease ($117 to $154 billion in 1994).

- As many as 28% of hospital admissions (more than 8 million per year) at a cost in excess of $47 billion annually appear to be due to drug-related morbidity and mortality.[2]
- It is estimated that 115 million physician visits per year (17.3% of all physician office visits), at an annual cost of approximately $7.5 billion, are due to drug-induced problems and therapeutic misadventures.[2,3]
- Approximately 140,000 Americans die annually from failure to consume drugs properly.
- Approximately 23% of nursing home admissions result from the inability of patients to manage medication use in the home.
- The compliance rate to prescribed antihypertensive therapy in patients diagnosed for at least 3 years is approximately 32%.
- The compliance rate to immunosuppressant therapy in outpatient organ transplant recipients is only 82%.
- Approximately 24% to 66% of antibiotic use in hospitals is either inappropriate or unnecessary as judged by expert panels of infectious disease physicians.
- Noncompliance of prescribed drug therapy produces a loss of more than 20,000,000 workdays per year.

These facts dramatically reveal, and place into perspective, the need for application of information included in *Patient Drug Facts*. This publication is designed to serve as a clear, concise, and current reference source and information tool for health care providers in optimizing pharmacotherapy, improving health outcomes, and minimizing drug-induced adverse events. The format and language of *Patient Drug Facts* is designed to present drug information in a user-friendly format.

Patient Drug Facts contains vital information on the most frequently prescribed and consumed prescription and nonprescription drugs. The hundreds of monographs provide product information on over 6500 generic and brand name drugs. Proper use of this reference has contributed and will continue to contribute, to improved drug therapy management and health outcomes.

Timothy R. Covington, PharmD, MS
Associate Editor

[1] Noncompliance with Medications: An Economic Tragedy With Important Implications for Health Care Reform. Baltimore, MD: The Task Force for Compliance, 1993.

[2] Johnson JA, Bootman JL. Drug-Related Morbidity and Mortality – A Cost-of-Illness Model. *Arch Intern Med* 1995;155(Oct 9):1949-1956.

[3] Schappert SM. National Ambulatory Medical Care Survey: 1991 Summary. Hyattsville, MD: National Center for Health Statistics, 1993 (No. 230).

Introduction

Patient drug information provides a dilemma. The health care community wishes to inform – not scare – and wants to spend quality time with patients. Whether the learning process takes place in a classroom, counseling session, or at the prescription counter, *Patient Drug Facts* can be instrumental.

Communication courses and teaching courses tell us we must set the stage for learning and remembering with our audience. The same is true for patient counseling. First, we must tell the patient what it is we plan to talk about (state our objectives). Then we must tell them what they need to know (provide instructions) and allow time for their questions and feedback. Lastly, we must repeat what we told them (restate the objectives). Ideally, the next time we see the patient we can ask them questions and reinforce the learning process.

Our goal in developing *Patient Drug Facts* is to make available a drug information counseling tool for health care providers. We want to provide these individuals with a guidebook for answering patient questions, for counseling and teaching patients, and for providing patient information.

Our Objectives for *Patient Drug Facts* are:

1. To provide information for health care providers to tell patients what they need to know about their medications.
2. To provide a standardized, concise format for patient instruction and learning in a classroom or patient counsulting session or at the prescription counter.

The National Council on Patient Information and Education (NCPIE) has set guidelines to help patients "get the answers." These guidelines provide us with the groundwork for our first objective. *Patient Drug Facts* provides the answers for the NCPIE questions and much more.

NCPIE Questions
1. What is the name of the drug and what is it supposed to do? **Type of Drug, How the Drug Works, Uses**
2. How and when do I take it – and for how long? **Guidelines for Use** (and prescription on product label)
3. What foods, drinks, other medicines, or activities should I avoid while taking this drug? **Precautions, Drug Interactions, Guidelines for Use**
4. Are there any side effects, and what do I do if they occur? **Precautions, Side Effects, Guidelines for Use**
5. Is there any written information available about this drug? **PDF monographs** can be copied and highlighted for an individual patient in the course of specific patient-related consultation.

In addition to answering the NCPIE questions, *Patient Drug Facts* contains an appendix for quick reference on necessary household medicines, oral dosage forms that should not be crushed or chewed, an international system of units, normal laboratory values, FDA pregnancy categories, poison center hotline, and drug names that look alike and sound alike.

Our second objective is to provide a standard, concise format for patient education and learning in a classroom or patient counseling session or at the prescription counter. The monographs are grouped together by therapeutic class. The product listings are located at the beginning of the monographs which allows the reader to immediately make an association between the trade name and the generic name of the drug. Common dosage forms and dosage strengths available to consumers are listed. Generic availability is also indicated. After the product list, the standardized presentation of information includes: Type of Drug, How the Drug Works, Uses, Drug Interactions, Side Effects, and Guidelines for Use.

The format is important in providing a guide for patient counseling. The *Patient Drug Facts* format outlines information for a brief patient encounter in a clear, concise manner. It provides the name of the drug, how it works, what it is used for, when it cannot be used, and guidelines for proper use. The information provided in the monographs reminds the patient counselor of important and unique characteristics of a particular drug or drug group (eg, the drug causes the urine to turn yellow or the undissolved capsule may appear in the stool).

We feel we have met our goal to develop a tool for health care providers to use during patient drug information counseling. *Patient Drug Facts* is adaptable for use in the classroom or at the prescription counter. As always, we are interested in your comments and suggestions for future updates and additions.

Guidelines For Use

Patient Drug Facts is a comprehensive drug information compendium organized by therapeutic class. A general table of contents, detailed chapter table of contents, a comprehensive alphabetical index and cross references enable the reader to quickly locate needed information. The following pages explain the organization and contents of *Patient Drug Facts* in detail. All readers are urged to review this information to ensure efficient and effective use of *Patient Drug Facts.*

Editorial Overview

The core of information for monographs in *Patient Drug Facts* is based on the *Drug Facts and Comparisons* database. We have included information on prescription and over-the-counter medications which are predominantly used in an outpatient environment (ie, drugs used specifically in a hospital environment are not included).

General prescribing information is presented in a standardized format and the technical language has been translated to assist the health care provider in effective communication with, and counseling of, patients.

Since the material has been written with the patient in mind, a monograph can be photocopied, highlighted, and used as a tool with an individual patient in the course of a specific patient-related consultation.

Editorial Panel

The Editorial Panel for *Patient Drug Facts* is an interdisciplinary group of established and respected clinicians and educators. The panel includes recognized experts in the fields of pharmacology, pharmacy practice and drug information. These experts provide direction for *Patient Drug Facts,* as well as write and review monograph material.

The *Drug Facts and Comparisons* Editorial Advisory Panel consists of physicians, pharmacologists, and pharmacists. This panel reviews monographs and provides editorial direction for the entire Facts and Comparisons database.

Organization

Patient Drug Facts is divided into chapters. The first page of each chapter has a detailed Table of Contents, including page references, of the information presented in that chapter. Each chapter is divided into therapeutic groups and subgroups according to the use of the drug. Products similar in content or use are listed together.

Index

The alphabetical index includes page references for drugs by their generic name, brand name, and therapeutic group names. Additionally, many synonyms and therapeutic uses for agents are included.

Appendix

The appendix provides supplementary listing for quick reference on the following topics:

The Home Medicine Cabinet – A suggested listing of the basic medicines and equipment patients should keep in their medicine chests.

Oral Dosage Forms That Should Not be Crushed or Chewed – A listing of drugs that must be swallowed whole to be effective.

Normal Laboratory Values – Guidelines for normal laboratory values.

Poison Center Hotline – National toll-free poison center hotline information.

Drug Names That Look Alike and Sound Alike – A listing of drug names that can easily be confused because of similar spellings or pronunciations.

Product Listings

Tables of individual products are found at the beginning of each monograph. Most of the products listed are protected by patent and their names are trademarked and registered. Listing of specific products is only an indication of availability on the market and does not constitute an endorsement or recommendation. Prescription products that contain identical amounts of active ingredients are listed together for comparison. **Listing of products together does not imply that they are therapeutically equivalent or legally interchangeable.** Drug product interchange is regulated by state law. Caution is particularly advised when comparing sustained release, timed release or repeat action dosage forms.

The format and components of the product listings are discussed below and illustrated on the opposite page.

① The therapeutic class and/or the generic titles appear at the beginning of the monograph. All drugs in a therapeutic class are listed in alphabetical order.

② Generic product availability is indicated in the last column.

③ Generic names of the products are indicated by bold-face print.

④ Brand name examples of the products are indicated in italics. The listing of brand name products has been included to provide examples of common names of products to help the patient identify the drug he/she is taking. While we have made a sincere attempt to include as many brand names as possible, we do not purport this listing as comprehensive. Brand name products that are identical in formulation will be listed together in alphabetical order. Products most similar in formulation are listed next to each other. This format makes it easy to compare identical, similar or related products.

⑤ Products are grouped by dosage form. Available strengths of the product are included.

⑥ Distribution status of products is indicated as *Rx* (prescription or legend), controlled substance status (*c-II, c-III,* etc) or *otc* (nonprescription or over-the-counter).

①

278 **ANTITUSSIVES – NONNARCOTIC**

Cough is a normal protective reflex. It helps clear mucus, irritants and other foreign matter from the throat, trachea and lungs. Caution is advised in attempting to suppress a productive cough (mucus is coughed up). The productive cough is essential to the removal of foreign debris. If mucus is not removed from the lungs, it may support growth of bacteria and make breathing more difficult. Moderate cough suppression may be used to reduce discomfort and allow sleep, but do not attempt to completely suppress a productive cough.

The dry, nonproductive cough is a good candidate for theapeutic cough suppression. If such coughs are persistent, bothersome or sleep disrupting, they may respond well to treatment with antitussives.

	Generic Name —③ *Brand Name Examples*	**Supplied As**	② **Generic Available**
Rx	**Benzonatate**		
	Tessalon Perles	**Capsules:** 100 mg	No
otc	**Dextromethorphan HBr**		
④	*Mediquell*	**Chewy squares:** 15 mg	No
	Hold, Sucrets Cough Control	**Lozenges:** 5mg	No
	Benylin DM[1], Congespirin for Children, Cremacoat 1[1], DM Cough[1], Pedia Care 1, Pertussin[1], St. Joseph Cough	⑤ **Syrup:** 5 mg/tsp, 7.5 mg/tsp, 10 mg/tsp, 15 mg/tsp	No
	Delsym[1]	**Liquid, sustained action:** Equivalent to 30 mg dextromethorphan HBr/tsp	No
	Diphenhydramine HCl		
⑥ *otc*	*Beldin[1], Benylin Cough[1], Bydramine Cough[1], Diphen Cough, Gen-D-phen[1], Hydramine Cough[1], Nordryl Cough[1]*	**Syrup:** 12.5 mg/tsp, 13.3 mg/tsp	Yes
Rx	*Hydramyn[1], Tusstat[1], Valdrene[1]*	**Syrup:** 12.5 mg/tsp, 13.3 mg/tsp	Yes
	Nonnarcotic Antitussive Combinations		
otc	*Spec-T[2]*	**Lozenges:** 10 mg dextromethorphan HBr and 10 mg benzocaine	No
otc	*Formula 44 Cough Control Disks*	**Lozenges:** 5 mg dextromethorphan HBr and 1.25 mg benzocaine	No
otc	*Vick's Cough Silencers[2]*	**Lozenges:** 2.5 mg dextromethorphan HBr and 1 mg benzocaine	No

[1] Contains alcohol.
[2] Contains the dye tartrazine.

Type of Drug:
Cough medicine; cough suppressants.

Drug Monographs

Patient counseling information is presented in the text of the drug monographs. General information on a group of closely related drugs may be presented in a group monograph (eg, Antibiotics — Cephalosporins). Information relating to a particular drug is presented in an individual monograph under the generic name of the drug (eg, Antianxiety — Meprobamate). All monographs are divided into sections identified with bold titles for ease in locating the desired information.

Drug Class

A brief statement describing the class of the drug or drugs represented in the monographs can be found in the **Drug Class** section. When appropriate, slang terms often used by patients may be included (eg, Diuretics, "water pills").

How the Drug Works

This section briefly describes, in simplified language, the mechanism of action of the drug(s) represented in the monograph. This section tells the patient basically how the drug works in the body. For detailed information on mechanisms of action, pharmacology and pharmacokinetics, refer to *Drug Facts and Comparisons.*

Uses

The Food and Drug Administration's (FDA) approved indications for the drug or drugs represented in the monograph are listed.

Occasionally, a drug may be prescribed by the doctor for a use not officially recognized by the FDA. These unofficial uses are listed under *Unlabeled Uses.*

Precautions

This section contains brief statements in simplified language derived from the Contraindications, Warnings and Precautions sections of appropriate drug literature.

Two important statements found in this section list conditions in which the drug or drugs in the monograph should be used with caution or not at all.

Do not use in the following situations:

This list specifies those disease states and conditions in which the drug should NOT be used. If the patient has one of the conditions listed, contact his or her doctor.

Use with caution in the following situations:

This list specifies conditions in which the use of the drug may be hazardous to the patient. Consider contacting the patient's doctor if the patient has one of the conditions listed.

Examples of other items covered in the Precautions section include:

- breastfeeding
- children
- diabetes
- elderly
- lab tests
- photosensitivity
- pregnancy
- sulfites
- superinfection
- tartrazine

Drug Interactions

A list of potential drug-drug and drug-food interactions is provided. Drugs are listed by drug class or generic name. An example drug product is provided.

fluoxetine *(Prozac)* . . . . generic name (only brand name available)

phenytoin (eg, *Dilantin*). . . . . generic name (one example of the brand name products available)

tricyclic antidepressants (eg, amitriptyline). . . . . drug class (one example of a generic drug in this drug class)

Side Effects

Side effects which have been reported are listed by organ system (eg, Digestive Tract, Nervous System). Occasionally, side effects specific to a drug or drug class are listed.

Guidelines for Use

This boxed section includes Patient Information available in drug literature. The statements included in this list should reflect standard "Caution Label" ("sticker") language. The guidelines section also highlights other significant information that is important to verbally communicate to the patient.

NUTRITIONALS

Vitamins

Recommended Dietary Allowances of Vitamins and Minerals, 3

Recommended Dietary Allowances of Vitamins and Minerals Chart, 5

Vitamin A, 7

Vitamin B_1 (Thiamine), 10

Vitamin B_2 (Riboflavin), 12

Vitamin B_3 (Nicotinic Acid/Niacin), 14

Vitamin B_5 (Calcium Pantothenate), 17

Vitamin B_6 (Pyridoxine), 18

Vitamin C (Ascorbic Acid), 20

Vitamin D, 23

Vitamin E, 27

Minerals and Electrolytes

Calcium, 29

Electrolyte Mixtures, Oral, 33

Fluoride, 35

Magnesium, 39

Potassium, 41

Zinc, 45

Vitamin Combinations

Vitamin A and D, 47

Vitamin B, 48

Vitamin B with C, 49

Vitamin B with Folic Acid, 51

Calcium and Vitamin D, 53

Nutritional Supplements

Amino Acids, 55

Amino Acid Combinations, 56

Bioflavonoids, 58

Fish Oils, 60

Levocarnitine, 63

Lipotropic Products, 65

Para-Aminobenzoic Acid (PABA), 67

RECOMMENDED DIETARY ALLOWANCES OF VITAMINS AND MINERALS

Recommended Dietary Allowances (RDA) are published by the Food and Nutrition Board, National Research Council-National Academy of Sciences, as a guide for nutritional problems and to provide standards of good nutrition for different age groups. They are revised periodically.

The RDA values are *not requirements;* they are *recommended* daily intakes of certain essential nutrients. Based on available scientific knowledge, they are believed to be adequate for known nutritional needs for most *healthy* people under usual environmental stresses. The recommended allowances vary for age and sex, with extra allowances for women during pregnancy and breastfeeding. The most commonly used RDA values (the "reference male" and the "reference female") are those of adults 23 to 50 years of age. With the exception of energy (kilocalories [kcal]), the RDA provide for individual requirement variations and prevent symptoms of clinical deficiency of 97% of the population.

RDA have been established for many essential nutrients; however, present knowledge of human nutritional needs of pantothenic acid and biotin is incomplete. Therefore, to ensure adequate nutrient intake, obtain the recommended allowances from as varied a selection of foods as possible.

Nutritionists suggest that dietary planning include regular intake of each of the four basic food groups:

Milk, cheese, dairy products — Minimum 2 servings/day.
Meat, poultry, fish, beans — Minimum 2 servings/day.
Vegetables, fruit — Minimum 4 servings/day.
Bread, cereal (whole-grain and enriched or fortified) — Minimum 4 servings/day.

Such a balance, in sufficient quantities, will provide approximately 1200 kcal, enough protein, and most of the vitamins and minerals required daily. A person may increase nutrient and energy intake by consuming larger quantities (or more servings/day) of the four basic food groups. Nutrient and energy intake may also be increased by selecting food from a fifth group, fats-sweets-alcohol, which provides mainly energy.

RDA quantities apply only to healthy people and are not intended to cover therapeutic nutritional requirements in disease or other abnormal states (eg, metabolic disorders, weight reduction, chronic disease, drug therapy). Although certain single nutrients in larger quantities may have pharmacologic actions, these are unrelated to nutritional functions. There is no convincing evidence that consuming excessive quantities of single nutrients will cure or prevent nonnutritional diseases.

RECOMMENDED DIETARY ALLOWANCES OF VITAMINS AND MINERALS

The "official" listings of United States Recommended Daily Allowances (US-RDAs) should not be confused with the RDA values. US-RDAs are derived from the 1968 RDA and serve as legal standards for nutritional labeling of food and dietary food and dietary supplement products controlled by the US Food and Drug Administration. Generally, they represent the higher value of the male or female RDA and are grouped into only three age brackets plus one category for pregnant or breastfeeding women. Prior to 1972, these allowances were erroneously listed as minimum daily requirements (MDR). A second fallacy perpetuated by the US-RDA labeling of foods is the implication that a food is defective if it does not contain all of the officially established nutrients in their full US-RDA quantities. No individual food is nutritionally complete, but several foods together should complement each other to provide maximal nutrient balance and to minimize naturally occurring toxic principles consumed from any individual foodstuff.

The RDAs for adult males and adult females are included in each individual vitamin monograph. The table on the following page presents the listing of vitamin and mineral RDA values for all age groups as published in *Recommended Dietary Allowances,* 10th Edition, National Academy of Sciences, Washington, D.C., 1989.

If you have any questions, consult your doctor, pharmacist, or health care provider.

RECOMMENDED DIETARY ALLOWANCES[1]													
Patient Parameters						Minerals							
Age (years) or Condition	Weight[2] (kg)	Weight[2] (lb)	Height[2] (cm)	Height[2] (in)	Protein g	Calcium mg	Phosphorus mg	Magnesium mg	Iron mg	Zinc mg	Iodine µg	Selenium µg
Infants												
0.0-0.5	6	13	60	24	13	400	300	40	6	5	40	10
0.5-1	9	20	71	28	14	600	500	60	10	5	50	15
Children												
1-3	13	29	90	35	16	800	800	80	10	10	70	20
4-6	20	44	112	44	24	800	800	120	10	10	90	20
7-10	28	62	132	52	28	800	800	170	10	10	120	30
Males												
11-14	45	99	157	62	45	1200	1200	270	12	15	150	40
15-18	66	145	176	69	59	1200	1200	400	12	15	150	50
19-24	72	160	177	70	58	1200	1200	350	10	15	150	70
25-50	79	174	176	70	63	800	800	350	10	15	150	70
51 +	77	170	173	68	63	800	800	350	10	15	150	70
Females												
11-14	46	101	157	62	46	1200	1200	280	15	12	150	45
15-18	55	120	163	64	44	1200	1200	300	15	12	150	50
19-24	58	128	164	65	46	1200	1200	280	15	12	150	55
25-50	63	138	163	64	50	800	800	280	15	12	150	55
51 +	65	143	160	63	50	800	800	280	10	12	150	55
Pregnant					60	1200	1200	320	30	15	175	65
Lactating – 1st 6 mo.					65	1200	1200	355	15	19	200	75
2nd 6 mo.					62	1200	1200	340	15	16	200	75

Reproduced from: *Recommended Dietary Allowances*, 10th edition, 1989, National Academy of Sciences, National Academy Press, Washington, DC.

[1] The allowances, expressed as average daily intakes over time, are intended to provide for individual variations among most normal persons as they live in the US under usual environmental stresses. Diets should be based on a variety of common foods in order to provide other nutrients for which human requirements have been less well defined.

[2] Weights and heights of Reference Adults are actual medians for the US population of the designated age, as reported by NHANES II. The median weights and heights of those under 19 years of age were taken from Hamill PV et al. *Am J Clin Nutr* 1979;32:607-29. The use of these figures does not imply that the height-to-weight ratios are ideal.

RECOMMENDED DIETARY ALLOWANCES[1]

Patient Parameters					Protein	Fat-Soluble Vitamins				Water-Soluble Vitamins						
Age (years) or Condition	Weight[2]		Height[2]		Protein	Vitamin A	Vitamin D	Vitamin E	Vitamin K	Ascorbic Acid (C)	Thiamine (B_1)	Riboflavin (B_2)	Niacin (B_3)	Pyridoxine (B_6)	Folate	Cyanocobalamin(B_{12})
	(kg)	(lb)	(cm)	(in)	g	µg RE[3]	IU[4]	IU[5]	µg	mg	mg	mg	mg	mg	µg	µg
Infants																
0.0-0.5	6	13	60	24	13	375	300	4	5	30	0.3	0.4	5	0.3	25	0.3
0.5-1	9	20	71	28	14	375	400	6	10	35	0.4	0.5	6	0.6	35	0.5
Children																
1-3	13	29	90	35	16	400	400	9	15	40	0.7	0.8	9	1	50	0.7
4-6	20	44	112	44	24	500	400	10	20	45	0.9	1.1	12	1.1	75	1
7-10	28	62	132	52	28	700	400	10	30	45	1	1.2	13	1.4	100	1.4
Males																
11-14	45	99	157	62	45	1000	400	15	45	50	1.3	1.5	17	1.7	150	2
15-18	66	145	176	69	59	1000	400	15	65	60	1.5	1.8	20	2	200	2
19-24	72	160	177	70	58	1000	400	15	70	60	1.5	1.7	19	2	200	2
25-50	79	174	176	70	63	1000	200	15	80	60	1.5	1.7	19	2	200	2
51 +	77	170	173	68	63	1000	200	15	80	60	1.2	1.4	15	2	200	2
Females																
11-14	46	101	157	62	46	800	400	12	45	50	1.1	1.3	15	1.4	150	2
15-18	55	120	163	64	44	800	400	12	55	60	1.1	1.3	15	1.5	180	2
19-24	58	128	164	65	46	800	400	12	60	60	1.1	1.3	15	1.6	180	2
25-50	63	138	163	64	50	800	200	12	65	60	1.1	1.3	15	1.6	180	2
51 +	65	143	160	63	50	800	200	12	65	60	1	1.2	13	1.6	180	2
Pregnant					60	800	400	15	65	70	1.5	1.6	17	2.2	400	2.2
Lactating – 1st 6 mo.					65	1300	400	18	65	95	1.6	1.8	20	2.1	280	2.6
2nd 6 mo.					62	1200	400	16	65	90	1.6	1.7	20	2.1	260	2.6

[3] Retinol equivalents. 1 retinol equivalent = 1 µg retinol or 6 µg β-carotene.
[4] As cholecalciferol. 10 µg cholecalciferol = 400 IU of vitamin D.
[5] α-Tocopherol equivalents. 1 mg d-α-tocopherol = α-TE = 1.49 IU.

	Generic Name *Brand Name Examples*	Supplied As	Generic Available
	Vitamin A		
otc	*Palmitate-A 5000, Vitamin A and Beta Carotene, Vitamin A Palmitate*	**Tablets:** 5000 IU, 10,000 IU, 15,000 IU, 25,000 IU	Yes
	Vitamin A	**Capsules:** 10,000 IU, 25,000 IU	Yes
Rx	*Vitamin A*	**Capsules:** 25,000 IU	Yes

For a complete listing of Recommended Dietary Allowances, see the RDA table.

Type of Drug:

Fat-soluble vitamin. Vitamin that can be stored by the body.

How the Drug Works:

Vitamin A is essential for vision (prevents night blindness), dental development, growth, hydrocortisone synthesis, reproduction, and normal skin.

Uses:

To treat or prevent vitamin A deficiency.

Precautions:

Do not use in the following situations:

allergy to vitamin A
hypervitaminosis A (overuse of vitamin A)
oral use in malabsorption syndrome

Kidney disease: Patients with chronic kidney failure may develop vitamin A toxicity.

Multiple vitamin deficiency: It is unusual for vitamin A deficiency to occur alone. Other vitamin supplements may be needed. Consult your pharmacist or doctor.

Acne: Taking large doses of vitamin A (100,000 to 300,000 IU/day) by mouth has not been shown to be effective in the treatment of acne. Topical vitamin A derivatives (retinoic acid [tretinoin] and isotretinoin) have been found to be effective.

Pregnancy: Adequate studies have not been done in pregnant women. Use only if clearly needed and potential benefits outweigh the possible hazards to the fetus. Safety of amounts over 5000 IU daily during pregnancy has not been established.

Breastfeeding: The US-RDA of vitamin A is 1300 mcg retinol equivalents in the first 6 months for nursing mothers and 1200 mg retinol equivalents in the second 6 months. Human milk supplies sufficient vitamin A for infants unless the mother's diet is inadequate.

Drug Interactions:

Tell your doctor or pharmacist if you are taking or if you are planning to take any over-the-counter or prescription medications with vitamin A. Doses of one or both drugs may need to be modified or a different drug may need to be prescribed. The following drugs and drug classes interact with vitamin A:

aminoglycosides (eg, neomycin)
mineral oil

Side Effects:

Every drug is capable of producing side effects. Many vitamin A users experience no, or minor, side effects. The frequency and severity of side effects depend on many factors including dose, duration of therapy, and individual susceptibility. Possible side effects include:

Acute Toxicity (occurs 8 to 12 hours after a large dose): Headache; nausea; vomiting; blurred or double vision; drowsiness; feeling of whirling motion; bulging fontanelle (soft spot) in infants.

The following are symptoms of hypervitaminosis A (toxicity after long-term use):

Digestive Tract: Stomach discomfort; vomiting; appetite loss; nausea.

Nervous System: Unusual tiredness; dizziness; irritability; headache; bulging eyes; drowsiness.

Skin: Cracking of lips or skin; hair loss; scaling; itching; redness; inflammation of tongue, lips, and gums; yellowing of skin and eyes; face inflammation; sticky skin.

Other: Slow growth; night sweats; bone and joint pain; swelling of legs and ankles; decreased menstrual periods; dry mucous membranes; eye inflammation; blurred vision.

Guidelines for Use:

- Dosage will be individualized.
- Most people on balanced diets do not need vitamin supplements. People with hepatic cirrhosis, biliary tract or pancreatic disease, sprue, cystic fibrosis, or digestive tract diseases who are unable to digest fats are at risk for vitamin A deficiency.
- *Recommended Dietary Allowances (RDAs)* —
  Adult males: 1000 mcg retinol equivalents
  Adult females: 800 mcg retinol equivalents
- Do not take more than the recommended doses.
- Notify your doctor if signs of overdosage occur: Nausea, vomiting, headache, bulging fontanelle (soft spot) in infants, dizziness, feeling of whirling motion, drowsiness, blurred vision.
- *Common sources of vitamin A* — Liver, sweet potatoes, carrots, dark green leafy vegetables, whole milk, butter, cheese, egg yolk, meat, fish, squash, cantalopes.
- *Other vitamin A sources* — Fortified foods, multivitamins, and cod liver oil. Vitamin A is stored in the liver. Consider all possible sources of vitamin A before taking a supplement. Doses of vitamin A over 25,000 IU daily should be taken only with a doctor's order.
- Store as directed on container or package.

If you have any questions, consult your doctor, pharmacist, or health care provider.

Generic Name *Brand Name Examples*	Supplied As	Generic Available
Thiamine HCl/Vitamin B_1		
Rx Thiamine HCl	**Injection:** 100 mg/mL	Yes
otc Betalin S	**Tablets:** 50 mg, 100 mg, 250 mg, 500 mg	Yes
otc Thiamilate	**Tablets, enteric coated:** 20 mg	No

For a complete listing of Recommended Dietary Allowances, see the RDA table.

Type of Drug:

Water-soluble vitamin. Vitamin not stored by the body.

How the Drug Works:

Thiamine (vitamin B_1) is important in carbohydrate (sugar and starch) metabolism, maintenance of normal growth, and transmission of nerve impulses.

Uses:

To treat or prevent thiamine deficiency (a severe form is called beriberi). Beriberi may cause vomiting, rapid heart rate, abnormal skin sensations in the hands and feet, loss of muscle strength, appetite loss, difficulty breathing, pounding in the chest, fluid retention, greenish stools, voice loss, and muscle wasting or rigidity.

Unlabeled Use(s): Oral thiamine has been used as a mosquito repellant; however, effectiveness has not been proven.

Precautions:

Do not use in the following situations: Allergy to thiamine.

Use with caution in the following situations: Wernicke-Korsakoff syndrome.

Multiple vitamin deficiencies: It is unusual for thiamine deficiency to occur alone. Other vitamin supplements may be needed. Consult your pharmacist or doctor.

Pregnancy: This drug appears to be safe for use during pregnancy. However, no drug should be used during pregnancy unless clearly needed. Use only in amounts recommended by your doctor.

Breastfeeding: It is not known whether thiamine appears in breast milk. Consult your doctor before you begin breastfeeding.

Side Effects:

Every drug is capable of producing side effects. Many thiamine users experience no, or minor, side effects. The frequency and severity of side effects depend on many factors including dose, duration of therapy, and individual susceptibility. Possible side effects include:

Nervous System: Weakness; restlessness.

Skin: Itching; rash; hives; sweating; bluish skin discoloration; tenderness or hardening of the skin at injection site (injection only).

Other: Feeling of warmth; nausea; fluid retention; tightness of throat; low blood pressure; fluid accumulation in the lungs; dizziness.

Guidelines for Use:

- Most people on balanced diets do not need vitamin supplements. People with excessive alcohol intake, long-term dialysis, malapsorption, excessive carbohydrate intake, excessive coffee or tea intake, appetite loss, chronic diarrhea, bilary disease, liver dysfunction, or hyperthyroidism are at risk for thiamine deficiency.
- Do not take enteric-coated tabets with dairy products.
- *Recommended Dietary Allowances (RDAs)* —
  Adult males: 1.2 to 1.5 mg
  Adult females: 1 to 1.1 mg
- *Common sources of thiamine* — Pork, liver, brewer's yeast, legumes, beef, milk, nuts, whole grains, enriched flour.
- Store at controlled room temperature (59° to 86°F). Protect from moisture.

If you have any questions, consult your doctor, pharmacist, or health care provider.

	Generic Name	Supplied As	Generic Available
otc	**Riboflavin/Vitamin B_2**	**Tablets:** 50 mg, 100 mg, 400 mg	Yes

For a complete listing of Recommended Dietary Allowances, see the RDA table.

Type of Drug:

Water-soluble vitamin. Vitamin not stored by the body.

How the Drug Works:

Riboflavin (vitamin B_2) acts in a variety of important metabolic processes in the body and promotes healthy skin and vision.

Uses:

To treat and prevent riboflavin deficiency. Symptoms of riboflavin deficiency include itching and burning eyes, lips, mouth, or tongue; sensitivity to light; sore throat; mouth or tongue inflammation; scrotal or vulval skin changes; skin inflammation; red eyes; cataract formation; dry lips and corners of the mouth; or scaly skin inflammation on the face and scalp.

Precautions:

Multiple vitamin deficiencies: It is unusual for riboflavin deficiency to occur alone. Other vitamins and protein may also be needed. Consult your pharmacist or doctor.

Pregnancy: Adequate, well-controlled studies have failed to demonstrate risk to the fetus. In doses that exceed RDA, risk cannot be ruled out. However, potential benefits to the mother may justify the potential risks to the fetus. Consult your doctor.

Breastfeeding: Riboflavin is excreted in breast milk. Consult your doctor before you begin breastfeeding.

Guidelines for Use:

- Most people on balanced diets do not need vitamin supplements. People with excessive alcohol intake, malabsorption, or poor diets are at risk for riboflavin deficiency.
- Dosage for treatment of deficiency states is 5 to 10 mg/day
- May cause a yellow discoloration of the urine when taken in large doses.
- *Recommended Dietary Allowances (RDAs)* —
  Males: 1.4 to 1.8 mg
  Females: 1.2 to 1.3 mg
- *Common sources of riboflavin* – Meats, poultry, fish, dairy products, broccoli, turnips, asparagus, spinach, enriched and fortified grains, cereals, and bakery products.
- Store at controlled room temperature (59° to 86°F). Protect from moisture.

If you have any questions, consult your doctor, pharmacist, or health care provider.

	Generic Name *Brand Name Examples*	Supplied As	Generic Available
Rx	**Nicotinic Acid/Niacin**[1]	**Capsules, sustained-release**: 500 mg	Yes
		Capsules, timed-release: 500 mg	Yes
Rx	*Niacor*	**Tablets:** 500 mg	Yes
otc	**Nicotinic Acid/Niacin**[1]	**Tablets**: 50 mg, 100 mg, 250 mg, 500 mg	Yes
		Tablets, sustained-release: 500 mg	Yes
		Tablets, timed-release: 250 mg, 500 mg	Yes
		Capsules, extended-release: 250 mg, 400 mg	Yes
		Capsules, sustained-release: 125 mg, 500 mg	Yes
		Capsules, timed-release: 250 mg, 500 mg	Yes
otc	*Slo-Niacin*	**Tablets, controlled-release**: 250 mg, 500 mg, 750 mg	Yes
otc	*Nicotinex*	**Elixir:** 50 mg/5 mg	No
otc	**Nicotinamide/Niacin-amide**	**Tablets:** 100 mg, 500 mg	Yes

[1] Some products may be available *Rx* according to distributor discretion.

For a complete listing of Recommended Dietary Allowances, see the RDA table.

Type of Drug:

Water-soluble vitamin. Vitamin not stored by the body. Nicotinamide (niacinamide) is chemically related to niacin.

How the Drug Works:

Niacin (nicotinic acid) is a biochemical entity involved in fat metabolism, tissue respiration, and energy production. Vitamins do not give people energy, even though they are involved in the energy production process in the body.

Niacin and nicotinamide both act as vitamins in the body. However, only niacin dilates blood vessels in the face, neck, and chest and lowers cholesterol and triglyceride levels in the blood.

Uses:

The following information pertains primarily to uses of niacin in doses greater than the Recommended Dietary Allowance (RDA).

To prevent or to treat niacin deficiency. Niacin requirements may be increased during periods of increased calorie use (recovery from illness or injury).

To prevent and to treat pellagra. Pellagra is rare. It occurs most frequently in alcoholics, the poorly-nourished elderly, and people on unusual diets. It also occurs in areas where much corn is eaten, because the niacin in corn is bound to indigestible constituents, making it unavailable for use by the body.

Precautions:

Do not use in the following situations:

allergy to niacin or any of its ingredients
bleeding, arterial
liver disease
peptic ulcer, active

Use with caution in the following situations:

alcoholics
angina, unstable
bleeding, arterial, history of
diabetes
gallbladder disease
gout
heart disease
jaundice, history of
liver disease, history of
MI, acute phase
peptic ulcer, history

Diabetes mellitus: Niacin may decrease glucose tolerance. Diet or blood sugar lowering drugs may have to be adjusted. Consult your doctor before taking niacin supplements.

Gout: Niacin may cause an increase in uric acid levels, possibly causing a gout attack.

Pregnancy: Adequate studies have not been done in pregnant women. Use doses in excess of the RDA only if clearly needed and potential benefits to the mother outweigh the possible hazards to the fetus.

Breastfeeding: Niacin appears in breast milk. Consult your doctor before you begin breastfeeding.

Children: Safety and efficacy in children have not been established in doses that exceed the RDA.

Lab tests may be required to monitor therapy. Tests may include lipids (cholesterol and triglycerides), blood glucose, and liver function tests.

Drug Interactions:

Tell your doctor or pharmacist if you are taking or if you are planning to take any over-the-counter or prescription medications with niacin. Doses of one or both drugs may need to be modified or a different drug may need to be prescribed. The following drugs and drug classes interact with niacin:

beta blockers (eg, propranolol)
HMG-CoA reductase inhibitors (eg, lovastatin)
sulfinpyrazone (eg, *Anturane*)

Side Effects:

Every drug is capable of producing side effects. Many niacin users experience no, or minor, side effects. The frequency and severity of side effects depend on many factors including dose, duration of therapy, and individual susceptibility. Possible side effects include:

Digestive Tract: Stomach distress or pain; nausea; vomiting; diarrhea; indigestion; activation of peptic ulcer.

Skin: Rash; hives; itching; dry skin; flushing; tingling of skin; sensation of warmth; thickening and brownish discoloration of the skin in bony folds.

Other: Headache; low blood pressure; dimming of vision; abnormal heart rhythms; liver dysfunction; lab test abnormalities; elevated blood sugar; yellowing of the skin or eyes; gout; vision changes.

Guidelines for Use:

- Most people on balanced diets do no need vitamin supplements.
- *Recommended Dietary Allowances (RDAs)* —
  Adult males: 15 to 20 mg
  Adult females: 13 to 15 mg
- *For hyperlipidemia* — Usual target dosage is 1 to 2 g 2 or 3 times daily. Do not exceed 6 g/day.
  For pellagra — Take up to 500 mg/day.
- *Niacinamide* — Usual dosage is 100 to 500 mg/day.
- *Sustained-, extended-, or timed-release products* — Take whole. Do not break, crush, or chew before swallowing.
- Do not substitute sustained-, extended-, or timed-release preparations for immediate-release (crystalline) nicotinic acid.
- May cause stomach upset. Take with meals.
- If dizziness occurs, avoid sudden changes in posture.
- Flushing appears frequently with oral therapy and generally begins 20 minutes after ingestion and lasts 30 to 60 minutes. Flushing is transient and will usually subside after 3 to 6 weeks of continued therapy. The flush response can be reduced by slowly increasing the dose (100 mg 3 times daily each week), administering with food or milk, or by administering either a nonsteroidal anti-inflammatory drug (eg, ibuprofen) or aspirin 60 minutes prior to niacin administration.
- Discontinue use and contact a doctor if any of the following symptoms occur: Persistent flu-like symptoms (nausea, vomiting, general unwell feeling); hives; loss of appetite; decreased urine output associated with dark-colored urine; muscle discomfort such as tender, swollen muscles or muscle weakness; irregular heartbeat; or dimming of vision.
- *Common sources of niacin* — Liver, meat, fish, chicken, nuts, legumes, green vegetables, yeast, potatoes, and whole-grain enriched cereals and breads.
- Lab tests may be required to monitor therapy. Be sure to keep appointments.
- Store at controlled room temperature (59° to 86°F).

If you have any questions, consult your doctor, pharmacist, or health care provider.

	Generic Name	Supplied As	Generic Available
otc	**Calcium Pantothenate/ Vitamin B_5**	**Tablets:** 100 mg (= to 92 mg pantothenic acid), 218 mg (= to 200 mg pantothenic acid), 545 mg (= to 500 mg pantothenic acid)	Yes

For a complete listing of Recommended Dietary allowances, see the RDA table.

Type of Drug:

Water-soluble vitamin. Pantothenic acid. Vitamin not stored by the body.

How the Drug Works:

Calcium pantothenate (vitamin B_5) in the formation and metabolism of carbohydrates (sugars), fatty acids, and hormones in the body.

Uses:

To treat pantothenic acid deficiency. Most people on regular diets do not need pantothenic acid supplements. Symptoms of deficiency are very rare and may include fatigue, headache, sleep disturbances, stomach cramps, vomiting, gas, muscle cramps, abnormal skin sensations in the arms and legs, and impaired coordination.

Precautions:

Multiple vitamin deficiencies: It is unusual for pantothenic acid deficiency to occur alone. Other vitamins may be needed; consult your pharmacist or doctor.

Pregnancy: This drug appears to be safe for use during pregnancy. However, no drug should be used during pregnancy unless clearly needed. Adequate studies have not been done in pregnant women taking doses that exceed the recommended daily allowance (RDA); therefore, use only if clearly needed and potential benefits to the mother outweight possible hazards to the fetus.

Breastfeeding: Pantothenic acid appears in breast milk. Consult your doctor before you begin breastfeeding.

Guidelines for Use:

- Most people on balanced diets do not need vitamin supplements.
- *Recommendation for adults* — An approximate dietary intake of 4 to 7 mg/day has been recommended.
- *Common sources of pantothenic acid* — Meat, poultry, fish, cereals, fruits, vegetables, milk, and egg yolks.
- Store at controlled room temperature (59° to 86°F). Protect from moisture.

If you have any questions, consult your doctor, pharmacist, or health care provider.

	Generic Name *Brand Name Examples*	Supplied As	Generic Available
	Pyridoxine/Vitamin B_6		
otc	*Nestrex*	**Tablets**: 25 mg	Yes
otc	*Vitamin B_6*	**Tablets**: 25 mg, 50 mg, 100 mg, 200 mg, 250 mg, 500 mg	Yes
otc	*Aminoxin*	**Tablets, enteric-coated**: 20 mg	No
Rx	*Pyridoxine HCl*	**Injection**: 100 mg/mL	Yes

For a complete listing of Recommended Dietary Allowances, see the RDA table.

Type of Drug:

Water-soluble vitamin. Vitamin not stored by the body.

How the Drug Works:

Pyridoxine acts in protein, carbohydrate, and fat metabolism in the body.

Uses:

To treat or prevent pyridoxine deficiency. Symptoms of a severe deficiency include dry, oily, or flaky skin around the eyes, nose, and mouth; mouth inflammation; abnormal blood counts; convulsions; irritability; or numbness or tingling in the hands or feet.

Precautions:

Do not use in the following situations: Allergy to pyridoxine.

Multiple vitamin deficiency: It is unusual for pyridoxine deficiency to occur alone. Other vitamin supplements may be needed; consult your pharmacist or doctor.

Abuse and dependence: Withdrawal symptoms (eg, loss of coordination, numbness of the hands or feet) may occur after suddenly stopping 200 mg/day doses taken for longer than 2 months.

Pregnancy: This drug appears to be safe for use during pregnancy. However, drugs should not be used during pregnancy unless clearly needed. Adequate studies have not been done in pregnant women taking doses that exceed the RDA; therefore, use only if clearly needed and potential benefits to the mother outweigh possible hazards to the fetus.

Breastfeeding: Pyridoxine appears in breast milk. Seizures in nursing infants have been reported. Consult your doctor before you begin breastfeeding.

Children: Safety and efficacy have not been established for use in children in doses that exceed the RDA.

Drug Interactions:

Tell your doctor or pharmacist if you are taking or if you are planning to take any over-the-counter or prescription medications with pyridoxine. Doses of one or both drugs may need to be modified or a different drug may need to be prescribed. The following drugs and drug classes interact with pyridoxine:

hydantoins (eg, phenytoin)
levodopa (eg, *Larodopa*)
phenobarbital (eg, *Solfoton*)
primidone (eg, *Mysoline*)

Side Effects:

Every drug is capable of producing side effects. Many pyridoxine users experience no, or minor, side effects. The frequency and severity of side effects depend on many factors including dose, duration of therapy, and individual susceptibility. Possible side effects include:

Skin: Numbness or tingling on skin or in fingers and toes; numbness around mouth; abnormal skin sensations.

Other: Unstable walk; awkwardness of hands; decreased sensation to touch, temperature, and vibration perception; drowsiness; clumsiness; sensitivity to light.

Guidelines for Use:

- Most people on balanced diets do not need vitamin supplements. Those on certain prescription drugs (eg, isoniazid, oral contraceptives, hydralazine); who are pregnant; who have kidney failure, liver disease, or malignancies; and chronic alcoholics are at risk for pyridoxine deficiency.
- *Recommended Dietary Allowances (RDAs)* —
  Adult males: 1.7 to 2 mg
  Adult females: 1.4 to 1.6 mg
- *Enteric-coated tablets* — Do not cut, crush, or chew. Swallow whole with a glass of water.
- *Common sources of pyridoxine* — Liver, eggs, meat, whole-grain breads and cereals, soybeans, vegetables, peanuts, walnuts, and corn.
- Store at controlled room temperature (59° to 86°F). Protect from moisture.

If you have any questions, consult your doctor, pharmacist, or health care provider.

	Generic Name *Brand Name Examples*	Supplied As	Generic Available
	Ascorbic Acid/Vitamin C		
otc	*Vitamin C*	**Tablets**: 250 mg, 500 mg, 1000 mg	Yes
otc	*Vitamin C*	**Capsules:** 750 mg	Yes
otc	*Cevi-Bid*	**Tablets, timed-release:** 500 mg, 1000 mg	Yes
otc	*N'ice Vitamin C Drops*	**Lozenges:** 60 mg	Yes
otc	*Cecon*	**Oral solution:** 100 mg/mL	Yes
otc	*Dull-C*	**Powder:** 1060 mg/g	Yes
otc	*Vita-C*	**Crystals:** 1000 mg/g	Yes
Rx	*Cenolate*	**Injection:** 500 mg/mL	Yes
otc	**Calcium Ascorbate**	**Tablets:** 500 mg	Yes
		Powder: 814 mg/g	Yes

For a complete listing of Recommended Dietary Allowances, see the RDA table.

Type of Drug:

Water-soluble vitamin with antioxidant properties. Vitamin not stored by the body.

How the Drug Works:

Vitamin C is involved with several functions in the body, including the following: Utilization of carbohydrates; formation of fats and proteins; maintenance of blood vessels; cell respiration; formation of connective tissues (eg, collagen); promotion of growth, tissue repair, and wound healing; aiding tooth and bone formation; increasing iron absorption; resistance to infections.

Uses:

To prevent and treat scurvy (vitamin C deficiency), characterized by slow wound healing, defects in tooth formation (children), faulty bone development (children), bleeding gums and loose teeth, irritability, easy bruising, joint pain, fatigue, and muscle weakness.

Scurvy is a rare condition in the US. It develops only when psychiatric illness, alcoholism, age, disease of the digestive system, food fads, poverty, or ignorance result in inadequate nutrition. It may also develop in infants whose formulas lack adequate vitamin C.

Unlabeled Use(s): Vitamin C may occasionally be used as a supplement in patients with chronic illnesses, infections, conditions with fever, burns, and certain types of blood disorders, and in infants or smokers. It may be used to improve the general health and well-being of institutionalized elderly patients; to promote healing after surgery, trauma, and fractures; to prevent the common cold; to treat asthma; and to decrease recovery time from cold sores, pressure sores, rectal polyps, and other lesions. It is also used as a urinary acidifier at high doses.

Precautions:

Use with caution in the following situations: Kidney stones or a history of kidney stones

Lab test interference: Vitamin C doses over 500 mg may cause false-negative urine sugar results in some tests. Also, vitamin C use 48 to 72 hours before certain types of tests for blood in the stool may cause false-negative results. Use with caution.

Drug interactions: Large doses (more than 2 g/day) may affect the pH of urine, making it more acidic. Changes in urine pH may cause the effects of other medications to be exaggerated (increased) or may decrease their effectiveness.

Kidney stone formation: Kidney stone formation with vitamin C is more likely if large doses are taken over long periods of time. Symptoms include severe flank pain associated with nausea and vomiting, difficult or painful urination, and blood in the urine.

Pregnancy: Adequate studies have not been done in pregnant women. Use only if clearly needed and potential benefits outweigh the possible hazards to the fetus.

Breastfeeding: Vitamin C appears in breast milk. Consult your doctor before you begin breastfeeding.

Tartrazine: Some of these products may contain the dye tartrazine (FD&C Yellow No. 5), which can cause allergic reactions in certain individuals. Check the package label when available or consult your pharmacist or doctor.

Drug Interactions:

Tell your doctor or pharmacist if you are taking or planning to take any over-the-counter or prescription medications with vitamin C. Doses of one or both drugs may need to be modified or a different drug may need to be prescribed. The following drugs and drug classes interact with vitamin C:

contraceptives, oral (eg,*Ortho-Novum*)
sulfonamides (eg,*Gantrisin*)
warfarin (eg, *Coumadin*)

Side Effects:

Every drug is capable of producing side effects. Many vitamin C users experience no, or minor, side effects. The frequency and severity of side effects depend on many factors, including dose, duration of therapy, and individual susceptibility. Possible side effects include:

Digestive Tract: Diarrhea; mouth sores; nausea; vomiting; stomach upset; heartburn.

Other: Kidney stones; fatigue; flushing; headache; sleeplessness; sleepiness.

Guidelines for Use:

- Most people on a balanced diet do not need vitamin supplements.
- *Recommended Dietary Allowances (RDAs)* —
  Adults: 60 mg
- *Tablets* — May discolor slightly. This does not affect potency.
- *Powder/Crystals* — Dissolve the recommended dose in a glass of water or juice.
- *Solution* — Add recommended dose to any desired liquid (eg, milk, juice).
- Total vitamin C intake includes the amounts taken in the diet, plus supplements. This total should not substantially exceed the RDA.
- Common sources of vitamin C – Strawberries, citrus fruit, tomatoes, potatoes, leafy vegetables, cabbage greens, and melons.
- Store at controlled room temperature (59° to 86°F). Keep containers tightly closed.

If you have any questions, consult your doctor, pharmacist, or health care provider.

	Generic Name *Brand Name Examples*	Supplied As	Generic Available
Rx	**Calcifediol**[1]		
	Calderol	**Capsules:** 20 mcg, 50 mcg	No
Rx	**Calcitriol**[1]		
	Rocaltrol	**Capsules:** 0.25 mcg, 0.5 mcg	No
	Rocaltrol	**Oral solution:** 1 mcg/mL	No
	Calcijex	**Injection:** 1 mcg/mL, 2 mcg/mL	No
otc	**Cholecalciferol (D_3)**[1]		
	Delta D3, Vitamin D3	**Tablets:** 400 IU, 1000 IU	Yes
Rx	**Dihydrotachysterol (DHT)**[2]		
	Hytakerol	**Capsules:** 0.125 mg	No
	DHT	**Tablets:** 0.125 mg, 0.2 mg, 0.4 mg	No
	DHT Intensol	**Solution:** 0.2 mg/mL	No
	Ergocalciferol (D_2)[1]		
otc	*Calciferol Drops*	**Solution:** 200 IU/drop	No
otc	*Drisdol*	**Solution:** 200 IU/drop	No
otc	*Delta-D2*	**Tablets:** 400 IU	Yes
Rx	*Drisdol*[3]	**Capsules:** 50,000 IU	No
Rx	*Calciferol*	**Injection, in oil:** 500,000 IU/mL	No
Rx	**Paricalcitol**[4]		
	Zemplar	**Injection:** 5 mcg/mL	No

[1] 1 mg = 40,000 IU.
[2] 1 mg DHT is approximately equal to 3 mg vitamin D_2, which is equal to 120,000 IU.
[3] Contains tartrazine.
[4] Synthetic vitamin D analog.

For a complete listing of Recommended Dietary Allowances, see the RDA table.

Type of Drug:

Fat-soluble vitamin. Essential vitamin that can be stored by the body. Natural supply of vitamin D depends largely upon exposure to the ultraviolet (UV) light of the sun.

How the Drug Works:

Vitamin D promotes proper absorption and use of calcium and phosphate by the body and normal bone development and maintenance. It also helps regulate parathyroid hormone levels and is involved in magnesium metabolism.

Uses:

As a dietary supplement (cholecalciferol).

To prevent and treat rickets, a vitamin D deficiency disease characterized by weak bones, deformed skeleton, bowed legs, deformed spine, "potbelly" appearance, sometimes flat feet, stunted growth, soft bones, and deformed joints (ergocalciferol, cholecalciferol).

To help regulate levels of parathyroid hormone (DHT, calcitriol, calcifediol, ergocalciferol, paricalcitol).

To prevent and treat postsurgical and other types of tetany (severe muscle spasms due to low calcium levels) (DHT).

To treat low calcium levels and bone disease in patients on chronic kidney dialysis (calcitriol, calcifediol, ergocalciferol).

Precautions:

Do not use in the following situations:

abnormal sensitivity to effects of vitamin D (eg, become toxic at lower doses)
allergy to vitamin D or any of its ingredients
high calcium levels
kidney function, decreased (ergocalciferol)
malabsorption syndrome (oral forms)
vitamin D toxicity

Use with caution in the following situations:

bone lesions
coronary artery disease (in elderly patients)
hypoparathyroidism
kidney disease
kidney stones

Hypercalcemia: Instruct patients to discontinue therapy immediately and contact their physician if signs or symptoms of high blood calcium develop. Symptoms may include the following: Weakness; headache; tiredness; vomiting; nausea; dry mouth; constipation; muscle pain; bone pain; metallic taste; increased urinary frequency; increased thirst; loss of appetite; weight loss; increased urinary frequency at night; eye inflammation; any other unusual symptoms.

Pregnancy: Adequate studies have not been done in pregnant women. Use only if clearly needed and potential benefits outweigh the possible hazards to the fetus.

Breastfeeding: Vitamin D is excreted in breast milk. Do not breastfeed while using calcitriol. Consult your doctor before using other vitamin D supplements during breastfeeding.

Children: Safety and effectiveness in children of doses exceeding the RDA and in children undergoing dialysis have not been established.

Lab tests will be required to monitor therapy. Tests may include blood calcium, magnesium, and phosphorus; kidney function; and urine tests.

Tartrazine: Some of these products may contain the dye tartrazine (FD&C Yellow No. 5), which can cause allergic reactions in certain individuals. Check the package label when available or consult your doctor or pharmacist.

Drug Interactions:

Tell your doctor or pharmacist if you are taking or planning to take any over-the-counter or prescription medications with vitamin D. Doses of 1 or both drugs may need to be modified or a different drug may need to be prescribed. The following drugs and drug classes interact with vitamin D.

cholestyramine (eg, *Questran*)
digitalis glycosides (eg, digoxin)
magnesium-containing antacids (eg, *Maalox*)
mineral oil
phosphate or vitamin D-related compounds
thiazide diuretics (eg, hydrochlorothiazide)
verapamil (eg, *Calan*)

Side Effects:

Every drug is capable of producing side effects. Many vitamin D users experience no, or minor, side effects. The frequency and severity of side effects depend on many factors, including dose, duration of therapy, and individual susceptibility. Possible side effects include:

Digestive Tract: Loss of appetite; stomach pain or cramps; constipation; digestive tract bleeding; excessive thirst; nausea; vomiting; dry mouth; metallic taste.

Nervous System: Weakness; irritability; headache; drowsiness.

Renal: Increased urinary frequency; increased urination at night.

Other: Muscle or bone pain; increased blood pressure; itching; runny nose; sensitivity to light; weight loss; decreased sex drive; pneumonia; chills; fever; flu-like symptoms; irregular heartbeat; fluid retention; increased body temperature; pounding in the chest.

Guidelines for Use:

- Dosage will be individualized. Do not change the dose or stop taking unless advised to do so by your doctor.
- *Recommended Dietary Allowances (RDAs)* —
  Adults (24 years of age or older): 200 IU
- *Calciferol in oil injection* - For intramuscular administration only. Do not administer intravenously or subcutaneously.
- *Common sources of vitamin D* – Fortified milk and milk products, eggs, fish liver oils (eg, cod oil), livers of animals that eat fish.
- The total amount of vitamin D taken each day includes both dietary intake and supplements. Do not take more than the RDA unless advised to do so by your doctor.
- Carefully measure liquid doses of vitamin D-containing products because some doseforms are very concentrated. Do not exceed recommended volume.
- Eating a balanced diet and periodic exposure to sunlight usually satisfies normal vitamin D requirements. Never use vitamin supplements as a substitute for a balanced diet.
- Compliance with dosage instructions, diet, and calcium supplementation are essential, especially in patients undergoing dialysis.
- Swallow tablets and capsules whole. Do not crush or chew.
- Drink plenty of fluids while taking vitamin D.
- Overdosage of any form of vitamin D is dangerous. Discontinue therapy and notify your doctor if any of the following occurs: Weakness, drowsiness, headache, metallic taste, loss of appetite, weight loss, nausea, vomiting, stomach pain or cramps, diarrhea, constipation, excessive thirst, excessive urine output, dry mouth, muscle or bone pain. These may be caused by high blood calcium levels.
- Avoid use of nonprescription drugs, including magnesium-containing antacids, multivitamins containing vitamin D, and natural products unless such use has been discussed with your doctor.
- Patients with digestive tract, liver, or biliary disease associated with vitamin D malabsorption require intramuscular administration of vitamin D.
- The effects of dihydrotachysterol can last for up to 1 month after stopping treatment. The effects of ergocalciferol can last for 2 or more months after stopping treatment.
- Avoid simultaneous use of mineral oil while taking vitamin D products.
- Lab tests may be required to monitor treatment. Be sure to keep appointments.
- Store at controlled room temperature (59° to 86°F). Protect from heat and light.

	Generic Name *Brand Name Examples*	Supplied As	Generic Available
otc	**Vitamin E**[1]		
	Dry E 400, E-Pherol	**Tablets:** 100 IU, 200 IU, 400 IU, 500 IU, 800 IU	Yes
	Vitamin E 400 I.U., Vitamin E 1000 I.U., Vita-Plus E	**Capsules:** 200 IU, 400 IU, 1000 IU	Yes
	d'ALPHA E 400 , d'ALPHA E 1000, E-400[2]*, Formula E-400, Mixed E 400, Mixed E 1000*	**Softgels:** 100 IU, 200 IU, 400 IU, 600 IU, 1000 IU	Yes
	Aquavit-E	**Drops:** 15 IU/0.3 mL	No
	Vitamin E	**Liquid:** 1150 IU/1.25 mL	Yes

[1] The exact number of IU per mg of vitamin E varies depending on the vitamin E source. One mg of vitamin E equals 0.9 to 1.5 IU of vitamin E.
[2] Also available with 50 mcg of selenium.

For a complete listing of Recommended Dietary Allowances, see the RDA table.

Type of Drug:

Fat-soluble vitamin; essential vitamin with antioxidant properties.

How the Drug Works:

Vitamin E prevents destructive "oxidation" reactions in the body. It helps red blood cells maintain their integrity, decreases platelet clumping, and may be an important biochemical component of certain human enzyme systems.

Uses:

A dietary supplement used to treat or prevent vitamin E deficiency.

Unlabeled Use(s): Occasionally doctors may prescribe vitamin E for premature infants to prevent bleeding in the brain and for those on oxygen therapy to reduce the possibility of lung and eye problems. It has also been used in cancer, skin problems, night leg cramps, sexual problems, heart disease, aging, premenstrual problems, and to increase athletic performance.

Precautions:

Do not use in the following situations: Intravenously.

Multiple vitamin deficiencies: It is unusual for vitamin E deficiency to occur alone. Other vitamins may be needed; consult your pharmacist or doctor.

Breastfeeding: Vitamin E appears in breast milk. Consult your doctor before you begin breastfeeding.

Drug Interactions:

Tell your doctor or pharmacist if you are taking or if you are planning to take any over- the-counter or prescription medications with vitamin E. Doses of 1 or both drugs may need to be modified or a different drug may need to be prescribed. Oral anticoagulants (eg, *Coumadin*) interact with vitamin E.

Side Effects:

Every drug is capable of producing side effects. Many vitamin E users experience no, or minor, side effects. The frequency and severity of side effects depend on many factors including dose, duration of therapy, and individual susceptibility. Possible symptoms of toxicity include: Nausea; gas; diarrhea; unusual tiredness or weakness; stomach cramps; headache; blurred vision; breast enlargement.

Guidelines for Use:

- Most people on balanced diets do not need vitamin supplements. People with cystic fibrosis or gastrointestinal diseases who are unable to digest or absorb fats, premature or underfed infants, and people with specific blood disorders may be at risk for vitamin E deficiency.
- *Recommended Dietary Allowances (RDAs)* —
  Adult males: 15 IU
  Adult females: 12 IU
- *Vitamin E drops* — Use included marked dropper to measure dose. Drops may be administered directly on the tongue or mixed with liquid (eg, milk, formula, juice) or semi-liquid food (eg, applesauce, cereal).
- Swallow capsules whole. Do not crush or chew.
- *Common sources of vitamin E* – Vegetable oils, seeds, corn, soy, margarine, leafy vegetables, milk, eggs, meat, whole wheat flour, and nuts. Consider all possible dietary sources of vitamin E before using a supplement.
- Store in a dry, air-tight container.

If you have any questions, consult your doctor, pharmacist, or health care provider.

	Generic Name *Brand Name Examples*	Supplied As (mg of elemental calcium/dose unit)	Generic Available
otc	**Calcium Glubionate** (6.5% Ca)		
	Calcionate, Calciquid	**Syrup:** 115 mg Ca/5 mL	No
otc	**Calcium Gluconate** (9.3% Ca)	**Tablets:** 50 mg Ca, 60 mg Ca, 90 mg Ca	Yes
		Powder: 89 mg Ca/g	Yes
otc	**Calcium Lactate** (13% Ca)	**Tablets:** 84 mg Ca	Yes
		Capsules: 96 mg Ca	
otc	**Calcium Citrate** (21% Ca)		
	Cal-Citrate, Citracal, Citracal Caplets + D	**Tablets:** 200 mg Ca, 250 mg Ca, 315 mg Ca	Yes
	Citracal Liquitab[1]	**Tablets, effervescent:** 500 mg Ca	No
otc	**Dibasic Calcium Phosphate Dihydrate** (23% Ca)	**Tablets:** 112 mg Ca	Yes
otc	**Tribasic Calcium Phosphate** (39% Ca)		
	Posture, Posture-D	**Tablets:** 600 mg Ca	No
	Posture-D	**Tablets, chewable:** 600 mg Ca	No
otc	**Calcium Carbonate** (40% Ca)	**Powder:** 800 mg Ca/g	Yes
	Cal-Carb Forte, Caltrate 600, Caltrate 600+D, Caltrate 600 Plus, Caltrate 600+Soy, Nephro-Calci, OsCal 250+D[2]*, OsCal 500*[2]*, OsCal 500+D*[2]*, Oysco 500*[2]*, Oyst-Cal 500*[2]*, Oyst-Cal-D*[2]*, Oyst-Cal-D 500*[2]*, Oystercal 500, Oystercal-D 250*	**Tablets:** 250 mg Ca, 500 mg Ca, 600 mg Ca	Yes
	Florical	**Tablets:** 145 mg Ca with 8.3 mg sodium fluoride	No

Generic Name *Brand Name Examples*	Supplied As (mg of elemental calcium/dose unit)	Generic Available
Alka-Mints, Amitone, Cal-Carb Forte, Cal-Mint, Cal-ciChew, Caltrate 600 Plus, Chooz[1]*, Dicarbosil, Malla-mint, OsCal, Rolaids*[2]*, Tums, Tums 500, Tums E-X*[2]*, Tums E-X Sugar Free, Tums Ultra*[2]	**Tablets, chewable:** 168 mg Ca, 200 mg Ca, 220 mg Ca, 260 mg Ca, 300 mg Ca, 340 mg Ca, 350 mg Ca, 400 mg Ca, 500 mg Ca, 600 mg Ca	Yes
Super Calcium 1200	**Capsules:** 600 mg Ca	No
Florical	**Capsules:** 145 mg Ca with 8.3 mg sodium fluoride	No

[1] Contains phenylalanine.
[2] Contains tartrazine.

The amount of calcium provided by a product varies with the calcium salt (formulation) contained in the product. For example, the salt calcium glubionate contains 6.5% calcium (Ca), while the calcium carbonate formulations are 40% Ca. The percentage of calcium represents elemental, or active calcium. Therefore, 1500 mg of calcium glubionate only contains 98 mg of elemental calcium, while 1500 mg of calcium carbonate contains 600 mg of elemental calcium.

For a complete listing of Recommended Dietary Allowances, see the RDA table.

Type of Drug:

Mineral; calcium supplement.

How the Drug Works:

Calcium is the fifth most abundant element in the body. The majority is in the bones. It is essential for normal development and maintenance of bones; normal functioning of nerves and muscles; normal heart functioning; normal blood clotting; and normal functioning of a variety of cells, glands, and enzyme systems.

Uses:

As a dietary supplement, especially at times when dietary intake may be inadequate (eg, children and teens, the elderly, during pregnancy and breastfeeding, after menopause, patients with kidney failure).

To treat and prevent calcium deficiency (eg, osteoporosis, rickets, osteomalacia, hypoparathyroidism).

To treat muscle cramps caused by low calcium levels.

Unlabeled Use(s): Doctors may occasionally prescribe calcium for high blood pressure in patients with calcium deficiency.

Precautions:

Do not use in the following situations:

high blood calcium levels
kidney stones
low blood phosphate levels

Use with caution in the following situations:

constipation
kidney disease (calcium citrate only)
low stomach acid levels (all except calcium lactate)

Pregnancy and breastfeeding: Do not take more than the RDA without first contacting your doctor.

Adequate calcium intake: Adequate calcium intake is particularly important during periods of bone growth in childhood and adolescence, and during pregnancy and breastfeeding. An adequate intake of calcium is also necessary in adults, especially those > 40 years of age, to help prevent the development of osteoporosis.

Vitamin D: Vitamin D facilitates the absorption of calcium from the digestive tract. A vitamin D deficiency can interfere with calcium balance in the body. This is a concern for the elderly because of limited exposure to the sun, reduced intake of dairy products, and decreased absorption because of the natural aging process. Consult your doctor before increasing vitamin D intake above the RDA.

Phenylketonuria: Some of these products contain phenylalanine. Check package label when available or consult your doctor or pharmacist.

Lab tests may be required to monitor therapy. Tests may include kidney function and calcium and phosphate blood levels.

Tartrazine: Some of these products contain tartrazine (FD&C Yellow No. 5), which may cause allergic reactions in certain individuals. Check package label when available or consult your doctor or pharmacist.

Drug Interactions:

Tell your doctor or pharmacist if you are taking or if you are planning to take any over-the-counter or prescription medications with calcium. Doses of one or both drugs may need to be modified or a different drug may need to be prescribed. The following drugs and drug classes interact with calcium:

atenolol (eg, *Tenormin*)
fiber (eg, bran)
iron salts (eg, *Feosol*)
hydantoins (eg, phenytoin)
quinolone antibiotics (eg, ciprofloxacin)
sodium polystyrene sulfonate (eg, *Kayexalate*)
tetracycline (eg, *Achromycin V*)
thiazide diuretics (eg, hydrochlorothiazide)
valproic acid (eg, *Depakote*)
verapamil (eg, *Calan*)

Side Effects:

Every drug is capable of producing side effects. Many calcium users experience no, or minor, side effects. The frequency and severity of side effects depend on many factors including dose, duration of therapy, and individual susceptibility. Possible side effects of high calcium levels include: Loss of appetite; nausea; vomiting; dry mouth; increased urination; constipation; stomach pain; thirst; confusion; delirium.

Guidelines for Use:

- Calcium products are confusing. Calcium salts and elemental, or active, calcium vary from product to product. Read the "Supplemental Facts" on the package to determine the serving size and amount of elemental calcium per serving.
- Divide total daily dose into 2 or 3 separate doses.
- Take with a glass of water with or after meals to increase absorption by the body.
- Make sure you are taking your RDA of vitamin D every day. If you are taking a multivitamin containing vitamin D you may not need a calcium product that also contains vitamin D. Do not exceed the RDA of vitamin D without consulting your doctor.
- Some tablets and capsules are larger than others. Ease of swallowing may be a consideration in product selection.
- *Chewable tablets* — Chew well before swallowing. May be followed with a glass of water.
- *Effervescent tablets* — Allow the tablet to stop fizzing before taking.
- Notify your doctor if loss of appetite, nausea, vomiting, constipation, stomach pain, dry mouth, thirst, or increased urination occurs.
- Do not take more than 2000 mg of elemental calcium daily (including calcium in diet, vitamins, and supplements), unless advised to do so by your doctor.
- *Recommended Dietary Allowances (RDA)* —
  Adult males: 1200 mg.
  Adult females: 1200 mg
- *Common sources of calcium* — Dairy products, calcium fortified foods, and some leafy green vegetables (eg, broccoli, kale, collards).
- Products derived from bonemeal or dolomite have been reported to contain toxic metals (eg, lead, arsenic, mercury). These products have been associated with problems involving the nervous system, digestive system, skin, and blood. Some health authorities suggest avoiding these products.

If you have any questions, consult your doctor, pharmacist, or health care provider.

	Brand Name Examples	Electrolyte content (mEq/L) Sodium	Potassium	Chloride	Citrate	Calories/ fl. oz.
otc	*Rehydralyte Solution*	75	20	65	30	3
otc	*Infalyte Oral Solution*	50	25	45	34	4.2
otc	*Pediatric Electrolyte Solution*	45	20	35	48	3
otc	*Gerber Pediatric Electrolyte Solution, Pedialyte Freezer Pops, Pedialyte Solution*	45	20	35	30	3

Type of Drug:

Electrolyte solutions and oral rehydration solutions.

How the Drug Works:

Used properly, mixtures with electrolytes, water, and sugar prevent dehydration (fluid loss) or achieve rehydration and maintain strength and a feeling of well-being. They contain sodium, chloride, potassium, and bicarbonate to replace depleted electrolytes and restore acid-base balance and sugar, which aids in sodium and water absorption by the body.

Uses:

For maintenance of water and electrolytes following corrective intravenous therapy for severe diarrhea, for maintenance to replace mild-to-moderate fluid loss when food and liquid intake are discontinued, and for the restoration of fluid and electrolytes lost in diarrhea and vomiting in infants and children.

Precautions:

Do not use in the following situations:

diarrhea, severe and continuing
kidney disease, severe
obstructed bowel
shock, prolonged
vomiting, severe and unremitting

Pregnancy and breastfeeding: A pregnant or breastfeeding woman should consult a doctor before using these products.

Guidelines for Use:

- Dosage will be individualized. Follow the package directions or your doctor's instructions when using these products.
- Use only the recommended volumes to avoid excessive electrolyte ingestion.
- Do not mix with other electrolyte-containing liquids (eg, milk, fruit juices, sports drinks).
- Store opened solutions in the refrigerator. Discard any remaining solution after 48 hours.

If you have any questions, consult your doctor, pharmacist, or health care provider.

	Generic Name *Brand Name Examples*	Supplied As	Generic Available
Rx	**Fluoride, Oral**	**Drops**: 0.125 mg/drop (from ≈ 0.275 mg sodium fluoride)	Yes
	Fluoritab, Luride Lozi-Tabs	**Tablets, chewable**: 0.25 mg (from 0.55 mg sodium fluoride)	No
	Fluoritab, Luride Lozi-Tabs, Pharmaflur 1.1	**Tablets, chewable**: 0.5 mg (from 1.1 mg sodium fluoride)	Yes
	Fluoritab, Flura-Loz, Luride Lozi-Tabs, Pharmaflur	**Tablets, chewable** 1 mg (from 2.2 mg sodium fluoride)	Yes
	Fluoritab	**Drops**: 0.25 mg/drop (from 0.55 mg sodium fluoride)	No
	Luride, Pediaflor	**Drops**: 0.5 mg /mL (from 1.1 mg sodium fluoride)	Yes
	Fluoride, Topical		
otc	*ACT[1], ACT for Kids, Fluorigard[1]*	**Rinse**: 0.02% (from 0.05% sodium fluoride)	No
otc	*Phos-Flur*	**Rinse**: 0.044% sodium fluoride, acidulated phosphate fluoride	No
Rx	*Fluorinse*	**Rinse**: 0.09% (from 0.2% sodium fluoride)	No
Rx	*Gel-Kam, PerioMed*	**Rinse**: 0.1% when diluted (from 0.63% stannous fluoride)	No
Rx	*PreviDent[2]*	**Rinse**: 0.2% neutral sodium fluoride	No
Rx	*Gel-Tin, Just for Kids, OMNI*	**Gel**: 0.1% (from 0.4% stannous fluoride)	No
otc	*Stop*	**Gel**: 0.1% (from 0.4% stannous fluoride)	No
Rx	*Karigel, Karigel Maintenance Neutral, PreviDent, SF 1.1%*	**Gel**: 0.5% (from 1.1% sodium fluoride)	No
Rx	*NeutraCare, Phos-Flur*	**Gel**: 0.5% (from 1.1% sodium fluoride and acidulated phosphate fluoride)	No
Rx	*Thera-Flur-N*	**Gel drops**: 0.5% (from 1.1% sodium fluoride)	No
Rx	*PreviDent 5000 Plus, SF 5000 Plus*	**Cream**: 1.1% sodium fluoride	No

[1] Contains tartrazine.
[2] Contains alcohol.

The amount of fluoride provided by a product varies with the fluoride salt (formulation) contained in the product. The table above lists the fluoride salts by the amount of fluoride contained in the formulation.

Type of Drug:

Mineral.

How the Drug Works:

Fluoride acts on teeth before (tablets, drops) and after (rinses, gels, creams) they erupt to make them more resistant to cavities by increasing tooth resistance to acid and bacteria decay.

Uses:

To help prevent cavities when water supplies are low in fluoride (≤ 0.7 parts per million [ppm]), to prevent decalcification under and around orthodontic brackets, and to control rampant dental decay after xerostomia (dry mouth)-producing radiotherapy of head and neck tumors.

Unlabeled Use(s): Occasionally doctors may prescribe sodium fluoride for osteoporosis.

Precautions:

Do not use in the following situations:

allergy to the drug or any of its ingredients
drinking water with a fluoride content over 0.7 ppm
low-sodium diet

Concurrent use with fluoridated drinking water: Fluoride tablets and drops provide systemic fluoride to the body. Fluoridated drinking water also provides systemic fluoride. Excessive fluoride ingestion can damage the teeth (dental fluorosis). Depending on the amount of fluoride in your drinking water (eg, 0.7 ppm), some of these products should not be used or the dose should be reduced. If you move from one community to another, fluoridation levels may change and dosage adjustments will need to be made. Check with your doctor or dentist. This is not a concern with topical fluoride products.

Gum tissues: Gum tissues may be sensitive to some flavors or to the alcohol contained in some of the topical products.

Pregnancy: There are no adequate and well-controlled studies in pregnant women. Use only if clearly needed and the potential benefits to the mother outweigh the possible risks to the fetus.

Breastfeeding: It is not known if fluoride appears in breast milk. Consult your doctor before you begin breastfeeding.

Children: Do not use drops or chewable tablets in children under 6 months of age. Consult your doctor before using a rinse in a child under 6 years of age. Use of a cream, rinse, or gel in pediatric patients should be supervised by an adult to prevent swallowing of the product. Do not use topical products in children under 6 years of age, unless advised to do so by your doctor.

Tartrazine: Some of these products may contain the dye tartrazine (FD&C Yellow No. 5), which can cause allergic reactions in certain individuals. Check package label when available or consult your doctor or pharmacist.

Drug Interactions:

Tell your doctor or pharmacist if you are taking or if you are planning to take any over-the-counter or prescription medications with fluoride. Doses of one or both drugs may need to be modified or a different drug may need to be prescribed. Dairy products and calcium supplements may interact with fluoride drops and tablets.

Side Effects:

Every drug is capable of producing side effects. Many fluoride users experience no, or minor, side effects. The frequency and severity of side effects depend on many factors including dose, duration of therapy, and individual susceptibility. Possible side effects include:

Other: Rash; gum irritation (topical products only).

Guidelines for Use:

- Use exactly as directed by your doctor or dental professional.
- Do not stop using or change the dose, unless advised to do so by your doctor.
- For best results, do not eat, drink, or rinse mouth for 30 minutes after topical application.
- Do not swallow topical doseforms.
- *Tablets and drops* — Do not eat or drink dairy products within 1 hour of administration. Take with meals if stomach upset occurs.
- *Tablets* — Dissolve in the mouth, chew, swallow whole, add to drinking water or fruit juice, or add to water for use in infant formulas or other nondairy food.
- *Drops* — Take orally, undiluted, or mix with fluids or nondairy food.
- *Cream* — Use once a day in place of your regular toothpaste, unless advised otherwise by your dentist. Brush thoroughly for 2 minutes, then spit out. Pediatric patients 6 to 16 years of age should rinse out their mouth thoroughly after use.
- *Gel* — Once daily, following brushing and flossing, apply with a toothbrush or mouth tray and allow to remain on teeth for 1 minute and then spit out. Pediatric patients 6 to 16 years of age should rinse out their mouth thoroughly after use.
- *Gel drops* — Apply once daily with applicators supplied by your dentist. Apply 4 to 8 drops as required to cover the inner surface of each applicator. Spread gel drops with tip of bottle. Place applicator over upper and lower teeth at the same time. Bite down lightly for 6 minutes. Remove applicators and rinse mouth. Clean applicators with cold water.
- *Rinse* — Use once daily or as directed by your dental professional. Most effective immediately after brushing and flossing just prior to bedtime. Vigorously swish between teeth for 1 minute. Spit out remaining solution. Do not swallow rinse. Do not dilute acidulated gels or rinses in a porcelain or glass container; use plastic.
- Notify your dentist if your teeth become spotted or stained.
- Fluoride helps to reduce cavity formation but does not replace good oral hygiene practices (eg, brushing, flossing). See your dental professional regularly.
- Store at controlled room temperature (59° to 86°F).

If you have any questions, consult your doctor, pharmacist, or health care provider.

	Generic Name *Brand Name Examples*	Supplied As	Generic Available
otc	**Magnesium Amino Acid Chelate**		
	Chelated Magnesium, Magnesium AA	**Tablets:** 100 mg	No
otc	**Magnesium Carbonate**		
	Mag-Carb	**Capsules:** 72 mg	No
otc	**Magnesium Chloride Hexahydrate**		
	Mag-SR, Slow-Mag	**Tablets, sustained release:** 64 mg	No
otc	**Magnesium Citrate**	**Tablets:** 100 mg	Yes
otc	**Magnesium Gluconate Dihydrate**		
	Almora, Magonate	**Tablets:** 27 mg	Yes
	Magtrate	**Tablets**: 29 mg	No
	Magonate	**Liquid**: 54 mg/5 mL	No
	Magonate Natal	**Liquid**: 3.52 mg/mL	No
	Magnesium Lactate		
	Mag-Tab SR	**Tablets, sustained release**: 84 mg	No
otc	**Magnesium Oxide**		
	Mag-Ox 400	**Tablets**: 241.3 mg	Yes
	Uro-Mag	**Capsules**: 84.5 mg	No

The amount of magnesium provided by a product varies with the magnesium salt (formulation) contained in the product. The table above lists the magnesium salts by the amount of magnesium contained in the formulation.

For a complete listing of Recommended Dietary Allowances, see the RDA table at the beginning of this chapter.

Type of Drug:

Electrolyte. Dietary supplement.

How the Drug Works:

Magnesium is needed for normal enzyme activity, muscle contraction, and nerve conduction.

Uses:

To reverse or prevent magnesium deficiency. Magnesium deficiency may occur due to prolonged diarrhea, vomiting, chronic alcoholism, malabsorption syndromes, hemodialysis, kidney disease, electrolyte abnormalities, or diuretic use.

Unlabeled Use(s): Occasionally doctors may prescribe pyridoxine/magnesium oxide combinations to prevent recurrence of calcium oxalate kidney stones.

Precautions:

Use with caution in the following situations: Kidney disease.

Drug Interactions:

Tell your doctor or pharmacist if you are taking or planning to take any over-the-counter or prescription medications with magnesium. Doses of one or both drugs may need to be modified or a different drug may need to be prescribed. The following drugs and drug classes interact with magnesium:

aminoquinolones (eg, chloroquine)
fluoroquinolones (eg, ciprofloxacin)
nitrofurantoin (eg, *Macrodantin*)
penicillamine (eg, *Cuprimine*)
tetracyclines (eg, oxytetracycline)

Side Effects:

Every drug is capable of producing side effects. Many magnesium users experience no, or minor, side effects. The frequency and severity of side effects depend on many factors including dose, duration of therapy and individual susceptibility. Possible side effects at high doses include diarrhea.

Guidelines for Use:

- Dosage will be individualized.
- Excessive doses may cause diarrhea and gastrointestinal irritation.
- *Recommended Dietary Allowances (RDAs)* —
  Adult males: 350 to 400 mg
  Adult females: 280 to 300 mg
- Swallow sustained-release tablets whole. Do not crush or chew.
- *Common sources of magnesium* — Bananas, avocados, roasted peanuts, legumes, unmilled grains, green vegetables.
- Magnesium-containing antacids may also be used as dietary supplements. See the Antacids monograph in the Gastrointestinal Drugs chapter.
- Store at controlled room temperature (59° to 86°F) in a dry place. Keep out of the reach of children.

If you have any questions, consult your doctor, pharmacist, or health care provider.

	Generic Name *Brand Name Examples*	Supplied As	Generic Available
Rx	**Potassium Chloride**		
	K+8, K+10, K-Dur 10, K-Dur 20, K-Tab, Kaon-Cl 10, Klor-Con 8, Klor-Con 10, Klotrix, Slow-K	**Tablets, controlled release:** 8 mEq, 10 mEq, 20 mEq	Yes
	K-Lyte/Cl, K-Lyte/Cl 50	**Effervescent tablets:** 25 mEq, 50 mEq	No
	Micro-K Extencaps, Micro-K 10 Extencaps	**Capsules, controlled release:** 8 mEq, 10 mEq	Yes
	Kaochlor[1]*, Kaochlor-SF, Kaon-Cl, Kay Ciel, Rum-K*	**Liquid:** 15 mEq/5 mL, 20 mEq/5 mL, 30 mEq/5 mL	Yes
	K-Lor, Kay Ciel, Klor-Con, Klor-Con/25	**Powder:** 20 mEq/packet, 25 mEq/packet	Yes
otc	**Potassium Gluconate**	**Tablets**: 2.1 mEq	Yes
otc	*Potassium 99*	**Tablets:** 2.5 mEq	Yes
otc	*K-99*	**Capsules:** 2.5 mEq	No
Rx	*Kaon Elixir*	**Liquid**: 20 mEq/15 mL	Yes
	Potassium Combinations[2]		
Rx	*Effer-K, K-Lyte DS, Klor-Con/EF*	**Effervescent tablets:** 25 mEq, 50 mEq	Yes
Rx	*Tri-K*	**Liquid:** 45 mEq/15 mL	No

[1] Contains tartrazine.
[2] As potassium gluconate, potassium acetate, potassium bicarbonate, or potassium citrate.

The amount of potassium provided by a product varies with the potassium salt (formulation) contained in the product. For example, the salt potassium chloride contains 13.4 mEq potassium per gram of salt, while potassium gluconate contains only 4.5 mEq potassium per gram of salt.

Type of Drug:

Essential electrolyte. Dietary supplement.

How the Drug Works:

Potassium is involved in many biochemical processes in the body. It is required for normal functioning of cells, nerve conduction, muscle contractions, kidney function, and acid-base balance.

Uses:

To treat or prevent hypokalemia (low potassium blood levels) when dietary intake is inadequate. Low potassium levels may also be caused by some diseases, severe or prolonged episodes of vomiting or diarrhea, or by certain medicines (eg, potassium-losing diuretics). Symptoms of low potassium levels include weakness, constipation, fatigue, or weakening of reflexes.

Precautions:

Do not use in the following situations:

- allergy to potassium supplements or any of their ingredients
- Addison's disease, untreated
- anticholinergic drugs, concurrent use
- conditions predisposing to high potassium levels (eg, dehydration, heat cramps)
- delay in passage through gastrointestinal tract (tablets only)
- high blood potassium levels
- kidney disease, severe

Use with caution in the following situations:

- digestive tract diseases
- kidney disease
- potassium-sparing diuretics, concurrent use (solid doseforms only)

Digestive tract disease: Solid doseforms, especially enteric-coated products, of potassium supplements should not be used by any patient who may have difficulty passing the tablet through the digestive tract. Some preparations may cause ulcers on the esophagus (food pipe), stomach, and intestines. Potassium supplementation should be taken as a liquid preparation by these individuals.

Heart patients: Too much or too little potassium can adversely affect the heart. Be sure that your doctor and pharmacist are aware of any heart medications you are taking.

Pregnancy: There are no adequate and well-controlled studies in pregnant women. Use only if clearly needed and potential benefits to the mother outweigh the possible hazards to the fetus.

Breastfeeding: Safety for use during breastfeeding has not been established. Consult your doctor before you begin breastfeeding.

Children: Safety and effectiveness in children have not been established.

Lab tests may be required to monitor therapy. Tests may include serum potassium levels, electrolytes, and electrocardiograms.

Tartrazine: Some of these products may contain the dye tartrazine (FD&C Yellow No. 5), which can cause allergic reactions in certain individuals. Check package label when available or consult your doctor or pharmacist.

Drug Interactions:

Tell your doctor or pharmacist if you are taking or planning to take any over-the-counter or prescription medications with potassium supplements. Doses of one or both drugs may need to be modified or a different drug may need to be prescribed. The following drugs and drug classes interact with potassium supplements:

- ACE inhibitors (eg, captopril, enalapril)
- anticholinergics (eg, *Banthine*) (solid doseforms only)
- potassium-sparing diuretics (eg, amiloride)
- salt substitutes

Side Effects:

Every drug is capable of producing side effects. Many potassium users experience no, or minor, side effects. The frequency and severity of side effects depend on many factors including dose, duration of therapy, and individual susceptibility. Possible side effects include:

Digestive Tract: Stomach pain or discomfort; nausea; vomiting; black, tarry stools; throat pain when swallowing; diarrhea; gas.

Nervous System: Confusion; unusual tiredness or weakness; anxiety.

Respiratory System: Shortness of breath; breathing difficulties.

Other: Tingling or numbness of hands, feet, or lips; feeling of heaviness or weakness of the arms or legs; high blood potassium levels; irregular heart rhythm.

Guidelines for Use:

- Dosage will be individualized.
- Do not stop taking or change the dose, unless advised to do so by your doctor.
- May cause stomach upset. Take after meals or with food and with a full glass of water or other liquid.
- Do not crush or chew tablets or capsules. Swallow whole.
- *Liquids, powders, and effervescent tablets* — Must be dissolved or diluted before using. The package label will recommend the amount (eg, 4 ounces) of cold water, juice, or other beverage in which the medicine should be dissolved or mixed. After thoroughly dissolving or mixing, drink slowly over a 5- to 10-minute period.
- *Wax matrix products* — Following the release of potassium chloride, the wax matrix of the tablets, which is not absorbable, is excreted in the stool. This is normal and no cause for concern.
- Do not use salt substitutes, which contain additional potassium, except on the advice of your doctor.
- Notify your doctor immediately if you experience tingling of the hands and feet; abnormal heartbeat; unusual tiredness or weakness; a feeling of heaviness in the arms or legs; severe vomiting; stomach pain or swelling; black, tarry stools; indigestion; or if you have trouble swallowing the tablets or capsules or they seem to stick in your throat.
- Over-the-counter (OTC) potassium products contain very little potassium and cannot be substituted for prescription-strength potassium products.
- Too much or too little potassium can adversely affect the heart. Be sure your doctor and pharmacist are aware of any heart medications you are taking.
- *Common sources of potassium* — Beef, veal, ham, chicken, turkey, fish, milk, bananas, dates, prunes, raisins, avocado, watermelon, cantaloupes, apricots, molasses, beans, yams, broccoli, brussel sprouts, lentils, potatoes, spinach.
- Lab tests may be required to monitor therapy. Be sure to keep appointments.
- Keep out of the reach of children.

If you have any questions, consult your doctor, pharmacist, or health care provider.

	Generic Name *Brand Name Examples*	Supplied As	Generic Available
otc	**Zinc Gluconate** (14.3% zinc)	**Tablets:** 10 mg, 15 mg, 30 mg, 50 mg, 100 mg	Yes
		Lozenges: 10.5 mg, 23 mg, 30 mg	Yes
	Zinc Sulfate (23% zinc)		
otc	*Orazinc 110, Zinc 15*	**Tablets:** 15 mg, 25 mg	No
otc	*Orazinc 220, Zinc-220*	**Capsules:** 50 mg	Yes
Rx	*Zincate*	**Capsules:** 50 mg	Yes

The amount of zinc provided by a product varies with the zinc salt (formulation) contained in the product. For example, the salt zinc sulfate contains 23% zinc and zinc gluconate contains 14.3% zinc. The table above lists the zinc products by the amount of zinc contained in the product.

For a complete listing of Recommended Dietary Allowances, see the RDA table at the beginning of this chapter.

Type of Drug:

Mineral; trace element.

How the Drug Works:

Zinc is needed for normal tissue growth and repair and for protein and carbohydrate metabolism.

Uses:

To treat or prevent zinc deficiency. Symptoms of zinc deficiency include appetite loss; growth retardation; impaired taste or smell; hair loss; dwarfism; rashes; skin lesions; swelling or inflammation of the mouth, tongue, or eyelids; hangnails; and impaired wound healing.

Unlabeled Use(s): Occasionally doctors may prescribe zinc for the common cold, acrodermatitis enteropathica (a severe digestive tract and skin disorder of early childhood), delayed wound healing, acne, rheumatoid arthritis, and senile dementia.

Precautions:

Do not use in the following situations: Allergy to zinc supplements or any of their ingredients.

Pregnancy: Because zinc deficiency is very rare, routine use of zinc supplementation during pregnancy is not recommended.

Breastfeeding: Breast milk concentrations of zinc decrease over time following delivery; extra dietary intake of zinc 7 mg/day for the first 6 months of breastfeeding and 4 mg/day during the second 6 months is recommended.

Children: Consult your doctor regarding use in children under 12 years of age.

Drug Interactions:

Tell your doctor or pharmacist if you are taking or planning to take any over-the-counter or prescription medications with oral zinc supplements. Doses of one or both drugs may need to be modified or a different drug may need to be prescribed. The following products interact with oral zinc supplements:

fluoroquinolones (eg, ciprofloxacin)
tetracyclines (eg, oxytetracycline)

Side Effects:

Every drug is capable of producing side effects. Many zinc users experience no, or minor, side effects. The frequency and severity of side effects depend on many factors including dose, duration of therapy, and individual susceptibility. Possible side effects include:

Digestive Tract: Nausea; vomiting.

Guidelines for Use:

- Dosage will be individualized.
- If stomach upset or nausea occurs, take with food or liquid.
- Avoid taking with foods high in bran, calcium, phosphorus, or phytate.
- Do not exceed the prescribed or recommended dose. Vomiting is likely to occur with doses over 2 g.
- *Recommended Dietary Allowance (RDA)* —
  Adults: 12 to 15 mg
- *Common sources of zinc* — Cooked dry beans, meat, eggs, liver, seafoods, wheat germ, whole grain products.
- Store at controlled room temperature (59° to 86°F). Protect from moisture. Keep out of the reach of children.

If you have any questions, consult your doctor, pharmacist, or health care provider.

	Vitamins A and D Combinations *Brand Name Examples*	Vitamin A (IU)	Vitamin D (IU)	Vitamin C (mg)
otc	*Vitamin A & D Tablets*	10,000/tablet	400/tablet	
otc	*Tri-Vi-Sol Drops, Vi-Daylin ADC Oral Solution*	1500/mL	400/mL	35/mL
otc	*Norwegian Cod Liver Oil Capsules*	1250/ capsule	≈ 130/ capsule	
otc	*Scott's Emulsion*	1250/5 mL	100/5 mL	
otc	*Cod Liver Oil USP, Norwegian Cod Liver Oil*	5000/5 mL 5000/5 mL 4600/5 mL	500/5 mL 400/5 mL 460/5 mL	

For a complete listing of Recommended Dietary Allowances, see the RDA table at the beginning of this chapter. For more information, see the Vitamin A and Vitamin D monographs in this chapter.

Type of Drug:
Vitamin combinations.

Uses:
Dietary supplement.

Guidelines for Use:

- Dosage will be individualized.
- Do not exceed the recommended dose, unless advised to do so by your doctor.
- Most people on regular diets do not need vitamin supplements.
- *Capsules* — Take with meals. Store in a cool, dry place.
- *Drops* — Administer directly into mouth using dropper, or mix with formula, fruit juice, cereal, or other food. Store at room temperature. Protect from light.
- *Emulsion* — Shake well before using. Store at room temperature.
- Keep out of the reach of children.

If you have any questions, consult your doctor, pharmacist, or health care provider.

	Vitamin B Combinations *Brand Name Examples*	B_1 (mg)	B_2 (mg)	B_3 (mg)	B_5 (mg)	B_6 (mg)	B_{12} (mcg)
otc	*Neurodep-Caps Capsules*	125				125	1000
otc	*B Complex Tablets*	25	25	100	25	25	25
otc	*Apatate Liquid, Apatate Tablets*	15				0.5	25
otc	*Orexin Chewable Tablets*	8.1				4.1	25
otc	*B-Complex and B-12 Tablets*	7	14	4.5			25
otc	*Super B Complex Capsules*	3	6	1			3
otc	*Gevrabon Liquid*	0.83	0.42	8.3	1.67	0.17	0.17
otc	*Brewers Yeast 500 Tablets*	0.4	0.1	1.2			
otc	*Natural Brewers Yeast 7½ grs Tablets*	0.12	0.04	0.4			

Content in the table above is given per serving of capsule, tablet, or teaspoon (5 milliliters). Products containing the greatest amount of Vitamin B_1 are listed first.

For a complete listing of Recommended Dietary Allowances, see the RDA table at the beginning of this chapter. For more information, see the Vitamin B monographs in this chapter.

Type of Drug:

Vitamin combinations.

Uses:

Dietary supplement.

Guidelines for Use:

- Dosage will be individualized.
- Do not exceed the recommended dose, unless advised to do so by your doctor.
- Most people on regular diets do not need vitamin supplements.
- Store at controlled room temperature (59° to 86°F). Protect from moisture.

If you have any questions, consult your doctor, pharmacist, or health care provider.

	Vitamin B with C Combinations *Brand Name Examples*	B_1 (mg)	B_2 (mg)	B_3 (mg)	B_5 (mg)	B_6 (mg)	B_{12} (mcg)	C (mg)
otc	*Optimum Stress Formula Capsules*[1,2]	75	37	150	75	45	25	600
otc	*Enviro-Stress Tablets*[1]	50	50	100	50	50	25	600
otc	*T-Vites Tablets*	25	25	150	25	25		100
otc	*ThexForte Caplets*	25	15	100	10	5		500
Rx	*B C w/Folic Acid Plus Tablets*[2]	20	20	100	25	25	50	500
otc	*Vicon-C Capsules, Viogen-C Capsules*	18	10	95	22	4		300
Rx	*Berocca Tablets*[1], *B-Plex Tablets*[1], *Strovite Tablets*[1,3]	15	15	100	18	4	5	500
otc	*Surbex-T Filmtabs*	15	10	100	20	5	10	500
otc	*Glutofac Caplets*[1]	15	10	50	20	50	12	300
otc	*Arcobee with C Caplets, Therapeutic B Complex with C Capsules*[3], *Vita-Bee w/C Captabs*	15	10	50	10	5		300
otc	*B-Complex plus C High Potency Timed-Release Tablets*	10	10	50	10	5	10	200
otc	*Surbex with C Filmtabs*	6	6	30	10	2.5	5	250
otc	*Nephro-Vite OTC Tablets*[1]	1.5	1.7	20	10	10	6	60
Rx	*Nephro-Vite Rx Tablets*[1]	1.5	1.7	20	10	10	6	60
Rx	*Nephrocaps Capsules*[1]	1.5	1.7	20	5	10	6	100

[1] Contains folic acid
[2] Contains iron (ferrous fumarate).
[3] Contains tartrazine.

Content in the table above is given per capsule or tablet. Products containing the greatest amount of Vitamin B_1 are listed first.

For a complete listing of Recommended Dietary Allowances, see the RDA table at the beginning of this chapter. For more information, see the Vitamin B and Vitamin C monographs in this chapter.

Precautions:

Tartrazine: Some of these products contain the dye tartrazine (FD&C Yellow No. 5), which can cause allergic reactions in some individuals. Check package label when available or consult your doctor or pharmacist.

Guidelines for Use:

- Most people on regular diets do not need vitamin supplements.
- Do not exceed the recommended dose, unless advised to do so by your doctor.
- Store at controlled room temperature (59° to 86°F) in a dry place.

If you have any questions, consult your doctor, pharmacist, or health care provider.

Vitamin B with Folic Acid Combinations

	Brand Name Examples	B_1 (mg)	B_2 (mg)	B_3 (mg)	B_5 (mg)	B_6 (mg)	B_{12} (mcg)	FA (mg)	Other content
otc	*Balanced B-100 Capsules, Super DEC B-100 Tablets, Vitamin B-100 Complex Tablets*	100	100	100	100	100	100	0.4	Biotin, choline, inositol, PABA
otc	*B-100 Ultra B Complex Timed-Release Tablets, Mega-B Tablets*	100	100	100	100	100	100	0.1	Biotin, choline, inositol, lecithin, PABA
otc	*Balanced B-50 Capsules, Super Quints B-50 Tablets*	50	50	50	50	50	50	0.4	Biotin, choline, inositol, PABA
otc	*B-50 Caps Capsules, B-50 Super B Complex Tablets*	50	50	50	50	50	50	0.1	Biotin, choline, inositol, lecithin, PABA
otc	*Quin B Strong B-25 Tablets*	25	25	100	25	25	25	0.4	Biotin, choline, inositol, PABA
otc	*Parvlex Tablets*	20	20	20	10	10	50	0.4	Copper, iron, manganese
otc	*Kobee Tablets*	10	10	50	10	10	10	0.4	Biotin, choline, inositol, PABA
otc	*B-Complex with Vitamin B-12 Tablets*	1.5	1.7	20	10	2	6	0.4	
otc	*Vitamin B12 with Folic Acid Tablets*						500	0.4	

Content in the table above given per tablet or 15 mL. Products containing the greatest amount of Vitamin B_1 are listed first.

For a complete listing of Recommended Dietary Allowances, see the RDA table. For more information, see the Vitamin B monographs in this chapter and the Folic Acid monograph in the Blood Modifiers chapter.

Type of Drug:

Vitamin and mineral combinations.

Uses:

Dietary supplement.

Guidelines for Use:

- Dosage will be individualized.
- Do not exceed the recommended dose, unless advised to do so by your doctor.
- Most people on regular diets do not need vitamin supplements.

If you have any questions, consult your doctor, pharmacist, or health care provider.

	Calcium and Vitamin D Combinations *Brand Name Examples*	Elemental Calcium (mg)	Vitamin D (IU)
otc	*Calcium 600 mg with D Tablets, Calcium 600 with Vitamin D Tablets, Caltrate 600+D Tablets*	600	200
otc	*Calcarb 600 with Vitamin D Tablets, Calcium 600-D Tablets, Posture D-Chewable Tablets, Posture D-Tablets*	600	125
otc	*Os-Cal 500+D Tablets*[1], *Parva-Cal 500 Tablets*	500	200
otc	*Calcium 500 mg with D Tablets*[1], *Oysco 500+D Tablets, Oyst-Cal-D 500 Tablets*[1], *Oystercal-D 500 Tablets*	500	125
otc	*Citrus Calcium+D Tablets*	315	200
otc	*Calcet Tablets*[1]	300	200
otc	*Os-Cal 250+D Tablets, Oyst-Cal-D Tablets*[1], *Oystercal-D 250 Tablets, Oysco D Tablets*	250	125
otc	*Parva-Cal 250 Tablets*	250	100
otc	*Dical-D Tablets*	117	133

[1] Contains tartrazine.

Content in the table above given per capsule or tablet. Products containing the greatest amount of elemental calcium are listed first.

A variety of calcium salts are available. Some are derived from natural products such as bone or oyster shell. Calcium carbonate and calcium phosphate products contain the highest amount of calcium per serving (≈ 40%). Calcium lactate and calcium gluconate contain the least amount of calcium per serving.

For a complete listing of Recommended Dietary Allowances, see the RDA table at the beginning of this chapter. For more information, see the Vitamin D monograph and the Calcium monograph in this chapter.

Type of Drug:

Vitamin and mineral combinations.

Uses:

Dietary supplement.

Precautions:

Tartrazine: Some of these products contain the dye tartrazine (FD&C Yellow No. 5), which can cause allergic reactions in certain individuals. Check package label when available or consult your doctor or pharmacist.

Guidelines for Use:

- Dosage will be individualized.
- Take in divided doses with meals to enhance absorption.
- Do not exceed the recommended dose, unless advised to do so by your doctor.
- Most people on regular diets do not need vitamin supplements.
- Store at room temperature (59° to 86°F). Keep out of the reach of children.

If you have any questions, consult your doctor, pharmacist, or health care provider.

	Generic Name	Supplied As	Generic Available
otc	**L-Lysine**	**Tablets:** 500 mg, 1000 mg	Yes
		Capsules: 500 mg	Yes

Type of Drug:

Essential amino acid (an amino acid required by the body). Nutritional supplement.

Uses:

To improve use of vegetable protein in the body.

Unlabeled Use(s): Occasionally doctors may recommend L-lysine for herpes simplex infections (eg, fever blisters).

Guidelines for Use:

- Dosage will be individualized.
- Do not exceed the recommended dose, unless advised to do so by your doctor.
- Most people on regular diets do not need nutritional supplements.
- Store at controlled room temperature (59° to 86°F). Protect from moisture. Keep out of the reach of children.

If you have any questions, consult your doctor, pharmacist, or health care provider.

NUTRITIONAL SUPPLEMENTS — AMINO ACID COMBINATIONS

	Brand Name Examples	Amino Acids	Vitamins/Minerals
otc	*A/G-Pro*	**Tablets:** 542 mg protein hydrolysate (45% amino acids), 50 mg L-lysine, 12.5 mg L-methionine	10.33 mg B_6, 6.7 mg vitamin C, with copper, iodine, iron, potassium, zinc, magnesium, manganese
otc	*Dequasine*	**Tablets:** 20 mg L-lysine, 50 mg L-cysteine, 150 mg dl-methionine, 50 mg N-acetylcysteine	200 mg vitamin C, with calcium, copper, iodine, iron, magnesium, molybendum, manganese, potassium, zinc
otc	*Jets*	**Tablets, chewable:** 300 mg L-lysine	25 mg vitamin C, 25 mcg B_{12}, 5 mg B_6, 10 mg B_1
otc	*NeuRecover-DA*	**Capsules:** 460 mg L-phenylalanine, 25 mg L-glutamine	333.3 IU vitamin A, 2.4 mg B_1, 0.85 mg B_2, 33 mg B_3, 15 mg B_5, 3 mg B_6, 5 mcg, B_{12}, 100 mg C, 5 IU E, with folic acid, biotin, calcium, chromiun, iron, magnesium, zinc
otc	*NeuRecover-SA*	**Capsules:** 250 mg L-phenylalanine, 150 mg L-tyrosine, 50 mg L-glutamine	167 mg vitamin B_1, 2.5 mg B_2, 16.6 mg B_3, 15 mg B_5, 3.3 mg B_6, 5 mcg B_{12}, 100 mg C, with folic acid, calcium, chromium, iron, magnesium, zinc
otc	*NeuroSlim*	**Capsules:** 500 mg D/L-phenylalanine, 15 mg L-glutamine, 25 mg L-tyrosine, 10 mg L-carnitine, 10 mg L-arginine pyroglutamate, 10 mg ornithine aspartate	0.33 mg vitamin B_1, 0.5 mg B_2, 3.3 mg B_3, 0.12 mg B_5, 0.33 mg B_6, 1 mcg B_{12}, 5 IU E, with biotin, folic acid, iron, zinc, chromium, selenium, calcium, iodine, copper, magnesium
otc	*PDP Liquid Protein*	**Liquid:** 15 g protein (from protein hydrolysate)/30 mL	

For a complete listing of Recommended Dietary Allowances, see the RDA table at the beginning of this chapter. For more information, see the Amino Acids monograph and the individual vitamin and mineral monographs in this chapter.

Type of Drug:

Dietary supplement.

Uses:

To prevent or treat a variety of rare deficiency disorders. Science-based clinical evaluations of safety and efficacy for inferred therapeutic value are lacking. Use with caution.

Guidelines for Use:

- Dosage will be individualized.
- Do not exceed the recommended dose, unless advised to do so by your doctor.
- Most people on regular diets do not need dietary supplements.

If you have any questions, consult your doctor, pharmacist, or health care provider.

	Brand Name Examples	Supplied As
otc	*C Factors "1000" Plus*	**Tablets:** 1000 mg vitamin C, 250 mg citrus bioflavonoids complex, 50 mg rutin, 20 mg hesperidin complex
otc	*Extra Potency Ester-C Plus*	**Tablets:** 1000 mg vitamin C, 200 mg citrus bioflavonoids complex, 25 mg acerola, 25 mg rutin, 25 mg rose hips, 125 mg calcium
otc	*Flavons*	**Tablets:** 500 mg citrus bioflavonoids
otc	*Pan-C 500*	**Tablets:** 100 mg hesperidin, 100 mg citrus bioflavonoids, and 500 mg vitamin C
otc	*Peridin-C*	**Tablets:** 150 mg hesperidin complex, 50 mg hesperidin methyl chalcone (bioflavonoids), and 200 mg vitamin C
otc	*Quercetin*	**Tablets:** 50 mg, 250 mg quercetin (from eucalyptus)
otc	*Rutin*	**Tablets:** 50 mg rutin
otc	*Span C*	**Tablets:** 300 mg citrus bioflavonoids, 200 mg vitamin C
otc	*Tri Super Flavons*	**Tablets:** 100 mg hesperidin, 900 mg citrus bioflavonoids
otc	*Ester-C Plus 500 mg Vegicaps*	**Capsules:** 500 mg vitamin C, 62 mg calcium, 25 mg citrus bioflavonoid complex, 10 mg acerola, 10 mg rose hips, 5 mg rutin
otc	*Ester-C Plus Multi-Mineral Formula Vegicaps*	**Capsules:** 425 mg vitamin C, 50 mg citrus bioflavonoid complex, 12.5 mg acerola, 12.5 mg rose hips, 5 mg rutin, 25 mg calcium, 13 mg magnesium, 12.5 mg potassium, 2.5 mg zinc
otc	*P-1000*	**Capsules:** 1000 mg lemon bioflavonoids complex

Type of Drug:

Water-soluble vitamins not stored by the body. Vitamin P. Citrus bioflavonoids.

Uses:

There is no established need for bioflavonoids in human nutrition, nor is there a recommended dietary allowance. There is little evidence that bioflavonoids are effective for any medical condition.

Guidelines for Use:

- Dosage will be individualized.
- Do not exceed the recommended dose, unless advised to do so by your doctor.
- Most people on regular diets do not need dietary supplements.
- *Common dietary sources of bioflavonoids* — Fruits, vegetables, nuts, seeds, grains, tea, wine.

If you have any questions, consult your doctor, pharmacist, or health care provider.

	Brand Name Examples	Fish oil (mg/capsule)	Omega-3 Fatty Acid Content EPA	DHA	Other Content
otc	*Mega-MaxEPA Capsules*	1275	225	150	2.5 IU vitamin C
otc	*Marine Lipid Concentrate Capsules*	1200	360	240	5 IU vitamin E
otc	*Sea-Omega 30 Capsules*	1200	180	140	2 IU vitamin E
otc	*Sea-Omega 50 Capsules*	1000	300	200	1 IU vitamin E
otc	*EPA Capsules*	1000	180	120	5 IU vitamin E
otc	*Max EPA Capsules*	1000	180	120	2 IU vitamin E
otc	*EPA Capsules, Optimal Omega Capsules*	1000	180	120	1 IU vitamin E
otc	*Omega-3 700 Capsules*	700	400	300	2 mg vitamin C, 2 IU vitamin E
otc	*Sam-EPA Capsules*	500	300	200	1 IU vitamin E

Cold-water fish oils contain large amounts of omega-3 polyunsaturated fatty acids (eg, eicosapentaenoic acid [EPA] and docosahexaenoic acid [DHA]).

Type of Drug:

Fish oils, omega-3 (N-3) polyunsaturated fatty acids; nutritional supplement.

How the Drug Works:

Omega-3 fatty acids appear to act on several factors which may contribute to the development of certain types of heart disorders (especially the development of fatty deposits in the heart blood vessels).

They possibly decrease the levels of fats in the blood by reducing the amount of fats produced by the liver, or by increasing the excretion of fats from the body.

Studies have indicated that diets high in omega-3 fatty acids may lower total cholesterol levels and very low-density lipoproteins (VLDL). However, some studies indicate that fish oils may actually raise LDL cholesterol levels. HDL cholesterol levels appear not to be affected as much as LDL levels.

Some studies indicate that fish oils may produce some anti-inflammatory effects by interfering with the normal inflammatory processes in the body.

It has been observed that fish oils may promote the development of beneficial prostaglandins. Prostaglandins are hormones made locally by tissues throughout the body. The fish oils seem to favor the development of protective types of prostaglandins, thereby helping to reduce chemical reactions in the body, which can contribute to blood clot and plaque formation, which, in turn, can clog blood vessels.

Uses:

To supplement the diet of people at early risk for heart diseases affecting the blood vessels of the heart (coronary artery disease). The American Heart Association recommends eating fish; however, it does not find justification for fish oil capsule supplements.

Unlabeled Use(s): Occasionally doctors may prescribe omega-3 fatty acids as adjunctive treatment for rheumatoid arthritis, psoriasis, and other inflammatory diseases.

Precautions:

Use with caution in the following situations:

anticoagulant (eg, warfarin) therapy, concurrent
aspirin use, concurrent
surgery, recent
type 2 diabetes mellitus

Pregnancy and breastfeeding: Do not use fish oil products until further information is available.

Children: Dot use fish oil products until further information is available.

Side Effects:

Every drug is capable of producing side effects. Many fish oil users experience no, or minor, side effects. The frequency and severity of side effects depend on many factors including dose, duration of therapy, and individual susceptibility. Diarrhea has been reported in patients taking 4 to 6 capsules daily.

Guidelines for Use:

- Dosage will be individualized.
- Do not exceed the recommended dose, unless advised to do so by your doctor.
- Consult your doctor if you plan to take large amounts of fish oils or you plan to take them for a long period of time.
- It is not known whether fish oils can reduce the incidence of heart disease. At this time, health authorities do not know whether or not fish oil supplements can be recommended as a measure for preventing heart disease or other diseases.
- People who consider taking fish oils to reduce their risks for heart disease should also make appropriate lifestyle changes. These include reduced intake of fats, cholesterol, salt, and alcohol in the diet; elimination of smoking; appropriate exercise; and control of blood pressure.
- Fish oil supplements do not replace prescription medicines that lower cholesterol (eg, lovastatin). Do not stop prescription cholesterol medicines when starting fish oil supplements, unless advised to do so by your doctor.

If you have any questions, consult your doctor, pharmacist, or health care provider.

	Generic Name *Brand Name Examples*	Supplied As	Generic Available
	Levocarnitine (L-Carnitine)		
otc	*L-Carnitine*	**Tablets**: 500 mg	Yes
otc	*L-Carnitine*	**Capsules:** 250 mg, 500 mg	Yes
Rx	*Carnitor*	**Tablets:** 330 mg	No
Rx	*Carnitor*	**Oral solution:** 100 mg/mL	No
Rx	*Carnitor*	**Injection:** 500 mg/2.5 mL, 1 g/5 mL	No

Type of Drug:

Amino acid derivative.

How the Drug Works:

Occurring naturally in the body, L-carnitine is needed by the body for energy metabolism and to properly use fats.

Uses:

To supplement the diet of people born with primary carnitine deficiency. Symptoms of primary carnitine deficiency include low blood sugar, lethargy, liver problems, heart problems, muscle weakness, neurologic disturbances, and impaired growth and development in infants.

Carnitor is used for the acute and chronic treatment of patients with internal metabolism errors that cause a secondary carnitine deficiency. It is also used for the prevention and treatment of carnitine deficiency in patients with end-stage kidney disease who are also undergoing dialysis.

Unlabeled Use(s): Occasionally doctors may prescribe L-carnitine for modifying abnormal plasma lipoprotein patterns.

Precautions:

Do not use in the following situations: Allergy to L-carnitine or any of its ingredients.

Kidney disease: Patients with kidney disease taking D, L-carnitine (not L-carnitine) have, on rare occasions, noted mild muscle weakness.

Pregnancy: There are no adequate and well-controlled studies in pregnant women. Use only if clearly needed and the potential benefits to the mother outweigh the possible risks to the fetus.

Breastfeeding: It is not known if L-carnitine appears in breast milk. Consult your doctor before you begin breastfeeding.

Lab tests may be required to monitor therapy. Tests include blood chemistries, vital signs, plasma L-carnitine concentrations, and overall clinical condition.

Side Effects:

Every drug is capable of producing side effects. Many L-carnitine users experience no, or minor, side effects. The frequency and severity of side effects depend on many factors including dose, duration of therapy, and individual susceptibility. Possible side effects include:

Digestive Tract: Nausea; vomiting; stomach cramps; diarrhea.

Other: Body odor.

Guidelines for Use:

- Dosage will be individualized.
- *Capsules and tablets* — Take on an empty stomach.
- *Oral solution* — Take alone or dissolve in drinks or liquid food. Consume slowly. Space doses evenly (eg, every 3 or 4 hours), preferably with or after meals.
- D, L-carnitine, sold in health food stores as vitamin B_T, inhibits L-carnitine and can cause a deficiency.
- Lab tests may be required to monitor therapy. Be sure to keep appointments.
- Store at controlled room temperature (59° to 86°F).

If you have any questions, consult your doctor, pharmacist, or health care provider.

	Generic Name *Brand Name Examples*	Supplied As	Generic Available
otc	**Choline**	**Tablets:** 250 mg, 300 mg, 500 mg, 650 mg	Yes
otc	**Choline Bitartrate**	**Capsules:** 350 mg	Yes
		Powder	Yes
otc	**Inositol**	**Tablets:** 250 mg, 650 mg	Yes
		Capsules: 500 mg	Yes
		Powder	Yes
otc	**Lipotropic Combinations**		
	Lecithin	**Capsules:** 400 mg, 500 mg, 1200 mg, 1360 mg	Yes
	PhosChol	**Capsules:** 900 mg	No
	Lecithin	**Granules**	Yes
	PhosChol	**Liquid:** 3000 mg/5 mL	No

The need for lipotropics in human nutrition has not been established. The lipotropic factors choline, inositol, and betaine have not been proven therapeutically valuable, although they have been used for treatment of liver disorders and disturbed fat metabolism.

Type of Drug:

Lipotropic.

How the Drug Works:

Lipotropic products increase the removal of, or decrease, fat deposits in the liver.

Uses:

To treat liver disorders and fat metabolism diseases.

Unlabeled Use(s): Occasionally doctors may prescribe choline for tardive dyskinesia, Huntington's chorea, Tourette's syndrome, Friedreich's ataxia, presenile dementia, fatty liver, cirrhosis, Alzheimer's disease, and eyelid spasms.

Side Effects:

Every drug is capable of producing side effects. Many lipotropic product users experience no, or minor, side effects. The frequency and severity of side effects depend on many factors including dose, duration of therapy, and individual susceptibility. Possible side effects for choline include: Depression; uncontrollable urination; fishy odor; nausea; vomiting; diarrhea; stomach discomfort.

NUTRITIONAL SUPPLEMENTS — LIPOTROPIC PRODUCTS

Guidelines for Use:

- Dosage will be individualized.
- Do not exceed the recommended dose, unless advised to do so by your doctor.
- Take with plenty of liquids.

If you have any questions, consult your doctor, pharmacist, or health care provider.

	Generic Name *Brand Name Examples*	Supplied As	Generic Available
otc	**Para-Aminobenzoic Acid (PABA)**	**Tablets:** 100 mg	Yes
Rx	**Potassium Para-Aminobenzoate (KPAB)**		
	Potaba	**Tablets:** 500 mg	No
		Capsules: 500 mg	No
		Powder (Envules): 2 g	No

Type of Drug:

Accessory food factor naturally associated with B-complex vitamins.

How the Drug Works:

A component of several important biochemical processes, PABA and KPAB, working by undefined mechanisms, may prevent or reduce inappropriate fibrosis (making of fibrous tissue). It has no nutrient value. It is not a true vitamin.

Uses:

KPAB only — To treat scleroderma, dermatomyositis, morphea, linear scleroderma, pemphigus, and Peyronie's disease.

Precautions:

Do not use in the following situations:

allergy to PABA or KPAB
sulfonamide anti-infective therapy, concurrent

Use with caution in the following situations:

appetite loss
kidney disease or impairment
nausea

Pregnancy: Adequate studies have not been done in pregnant women. Use only if clearly needed and potential benefits outweigh the possible hazards to the fetus.

Breastfeeding: It is not known if PABA appears in breast milk. Consult your doctor before you begin breastfeeding.

Drug Interactions:

Tell your doctor or pharmacist if you are taking or if you are planning to take any over-the-counter or prescription medications with PABA or KPAB. Doses of one or both drugs may need to be modified or a different drug may need to be prescribed. The following drugs and drug classes interact with PABA or KPAB.

dapsone
sulfonamides (eg, sulfisoxazole)

Side Effects:

Every drug is capable of producing side effects. Many PABA or KPAB users experience no, or minor, side effects. The frequency and severity of side effects depend on many factors including dose, duration of therapy, and individual susceptibility. Possible side effects include:

Digestive Tract: Loss of appetite; nausea; vomiting; stomach upset.

Other: Fever; itching; rash; decreased white blood cell count; liver toxicity.

Guidelines for Use:

- Average adult daily dosage is 12 g, given in 4 to 6 separate doses. Six (6) tablets or capsules can be given 4 times daily, usually with meals and at bedtime with a snack. Tablets, capsules, and powder (envules) must be taken with an adequate amount of liquid or food to prevent stomach upset. Envules contain 2 g of potassium para-aminobenzoate powder each. Six (6) envules are given for a total of 12 g daily.
- Take with food to minimize stomach upset.
- If a dose is missed, take it as soon as possible. If several hours have passed or if it is nearing time for the next dose, do not double the dose in order to catch up, unless advised to do so by your doctor. If more than one dose is missed, or it is necessary to establish a new dosage schedule, contact your doctor or pharmacist.
- If loss of appetite or nausea occurs, stop therapy until you are eating normally again.
- Although not a vitamin, this food factor is found naturally associated with B-complex vitamins. Small amounts are found in cereal, eggs, milk, and meats.

If you have any questions, consult your doctor, pharmacist, or health care provider.

Iron-Containing Products, 71

Iron Combinations
Iron with Vitamin C, 75
Iron with Vitamins, 76
Iron with Vitamin B_{12} and Intrinsic Factor, 77

Folic Acid, 81

Leucovorin, 83

Vitamin B_{12}, 85

Dipyridamole, 88

Ticlopidine HCl, 90

Glycosaminoglycan Anticoagulants
Danaparoid Sodium, 93

Antiplatelet Agents
Dipyridamole and Aspirin, 95

Heparin, 98

Enoxaparin Sodium, 101

Dalteparin Sodium, 104

Ardeparin Sodium, 107

Anticoagulants
Tinzaparin Sodium, 109

Coumarin Derivatives, 111

Thrombolytic Agents, 116

Clopidogrel Bisulfate, 119

Pentoxifylline, 122

Phytonadione (Vitamin K), 124

Sodium Phenylbutyrate, 126

Epoetin Alfa, 128

Colony Stimulating Factor
Filgrastim, 131
Sargramostim, 134

Generic Name *Brand Name Examples*	Supplied As	Generic Available
otc **Ferrous Sulfate**		
Feratab, Mol-Iron	**Tablets:** 195 mg, 300 mg, 324 mg	Yes
Fero-Gradumet Filmtab	**Tablets, timed release:** 525 mg	No
Ferospace	**Capsules:** 250 mg	Yes
Fer-In-Sol[1]	**Syrup:** 90 mg/tsp	No
Feosol[1]	**Elixir:** 220 mg/tsp	Yes
Fen-gen-sol[1], *Fer-In-Sol*[1], *Fer-Iron*[1]	**Drops:** 75 mg/0.6 mL	Yes
otc **Ferrous Sulfate Exsiccated**		
Feosol	**Tablets:** 200 mg	No
Slow FE	**Tablets, slow release:** 160 mg	No
Fer-In-Sol	**Capsules:** 190 mg	No
Feosol, Ferralyn Lanacaps, Ferra-TD	**Capsules, timed release:** 159 mg, 250 mg	Yes
otc **Ferrous Gluconate**		
Fergon, Ferralet	**Tablets:** 300 mg, 320 mg, 325 mg	Yes
Ferralet Slow Release	**Tablets, sustained release:** 320 mg	No
Simron	**Capsules:** 86 mg	No
Fergon[1]	**Elixir:** 300 mg/tsp	No
otc **Ferrous Fumarate**		
Femiron, Ferretts, Fumasorb, Fumerln, Hemocyte, Ircon, Nephro-Fer	**Tablets:** 63 mg, 106 mg, 195 mg, 200 mg, 324 mg, 325 mg, 350 mg	Yes
Feostat	**Tablets, chewable:** 100 mg	No
Span-FF	**Capsules, controlled release:** 325 mg	No
Feostat	**Suspension:** 100 mg/tsp	No
Feostat	**Drops:** 45 mg/0.6 mL	No

	Generic Name *Brand Name Examples*	Supplied As	Generic Available
otc	**Polysaccharide-Iron Complex**		
	Niferex	**Tablets:** 50 mg iron	No
	Hytinic, Niferex-150, Nu-Iron 150	**Capsules:** 150 mg iron	No
	Niferex [1,2,3], *Nu-Iron* [1,2]	**Elixir:** 100 mg iron/tsp	No
otc	**Modified Iron Products**		
	Fermalox	**Tablets:** 200 ferrous sulfate, 100 mg magnesium hydroxide, 100 mg aluminum hydroxide	No
	Ferocyl, Ferro-Sequels	**Tablets, sustained release:** 150 mg ferrous fumarate, 100 mg docusate sodium	No
	Ferro-Docusate T.R., Ferro-Dok TR, Ferro-DSS S.R.	**Capsules, timed released:** 150 mg ferrous fumarate, 100 mg docusate sodium	No

[1] Contains alcohol.
[2] Sugar free.
[3] Dye free.

The amount of elemental iron provided by a product varies with the iron salt (formulation) contained in the product. For example, ferrous sulfate contains 20% elemental iron and ferrous gluconate contains 11.6% elemental iron. The above table lists the amount of iron salts (not elemental iron). Iron is also available in combination with other vitamins and minerals and by injection (eg, iron dextran). For a complete listing of Recommended Dietary Allowances, see p. 4.

Type of Drug:

Iron supplements.

How the Drug Works:

Iron, a mineral found in some foods, is needed to make hemoglobin, a component of red blood cells. Hemoglobin allows red blood cells to carry oxygen throughout the body.

Uses:

To prevent or treat iron deficiency anemia.

Unlabeled Use(s): Occasionally doctors may prescribe iron supplementation for patients receiving epoetin therapy.

Precautions:

Do not use in the following situations:

allergy to any ingredients in these products
iron overload (eg, hemachromatosis)
non-iron deficiency anemias or blood disorders (eg, hemolytic anemia)
normal iron balance

Use with caution in the following situations:

chronic fatigue of unknown cause
enteritis (inflammation of small intestine)
peptic ulcer
ulcerative colitis

Occult blood tests: Iron products may skew results of occult blood tests.

Children: Children are particularly sensitive to accidental overdoses of iron-containing products. Immediately report any suspected overdoses to your local Poison Control Center.

Tartrazine: Some of these products may contain the dye tartrazine (FD&C Yellow No. 5) which can cause allergic reactions in certain individuals. Check package label when available or consult your doctor or pharmacist.

Sulfites: Some of these products may contain sulfite preservatives which can cause allergic reactions in certain individuals (eg, asthmatics). Check package label when available or consult your doctor or pharmacist.

Drug Interactions:

Tell your doctor or pharmacist if you are taking or if you are planning to take any over-the-counter or prescription medications while taking this medicine. Doses of one or both drugs may need to be modified or a different drug may need to be prescribed. The following drugs and drug classes interact with this medicine.

antacids (eg, *Maalox)*
chloramphenicol *(Chloromycetin)*
cimetidine *(Tagamet)*
fluorquinolones (eg, *Cipro)*
levodopa (eg, *Dopar)*
methyldopa (eg, *Aldomet)*
penicillamine (eg, *Cuprimine)*
tetracyclines (eg, *Achromycin V)*
vitamin C

Side Effects:

Every drug is capable of producing side effects. Many patients experience no, or minor, side effects. The frequency and severity of side effects depend on many factors including dose, duration of therapy and individual susceptibility. Possible side effects include:

Iron Overdose: Unexplained tiredness; nausea; vomiting; abdominal pain; black, tarry stools; weak, rapid pulse; decreased blood pressure; dehydration; coma; fast breathing.

Digestive Tract: Stomach upset; appetite loss; nausea; vomiting; constipation; diarrhea; dark stools; staining of teeth (liquids only).

Guidelines for Use:

- Certain foods (eg, eggs, milk, coffee, tea) may decrease iron absorption. Take on an empty stomach with water. However, if stomach upset occurs, take after meals or with food.
- Do not chew or crush sustained-release preparations.
- Avoid taking antacids, fluoroquinolones or tetracycline at the same time. Allow 1 to 2 hours between iron and the antacid or antibiotics.
- Drink liquid iron preparations mixed in water or juice and through a straw to prevent staining of teeth.
- Medication may cause black stools, constipation or diarrhea.
- Discontinue medication and contact your doctor immediately if you experience unexplained tiredness, nausea, vomiting, abdominal pain, black tarry stools, weak rapid pulse, decreased blood pressure or dehydration.
- If a dose is missed, take it as soon as possible. If several hours have passed or if it is nearing time for the next dose, do not double the dose in order to "catch up" (unless advised to do so by your doctor). If more than one dose is missed or it is necessary to establish a new dosage schedule, contact your doctor or pharmacist.
- *Recommended Dietary Allowances(RDA)* — Adults: males and females over 50 years of age, 10 mg; females 11-50 years of age, 15 mg; pregnancy, 30 mg (if this increased requirement cannot be met by ordinary diets, the use of supplemental iron may be recommended); breastfeeding, 15 mg.
- *Common sources of iron:* Meat, eggs, vegetables, fortified or enriched cereals.
- In a true iron deficiency state, iron doses are higher than the RDA. Discuss the desired dose and duration of therapy with your doctor if you are iron deficient.

If you have any questions, consult your doctor, pharmacist, or health care provider.

	Iron with Vitamin C *Brand Name Examples*	Iron (mg)	Vitamin C Ascorbic Acid (mg)	Vitamin C Sodium Ascorbate (mg)
otc	*Vitron-C-Plus Tablets*	132	250	
otc	*Ferancee-HP Tablets*	110	600	
otc	*Hemaspan Tablets*[2]	110	200	
otc	*Fero-Grad-500 Filmtabs*[2]	105		500
otc	*Fe-O.D. Tablets*[2]	100	500	
otc	*Ferancee Tablets*[1,3]	67	150	
otc	*Vitron-C Tablets*[3]	66	125	
otc	*Ferromar Caplets* [2]	65	200	
otc	*Irospan Capsules*[2], *Irospan Tablets*[2]	60	150	
otc	*Niferex w/Vitamin C Tablets*[3]	50	100	169
otc	*Mol-Iron w/Vitamin C Tablets*	39	75	

[1] Contains the dye tartrazine.
[2] Timed release.
[3] Chewable.

For more information, see Iron-Containing Products, p. 55, and individual drug monographs. Products containing the greatest amount of iron are listed first.

Content given per capsule or tablet.

If you have any questions, consult your doctor, pharmacist, or health care provider.

IRON COMBINATIONS — IRON WITH VITAMINS

Content given per capsule or tablet. Products containing the greatest amount of elemental iron are listed first.

	Iron with Vitamins *Brand Name Examples*	Elemental Iron (mg)	Vitamin B_{12} (mcg)	Vitamin C (mg)	Folic Acid (mg)
otc	*Tolfrinic Tablets*	200	25	100	
Rx	*Fe-Tinic 150 Forte Capsules, Niferex-150 Forte Capsules*	150	25		1
otc	*Iberet Filmtabs*[1]	150	25	150	
Rx	*Hemocyte-F Tablets*	106			1
Rx	*Hemocyte Plus Tablets*	106	15	200	1
Rx	*Iberet-Folic-500 Filmtabs*[1]	105	25	500	0.8
Rx	*Fero-Folic-500 Filmtabs*[1]	105		500	0.8
otc	*Generet-500 Tablets*[1], *Iberet-500 Filmtabs*[1]	105	25	500	
otc	*Iron-Folic 500 Tablets*[1]	105	25	500	0.8
otc	*Ircon-FA Tablets*	82			0.8
Rx	*Fumatinic Capsules* [2]	66	5	60	
Rx	*Nephron FA Tablets* [3]	66	6	40	1
otc	*Parvlex Tablets*	29	50	50	0.4

[1] Controlled release.
[2] Extended release with a trace amount of intrinsic factor.
[3] Contains 75 mg docusate sodium.

If you have any questions, consult your doctor, pharmacist, or health care provider.

	Iron with Vitamin B_{12} and Intrinsic Factor *Brand Name Examples*	Iron (mg)	B_{12} (mcg)	IFC (mg)	B_1 (mg)	B_2 (mg)	B_3 (mg)	C (mg)	Folic Acid (mg)
Rx	*TriHemic 600 Tablets*[1]	115	25	75				600	1
Rx	*Chromagen Capsules*[4]	66	10					250	
Rx	*Contrin Capsules, Ferotrinsic Capsules, Livitrinsic-f Capsules, Trinsicon Capsules, Tri-Tinic Capsules*	36.3	15	240				75	0.5
Rx	*Lextron ferrous Pulvules*	35	2	50	1	0.25			
Rx	*Livitamin w/Intrinsic Factor Capsules*[6]	33	5		3	3	10	100	
Rx	*Lextron Pulvules*	30	2	50	1	0.25			

[1] Contains 50 mg docusate sodium and 30 IU vitamin E.
[2] Contains 50 mg desiccated liver, 0.9 mg vitamin B_5, 1.6 mg vitamin B_6, calcium, copper, iodine, potassium, magnesium, manganese, molybdenum and phosphorus.
[3] Contains NF unit vitamin B_{12} with IFC, 10 mg vitamin B_5, 1 mg vitamin B_6 and copper.
[4] Contains 100 mg desiccated stomach substance.
[5] Contains NF unit B_{12} with IFC.
[6] Contains 150 mg desiccated liver, NF unit B_{12} with IFC, 2 mg vitamin B_5, 3 mg vitamin B_6 and copper.

These products contain Intrinsic Factor derived from stomach extract to promote the absorption of vitamin B_{12}. Although previously used to treat anemias responding to oral therapy, injectable cobalamin is preferred for B_{12} deficiencies, including pernicious anemia. Content given per capsule or tablet. Products containing the greatest amount of iron are listed first.

	Iron with Vitamin B_{12} and Intrinsic Factor *Brand Name Examples*	Elemental Iron (mg)	B_{12} (mcg)	IFC (mg)	B_1 (mg)	B_2 (mg)	B_3 (mg)	C (mg)	Folic Acid (mg)
Rx	*TriHemic 600 Tablets*[1]	115	25	75				600	1
Rx	*Contrin Capsules, Foltrin Capsules, Trinsicon Capsules*	110	15	240				75	0.5
Rx	*Chromagen Capsules*	66	10	*2				250	

[1] Contains 50 mg docusate sodium and 30 IU vitamin E.
[2] Contains 100 mg desiccated stomach substance.

Type of Drug:

Dietary and therapeutic supplement.

Uses:

To prevent and treat iron deficiency or iron deficiency anemia associated with certain nutritional deficiencies (eg, vitamin B_{12}).

Ascorbic acid (vitamin C) may enhance the absorption of some forms of iron.

Precautions:

Do not use in the following situations:

- allergy to any ingredients in these products
- iron overload (eg, hemochromatosis)
- non-iron deficiency anemias or blood disorders (eg, hemolytic anemia)
- normal iron balance

Use with caution in the following situations:

- chronic fatigue of unknown cause
- enteritis (inflammation of intestine)
- peptic ulcer
- ulcerative colitis

Occult blood tests: Iron products may skew results of occult blood tests.

Children: Children are particularly sensitive to accidental overdoses of iron-containing products. Immediately report any suspected overdoses to your local Poison Control Center.

Drug Interactions:

Tell your doctor or pharmacist if you are taking or if you are planning to take any over-the-counter or prescription medications while taking this medicine. Doses of one or both drugs may need to be modified or a different drug may need to be prescribed. The following drugs and drug classes interact with this medicine.

- antacids (eg, *Maalox*)
- chloramphenicol (*Chloromycetin*)
- cimetidine (eg, *Tagamet*)
- fluoroquinolones (eg, ciprofloxacin)
- levodopa (eg, *Dopar*)
- methyldopa (eg, *Aldomet*)
- penicillamine (eg, *Cuprimine*)
- tetracyclines (eg, doxycycline)
- vitamin C

Side Effects:

Every drug is capable of producing side effects. Many patients experience no, or minor, side effects. The frequency and severity of side effects depend on many factors including dose, duration of therapy, and individual susceptibility. Possible side effects include:

Iron Overdose: Unexplained tiredness; nausea; vomiting; abdominal pain; black, tarry stools; weak, rapid pulse; decreased blood pressure; dehydration; coma; fast breathing.

Digestive Tract: Stomach upset; appetite loss; nausea; vomiting; constipation; diarrhea; dark stools.

IRON WITH VITAMIN B_{12} AND INTRINSIC FACTOR

Guidelines for Use:

- Take on an empty stomach with water. If stomach upset occurs, take after meals or with food. Do not chew or crush sustained release preparations. Sustained release products may be better tolerated.
- Avoid taking antacids, cholestyramine, or tetracycline at the same time. Take 1 hour before or 2 hours after the antacid, cholestyramine, or tetracycline.
- Medication may cause black stools, constipation, nausea, vomiting, pain, or diarrhea. Inform your doctor if any of these occur and are intolerable.
- *Recommended Dietary Allowances (RDA) for Iron —*
  Adult males: 10 mg.
  Adult females: 15 mg if menstruating, 10 mg if not menstruating.
  During pregnancy: 30 mg. If this increased requirement cannot be met by
  ordinary diets, the use of supplemental iron may be recommended.
  During breastfeeding: 15 mg.
- In a true iron deficiency state, iron doses are higher than the RDA. Discuss the desired dose and duration of therapy with your doctor if you are iron-deficient.
- Accidental overdose of iron-containing products is a leading cause of fatal poisoning in children. Keep these products out of reach of children. In case of accidental overdose, call a poison control center immediately.
- Sustained release iron products may not be as effective as regular release products due to delayed absorption of iron.
- Lab tests may be required to monitor therapy. Be sure to keep appointments.
- Store at room temperature (59° to 86°F) in a tightly closed container.

If you have any questions, consult your doctor, pharmacist, or health care provider.

	Generic Name *Brand Name Examples*	Supplied As	Generic Available
	Folic Acid[1]		
otc	*Folic Acid*	**Tablets:** 0.4 mg, 0.8 mg	Yes
Rx	*Folic Acid*	**Tablets:** 1 mg	Yes
Rx	*Folvite*	**Injection:** 5 mg/mL	Yes

Type of Drug:
Folate; folacin; pteroylglutamic acid.

How the Drug Works:
Folic acid stimulates the production of red and white blood cells and platelets (used in clotting). Folic acid acts on megaloblastic bone marrow to produce a normoblastic marrow.

Uses:
To treat anemia (low red blood cell count) caused by folic acid deficiency due to digestive disorders (eg, sprue), poor diet, pregnancy, infancy, or childhood. Folic acid is rarely taken alone.

Precautions:
Do not use in the following situations: Allergy to folic acid or any of its ingredients.

Use with caution in the following situations:
alcoholism
anemia due to vitamin B_{12} deficiency
epilepsy controlled with phenytoin, primidone, or phenobarbital
non-folic acid deficiency anemias (eg, pernicious anemia)

Pregnancy: Folic acid is often prescribed during pregnancy and is safe when used as directed. Folic acid requirements are markedly increased during pregnancy, and deficiency will likely result in fetal damage.

Breastfeeding: Folic acid appears in breast milk. Usually, amounts present in breast milk are adequate to fulfill infant requirements, but the lactating mother may require folic acid supplementation. Consult your doctor before you begin breastfeeding.

Drug Interactions:
Tell your doctor or pharmacist if you are taking or if you are planning to take any over-the-counter or prescription medications with folic acid. Doses of one or both drugs may need to be modified or a different drug may need to be prescribed.

alcohol
antimetabolites (eg, methotrexate)
barbiturates (eg, phenobarbital)
hydantoins (eg, phenytoin)
nitrofurantoin (eg, *Furadantin*)
primidone (eg, *Mysoline*)
pyrimethamine (eg, *Daraprim*)

Side Effects:

Every drug is capable of producing side effects. Many folic acid users experience no, or minor, side effects. The frequency and severity of side effects depend on many factors including dose, duration of therapy, and individual susceptibility. Possible side effects include: Difficulty breathing; itching; skin redness or rash; general body discomfort; flushing.

In higher doses (15 mg/day), additional possible side effects include: Loss of appetite; nausea; stomach bloating or swelling; gas; bitter or bad taste; altered sleep patterns; difficulty in concentrating; irritability; overactivity; excitement; depression; confusion; impaired judgment; decreased vitamin B_{12} levels (in patients receiving prolonged therapy).

Guidelines for Use:

- Take only when recommended by your doctor.
- *Treatment of Anemia –*
  Usual therapeutic (treatment) dose for anemia: Up to 1 mg daily.
  Usual maintenance dose once amenia has been corrected:
  Infants: 0.1 mg/day.
  Children under 4 years of age: Up to 0.3 mg/day.
  Adults and children over 4 years of age: 0.4 mg/day.
  Pregnant and breastfeeding women: 0.8 mg/day.
- In the presence of alcoholism, hemolytic anemia, anticonvulsant therapy, or chronic infection, the maintenance dose may need to be increased.
- Except during pregnancy and lactation, folic acid should not be given in doses > 0.4 mg/day until pernicious anemia has been ruled out.
- Oral administration is preferred. Intramuscular, intravenous, and subcutaneous routes may be used if the disease is severe, or if oral absorption is impaired.
- Store at room temperature (59 to 86°F). Protect from light and moisture.

If you have any questions, consult your doctor, pharmacist, or health care provider.

	Generic Name *Brand Name Examples*	Supplied As	Generic Available
	Leucovorin Calcium[1]		
Rx	*Wellcovorin*	**Tablets:** 5 mg, 10 mg, 15 mg, 25 mg	Yes

[1] This product is also available as an injection.

Type of Drug:

Folic acid derivative; folinic acid, citrovorum factor.

How the Drug Works:

Leucovorin is a faster acting and more potent form of folic acid. It interferes with the harmful action of folic acid-inhibiting drugs such as methotrexate.

Uses:

Tablets and injection: To lessen the toxicity and counteract the adverse effects of large doses of some drugs that are folic acid antagonists (eg, methotrexate).

Injection: To treat anemias due to folic acid deficiency when oral folic acid therapy is not possible.

Precautions:

Do not use in the following situations:

pernicious anemia and other anemias due to a vitamin B_{12} deficiency

Pregnancy: Adequate studies have not been done in pregnant women. Use only if clearly needed and potential benefits outweigh the possible hazards to the fetus.

Breastfeeding: It is not known if leucovorin appears in breast milk. Consult your doctor before you begin breastfeeding.

Lab tests may be required during treatment with leucovorin. Tests may include complete blood counts, electrolyte and liver function tests.

Drug Interactions:

Tell your doctor or pharmacist if you are taking or if you are planning to take any over-the-counter or prescription medications with leucovorin. Doses of one or both drugs may need to be modified or a different drug may need to be prescribed. The following drugs and drug classes interact with leucovorin.

anticonvulsants (eg, phenytoin)
fluorouracil (*Adrucil*)
methotrexate (*Mexate*)

Side Effects:

Every drug is capable of producing side effects. Many leucovorin users experience no, or minor, side effects. The frequency and severity of side effects depend on many factors including dose, duration of therapy and individual susceptibility. Possible side effects include: Allergic reactions (eg, difficulty breathing, itching, skin redness/rash).

Guidelines for Use:

- Take only under medical supervision.
- Itching, rash, difficult breathing or other signs of hypersensitivity should be reported immediately.

If you have any questions, consult your doctor, pharmacist, or health care provider.

Generic Name	Supplied As	Generic Available
otc **Vitamin B_{12}**[1, 2]	**Tablets:** 25 mcg, 50 mcg, 100 mcg, 250 mcg, 500 mcg, 1000 mcg	Yes
	Nasal gel: 400 mcg/unit	No

[1] This product is also available as an injection *(Rx).*
[2] Some products may be available sugar free.

For a complete listing of Recommended Dietary Allowances, see p. 4.

Type of Drug:

Water-soluble vitamin. Vitamin that can be stored by the body. Vitamin B_{12} includes cyanocobalamin and hydroxocobalamin.

How the Drug Works:

Vitamin B_{12} is needed for normal growth and reproduction of red blood cells, muscle and nerve tissue. It is usually adequately provided by the diet.

Uses:

To treat diagnosed vitamin B_{12} deficiency that may be due to pernicious anemia, inadequate diet, digestion disorders (sprue), trauma, surgery, cancer or infections.

Vitamin B_{12} requirements may increase during pregnancy, in vegetarians, after blood loss, during illnesses involving the liver and kidneys, in hemolytic anemia and in thyrotoxicosis.

Unlabeled Use(s): Occasionally doctors may prescribe hydroxocobalamin for cyanide poisoning associated with sodium nitroprusside.

Precautions:

Do not use in the following situations:

- allergy to cobalt
- allergy to vitamin B_{12} or any component of the formulation

Use with caution in the following situations:

- bone marrow suppressant drugs (eg, chloramphenicol)
- folic acid deficiency
- infection
- iron deficiency
- Leber's disease
- polycythemia vera
- uremia

Eye problems: Use of vitamin B_{12} may worsen Leber's disease, a rare hereditary eye condition.

Single deficiency (vitamin B_{12} alone) is rare. Expect multiple vitamin deficiency in any dietary deficiency.

Pregnancy: Adequate studies have not been done in pregnant women. However, B_{12} is an essential vitamin and needs are increased during pregnancy.

Breastfeeding: Vitamin B_{12} appears in breast milk. Consult your doctor before you begin breastfeeding.

Lab tests During treatment with vitamin B_{12}, it may be necessary to have lab tests to determine progress of therapy.

Drug Interactions:

Tell your doctor or pharmacist if you are taking or if you are planning to take any over-the-counter or prescription medications (including folic acid) while taking this medicine. Doses of one or both drugs may need to be modified or a different drug may need to be prescribed. The following drugs and drug classes interact with this medicine.

alcohol (excessive intake)
aminosalicylic acid *(P.A.S. Sodium)*
chloramphenicol (*Chloromycetin*)
colchicine
omeprazole *(Prilosec)*

Side Effects:

Every drug is capable of producing side effects. Many patients experience no, or minor, side effects. The frequency and severity of side effects depend on many factors including dose, duration of therapy and individual susceptibility. Possible side effects include:

Injectable vitamin B_{12} : Discomfort following injection; pain at injection site; blood clots in arms or legs; breathing difficulties; congestive heart failure; anaphylactic shock; death.

Skin: Rash; itching; hives; bruising.

Other: Fever; vision difficulties; feeling of swelling of the entire body; mild diarrhea; abnormal blood counts.

Guidelines for Use:

- *Recommended Dietary Allowances (RDA)* —
  Adult males: 2 mcg
  Adult females: 2 mcg
  Pregnant women: 2.2 mcg
  Breastfeeding women: 2.6 mcg
  Infants and children: 0.3 to 2 mcg
  Doses larger than the RDA are used to treat vitamin B_{12} deficiency.
- A well-balanced diet is necessary. Correct poor eating habits. Strict vegetarian diets containing no animal products (including milk products and eggs) do not supply vitamin B_{12}. Vegetarians should take vitamin B_{12} regularly.
- *Common source of vitamin B_{12}* — Meat, liver.
- Although oral dosing of vitamin B_{12} is convenient, injections may be required.
- Initially, vitamin B_{12} may be given daily.
- In some cases, vitamin B_{12} must be continued indefinitely to prevent return of the anemia and to prevent damage to the central nervous system.
- Folic acid is sometimes taken with vitamin B_{12} but is not a substitute for it. In pernicious anemia, folic acid may effectively return the blood profile to normal while nerve damage due to vitamin B_{12}deficiency progresses.

If you have any questions, consult your doctor, pharmacist, or health care provider.

DIPYRIDAMOLE

	Generic Name *Brand Name Example*	Supplied As	Generic Available
	Dipyridamole		
Rx	*Persantine*	**Tablets:** 25 mg, 50 mg, 75 mg	Yes

Type of Drug:

An antiplatelet agent (platelet adhesion inhibitor).

How the Drug Works:

Dipyridamole prevents blood clots from forming by preventing platelets from clumping together. Platelets are parts of the blood that aid in clot formation.

Uses:

Given with oral anticoagulants (eg, warfarin) to prevent clot formation after heart valve surgery.

Unlabeled Use(s): Occasionally doctors may prescribe dipyridamole with aspirin to prevent heart attacks and reduce heart attack damage.

Precautions:

Hypotension (low blood pressure): Dipyridamole may aggravate lightheadedness in people with low blood pressure. Be cautious when rising from sitting or lying.

Pregnancy: Studies in pregnant women or in animals have been judged not to show a risk to the fetus. However, no drug should be used during pregnancy unless clearly needed.

Breastfeeding: Dipyridamole appears in breast milk. Consult your doctor before you begin breastfeeding.

Children: Safety and effectiveness have not been established in children under 12 years of age.

Drug Interactions:

Tell your doctor or pharmacist if you are taking or if you are planning to take any over-the-counter or prescription medications (especially adenosine) while taking this medicine. Drug doses may need to be modified or a different drug prescribed.

Side Effects:

Every drug is capable of producing side effects. Many patients experience no, or minor, side effects. The frequency and severity of side effects depend on many factors including dose, duration of therapy and individual susceptibility. Possible side effects include:

Digestive Tract: Stomach ache; diarrhea; nausea; vomiting.

Other: Dizziness; lightheadedness; fainting; headache; rash; flushing; itching.

Guidelines for Use:

- Take exactly as directed. Do not stop taking this medicine except on your doctor's advice.
- Take without regard to food.
- If a dose is missed, take it as soon as possible. If several hours have passed or if it is nearing time for the next dose, do not double the dose in order to "catch up." Contact your doctor or pharmacist.
- If using this medicine in combination with oral anticoagulants (eg, warfarin), do not take aspirin unless directed by your doctor.

If you have any questions, consult your doctor, pharmacist, or health care provider.

	Generic Name *Brand Name Example*	Supplied As	Generic Available
Rx	**Ticlopidine HCl**		
	Ticlid	**Tablets:** 250 mg	Yes

Type of Drug:

Antiplatelet agent.

How the Drug Works:

Ticlopidine prevents blood clots from forming and reduces the risk of strokes caused by blood clots by preventing platelets from clumping together. Platelets are components of the blood that aid in clot formation.

Uses:

To reduce the risk of stroke caused by blood clots in patients who have experienced stroke precursors (eg, transient ischemic attacks, transient blindness, or minor stroke), and in patients who have had a completed stroke caused by a blood clot. It is used in patients who are intolerant or allergic to aspirin therapy or have failed aspirin therapy for stroke prevention.

Unlabeled Use(s): Occasionally doctors may prescribe ticlopidine to improve blood flow in the lower extremities; reduce neurological deficit in patients with subarachnoid hemorrhage; as an aid in surgery; and treatment of sickle cell disease or glomerulonephritis. Such use has not been well established through objective clinical trials.

Precautions:

Do not use in the following situations:

allergy to ticlopidine or any of its ingredients
blood clotting disorders or active bleeding (eg, low white blood cell count, decreased blood platelets, bleeding peptic ulcer, or bleeding in the brain)
liver disease, severe

Use with caution in the following situations:

gastrointestinal bleeding
kidney disease
liver disease
trauma, surgery, or pathological conditions that increase risk of bleeding
ulcers (gastric or intestinal)

Pregnancy: Adequate studies have not been done in pregnant women. Use only if clearly needed and potential benefits to the mother outweigh the possible hazards to the fetus.

Breastfeeding: It is not known if ticlopidine appears in breast milk. Because of the potential for adverse effects, a decision should be made whether to discontinue nursing or the drug, taking into account the importance of the drug to the mother. Consult your doctor.

Children: Safety and effectiveness have not been established.

Lab tests are required during treatment with ticlopidine. Tests may include complete blood counts, white cell differentials, platelet counts, and liver function tests.

Drug Interactions:

Tell your doctor or pharmacist if you are taking or if you are planning to take any over-the-counter or prescription medications with ticlopidine. Doses of one or both drugs may need to be modified or a different drug may need to be prescribed. The following drugs and drug classes interact with ticlopidine:

antacids
aspirin
carbamazepine (eg, *Tegretol*)
cimetidine (eg, *Tagamet)*
cyclosporine (eg, *Sandimmune*)
digoxin (eg, *Lanoxin)*
ginkgo biloba
NSAIDs (eg, ibuprofen)
phenytoin (eg, *Dilantin)*
propranolol (eg, *Inderal)*
theophylline (eg, *Theo-Dur)*

Side Effects:

Every drug is capable of producing side effects. Many ticlopidine users experience no, or minor, side effects. The frequency and severity of side effects depend on many factors including dose, duration of therapy, and individual susceptibility. Possible side effects include:

Digestive Tract: Diarrhea; nausea; indigestion; stomach pain; vomiting; gas; appetite loss.

Skin: Rash; bruising; itching, subcutaneous bleeding.

Other: Dizziness; abnormal blood counts; abnormal liver function or other lab tests, yellow skin or eyes; dark urine; light-colored stool.

Guidelines for Use:

- The usual recommended dosage is 250 mg taken twice daily.
- Do not stop taking or change the dose unless advised to do so by your doctor.
- Take ticlopidine with food or just after eating to minimize stomach discomfort and optimize absorption.
- Contact your doctor immediately if you experience any signs of infection such as fever, chills, or sore throat.
- It may take longer than usual to stop bleeding when taking ticlopidine. Report any unusual bleeding, bruising, or dark-colored stools to your doctor.
- Tell your dentist or doctor that you are taking ticlopidine before any surgery is scheduled (including tooth extraction) and before any new drug is prescribed.
- Notify your doctor promptly if you experience severe or persistent diarrhea, seizures, rashes, bleeding beneath the skin, pale color, weakness on a side of the body, or any signs of liver damage such as yellow skin or eyes, dark urine, or light-colored stool.
- Lab tests will be required to monitor therapy. Be sure to keep appointments.
- Store at controlled room temperature (59° to 86°F).

If you have any questions, consult your doctor, pharmacist, or health care provider.

	Generic Name *Brand Name Examples*	Supplied As	Generic Available
	Danaparoid Sodium		
Rx	*Orgaran*[1]	**Injection:** 0.6 mL ampules, 0.8 mL disposable syringes	No

[1] Contains sulfites.

Type of Drug:

Glycosaminoglycuronan antithrombotic agent.

How the Drug Works:

Danaparoid prevents fibrin formation needed for blood clot development.

Uses:

For prevention of deep vein thrombosis (clotting), which may lead to clotting of the lung vessels in patients having elective hip replacement surgery.

Unlabeled Use(s): Occasionally doctors may prescribe danaparoid sodium to prevent blood clots during hemodialysis or cardiovascular operations; to treat pregnant women at high risk of forming blood clots.

Precautions:

Do not use in the following situations:

- tendency for spontaneous bleeding (ie, hemophiliac)
- active bleeding including hemorrhagic stroke
- allergy to drug or sulfites
- allergy to pork products

Use with caution in the following situations:

- active ulcer, stomach disease
- bleeding disorders
- during administration of anticoagulants and platelet inhibitors
- high blood pressure, uncontrolled
- impaired kidney function
- inflammation of the heart wall caused by bacteria
- menstrual bleeding disorders
- shortly after brain, spinal or eye surgery
- stroke, non-hemorrhagic

Pregnancy: There are no adequate and well controlled studies in pregnant women. No drug should be used during pregnancy unless clearly needed.

Breastfeeding: It is not known if danaparoid sodium appears in breast milk. Consult your doctor before you begin breastfeeding.

Children: Safety and effectiveness in children have not been established.

Lab tests are recommended during treatment. Be sure to keep appointments.

Sulfites: This product contains a sulfite preservative that can cause severe allergic reactions in certain individuals (eg, asthmatics).

Drug Interactions:

Tell your doctor or pharmacist if you are taking or planning to take any over-the-counter or prescription medications while taking this medicine. Doses of one or both drugs may need to be modified or a different drug may need to be prescribed. Oral anticoagulants (eg, warfarin sodium) and platelet inhibitors (ASA, dipyridamole) interact with this medicine.

Side Effects:

Every drug is capable of producing side effects. Many patients experience no, or minor, side effects. The frequency and severity of side effects depend on many factors including dose, duration or therapy and individual susceptibility. Possible side effects include:

Digestive Tract: Nausea; constipation; vomiting.

Nervous System: Sleeplessness; dizziness.

Circulatory System: Bleeding; anemia.

Urinary and Reproductive Tract: Urinary tract infection; urinary retention.

Skin: Rash; itching.

Other: Fever; injection site pain; joint disorder; headache; weakness; swelling in arms and legs; pain; infection.

Guidelines for Use:

- This medicine will be administered by a healthcare provider.
- Injection is subcutaneous for 7 to 14 days. It is started just prior to surgery.
- If easy bruising or bleeding occurs or if there is a fall in blood pressure, contact your physician.
- The injection contains sodium sulfite which may cause allergic-type reactions, including life-threatening or less severe asthmatic episodes in certain susceptible people.
- Periodic lab tests or exams will be required to monitor treatment. Tests will include complete blood counts (eg, platelet count and stool occult blood tests).
- Store ampules at room temperature (36° to 86°F) and syringes under refrigeration (36° to 46°F). Protect from light.

If you have any questions, consult your doctor, pharmacist, or health care provider.

	Generic Name *Brand Name Example*	Supplied As	Generic Available
Rx	**Dipyridamole and Aspirin**		
	Aggrenox	**Capsules, extended-release**: 200 mg	No

Type of Drug:
Combination antiplatelet agent.

How the Drug Works:
Aspirin and dipyridamole work together to prevent blood clots from forming by preventing platelets from clumping together. Platelets are parts of the blood that aid in clot formation.

Uses:
To reduce the risk of stroke in patients who have had transient ischemia of the brain or complete ischemic stroke because of blood clots.

Precautions:
Do not use in the following situations:
allergy to dipyridamole, aspirin, NSAIDs, or any of their ingredients
asthma, nasal polyps, or rhinitis syndrome
sinus infection or inflammation
viral infections with or without fever, children or teenagers

Use with caution in the following situations:
alcohol use
bleeding abnormalities
coronary artery disease
gastrointestinal bleeding or ulcers
kidney disease
liver disease
low blood pressure
peptic ulcer disease

Reye syndrome: There is a risk of Reye syndrome in children and teenagers when usingaspirin in certain viral illnesses. Do not use in children or teenagers with viral infections with or without fever.

Pregnancy: There are no adequate and well-controlled studies in pregnant women. Use only when clearly needed and potential benefits to the mother outweigh the possible hazards to the fetus. Avoid the combination in the third trimester of pregnancy because of the aspirin component.

Breastfeeding: Dipyridamole and aspirin are excreted in breast milk in low concentrations. Use caution when breastfeeding during therapy. Consult your doctor.

Children: Safety and effectiveness in children have not been established. This product is not recommended in children and teenagers because of the aspirin component.

Lab tests may be required during treatment. Tests include liver and kidney function, blood counts, urine tests, and bleeding tests.

Drug Interactions:

Tell your doctor or pharmacist if you are taking or if you are planning to take any over-the-counter or prescription medications or dietary supplements with dipyridamole and aspirin. Doses of one or both drugs may need to be modified or a different drug may need to be prescribed. The following drugs and drug classes interact with dipyridamole and aspirin:

- ACE inhibitors (eg, captopril)
- acetazolamide (eg, *Diamox*)
- adenosine (*Adenocard*)
- anticoagulants (eg, warfarin)
- beta-blockers (eg, propranolol)
- cholinesterase inhibitors (eg, tacrine)
- diuretics (eg, furosemide)
- heparin
- hypoglycemics, oral (eg, sulfonylureas)
- methotrexate (eg, *Rheumatrex*)
- NSAIDs (eg, ibuprofen)
- phenytoin (eg, *Dilantin*)
- uricosuric agents (eg, probenecid)
- valproic acid (eg, *Depakene*)

Side Effects:

Every drug is capable of producing side effects. Many dipyridamole and aspirin users experience no, or minor, side effects. The frequency and severity of side effects depend on many factors including dose, duration of therapy, and individual susceptibility. Possible side effects include:

Nervous System: Headache; forgetfulness; convulsions; confusion; drowsiness; dizziness; fatigue; fainting; weakness.

Digestive Tract: Stomach pain; indigestion; heartburn; nausea; vomiting; diarrhea; appetite loss; dark or bloody stools; rectal bleeding; stomach bleeding; hemorrhoids.

Other: Unusual bleeding or bruising; nosebleed; anemia; joint, chest, muscle, or back pain; joint disease; arthritis; rash; itching; hives; general body discomfort; coughing; upper respiratory tract infection; accidental injury; heart failure; abnormal tissue growth.

Guidelines for Use:

- Dosage is individualized. Take exactly as prescribed.
- Swallow capsules whole. Do not crush or chew.
- Take with food if stomach upset occurs.
- Do not interchange with individual components of aspirin and dipyridamole.
- If a dose is missed, take it as soon as possible. If several hours have passed or if it is nearing time for the next dose, do not double the dose to catch up, unless advised by your doctor. If more than one dose is missed or it is necessary to establish a new dosage schedule, consult your doctor or pharmacist.
- Patients who consume 3 or more alcoholic drinks every day are at a higher risk of gastrointestinal bleeding while taking aspirin.
- Do not use in children or teenagers with viral infections with or without fever because of the risk of Reye syndrome with associated use of aspirin in certain viral illnesses.
- Do not use other aspirin-containing products unless advised by your doctor.
- Notify your doctor if you are pregnant, become pregnant, planning to become pregnant, or are breastfeeding.
- Contact your doctor immediately if you experience signs and symptoms of gastrointestinal side effects (eg, severe or persistant stomach pain, heartburn, nausea, vomiting) or gastrointestinal bleeding (eg, bloody vomit, dark tarry stools).
- Aspirin is contraindicated in patients with known allergy to NSAIDs and in patients with asthma, rhinitis, and nasal polyps.
- Lab tests may be required to monitor treatment. Be sure to keep appointments.
- Store at room temperature (59° to 86°F) in a dry place.

If you have any questions, consult your doctor, pharmacist, or health care provider.

	Generic Name *Brand Name Examples*	Supplied As	Generic Available
Rx	**Heparin Sodium**		Yes
	Heparin Sodium, Unit-Dose	**Injection:** 1000 units/dose; 2500 units/dose; 5000 units/dose; 7500 units/dose; 10,000 units/dose; 20,000 units/dose	
	Heparin Sodium, Multiple Dose Vials	**Injection:** 1000 units/mL; 5,000 units/mL; 10,000 units/mL; 20,000 units/mL; 40,000 units/mL	Yes
	Heparin Sodium, Single Dose Ampules and Vials	**Injection:** 1000 units/mL; 5000 units/mL; 10,000 units/mL; 20,000 units/mL	Yes

Type of Drug:

Injectable anticoagulant; "blood thinner."

How the Drug Works:

Heparin blocks the formation of fibrin (the framework for blood clots), thereby preventing blood clots from forming. It will not dissolve already-formed blood clots, but will prevent them from becoming larger.

Uses:

To prevent blood clots from forming in veins or reaching the lungs.

To treat the extension of existing blood clots in veins, arteries, lungs or heart.

To prevent blood-clotting complications of arterial and heart surgery, blood transfusions, artificial circulation (eg, heart-lung device), dialysis procedures and blood samples for laboratory purposes.

Unlabeled Use(s): To reduce the risk of heart attack or stroke; to decrease angina attacks.

Precautions:

Do not use in the following situations:

absence of blood coagulation tests (full-dose heparin only)
allergy to heparin
bleeding, uncontrolled
intramuscular injection (IM)
low platelet count, severe

Use with caution in the following situations:

arteriosclerosis (hardening of the arteries)
bleeding disorders (eg, hemophilia)
brain, spinal or eye surgery
cancer
diabetes
fever
heart problems (eg, aneurysm)
high blood pressure
increased lipoproteins (type III hyperlipidemia)
infections
kidney disease
liver disease
menstruation
spinal tap/anesthesia, immediately following surgery
ulcers
women over 60 years of age

Allergy: Heparin is derived from animal tissue. Use with caution if there is a history of allergies.

Pregnancy: Adequate studies have not been done in pregnant women, or animal studies may have shown a risk to the fetus. Use only if clearly needed and potential benefits outweigh the possible hazards to the fetus. Heparin does not cross the placenta, but bleeding problems can occur.

Breastfeeding: Heparin does not appear in breast milk. Consult your doctor before you begin breastfeeding.

Children: Safety and effectiveness has not been established in newborns.

Lab tests are used to monitor treatment. Examples of lab tests used include: Partial Thromboplastin Time (PTT), Activated Coagulation Time (ACT), Activated Partial Thromboplastin Time (APTT), platelet count, hematocrit, potassium and occult blood tests for the stool and urine.

Drug Interactions:

Tell your doctor or pharmacist if you are taking or if you are planning to take any over-the-counter or prescription medications while taking this medicine. Doses of one or both drugs may need to be modified or a different drug may need to be prescribed.The following drugs and drug classes interact with this medicine.

antihistamines (eg, *Benadryl)*
aspirin
cephalosporins (eg, cefaclor)
dextran (eg, *Macrodex)*
digitalis (eg, digoxin)
dipyridamole (*Persantine)*
hydroxychloroquine (*Plaquenil)*
ibuprofen (eg, *Motrin)*
indomethacin (eg, *Indocin)*
nicotine (smokers)
nitroglycerin IV (eg, *Nitrostat IV)*
oral anticoagulants (eg, warfarin)
penicillins
tetracyclines (eg, *Sumycin)*

Side Effects:

Every drug is capable of producing side effects. Many patients experience no, or minor, side effects. The frequency and severity of side effects depend on many factors including dose, duration of therapy and individual susceptibility. Possible side effects include:

Digestive Tract: Nausea; vomiting; stomach pain; tarry stools.

Circulatory System: Hemorrhaging (bleeding); chest pain; increased blood pressure.

Respiratory System: Asthma; runny nose; difficulty breathing/swallowing.

Skin: Hives; itching; burning; irritation; mild pain, redness/bruising at injection site; hair loss; unusual bleeding or bruising; discoloration.

Other: Chills; fever; tearing; joint pain; painful sustained erection; headache; abnormal blood counts; shock; paralysis; swelling; osteoporosis (long-term use).

Guidelines for Use:
- Given by injection, usually by health professionals.
- Given continuously or intermittently intravenously (IV) or subcutaneously (SC) several times daily. Intramuscular (IM) use is to be avoided.
- Report any unusual bleeding/bruising, itching, chills, fever or difficulty breathing to your doctor immediately.
- Avoid alcohol while using this medicine.
- Lab tests are required to monitor therapy. Keep appointments.
- Store at room temperature.

If you have any questions, consult your doctor, pharmacist, or health care provider.

Generic Name *Brand Name Example*	Supplied As	Generic Available
Rx **Enoxaparin Sodium**		
Lovenox	**Injection:** 30 mg/0.3 mL, 40 mg/0.4 mL, 60 mg/0.6 mL, 80 mg/0.8 mL, 100 mg/mL	No

Type of Drug:

Low molecular weight heparin (LMWH); injectable anticoagulant; "blood thinner."

How the Drug Works:

Enoxaparin is a low molecular weight heparin ("blood thinner") that prevents blood clots from forming.

Uses:

For the prevention of deep vein thrombosis (DVT), which may lead to pulmonary embolism (PE) (blood clots in the lung) in patients undergoing hip replacement surgery, during and following hospitalization for knee replacement surgery or abdominal surgery in patients who are at risk for blood clotting complications. Patients at risk include those who are > 40 years of age, obese, undergoing surgery under general anesthesia lasting > 30 minutes, or who have additional risk factors such as cancer or a history of DVT or PE.

In conjunction with warfarin sodium (eg, *Coumadin*) for inpatient treatment of acute DVT with and without PE or outpatient treatment of acute DVT without PE.

For the prevention of ischemic complications of unstable angina and non-Q-wave myocardial infarction when coadministered with aspirin.

Precautions:

Do not use in the following situations:

allergy to any other low molecular weight heparin
allergy to enoxaparin or any of its ingredients
allergy to heparin
allergy to pork products
bleeding, active major
thrombocytopenia (low platelet count) with positive test for antiplatelet antibody

Use with caution in the following situations:

bleeding disorders
diabetic retinopathy
elderly
endocarditis, bacterial
gastrointestinal disease (eg, ulcers or bleeding)
heparin-induced thrombocytopenia, history of
high blood pressure, severe and uncontrolled
kidney disease
stroke, hemorrhagic
surgery, recent (brain, spine, or eye)

Pregnancy: There are no adequate and well-controlled studies in pregnant women. Use only if clearly needed and the potential benefits to the mother outweigh the possible risks to the fetus.

Breastfeeding: It is not known if enoxaparin appears in breast milk. Consult your doctor before you begin breastfeeding.

Children: Safety and effectiveness in children have not been established.

Lab tests may be required to monitor therapy. Tests may include complete blood counts, urinalysis, and stool occult blood tests.

Drug Interactions:

Tell your doctor or pharmacist if you are taking or planning to take any over-the-counter or prescription medications or dietary supplements while taking this medicine. Doses of one or both drugs may need to be modified or a different drug may need to be prescribed. The following drugs and drug classes interact with this medicine:

anticoagulants, oral (eg, warfarin)
platelet inhibitors (eg, aspirin, NSAIDs)

Side Effects:

Every drug is capable of producing side effects. Many patients experience no, or minor, side effects. The frequency and severity of side effects depend upon many factors including dose, duration of therapy, and individual susceptibility. Possible side effects include:

Other: Pain, redness, hardness, or bruising at the injection site; heavy or unusual bleeding or bruising; black stools; fever; nausea; swelling of the arms or legs; abnormal blood counts; lab test abnormalities; blood in the urine.

Guidelines for Use:

- Dosage is individualized.
- Do not stop taking or change the dose unless advised to do so by your doctor.
- This medicine is administered once or twice daily. When it is started and how long therapy lasts depends on many factors, including the condition being treated. Your health care provider will advise you on how often to administer and for how long.
- Follow the storage, preparation, and administration techniques taught to you by your health care provider.
- Injections are given around the abdomen.
- Do not rub or massage the injection site after completing the injection. Excessive bruising may occur.
- Administer subcutaneously (SC) (beneath the skin) only; do not administer intramuscularly (IM) or intravenously (IV).
- Change the injection site with each dose.
- If a dose is missed, inject as soon as possible. If > 6 hours have passed or if it is nearing time for the next dose, do not double the dose to catch up, unless advised to do so by your doctor. If more than one dose is missed or it is necessary to establish a new dosing schedule, contact your doctor or pharmacist.
- If excessive bruising occurs at the injection site, it may be lessened by an ice cube massage of the site prior to injection.
- Contact your doctor if you experience bleeding, unusual bruising, dizziness, lightheadedness, itching, rash, fever, swelling of the arms or legs, or difficulty breathing.
- Do not use or substitute any other blood thinner or low molecular weight heparin without first checking with your doctor.
- Do not use if solution is discolored or contains particles.
- Lab tests may be required to monitor therapy. Be sure to keep appointments.
- Store at controlled room temperature (59° to 77°F).

If you have any questions, consult your doctor, pharmacist, or health care provider.

	Generic Name *Brand Name Example*	Supplied As	Generic Available
Rx	**Dalteparin Sodium**		
	Fragmin	**Injection:** 2500 IU (16 mg/ 0.2 mL), 5000 IU (32 mg/ 0.2 mL), 10,000 IU (64 mg/mL)	No

Type of Drug:

Low molecular weight heparin (LMWH); injectable anticoagulant; "blood thinner."

How the Drug Works:

Dalteparin is a low molecular weight heparin ("blood thinner") that prevents blood clots from forming. It will not dissolve already-formed blood clots but may keep them from becoming bigger and breaking loose (embolus).

Uses:

For the prevention of ischemic complications of unstable angina and non-Q-wave myocardial infarction when coadministered with aspirin.

For prevention of deep vein thrombosis (DVT), which may lead to pulmonary embolism (PE) (blood clotting in the lung), in patients undergoing hip replacement surgery or in patients undergoing abdominal surgery who are at risk for blood clotting complications. Patients at risk include those who are > 40 years of age, obese, undergoing surgery under general anesthesia lasting > 30 minutes, or who have additional risk factors such as cancer or a history of DVT or PE.

Unlabeled Use(s): For anticoagulation in venous and arterial thromboembolic complications.

Precautions:

Do not use in the following situations:

allergy to dalteparin or any of its ingredients
allergy to heparin
allergy to pork products
bleeding, active major
thrombocytopenia (low platelet counts) with positive test for antiplatelet antibody

Use with caution in the following situations:

bleeding disorders
endocarditis, bacterial
gastrointestinal disease (eg, ulcers or bleeding)
heparin-induced thrombocytopenia, history of
high blood pressure, severe uncontrolled
kidney disease
retinopathy, hypertensive or diabetic
liver disease
stroke
surgery, recent (brain, spine, or eye)

Pregnancy: There are no adequate and well-controlled studies in pregnant women. Use only if clearly needed and the potential benefits to the mother outweigh the possible risks to the fetus. The multiple-dose vial of *Fragmin* contains benzyl alcohol. Do not use during pregnancy.

Breastfeeding: It is not known if dalteparin appears in breast milk. Consult your doctor before you begin breastfeeding.

Children: Safety and effectiveness in children have not been established.

Lab tests may be required to monitor therapy. Tests may include complete blood counts, urinalysis, and stool occult blood tests.

Drug Interactions:

Tell your doctor or pharmacist if you are taking or planning to take any over-the-counter or prescription medications or dietary supplements while taking this medicine. Doses of one or both drugs may need to be modified or a different drug may need to be prescribed. The following drugs and drug classes interact with this medicine:

anticoagulants, oral (eg, warfarin)
platelet inhibitors (eg, aspirin, dipyridamole, NSAIDs, ticlodipine)

Side Effects:

Every drug is capable of producing side effects. Many patients experience no, or minor, side effects. The frequency and severity of side effects depend on many factors including dose, duration of therapy, and individual susceptibility. Possible side effects include:

Other: Heavy or unusual bleeding; pain or bruising at the injection site; black stools; rash; fever; abnormal blood counts.

Guidelines for Use:

- Dosage is individualized.
- Do not stop taking or change the dose unless advised to do so by your doctor.
- This medicine is administered once or twice daily. When it is started and how long therapy lasts depends on many factors, including the condition being treated.
- Follow the storage, preparation, and administration techniques taught to you by your health care provider.
- Administer subcutaneously (SC) (beneath the skin); do not administer intramuscularly (IM) or intravenously (IV).
- Injections are typically given around the navel or into the upper thigh or buttocks. Change the injection site with each dose.
- If excessive bruising occurs at the injection site, it may be lessened by an ice cube massage of the site before injection.
- Do not rub or massage the injection site after completing the injection. Excessive bruising may occur.
- Do not use if solution is discolored or contains particles.
- If a dose is missed, inject as soon as possible. If > 12 hours have passed or if it is nearing time for the next dose, do not double the dose to catch up, unless advised to do so by your doctor. If more than one dose is missed or it is necessary to establish a new dosing schedule, contact your doctor or pharmacist.
- Contact your doctor if you experience bleeding, bruising, dizziness, lightheadedness, itching, rash, fever, swelling of the arms or legs, or difficulty breathing.
- Do not use or substitute any other blood thinner or low molecular weight heparin without first checking with your doctor.
- Lab tests may be required to monitor therapy. Be sure to keep appointments.
- Store at controlled room temperature (68° to 77°F).

If you have any questions, consult your doctor, pharmacist, or health care provider.

	Generic Name *Brand Name Examples*	Supplied As	Generic Available
Rx	**Ardeparin Sodium** *Normiflo*	**Injection:** 5,000 anti-Xa U/ 0.5 mL; 10,000 anti-Xa U/ 0.5 mL	No

Type of Drug:

Low molecular weight heparin.

How the Drug Works:

Inhibits reactions that lead to blood clots.

Uses:

For the prevention of blood clots in deep veins, which may lead to pulmonary embolism, following knee replacement surgery.

Precautions:

Do not use in the following situations:

- allergy to the drug or pork products
- bleeding, active major
- decreased blood platelets

Use with caution in the following situations:

- active gastrointestinal pathology
- allergy to methylparaben, propylparaben or metabisulfate
- bacterial endocarditis
- bleeding diathesis
- bleeding disorders, congenital or acquired
- epidural anesthesia
- gastric bleeding, recent
- high blood pressure, severe uncontrolled
- kidney failure, severe
- liver disease, severe
- platelet defects
- platelet inhibitor treatment
- retinal disease, high blood pressure or diabetic
- spinal puncture
- spinal anesthesia
- stroke, hemorrhagic
- surgery, after brain, spinal or eye

Ardeparin cannot be used interchangeably with sodium heparin or other low molecular weight heparins.

Pregnancy: Adequate studies have not been done in pregnant women. Use only if clearly needed and potential benefits outweigh the possible hazards to the fetus.

Breastfeeding: It is not known if ardeparin appears in breast milk. Consult your doctor before you begin breastfeeding.

Children: Safety and effectiveness in children have not been established.

Lab tests or exams may be required to monitor treatment. Be sure to keep appointments. Tests may include blood counts.

Sulfites: Contains metabisulfite preservatives that can cause allergic reactions in certain individuals (eg, asthmatics). Check package label when available or consult your doctor or pharmacist.

Drug Interactions:

Tell your doctor or pharmacist if you are taking or planning to take any over-the-counter or prescription medications with ardeparin sodium. Doses of one or both drugs may need to be modified or a different drug may need to be prescribed. The following drugs and drug classes interact with ardeparin.

anticoagulants (eg, warfarin)
aspirin
NSAIDs (eg, ibuprofen)
platelet inhibitors

Side Effects:

Every drug is capable of producing side effects. Many ardeparin users experience no, or minor, side effects. The frequency and severity of side effects depend on many factors including dose, duration of therapy and individual susceptibility. Possible side effects include:

Digestive Tract: Vomiting; vomiting of blood; black vomit; nausea; bloody, black or tarry stool.

Nervous System: Cerebrovascular accident; dizziness; headache; sleeplessness.

Circulatory System: Bleeding; decreased blood platelets; unusual bruising; anemia; chest pain.

Skin: Rash; itching; hives; bruises.

Other: Nosebleed; difficulty breathing; blood in urine; fever; joint pain; bruising; bleeding; swelling, inflammation or pain at injection site; swelling of arms and legs.

Guidelines for Use:

- Administer SC. Do not administer IM or IV.
- Do not use interchangeably with other low molecular weight heparins.
- Do not mix with other injectables or infusions.
- Rotate injection sites.
- Dose is based on weight and administered every 12 hours.
- Do not rub injection site after completing the injection.
- Begin treatment in the evening of the day of surgery or the following morning and continue for up to 14 days or until patient is fully ambulatory.
- Do not use if discolored or if particulate matter is noted in syringe.
- Store at room temperature (59° to 77°F).

If you have any questions, consult your doctor, pharmacist, or health care provider.

	Generic Name *Brand Name Example*	Supplied As	Generic Available
Rx	**Tinzaparin Sodium**		
	Innohep[1]	**Injection**: 20,000 IU/mL	No

[1] Contains sodium metabisulfite and benzyl alcohol.

Type of Drug:

Injectable anticoagulant; "blood thinner."

How the Drug Works:

Tinzaparin inhibits reactions that lead to the clotting of blood, including the formation of fibrin clots. It acts as a potent co-inhibitor of several activated coagulation factors, especially factors Xa and IIa (thrombin). The primary inhibitory activity is mediated through the plasma protease inhibitor, antithrombin.

Uses:

For the treatment of acute symptomatic deep vein thrombosis (DVT) with or without pulmonary embolism (PE) when administered in conjuction with warfarin sodium.

Precautions:

Do not use in the following situations:

active major bleeding
allergy to heparin, benzyl alcohol, sulfites, or pork products
allergy to tinzaparin or any of its ingredients
heparin-induced thrombocytopenia, active or history of

Use with caution in the following situations:

amyloidosis
angiodysplasic gastrointestinal disease
bacterial endocarditis
congenital or aquired bleeding disorders
gastrointestinal disease, ulcerative
high blood pressure, severe or uncontrolled
kidney disease
liver disease
platelet inhibitor use, concomitant
stroke, hemorrhagic

Surgery: Use caution when administering tinzaparin shortly after brain, spinal, or ophthalmological surgery.

Pregnancy: There are no adequate and well-controlled studies in pregnant women. Use only if clearly needed and the potential benefits to the mother outweigh the possible hazards to the fetus.

Breastfeeding: It is not known whether tinzaparin is excreted in breast milk. Consult your doctor before you begin breastfeeding.

Children: Safety and effectiveness in children have not been established.

Lab tests will be required periodically during treatment. Tests may include platelet counts, hemotocrit counts, hemoglobin counts, and stool tests.

Drug Interactions:

Tell your doctor or pharmacist if you are taking or planning to take any over-the-counter or prescription medication or dietary supplements with tinzaparin. Doses of one or both drugs may need to be modified or a different drug may need to be prescribed. The following drugs and drug classes interact with tinzaparin:

dextran 1 (*Promit*)
dipyridamole (eg, *Persantine*)
NSAIDs (eg, ketorolac tromethamine)
salicylates (eg, aspirin)
sulfinpyrazone (eg, *Anturane*)
thrombolytic agents (eg, alteplase)
warfarin (eg, *Coumadin*)

Side Effects:

Every drug is capable of producing side effects. Many tinzaparin users experience no, or minor, side effects. The frequency and severity of side effects depend on many factors including dose, duration of therapy, and individual susceptibility. Possible side effects include:

Hematologic: Abnormal blood counts; blood in urine; anemia; decreased blood platelets; rectal bleeding; nosebleeds; cerebral bleeding; gastrointestinal bleeding; blood in the joints; vomiting of blood; bloody stools; unusual bleeding or bruising; abdominal bleeding; vaginal bleeding; wound bleeding; eye bleeding; coughing up blood; increased aminotransferase levels.

Digestive Tract: Gas; gastrointestinal disorder; indigestion; constipation; diarrhea; abdominal pain; vomiting; nausea.

Circulatory System: Fast heartbeat; chest pain; changes in blood pressure.

Skin: Rash; hives; skin disorder; itching; flushing or redness; skin inflammation; injection site reaction.

Other: Fever; dizziness; headache; difficulty breathing; respiratory disorder; pneumonia; liver disorder; persistant erection; sleeplessness; confusion; healing impairment; urinary retention; painful or difficult urination; urinary tract infection; inflammation of the veins with clot formation.

Guidelines for Use:

- This medicine will be prepared and administered by your health care provider in a medical setting.
- Dosage is individualized.
- Inform your doctor if you are pregnant, become pregnant, planning to become pregnant, or are breastfeeding.
- Inform you doctor if you suffer from a bleeding disorder, uncontrolled arterial high blood pressure, or a history of recent gastrointestinal ulceration, diabetic retinopathy, and hemorrhage.
- Contact your doctor if any side effect becomes bothersome.

If you have any questions, consult your doctor, pharmacist, or health care provider.

	Generic Name *Brand Name Examples*	Supplied As	Generic Available
	Anisindione		
Rx	*Miradon*	**Tablets:** 50 mg	No
Rx	*Dicumarol*	**Tablets:** 25 mg	Yes
	Warfarin Sodium		
Rx	*Coumadin*	**Tablets:** 1 mg, 2 mg, 2.5 mg, 4 mg, 5 mg, 7.5 mg, 10 mg	No
Rx	*Coumadin*	**Injection:** 2 mg/mL	No

All of the products listed on this table are coumarin derivatives; however, they or their brand names are not interchangeable. For examplo, dicumarol cannot be used for anisindione, or coumadin cannot be used for generic warfarin. Daily dose may vary depending on individual needs. Do not adjust the dose without consulting your pharmacist or doctor.

Type of Drug:

Coumarin; anticoagulants, anti-clotting drugs; warfarin, blood thinners.

How the Drug Works:

Coumarin prevents the liver from making substances needed to form blood clots. Anticoagulants are often given after stopping injectable heparin. Anticoagulants will not dissolve already-formed blood clots or repair tissue damage caused by blood clots.

Uses:

To prevent or treat blood clots in veins.

To prevent or treat blood clots in the lungs.

To prevent blood clots associated with atrial fibrillation.

Warfarin — To reduce the risk of recurrence of a heart attack or a stroke after a heart attack, and to prevent blood clots after heart valve replacement or in patients with damaged heart valves.

Anisindione, dicumarol — To treat coronary blockage.

Unlabeled Use(s): Occasionally doctors may prescribe anticoagulants to prevent heart attack or symptoms which precede stroke. Warfarin has also been prescribed with cancer drugs and radiation for treatment of small cell lung cancer.

Precautions:

Do not use in the following situations:

abnormal bleeding, history
abortion, threatened
alcoholism
allergy to this medicine
anesthesia, spinal
aneurysm
arthritis (anisindione only)
bleeding (eg, hemophilia, ulcers, genital or respiratory bleeding)
blood disease (anisindione only)
bruising

cancer, abdominal (dicumarol, anisindione)
colitis, ulcerative (anisindione only)
diverticulitis (anisindione only)
drainage (anisindione only)
emaciation (excessive leanness)
endocarditis, bacterial
high blood pressure, severe
inflammation or fluid around the heart
intrauterine device (IUD) insertion
kidney disease, serious (dicumarol, anisindione)
leukemia (anisindione only)
liver disease, serious (dicumarol, anisindione)
malnutrition (anisindione only)
polycythemia vera (eg, increase in blood volume) (anisindione only)
preeclampsia or eclampsia
pregnancy
prostate surgery
psychotic mental disorder
senility, unsupervised
spinal tap (puncture)
stroke, recent
surgery of eye, brain or central nervous system or resulting in large open surfaces
surgery, major
uncooperative patients
vitamin C deficiency (anisindione only)
vitamin K deficiency (dicumarol, anisindione)
wounds, open

Use with caution in the following situations:

absorption problems
allergic or anaphylactic disorders, severe
anemia, severe
antibiotic therapy
biliary tract abnormalities (anisindione only)
blood clots, recent
catheter use
congestive heart failure
dental procedures
diabetes, severe
diarrhea
drainage tubes, use (dicumarol only)
elderly
fever (anisindione, dicoumerol)
gastrointestinal bleeding, history
heart attack, recent
heart rhythm problems
high blood pressure
high cholesterol (anisindione only)
high triglycerides (anisindione only)
hyperthyroidism (anisindione only)
infections
injections, intramuscular
intestinal flora disturbances
jaundice (anisindione only)
kidney disease
liver disease
menstruation
polycythemia vera (increase in blood volume) (warfarin, dicumarol)
postpartum (after childbirth) (dicumarol only)
preparatory bowel sterilization (anisindione only)
protein C deficiency
protein C resistance
stomach bleeding, history of
stroke, history of
surgery with large exposed raw surfaces
surgery, recent
surgery/trauma, with potential internal bleeding
tuberculosis, active (dicumarol only)
vascular damage (anisindione only)
vasculitis (warfarin, dicumarol)
X-ray therapy (anisindione only)

Lab tests: Treatment with anticoagulants may be different with each patient. Dosage is controlled by lab tests. Tests may include kidney or liver function tests, prothrombin time (protime, PT) or INR (Interactional Normalized Ratio). Testing may be daily in the beginning of treatment. Once the dosage is stabilized, testing is every 4 to 6 weeks. Be sure to keep appointments.

Pregnancy: Do not use during pregnancy. The risk of use in a pregnant woman clearly outweighs any possible benefit.

Breastfeeding: Anticoagulants appear in breast milk. Nursing is not recommended while using anticoagulants.

Children: Safety and effectiveness have not been established.

Elderly: Elderly patients may be more sensitive to these agents.

Drug Interactions:

Tell your doctor or pharmacist if you are taking or if you are planning to take any over-the-counter or prescription medications while taking this medicine. Doses of one or both drugs may need to be modified or a different drug may need to be prescribed. The following drugs and drug classes interact with this medicine.

acetaminophen (eg, *Tylenol*)
adrenocortical steroids (eg, corticotropin)
alcohol
allopurinol (eg, *Zyloprim*)
aminoglutethimide (*Cytadren*)
aminoglycosides, oral (eg, neomycin)
aminosalicylic acid (*Pasar*)
amiodarone (*Cordarone*)
anabolic steroids (eg, oxandrolone)
androgens (eg, testosterone)
anesthetics, inhalation
antacids
antihistamines (eg, terfenadine)
azole antifungal agents (eg, metronidazole)
barbiturates (eg, phenobarbital)
beta blockers (eg, propranolol)
carbamazepine (eg, *Tegretol*)
cephalosporins (eg, cefaclor)
chloral hydrate
chloramphenicol (*Chloromycetin*)
chlordiazepoxide (eg, *Librium*)
chlorpropamide (eg, *Diabinese*)
cholestyramine (eg, *Questran*)
chymotrypsin (*Catarase*)
cimetidine (eg, *Tagamet*)
clofibrate (eg, *Atromid-S*)
contraceptives, oral (eg, *Ortho-Novum*)
corticosteroids (eg, prednisone)
cyclophosphamide (eg, *Cytoxan*)
dextran (eg, *Gentran*)
dextrothyroxine (*Choloxin*)
diazoxide (*Proglycam*)
dicloxacillin (eg, *Dynapen*)
diflunisal (*Dolobid*)
dipyridamole (*Persantine*)
disopyramide (eg, *Norpace*)
disulfiram (eg, *Antabuse*)
diuretics (eg, thiazides)
erythromycin (eg, *E-Mycin*)
estrogens (eg, estradiol)
ethacrynic acid (*Edecrin*)
ethchlorvynol (*Placidyl*)
etretinate (*Tegison*)
fenoprofen (eg, *Nalfon*)
fluorouracil (eg, *Adrucil*)
gemfibrozil (*Lopid*)
glucagon
glutethimide
griseofulvin (eg, *Grisactin*)
haloperidol (eg, *Haldol*)
hydantoins (eg, phenytoin)
hydrochloroquine (*Plaquenil*)
influenza vaccine
ifosfamide (*Ifex*)
isoniazid (eg, *Nydrazid*)
lovastatin (*Mevacor*)

magnesium salts (eg, *Milk of Magnesia)*
MAO inhibitor antidepressants (eg, phenelzine)
mefenamic acid (*Ponstel*)
meprobamate (eg, *Meprospan*)
methyldopa (eg, *Aldomet*)
methylphenidate (eg, *Ritalin*)
mineral oil
mitotane (*Lysodren*)
moricizine (*Ethmozine*)
nalidixic acid (*NegGram*)
nonsteroidal anti-inflammatory agents (eg, ibuprofen)
omeprazole (*Prilosec*)
paraldehyde (*Paral*)
penicillins (eg, amoxcillin)
pentoxifylline (*Trental*)
primadone (*Mysoline*)
propafenone (*Rythmol*)
propoxyphene (eg, *Darvon*)
quinidine (eg, *Quinora*)
quinine
quinolones (eg, ciprofloxacin)
rifamycins (eg, rifampin)
ranitidine (eg, *Zantac*)
salicylates (eg, aspirin)
serotonin reputake inhibitor antidepressants (eg, fluoxetine)
spironolactone (eg, *Aldactone*)
sucralfate (*Carafate*)
sulfonamides, (eg, sulfamethoxazole/trimethoprim)
sulfinpyrazone (eg, *Anturane*)
tamoxifen (*Nolvadex*)
tetracyclines (eg, doxycycline)
thioamines (eg, propylthiouracil)
thiopurines (eg, azathioprine)
thrombolytic agents (eg, alteplase)
thyroid hormones (eg, levothyroxine)
ticlopidine (*Ticlid*)
tolbutamide (eg, *Orinase*)
trazodone (eg, *Desyrel*)
tricyclic antidepressants (eg, amitriptyline)
valproic acid (eg, *Depakene*)
vitamin C
vitamin E
vitamin K

Side Effects:

Every drug is capable of producing side effects. Many patients experience no, or minor, side effects. The frequency and severity of side effects depend on many factors including dose, duration of therapy and individual susceptibility. Possible side effects include:

Hemorrhage: Bloody or tarry stools; blood in urine; red or dark urine; excessive
menstrual bleeding; unusual bleeding or bruising.

Digestive Tract: Diarrhea; nausea; vomiting; stomach pain; mouth sores; appetite loss.

Skin: Dermatitis; hives; purple toes; gangrene.

Other: Hair loss; yellowing of skin or eyes; fever; chills; chest, abdomen or joint pain; shortness of breath; difficulty breathing or swallowing; swelling; shock; paralysis; headache; drowsiness; sore throat; blurred vision; orange-red discoloration of urine; inability to urinate (anisindione only); sustained and painful erection.

Guidelines for Use:

- Use exactly as prescribed. Strict adherence to prescribed dosage schedule is necessary.
- Dosing is individualized and may have to be frequently adjusted based on lab test results.
- *Injection* — Follow the injection procedure taught to you by your health care provider.
- If a dose is missed, take it as soon as possible. If several hours have passed or if it is nearing time for the next dose, do not double the dose to catch up, unless advised by your doctor. If more than one dose is missed, contact your doctor or pharmacist.
- Do not take or discontinue any other medication except on advice of your pharmacist or doctor.
- Avoid alcohol, aspirin, topical pain killers, large amounts of green leafy vegetables, or drastic changes in dietary habits.
- Inform your doctor if you are pregnant, become pregnant, are planning to become pregnant, or if you are breastfeeding.
- Contact your doctor if you experience diarrhea, infection, fever, pain, swelling, discomfort, prolonged bleeding from cuts, increased menstrual flow or vaginal bleeding, blood in urine, nosebleeds, bleeding from gums when brushing, other unusual bleeding or bruising, red or dark brown urine, red or tar black stools, purple toes, toe pain or tenderness, rash, ulcers, or hair loss.
- *Anisindione* — Contact your doctor if you experience excessive fatigue, chills, fever, or sore throat.
- Contact your doctor before undergoing dental work or elective surgery.
- Warfarin may cause a red-orange discoloration of urine.
- All of the products listed on this table are coumarin derivatives; however, they are not interchangeable.
- Lab tests will be required to monitor therapy. Be sure to keep appointments.
- *Injection* — Visually inspect solution for particles or discoloration.
- Store reconstituted injection solution at room temperature (59° to 86°F). Do not refrigerate. Use within 4 hours. Discard any unused solution.
- Store tablets at room temperature (59° to 77°F) in a tight, light-resistant container.

If you have any questions, consult your doctor, pharmacist, or health care provider.

	Generic Name *Brand Name Examples*	Supplied As	Generic Available
Rx	**Alteplase, Recombinant**		
	Activase	**Powder for injection, lyophilized**: 50 mg/vial,[1] 100 mg/vial[1]	No
Rx	**Anistreplase**		
	Eminase	**Powder for injection, lyophilized**: 30 units	No
Rx	**Reteplase, Recombinant**		
	Retavase	**Powder for injection, lyophilized**: 18.1 mg reteplase[2]	No
Rx	**Streptokinase**		
	Streptase	**Powder for injection, lyophilized**: 250,000 IU, 750,000 IU, 1,500,000 IU	No
Rx	**Tenecteplase**		
	TNKase	**Powder for injection, lyophilized**: 50 mg[1]	No

[1] Contains L-arginine, phosphoric acid, polysorbate 80.
[2] Contains L-arginine.

Type of Drug:

Blood clot dissolvers.

How the Drug Works:

Thrombolytic agents dissolve blood clots and restore blood circulation to affected body tissue.

Uses:

To dissolve blood clots, including those blocking coronary arteries in acute heart attacks.

Alteplase: To help manage acute ischemic strokes in adults to reduce the chances of disability, or to reduce the incidence of congestive heart failure (CHF) and death due to heart attack.

Streptokinase: To dissolve large blood clots in legs.

Unlabeled Use(s): Occasionally doctors may prescribe alteplase for the treatment of unstable angina pectoris (chest pain).

Precautions:

Do not use in the following situations:

abnormal bleeding conditions
allergy to the thrombolytic agent or any of its ingredients
bleeding into or around the brain
brain aneurysm
brain cancer
cardiopulmonary resuscitation (CPR), recent
cerebrovascular accident (stroke), history of
high blood pressure, severe, uncontrolled
internal bleeding
low platelet count
seizures at onset of stroke
stroke, previous (within 2 to 3 months)
surgery or trauma to head or spine (within 2 to 3 months)

Use with caution in the following situations:

bacterial endocarditis
black or tarry stools
bleeding
blood clot in heart chamber
brain blood vessel disease
childbirth
diabetic bleeding retinopathy
gastrointestinal bleeding, recent
genitourinary bleeding, recent
high blood pressure
infections involving the heart
kidney disease
liver disease
major surgery or trauma, recent
older than 75 years of age
pregnancy
readministration (alteplase, anistrepalse, streptokinase, tenecteplase only)
stroke, history of

Abnormal heartbeats: Use of thrombolytic agents to dissolve clots in coronary arteries (acute heart attack) may result in abnormal heartbeat. Heart rate will need to be monitored during and following therapy.

Pregnancy: Safety for use during pregnancy has not been established. Use only if clearly needed and the potential benefits to the mother outweigh the possible hazards to the fetus.

Breastfeeding: It is not known if thrombolytic agents appear in breast milk. Consult your doctor before you begin breastfeeding.

Children: Safety and effectiveness have not been established.

Lab tests will be required to monitor therapy. Tests may include platelet counts, thrombin time (TT), activated partial thromboplastin time (APTT), prothrombin time (PT), fibrinogen levels, hematocrit counts, as well as the monitoring of blood pressure, heart rate and rhythm, and other vital signs (eg, respirations, temperature).

Drug Interactions:

Tell your doctor or pharmacist if you are taking or will be taking any over-the-counter or prescription medications or dietary supplements while taking a thrombolytic agent. Doses of one or both drugs may need to be modified or a different drug may need to be prescribed. The following drugs and drug classes interact with thrombolytic agents:

anticoagulants (eg, warfarin)
antiplatelet agents (eg, *Persantin*)
aspirin
heparin (eg, *Hep-Lock*)
indomethacin (eg, *Indocin*)

Side Effects:

Every drug is capable of producing side effects. Many thrombolytic agent users experience no, or minor, side effects. The frequency and severity of side effects depend on many factors including dose, duration of therapy, and individual susceptibility. Possible side effects include:

Bleeding: Bleeding at puncture and incision sites; bleeding from rectum, stomach, lungs, gums, mouth, nose, or urinary tract.

Digestive Tract: Nausea; vomiting.

Circulatory System: Internal bleeding; irregular heartbeat; changes in blood pressure.

Skin: Rash; unusual bruising.

Other: Fever; chills; difficult or fast breathing; back pain.

Guidelines for Use:

- This medicine will be prepared and administered intravenously (into a vein) by your health care provider in a medical setting.
- Dosage is individualized.
- Effectiveness depends on how quickly the drug is given.
- Bleeding is a common side effect of thrombolytic agent therapy.
- Notify your doctor immediately if you experience fever, shivering, chills, rash, hives, swelling, or difficult or rapid breathing.

If you have any questions, consult your doctor, pharmacist, or health care provider.

	Generic Name *Brand Name Examples*	Supplied As	Generic Available
Rx	**Clopidogrel Bisulfate** *Plavix*	**Tablets:** 75 mg	No

Type of Drug:

An antiplatelet agent.

How the Drug Works:

Clopidogrel prevents blood clots from forming by preventing platelets from clumping together. Platelets are components of the blood that aid in clot formation.

Uses:

Reduction of heart attack, stroke and vascular death in patients with atherosclerosis (hardening of the arteries).

Precautions:

Do not use in the following situations:

allergy to clopidogrel or any of its ingredients
any bleeding disorder (eg, bleeding peptic ulcer or brain bleeding)
GI bleeding

Use with caution in the following situations:

asprin use
liver disease
nonsteroidal anti-inflammatory agent use
trauma, surgery or pathological conditions that increase risk of bleeding
ulcers, GI; duodenal

Pregnancy: Studies in pregnant women have not shown a risk to the fetus. However, no drug should be used during pregnancy unless clearly needed.

Breastfeeding: It is not known if clopidogrel appears in breast milk. Consult your doctor before you begin breastfeeding.

Children: Safety and effectiveness in children have not been established.

Lab tests may be required during treatment with clopidogrel. Tests may include: Complete blood counts, white cell differentials.

Drug Interactions:

Tell your doctor or pharmacist if you are taking or if you are planning to take any over-the-counter or prescription medications with clopidogrel. Doses of one or both drugs may need to be modified or a different drug may need to be prescribed. The following drugs and drug classes interact with clopidogrel.

aspirin
fluvastatin (*Lescol*)
heparin
phenytoin (eg, *Dilantin*)
NSAIDS (eg, ibuprofen)
tamoxifen (*Nolvadex*)
tolbutamide (*Orinase*)
torsemide (*Demadex*)
warfarin (eg, *Coumadin*)

Side Effects:

Every drug is capable of producing side effects. Many clopidogrel users experience no, or minor, side effects. The frequency and severity of side effects depend on many factors including dose, duration of therapy and individual susceptibility. Possible side effects include:

Digestive Tract: GI bleeding; stomach pain; indigestion; diarrhea; nausea; constipation; vomiting.

Nervous System: Headache; dizziness; depression; fainting; decreased sensitivity to stimulation; nerve pain; abnormal skin sensations; feeling of whirling motion; anxiety; sleeplessness.

Circulatory System: High blood pressure; anemia; high blood cholesterol levels; pounding in the chest (palpitations); heart failure; abnormal heart rhythms; decreased platelets and white blood cells.

Respiratory System: Upper respiratory tract infection; difficulty breathing; sinus infection; bronchitis; coughing; congested or runny nose; pneumonia.

Skin: Rash; itching; inflamed skin; easy bruising.

Other: Accidental injury; flu-like symptoms; pain; fatigue; swelling; chest or joint pain; back pain; red or purple spots/patches under the skin (caused from unusual bleeding or bruising); nosebleed; urinary tract infection; weakness; hernia; leg cramps; gout; high blood uric acid levels; joint problems; cataracts; inflammation, redness of eye; bladder inflammation; increased liver enzymes.

Guidelines for Use:

- Usual dose is 75 mg once daily.
- May be taken with or without food. Take with food if stomach upset occurs.
- If a dose is missed, take it as soon as possible. If several hours have passed or if it is nearing time for the next dose, do not double the dose in order to "catch up" (unless advised to do so by your doctor). If more than one dose is missed or it is necessary to establish a new dosage schedule, contact your doctor or pharmacist. Use exactly as prescribed.
- It may take longer than usual to stop bleeding when taking clopidogrel. Report any unusual bleeding (eg, bruising, nosebleed, blood in urine or stools) or dark-colored stools to your doctor.
- Contact your doctor immediately if you experience any signs of infection such as fever, chills or sore throat.
- Contact your doctor if rash, difficulty breathing or irregular heartbeat occurs.
- Tell your dentist and doctor that you are taking clopidogrel before any surgery is scheduled and before any new drug is prescribed.
- Discontinue clopidogrel 7 days before any surgery or procedure in which antiplatelet effects are not wanted.
- Inform your doctor if you are pregnant, become pregnant, are planning to become pregnant or if you are breastfeeding.
- Store at room temperature.

If you have any questions, consult your doctor, pharmacist, or health care provider.

	Generic Name *Brand Name Examples*	Supplied As	Generic Available
	Pentoxifylline		
Rx	*Trental*	**Tablets, controlled release:** 400 mg	No

Type of Drug:

Hemorrheologic agent; a drug that improves blood flow.

How the Drug Works:

Pentoxifylline improves blood flow by reducing the thickness of the blood and improving red blood cell flexibility.

Uses:

To treat circulatory conditions in the arms and legs (eg, intermittent claudication) that cause discomfort. It does not, however, cure these conditions.

Unlabeled Use(s): Occasionally doctors may prescribe pentoxifylline for cerebrovascular problems, circulatory and problems caused by diabetes, leg ulcers, sickle cell anemia, strokes, high altitude sickness, hearing problems, eye circulation disorders and Reynaud's syndrome.

Precautions:

Do not use in the following situations:
allergy to pentoxifylline, caffeine, theophylline or theobromine
cerebral and/or retinal bleeding

Use with caution in the following situations:
arteriosclerosis (hardening of the arteries)
kidney disease
peptic ulcers
surgery, recent

Pregnancy: Adequate studies have not been done in pregnant women, or animal studies may have shown a risk to the fetus. Use only if clearly needed and potential benefits outweigh the possible hazards to the fetus.

Breastfeeding: Pentoxifylline appears in breast milk. Consult your doctor before you begin breastfeeding.

Children: Safety and effectiveness in children have not been established.

Lab tests or exams may be required to monitor therapy. Be sure to keep appointments. Tests may include prothrombin time and exams for bleeding (eg, hematocrit/hemoglobin).

Drug Interactions:

Tell your doctor or pharmacist if you are taking or planning to take any over-the-counter or prescription medications while taking this medicine. Doses of one or both drugs may need to be modified or another drug may need to be prescribed. The following drugs and drug classes interact with this medicine:

anticoagulants, oral (eg, warfarin)
theophylline (eg, *Slo-Phyllin*)

Side Effects:

Every drug is capable of producing side effects. Many patients experience no, or minor, side effects. The frequency and severity of side effects depend on many factors including dose, duration of therapy and individual susceptibility. Possible side effects may include:

Digestive Tract: Stomach ache; nausea; vomiting; indigestion.

Nervous System: Dizziness; headache.

Guidelines for Use:

- Use exactly as prescribed.
- Take 1 tablet, three times daily with meals. A lower dose may be necessary if side effects occur. Consult your doctor.
- Do not crush, chew or break tablet.
- If a dose is missed, take it as soon as possible. If several hours have passed or if it is nearing time for the next dose, do not double the dose in order to "catch up" (unless advised to do so by your doctor). If more than one dose is missed or it is necessary to establish a new dosage schedule, contact your doctor or pharmacist.
- Improvement may take 2 to 4 weeks to notice and up to 8 weeks for maximum relief.
- If severe indigestion, nausea, vomiting, nervousness, dizziness or headache occur, contact your doctor immediately.
- May cause dizziness. Use caution while driving or performing other tasks requiring alertness, coordination or physical dexterity.
- Store at room temperature (59° to 86°F). Protect from light.

If you have any questions, consult your doctor, pharmacist, or health care provider.

	Generic Name *Brand Name Examples*	Supplied As	Generic Available
	Phytonadione		
Rx	*Mephyton*	**Tablets:** 5 mg	No
Rx	*AquaMEPHYTON*	**Injection:** 2 mg/mL, 10 mg/mL	Yes

Type of Drug:

Antihemorrheologic; antibleeding agent.

How the Drug Works:

Phytonadione stimulates the production of certain factors needed for blood to clot.

Uses:

To treat certain bleeding disorders caused by a lack of vitamin K or interference with the way vitamin K works.

Precautions:

Do not use in the following situations: Allergy to this medicine.

Use with caution in the following situations: Anticoagulant use, liver disease.

Injection: Phytonadione should be given under the skin or in the muscle. Injection into the vein (IV) may lead to shock, heart attack, stopped breathing and death. IV injection should only be used when the other methods are not possible and the serious risk involved is considered justified.

Pregnancy: Adequate studies have not been done in pregnant women, or animal studies may have shown a risk to the fetus. Use only if clearly needed and potential benefits outweigh the possible risk to the fetus.

Breastfeeding: Phytonadione appears in breast milk. Consult your doctor.

Children: Safety and effectiveness have not been established. Certain blood and liver problems in infants may be related to phytonadione use. Do not exceed recommended dosage.

Lab tests will be required. Tests may include prothrombin time monitoring.

Drug Interactions:

Tell your doctor or pharmacist if you are taking or will be taking any other medications. Doses need to be adjusted or a different drug may need to be prescribed. Anticoagulants (eg, warfarin) and mineral oil interact with this medicine.

Side Effects:

Every drug is capable of producing side effects. Many patients experience no, or minor, side effects. The frequency and severity of side effects depend on many factors including dose, duration of therapy and individual susceptibility. Possible side effects include: Temporary flushing and taste changes; pain, swelling and tenderness at the injection site; allergic reactions.

Guidelines for Use:

- Results are not immediate.
- Store at room temperature. Protect from light.

If you have any questions, consult your doctor, pharmacist, or health care provider.

Generic Name *Brand Name Examples*	Supplied As	Generic Available
Rx **Sodium Phenylbutyrate**		
Buphenyl	**Tablets:** 500 mg	No
Buphenyl	**Powder:** 3.2 g/tsp, 9.1 g/tbsp	No

Type of Drug:

Urea cycle disorder treatment.

How the Drug Works:

Sodium phenylbutyrate forms a substance needed for the elimination of nitrogen waste (ammonia) from the body.

Uses:

Adjunctive therapy for chronic management of patients with urea cycle disorder and in infants with enzymatic deficiencies that result in elevated levels of ammonia in the blood.

Precautions:

Do not use in the following situations:

to manage acute elevated ammonia blood levels

Use with caution in the following situations:

congestive heart failure (CHF)
kidney disease
liver disease
nerve impairment
sodium retention causing fluid retention (edema, swelling, water retention)

Pregnancy: Adequate studies have not been done in pregnant women, or animal studies may have shown a risk to the fetus. Use only if clearly needed and the potential benefits outweigh the possible hazards to the fetus.

Breastfeeding: It is not known if sodium phenylbutyrate appears in breast milk. Consult your doctor before you begin breastfeeding.

Children: Use of the tablets in newborns, infants and children under 44 lbs is not recommended.

Lab tests will be required to monitor therapy. Tests may include: Blood counts and ammonia and amino acid blood levels.

Drug Interactions:

Tell your doctor or pharmacist if you are taking or planning to take any over-the-counter or prescription medication while taking this medicine. Doses of one or both drugs may need to be modified or a different drug may need to be prescribed. The following drugs and drug classes interact with this medicine:

corticosteroids (eg, prednisone)
haloperidol (eg, *Haldol*)
probenecid (eg, *Benemid*)
valproate (eg, *Depakote*)

Side Effects:

Every drug is capable of producing side effects. Many patients experience no, or minor, side effects. The frequency and severity of side effects depend upon many factors including dose, duration of therapy and individual susceptibility. Possible side effects include:

Digestive Tract: Stomach pain; nausea; vomiting; constipation; rectal bleeding; appetite loss; peptic ulcers.

Nervous System: Depression; drowsiness; fatigue; lightheadedness; headache.

Circulatory System: Anemia; abnormal heartbeat.

Other: Menstrual problems; body odor; bad taste; fainting; weight gain; rash; swelling; kidney problems; abnormal lab tests.

Guidelines for Use:

- Use exactly as prescribed.
- *Tablets* — Take in equally divided amounts three times daily with meals.
- *Powder* — Take in equally divided amounts with each meal or feeding, four to six times daily. Mix with food (solid or liquid). Avoid acidic drinks. Shake lightly before use.
- If a dose is missed, take it as soon as possible. If several hours have passed or if it is nearing time for the next dose, do not double the dose in order to "catch up" (unless advised to do so by your doctor). If more than one dose is missed or it is necessary to establish a new dosage schedule, contact your doctor or pharmacist.
- A special diet will be needed to derive the most benefit in using this drug.
- Sodium phenylbutyrate may have to be taken all your life unless liver transplantation is chosen.
- May cause drowsiness, fatigue, fainting or lightheadedness. Use caution while driving or performing other tasks that require alertness, coordination or physical dexterity.
- Contact your doctor immediately if decreased mental awareness, vomiting, combativeness, slurred speech, unstable gait, unconsciousness or fever occurs.
- Store at room temperature (59° to 86°F). Keep bottle tightly closed.

If you have any questions, consult your doctor, pharmacist, or health care provider.

Generic Name *Brand Name Examples*		Supplied As	Generic Available
	Epoetin Alfa		
Rx	*Epogen, Procrit*	**Injection:** 2000 units, 3000 units, 4000 units, 10,000 units	No

Type of Drug:
Blood modifier; antianemia.

How the Drug Works:
Epoetin alfa is a protein produced by the kidney which stimulates red blood cell production.

Uses:
To raise or maintain red blood cell levels and decrease the need for blood transfusions in patients with anemia associated with chronic kidney failure or on zidovudine (AZT) therapy for HIV.

To raise red blood cell levels and decrease the need for blood transfusions in patients with non-myeloid cancer who develop anemia because of chemotherapy. It is intended for patients who will be receiving chemotherapy for at least 2 months.

Unlabeled Use(s): Occasionally doctors may prescribe epoetin alfa to increase a patient's own red blood cell production to use for transfusion for that patient during elective surgery.

Precautions:
Do not use in the following situations:
allergy to this medicine, mammalian (animal) cell-derived products or human albumin
high blood pressure, uncontrolled

Use with caution in the following situations:
anemia due to iron or folate deficiencies, hemolysis or gastrointestinal bleeding (eg, HIV-infected patients and cancer patients)
anemia, severe (chronic kidney failure)
blood disease
high blood pressure, preexisting
low cholesterol, apoprotein B or triglycerides
porphyria
seizures
vascular disease, preexisting

Pregnancy: Adequate studies have not been done in pregnant women, or animal studies may have shown a risk to the fetus. Use only if clearly needed and potential benefits outweigh the possible hazards to the fetus.

Breastfeeding: It is not known if epoetin alfa appears in breast milk. Consult your doctor before you begin breastfeeding.

Children: Safety and effectiveness in children have not been established.

Lab tests will be required to monitor therapy. Be sure to keep appointments. Tests may include: Blood pressure; blood and platelet counts; bleeding time; kidney function tests; fluid and electrolyte tests; serum chemistry; iron evaluation tests.

Drug Interactions:

Tell your doctor or pharmacist if you are taking or planning to take any over-the-counter or prescription medications while taking this medicine. Doses of one or both drugs may need to be modified or a different drug may need to be prescribed.

Side Effects:

Every drug is capable of producing side effects. Some patients experience no, or minor, side effects. The frequency and severity of side effects de end upon man factors including dose, duration of therapy and individual susceptibility. Possible side effects include:

Digestive Tract: Nausea; vomiting; diarrhea.

Nervous System: Headache; fatigue; weakness; dizziness; seizures; abnormal skin sensations.

Circulatory System: High blood pressure; chest pain; blood clots (eg, swelling of the lower legs).

Respiratory System: Congestion; shortness of breath; cough; upper respiratory infection.

Other: Joint or trunk pain; fluid retention; pain or tenderness at injection site; rash; fever.

Guidelines for Use:

- Follow patient instructions provided with the medicine exactly.
- Follow the injection procedure taught to you by your healthcare provider.
- Do not administer with other injections.
- Use this medicine three times weekly. Your doctor will make any necessary dosage adjustments.
- If a dose is missed, inject it as soon as possible. If several hours have passed or if it is nearing time for the next dose, do not double the dose in order to "catch up" (unless advised to do so by your doctor). If more than one dose is missed, contact your doctor or pharmacist.
- Continue to follow the diet and/or dialysis prescribed by your doctor, even if you start to feel better.
- *High blood pressure* — It is important to follow the blood pressure and diet restrictions established by your doctor while taking this medicine.
- Discontinue use and contact your doctor immediately at the first appearance of rash or other signs of allergic reactions (eg, hives).
- Do not reuse needles or syringes. Dispose of used needles and syringes in the puncture-resistant container provided with your medication as directed by your doctor.
- Contraceptive measures (birth control) are recommended during treatment.
- May cause dizziness or seizures. Use caution when driving or performing other tasks requiring alertness, coordination or physical dexterity.
- Visually inspect solution for particles or discoloration before use.
- *Single-dose vials(1 mL)* — Contains no preservatives. Use only one dose per vial. Discard any unused portions.
- *Multi-dose vials (2 mL)* — Contains preservatives. Discard 21 days after first use.
- Refrigerate at 36° to 46°F. Do not freeze or shake.

If you have any questions, consult your doctor, pharmacist, or health care provider.

Generic Name / *Brand Name Examples*	Supplied As	Generic Available
Filgrastim		
Rx *Neupogen*	**Injection:** 300 mcg/mL	No

Type of Drug:

Granulocyte colony or white blood cell stimulating factor.

How the Drug Works:

Filgrastim is a glycoprotein that stimulates the production of neutrophils (white blood cells) in the bone marrow.

Uses:

To decrease the incidence of infections due to neutropenia (low white blood cell counts) with fever in cancer patients who are receiving immunity suppressing anticancer drugs.

To reduce the duration of neutropenia and its symptoms (eg, fever, infections, mouth/throat ulcers) in cancer patients undergoing chemotherapy followed by bone marrow transplantation.

For chronic use to reduce the incidence and duration of the symptoms of neutropenia (eg, fever, infections, oropharyngeal ulcers) in patients with severe chronic neutropenia (SCN).

Unlabeled Use(s): Occasionally doctors may prescribe filgrastim for AIDS, aplastic anemia, hairy cell leukemia or developmental defects of the spinal cord.

Precautions:

Do not use in the following situations:

allergy to filgrastim, *E. coli*-derived proteins or any ingredient of this medicine

Use with caution in the following situations:

chemotherapy
heart conditions
myeloid cancer (bone marrow)
neutropenia (non-SCN)
neutrophil-releasing agents (eg, lithium)
platelet-lowering agents (eg, chlorambucil)
radiation therapy

Allergic reactions are rare, but have been reported usually within 30 minutes of coadministration. Reactions may include rash, itching, facial swelling, difficulty breathing, low blood pressure or fast heartbeat.

Pregnancy: Adequate studies have not been done in pregnant women, or animal studies may have shown a risk to the fetus. Use only if clearly needed and potential benefits outweigh the possible hazards to the fetus.

Breastfeeding: It is not known if filgrastim is excreted in breast milk. Consult your doctor before you begin breastfeeding.

Children: Safety and effectiveness in neonates and children with autoimmune neutropenia of infancy have not been established. Serious long-term risks from daily filgrastim have not been identified in children between 4 months and 17 years of age with severe chronic neutropenia.

Lab tests will be required. Be sure to keep appointments. Tests may include: Blood, neutrophil and platelet counts; bone marrow tests.

Drug Interactions:

Tell your doctor or pharmacist if you are taking or planning to take any over-the-counter or prescription medications while taking this medicine. Doses of one or both drugs may need to be modified or a different drug may need to be prescribed. The following drugs and drug classes interact with this medicine.

neutrophil-releasing agents (eg, lithium)
platelet-lowering agents (eg, chlorambucil)

Side Effects:

Every drug is capable of producing side effects. Many patients experience no, or minor side effects. The frequency and severity of side effects depend on many factors including dose, duration of therapy and individual susceptibility. Possible side effects include:

Digestive Tract: Nausea; vomiting; diarrhea; appetite loss; inflammation of the mouth or mucous membranes; constipation; stomach pain or tenderness.

Other: Bone pain; hair loss; fever; fatigue; difficulty breathing; cough; headache; weakness; rash; chest pain; changes in blood pressure; sore throat; general body pain; abnormal lab tests; nosebleed; itching; facial swelling; fast heartbeat.

Guidelines for Use:

- Follow the patient instructions provided with the medicine exactly.
- Follow injection procedure taught to you by your healthcare provider.
- If a dose is missed, inject it as soon as possible. If several hours have passed or if it is nearing time for the next dose, do not double the dose in order to "catch up" (unless advised to do so by your doctor). If more than one dose is missed or it is necessary to establish a new dosage schedule, contact your doctor or pharmacist.
- Do not stop using this medicine or change the dose without checking with your doctor; this could have serious adverse effects.
- If fever, chills, infection, rash, difficulty breathing, wheezing, low blood pressure or fast heartbeat occurs, contact your doctor immediately.
- Do not reuse needles or syringes. Dispose of needles and syringes in the puncture-resistant containers provided with your medication as directed by your doctor.
- Lab tests will be required. Be sure to keep appointments.
- Visually inspect solution for particles or discoloration before use.
- Refrigerate at 36° to 46°F. Do not freeze or shake. Before injection, filgrastim may be allowed to reach room temperature for a maximum of 24 hours. Discard any solution left at room temperature after 24 hours. Throw out any unused solution.

If you have any questions, consult your doctor, pharmacist, or health care provider.

	Generic Name *Brand Name Examples*	Supplied As	Generic Available
	Sargramostim		
Rx	*Leukine*	**Injection:** 250 mcg, 500 mcg	No

Type of Drug:

Granulocyte colony or white blood cell stimulating factor.

How the Drug Works:

Sargramostim is a glycoprotein that stimulates the production of neutrophils (white blood cells) in the bone marrow.

Uses:

For use after induction of chemotherapy in patients 55 years of age or older with acute myelogenous leukemia (AmL) to shorten time to neutrophil recovery to lower the risks of severe and life-threatening infections.

To accelerate bone marrow recovery in patients with non-Hodgkin's lymphoma (NHL), acute lymphoblastic leukemia (ALL) and Hodgkin's disease undergoing bone marrow transplantation (BMT).

For bone marrow transplant patients in whom engraftment of bone marrow is delayed or fails.

Unlabeled Use(s): Occasionally doctors may prescribe sargramostim to increase white blood cell counts in patients with developmental defects of the spinal cord or in AIDS patients receiving zidovudine (AZT); to decrease the low white blood cell counts secondary to immunity depressing chemotherapy and decrease low immunity in preleukemic patients; to correct low white blood cell counts in aplastic anemia patients; and to decrease transplantation-associated organ system damage, particularly in the liver and kidney.

Precautions:

Do not use in the following situations:

allergy to sargramostim, yeast-derived products or any ingredient of this medicine
chemotherapy, current
immature white blood cells in the bone marrow or peripheral blood, excessive radiation therapy, current

Use with caution in the following situations:

chemotherapy, previous
congestive heart failure (CHF)
fluid retention
heart disease
hypoxia (low oxygen level in the blood)
kidney disease
liver disease
lung disease
lung infiltrates
myeloid (bone marrow) cancer
radiation therapy, previous

Pregnancy: Adequate studies have not been done in pregnant women, or animal studies may have shown a risk to the fetus. Use only if clearly needed and potential benefits outweigh the possible risk to the fetus.

Breastfeeding: It is not known if sargramostim appears in breast milk. Consult your doctor before you begin breastfeeding.

Children: Safety and effectiveness in children have not been established.

Lab tests will be required to monitor therapy. Be sure to keep appointments. Tests may include: Blood and platelet counts; liver and kidney tests.

Drug Interactions:

Tell your doctor or pharmacist if your are taking or planning to take any over-the-counter or prescription medication while taking this medicine. Doses of one or both drugs may need to be modified or a different drug may need to be prescribed. The following drugs and drug classes interact with this medicine.

corticosteroids (eg, hydrocortisone)
lithium (eg, *Eskalith)*

Side Effects:

Every drug is capable of producing side effects. Many patients have no, or minor, side effects. The frequency and severity of side effects depend on many factors including dose, duration of therapy and individual susceptibility. Possible side effects include:

Digestive Tract: Nausea; vomiting; diarrhea; appetite loss; gastrointestinal upset or bleeding; inflammation of the mouth; stomach pain or bloating; indigestion; bloody vomit or stools; difficulty swallowing; constipation.

Nervous System: Weakness; general body discomfort; nervous system disorder; headache; abnormal skin sensations; sleeplessness; anxiety.

Circulatory System: Blood disorder; chest pain; changes in blood pressure; unusual bleeding/bruising; heart problems

Respiratory System: Difficulty breathing; lung disorder; sore throat; runny nose.

Skin: Hair loss; rash; itching; skin disorders.

Other: Fever; chills; infection; weight changes; allergic reactions; sweating; mucous membrane disorder; fluid retention; swelling of the arms and legs; blood poisoning; yellowing of skin or eyes; urinary tract disorder; abnormal kidney function; joint, bone, back or muscle pain; nosebleed; abnormal lab tests; abnormal blood counts; blood in urine.

Guidelines for Use:

- Follow patient instruction provided with this medicine exactly.
- Follow the injection procedure taught to you by your healthcare provider.
- If a dose is missed, inject it as soon as possible. If several hours have passed or if it is nearing time for the next dose, do not double the dose in order to "catch up" (unless advised to do so by your doctor). If more than one dose is missed or it is necessary to establish a new dosage schedule, contact your doctor or pharmacist.
- If rash, difficulty breathing, flushing, dizziness or lightheartedness, fainting or fast heartbeat occurs, contact your doctor immediately.
- Visually inspect solution for particles or discoloration.
- Do not mix with any other medicines.
- If the powder is reconstituted with a:
  Solution without preservatives — Use with 6 hours after reconstitution. Discard any unused portion.
  Solution with preservatives — May be stored for up to 20 days prior to use.
- Refrigerate the powder, reconstituted solution and diluted solution at 36° to 46°F. Do not freeze or shake.

If you have any questions, consult your doctor, pharmacist, or health care provider.

Octreotide Acetate, 139

Sex Hormones
- Anabolic Steroids, 142
- Mifepristone, 146
- Androgens, 149
- Androgen Inhibitors – Finasteride, 153
- Estrogens, 156
- Estrogen Combinations, 161
- Selective Estrogen Receptor Modulator, 164
- Progestins, 166
- Contraceptive Methods, 170
- Contraceptives, 172
- Medroxyprogesterone Acetate/Estradiol Cypionate, 174
- Oral Contraceptives, 177
- Emergency Contraceptives, 186
- Contraceptive Systems – Intrauterine Progesterone, 189
- Contraceptive Systems – Levonorgestrel Implant, 192
- Contraceptive Systems – Levonorgestrel-Releasing Intrauterine, 195
- Contraceptive Transdermal Systems – Norelgestromin/Ethinyl Estradiol, 199

Fertility Agents
- Choriogonadotropin Alfa, 202
- Chorionic Gonadotropin, 204
- Urofollitropin, 207
- Follitropin Alfa, 209
- Follitropin Beta, 212
- Clomiphene Citrate, 214
- Menotropins, 217

Danazol, 220

Nafarelin Acetate, 223

Posterior Pituitary Hormones
- Desmopressin Acetate, 226

Growth Hormones
- Somatrem, 229
- Somatropin, 231

Adrenal Cortical Steroids
- Corticotropin, 235
- Glucocorticoids, 239
- Corticosteroids, Topical, 247
- Corticosteroid Combinations, Topical, 254
- Mineralocorticoid, 258

Adrenal Steroid Inhibitors
- Aminoglutethimide, 262

Antidiabetic Agents
- Insulin, 264
- Alpha-Glucosidase Inhibitors, 272
- Thiazolidinediones, 275
- Sulfonylureas, 278
- Meglitinides, 283
- Metformin, 286
- Glyburide/Metformin, 289

Glucose Elevating Agents
- Glucagon, 292

Thyroid Drugs
- Antithyroid Agents, 294
- Iodine Products, 297
- Thyroid Hormones, 299

Calcitonin, 302

Bisphosphonates, 305

Imiglucerase, 309

	Generic Name *Brand Name Examples*	Supplied As	Generic Available
Rx	**Octreotide Acetate** *Sandostatin*	**Injection:** 0.05 mg/mL, 0.1 mg/mL, 0.2 mg/mL, 0.5 mg/mL, 1 mg/mL	No

Type of Drug:

Synthetic hormone closely related to the natural hormone somatostatin (growth hormone inhibitor).

How the Drug Works:

Octreotide reduces blood levels of a variety of hormones (eg, growth hormone) and chemical messengers (eg, gastrin).

Uses:

To reduce the blood levels of growth hormone and IGF-I in patients with acromegaly who have had inadequate response to or cannot be treated with surgical resection, pituitary irradiation and bromocriptine mesylate at maximally tolerated doses. The goal is to achieve normalization of growth hormone and IGF-I levels.

To treat symptoms of patients with metastatic carcinoid tumors where it suppresses or inhibits severe diarrhea and flushing episodes.

Treatment of the profuse watery diarrhea associated with vasoactive intestinal peptide (VIP) tumors.

Unlabeled Use(s): Occasionally doctors may prescribe this medicine to reduce output from gastrointestinal or pancreatic sores; treat variceal bleeding, diarrheal states associated with a variety of conditions, irritable bowel syndrome, dumping syndrome, enteric fistula, pancreatitis, pancreatic surgery, glucagonoma, insulinoma, gastrinoma (Zollinger-Ellison syndrome), intestinal obstruction, local radiotherapy, thyrotropin- and TSH-secreting tumors; for chronic pain management, antineoplastic (anti-cancer) therapy or to decrease insulin requirements in diabetes mellitus.

Precautions:

Do not use in the following situations:
sensitivity to any component of this medicine

Use with caution in the following situations:
diabetes
kidney disease

Pregnancy: Studies in pregnant women or in animals have been judged not to show a risk to the fetus. However, no drug should be used during pregnancy unless clearly needed.

Breastfeeding: It is not known if octreotide appears in breastmilk. Consult your doctor before you begin breastfeeding.

Elderly: Lower doses may be necessary.

Lab tests may be required to monitor therapy. Lab tests may include blood tests and thyroid function tests.

Drug Interactions:

Tell your doctor or pharmacist if you are taking or if you are planning to take any over-the-counter or prescription medications or dietary supplements while taking this medicine. Doses of one or both drugs may need to be modified or a different drug may need to be prescribed. The following drugs and drug classes may interact with this medicine.

- beta blockers (eg, propranolol)
- calcium channel blockers (eg, nifedipine)
- cyclosporine (eg, *Sandimmune*)
- drugs to control fluid and electrolyte balance
- hypoglycemic agents, oral (eg, sulfonylureas)
- insulin

Side Effects:

Every drug is capable of producing side effects. Many patients experience no, or minor, side effects. The frequency and severity of side effects depend on many factors including dose, duration of therapy and individual susceptibility. Possible side effects include:

Digestive Tract: Diarrhea; loose stools; nausea; stomach pain; vomiting; gas; bloating; constipation.

Nervous System: Headache; dizziness; tiredness; weakness; depression.

Circulatory System: Slow or irregular heart rate.

Skin: Injection site pain or bruising; swelling; itching; hair loss; bruising; flushing.

Other: Gallbladder problems, especially stones or biliary sludge; back or joint pain; cold or flu symptoms; visual problems; blurred vision; frequent urination; urinary tract infection; changes in blood sugar levels; underactive thyroid; goiter.

Guidelines for Use:

- Use exactly as prescribed.
- Follow the injection procedures taught to you by your healthcare provider. Use proper technique; inject deep under the skin, NOT into muscle. Rotate injection sites.
- If a dose is missed, inject it as soon as possible. If several hours have passed or if it is nearing time for the next dose, do not double the dose in order to "catch up" (unless advised to do so by your doctor). If more than one dose is missed or it is necessary to establish a new dosage schedule, contact your doctor or pharmacist.
- *Diabetics* — Insulin requirements may increase or decrease. Be prepared to monitor blood sugar more often.
- May cause dizziness. Use caution when driving or performing other tasks requiring alertness, coordination or physical dexterity.
- Lab tests may be required to monitor therapy. Be sure to keep appointments.
- Visually inspect solution for particles or discoloration before use.
- *Ampules* — Open just prior to administration. Discard any unused portion.
- *Vials* — Discard any unused portion within 14 days of first use.
- Store at room temperature (70°-86°F) away from light, for up to 14 days. For prolonged storage, store in the refrigerator (36°-46°F) away from light. Solution may be warmed to room temperature naturally. Do not warm artificially.

If you have any questions, consult your doctor, pharmacist, or health care provider.

	Generic Name *Brand Name Examples*	Supplied As	Generic Available
c-III	**Nandrolone Decanoate**		
	Deca-Durabolin[1]	**Injection (in oil):** 50 mg/mL, 100 mg/mL, 200 mg/mL	No
c-III	**Oxandrolone**		
	Oxandrin	**Tablets:** 2.5 mg	No
c-III	**Oxymetholone**		
	Anadrol-50	**Tablets:** 50 mg	No
c-III	**Stanozolol**		
	Winstrol	**Tablets:** 2 mg	No

[1] Contains benzyl alcohol.

All of the products listed in the preceding table are anabolic steroids; however, they are not interchangeable. For example, oxandrolone cannot be used for oxymetholone. Daily dose may vary depending on individual needs. Do not change the dose without consulting your pharmacist or doctor.

Type of Drug:

Synthetic hormones (anabolic steroids) closely related to the androgen testosterone (male sex hormone).

How the Drug Works:

Anabolic steroids promote body tissue-building processes and reverse destructive tissue-depleting processes. They also decrease normal testosterone production by the testicles.

Uses:

Nandrolone and oxymetholone — To treat certain types of anemia.

Oxandrolone — To treat weight loss due to severe illness, following extensive surgery, and in some patients who, without definite reasons, fail to gain or maintain normal weight.

To relieve bone pain caused by osteoporosis (brittle bones).

To prevent the breakdown of protein associated with prolonged corticosteroid (eg, prednisone) use.

Stanozolol — To decrease the frequency and severity of hereditary angioedema attacks.

Unlabeled Use(s): Occasionally doctors may prescribe oxandrolone for alcoholic hepatitis, short stature associated with Turner syndrome, HIV wasting syndrome, and HIV-associated muscle weakness.

Precautions:

Do not use in the following situations:

allergy to the anabolic steroid or any of its ingredients
breast cancer, females with excess calcium in blood or males
for enhancement of physical appearance or athletic performance
hypercalcemia (excess calcium in blood) (oxandrolone only)
liver disease, severe (oxymetholone only)
nephrosis
pregnancy
prostate gland cancer

Use with caution in the following situations:

diabetes
elderly males
heart disease
hyperlipidemia
kidney disease
liver disease
migraine
seizure disorder (eg, epilepsy)

Athletic performance: Anabolic steroids have not been shown to enhance athletic ability. An athlete's motivation to use steroids includes: Increased muscle mass and strength; decreased muscle recovery time, allowing more frequent weight training; decreased healing time after muscle injury; increased aggressiveness. The increase in muscle size and weight gain is partially attributed to increased sodium and water retention. The serious health hazards associated with anabolic steroids minimize any real or perceived gain in performance. Effects of these agents may persist for up to 6 months after the last dose. Adverse effects may be serious and irreversible.

Benzyl alcohol: Some of these products contain benzyl alcohol, which has been associated with fatal "gasping syndrome" in premature infants. Consult your doctor or pharmacist.

Edema: Edema (swelling), with or without congestive heart failure, may occur. Use with caution in patients with heart, kidney, or liver disease; epilepsy; migraine; or other conditions that may be aggravated by fluid retention. In addition to discontinuation of the drug, diuretic therapy may be required.

High serum cholesterol: Anabolic steroids may lower high-density lipoprotein (HDL) ("good" cholesterol) and raise low-density lipoprotein (LDL) ("bad" cholesterol). This effect may increase the risk of atherosclerosis (hardening of the arteries) and coronary artery disease.

Leukemia: Leukemia has been observed in patients with aplastic anemia treated with oxymetholone, but the role of oxymetholone is unclear.

Liver disease: Liver cysts and tumors have occurred during treatment with anabolic steroids. They are often not recognized until a life-threatening condition develops. Stopping the medicine usually results in shrinking or complete disappearance of the lesions.

Males after puberty: Anabolic steroids may inhibit function of the testes, aggravate acne, decrease sperm count, promote development of breast tissue, cause the testes to shrink, and lead to impotence.

Women: Anabolic steroids may produce irreversible virilization (eg, deepening of voice, unusual hair growth, enlargement of the clitoris) in females. Women should be carefully monitored and drug therapy stopped at the first sign of virilization (eg, menstrual irregularities).

Pregnancy: Do not use during pregnancy. The risk of use in a pregnant woman clearly outweighs any possible benefit. Anabolic steroids may cause masculinization of the female fetus.

Breastfeeding: It is not known if anabolic steroids appear in breast milk. Because of the potential for serious adverse effects, decide whether to discontinue nursing or the drug. Consult your doctor before you begin breastfeeding.

Children: The adverse effects of use in young children are not fully understood. Anabolic steroids may interfere with growth to normal adult height. Use with caution.

Elderly: Anabolic steroids may increase risk of prostate enlargement or prostate cancer. Use with caution.

Lab tests may be required to monitor therapy. Tests may include liver function, blood calcium levels, cholesterol levels, and hemoglobin tests.

Drug Interactions:

Tell your doctor or pharmacist if you are taking or if you are planning to take any over-the-counter or prescription medications or dietary supplements while taking an anabolic steroid. Doses of one or both drugs may need to be modified or a different drug may need to be prescribed. Anticoagulants (eg, warfarin) interact with anabolic steroids.

Side Effects:

Every drug is capable of producing side effects. Many anabolic steroid users experience no, or minor, side effects. The frequency and severity of side effects depend on many factors including dose, duration of therapy, and individual susceptibility. Possible side effects include:

Males (before puberty): Increased size of penis; increased frequency of erections.

Males (after puberty): Breast enlargement; changes in sex drive; impotence; persistent, painful erections; shrinking of testes; decreased semen volume; bladder irritation; inhibition of testicular function.

Females: Excessive growth of body hair; hoarseness or deepening of the voice; enlargement of the clitoris; changes in sex drive; changes in menstruation; male pattern baldness.

Digestive Tract: Nausea; vomiting; diarrhea.

Nervous System: Sleeplessness; dependency; depression; excitability.

Skin: Yellowing of the skin or eyes; acne.

Other: Fluid retention; ankle swelling; electrolyte imbalance; abnormal cholesterol levels; abnormal lab tests; liver disease; elevated blood sugar.

Guidelines for Use:

- Dosage is individualized. Take exactly as prescribed.
- Do not change the dose or stop taking, unless advised by your doctor.
- The injectable form of nandrolone will usually be prepared and administered by your health care provider in a medical setting.
- May cause nausea or gastrointestinal upset.
- *Diabetic patients* — Glucose tolerance may be altered. Monitor blood sugar closely and report any changes to your doctor.
- *Seizure disorders* — Epileptic patients may note an increase in seizure frequency; notify your doctor if this occurs.
- Notify your doctor if you experience nausea, vomiting, yellowing of skin color, or ankle swelling.
- Female patients should notify their doctor if they experience hoarseness, deepening of the voice, changes in body hair growth, menstrual changes, male-pattern baldness, or acne.
- Male patients should notify their doctor if they experience too frequent or persistent erections of the penis or development or worsening of acne.
- Tell your doctor if you are pregnant, planning to become pregnant, or breastfeeding.
- Do not use to enhance physical appearance or athletic performance.
- Effects of anabolic steroids may persist for up to 6 months after the last dose; some adverse effects are irreversible.
- Maximum benefit may not be reached for several months.
- Lab tests may be required to monitor therapy. Be sure to keep appointments.
- Store tablets at controlled room temperature (59° to 86°F).

If you have any questions, consult your doctor, pharmacist, or health care provider.

	Generic Name *Brand Name Example*	Supplied As	Generic Available
Rx[1]	**Mifepristone**		
	Mifeprex	**Tablets**: 200 mg	No

[1] Mifepristone will be supplied only to licensed physicians who sign and return a Prescriber's Agreement.

Type of Drug:

Uterine-active agent; abortifacient.

How the Drug Works:

The hormone progesterone acts on the uterus in a pregnant woman to help maintain the pregnancy. Mifepristone blocks the action of progesterone on the uterus, resulting in termination of pregnancy.

Uses:

For the medical termination of intrauterine pregnancy through 49 days of pregnancy. For purposes of this treatment, pregnancy is dated from the first day of the last menstrual period in a presumed 28-day cycle with ovulation occurring at mid-cycle. The duration of pregnancy may be determined from menstrual history and by clinical examination.

Unlabeled Use(s): Occasionally, doctors may prescribe mifepristone for postcoital contraception, intrauterine fetal death, unresectable meningioma, endometriosis, and Cushing's syndrome.

Precautions:

Do not use in the following situations:

adnexal mass, undiagnosed
adrenal failure, chronic
allergy to mifepristone or any of its ingredients
allergy to misoprostol or any other prostaglandin
anticoagulant therapy, concurrent
bleeding disorder
corticosteroid therapy, concurrent long-term
ectopic pregnancy, confirmed or suspected
inadequate access to medical facilities equipped to provide emergency treatment
intrauterine device (IUD) in place
porphyrias, inherited

Use with caution in the following situations: Patient is over 35 years of age and smokes 10 or more cigarettes/day.

Incomplete abortion: If mifepristone results in incomplete abortion, surgical intervention may be necessary.

Pregnancy: Mifepristone is indicated for use in the termination of pregnancy (through 49 days of pregnancy) and has no other approved indication for use during pregnancy. Birth defects may occur if treatment fails and pregnancy is allowed to go to term.

Breastfeeding: It is not known if mifepristone appears in breast milk. Consult your doctor before you begin breastfeeding.

Children: Safety and effectiveness in children have not been established.

Drug Interactions:

Tell your doctor or pharmacist if you are taking or planning to take any over-the-counter or prescription medications or dietary supplements while taking mifepristone. Doses of one or both drugs may need to be modified or a different drug may need to be prescribed. The following drugs or drug classes interact with mifepristone:

- carbamazepine (eg, *Tegretol*)
- dexamethasone (eg, *Decadron*)
- erythromycin (eg, *E.E.S.*)
- grapefruit juice
- itraconazole (*Sporanox*)
- ketoconazole (eg, *Nizoral*)
- phenobarbital
- phenytoin (eg, *Dilantin*)
- rifampin (eg, *Rifadin*)
- St. John's Wort

Side Effects:

Every drug is capable of producing side effects. Many mifepristone users experience no, or minor, side effects. The frequency and severity of side effects depend on many factors including dose, duration of therapy, and individual susceptibility. Possible side effects include:

Nervous System: Headache; dizziness; sleeplessness; anxiety; fainting; fatigue; weakness.

Digestive Tract: Stomach pain or cramping; indigestion; nausea; vomiting; diarrhea.

Urinary and Reproductive Tract: Uterine cramping and bleeding; vaginitis; pelvic pain.

Other: Abnormal blood counts; back pain; fever; leg pain; sinus congestion; viral infection; rigors (eg, chills, shaking).

Guidelines for Use:

- Treatment with mifepristone and misoprostol for the termination of pregnancy requires 3 office visits. Mifepristone may be administered only in a clinic, medical office, or hospital, by or under the supervision of a physician able to assess how far the pregnancy has progressed and to diagnose ectopic pregnancies.
- Mifepristone should not be used by any patient who may be unable to understand the effects of the treatment procedure or follow the regimen. Each patient must understand the following:
  The necessity of completing the treatment schedule, including a follow-up visit about 14 days after taking mifepristone;
  that vaginal bleeding and uterine cramping probably will occur;
  that prolonged or heavy vaginal bleeding is not proof of a complete abortion;
  that if the treatment fails, there is a risk of fetal abnormalities;
  that incomplete abortions are managed by surgical procedures;
  the steps to take in an emergency situation, including precise instructions and a telephone number that can be called if she has any problems or concerns.
- *Day 1* — Patients must read the medication guide and read and sign the patient agreement before mifepristone is taken. Three 200 mg tablets (600 mg) of mifepristone are taken in a single oral dose.
- *Day 3* — The patient returns to the health care provider 2 days after taking mifepristone. Unless abortion has occurred and has been confirmed by clinical examination or ultrasonographic scan, the patient takes two 200 mcg tablets (400 mcg) of misoprostol orally. During the period immediately following the administration of misoprostol, the patient may need medication for cramps or gastrointestinal symptoms. The patient instructions should be given on what to do if significant discomfort, excessive bleeding, or other adverse reactions occur and a phone number to call if she has questions following the administration of misoprostol. In addition, the patient should have the name and phone number of the physician who will be handling emergencies.
- *Day-14, post-treatment examination* — Patients will return for a follow-up visit about 14 days after taking the mifepristone. The visit is very important to confirm by clinical examination or ultrasonographic scan that a complete termination of pregnancy has occurred. Patients who have an ongoing pregnancy at this visit have a risk of fetal malformation resulting from the treatment. Surgical termination is recommended to manage mifepristone treatment failures.
- Another pregnancy can occur following termination of pregnancy and before resumption of normal menses. Contraception can be initiated as soon as the termination of the pregnancy has been confirmed, or before resuming sexual intercourse.

If you have any questions, consult your doctor, pharmacist, or health care provider.

	Generic Name *Brand Name Examples*	Supplied As	Generic Available
C-III	**Fluoxymesterone**		
	Halotestin	**Tablets:** 2 mg, 5 mg, 10 mg	Yes
C-III	**Methyltestosterone**	**Tablets, buccal:** 10 mg	Yes
	Android	**Tablets:** 10 mg, 25 mg	Yes
	Android, Testred, Virilon	**Capsules:** 10 mg	No
C-III	**Testosterone (in Aqueous Suspension)**	**Injection:** 25 mg/mL, 50 mg/mL, 100 mg/mL	Yes
C-III	**Testosterone Cypionate (in Oil)**		
	Depo-Testosterone, Depotest 100, Depotest 200	**Injection:** 100 mg/mL, 200 mg/mL	Yes
C-III	**Testosterone Enanthate (in Oil)**		
	Delatestryl, Everone 200	**Injection:** 100 mg/mL, 200 mg/mL	Yes
C-III	**Testosterone Propionate (in Oil)**	**Injection:** 100 mg/mL	Yes
C-III	**Testosterone Pellets**		
	Testopel	**Pellets:** 75 mg	No
C-III	**Testosterone Transdermal**		
	Androderm, Testoderm, Testoderm TTS	**Transdermal System:** 2.5 mg, 4 mg, 5 mg, 6 mg/24 hours	No

All of the products listed on this table are androgens; however, they are not interchangeable. For example, methyltestosterone cannot be used for fluoxymesterone. Daily dose may vary depending on individual needs.

Type of Drug:

Male hormones.

How the Drug Works:

Testosterone is the primary natural androgen (male sex hormone) produced by the testes. Androgens promote normal growth and development of male sex organs (eg, prostate, seminal vesicles, penis, scrotum) and affect fertility. They also produce the distinctive male characteristics of hair distribution, voice depth, fat distribution, and muscle development. Androgens contribute to growth during adolescence.

Uses:

To treat testosterone deficiency. Prolonged treatment is required to maintain male sex characteristics.

For hormone deficiency due to developmental defects of the testes.

To treat delayed male puberty (brief treatment with low doses) in carefully selected patients.

To treat male impotence caused by androgen deficiency (methyltestosterone only).

Used for breast pain and swelling in women immediately after childbirth. Also used as secondary therapy in postmenopausal women for advanced, inoperable breast cancer that has spread to other areas, including bone.

Unlabeled Use(s): Testosterone enanthate has been studied for male contraception.

Precautions:

Do not use in the following situations:

- allergy to androgens, mercury compounds, or patch materials
- cancer of the prostate gland or breast tissue (men)
- females (*Androderm* and *Testoderm* only)
- heart disease, serious
- kidney disease, serious
- liver disease, serious
- pregnancy

Use with caution in the following situations:

- breast cancer (women)
- breast development, abnormal (men)
- calcium blood level, increased (children)
- delayed puberty, healthy males
- elderly males
- epilepsy
- heart, liver or kidney disease
- high cholesterol
- migraine

Males frequently experience breast swelling or development. Reduced sperm counts may occur after prolonged use.

Women may show signs of masculinization: Deepening of voice, hair growth, acne, increased size of clitoris, menstrual changes. These symptoms usually follow high doses of androgens and should be tolerated during treatment for advanced breast cancer. Treatment may have to be discontinued. Consult your doctor. (The transdermal systems have not been tested in women and should not be used by women.)

Product interchange: Do not try to substitute short-acting and long-acting testosterone products. These products are not considered to be interchangeable.

Athletic performance/physical appearance: Androgens are not safe and effective for enhancement of athletic performance or physical appearance; use could produce serious adverse effects.

Fluid retention: Since androgens may cause fluid retention, use with caution in epilepsy, migraine, and heart, liver or kidney disease.

Pregnancy: Do not use during pregnancy. The risk of use in a pregnant woman clearly outweighs any possible benefit. Androgens may masculinize a female fetus.

Breastfeeding: It is not known if androgens appear in breast milk. Consult your doctor before you begin breastfeeding.

Children: Androderm has not been tested in males under 15 years of age. *Testoderm* has not been tested in males under 18 years of age. Use other androgens very cautiously in children under 18 years of age. Androgens may stop or stunt the growth process.

Elderly: Use with caution in elderly males. Androgens may increase risk of prostate enlargement or prostate cancer. An increase in sex drive may occur.

Lab tests may be required to monitor therapy. Be sure to keep appointments.

Tartrazine: Some of these products may contain the dye tartrazine (FD&C Yellow No. 5) which can cause allergic reactions in certain individuals. Check package label when available or consult your doctor or pharmacist.

Drug Interactions:

Tell your doctor or pharmacist if you are taking or if you are planning to take any over-the-counter or prescription medications or dietary supplements while taking this medicine. Doses of one or both drugs may need to be modified or a different drug may need to be prescribed.The following drugs and drug classes interact with this medicine.

- anticoagulants, oral (eg, *Coumadin)*
- blood-sugar-lowering agents (eg, *Diabinese)*
- imipramine (eg, *Tofranil)*
- insulin

Side Effects:

Every drug is capable of produci ng side effects. Many patients experience no, or minor, side effects. The frequency an severity of side effects depend on many factors including dose, duration of therapy and individual susceptibility. Possible side effects include:

Female – Irregular menstruation; absence of menstruation; deepening voice; enlargement of clitoris; changes in sex drive.

Male – Breast tenderness, swelling or development; decreased sperm count; erection problems (pain, frequency, increased duration); changes in sex drive; itching, blisters, bruising, hardening, redness, discomfort or irritation (patch only); enlargement of the prostate.

Nervous System: Headache; anxiety; depression; sleep disorders; memory loss; abnormal skin sensations.

Skin: Excessive growth of body hair; loss of scalp hair; acne; oily skin; changes in skin color (yellowing); rash; irritation (patch only).

Other: Fluid retention (edema); ankle swelling; nausea; pain at injection or implantation site; increased cholesterol; liver problems; vomiting; dilated pupils; abnormal bleeding or bruising; inflammation of the mouth (tablets only); stroke; black or tarry stools; urinary tract infection.

Guidelines for Use:

- *Oral tablets* — May cause stomach upset.
- *Buccal tablets* — Do not swallow. Allow to dissolve between the gum and cheek. Avoid eating, drinking or smoking while tablet is in place.
- Notify your doctor if nausea, vomiting, swelling of the extremities (edema), prolonged or painful erections, or yellowing of the skin or eyes occurs.
- *Female patients* — Notify your doctor if hoarseness, deepening of the voice, hair growth changes, acne, menstrual irregularities or suspected pregnancy occur.
- Androgens are not effective and may be dangerous if used for fractures, surgery, convalescence, bleeding of the uterus or enhancement of athletic performance or physical appearance.
- *Brand interchange* — Do not change from one brand of these drugs to another without consulting your pharmacist or doctor.
- *Testosterone injections* — Shake well before using. Administer into buttock muscle only. Effects of *enanthate* and *cypionate* injections last about 4 weeks.
- *Transdermal systems* — Read patient instructions. Store at room temperature (59°-86° F) in provided pouch until ready to use. Carefully discard used patches to prevent accidental application or ingestion by others (eg, children, pets).
  Androderm : Place on clean dry non-scrotal skin (eg, back, abdomen, upper arm, thigh) every night. Rotate application sites, allowing 7 days between applications to the same site. Site should not be oily, damaged or irritated. Patch does not need to be removed during sexual intercourse or while bathing.
  Testoderm: Place on clean, dry scrotal skin. Scrotal hair should be dry-shaved for best contact. Do not use depilatories (chemical hair removers). System should be worn 22-24 hours, but can be removed for swimming or bathing and then reapplied. Lab tests should be made after 3 to 4 weeks of use.
- *Pellet implantation* — Report any unusual irritation or infection at the implant site. If treatment is discontinued, the pellets will have to be removed.
- Female sexual partners of male testosterone patients should contact a doctor if the following occur: changes in body hair distribution or increased acne.
- Do not alter the dose unless directed by your doctor.
- Diabetics may require insulin dose adjustments. Consult your doctor.
- Lab tests or exams may be necessary. Be sure to keep appointments.
- Store tablets in a closed container at room temperature.
- Avoid freezing injectable products.

If you have any questions, consult your doctor, pharmacist, or health care provider.

	Generic Name *Brand Name Example*	Supplied As	Generic Available
Rx	**Finasteride**		
	Proscar	**Tablets:** 5 mg	No
	Propecia	**Tablets:** 1 mg	No

Type of Drug:

An enzyme inhibitor.

How the Drug Works:

Finasteride inhibits the production of androgen, a hormone that is involved in the development of the prostate and male pattern baldness. By reducing the amount of androgen, finasteride helps relieve urinary symptoms often associated with overdevelopment of the prostate and appears to interrupt processes leading to male pattern hair loss.

Overdevelopment or enlargement of the prostate is also known as benign prostatic hyperplasia (BPH).

Male pattern baldness is hair loss on the crown of the head or the front scalp area.

Uses:

Proscar — To treat symptomatic benign prostatic hyperplasia (BPH); to reduce the risk of acute urinary retention; to reduce the need for prostate surgery.

Propecia — To treat male pattern hair loss in men 18 to 41 years of age. Effectiveness with other types of hair loss has not been determined.

Finasteride is not indicated for use in women or children.

Unlabeled Use(s): Finasteride is being investigated as therapy following prostate surgery, prevention of the progression of first-stage prostate cancer, and treatment of acne and abnormal hair growth.

Precautions:

Do not use in the following situations:

allergy to any ingredient of the formulation
breastfeeding
children
pregnancy
women

Use with caution in the following situations:

liver disease
obstructive uropathy
urinary difficulty/blockage, major

Pregnancy: Do not use during pregnancy. The risk of use in a pregnant woman clearly outweighs any possible benefit. Finasteride is not indicated for use in women.

Breastfeeding: It is not known if finasteride appears in breast milk; however, it is not indicated for use in women. Consult your doctor before you begin breastfeeding.

Children: Safety and effectiveness in children have not been established; however, finasteride is not indicated for use in children.

Lab tests may be required during treatment with finasteride.

Drug Interactions:

Tell your doctor or pharmacist if you are taking or if you are planning to take any over-the-counter or prescription medications or dietary supplements with finasteride. Doses of one or both drugs may need to be modified or a different drug may need to be prescribed.

Side Effects:

Every drug is capable of producing side effects. Many finasteride users experience no, or minor, side effects. The frequency and severity of side effects depend on many factors including dose, duration of therapy and individual susceptibility. Possible side effects include impotence, decreased sex drive, decreased amount of ejaculate, allergic reactions including lip swelling, rash and breast tenderness (male).

Guidelines for Use:

- Read the patient information insert before beginning therapy.
- *Male pattern baldness* — Recommended dose is 1 mg once a day. Continued use is recommended to sustain benefit. Stopping treatment can reverse results within 12 months.
- *Benign prostatic hyperplasia (BPH)* — Recommended dose is 5 mg once a day. Six to twelve months of treatment may be necessary to determine response.
- Take without regard to meals.
- Women who are pregnant or may become pregnant should not handle broken or crushed tablets because of the potential for absorption and potential risk to male fetus. Similarly, when a male patient's sexual partner is or may become pregnant, the patient should either avoid exposure of his partner to semen or he should discontinue finasteride.
- The amount of ejaculate may be decreased. This should not interfere with normal sexual function. However, impotence (erectile dysfunction) and decreased sex drive may occur.
- Protect from light and moisture. Keep container tightly closed. Store at room temperature below 86°F.

If you have any questions, consult your doctor, pharmacist, or health care provider.

Generic Name *Brand Name Examples*	Supplied As	Generic Available
Rx **Conjugated Estrogens**		
Premarin	**Tablets:** 0.3 mg, 0.625 mg, 0.9 mg, 1.25 mg, 2.5 mg	No
Premarin	**Vaginal cream:** 0.625 mg/g	No
Premarin Intravenous	**Injection:** 25 mg/vial	No
Rx **Dienestrol**		
Ortho Dienestrol	**Vaginal cream:** 0.01%	No
Rx **Esterified Estrogens**		
Estratab, Menest	**Tablets:** 0.3 mg, 0.625 mg, 1.25 mg, 2.5 mg	No
Rx **Estradiol**		
Estrace, Gynodiol	**Tablets:** 0.5 mg, 1 mg, 1.5 mg, 2 mg[1]	Yes
Estrace	**Vaginal cream:** 0.01%	No
Alora, Climara, Esclim, Estraderm, FemPatch, Vivelle, Vivelle-Dot	**Transdermal system (patch):** 0.025 mg/day, 0.0375 mg/day, 0.05 mg/day, 0.075 mg/day, 0.1 mg/day	Yes
Estring	**Ring**: 2 mg	No
Rx **Estradiol Cypionate in Oil**		
Depo-Estradiol, Depogen	**Injection:** 5 mg/mL	Yes
Rx **Estradiol Hemihydrate**		
Vagifem	**Vaginal tablets**: 25 mcg	No
Rx **Estradiol Valerate in Oil**		
Delestrogen, Valergen 20, Valergen 40	**Injection:** l0 mg/mL, 20 mg/mL, 40 mg/mL	Yes
Rx **Estrone Aqueous**		
Kestrone 5	**Injection:** 5 mg/mL	Yes
Rx **Estropipate (Piperazine Estrone Sulfate)**		
Ogen, Ortho-Est	**Tablets:** 0.625 mg, 1.25 mg, 2.5 mg	Yes
Ogen	**Vaginal cream:** 1.5 mg/g	No
Rx **Ethinyl Estradiol**		
Estinyl	**Tablets:** 0.02 mg[1], 0.05 mg	No

	Generic Name *Brand Name Examples*	Supplied As	Generic Available
Rx	**Synthetic Conjugated Estrogens, A**		
	Cenestin	**Tablets:** 0.625 mg, 0.9 mg	No

[1] *Estrace* 2 mg and *Estinyl* 0.02 mg contain the dye tartrazine.

All of the products listed in the previous table are estrogens; however, they are not interchangeable without dosage adjustments. For example, estradiol cannot be substituted for conjugated estrogens without changing the dose. Daily dose may vary depending on individual needs. Do not adjust the dose without consulting your pharmacist or doctor.

Type of Drug:

Female hormones; estrogens.

How the Drug Works:

Estrogens represent a group of several female hormones. The ovary produces and releases several natural estrogens until menopause occurs. All estrogens produce similar effects. They play a key role in the development and normal function of the reproductive system (including the vagina, uterus, fallopian tubes, and breasts) and secondary sex characteristics (eg, pubic hair) of women. Estrogens also assist in development and maintenance of strong bones.

Uses:

To treat hot flashes associated with menopause.

To treat vulval, vaginal, and lower urinary tract tissue breakdown, drying, and thinning following menopause. Estrogen supplements may prevent or decrease complications.

To treat *kraurosis vulvae*, a condition involving the breakdown and drying of the external female genitalia (vulval area).

For estrogen replacement therapy after a failure of the ovaries due to menopause, disease, or surgical removal.

To treat advanced androgen-dependent cancer of the prostate gland in men.

To relieve the symptoms of breast cancer in selected men and women with metastatic disease.

Conjugated estrogens, injection: To treat abnormal uterine bleeding caused by hormone imbalance.

Estradiol tablets and transdermal system (patch): To prevent osteoporosis (brittle bones) related to a lack of estrogen after menopause. Therapy should be accompanied by a balanced diet, adequate daily calcium either through the diet or calcium supplements, adequate vitamin D, and weight-bearing exercises.

Unlabeled Use(s): Ethinyl estradiol has been used for treating Turner's syndrome.

Precautions:

Do not use in the following situations:

allergy to estrogens or any of their ingredients
blood clots, active
blood clots, history of with previous estrogen use
breast cancer, known or suspected
estrogen-dependent cancer, known or suspected
genital bleeding, abnormal undiagnosed
pregnancy, known or suspected

Use with caution in the following situations:

asthma
blood clots, risk factors or a history of
bone disease, metabolic
breast cancer, family history of, history of, or active
breast nodules
depression, history of
diabetes
endometrial cancer
endometriosis
epilepsy
fibrocystic breast disease
gallbladder disease
heart disease
high blood pressure
high blood calcium levels
immobilization, prolonged
jaundice, history of with pregnancy
kidney disease
liver disease
mammogram, abnormal
migraine headaches
narrow, short, or constricted vagina (estradiol ring only)
porphyria
stroke, history of
surgery
uterine cancer, history of
uterine fibroids, preexisting

Blood Clots: There is an increased risk of blood clots in men receiving estrogens for prostate cancer, in women using estrogens for postpartum breast engorgement, and in those taking oral contraceptives in general.

Cancer Risk: Estrogens may increase the risk of endometrial (lining of the uterus) cancer in postmenopausal women. Have regular physical examinations and contact your doctor if you experience persistent or recurrent abnormal vaginal bleeding.

Concurrent progestin therapy: A progestin agent is frequently added to long-term estrogen regimens in women who have a uterus. The addition of a progestin reduces the risk of estrogen-induced cancer of the uterus.

History/physical exam: Before beginning estrogen therapy, a complete medical and family history should be performed. Examinations every 12 months should include blood pressure tests, abdomen and pelvic organ examinations, and a Pap test (once a year). Patients should examine their breasts for lumps on a monthly basis. Women older than 40 years of age who take estrogens should have regular mammograms.

Pregnancy: Do not use during pregnancy. The risk of use in a pregnant woman clearly outweighs any possible benefit. Urinary system problems and testicular cancer have occurred in sons of women given diethylstilbestrol (DES) (not available in the US) during pregnancy. Daughters of women given DES during their pregnancy have shown an increased risk of developing vaginal or cervical cancer.

Breastfeeding: It is not known if estrogens appear in breast milk. Consult your doctor before you begin breastfeeding.

Children: Safety and effectiveness in children have not been established. Use with extreme caution in young patients who are still growing. Estrogens may interfere with normal bone development.

Tartrazine: Some of these products may contain the dye tartrazine (FD&C Yellow No. 5), which can cause allergic reactions in certain individuals. Check package label when available or consult your doctor or pharmacist.

Drug Interactions:

Tell your doctor or pharmacist if you are taking or if you are planning to take any over-the-counter or prescription medications or dietary supplements while taking this medicine. Doses of one or both drugs may need to be modified or a different drug may need to be prescribed. The following drugs and drug classes interact with this medicine:

barbiturates (eg, phenobarbital)
corticosteroids (eg, prednisone)
hydantoins (eg, phenytoin)
rifampin (eg, *Rifadin*)
topiramate (*Topamax*)

Side Effects:

Every drug is capable of producing side effects. Many patients experience no, or minor, side effects. The frequency and severity of side effects depend on many factors including dose, duration of therapy, and individual susceptibility. Possible side effects include:

Urinary and Reproductive Tract: Change in menstrual flow; abnormal vaginal bleeding; vaginal discomfort or pain; vaginal infection; unusual vaginal secretions; painful menstruation; absence of menstruation during or after treatment; premenstrual-like syndrome; increased size of uterine fibroids; urinary tract infection symptoms.

Digestive Tract: Nausea; vomiting; stomach pain or cramps; bloating; pancreatitis; diarrhea; gas; enlarged stomach; constipation; indigestion.

Nervous System: Headache; migraine; dizziness; depression; weakness; unusual, jerky body movements; sleeplessness; emotional instability; anxiety; nervousness.

Skin: Rash; hives; itching; skin discoloration, particularly on the face; scalp hair loss; excessive growth of body or facial hair.

Local: Pain at the injection site; redness; irritation or itching at patch application site.

Other: Intolerance to contact lenses; weight changes; breast tenderness or enlargement; breast milk secretion; sudden vision problems; abnormal blood glucose levels; swelling; high blood pressure; changes in sex drive; yellowing of skin or eyes; swelling of the arms or legs; vertigo (feeling of whirling motion); cough; abnormal lab tests; gallbladder disease; blood clots; steepening of corneal curvature; reduced carbohydrate tolerance; liver tumor development; runny nose; back, joint, muscle, or bone pain; sore throat; flu-like symptoms; hot flushes; palpitations (pounding in the chest); leg cramps; abnormal skin sensations.

Guidelines for Use:

- Dosage is individualized.
- Carefully read the patient package insert available with your medicines.
- The lowest dose that will control symptoms should be chosen and medication should be discontinued as soon as possible.
- Notify your doctor immediately if you experience pain in the groin, calves, or chest; sudden shortness of breath; abnormal vaginal bleeding; missed menstrual period or suspected pregnancy; lumps in the breast; severe headache; dizziness; fainting; changes in vision or speech; weakness or numbness in an arm or leg; stomach pain, swelling, or tenderness; yellowing of the skin or eyes; severe depression; severe vomiting; or coughing up blood.
- Fluid retention caused by estrogens may aggravate asthma, epilepsy, migraine, heart disease, or kidney disease. Use with caution if you have any of these conditions.
- If a dose is missed, take it as soon as possible. If several hours have passed or if it is nearing time for the next dose, do not double the dose in order to catch up, unless advised to do so by your doctor. If several doses are missed, or it is necessary to establish a new dosage schedule, contact your doctor or pharmacist.
- While taking estrogens, it is important to visit your doctor at least once a year for a check-up. If members of your family have had breast cancer or if you have ever had breast lumps, you may need to have more frequent breast exams.
- Approximately every 6 months, you and your doctor should reevaluate whether or not you need to continue estrogen therapy.
- *Diabetic patients* — Glucose tolerance may be decreased. Monitor blood sugar closely and report changes to your doctor.
- When using estrogens to treat hot flashes and other symptoms of menopause, the dose may need to be changed occasionally. Discuss your symptoms with your doctor.
- Inform your doctor if you are pregnant, become pregnant, or are planning to become pregnant or if you are breastfeeding.
- Do not share your medicine with anyone else.
- *Brand interchange* — Do not change from one brand of these drugs to another without consulting your pharmacist or doctor. Products manufactured by different companies may not be equally effective and will require different doses.
- *Injections* — Visually inspect solutions for particles or discoloration. If you are self-administering, carefully follow the storage, preparation, and administration instructions provided by your health care provider.
- *Transdermal system (patch)* — Apply immediately after opening the pouch and removing the protective liner. Press firmly in place with the palm of the hand for ≈ 10 seconds. Make sure there is good contact, especially around the edges. Avoid touching the sticky side of the patch with your fingers.
  Place adhesive side of the system on a clean, dry area of the skin on the trunk of the body that is not exposed to sunlight, preferably the buttocks or the abdomen. Do not apply to the breasts.

Guidelines for Use (cont.):

- *Transdermal system (patch)* (cont.) — When it is time to change the patch, remove the old patch and discard. Apply a new patch on a different skin site.
  Rotate the application site with an interval of at least 1 week between applications to a particular site. The area selected should not be oily, damaged, or irritated. Avoid the waistline since tight clothing may rub the system off. Application to areas where sitting would dislodge the system should also be avoided.
  In the unlikely event that a system should fall off, the same system may be reapplied. If necessary, apply a new system. In either case, continue the original treatment schedule. If a rash or irritation develops at an application site, remove the patch and reapply at a different site. Contact your doctor if rash or irritation continues with each patch application.
  Contact with water while bathing, swimming, or showering will not affect the patch.
- *Vaginal creams* — Fill the applicator provided with the prescribed amount of cream. Insert the applicator high into the vagina. After use, clean applicator by removing the plunger from the barrel. Wash with mild soap and warm water. Do not boil or use hot water.
  Cream exposure has been reported to weaken latex condoms. The potential for creams to weaken and contribute to the failure of condoms, diaphragms, or cervical caps made of latex or rubber should be considered.
- *Vaginal ring* — Press the ring into an oval shape and insert as deeply as possible into the upper one-third of the vaginal vault. The ring will remain in place continuously for 3 months, after which it is removed and, if appropriate, replaced by a new ring.
  The exact position of the ring is not critical, although if you feel discomfort, it is probably not far enough inside the vagina. You should not feel the ring when it is in place and it should not interfere with sexual intercourse.
  Some women have experienced moving or gliding of the ring in the vagina. Instances of the ring being expelled from the vagina in connection with moving the bowels, strain, or constipation have been reported. If this occurs, the ring can be rinsed in lukewarm water and reinserted into the vagina.
  The ring should be removed if another intravaginally administered medication is being used.
  The ring may be removed by hooking a finger through the ring and pulling it out.
  Contact your doctor if signs of vaginal irritation develop.
- *Calcium* — If you are taking calcium supplements as part of the treatment to prevent osteoporosis, check with your doctor about the amounts recommended.
- *Storage* — Before reconstitution, store the conjugated estrogens injection in the refrigerator (36° to 46°F). Use the reconstituted solution within a few hours. Reconstituted solution is stable for 60 days in the refrigerator. All other doseforms can be stored at controlled room temperature (59° to 86°F).

	Brand Name Examples	Estrogen	Progestin	Androgen
Rx	*Depo-Testadiol* injection, *Depotestogen* injection	2 mg estradiol cypionate/mL		50 mg testosterone cypionate/mL
Rx	*Estratest* tablets	1.25 mg esterified estrogens		2.5 mg methyltestosterone
Rx	*Estratest H.S.* tablets	0.625 mg esterifiod estrogens		1.25 mg methyltestosterone
Rx	*Prempro* tablets	0.625 mg conjugated estrogens	2.5 mg medroxyprogesterone acetate	
Rx	*Prempro* tablets	0.625 mg conjugated estrogens	5 mg medroxyprogesterone acetate	
Rx	*Premphase* tablets	0.625 mg conjugated estrogens (days 1-14)		
		0.625 mg conjugated estrogens (days 15-28)	5 mg medroxyprogesterone acetate (days 15-28)	
Rx	*femhrt* tablets	5 mcg ethinyl estradiol	1 mg norethindrone acetate	
Rx	*Activella* tablets	1 mg estradiol	0.5 mg norethindrone acetate	
Rx	*Ortho-Prefest* tablets	1 mg estradiol (days 1-3)		
		1 mg estradiol (days 4-6)	0.09 mg norgestimate (days 4-6)	

	Brand Name Examples	Estrogen	Progestin	Andro-gen
Rx	*Combipatch* 9 cm^2 trans-dermal patch	0.05 mg estradiol/ day	0.14 mg norethindrone acetate/day	
	Combipatch 16 cm^2trans-dermal patch	0.05 mg estradiol/ day	0.25 mg norethindrone acetate/day	

For complete information, see the Estrogens, Progestins, and Androgens monographs in this chapter.

Type of Drug:

Combination hormone products.

Uses:

Estrogen and androgen combinations: To treat moderate to severe vasomotor symptoms associated with menopause (feeling of warmth in the face, neck, or chest or sudden intense episodes of heat and sweating throughout the body) in patients who have not improved with treatment of estrogens alone.

To treat vulvar and vaginal atrophy associated with menopause.

Estrogen and progestin combinations: To treat moderate to severe vasomotor symptoms associated with menopause (feeling of warmth in the face, neck, or chest or sudden intense episodes of heat and sweating throughout the body) in patients who have not improved with treatment of estrogens alone.

To treat vulvar and vaginal atrophy associated with menopause (*femhrt* excluded).

To prevent osteoporosis (*Combi-Patch* excluded).

To treat low estrogen conditions caused by diseases such as hypogonadism or primary ovarian failure.

Unlabeled Use(s): There is no adequate evidence that estrogens are effective for nervous symptoms or depression that might occur during menopause and they should not be used to treat these conditions.

Guidelines for Use:

- Dosage is individualized. Take exactly as prescribed.
- Do not change the dose or stop taking, unless directed by your doctor.
- Carefully read the patient package insert available with your medicine.
- Fluid retention may aggravate asthma, epilepsy, migraine, heart disease or kidney disease. Use with caution in these conditions.
- *Brand interchange* — Do not change from one brand of these drugs to another without consulting your pharmacist or doctor. Products manufactured by different companies may not be equally effective.
- If a dose is missed, take it as soon as possible. If several hours have passed or if it is nearing time for the next dose, do not double the dose to catch up, unless advised by your doctor. If more than one dose is missed, or it is necessary to establish a new dosage schedule, contact your doctor or pharmacist.
- Store as directed by package labeling.

If you have any questions, consult your doctor, pharmacist, or health care provider.

	Generic Name *Brand Name Example*	Supplied As	Generic Available
Rx	**Raloxifene HCl**		
	Evista	**Tablets:** 60 mg	No

Type of Drug:

Selective estrogen receptor modulator (SERM).

How the Drug Works:

Raloxifene binds to estrogen receptors producing estrogen-like effects on some tissues and organs. Raloxifene reduces bone loss (prevents brittle bones) and elevated LDL ("bad") cholesterol values associated with menopause or hysterectomy (ovarian removal). However, unlike estrogen, raloxifene lacks estrogen-like effects on the uterus and breasts and does not reduce or eliminate hot flushes.

Uses:

For the treatment and prevention of osteoporosis (brittle bones) in postmenopausal women.

Precautions:

Do not use in the following situations:

- allergy to raloxifene or any of its ingredients
- blood clotting in legs, lungs, or eyes, history of
- estrogen therapy, concurrent
- immobilization, prolonged (postsurgical recovery, prolonged bed rest)
- pregnancy
- premenopausal women

Use with caution in the following situations:

- breast abnormality, unexplained
- breast cancer, history of
- cholesterol-lowering agent therapy, concurrent
- liver disease
- uterine bleeding, unexplained

Pregnancy: Do not use during pregnancy. The risk of use in a pregnant woman clearly outweighs any possible benefit.

Breastfeeding: It is not known if raloxifene appears in breast milk. Do not use this drug while nursing.

Children: Raloxifene should not be used in pediatric patients.

Drug Interactions:

Tell your doctor or pharmacist if you are taking or planning to take any over-the-counter or prescription medications or dietary supplements while taking raloxifene. Doses of one or both drugs may need to be modified or a different drug may need to be prescribed. The following drugs and drug classes interact with raloxifene:

- cholestyramine (eg, *Questran*)
- diazepam (eg, *Valium*)
- diazoxide (*Proglycem*)
- warfarin (eg, *Coumadin*)

Side Effects:

Every drug is capable of producing side effects. Many raloxifene users experience no, or minor, side effects. The frequency and severity of side effects depend on many factors including dose, duration of therapy, and individual susceptibility. Possible side effects include:

Digestive Tract: Nausea; indigestion; vomiting; gas; stomach disorder; diarrhea.

Nervous System: Migraine; depression; sleeplessness; fainting; nerve pain; headache; loss of sensitivity to touch; vertigo (feeling of whirling motion).

Respiratory System: Nasal congestion; sore throat; sinusitis; increased cough; pneumonia; voice loss; bronchitis.

Urinary and Reproductive Tract: Vaginal inflammation; urinary tract infection; bladder inflammation; white vaginal discharge; uterine wall abnormality; breast pain; vaginal bleeding; urinary tract disorder.

Skin: Rash; sweating.

Other: Leg cramps; infection; hot flushes; flu-like syndrome; chest pain; fever; fluid retention; swelling of arms or legs; joint and muscle pain; joint swelling; weight gain; varicose vein; tendon disorder; eye inflammation.

Guidelines for Use:

- Read patient package insert before beginning raloxifene therapy and re-read upon prescription renewal.
- Dosage is individualized. Take exactly as prescribed.
- Do not stop taking or change the dose unless directed by your doctor.
- Take this medicine once a day without regard to meals.
- If you miss a dose, start taking the medicine again as soon as possible on your normal schedule. You do not have to make up for the missed dose.
- Take raloxifene as long as your doctor prescribes it.
- Contact your doctor if you experience swelling of hands, feet, or legs, abnormal vaginal bleeding, or breast pain or enlargement.
- Inform your doctor if you are pregnant, become pregnant, plan to become pregnant, or are breastfeeding.
- Notify your doctor immediately if you experience pain in calves or leg swelling, sudden chest pain, shortness of breath, coughing blood, or changes in vision.
- Discontinue therapy 72 hours before and during prolonged immobilization such as postsurgical recovery and prolonged bed rest. Avoid prolonged restriction of movement during travel because of increased blood clotting risks.
- Raloxifene does not reduce hot flashes or flushes associated with menopause or estrogen deficiency. Hot flashes may occur upon beginning therapy.
- Take additional calcium and vitamin D if daily dietary intake is inadequate. Consider weight-bearing exercise and reduction of cigarette smoking and alcohol consumption.
- Store at room temperature (59° to 86°F).

If you have any questions, consult your doctor, pharmacist, or health care provider.

	Generic Name *Brand Name Examples*	Supplied As	Generic Available
Rx	**Hydroxyprogesterone Caproate**		
	Hylutin	**Injection:** 125 mg/mL, 250 mg/mL	Yes
Rx	**Medroxyprogesterone Acetate**		
	Amen, Curretab, Cycrin, Provera	**Tablets:** 2.5 mg, 5 mg, 10 mg	Yes
Rx	**Megestrol Acetate**		
	Megace	**Suspension:** 40 mg/mL	No
Rx	**Norethindrone Acetate**		
	Aygestin	**Tablets:** 5 mg	No
Rx	**Progesterone**		
	Crinone	**Gel, vaginal:** 45 mg (4%), 90 mg (8%)/applicator	No
	Progesterone in oil	**Injection:** 50 mg/mL	Yes
	Prometrium	**Capsules:** 100 mg	No

All of the products listed on this table are progestins; however, they are not interchangeable. For example, norethindrone cannot be used for medroxyprogesterone. Daily dose may vary depending on individual needs. Do not adjust the dose without consulting your doctor or pharmacist.

Type of Drug:

Female sex hormone.

How the Drug Works:

Progesterone is the primary progestin produced by the body. Progestins prepare the uterus for implantation of a fertilized egg. They are also needed for the maintenance of pregnancy once implantation occurs. At normal doses they inhibit the secretion of pituitary hormones, thus preventing ovulation. They may also inhibit spontaneous uterine contractions.

Uses:

To treat amenorrhea (absence of menstrual flow) and secondary amenorrhea.

To treat abnormal bleeding from the uterus.

To treat endometriosis.

As a test for endogenous estrogen production (hydroxyprogesterone caproate injection only).

For appetite enhancement in HIV-infected patients (megestrol acetate suspension only).

To treat infertility as part of Assisted Reproductive Technology (progesterone gel only).

Unlabeled Use(s): Occasionally doctors may prescribe progesterone suppositories to treat premenstrual syndrome (PMS), to decrease spontaneous abortions, and to improve fertility. Other forms of progesterone have been used to treat premature labor and with estrogen replacement therapy for menopause. Medroxyprogesterone acetate may be prescribed to treat menopausal symptoms. Megestrol may be prescribed for the treatment of endometrial and breast cancers. Norethindrone has been prescribed for women after menopause who have an overactive parathyroid gland associated with increased blood levels of calcium.

Precautions:

Do not use in the following situations:

allergy to any ingredient of this medicine
blood clots, current or history
breast cancer, known or suspected
cerebral hemorrhage, current or history
genital cancer, known or suspected
liver disease
miscarriage (physician suspects some tissue is still in uterus)
missed abortion
pregnancy, known or suspected
pregnancy test
vaginal bleeding, undiagnosed

Use with caution in the following situations:

asthma
depression
diabetes
epilepsy
heart disease
kidney disease
migraine
weight loss (megestrol only)

Eyes: Discontinue medication pending an eye exam if there is a loss or change in your vision, protrusion of the eyes, double vision, or migraines.

Physical exams should include self-examination of breasts (monthly), pelvic examination, and Pap smear test (yearly). Consult your doctor in all cases of unusual vaginal bleeding.

Blood clot disorders occasionally occur. Notify your doctor if you experience any of the following: Pain in the calves or chest; abnormal vaginal bleeding; sudden shortness of breath; coughing blood; sudden severe headache or vomiting; dizziness; fainting; visual or speech disturbances; weakness or numbness in an arm or leg; breast lumps; yellowing of skin or eyes.

Pregnancy: Use during pregnancy is not recommended. Progestin used during the first 4 months of pregnancy may cause masculinization of the female fetus as well as congenital heart and liver defects. Progesterone gel may be used during the first 12 weeks of pregnancy to maintain the pregnancy.

Breastfeeding: Progestins appear in breast milk. Consult your doctor before you begin breastfeeding. Medroxyprogesterone may increase milk production and duration of production when taken after delivery.

Drug Interactions:

Tell your doctor or pharmacist if you are taking or if you are planning to take any over-the-counter or prescription medications or dietary supplements while taking this medicine. Doses of one or both drugs may need to be modified or a different drug may need to be prescribed. Aminoglutethimide (*Cytadren*) interacts with medroxyprogesterone. Ketoconazole (*Nizoral*) interacts with progesterone.

Side Effects:

Every drug is capable of producing side effects. Many patients experience no, or minor, side effects. The frequency and severity of side effects depend on many factors including dose, duration of therapy, and individual susceptibility. Possible side effects include:

Urinary and Reproductive Tract: Change in menstrual flow; spotting; vaginal bleeding at abnormal times; unusual vaginal secretions; changes in cervical erosion; amenorrhea (absence of menstrual flow); bladder problems; genital infection; genital itching; impotence; decreased sex drive; pain during intercourse; breast pain; breast enlargement; urinary tract infection.

Digestive Tract: Nausea; constipation; vomiting; bloating; stomach pain; diarrhea;appetite changes; gas.

Nervous System: Depression; sleeplessness; drowsiness; nervousness; headache; dizziness; fatigue; numbness in an arm or leg; mood swings; irritability.

Skin: Discoloration of the skin; itching; rash; hives; acne; excessive hair growth; hair loss.

Local: Pain, irritation, and discomfort at the injection site.

Other: Fluid retention (edema); weight changes; high blood pressure; high blood sugar; fever; vision changes; upper respiratory tract infection; sinus infection; shortness of breath; pneumonia; viral infection; muscle, leg, back, chest, or joint pain; yellowing of skin or eyes; body pain; flu symptoms.

Guidelines for Use:

- Use exactly as prescribed.
- Patient package inserts are available with most of these products. However, they are not required to be dispensed to cancer patients.
- *Oral dosage forms* — Take with food if stomach upset occurs.
- If a dose is missed, take it as soon as possible. If several hours have passed or if it is nearing time for the next dose, do not double the dose in order to catch up (unless advised to do so by your doctor). If more than one dose is missed, or it is necessary to establish a new dosage schedule, contact your doctor or pharmacist.
- Physical exams should include self-examination of breasts (monthly), pelvic examination, and Pap smear test (yearly). Consult your doctor in all cases of unusual vaginal bleeding.
- *Diabetic patients* — Glucose tolerance may be decreased. Monitor blood sugar closely and report any abnormal results to your doctor.
- *Progesterone gel* — Notify your doctor immediately if any of the following occurs: Pain in the calves or chest; abnormal vaginal bleeding; sudden shortness of breath; coughing blood; sudden severe headache or vomiting; dizziness; fainting; visual or speech disturbances; weakness or numbness in an arm or leg; breast lumps; yellowing of skin or eyes.
- Dizziness may occur in some patients. Use caution when driving a motor vehicle or operating machinery.
- Inform your doctor if you are pregnant, become pregnant, are planning to become pregnant, or if you are breastfeeding.
- *Fluid retention* caused by progestins may aggravate asthma, epilepsy, migraine, heart disease, or kidney disease. Use with caution in these conditions.
- *Brand interchange* — Do not change from one brand of these drugs to another without consulting your doctor or pharmacist. Products manufactured by different companies may not be equally effective.
- *Progesterone gel* — Follow directions for preparation and use of the disposable applicator. Store at room temperature. Do not use after the printed expiration date.

If you have any questions, consult your doctor, pharmacist, or health care provider.

For more information on individual methods, see Oral Contraceptives, IUD, Levonorgestrel Implants and Spermicides monographs.

The following table gives ranges of pregnancy rates reported for various means of contraception. *The effectiveness of these means of contraception (except IUD, medroxyprogesterone injection, levonorgestrel implants, vasectomy, and tubal ligation) depends upon the degree of adherence to the method.*

Pregnancy Rates for Various Means of Contraception (%)[1]		
Method of Contraception	Typical[2]	Lowest[3]
Oral Contraceptives		
Combination	5	≤ 1
Progestin-only	5	≤ 1
Mechanical/Chemical		
Cervical cap[4]		
Multiparous	40	26
Nulliparous	20	9
Condoms without spermicide	14	3
Diaphragm[4]	20	6
Female condom	21	5
IUD	≤ 1 to 2	≤ 1 to 1.5
Levonorgestrel implants	≤ 1	≤ 1
Medroxyprogesterone injection	≤ 1	≤ 1
Spermicide alone	26	6
Vaginal sponge[5]		
Multiparous	40	20
Nulliparous	20	9
Rhythm (all types)	25	1 to 9
Vasectomy/Tubal Ligation	≤ 1	≤ 1

Pregnancy Rates for Various Means of Contraception (%)[1]		
Method of Contraception	Typical[2]	Lowest[3]
Withdrawal	19	4
No contraception	85	85

[1] During first year of continuous use.
[2] A "typical" couple who initiated a method that was either not always used correctly or was not used with every act of sexual intercourse, and who experienced an accidental pregnancy.
[3] The method of birth control was always used correctly with every act of sexual intercourse but the couple still experienced an accidental pregnancy.
[4] Used with spermicide.
[5] Contains spermicide.

If you have any questions, consult your doctor, pharmacist, or health care provider.

	Generic Name *Brand Name Example*	Supplied As	Generic Available
Rx	**Medroxyprogesterone Acetate**		
	Depo-Provera	**Injection:** 150 mg/mL	No

Type of Drug:

Female hormone; birth control injection; contraceptive injection.

How the Drug Works:

This hormone, when administered at the recommended dose, prevents ovulation by suppressing the follicle stimulating hormone (FSH) and the luteinizing hormone (LH). These changes result in endometrial thinning.

Uses:

To prevent pregnancy. It is a long-term injectable contraceptive in women when administered at 3-month intervals.

Precautions:

Do not use in the following situations:

allergy to any component of the formulation
breast cancer, known or suspected
clotting disorder, current or history of
liver disease
pregnancy, known or suspected
stroke, current or history of
vaginal bleeding, undiagnosed abnormal

Use with caution in the following situations:

asthma
depression
diabetes
epilepsy
heart disease
jaundice (yellowing of skin or eyes)
kidney disease
migraine

Use of injectable medroxyprogesterone may be associated with an increased risk of the following:

blood clots
ectopic pregnancy
osteoporosis
visual disorders

Eye problems: Do not readminister pending examination if there is a sudden partial or complete loss of vision or if there is a sudden onset of eyeball protrusion, double vision or migraine. Consult your doctor if you experience any of these.

Pregnancy: Do not use during pregnancy. The risk of use in a pregnant woman clearly outweighs any possible benefit.

Breastfeeding: Medroxyprogesterone appears in breast milk. Consult your doctor before you begin breastfeeding.

Drug Interactions:

Tell your doctor or pharmacist if you are taking or if you are planning to take any over-the-counter or prescription medications or dietary supplements with medroxyprogesterone. Doses of one or both drugs may need to be modified or a different drug may need to be prescribed. Aminoglutethimide (*Cytadren*) interacts with medroxyprogesterone.

Side Effects:

Every drug is capable of producing side effects. Many medroxyprogesterone users experience no, or minor, side effects. The frequency and severity of side effects depend on many factors including dose, duration of therapy and individual susceptibility. Possible side effects include:

Urinary and Reproductive Tract: Menstrual irregularities; decreased sex drive; failure to experience orgasm; vaginal infection; pelvic pain; breast pain; vaginal discharge.

Digestive Tract: Stomach pain/discomfort; nausea; bloating.

Nervous System: Headache; nervousness; dizziness; weakness; depression; sleeplessness.

Other: Weight changes; backache; leg cramps; acne; no hair growth or hair loss; rash; edema (fluid retention); hot flashes.

Guidelines for Use:

- Patient labeling available with product.
- Menstrual cycle may be disrupted and irregular when beginning treatment. This should decrease to the point of an absence of menstruation as treatment continues.
- Notify your doctor if there is a sudden partial or complete loss of vision, double vision or if migraine occurs.

If you have any questions, consult your doctor, pharmacist, or health care provider.

	Generic Name *Brand Name Example*	Supplied As	Generic Available
Rx	**Medroxyprogesterone Acetate/Estradiol Cypionate**		
	Lunelle	**Injection**: 25 mg/5 mg per 0.5 mL	No

Type of Drug:

Female hormone; monthly birth control injection; monthly contraceptive injection.

How the Drug Works:

This drug prevents ovulation by inhibiting the release of certain hormones. Other effects that enhance contraceptive effectiveness include a thickening of cervical mucus (decreases sperm penetration) and thinning of the endometrium (retards implantation of a fertilized egg).

Uses:

To prevent pregnancy.

Precautions:

Do not use in the following situations:

- allergy to any component of the formulation
- breast, endometrial, or other estrogen-dependent cancer, known or suspected
- cerebral vascular disease
- clotting disorder, current or history of
- coronary artery disease
- diabetes with vascular involvement
- heart disease, valvular
- high blood pressure, severe
- jaundice associated with pregnancy or hormonal contraceptive use, history of
- liver disease
- migraine headaches with neurological symptoms
- pregnancy, known or suspected
- smoking, heavy (15 or more cigarettes/day) and older than 35 years of age
- stroke or history of stroke
- vaginal bleeding, undiagnosed abnormal

Use with caution in the following situations:

- depression, history of
- diabetes
- gallbladder disease
- high cholesterol levels

Use may be associated with an increased risk of the following:

- blood clots
- gallbladder disease
- heart disease
- hypertriglyceridemia
- liver disease
- osteoporosis
- stroke
- visual disorders

Pregnancy: Do not use during pregnancy. The risk of use in a pregnant woman clearly outweighs any possible benefit.

Breastfeeding: It is not known if medroxyprogesterone/estradiol cypionate appears in breast milk. Consult your doctor before you begin breastfeeding.

Children: Safety and effectiveness have been established in women of reproductive age. Safety and effectiveness are expected to be the same for postpubertal adolescents ≥ 16 years of age. Use before the first menstruation is not indicated.

Drug Interactions:

Tell your doctor or pharmacist if you are taking or planning to take any over-the-counter or prescription medications or dietary supplements with this medicine. Doses of one or both drugs may need to be modified or a different drug may need to be prescribed. The following drugs or drug classes interact with this medicine:

acetaminophen (eg, *Tylenol*)
aminoglutethimide (*Cytadren*)
antibiotics (eg, tetracycline)
anticonvulsants (eg, phenytoin)
ascorbic acid (vitamin C)
clofibrate (*Atromid-S*)
cyclosporine (eg, *Neoral*)
morphine (eg, *MS Contin*)
phenylbutazone
prednisolone (eg, *Prelone*)
rifampin (eg, *Rifadin*)
salicylic acid (eg, *Panscol*)
St. John's wort (hypericum perforatum)
temazepam (eg, *Restoril*)
theophylline (eg, *Slo-Phyllin*)

Side Effects:

Every drug is capable of producing side effects. Many patients experience no, or minor, side effects. The frequency and severity of side effects depend on many factors including dose, duration of therapy, and individual susceptibility. Possible side effects include:

Nervous System: Headache; depression; emotional lability; dizziness; nervousness.

Urinary and Reproductive Tract: Changes in menstrual bleeding (eg, frequent, irregular, prolonged, infrequent, or absence of bleeding); vaginal yeast infection.

Other: Increased blood pressure; weight gain; fluid retention; visual changes or changes in contact lens tolerance; breast tenderness or pain; stomach pain; acne; hair loss; decreased sex drive; nausea.

Guidelines for Use:

- Carefully read the patient labeling available with the product.
- The first intramuscular (IM; into the muscle) injection is given within the first 5 days of the onset of a normal menstrual period, within 5 days of a complete first trimester abortion, or at least 4 weeks postpartum if you are not breastfeeding. If you are breastfeeding, the first injection is administered at least 6 weeks postpartum.
- The second and subsequent injections are administered monthly (28 to 30 days) after the previous injection, not to exceed 33 days. If the patient has not adhered to the prescribed schedule, pregnancy should be considered and she should not receive another injection until pregnancy is ruled out. Shortening the injection interval could lead to a change in menstrual pattern. Do not use bleeding episodes to guide the injection schedule.
- If a patient misses 2 consecutive periods, pregnancy should be considered before initiating or continuing injections.
- Menstrual cycle may be disrupted and irregular when beginning treatment. Notify your doctor if abnormal bleeding persists or is severe.
- Notify your doctor if you experience a sudden partial or complete loss of vision, double vision, yellowing of the skin or eyes, chest pain, pain in the legs, dizziness, or migraines.
- Medroxyprogesterone/estradiol cypionate injection does not protect against HIV (the virus that causes AIDS) or any other sexually transmitted diseases.
- When switching from other contraceptive methods, the injection should be given in a manner that ensures continuous contraceptive coverage based on the mechanism of action of both methods (eg, patients switching from oral contraceptives should have their first injection within 7 days after taking their last active pill).

If you have any questions, consult your doctor, pharmacist, or health care provider.

	Brand Name Examples	Estrogen (mcg)	Progestin (mg)
Rx	**Monophasic**		
	Necon 1/50, Nelova 1/50M, Norinyl 1+50, Ortho-Novum 1/50	50 mestranol	1 norethindrone
	Ovcon 50	50 ethinyl estradiol	1 norethindrone
	Demulen 1/50, Zovia 1/50E	50 ethinyl estradiol	1 ethynodiol diacetate
	Ovral	50 ethinyl estradiol	0.5 norgestrel
	Necon 1/35, Nelova 1/35E, Norethindrone and Ethinyl Estradiol, Norinyl 1+35, Ortho-Novum 1/35	35 ethinyl estradiol	1 norethindrone
	Brevicon, Modicon, Necon 0.5/35, Nelova 0.5/35E, Norethindrone and Ethinyl Estradiol	35 ethinyl estradiol	0.5 norethindrone
	Ovcon 35	35 ethinyl estradiol	0.4 norethindrone
	Ortho-Cyclen	35 ethinyl estradiol	0.25 norgestimate
	Demulen 1/35, Zovia 1/35E	35 ethinyl estradiol	1 ethynodiol diacetate
	Loestrin 1.5/30, Loestrin Fe 1.5/30[1]	30 ethinyl estradiol	1.5 norethindrone acetate
	Lo/Ovral, Low-Ogestrel	30 ethinyl estradiol	0.3 norgestrel
	Levlen, Levora, Nordette	30 ethinyl estradiol	0.15 levonorgestrel
	Apri, Desogen, Desogestrel and Ethinyl Estradiol, Ortho-Cept	30 ethinyl estradiol	0.15 desogestrel
	Loestrin 1/20, Loestrin Fe 1/20[1]	20 ethinyl estradiol	1 norethindrone acetate
	Alesse, Levlite	20 ethinyl estradiol	0.1 levonorgestrel
Rx	**Biphasic**		
	Jenest, Necon 10/11, Nelova 7/14, Nelova 10/11, Norethindrone and Ethinyl Estradiol (7/14), Norethindrone and Ethinyl Estradiol (10/11), Ortho-Novum 10/11		
	Phase 1	35 ethinyl estradiol	0.5 norethindrone
	Phase 2	35 ethinyl estradiol	1 norethindrone

Brand Name Examples	Estrogen (mcg)	Progestin (mg)
Rx **Biphasic**		
Mircette		
Phase 1	20 ethinyl estradiol	0.15 desogestrel
Phase 2	10 ethinyl estradiol	
Rx **Triphasic**		
Tri-Norinyl		
Phase 1	35 ethinyl estradiol	0.5 norethindrone
Phase 2	35 ethinyl estradiol	1 norethindrone
Phase 3	35 ethinyl estradiol	0.5 norethindrone
Ortho-Novum 7/7/7		
Phase 1	35 ethinyl estradiol	0.5 norethindrone
Phase 2	35 ethinyl estradiol	0.75 norethindrone
Phase 3	35 ethinyl estradiol	1 norethindrone
Ortho Tri-Cyclen		
Phase 1	35 ethinyl estradiol	0.18 norgestimate
Phase 2	35 ethinyl estradiol	0.215 norgestimate
Phase 3	35 ethinyl estradiol	0.25 norgestimate
Tri Levlen, Triphasil, Trivora		
Phase 1	30 ethinyl estradiol	0.05 levonorgestrel
Phase 2	40 ethinyl estradiol	0.075 levonorgestrel
Phase 3	30 ethinyl estradiol	0.125 levonorgestrel
Estrostep, Estrostep Fe[1]		
Phase 1	20 ethinyl estradiol	1 norethindrone acetate
Phase 2	30 ethinyl estradiol	1 norethindrone acetate
Phase 3	35 ethinyl estradiol	1 norethindrone acetate
Rx **Progestin Only**		
Micronor, Nor-QD	none	0.35 norethindrone
Ovrette [2]	none	0.075 norgestrel

[1] Seven tablets in the 28-day package contain 75 mg ferrous fumarate (iron) per tablet.
[2] Contains tartrazine.

All of the products listed in the table are oral contraceptives; however, they are not interchangeable. For example, *Lo/Ovral* cannot be used for *Ortho-Novum*. Daily doses may vary depending on individual needs. Do not adjust the dose without consulting your pharmacist or doctor.

Type of Drug:

Oral contraceptives. Birth-control pills, "the pill." POPs, "mini-pill" (progestin only).

How the Drug Works:

There are two different types of birth-control pills: Combination pills and progestin-only pills (POPs).

The *combination pill* contains the hormones estrogen and progestin. It prevents pregnancy by preventing ovulation, altering cervical mucous to inhibit sperm and decrease the chances of fertilization if an egg is released, and altering the lining of the uterus to prevent implantation of a fertilized egg.

There are three kinds of combination pills. The *monophasic* pill has the same dose of estrogen and progestin in each pill. The *biphasic* and *triphasic* pills have varying amounts of hormones. This produces an effect that more closely resembles the normal hormone cycle of the body. All of the biphasic pills (except *Mircette*) contain the same amount of estrogen in each pill. The progestin present is lower in the first half of the menstrual cycle than during the second half. The triphasic pill may contain differing amounts of both estrogen and progestin in the monthly cycle.

POPs contain only progestin. They appear to prevent pregnancy by causing changes in the cervical mucus and the inner lining of the uterus. These changes inhibit sperm from fertilizing the egg and prevent implantation should fertilization occur. POPs prevent ovulation in some women.

Uses:

To prevent pregnancy. Oral contraceptives are highly effective. Less than 1 of 100 women taking the oral contraceptives for 1 year become pregnant. Some of the pregnancies are not due to failure of the pill but to a failure of the user to take the pill properly (eg, missed doses). Approximately 3 of 100 women taking POPs for 1 year become pregnant.

Because of an association between estrogen use and the risk of blood clots, the estrogen dose in the combination pill should be as low as possible. Women should discuss this matter with their doctors.

Ortho Tri-Cyclen — Also indicated for the treatment of moderate acne in women 15 years of age or older who have no known contraindications to oral contraceptive therapy, desire contraception, have had their first menstruation, and are unresponsive to topical anti-acne medications.

Unlabeled Use(s): Occasionally doctors may prescribe oral contraceptives as a postcoital contraceptive or "morning-after" pill. See the Emergency Contraceptives monograph in this chapter.

Precautions:

Do not use in the following situations:

allergy to the oral contraceptive or any of its ingredients
angina pectoris (chest pain)
blood clots in the deep veins of the legs, active or history of
blood clotting disorder
cancer of breast, cervix, uterus, or vagina; known or suspected
cerebrovascular disease
coronary artery disease
estrogen-dependent growths, known or suspected
heart attack, history of
jaundice (yellowing of skin or eyes) during pregnancy or during previous use of oral contraceptives
liver disease or tumors
pregnancy, known or suspected
stroke, history of
thromboembolic disorders, active or history of
vaginal bleeding, undiagnosed or abnormal

Use with caution in the following situations:

abnormal breast x-ray or mammogram
breast nodules
depression, history of
diabetes or prediabetes
epilepsy
fibroids
gallbladder disease
headaches
heart disease
high blood pressure
hyperlipidemia (increased cholesterol or triglycerides)
kidney disease
menstrual flow, absent or irregular, history of
migraine
porphyria
smoker, current
surgery

Risk factors: All of the following are considered risk factors. The likelihood of side effects from oral contraceptives multiplies with each additional risk factor.

coronary artery disease, family history of
diabetes
high blood pressure
high cholesterol or triglycerides
jaundice, active or history of
older than 35 years of age
long term use (over 10 years)
smoking 15 or more cigarettes/day

Increased risk: Use of oral contraceptives is associated with an increased risk of the following:

blood clots
cerebral hemorrhage
decreased glucose tolerance
depression
fluid retention
gallbladder disease
headache
heart attack
high blood pressure
liver tumors
menstrual bleeding irregularities
stroke
vascular disease
visual disorders

Cigarette smoking: Cigarette smoking increases the risk of serious cardiovascular side effects from oral contraceptive use. The risk increases with age and with heavy smoking (15 or more cigarettes/day) and is quite marked in women over 35 years of age. Women who use oral contraceptives should not smoke.

Contact lens wearers: If you develop changes in vision or lens tolerance, contact your eye-care specialist. Consider temporarily or permanently stopping contact lens wear.

Diabetics: Oral contraceptives may cause decreased glucose tolerance. Monitor blood sugar closely and report changes to your doctor.

Eye problems: Discontinue use and notify your doctor if you experience double vision, unexplained loss of vision, or other vision changes.

Side effects: Side effects noted during initial cycles are usually related to the potency of the estrogen or progestin in the product and may be transient. If side effects continue, discuss changing products (different estrogen/progestin potency) with your doctor.

Use preceding pregnancy: Women who discontinue oral contraceptives with the intent of becoming pregnant should use an alternate form of contraception for approximately 3 months before attempting to conceive.

Pregnancy: Do not use during pregnancy. The risk of use in a pregnant woman clearly outweighs any possible benefit.

Breastfeeding: Oral contraceptives appear in breast milk. They may decrease both the quantity and quality of breast milk. Do not use until the infant is weaned.

Children: Safety and effectiveness have been established in women of reproductive age. Safety and effectiveness are expected to be the same for postpubertal adolescents 16 years of age or younger. Use of this product before the first menstruation is not indicated.

Tartrazine: Some of these products may contain the dye tartrazine (FD&C Yellow No. 5), which can cause allergic reactions in certain individuals. Check package label when available or consult your pharmacist or doctor.

Drug Interactions:

Tell your doctor or pharmacist if you are taking or planning to take any over-the-counter or prescription medications or dietary supplements with oral contraceptives. Doses of one or both drugs may need to be modified or a different drug may need to be prescribed. The following drugs and drug classes interact with oral contraceptives:

antibiotics (eg, penicillins, tetracyclines)
anticoagulants (eg, warfarin)
azole antifungal agents (eg, fluconazole, itraconazole)
barbiturates (eg, phenobarbital)
benzodiazepines (eg, diazepam)
beta blockers (eg, propranolol)
caffeine
carbamazepine (eg, *Tegretol*)
corticosteroids (eg, prednisone)
felbamate (*Felbatol*)
griseofulvin (eg, *Grisfulvin*)
hydantoins (eg, phenytoin)
penicillin V (eg, *Beepen-VK*)
phenylbutazone (not available in the US)
primidone (eg, *Mysoline*)
protease inhibitors (eg, nelfinavir, ritonavir)
rifampin (eg, *Rifadin*)
selegiline (eg, *Eldepryl*)
tetracyclines (eg, doxycycline)
theophyllines (eg, aminophylline)
troleandomycin (*Tao*)

Side Effects:

Every drug is capable of producing side effects. Many oral contraceptive users experience no, or minor, side effects. The frequency and severity of side effects depend on many factors including dose, duration of therapy, and individual susceptibility. Possible side effects include:

Serious: Blood clots; stroke; high blood pressure; heart attack; gallbladder disease; liver problems; changes in vision.

Urinary and Reproductive Tract: Change in menstrual flow; vaginal bleeding at abnormal times; absence of menstrual bleeding; spotting; temporary infertility after discontinuing drug; unusual vaginal secretions; vaginal fungal infection; change in cervical erosion or secretion.

Digestive Tract: Nausea; vomiting; stomach cramps; bloating.

Nervous System: Migraine; depression; headache; dizziness.

Skin: Spotty skin discoloration; rash; light sensitivity.

Other: Breast changes, tenderness, or enlargement; breast secretions; decrease in breast milk when given after childbirth; contact lens intolerance; change in corneal curvature; fluid retention; weight changes; reduced tolerance to carbohydrates; elevated blood sugar (diabetic patients); yellowing of skin or eyes; hypertriglyceridemia.

Guidelines for Use:

- Carefully read the patient package insert available with the product.
- Your doctor or health care provider will take a medical and family history and examine you before prescribing oral contraceptives. The physical examination may be delayed to another time if you request it and your doctor believes that it is a good medical practice to postpone it. You should be reexamined at least once a year while taking oral contraceptives.
- Take exactly as directed at intervals not greater than 24 hours. Take regularly with a meal or at bedtime. Strictly adhere to the dosage schedule for maximum effectiveness.
- Notify your doctor immediately if you experience pain in the groin or calves; sharp or crushing chest pain; heaviness in the chest; sudden shortness of breath; abnormal vaginal bleeding; missed menstrual period or suspected pregnancy; lumps in the breast; sudden severe headache, dizziness, or fainting; vision or speech disturbances; weakness or numbness in an arm or leg; severe stomach pain or tenderness in the stomach area; yellowing of the skin or eyes (especially if accompanied by fever, fatigue, loss of appetite, dark-colored urine, or light-colored bowel movements); severe depression; contact lens intolerance; coughing up blood; vomiting; sudden partial or complete loss of vision; difficulty sleeping; weakness; lack of energy; fatigue; or mood changes.
- Notify your doctor if you miss 2 consecutive menstrual periods. Oral contraceptive use should be discontinued until pregnancy is ruled out.
- If you experience vomiting or diarrhea, your oral contraceptive may not be as effective. Use a backup contraceptive method (eg, condoms, spermicide) until you speak with your doctor or pharmacist.
- May cause spotting, breakthrough bleeding, or nausea, especially during the first months of therapy. If this continues past the second month, notify your doctor.
- Fluid retention caused by oral contraceptives may aggravate seizure disorders; migraine; asthma; and heart, liver, or kidney disease. Use with caution in these situations.
- Report side effects to your doctor. Numerous combinations of oral contraceptives are available. Changes may be necessary to find the best one for you.
- If you have trouble remembering to take your oral contraceptive, talk to your doctor about how to make pill-taking easier or about using another method of contraception.
- Use an additional form of birth control for at least the first week after you begin taking oral contraceptives.
- *Diabetic patients* — Glucose tolerance may be decreased. Monitor blood sugar closely and report changes to your doctor.
- Oral contraceptives do not protect against HIV (the virus that causes AIDS) or any other sexually transmitted diseases.
- Lab tests may be required to monitor therapy. Be sure to keep appointments.

Guidelines for Use (cont.):

- Store at room temperature (59° to 77°F).
- *How to take the combination pill* —

  Sunday-Start packaging: If the instructions recommend starting the regimen on Sunday, take the first tablet on the first Sunday after menstruation begins. If menstruation begins on Sunday, take the first tablet on that day.

  21-Day regimen: For day 1 start, count the first day of menstrual bleeding as day 1. Take 1 tablet daily for 21 days, then no tablets are taken for 7 days; whether bleeding has stopped or not, start a new course of 21 days followed by 7 days off. Withdrawal flow will normally occur approximately 3 days after the last tablet is taken. Follow the schedule whether flow occurs as expected, or whether spotting or breakthrough bleeding occurs during the cycle.

  28-Day regimen: To eliminate the need to count the days between cycles, some products contain 7 inert or iron-containing tablets to permit continuous daily dosage during the entire 28-day cycle. Take the 7 inert or iron-containing tablets on the last 7 days of the cycle.

  Biphasic and triphasic pills: Follow the instructions on the dispensers or packs; these are clearly marked (ususally with arrows), indicating where to start on the regimen and in what order to take the pills, along with the appropriate week numbers. If there is any question, detailed instructions are provided in the specific package insert. As with the monophasic pills, 1 tablet is taken each day; however, as the color or shape of the tablet changes, the strength of the tablet also changes (ie, the estrogen/progestin ratio varies).
- *Missed dose: Combination pill* — Although ovulation is not likely to occur if only 1 tablet is missed, the possibility of spotting or bleeding is increased. The possibility of ovulation occurring increases each day that tablets are missed, especially if 2 or more consecutive tablets are missed. Any time 1 or more active tablets are missed, use an additional method of contraception until tablets have been taken for 7 consecutive days. If you forget to take 1 or more tablets, the following is suggested:

  One tablet: Take it as soon as remembered, or take 2 tablets the next day; alternatively, take 1 tablet, discard the other missed tablet, and continue as scheduled and use another form of contraception until menstruation.

  Two consecutive tablets: Take 2 tablets as soon as remembered with the next pill at the usual time, or take 2 tablets daily for the next 2 days, then resume the regular schedule. Use an additional method of contraception for the 7 days after pills are missed, preferably for the remainder of the cycle. If 2 active pills are missed in a row in the third week and you are a Sunday starter, 1 pill should be taken every day until Sunday. On Sunday, the rest of the pack should be discarded and a new pack of pills started that same day. If 2 active pills are missed in a row in the third week and you are a day 1 starter, the rest of the pill pack should be discarded and a new pack started that same day. Menstruation may not occur this month, but this is expected. However, if menstruation does not occur 2 months in a row, contact your doctor or health care professional to discuss the possibility of pregnancy.

Guidelines for Use (cont.):

- *Missed dose: Combination pill* (cont.) — *Three consecutive tablets:* If you are a Sunday starter, you should continue taking 1 pill every day until Sunday. On Sunday, the rest of the pack should be discarded and a new pack of pills started that same day. If you are a day 1 starter, the rest of the pill pack should be discarded and a new pack started that same day. Menstruation may not occur this month, but that is expected. However, if menstruation does not occur 2 months in a row, contact your doctor or health care professional to discuss the possibility of pregnancy. Pregnancy may result from sexual intercourse during the 7 days after the pills are missed. Use another form of contraception (eg, condoms, spermicide) as a backup method for those 7 days.
- *How to take POPs* — Take 1 tablet every day at the same time. Administration is continuous, with no interruption between pill packs. Every time a pill is taken late, and especially if a pill is missed, pregnancy is more likely.
- *Missed dose: POPs* — If you are more than 3 hours late or miss 1 or more tablet, take the missed pill as soon as you remember, then go back to taking the pill at the regular time, but be sure to use a backup method (eg, condom, spermicide) every time you have sexual intercourse for the next 48 hours.
- *Switching pills* — If you are switching from the combination pills to POPs, take the first POP the day after the last active combination pill is taken. Do not take any of the 7 inactive pills from the combination pill pack. Many women have irregular periods after switching to POPs. This is normal. If you are switching from POPs to the combination pills, take the first active combination pill on the first day of menstruation, even if the POP pack is not finished. If you are switching to another brand of POP, start the new brand at any time.
- *Missed menstruation* — If prescribed dosage regimen has not been followed, consider possible pregnancy. Stop taking the drug until pregnancy has been ruled out. If the prescribed regimen has been followed and 2 consecutive periods are missed, rule out the possibility of pregnancy before continuing the regimen. After several months of treatment, the menstrual flow may reduce to a point of virtual absence. This may occur as a result of medication and is not an indication of pregnancy.

If you have any questions, consult your doctor, pharmacist, or health care provider.

	Generic Name *Brand Name Examples*	Supplied As	Generic Available
Rx	**Ethinyl Estradiol/ Levonorgestrel**		
	Preven	**Tablets**: 50 mcg ethinyl estradiol, 0.25 mg levonorgestrel	No
Rx	**Levonorgestrel**		
	Plan B	**Tablets**: 0.75 mg	No

Type of Drug:

Sex hormones; emergency contraceptives; emergency contraceptive pills (ECPs).

How the Drug Works:

The exact mechanism of action is not known. ECPs may prevent pregnancy by inhibiting ovulation, altering transport of sperm or eggs to prevent fertilization, or altering the uterine environment to prevent implantation should fertilization occur.

Uses:

For the prevention of pregnancy following unprotected intercourse or a known or suspected contraceptive failure. Use of the ECPs should begin as soon as possible, but within 72 hours of intercourse.

Precautions:

Do not use in the following situations:

Preven and Plan B —

allergy to the drug or any of its ingredients
pregnancy, known or suspected
vaginal bleeding, abnormal or undiagnosed

Preven only —

blood clots in the deep leg veins, current or history of
blood clots in the lungs, current or history of
breast cancer, history of
breast cancer, known or suspected
cerebrovascular accidents, history of
diabetes with vascular involvement
headaches, severe (including migraine)
heart disease, ischemic
heavy smoking (more than 15 cigarettes/day) and more than 35 years of age
high blood pressure, severe
liver disease, active
liver tumors
major surgery with prolonged immobilization
stroke, current or history of
valvular heart disease with complications

Use with caution in the following situations:

diabetes
headaches
high blood pressure

Pregnancy: Do not use during pregnancy. The risk of use in a pregnant woman clearly outweighs any possible benefit.

Breastfeeding: Levonorgestrel and ethinyl estradiol appear in breast milk. Consult your doctor before you begin breastfeeding.

Children: Safety and effectiveness have been established in women of reproductive age. Safety and effectiveness are expected to be the same for postpubertal adolescents 16 years of age or younger. Use of this product before the onset of first menstruation is not indicated.

Drug Interactions:

Tell your doctor or pharmacist if you are taking or planning to take any over-the-counter or prescription medications or dietary supplements while taking emergency contraceptives. Doses of one or both drugs may need to be modified or a different drug may need to be prescribed. The following drugs and drug classes interact with emergency contraceptives:

barbiturates (eg, phenobarbital)
carbamazepine (eg, *Tegretol*)
hydantoins (eg, phenytoin)
griseofulvin (eg, *Grisactin*)
rifampin (eg, *Rifadin*)
primidone (eg, *Mysoline*)
protease inhibitors (eg, nelfinavir)
selegiline (eg, *Eldepryl*)

Side Effects:

Every drug is capable of producing side effects. Many emergency contraceptive users experience no, or minor, side effects. The frequency and severity of side effects depend on many factors including dose, duration of therapy, and individual susceptibility. Possible side effects include:

Digestive Tract: Nausea; vomiting; stomach pain or cramps.

Other: Headaches; dizziness; menstrual irregularities; breast tenderness; fatigue.

Guidelines for Use:

- Carefully read the patient package insert available with this product.
- Emergency contraceptives can be used at any time during the menstrual cycle.
- Take 1 (*Plan B)* or 2 (*Preven*) tablets as soon as possible, but no later than 72 hours after unprotected intercourse. Take the second dose of 1 (*Plan B)* or 2 (*Preven*) tablets 12 hours after the first dose.
- If vomiting occurs within 1 hour of taking either dose of the medication, notify your doctor to discuss whether to repeat that dose and whether to take an antinausea medication before taking the dose again.
- Nausea occurs frequently. It is usually mild and stops within a few hours, but may continue for up to 1 or 2 days.
- *Preven* — The *Preven* emergency contraceptive kit contains a pregnancy test. This test can be used to verify an existing pregnancy resulting from intercourse that occurred earlier in the current menstrual cycle or the previous cycle. If a positive pregnancy test is obtained, contact your doctor and do not take the pills in the kit.
- Notify your doctor immediately if you experience sharp or crushing chest pain, coughing up blood, sudden shortness of breath, pain in a calf, heaviness in the chest, sudden severe headache, vomiting, dizziness, fainting, vision or speech disturbance, weakness, numbness in an arm or leg, sudden partial or complete loss of vision, or severe pain or tenderness in the stomach area.
- Emergency contraceptives are not to be used for ongoing pregnancy protection and should not be used as a woman's routine form of contraception.
- Taking more emergency contraceptive pills than prescribed does not further reduce the risk of pregnancy, but does increase the risk of nausea and vomiting.
- Emergency contraceptives do not protect against HIV (the virus that causes AIDS) or any other sexually transmitted diseases.
- A 3-week follow-up visit with your doctor or health care provider is recommended.
- Store at controlled room temperature (59° to 86°F).

If you have any questions, consult your doctor, pharmacist, or health care provider.

	Generic Name *Brand Name Example*	Supplied As	Generic Available
Rx	**Progesterone**		
	Progestasert	**Intrauterine System**: 38 mg reservoir	No

Type of Drug:

Progestin-containing intrauterine birth-control device; IUD.

How the Drug Works:

The exact mechanism of action is not known. It is believed that the system inhibits sperm and alters the uterine environment to prevent implantation should fertilization occur.

Uses:

To prevent pregnancy for up to 1 year in women who have had at least one child, are in a stable, mutually monogamous relationship, and have no history of pelvic inflammatory disease (PID).

Unlabeled Use(s): Occasionally doctors may prescribe IUDs for excessive and prolonged menstrual bleeding.

Precautions:

Do not use in the following situations:

abnormal pap smear
cervical cancer, known or suspected
ectopic pregnancy, predisposal to or history of
genital actinomycosis
incomplete involution of uterus following abortion or childbirth
increased susceptibility to infections (eg, leukemia, diabetes, steroid therapy, immunosuppression)
infected abortion
inflammation of the cervix
inflammation of the vagina
IUD still in place
IV drug abuse
multiple sexual partners, either partner
pelvic inflammatory disease, history or presence of, or predisposing factors to
pelvic surgery, history of
postpartum endometritis (inflammation of uterine lining)
pregnancy, known or suspected
sexually transmitted disease, history or presence of
shunt, systemic pulmonary
uterine cancer, known or suspected
uterine cavity distortion
vaginal bleeding, undiagnosed abnormal

Use with caution in the following situations:

anemia
anticoagulant therapy, concurrent
blood clotting disorder
congenital heart condition
excessive or prolonged menstrual bleeding, history of

Continuation of pregnancy: If pregnancy occurs while the IUD is in place and the pregnancy is continued without removing the IUD, there may be an increased risk of birth defects, miscarriage, infection, or premature labor and delivery. During pregnancy, report any of the following to your doctor immediately: Flu-like symptoms, fever, chills, stomach cramps and pain, vaginal bleeding or discharge.

Ectopic pregnancy: Although the IUD acts to prevent normal pregnancy, it does not prevent ovulation or ectopic pregnancy. Therefore, a pregnancy that occurs with an IUD in place is more likely to be ectopic. Ectopic pregnancies are potentially fatal and have been associated with complications leading to loss of fertility. Discuss symptoms of ectopic pregnancy with your doctor.

Pelvic inflammatory disease (PID): An increased risk of PID associated with IUD use has been reported. The highest rate occurs shortly after insertion and up to 4 months thereafter. PID can result in tubal damage, affect fertility, or cause predisposition to ectopic pregnancy. Discuss symptoms of PID and ectopic pregnancy with your doctor.

Embedment: Partial penetration or lodging of an IUD in the uterine lining has occurred. This can result in difficult removal or IUD fragmentation that may require surgical removal.

Pregnancy: Long-term effects on the fetus are unknown. If pregnancy is suspected, consult your doctor. Risks of an infected abortion may be increased if pregnancy occurs with a system in place. This is more likely to occur in the second trimester. If pregnancy occurs with the system in place, the system must be removed and termination of the pregnancy must be considered.

Breastfeeding: Oral progestins appear in breast milk. It is not known if the IUD affects breast milk or breastfeeding. Consult your doctor before you begin breastfeeding.

Drug Interactions:

Tell your doctor or pharmacist if you are taking or if you are planning to take any over-the-counter or prescription medications or dietary supplements with IUDs. Doses of one or both drugs may need to be modified or a different drug may need to be prescribed. Anticoagulants (eg, warfarin) increase the risk of bleeding from the IUD insertion site.

Side Effects:

Every drug is capable of producing side effects. Many IUD users experience no, or minor, side effects. The frequency and severity of side effects depend on many factors including duration of therapy, and individual susceptibility. Possible side effects include:

Urinary and Reproductive Tract: Inflammation of the uterine lining; miscarriage; septic abortion; perforation of uterus and cervix; pelvic infection; cervical erosion; inflammation of the vagina; vaginal discharge; ectopic pregnancy; uterine embedment; difficult removal; complete or partial expulsion of the IUD; vaginal bleeding at abnormal times; prolonged menstrual bleeding; lack of or delayed menstrual bleeding; pelvic pain and cramping; painful menstruation; difficult or painful intercourse; fragmentation of IUD; tuboovarian abscess; tubal damage; fetal damage; birth defects; intrauterine pregnancy.

Digestive Tract: Perforation into the abdomen followed by peritonitis; abdominal adhesions; stomach pain; intestinal penetration; intestinal obstruction; local inflammatory reaction with abscess formation and erosion of adjacent organs; cystic masses in the pelvis.

Circulatory System: Decreased heart rate during insertion or removal; blood poisoning; anemia.

Other: Fainting during insertion or removal; backache.

Guidelines for Use:

- The patient information leaflet must be read and each section initialed by the patient.
- The Informed Choice Statement must be signed by the patient and by her doctor.
- A complete medical history and examination, including tests for chlamydia and gonorrhea, is required prior to insertion. The IUD should not be inserted immediately following childbirth or abortion.
- To prevent insertion in the presence of pregnancy, the system should be inserted during or shortly following menstruation.
- Reexamination is necessary within 3 months after the first postinsertion menstrual period and at 12 months for removal of the system. Normal pregnancy can occur after system removal, unless another system is inserted or other forms of contraception are started.
- Bleeding and cramps may occur during the first few weeks after insertion. Notify your doctor if symptoms continue or are severe.
- Notify your doctor immediately if you suspect you may be pregnant.
- Notify your doctor if you experience unusual, abnormal, or excessive vaginal bleeding; unusual or odorous vaginal discharge; fever; flu-like symptoms; genital sores; delayed or missed menstruation; pain during sexual intercourse; chills; pelvic pain or tenderness associated with fainting or the urge to defecate; unexplained shoulder pain; or stomach pain, cramping, or tenderness.
- If you notice the threads attached to the IUD, notify your doctor. Do not pull on the threads.
- Intrauterine progesterone does not protect against HIV (the virus that causes AIDS) or any other sexually transmitted diseases.

If you have any questions, consult your doctor, pharmacist, or health care provider.

	Generic Name *Brand Name Example*	Supplied As	Generic Available
Rx	**Levonorgestrel**		
	Norplant System	**Implants:** 6 each containing 36 mg (216 mg total)	No

Type of Drug:

Long-term (less than 5 years), reversible birth-control system; progestin-containing contraceptive system.

How the Drug Works:

Levonorgestrel appears to prevent pregnancy by preventing ovulation. It also causes changes in the inner lining of the uterus, preventing implantation should fertilization occur.

Uses:

To prevent pregnancy for up to 5 years. The implants should be removed by the end of the fifth year; new implants may be inserted at that time if continuing contraceptive protection is desired. Approximately 0.2 (patients weighing less than 110 lbs) to 8.5 (patients weighing 154 lbs or more) of 100 women using levonorgestrel implants become pregnant. The effectiveness of this method is not dependent on proper use, but does appear to vary in accordance with body weight.

Precautions:

Do not use in the following situations:

- allergy to levonorgestrel or any of its ingredients
- blood clotting disorder
- breast cancer, known or suspected
- idiopathic intracranial hypertension, history of
- liver disease, acute
- liver tumors, benign or malignant
- pregnancy, known or suspected
- vaginal bleeding, undiagnosed abnormal

Use with caution in the following situations:

- depression, history of
- diabetes or prediabetes
- hyperlipidemia (increased cholesterol or triglycerides)

Contact lens wearers: If you develop changes in vision or lens tolerance, contact your eye care specialist. Consider temporarily or permanently stopping contact lens wear.

Delayed follicular atresia: If the development of an ovarian follicle occurs, growth beyond the size attained in a normal cycle may occur. These enlarged follicles cannot be distinguished clinically from ovarian cysts. Usually they will spontaneously disappear; rarely, they may twist or rupture, possibly requiring surgery.

Ectopic pregnancy: Ectopic pregnancies have occurred among levonorgestrel implant users, although studies have shown no increase in the rate per year as compared with users of no method of contraception or of intrauterine progesterone (IUDs). The risk may increase with duration of use and possibly with the increased weight of the user.

Impaired liver function: If jaundice (yellowing of skin or eyes) develops, removal of the implants should be considered. Steroid hormones may be poorly metabolized in patients with impaired liver function.

Fluid retention: Steroid contraceptives may cause fluid retention. Therefore, they should be used with caution in patients with conditions that might be aggravated by fluid retention (eg, high blood pressure, heart failure).

Pregnancy: Do not use during pregnancy. The risk of use in a pregnant woman clearly outweighs any possible benefit.

Breastfeeding: Levonorgestrel appears in breast milk. Consult your doctor before you begin breastfeeding.

Children: Safety and effectiveness have been established in women of reproductive age. Safety and effectiveness are expected to be the same for postpubertal adolescents 16 years of age or younger. Use of this product before the onset of first menstruation is not indicated.

Drug Interactions:

Tell your doctor or pharmacist if you are taking or if you are planning to take any over-the-counter or prescription medications or dietary supplements with levonorgestrel implants. Doses of one or both drugs may need to be modified or a different drug may need to be prescribed. The following drugs and drug classes interact with levonorgestrel implants:

carbamazepine (eg, *Tegretol*)
phenytoin (eg, *Dilantin*)
rifampin (eg, *Rifadin*)

Side Effects:

Every drug is capable of producing side effects. Many levonorgestrel implant users experience no, or minor, side effects. The frequency and severity of side effects depend on many factors including duration of therapy and individual susceptibility. Possible side effects include:

Insertion site reactions: Pain; swelling; bruising; infection; blistering; ulceration; itching; skin sloughing; excessive scarring; discoloration; arm pain; numbness and tingling; nerve injury; removal difficulties; vein inflammation.

Urinary and Reproductive Tract: Change (typically a decrease) in menstrual flow; spotting; lack of menstrual bleeding; breast pain; breast discharge; inflammation of the vagina or cervix; vaginal discharge; enlarged ovarian follicles; prolonged, frequent, or irregular menstrual bleeding.

Digestive Tract: Nausea; vomiting; appetite changes; stomach ache.

Nervous System: Headache; anxiety; depression; nervousness; dizziness.

Other: Acne; skin inflammation; weight gain; excessive hair growth; scalp hair loss; abnormal lab tests; pain; fluid retention; rash; idiopathic intracranial hypertension; adnexal enlargement.

Also consider all side effects for combination (estrogen/progestin) oral contraceptives when using levonorgestrel implant. See the Oral Contraceptives monograph in this chapter.

Guidelines for Use:

- Carefully read the patient package insert available with this product.
- Capsules will be inserted beneath the skin of the upper arm.
- Capsules should be implanted or removed only by a health care professional thoroughly instructed in the insertion and removal technique.
- Pregnancy must be ruled out prior to insertion. Conduct pregnancy tests whenever pregnancy is suspected. If pregnancy occurs, the implants must be removed.
- Insertion of the levonorgestrel implants should be performed during the first 7 days after the beginning of menstruation or immediately following an abortion. If performed at any other time during the cycle, a nonhormonal contraceptive method (eg, condom, diaphragm) should be used for the remainder of that cycle. Insertion is not recommended until 6 weeks after childbirth in breastfeeding women.
- Removal of the implants should be considered in women who will be immobilized for a prolonged period of time due to surgery or illness.
- Implants must be removed at the end of the 5-year period. If new implants are not inserted at the same time, the patient's previous level of fertility will return and pregnancy can occur at any time.
- Some change in menstruation patterns can be expected, especially during the first year.
- Notify your doctor if you experience stomach or pelvic pain, persistent headache, visual disturbances, depression, or yellowing of the skin or eyes.
- *Diabetic patients* — Levonorgestrel implants may alter glucose tolerance. Monitor your blood glucose closely.
- Bruising may occur at the implant site during insertion or removal. Darkening of the skin over the implant site may occur in some women but is usually reversible upon removal.
- Levonorgestrel implants do not protect against HIV infection (the virus that causes AIDS) or any other sexually transmitted diseases.

If you have any questions, consult your doctor, pharmacist, or health care provider.

	Generic Name *Brand Name Example*	Supplied As	Generic Available
Rx	**Levonorgestrel**		
	Mirena	**Intrauterine system**: T-shaped unit containing a reservoir of 52 mg levonorgestrel covered by a silicone membrane	No

Type of Drug:

Levonorgestrel-releasing intrauterine system (LRIS).

How the Drug Works:

How LRIS works to prevent pregnancy is not fully understood. The system may inhibit ovulation, alter the transport of sperm or eggs to prevent fertilization, or alter the lining of the uterus to prevent egg implantation should fertilization occur.

Uses:

For intrauterine contraception for up to 5 years. Thereafter, if continued contraception is desired, the system should be replaced or alternative forms of contraception used.

LRIS is recommended for women who have had at least 1 child, are in a stable, mutually monogamous relationship, have no history of pelvic inflammatory disease (PID), and have no history of ectopic pregnancy or condition that would predispose to ectopic pregnancy.

Precautions:

Do not use in the following situations:

abnormal, unresolved Pap smear
allergy to the intrauterine system or any of its components
breast cancer, known or suspected
cervical cancer, known or suspected
cervicitis or vaginitis, untreated (including bacterial vaginosis or other lower genital tract infections until infection is controlled)
conditions associated with increased susceptibility to infections (eg, leukemia, AIDS, IV drug abuse)
ectopic pregnancy, history of or predisposition to
genital actinomycosis
genital bleeding of unknown etiology
infected abortion in the previous 3 months
intrauterine device already in place
liver disease, acute
liver tumor, benign or malignant
multiple sexual partners, patient or patient's partner
pelvic inflammatory disease (PID), acute or a history of unless there has been a subsequent intrauterine pregnancy
postpartum endometriosis in the past 3 months
pregnancy or suspicion of pregnancy
uterine irregularity (including fibroids if they distort the uterine cavity)
uterine cancer, known or suspected

Use with caution in the following situations:

anticoagulant therapy, concurrent	congenital heart disease
coagulopathy (bleeding disorder)	diabetes
	valvular heart disease

Intrauterine pregnancy: If a patient becomes pregnant with the LRIS in place, and if the LRIS cannot be removed or the patient chooses not to have it removed, she should be warned that failure to remove the LRIS increases the risk of miscarriage, sepsis, premature labor, and premature delivery. She should be monitored closely and advised to report immediately any flu-like symptoms, fever, chills, cramping, pain, bleeding, vaginal discharge, or leakage of fluid. When pregnancy continues with the LRIS in place, long-term effects on the offspring are unknown. Congenital anomalies have occurred infrequently when the LRIS has been in place during pregnancy.

Irregular bleeding and amenorrhea: LRIS can alter the bleeding pattern. During the first 3 to 6 months of LRIS use, the number of bleeding and spotting days may be increased and bleeding patterns may be irregular. Thereafter, the number of bleeding and spotting days usually decreases, but bleeding patterns may remain irregular. If bleeding irregularities develop during prolonged treatment, appropriate diagnostic measures should be taken to rule out other causes.

Amenorrhea (absence of menstrual flow) develops in approximately 20% of LRIS users by 1 year. The possibility of pregnancy should be considered if menstruation does not occur within 6 weeks of the onset of previous menstruation. Once pregnancy has been excluded, repeated pregnancy tests are not necessary in amenorrheic subjects unless indicated by other signs of pregnancy or by pelvic pain.

Pelvic inflammatory disease (PID): Use of IUDs had been associated with an increased risk of PID. All women who choose the LRIS must be informed prior to insertion about the possibility of PID and that PID can cause tubal damage leading to ectopic pregnancy or infertility, or in infrequent cases can necessitate hysterectomy, or can cause death. Women who have ever had PID are at an increased risk for a recurrence or reinfection. Symptoms of PID include the development of menstrual disorders (eg, prolonged or heavy bleeding), unusual vaginal discharge, stomach or pelvic pain or tenderness, pain during sexual intercourse, chills, and fever. The highest risk of PID occurs shortly after insertion (usually within the first 20 days thereafter). A decision to use the LRIS must include consideration of the risks of PID.

Pregnancy: Do not use during pregnancy. The risk of use in a pregnant woman outweighs any possible benefit.

Breastfeeding: Levonorgestrel appears in the breast milk of women using LRIS. There is an increased risk of intrauterine perforation in women who are lactating. Consult your doctor before you begin breastfeeding.

Children: Safety and effectiveness have been established in women of reproductive age. Use of LRIS before the onset of menstruation is not indicated.

Lab tests and exams will be required before and during therapy. Tests include a pelvic examination, Pap smear, tests for genital disease (eg, gonorrhea, chlamydia), and a pregnancy test.

Drug Interactions:

Tell your doctor or pharmacist if you are taking or planning to take any over-the-counter or prescription medications or dietary supplements with LRIS. Doses of one or both drugs may need to be modified or a different drug may need to be prescribed. To date, there have been no drug interactions reported.

Side Effects:

Every drug is capable of producing side effects. Many LRIS users experience no, or minor, side effects. The frequency and severity of side effects depend on many factors including dose, duration of therapy, and individual susceptibility. Possible side effects include:

Circulatory System: Fainting or abnormal heartbeat during insertion or removal; high blood pressure.

Nervous System: Headache; depression; nervousness; migraine.

Skin: Acne; skin disorder; hair loss; eczema.

Digestive Tract: Stomach pain; nausea; vomiting.

Urinary and Reproductive Tract: Enlarged follicles; ectopic pregnancy; septic abortion; PID; irregular or prolonged bleeding; spotting; cramping; absence of menstruation; perforation; partial penetration or embedment; ovarian cysts; vaginal discharge; vaginal inflammation; painful menstruation; abnormal Pap smear; cervical inflammation.

Other: Upper respiratory tract infection; sinus inflammation; sepsis; back or breast pain; weight gain; decreased sex drive; failed insertion; anemia; pain during sexual intercourse.

Guidelines for Use:

- Read the patient package insert provided before insertion of the LRIS.
- A complete medical history and examination will be required before LRIS insertion. A follow-up examination is required within 3 months of insertion.
- LRIS must be replaced every 5 years because contraceptive effectiveness after 5 years has not been established.
- Some vaginal bleeding, such as irregular or prolonged bleeding or spotting, or cramps may occur during the first few weeks after insertion. Notify your doctor if your symptoms continue or are severe.
- Notify your doctor immediately if you experience abnormal vaginal bleeding or pain, odorous vaginal discharge, fever, genital lesions or sores, migraine with or without vision loss, exceptionally severe headaches, yellowing of the skin or eyes, or increased blood pressure.
- Notify your doctor immediately if you suspect you may be pregnant.
- Women who currently have or have had breast cancer should not use hormonal contraception because breast cancer is a hormone-sensitive tumor.
- Patients with diabetes should closely monitor their blood glucose. Levonorgestrel may affect glucose tolerance.
- To check the location of the LRIS, reach to the top of the vagina with a clean finger after each menstrual period and feel the threads. Do not pull on the threads. If you feel more of the LRIS than just the threads or if you cannot feel the threads at all, the LRIS may not be in the right place, Contact your doctor immediately.
- Contraceptive effectiveness of the LRIS is lost if the system is displaced or expelled.
- Tampons can be used safely while the LRIS is in place.
- LRIS does not protect against HIV (the virus that causes AIDS) or any other sexually transmitted diseases.
- About 8 out of 10 women who wish to become pregnant conceive within 12 months after removal of the LRIS.
- Lab tests and exams will be required before and during therapy. Be sure to keep appointments.

If you have any questions, consult your doctor, pharmacist, or health care provider.

Generic Name *Brand Name Example*	Supplied As	Generic Available
Rx **Norelgestromin/Ethinyl Estradiol**		
Ortho Evra	**Transdermal patch**: 20 cm^2, 6 mg norelgestromin, 0.75 mg ethinyl estradiol	No

Type of Drug:

Combination contraceptive drug.

How the Drug Works:

Norelgestromin is the active form of the progestin norgestimate found in some oral contraceptives. Ethinyl estradiol is an estrogen. Together, norelgestromin and ethinyl estradiol inhibit ovulation, change cervical mucus, and alter the endothelium (uterine lining).

Uses:

To prevent pregnancy.

Precautions:

Do not use in the following situations:

abnormal genital bleeding
allergy to norelgestromin/ethinyl estradiol or any of its ingredients
artery disease
breast cancer
cerebrovascular disease (stroke)
chest pain
diabetes with kidney, eye, nerve, or blood vessel complications
emergency contraception use
estrogen-dependent neoplasia
headaches with neurological symptoms
heart disease
high blood pressure, severe
jaundice
liver disease
pregnancy
prolonged bed rest following major surgery
thromboembolic disorders
thrombophlebitis (blood clots in legs, lungs, or eyes)

Use with caution in the following situations:

cigarette smoking
conditions made worse by edema
depression
lipid disorders

Combination hormonal contraceptive risks: Women who use combination hormonal contraceptives have an increased risk of several serious conditions including myocardial infarction, thromboembolism, stroke, liver tumors, cancer, and gallbladder disease.

Pregnancy: Do not use during pregnancy. The risk of use in a pregnant woman clearly outweighs any possible benefit.

Breastfeeding: Norelgestromin/ethinyl estradiol appears in breast milk. Do not breastfeed while taking this medicine.

Children: Safety and effectiveness in children younger than 16 years of age have not been established.

Drug Interactions:

Tell your doctor or pharmacist if you are taking or if you are planning to take any over-the-counter or prescription medications or dietary supplements while using norelgestromin/ethinyl estradiol. Doses of one or both drugs may need to be modified or a different drug may need to be prescribed. The following drugs and drug classes interact with norelgestromin/ethinyl estradiol:

acetaminophen (eg, *Tylenol*)
antibiotics (eg, ampicillin)
anticonvulsants (eg, phenytoin)
antifungals (eg, griseofulvin)
atorvastatin (eg, *Lipitor*)
barbiturates (eg, phenobarbital)
carbamazepine (eg, *Tegretol*)
clofibric acid
cyclosporine (eg, *Sandimmune*)
felbamate (eg, *Felbatol*)
morphine
oxcarbazepine (eg, *Trileptal*)
phenylbutazone
prednisolone (eg, *Prelone*)
protease inhibitors
rifampin (eg, *Rifadin*)
salicylic acid
St. John's wort
theophylline (eg, *Theochron*)
topiramate (eg, *Topamax*)

Side Effects:

Every drug is capable of producing side effects. Many norelgestromin/ethinyl estradiol users experience no, or minor, side effects. The frequency and severity of side effects depend on many factors including dose, duration of therapy, and individual susceptibility. Possible side effects include:

Digestive Tract: Nausea; vomiting; cramps; bloating.

Circulatory System: Thrombophlebitis (leg clots); venous thrombosis; arterial thromboembolism; myocardial infarction (heart attack); increased blood pressure.

Nervous System: Stroke; brain clots; depression.

Other: Gallbladder disease; pulmonary embolism (lung clots); liver tumors; retinal thrombosis; mesenteric thrombosis; breakthrough bleeding; spotting; change in menstrual flow; temporary infertility after discontinuation of treatment; swelling of legs; patchy pigmentation of skin; breast tenderness or enlargement; nipple discharge; increased or decreased weight; jaundice; migraine; rash; decreased carbohydrate tolerance; vaginal fungal infections; intolerance to contact lenses; application site reaction; upper respiratory infection; menstrual cramps; emotional lability.

Guidelines for Use:

- Use exactly as prescribed.
- This medicine does not protect against HIV or any other sexually transmitted disease.
- A woman is not protected from pregnancy if she has more than 7 patch-free days. Use backup contraception (eg, condoms, spermicides, diaphragm) for the first week of the new cycle.
- Contact lens wearers may develop visual changes or changes in lens tolerance. See your doctor.
- The system uses a 28-day cycle. Apply a new patch each week for 3 weeks (21 total days). Week 4 is patch-free.
- Every patch should be applied on the same day of the week.
- Apply the patch to clean, dry, healthy skin on buttock, abdomen, upper outer arm, or upper torso.
- If a patch is partially or completely detached for 24 hours or more, or if the woman doesn't know how long the patch was detached, she may not be protected from pregnancy. Remove the old patch and start a new cycle by applying a new patch. Use backup contraception (eg, condoms, spermicides, diaphragm) for the first week of the new cycle.
- Do not apply makeup, creams, lotions, or powders to the skin where the patch is or will be placed.
- Lab tests may be required. Be sure to keep appointments.
- Store at room temperature.

If you have any questions, consult your doctor, pharmacist, or health care provider.

	Generic Name *Brand Name Example*	Supplied As	Generic Available
Rx	**Choriogonadotropin Alfa**		
	Ovidrel	**Powder for injection:** 250 mcg	No

Type of Drug:

Fertility drug.

How the Drug Works:

Choriogonadotropin alfa contains some of the same proteins that are in the naturally occurring hormones human chorionic gonadotropin (hCG), follicle stimulating hormone (FSH), and leutinizing hormone (LH).

Uses:

For use in women in assisted reproductive technology (ART) programs. Choriogonadotropin alfa is given when monitoring indicates that the follicles have developed adequately. Choriogonadotropin alfa induces ovulation.

To bring about ovulation and pregnancy in infertile patients with irregular cycles.

Precautions:

Do not use in the following situations:

- abnormal uterine bleeding of undetermined origin
- adrenal dysfunction, uncontrolled
- allergy to this medicine or any of its ingredients
- allergy to hCG preparations
- kidney disease
- liver disease
- ovarian cyst
- ovarian enlargement
- pituitary tumor
- pregnancy
- primary ovarian failure
- thyroid disfunction, uncontrolled
- tumors (sex hormone dependent tumors of reproductive tract and accessory organs)

Ovarian enlargement/hyperstimulation: Choriogonadotropin alfa may cause ovarian enlargement or ovarian hyperstimulation syndrome (OHSS). OHSS can develop rapidly (within 24 hours to several days) and can become a serious medical event. Contact your doctor immediately if you experience severe pelvic pain, nausea, vomiting, and weight gain.

Multiple births: Choriogonadotropin alfa treatment has been associated with multiple births. Consult your doctor.

Pregnancy: Do not use during pregnancy. The risk of use in a pregnant woman clearly outweighs any possible benefit.

Breastfeeding: It is not known if choriogonadotropin alfa appears in breast milk. Do not breastfeed while taking this medicine.

Children: Safety and effectiveness in children have not been established.

Lab tests will be required to monitor therapy.

Drug Interactions:

Tell your doctor or pharmacist if you are taking or planning to take any over-the-counter or prescription medications or dietary supplements while taking choriogonadotropin alfa. Doses of one or both drugs may need to be modified or a different drug may need to be prescribed.

Side Effects:

Every drug is capable of producing side effects. Many choriogonadotropin alfa users experience no, or minor, side effects. The frequency and severity of side effects depend on many factors including dose, duration of therapy, and individual susceptibility. Possible side effects include:

Digestive Tract: Stomach pain; nausea; vomiting.

Other: Injection site pain; bruising; post-operative pain.

Guidelines for Use:

- This medicine is injected subcutaneously (SC; under the skin). Use exactly as prescribed.
- Follow the injecting procedure taught to you by your health care provider.
- Visually inspect the solution. Do not use if discolored or contains particles.
- Overstimulation of the ovary may occur (ovarian hyperstimulation syndrome; OHSS). Contact your doctor immediately if you experience severe pelvic pain, nausea, vomiting, or weight gain.
- Use immediately after reconstitution. Discard unused solution.
- Lab tests will be required to monitor therapy. Be sure to keep appointments.
- Store vials at controlled room temperature (68° to 77°F) or refrigerate (36° to 46°F). Protect from light.

If you have any questions, consult your doctor, pharmacist, or health care provider.

FERTILITY AGENTS — CHORIONIC GONADOTROPIN

	Generic Name *Brand Name Examples*	Supplied As	Generic Available
Rx	**Chorionic Gonadotropin**		
	Pregnyl[1]	**Powder for injection:** 10,000 units/vial	Yes
	Profasi[1]	**Powder for injection:** 2000 units/vial; 5000 units/vial; 10,000 units/vial	No

[1] Contains benzyl alcohol.

Type of Drug:

HCG (human chorionic gonadotropin); hormone that stimulates the ovaries and testes.

How the Drug Works:

This hormone is produced by the human placenta. Its action is identical to the luteinizing hormone (LH) secreted from the pituitary gland. It also has a small degree of follicle stimulating hormone (FSH) activity. HCG has different uses in men and women. In men, HCG stimulates sex glands, specifically the cells in the testicles, to stimulate their growth and development and produce androgens (eg, testosterone). HCG also causes the development of secondary sex characteristics and may cause the testicles to drop. In women, HCG stimulates the ovaries to produce progesterone.

Uses:

Men: To stimulate testicular descent in prepubescent males whose testicles have not dropped or descended. Usually given to males between 4 and 9 years of age.

For selected cases of hypogonadism caused by pituitary deficiency.

To assist in the development of secondary sex characteristics in cases of hormone deficiency.

Women: To promote ovulation. HCG is used in combination with other medications.

Precautions:

Do not use in the following situations:

- allergy to chorionic gonadotropin or any of its ingredients
- early puberty
- pregnancy
- prostate cancer
- some types of cancers (eg, androgen dependent)

Use with caution in the following situations:

- asthma
- epilepsy
- heart disease
- kidney disease
- migraine

Early puberty: In young males using HCG to cause the testes to drop, early puberty can occur. Discontinue use if signs of early puberty (eg, enlargement of penis or testes, development of pubic hair, aggressive behavior) occur.

Multiple births: Pregnancies following therapy with HCG and menotropins resulted in 80% single births and 15% twin births; 5% of pregnancies resulted in 3 or more fetuses.

Fluid retention: Since androgens may cause fluid retention, use HCG with caution in patients with epilepsy, migraine, asthma, heart, or kidney disease.

Pregnancy: Do not use during pregnancy. The risk of use in a pregnant women clearly outweighs any possible benefit.

Breastfeeding: It is not known if chorionic gonadotropin appears in breast milk. Consult your doctor before you begin breastfeeding.

Children: Safety and effectiveness in children younger than 4 years of age have not been established.

Lab tests may be required to monitor treatment.

Drug Interactions:

Tell your doctor or pharmacist if you are taking or planning to take any over-the-counter or prescription medications or dietary supplements with chorionic gonadotropin. Doses of one or both drugs may be modified or a different drug may need to be prescribed.

Side Effects:

Every drug is capable of producing side effects. Many chorionic gonadotropin users experience no, or minor, side effects. The frequency and severity of side effects depend on many factors including dose, duration of therapy, and individual susceptibility. Possible side effects include:

Men only: Acne; enlargement or redness of penis or testes; early growth of pubic hair; rapid increase in height; breast tenderness or swelling.

Women only: Stomach pain; pelvic pain; multiple births.

Nervous System: Headache; irritability; restlessness; depression; fatigue; aggressive behavior.

Other: Fluid retention (edema); pain at injection site; redness; rash; hives; stroke; difficulty breathing; shortness of breath.

Guidelines for Use:

- Dosage is individualized. Take exactly as prescribed.
- Do not change the dose or stop taking, unless directed by your doctor.
- HCG has not been demonstrated to be effective in the treatment of obesity. HCG has no known effect on fat mobilization, appetite, sense of hunger, or body fat distribution.
- Inject intramusculraly (IM; into a muscle) only.
- If a dose is missed, inject it as soon as possible. If several hours have passed or it is nearing time for the next dose, do not double the dose to catch up, unless advised to do so by your doctor. If more than one dose is missed or it is necessary to establish a new dosage schedule, contact your doctor or pharmacist.
- Visually inspect solution for particles or discoloration before use.
- Lab tests may be required to monitor therapy. Be sure to keep appointments.
- Store dry powder at room temperature (59° to 86°F). After reconstitution (mixing), refrigerate at 36° to 46°F and use within 60 days.
- *Women —*
  HCG must be given following menotropins when tests indicate mature follicles are present (changes in vaginal smear or in cervical mucus, urinary estrogen test).
  Ovulation is confirmed by testing for progesterone production (rise in basal temperature, change in cervical mucus, etc).
  The couple should have intercourse daily, beginning on the day prior to HCG administration, until ovulation occurs. Take care to ensure insemination.
  During treatment with menotropins and HCG and for 2 weeks after treatment, patients must be examined by a doctor at least every other day.
  Monitor for signs of pregnancy. If pregnancy is suspected, contact your doctor.
  Multiple pregnancy is possible and poses potential hazards.
- *Men —*
  HCG is first used alone. Then menotropins and HCG are used together to stimulate sperm production.

If you have any questions, consult your doctor, pharmacist, or health care provider.

	Generic Name *Brand Name Examples*	Supplied As	Generic Available
Rx	**Urofollitropin**		
	Metrodin	**Injection:** 75 IU FSH activity/ amp, 150 IU FSH activity/ amp	No

Type of Drug:

Gonadotropin; hormone which stimulates the ovaries.

How the Drug Works:

Stimulates eggs in the ovaries to fully develop before ovulation.

Uses:

To induce ovulation in infertile women with polycystic ovarian syndrome (PCO) and who have not responded to clomiphene citrate (eg, *Clomid*, *Serophene*). Urofollitropin is used in combination with HCG.

Urofollitropin and HCG may be used to stimulate the development of multiple eggs in patients participating in an in vitro fertilization program.

Precautions:

Do not use in the following situations:

- adrenal disorders, uncontrolled
- allergy to this drug
- bleeding, abnormal
- infertility (other than not ovulating)
- intracranial lesion (eg, pituitary tumor)
- ovarian cysts or enlargement
- ovary failure, primary
- pregnancy
- thyroid disorder, uncontrolled

Multiple births: Pregnancies following therapy with HCG and urofollitropin resulted in 83% single births; 17% of pregnancies produced two or more fetuses.

Before therapy: Women must have a thorough pelvic exam and testing of the endocrine glands. A cervical dilation and curettage (D and C) must be done before beginning therapy if there is abnormal uterine bleeding or other signs of endometriosis. The partner's fertility potential must also be evaluated by a doctor.

Ovarian enlargement: Mild to moderate uncomplicated ovarian enlargement, which may be accompanied by abdominal bloating or pain, occurs in approximately 20% of patients treated with urofollitropin and HCG. It usually regresses without treatment within 2 or 3 weeks. If significant ovarian enlargement occurs after ovulation, do not engage in sexual intercourse.

Pregnancy: Do not use during pregnancy. The risk of use in a pregnant women clearly outweighs any possible benefit.

Breastfeeding: It is not known if urofollitropin appears in breast milk. Consult your doctor before you begin breastfeeding.

Lab tests may be required to monitor therapy. Be sure to keep appointments.

Side Effects:

Every drug is capable of producing side effects. Many patients experience no, or minor, side effects. The frequency and severity of side effects depend on many factors including dose, duration of therapy and individual susceptibility. Possible side effects include:

Digestive Tract: Nausea; vomiting; diarrhea; stomach cramps; weight gain.

Urinary and Reproductive Tract: Bloating; severe pelvic pain.

Skin: Rash, pain, swelling or irritation at injection site; dry skin; hair loss; hives.

Other: Chills; muscle and joint pain; headaches; fatigue; difficulty breathing; general body discomfort; decreased urination; breast tenderness; pain; stroke; blood clots (eg, swelling of the lower legs); multiple births.

Guidelines for Use:

- Use exactly as prescribed.
- Visually inspect solution for discoloration or particles. Use immediately after reconstitution (mixing). Discard any unused portion.
- Inject into muscle only.
- If a dose is missed, inject it as soon as possible. If several hours have passed or if it is nearing time for the next dose, do not double the dose in order to "catch up" (unless advised to do so by your doctor). If more than one dose is missed or it is necessary to establish a new dosage schedule, contact your doctor or pharmacist.
- Discontinue use and contact your doctor immediately if any of the following occur: severe pelvic pain, bloating, nausea, vomiting, diarrhea, weight gain, difficulty breathing or decreased urination.
- HCG must be given following urofollitropin when tests indicate mature follicles are present (changes in vaginal smear or in cervical mucus, urinary estrogen test).
- Ovulation is confirmed by testing for progesterone production (rise in basal temperature, change in cervical mucus, etc).
- The couple should have intercourse daily, beginning on the day prior to HCG administration, until ovulation occurs. Take care to ensure insemination. However, intercourse should be prohibited in patients in whom significant ovarian enlargement occurs after ovulation.
- During treatment with urofollitropin and HCG and for 2 weeks after treatment, patients must be examined by a doctor at least every other day.
- Monitor for signs of pregnancy. If pregnancy is suspected, contact your doctor.
- Multiple pregnancy is possible and poses potential hazards.
- Store refrigerated or at room temperature (37°-77° F). Protect from light.

If you have any questions, consult your doctor, pharmacist, or health care provider.

	Generic Name *Brand Name Example*	Supplied As	Generic Available
Rx	**Follitropin Alfa**		
	Gonal-F	**Powder for injection:** 37.5 IU,[1] 75 IU,[1] 150 IU[1]	No

[1] Contains 30 mg sucrose.

Type of Drug:

Gonadotropin; hormone that stimulates the ovaries; fertility drug.

How the Drug Works:

Follitropin alfa stimulates the ovaries to produce eggs.

Uses:

For the induction of ovulation and pregnancy in women whose ovaries still work but cannot form eggs (ovulate), and as a result, are not fertile (unable to become pregnant).

To stimulate the development of mutiple follicles in ovulatory patients undergoing Assisted Reproductive Therapy (ART) (eg, in vitro fertilization).

Precautions:

Do not use in the following situations:

- adrenal dysfunction, uncontrolled
- allergy to follitropin alfa or any of its ingredients
- follicle stimulating hormone, high levels of
- lesion, organic intracranial (eg, pituitary tumor)
- ovarian cyst or enlargement
- pregnancy
- thyroid disease, uncontrolled
- tumors, sex hormone dependent
- uterine bleeding, abnormal

Multiple births: Reports of multiple births have been associated with follitropin alfa treatment. Discuss this with your doctor before starting therapy.

Overstimulation of the ovary: Mild to moderate ovarian enlargement, with or without bloating or stomach pain, may occur and generally goes away within 2 or 3 weeks after discontinuing this medicine. All patients who experience bloating or stomach pain should be examined for ovarian enlargement. If significant ovarian enlargement occurs after ovulation, do not engage in sexual intercourse.

Respiratory complications: Serious respiratory conditions (eg, difficulty breathing, worsening of asthma) and blood clotting have been reported.

Pregnancy: Do not use during pregnancy. The risk of use in a pregnant woman clearly outweighs any possible benefit.

Breastfeeding: It is not known if follitropin alfa appears in breast milk. Consult your doctor before you begin breastfeeding.

Children: Safety and effectiveness in children have not been established.

Lab tests will be required during treatment. Tests may include blood hormone levels, ultrasound, and body temperature measurement.

Side Effects:

Every drug is capable of producing side effects. Many follitropin alfa users experience no, or minor, side effects. The frequency and severity of side effects depend on many factors including dose, duration of therapy, and individual susceptibility. Possible side effects include:

Digestive Tract: Stomach pain; nausea; gas; diarrhea; vomiting; indigestion; enlarged stomach; loss of appetite; thirst.

Nervous System: Headache; dizziness; drowsiness; anxiety; nervousness.

Respiratory System: Upper respiratory infection; congested or runny nose; sore throat; difficulty breathing; coughing; sinus headache; head congestion.

Urinary and Reproductive Tract: Bleeding between periods; ovarian cyst; breast pain; ovarian hyperstimulation; painful menstruation; ovarian disorder; cervix lesion; menstrual disorder; pelvic pain; unusual vaginal discharge; vaginal bleeding; urinary tract infection; genital fungal infection; genital itching.

Other: Back pain; muscle pain; flu-like symptoms; fever; acne; unstable emotions; injection site pain; weight gain; abnormal skin sensations; fatigue; low blood pressure.

Guidelines for Use:

- Dosage is individualized. Take exactly as prescribed.
- Carefully follow the preparation and administration techniques taught to you by your health care provider.
- Visually inspect the solution for discoloration or particles. Use immediately after reconstitution (mixing). Discard any unused portion.
- For subcutaneous (beneath the skin) injection only.
- Treatment with this drug requires close monitoring for overstimulation of the ovary. Contact your doctor immediately if you experience difficulty breathing, severe pelvic pain, nausea, vomiting, weight gain, stomach pain or bloating, diarrhea, or infrequent urination.
- The couple should have sexual intercourse daily, beginning on the day prior to human chorionic gonadotropin (HCG) administration, until ovulation occurs. Take care to ensure insemination. However, intercourse should be prohibited in patients in whom significant ovarian enlargement occurs after ovulation.
- Multiple pregnancy is possible and poses potential hazards.
- Other causes of infertility, as well as pregnancy, will be exluded before this medicine is used.
- Monitor signs of pregnancy. If pregnancy is suspected, contact your doctor.
- Lab tests will be required to monitor treatment. Be sure to keep appointments.
- Store in refrigerator or at room temperature (36° to 77°F). Protect from light.

If you have any questions, consult your doctor, pharmacist, or health care provider.

	Generic Name *Brand Name Example*	Supplied As	Generic Available
Rx	**Follitropin Beta**		
	Follistim[1]	**Powder for injection:** 75 IU	No

[1] Contains 25 mg sucrose.

Type of Drug:

Gonadotropin; hormone that stimulates the ovaries; fertility drug.

How the Drug Works:

Follitropin beta stimulates the ovaries to produce eggs.

Uses:

For the induction of ovulation and pregnancy in women whose ovaries still work but cannot form eggs (ovulate) and as a result, are not fertile (unable to become pregnant).

To stimulate the development of mutiple follicles in ovulatory patients undergoing Assisted Reproductive Therapy (ART) (eg, in vitro fertilization).

Precautions:

Do not use in the following situations:

adrenal dysfunction, uncontrolled
allergy to follitropin beta or any of its ingredients
follicle stimulating hormone, high levels
ovarian cyst or enlargement
pregnancy
thyroid disease, uncontrolled
tumors of the ovary, breast, uterus, hypothalamus, or pituitary gland
uterine bleeding, irregular or heavy of unknown cause

Multiple births: Reports of multiple births have been associated with follitropin beta treatment. Discuss this with your doctor before starting therapy.

Ovarian Hyperstimulation Syndrome (OHSS): Mild to moderate ovarian enlargement, with or without bloating or stomach pain, may occur and generally goes away within 2 or 3 weeks after discontinuing this medicine. All patients who experience bloating or stomach pain should be examined for ovarian enlargement. If significant ovarian enlargement occurs after ovulation, do not engage in sexual intercourse.

Respiratory complications: Serious respiratory conditions (eg, difficulty breathing, worsening of asthma) and blood clotting have been reported.

Pregnancy: Do not use during pregnancy. The risk of use in a pregnant woman clearly outweighs any possible benefit.

Breastfeeding: It is not known if follitropin beta appears in breast milk. Consult your doctor before you begin breastfeeding.

Children: Safety and effectiveness in children have not been established.

Lab tests will be required during treatment. Tests may include blood hormone levels, ultrasound, and body temperature measurement.

Side Effects:

Every drug is capable of producing side effects. Many follitropin beta users experience no, or minor, side effects. The frequency and severity of side effects depend on many factors including dose, duration of therapy, and individual susceptibility. Possible side effects include:

Digestive Tract: Stomach pain; bloating; nausea; vomiting; diarrhea.

Urinary and Reproductive Tract: Miscarriage; ovarian hyperstimulation; ectopic pregnancy; ovarian cyst; pelvic pain; breast tenderness; heavy or irregular vaginal bleeding; infrequent urination.

Skin: Dry skin; rash; hair loss; hives.

Other: Rapid heart beat; fast or difficult breathing; headache; dizziness; muscle or joint pain; aches; body discomfort; fever; chills; flu-like symptoms; injection site pain; weight gain.

Guidelines for Use:

- Dosage is individualized. Take exactly as prescribed.
- Visually inspect the solution for discoloration or particles. Use immediately after reconstitution (mixing). Discard any unused portion.
- Carefully follow the preparation and administration technique taught to you by your health care provider.
- For subcutaneous (beneath the skin) or intramuscular (into a muscle) injection only.
- Treatment with this drug requires close monitoring for overstimulation of the ovary. Contact your doctor immediately if you experience difficulty breathing, severe pelvic pain, nausea, vomiting, weight gain, stomach pain or bloating, diarrhea, or infrequent urination.
- The couple should have intercourse daily, beginning on the day prior to human chorionic gonadotropin (HCG) administration, until ovulation occurs. Take care to ensure insemination. However, intercourse should be prohibited in patients in whom significant ovarian enlargement occurs after ovulation.
- Multiple pregnancy is possible and poses potential hazards.
- Other causes of infertility will be excluded before this medicine is used.
- Monitor for signs of pregnancy before and during treatment. If pregnancy is suspected, contact your doctor.
- Lab tests will be required to monitor treatment. Be sure to keep appointments.
- Store in refrigerator or at room temperature (36° to 77°F). Protect from light.

If you have any questions, consult your doctor, pharmacist, or health care provider.

Generic Name *Brand Name Examples*	Supplied As	Generic Available
Rx **Clomiphene Citrate** *Clomid, Milophene, Serophene*	**Tablets:** 50 mg	Yes

Type of Drug:

Ovulation stimulant.

How the Drug Works:

Clomiphene produces a "false signal" that estrogen levels are low. The body responds by increasing the secretion of hormones (eg, gonadotropins) from the pituitary gland. These hormones stimulate the ovaries, causing the ovarian follicle to mature and results in ovulation (release of the egg). Clomiphene is not a steroid.

Effectiveness is documented but unpredictable. In 11 studies conducted between 1964 and 1978, pregnancy occurred in 30.6% of 5413 women with ovulation problems who received clomiphene.

Uses:

To treat female infertility when the patient desires pregnancy, the sexual partner is fertile and potent, and the patient has normal liver function and normal estrogen levels.

Ovulatory dysfunction (infertility) due to thyroid or adrenal conditions will not respond to clomiphene.

Unlabeled Use(s): Occasionally doctors may prescribe clomiphene citrate for male infertility.

Precautions:

Do not use in the following situations:

adrenal disorders, uncontrolled
intracranial lesion (eg, pituitary tumor)
liver disease, history
ovarian cyst or enlargement
pregnancy
thyroid disorders, uncontrolled
bleeding disorder, undiagnosed
uterine bleeding, abnormal

Multiple births: The risk of a multiple pregnancy is increased approximately 6 times when clomiphene is given. In 2369 pregnancies associated with clomiphene therapy, 92.1% were single and 6.9% were twins. The remainder resulted in triplets or more. Of the multiple pregnancies, 96% to 99% were live births.

Eyes: Blurring or other visual symptoms may occur. Use caution while driving or operating machinery, especially in variable light. If visual symptoms occur, discontinue treatment and call your doctor about a complete eye evaluation.

Before therapy: A complete pelvic examination is mandatory prior to treatment and repeated before each course. Clomiphene is not used in the presence of an ovarian cyst; further enlargement may occur. Other lab tests may also be required.

Overstimulation of the ovary: To reduce the risk of abnormal ovarian enlargement, use the lowest effective dose. Mild to moderate ovarian enlargement, with or without bloating or stomach pain, may occur and generally goes away within 2 or 3 weeks after discontinuing this medicine. All patients who experience bloating or stomach pain should be examined for ovarian enlargement. If significant ovarian enlargement occurs after ovulation, do not engage in sexual intercourse.

Pregnancy: Do not use during pregnancy. The risk of use in a pregnant woman clearly outweighs any possible benefit. Consult your doctor if pregnancy is suspected. Clomiphene may be linked to birth defects.

Side Effects:

Every drug is capable of producing side effects. Many patients experience no, or minor, side effects. The frequency and severity of side effects depend on many factors including dose, duration of therapy and individual susceptibility. Possible side effects include:

Eyes or Ocular: Blurred vision; blurred spots or flashes of light.

Digestive Tract: Nausea; vomiting; diarrhea; stomach or pelvic pain; bloating.

Nervous System: Headache; dizziness; lightheadedness; nervousness; vertigo (feeling of whirling motion).

Other: Multiple pregnancy; hot flushes; flushing; abnormal uterine bleeding; breast tenderness.

Guidelines for Use:

- Use exactly as prescribed.
- Each course of clomiphene should be started on or about the 5th day of the menstrual cycle. Wait 30 days between courses.
- If a dose is missed, take it as soon as possible. If several hours have passed or if it is nearing time for the next dose, do not double the dose in order to "catch up" (unless advised to do so by your doctor). If more than one dose is missed or it is necessary to establish a new dosage schedule, contact your doctor or pharmacist.
- Properly timed intercourse is important for good results.
- Intercourse should be prohibited in patients in whom significant ovarian enlargement occurs after ovulation.
- Notify your doctor immediately if bloating, stomach or pelvic pain, blurred vision, yellowing of skin or eyes, hot flushes, breast discomfort, headache, difficulty breathing, decreased urination, nausea or vomiting occurs.
- May cause dizziness, lightheadedness and visual disturbances. Use caution while driving or performing tasks requiring alertness, particularly in variable lighting.
- Multiple pregnancy is possible and poses potential hazards.
- The likelihood of conception diminishes with each succeeding course of therapy. If pregnancy has not been achieved after three courses of treatment, further treatment is not recommended. Long-term cyclic therapy is not recommended.
- Do not use this medicine if you are pregnant or think you might be pregnant. To avoid taking this medicine during early pregnancy, record your basal body temperature throughout all treatment menstrual cycles and see your doctor to determine whether ovulation occurs.
- Store at room temperature (59°-86°F) away from heat, light and moisture.

If you have any questions, consult your doctor, pharmacist, or health care provider.

Generic Name *Brand Name Example*	Supplied As	Generic Available
Rx **Menotropins**		
Humegon, Pergonal	**Injection:** 75 IU FSH activity and 75 IU LH activity/amp, 150 IU FSH activity and 150 IU LH activity/amp	No

Type of Drug:

Gonadotropins; hormones which stimulate the ovaries or testes.

How the Drug Works:

Menotropins are a combination of follicle stimulating hormone (FSH) and luteinizing hormone (LH). In women, menotropins help the ovaries produce mature eggs. Human chorionic gonadotropin (HCG) must follow menotropins to stimulate ovulation. Menotropins induce sperm formation (spermatogenesis) in men who have a low sperm count due to decreased function of the pituitary gland.

Uses:

To induce ovulation in women who do not ovulate, yet who also do not have primary ovarian failure. Menotropins are used in combination with HCG.

Menotropins and HCG may be used to stimulate the development and release of multiple eggs in patients participating in an in vitro fertilization program.

To stimulate spermatogenesis in men.

Precautions:

Do not use in the following situations:

Women—

adrenal disorders, uncontrolled
allergy to this medicine
bleeding, abnormal
infertility (other than not ovulating)
intracranial lesion (eg, pituitary tumor)
ovarian cysts
ovary failure, primary
pregnancy
thyroid disorders, uncontrolled

Men—

infertility (other than low sperm count)
pituitary function, normal
testes, primary failure

Multiple births: Pregnancies following therapy with HCG and menotropins resulted in 80% single births, 15% twin births and 5% of pregnancies resulted in three or more fetuses.

Before therapy: Women must have a thorough pelvic exam and testing of the endocrine glands. A cervical dilation and curettage (D and C) must be done before beginning therapy if there is abnormal uterine bleeding or other signs of endometriosis. The partner's fertility potential must also be evaluated by a doctor. Men should have their pituitary gland function evaluated.

Overstimulation of the ovary: To reduce the risk of abnormal ovary enlargement, use the lowest effective dose. Mild to moderate ovarian enlargement, with or without bloating or stomach pain, may occur and generally goes away within 2 or 3 weeks after discontinuing this medicine. All patients who experience bloating or stomach pain should be examined for ovarian enlargement. If significant ovarian enlargement occurs after ovulation, do not engage in sexual intercourse.

Pregnancy: Do not use during pregnancy. The risk of use in a pregnant woman clearly outweighs any possible benefit.

Breastfeeding: It is not known if menotropins appear in breast milk. Consult your doctor before you begin breastfeeding.

Lab tests may be required to monitor therapy. Be sure to keep appointments.

Side Effects:

Every drug is capable of producing side effects. Many patients experience no, or minor, side effects. The frequency and severity of side effects depend on many factors including dose, duration of therapy and individual susceptibility. Possible side effects include:

Digestive Tract: Nausea; vomiting; diarrhea; stomach cramps.

Other: Bloating; stomach pain; pelvic pain; ovarian cysts; ectopic pregnancy; fever; chills; breast enlargement or pain (men); rash; multiple births; muscle and joint pain; pain, rash, swelling or irritation at injection site; headache; dizziness; excitation; difficult or quick, shallow breathing; rapid heartbeat; general body discomfort; swelling of the lower legs.

Guidelines for Use:

- Use exactly as prescribed.
- Inject into muscle only
- Visually inspect the solution for discoloration or particles. Use immediately after reconstitution (mixing). Discard any unused portion.
- If a dose is missed, inject it as soon as possible. If several hours have passed or if it is nearing time for the next dose, do not double the dose in order to "catch up" (unless advised to do so by your doctor). If more than one dose is missed or it is necessary to establish a new dosage schedule, contact your doctor or pharmacist.
- Discontinue use and contact your doctor immediately if any of the following occur: severe pelvic pain, bloating, nausea, vomiting, diarrhea, weight gain, difficulty breathing or decreased urination.
- Store refrigerated or at room temperature (37°-77° F). Protect from light.
- *Women—*
  HCG must be given following menotropins when tests indicate mature eggs are present (changes in vaginal smear or cervical mucus, urinary estrogen test).
  Ovulation is confirmed by testing for progesterone production (rise in basal temperature, change in cervical mucus, etc).
  The couple should have intercourse daily, beginning on the day prior to HCG administration, until ovulation occurs. Take care to ensure insemination.
  Intercourse should be prohibited in patients in whom significant ovarian enlargement occurs after ovulation.
  During treatment with menotropins and HCG and for 2 weeks after treatment, patients must be examined by a doctor at least every other day.
  Multiple pregnancy is possible and poses potential hazards.
- *Men—*
  HCG is first used alone prior to treatment with both menotropins and HCG.

If you have any questions, consult your doctor, pharmacist, or health care provider.

	Generic Name *Brand Name Example*	Supplied As	Generic Available
Rx	**Danazol**		
	Danocrine	**Capsules:** 50 mg, 100 mg, 200 mg	Yes

Type of Drug:

Synthetic hormone; synthetic androgen.

How the Drug Works:

Danazol blocks the release of gonadotropin, a hormone secreted from the pituitary gland. The result of this blocking effect is to depress the output of two other hormones, FSH (follicle stimulating hormone) and LH (luteinizing hormone). FSH and LH are important in many functions of the sex glands, including ovulation.

Uses:

To treat endometriosis (an abnormal condition involving the inner lining of the uterus).

To treat fibrocystic breast disease (cysts or lumps in the breast).

To treat hereditary angioedema (swelling of the abdominal organs and tissue, extremities, face and airway).

Unlabeled Use(s): Occasionally doctors may prescribe danazol for early puberty, development of breasts (in males) and heavy menstrual flow. It has also been studied for the treatment of anemia.

Precautions:

Do not use in the following situations:

breastfeeding
genital bleeding, undiagnosed abnormal
heart disease, severe
kidney disorders, severe
liver disorders, severe
pregnancy
porphyria (anemia, certain types)

Use with caution in the following situations:

breast cancer
epilepsy
migraine

Fluid retention: Danazol can cause fluid retention which may aggravate epilepsy, migraine, heart or kidney disease. Use with caution.

Diabetes: Insulin requirements may increase. Abnormal glucose (sugar) tolerance tests may be seen. Monitor urine and blood sugar levels.

Women: Those taking danazol may experience masculinizing effects: Acne, edema (fluid retention), increased hair growth, decrease in breast size, deepening of the voice, oily skin or hair, weight gain and enlargement of the clitoris. These effects may not go away when the drug is stopped.

Men: In males (especially teenagers) receiving danazol, semen should be checked every 3 to 4 months.

Pregnancy: Do not use during pregnancy. The risk of use in a pregnant woman clearly outweighs any possible benefit. Masculinization of a female fetus may occur.

Breastfeeding: Do not use during breastfeeding.

Children: Safety and effectiveness in children have not been established.

Lab tests may be required to monitor treatment. Be sure to keep appointments.

Drug Interactions:

Tell your doctor or pharmacist if you are taking or if you are planning to take any over-the-counter or prescription medications or dietary supplements while taking this medicine. Doses of one or both drugs may need to be modified or a different drug may need to be prescribed.The following drugs and drug classes interact with this medicine.

insulin
carbamazepine (eg, *Tegretol*)
warfarin (eg, *Coumadin*)

Side Effects:

Every drug is capable of producing side effects. Many patients experience no, or minor, side effects. The frequency and severity of side effects depend on many factors including dose, duration of therapy and individual susceptibility.

If you experience any effects different from those listed, do not hesitate to contact your doctor or pharmacist. It could be a sign of a "rare" or unusual side effect that will need to be dealt with. Possible side effects include:

Masculinizing Effects – Acne; fluid retention (edema); decrease in breast size; deepening of the voice; mild abnormal growth of fine body hair; oily skin or hair; weight gain; menstrual changes/pain; hair loss; hoarseness; sore throat.

Signs of a Low Level of the Female Hormone Estrogen – Flushing; sweating; vaginitis (itching, dryness, burning and vaginal bleeding); nervousness; emotional instability; decrease in breast size.

Men – Reduction in sperm count; semen changes.

Guidelines for Use:

- Use exactly as prescribed.
- Notify your doctor if masculinizing effects occur (eg, abnormal growth of facial or fine body hair, deepening of the voice).
- Notify your doctor if headache, breast swelling, nausea, vomiting, visual disturbances or yellowing of the skin or eyes occurs.
- If a dose is missed, take it as soon as possible, If several hours have passed or if it is nearing time for the next dose, do not double the dose in order to "catch up" (unless advised to do so by your doctor). If more than one dose is missed or it is necessary to establish a new dosage schedule, contact your doctor or pharmacist.
- Lab tests may be required to monitor treatment. Be sure to keep appointments.
- Store in a tightly-closed container at room temperature.
- *Females—*
  Begin treatment during menstruation.
  Use nonhormonal contraceptive measures (eg, condom, diaphragm) during therapy. Discontinue use if pregnancy is suspected.
  It is essential that therapy for endometriosis continues uninterrupted for 3-6 months. May extend to 9 months.

If you have any questions, consult your doctor, pharmacist, or health care provider.

Generic Name *Brand Name Example*	Supplied As	Generic Available
Rx **Nafarelin Acetate**		
Synarel	**Nasal solution:** 2 mg/mL	No

Type of Drug:

Synthetic hormone.

How the Drug Works:

Nafarelin is similar to a gonadotropin releasing hormone. It stimulates the release of the pituitary hormones, luteinizing hormone and follicle stimulating hormone. These hormones stimulate the ovaries to produce estrogen and progestogen. Stimulation of the pituitary gland decreases over time.

Tissues and organs dependent on secretion of gonadal hormones (estrogen and progestogen) to function, including the uterine lining (endometrium), will become less active after about 4 weeks of twice daily therapy. This causes a decrease in the symptoms of endometriosis (eg, pelvic pain, menstrual cramps, painful intercourse).

Uses:

For the management of endometriosis in women 18 years and older for a period not to exceed 6 consecutive months of therapy. Also used for the treatment of central precocious puberty (CPP) in children of both sexes.

Precautions:

Do not use in the following situations:

allergy to the drug or to gonadotropin releasing hormone-type drugs
breastfeeding
pregnancy
vaginal bleeding, undiagnosed abnormal

Use with caution in the following situations:

alcohol/tobacco use, chronic
corticosteroid or anticonvulsant therapy, concurrent
menstruation
osteoporosis, family history
runny nose, chronic

Pregnancy: Do not use during pregnancy. The risk of use in a pregnant woman clearly outweighs any possible benefit.

Breastfeeding: It is not known if nafarelin acetate appears in breast milk. Use in nursing mothers is not recommended.

Drug Interactions:

Tell your doctor or pharmacist if you are taking or if you are planning to take any over-the-counter or prescription medications or dietary supplements while taking this medicine. Doses of one or both drugs may need to be modified or a different drug prescribed. Topical nasal decongestants (eg, *Afrin*) interact with this medicine.

Side Effects:

Every drug is capable of producing side effects. Many patients experience no, or minor, side effects. The frequency and severity of side effects depend on many factors including dose, duration of therapy and individual susceptibility. Possible side effects include:

Nervous System: Depression; headache; sleeplessness; emotional instability.

Respiratory System: Shortness of breath; chest pain.

Skin: Acne; body odor; excessive pubic or other hair growth; excessively oily skin; rash; hives; itching.

Other: Weight changes; edema (fluid retention); nasal irritation; hot flashes; vaginal dryness; change in breast size; change in breast size; change in sex drive; muscle pain; vaginal bleeding; lack of menstruation; possible elevation of serum triglycerides and cholesterol; white or brownish vaginal discharge; ovarian cysts; runny nose; abnormal lab tests.

Guidelines for Use:

- Use exactly as prescribed and follow patient information provided with the product.
- Avoid sneezing during or immediately following administration.
- Tilt head back slightly while administering this medicine.
- If using more than one spray in each nostril, wait 30 seconds between sprays.
- If the use of a topical nasal decongestant is necessary during treatment with nafarelin, do not use the decongestant until at least 2 hours after taking nafarelin.
- If a dose is missed, inhale it as soon as possible. If several hours have passed or if it is nearing time for the next dose, do not double the dose in order to "catch up" (unless advised to do so by your doctor). If more than one dose is missed or it is necessary to establish a new dosage schedule, contact your doctor or pharmacist.
- Store upright at room temperature. Protect from light.
- *For endometriosis* —
  Treatment should begin between the 2nd and 4th day of the menstrual period.
  Usual dose is one spray (about 200 mcg) into one nostril in the morning and one spray into the other nostril in the evening.
  When used regularly at the recommended dose, nafarelin usually inhibits ovulation and stops menstruation. However, use of the drug should not be considered a reliable form of contraception. Nonhormonal contraceptive measures (eg, condom, diaphragm) should be used during therapy.
  Do not use if pregnancy is suspected or if you are breastfeeding, experiencing undiagnosed vaginal bleeding or if you are allergic to any of the ingredients of this medicine.
  May cause breakthrough bleeding if doses are missed. However, if regular menstruation persists, notify your doctor.
  The usual course of therapy is 6 months. Retreatment is not currently recommended.
- *For central precocious puberty* —
  Usual dose is two sprays (about 400 mcg) into each nostril in the morning (four sprays total) and two sprays into each nostril in the evening (four sprays total).
  During the first month of treatment, some signs of puberty may occur. If this does not resolve within the first 2 months of treatment, contact your doctor.

If you have any questions, consult your doctor, pharmacist, or health care provider.

	Generic Name *Brand Name Examples*	Supplied As	Generic Available
Rx	**Desmopressin Acetate**		
	DDAVP	**Tablet:** 0.1 mg, 0.2 mg	No
	DDAVP, *Stimate*	**Nasal Solution:** 0.1 mg/mL, 1.5 mg/mL	No
	DDAVP	**Injection:** 4 mcg/mL	Yes

Type of Drug:

Human antidiuretic hormone (ADH).

How the Drug Works:

A hormone which makes the kidneys reabsorb (retain) water and increases the concentration/activity of certain blood factors necessary for normal blood clotting.

Uses:

DDAVP: As antidiuretic hormone replacement therapy in the management of central cranial diabetes insipidus and for temporary excessive urination and excessive thirst following head injury or surgery in the pituitary region. This will allow return to a more normal lifestyle with decreased urinary frequency and nighttime urination.

To treat nighttime bed-wetting (nasal solution only). May be used alone or in combination with behavioral conditioning or other nonmedicinal intervention.

To control bleeding in hemophilia A patients during and after surgery, and to stop spontaneous or trauma-induced bleeding in hemophilia A patients (injection only).

To control bleeding in patients with mild to moderate von Willebrand's disease (Type I) during and after surgery, and to stop spontaneous or trauma-induced bleeding in patients with von Willebrand's disease (injection only).

Stimate: To stop spontaneous or trauma-induced bleeding in patients with hemophilia A or mild to moderate von Willebrand's disease (Type I).

Unlabeled Use(s):

Nasal solution – To treat chronic autonomic failure (eg, nighttime bed-wetting, over-night weight loss and morning dizziness or lightheadedness when rising from a sitting or lying position).

Precautions:

Do not use in the following situations:

allergy to this medicine

Use with caution in the following situations:

blood clots
coronary artery insufficiency

fluid electrolyte imbalance (eg, cystic fibrosis)
hemophilia A, severe
high blood pressure
nasal blockage/obstruction (nasal solution only)
von Willebrand's disease (Type I), severe

Water intoxication: Very young and elderly patients should drink only enough fluids to satisfy thirst in order to decrease the potential occurrence of water intoxication (over-load) and salt depletion in the blood.

Long-term use: There have been reports of reduced responsiveness or duration of effect in patients using the drug for more than 6 months. Consult your doctor if such changes occur.

Pregnancy: Studies in pregnant women or in animals have been judged not to show a risk to the fetus. However, no drug should be used during pregnancy unless clearly needed.

Breastfeeding: It is not known if desmopressin acetate appears in breast milk. Consult your doctor before you begin breastfeeding.

Children: Infants and children need careful fluid intake restrictions to prevent possible salt depletion in the blood and water intoxication (overload). Nasal solution has been used safely and is modestly effective for short-term use (4 - 8 weeks) in children 6 years of age and older for the treatment of nighttime bed-wetting. Do not use injection in children under 3 months of age or the nasal solution in children under 11 months of age in the treatment of hemophilia A or von Willebrand's disease. Safety and effectiveness have not been established in children under 12 years of age (injection) or under 3 months of age (nasal solution) with diabetes insipidus. Desmopressin tablets have been used safely in children 4 years of age and older for periods of up to 44 months.

Lab tests may be necessary to monitor therapy. Be sure to keep appointments.

Drug Interactions:

Tell your doctor or pharmacist if you are taking or if you are planning to take any over-the-counter or prescription medications or dietary supplements while taking this medicine. Doses of one or both drugs may need to be modified or a different drug may need to be prescribed. The following drugs and drug classes interact with this medicine.

blood pressure elevating agents (eg, epinephrine)
carbamazepine (eg, *Tegretol*)
chlorpropamide (*Diabinese*)

Side Effects:

Every drug is capable of producing side effects. Many patients experience no, or minor, side effects. The frequency and severity of side effects depend on many factors including dose, duration of therapy and individual susceptibility. Possible side effects include:

DDAVP nasal solutions – Headache; runny nose; nausea; stomach cramps; vaginal pain; high blood pressure; facial flushing; nosebleed; sore throat; cough; difficulty breathing.

DDAVP injection – Redness, swelling or burning at injection site; headache; runny nose; nausea; stomach cramps; vaginal pain; high blood pressure; facial flushing.

Stimate nasal solution – Sleepiness; dizziness; itchy or light-sensitive eyes; sleeplessness; chills; warm feeling; pain; chest pain; palpitations (pounding in the chest); fast heartbeat; indigestion; fluid retention; vomiting; agitation; genital inflammation; difficulty breathing.

Guidelines for Use:

- Read and follow patient instructions carefully and use exactly as prescribed.
- If a dose is missed, take or use it as soon as possible. If several hours have passed or if it is nearing time for the next dose, do not double the dose in order to "catch up" (unless advised to do so by your doctor). If more than one dose is missed or it is necessary to establish a new dosage schedule, contact your doctor or pharmacist.
- If bleeding is not controlled or worsens, contact your doctor.
- Contact your doctor if headache, shortness of breath, heartburn, nausea, stomach cramps or vaginal pain occurs.
- *Nasal solutions* — For nasal use only. Use one spray per nostril. If used before surgery, administer 2 hours before the scheduled procedure.
- *Stimate* —
  Spray pump must be primed before the first use. To prime the pump, press down 4 times. The pump will stay primed for 1 week if refrigerated. Reprime the pump after 1 week if not used.
  Discard any solution remaining after 25 doses since the amount delivered thereafter may be less than the required dose. Do not transfer the remaining solution to another bottle.
- *Storage* —
  Refrigerate nasal solutions and injection at 36° to 46°F. When travelling, closed nasal solution containers may be kept at room temperature (72°F) for up to 3 weeks.
  Store tablets at room temperature (59° to 86°F) protected from heat and light.

If you have any questions, consult your doctor, pharmacist, or health care provider.

	Generic Name *Brand Name Examples*	Supplied As	Generic Available
Rx	**Somatrem**		
	Protropin	**Injection:** 5 mg (approx. 15 IU), 10 mg (approx. 30 IU)	No

Type of Drug:

Growth Hormone.

How the Drug Works:

Mimics actions of naturally occurring growth hormone; stimulates growth of bone, tissues, blood cells and internal organs.

Uses:

For the long-term treatment of children who have growth failure due to a lack of adequate endogenous growth hormone secretion.

Precautions:

Do not use in the following situations:
closed epiphyses (end of growth of arm and leg bones)
tumor growth
allergy to benzyl alcohol

Use with caution in the following situations:
glucose intolerance
brain lesion
endocrine problems (diabetes)
intracranial hypertension
scoliosis

Benzyl alcohol is used in the diluent of this product as a preservative and has been associated with toxicity in newborns. When administering somatrem to newborns, reconstitute with Sterile Water for Injection.

Pregnancy: Adequate studies have not been done in pregnant women; animal studies may have shown a risk to the fetus. Use only if clearly needed and if potential benefits outweigh the possible hazards to the fetus.

Breastfeeding: It is not known if somatrem appears in breast milk. Consult your doctor before you begin breastfeeding.

Lab tests and examinations will be required periodically to monitor treatment. Be sure to keep appointments. Tests may include eye examinations and thyroid function tests. In addition, testing for antibodies to human growth hormone may be performed in patients not responding to therapy.

Drug Interactions:

Tell your doctor or pharmacist if you are taking or planning to take any over-the-counter or prescription medications or dietary supplements while taking this medicine. Doses of one or both drugs may need to be modified or a different drug may need to be prescribed. The following drugs and drug classes interact with this medicine: Glucocorticoids (eg, prednisone).

Side Effects:

Every drug is capable of producing side effects. Many patients experience no, or minor, side effects. The frequency and severity of side effects depend on many factors including dose, duration of therapy and individual susceptibility. Possible side effects include: Injection site reactions; swelling; carpal tunnel syndrome.

Guidelines for Use:

- Take as directed by your doctor. The weekly dose varies depending on individual needs. Do not adjust the dose or stop taking the medication without consulting your pharmacist or doctor.
- Follow the preparation and injection procedure taught to you by your healthcare provider if you choose to administer the medicine at home. Rotate injection sites.
- Dispose of used equipment (eg, needles and syringes) in an appropriate container as instructed. Do not reuse needles or syringes.
- Patient instructions for use are enclosed with each package; follow instructions exactly.
- If local or systemic allergic reactions occur, contact your doctor.
- Report these symptoms to your physician: Limping; hip or knee pain; injection site reactions.
- Glucocorticoid therapy may inhibit the growth promoting effect of somatrem; if this therapy is required the doses must be carefully adjusted.
- Benzyl alcohol as a preservative in Bacteriostatic Water for Injection has been associated with toxicity in newborns. When administering somatrem to newborns, reconstitute with Sterile Water for Injection.
- Lab tests or exams will be required periodically to monitor treatment. These may include eye examinations and thyroid function tests. In addition, tests for antibodies to human growth hormone may be carried out in patients failing to respond to therapy.
- Store somatrem before and after reconstitution under refrigeration (36° to 46°F). Use reconstituted solution within 14 days. Avoid freezing. Do not use if cloudy.

If you have any questions, consult your doctor, pharmacist, or health care provider.

Generic Name *Brand Name Examples*	Supplied As	Generic Available
Rx **Somatropin**		
Genotropin[1]	**Powder for Injection, lyophilized:** 1.5 mg (≈ 4 IU/mL) 5.8 mg (≈ 15 IU/mL) 13.8 mg (≈ 36 IU/mL)	No
Norditropin	**Powder for Injection, lyophilized:** 4 mg (≈ 12 IU)/vial 8 mg (≈ 24 IU)/vial	No
Nutropin[2]	**Powder for Injection, lyophilized:** 5 mg (≈ 15 IU)/vial 10 mg (≈ 30 IU)/vial	No
Humatrope[3]	**Powder for Injection, lyophilized:** 5 mg (15 IU)/vial	No
Serostim	**Powder for Injection, lyophilized:** 5 mg (≈ 15 IU)/vial 6 mg (≈18 IU)/vial	No
Nutropin AQ	**Injection:** 10 mg (≈ 30 IU)/ vial	No

[1] Contains m-cresol in diluent.
[2] Contains benzyl alcohol in diluent.
[3] Contains m-cresol and glycerin in diluent.

Type of Drug:

Growth hormone.

How the Drug Works:

Mimics actions of naturally occuring growth hormone; stimulates growth of bone, tissues, blood cells and internal organs.

Uses:

Growth failure associated with chronic kidney insufficiency until time of transplantation (*Nutropin, Nutropin AQ*).

Growth failure (except *Serostim*).

Turner syndrome (*Nutropin* only).

AIDS wasting or cachexia (*Serostim* only).

Somatotropin deficiency syndrome (*Humatrope* only).

Unlabeled Use(s): Occasionally doctors may prescribe growth hormones for short children due to intrauterine growth retardation.

Precautions:

Do not use in the following situations:

- active tumor growth (discontinue therapy if this develops)
- allergy to benzyl alcohol (diluent supplied with *Nutropin*)
- allergy to growth hormone and constituents
- allergy to m-cresol or glycerin in certain formulations
- closed epiphyses (end of growth of arm and leg bones)

Use with caution in the following situations:

- acute pancreatitis
- brain injury or tumor
- carpal tunnel syndrome (*Serostim*)
- diabetes mellitus
- ear disorders (*Nutropin*)
- glucose intolerance (except *Norditropin*, *Humatrope*)
- hip problems, hip or knee pain
- HIV infection
- hypothyroidism
- intracranial hypertension
- kidney transplant or insufficiency
- scoliosis or other skeletal abnormalities
- skin lesions
- swelling of hands and feet (*Serostim*)

Pregnancy:

Serostim, Genotropin – Studies in pregnant women or in animals have been judged not to show a risk to the fetus. However, no drug should be used during pregnancy unless clearly needed.

Nutropin, Nutropin AQ, Humatrope, Norditropin – Adequate studies have not been done in pregnant women; animal studies may have shown a risk to the fetus. Use only if clearly needed and potential benefits outweigh the possible hazards to the fetus.

Breastfeeding: It is not known if somatropin appears in breast milk. Consult your doctor before you begin breastfeeding.

Children:

Serostim – Safety and effectiveness in children with AIDS have not been established.

Benzyl alcohol – Benzyl alcohol as a preservative in Bacteriostatic Water for Injection, USP has been associated with toxicity in newborns. When administering somatropin to newborns, reconstitute with Sterile Water for Injection.

Drug Interactions:

Tell your doctor or pharmacist if you are taking or planning to take any over-the-counter or prescription medications or dietary supplements while taking this medicine. Doses of one or both drugs may need to be modified or a different drug may need to be prescribed. The following drugs and drug classes interact with this medicine:

- Glucocorticoid therapy (except *Serostim*)
- Corticosteroids (eg, cortisone)
- Sex steroids
- Anticonvulsants (eg, phenytoin)
- Cyclosporine (eg, *Sandimmune*)

Side Effects:

Every drug is capable of producing side effects. Many patients experience no, or minor, side effects. The frequency and severity of side effects depend on many factors including dose, duration of therapy and individual susceptibility. Possible side effects include: High blood pressure; headache; high sugar in blood; antibody development; muscle pain; weakness; glucose in urine; swelling; swelling in arms and legs; breast growth; joint pain; nausea; stomach pain; vomiting; injection site reactions; leukemia.

Nutropin – Eye pain; visual changes; injection site pain; carpal tunnel syndrome; wrist pain.

Genotropin – Loss of skin fat; blood in urine.

Humatrope – Abnormal skin sensation; pain; runny nose; back pain; acne; joint disorder; flu syndrome; increased cough; decreased sensitivity to touch; respiratory disorder; sore throat.

Serostim – Musculoskeletal discomfort; fever; swelling of hands or feet; diarrhea; nerve disease; increased sweating; appetite loss; fast heartbeat; tiredness; abnormal blood counts; protein in urine; lymph node swelling; sleeplessness; carpal tunnel syndrome.

Guidelines for Use:

- Take as directed by your doctor. The daily dose varies depending on individual needs. Do not adjust the dose without consulting your pharmacist or doctor.
- Follow injection procedure taught to you by your healthcare provider. Follow instructions on patient information insert. Rotate injection sites.
- Report these symptoms to the doctor: Limping; hip or knee pain; headache; weakness; muscle pain; swelling; injection site reactions.
- If local or systemic allergic reactions occur, contact your doctor.
- Lab tests and examinations will include: Blood sugar; eye exams; thyroid function tests; antibody testing; nutritional tests (*Serostim* only). Keep appointments.
- Storage:
  Serostim: Store unopened vials at room temperature (59° to 86°F) and reconstituted solution under refrigeration for no longer than 24 hours.
  Genotropin, Humatrope, Nutropin: Store unopened vials/cartridges under refrigeration (36° to 46°F); store reconstituted solutions under refrigeration (36° to 46°F) for up to 14 days except 1.5 mg cartridge of *Genotropin* which must be used within 24 hours.
  Nutropin AQ: Store under refrigeration (36° to 46°F). Must be used within 28 days once opened.
  Avoid freezing.
- Do not use if cloudy.

If you have any questions, consult your doctor, pharmacist, or health care provider.

	Generic Name *Brand Name Examples*	Supplied As	Generic Available
Rx	**Repository Corticotropin (ACTH)**		Yes
	H.P. Acthar Gel	**Repository injection:** 80 units/mL	
Rx	**Cosyntropin**		No
	Cortrosyn	**Powder for injection, lyophilized:** 0.25 mg/vial	

Type of Drug:

Natural (corticotropin, ACTH) and synthetic (cosyntropin) adrenocorticotropic hormone.

How the Drug Works:

Corticotropin (ACTH) is secreted by the pituitary gland. It stimulates the adrenal cortex to produce and secrete adrenocortical hormones (corticosteroids, glucocorticoids). A functioning adrenal gland is necessary for corticotropin to work.

Uses:

Corticotropin and cosyntropin: Diagnostic testing of adrenal gland function.

Corticotropin: Although corticosteroid (eg, prednisone) therapy is the treatment of choice, ACTH may be used instead in the following disorders: Thyroid gland inflammation; high blood calcium levels due to cancer; acute worsening of multiple sclerosis; tuberculosis meningitis; trichinosis with brain or heart involvement; and treatment of glucocorticoid-responsive rheumatic, collagen, skin, allergic, kidney, eye, respiratory, blood, digestive tract disorders, and cancer.

Unlabeled Use(s): Occasionally ACTH is used to treat infantile spasms.

Precautions:

Do not use in the following situations:

Corticotropin –
- adrenocortical hyperfunction
- allergy to pork
- congestive heart failure (CHF)
- fungal infection, systemic
- herpes simplex infection in the eye
- high blood pressure (IV administration)
- live virus vaccine (eg, MMR), concurrent
- osteoporosis (brittle bones)
- primary adrenocortical insufficiency
- scleroderma (hardened or thickened skin)
- surgery, recent
- trauma
- ulcer, presence or history

Cosyntropin –
- allergy to cosyntropin

Use with caution in the following situations:

- abscess
- cirrhosis
- diabetes
- diverticulitis
- infection
- kidney disease
- liver disease
- myasthenia gravis
- psychological problems
- thyroid function, decreased
- tuberculosis, history

Diabetes: The requirement for insulin or oral sulfonylureas may be increased in diabetic patients receiving corticotropin.

Electrolytes: Corticotropin can increase blood pressure, potassium and calcium excretion, and cause salt and water retention. Dietary salt restriction and potassium supplements may be necessary.

Pregnancy: There are no adequate and well-controlled studies in pregnant women. Use only if clearly needed and potential benefits to the mother outweigh the possible hazards to the fetus.

Breastfeeding: It is not known if corticotropin or cosyntropin appears in breast milk. Consult your doctor before you begin breastfeeding.

Children: Prolonged use of corticotropin in children inhibits skeletal bone growth. If use is necessary, the drug should be given intermittently at the lowest effective dose and the child should be closely watched.

Drug Interactions:

Tell your doctor or pharmacist if you are taking or if you are planning to take any over-the-counter or prescription medications or dietary supplements with adrenal cortical steroids. Doses of one or both drugs may need to be modified or a different drug may need to be prescribed. The following drugs and drug classes interact with adrenal cortical steroids.

- amphotericin B (eg, *Fungizone*)
- antidiabetic agents (eg, insulin, glyburide)
- aspirin
- diuretics (eg, hydrochlorothiazide)

Side Effects:

Every drug is capable of producing side effects. Many corticotropin users experience no, or minor, side effects. The frequency and severity of side effects depend on many factors including dose, duration of therapy, and individual susceptibility. Possible side effects of corticotropin include:

Fluid and Electrolyte Disturbances: Sodium and fluid retention; potassium and calcium loss; hypokalemic alkalosis.

Digestive Tract: Nausea; vomiting; ulceration of esophagus; inflammation of the pancreas; peptic ulcer; stomach bloating.

Nervous System: Vertigo (feeling of whirling motion); headache; euphoria; sleeplessness; mood swings; depression; seizures; dizziness; psychic symptoms; increased intracranial pressure with papilledema.

Circulatory System: High blood pressure; congestive heart failure.

Skin: Impaired wound healing; increased sweating; excessive pigmentation of skin; thin, fragile skin; facial redness; acne; excessive body hair growth; rash; unusual bruising; suppression of skin test reactions; facial swelling; small red spots under the skin.

Other: Infection; menstrual irregularities; suppression of growth in children; cataracts; glaucoma; muscle weakness; loss of muscle mass; osteoporosis (brittle bones); abscess; increased intraocular pressure; shock; aseptic necrosis of femoral and humeral heads; vertebral compression fractures; pathologic fracture of long bones; secondary adrenocortical and pituitary unresponsiveness (particularly in times of stress, as in trauma, surgery, or illness); decreased carbohydrate tolerance; manifestations of latent diabetes mellitus; development of cushingoid state; increased requirements for insulin or blood-sugar-lowering agents in diabetic patients; protrusion of one or both eyeballs; negative nitrogen balance due to protein breakdown.

Guidelines for Use:

Corticotropin —

- Dosage will be individualized according to the condition being treated and the general medical condition of the patient. The usual dosage of repository corticotropin is 40 to 80 units given intramuscularly (IM) or subcutaneously (SC) every 24 to 72 hours. In the treatment of multiple sclerosis, daily IM doses of 80 to 120 units for 2 to 3 weeks may be administered.
- For IM or SC use only; intravenous (IV) administration is contraindicated.
- If self-administering, carefully follow the preparation, administration, and disposal techniques taught to you by your health care provider.
- Warm to room temperature before using.
- Treatment for acute gouty arthritis should be limited to a few days. Since rebound attacks may occur when corticotropin is discontinued, conventional concomitant antigout therapy should be administered during corticotropin treatment and for several days after it is stopped.
- Corticotropin may mask signs of infection. There may be decreased resistance and inability to localize infection when corticotropin is used.
- *Diabetics:* Insulin or oral blood-sugar-lowering agent requirements may increase.
- Notify your doctor if marked fluid retention, muscle weakness, abdominal pain, seizures, headache, dizziness, nausea, vomiting, shock, or skin reactions occur.
- Avoid immunization with live vaccines (eg, MMR) when receiving corticotropin.
- Sudden withdrawal after prolonged use may lead to recurrent disease symptoms which make it difficult to withdraw the medication. It may be necessary to slowly lower the dose and increase the injection interval to gradually discontinue the medication.
- Lab tests or exams may be required to monitor therapy. Be sure to keep appointments.
- Store in the refrigerator (36° to 46°F).

Cosyntropin —

- Cosyntropin will be administered by your health care provider. It is for IV or IM use only as a diagnostic agent.

If you have any questions, consult your doctor, pharmacist, or health care provider.

	Generic Name *Brand Name Examples*	Supplied As	Generic Available
Rx	**Betamethasone**		
	Celestone	**Tablets:** 0.6 mg	No
	Celestone[1]	**Syrup:** 0.6 mg/5 mL	No
Rx	**Betamethasone Sodium Phosphate**		
	Celestone Phosphate [2]	**Injection:** 4 mg/mL	No
Rx	**Betamethasone Sodium Phosphate and Betamethasone Acetate**		
	Celestone Soluspan	**Injection:** 3 mg betamethasone acetate and 3 mg betamethasone sodium phosphate/mL	No
Rx	**Cortisone Acetate**	**Tablets:** 5 mg, 10 mg, 25 mg	Yes
Rx	**Dexamethasone**		
	Decadron, Dexameth	**Tablets:** 0.25 mg, 0.5 mg, 0.75 mg, 1 mg, 1.5 mg, 2 mg, 2.5 mg, 4 mg, 6 mg	Yes
	Dexameth[1]	**Elixir**: 0.5 mg/5 mL	Yes
	Dexamethasone	**Oral solution:** 0.5 mg/5 mL	Yes
	Dexamethasone Intensol[1]	**Oral solution:** 1 mg/mL	Yes
Rx	**Dexamethasone Acetate**		
	Cortastat LA[2], *Dalalone D.P.*[2], *Dalalone L.A.*[2], *Decaject-L.A.*[2], *Solurex-LA*	**Injection:** 8 mg/mL, 16 mg/mL	Yes
Rx	**Dexamethasone Sodium Phosphate**		
	Cortastat [2], *Cortastat 10* [2], *Dalalone* [2], *Decadron Phosphate* [2], *Decaject* [2], *Solurex*	**Injection:** 4 mg/mL, 10 mg/mL, 20 mg/mL, 24 mg/mL	Yes
Rx	**Hydrocortisone (Cortisol)**		
	Cortef, Hydrocortone	**Tablets:** 5 mg, 10 mg, 20 mg	Yes
	Cortenema	**Retention enema**: 100 mg/60 mL	Yes
Rx	**Hydrocortisone Acetate**	**Injection:** 50 mg/mL	Yes
	Cortifoam	**Aerosol (intrarectal foam):** 90 mg/applicatorful	No

	Generic Name *Brand Name Examples*	Supplied As	Generic Available
Rx	**Hydrocortisone Cypionate**		
	Cortef	**Oral suspension**: 10 mg/5 mL	No
Rx	**Hydrocortisone Sodium Phosphate**		
	Hydrocortone Phosphate [2]	**Injection:** 50 mg/mL	No
Rx	**Hydrocortisone Sodium Succinate**		
	Solu-Cortef [3]	**Injection:** 100 mg/vial, 250 mg/vial, 500 mg/vial, 1000 mg/vial	No
Rx	**Methylprednisolone**		
	Medrol	**Tablets:** 2mg, 4mg, 8mg, 16 mg, 24 mg, 32 mg	Yes
Rx	**Methylprednisolone Acetate**		
	depMedalone 40, depMedalone 80, Depoject-40, Depoject-80, Depo-Medrol, Depopred, Methacort 40, Methacort 80	**Injection:** 20 mg/mL, 40 mg/mL, 80 mg/mL	Yes
Rx	**Methylprednisolone Sodium Succinate**		
	Solu-Medrol [3]	**Injection:** 40 mg/vial, 125 mg/vial, 500 mg/vial, 1000 mg/vial, 2000 mg/vial	No
Rx	**Prednisone**	**Oral solution:** 5 mg/5 mL	Yes
	Deltasone, Meticorten, Sterapred	**Tablets:** 1 mg, 2.5 mg, 5 mg, 10 mg, 20 mg, 50 mg	Yes
	Prednisone Intensol Concentrate[1]	**Oral solution:** 5 mg/mL	Yes
Rx	**Prednisolone**	**Tablets:** 5 mg	Yes
	Prelone[1]	**Syrup:** 5 mg/5 mL, 15 mg/5 mL	Yes
Rx	**Prednisolone Acetate**		
	Key-Pred, Predalone 50	**Injection:** 25 mg/mL, 40 mg/mL, 50 mg/mL, 100 mg/mL	Yes
Rx	**Prednisolone Sodium Phosphate**		
	Pediapred	**Oral solution:** 5 mg/5 mL	No

	Generic Name *Brand Name Examples*	Supplied As	Generic Available
Rx	**Triamcinolone**		
	Aristocort	**Tablets:** 1 mg, 2 mg, 4 mg, 8 mg	No
Rx	**Triamcinolone Acetonide**		
	Clinalog, Kenaject, Kenalog-10, Kenalog-40, Triam-A, Triamonide 40	**Injection:** 10 mg/mL, 40 mg/mL	Yes
Rx	**Triamcinolone Diacetate**		
	Aristocort Forte[3], *Aristocort Intralesional, Clinacort, Triamcin, Triam Forte, Tristoject*	**Injection:** 25 mg/mL, 40 mg/mL	Yes
Rx	**Triamcinolone Hexacetonide**		
	Aristospan Intralesional, Aristospan Intra-articular	**Injection:** 5 mg/mL, 20 mg/mL	No

[1] Contains alcohol.
[2] Contains sulfites.
[3] Contains benzyl alcohol.

Type of Drug:

Adrenal cortical steroids; glucocorticoids; anti-inflammatory steroids; corticosteroids.

How the Drug Works:

The naturally occurring adrenal cortical steroids have both anti-inflammatory (glucocorticoid) and salt-retaining (mineralocorticoid) activity. The synthetic adrenal cortical steroids have much greater anti-inflammatory (glucocorticoid) than salt-retaining activity. The glucocorticoids cause varied effects, including modifying the body's immune response.

The naturally occurring compounds, hydrocortisone and cortisone, are used as replacement therapy when the adrenal cortex is not functioning properly. The synthetic compounds can also be used as replacement therapy in adrenocortical deficiency states, but are more often used for their potent anti-inflammatory action.

Uses:

To treat primary or secondary adrenal cortex insufficiency (lack of function). Hydrocortisone or cortisone are the drugs of choice. Synthetic agents may be used in combination with mineralocorticoids.

To treat hypercalcemia (high calcium levels) associated with cancer.

To treat rheumatic disorders (eg, bursitis, tenosynovitis, gouty arthritis, rheumatoid arthritis, osteoarthritis). Use must be short term and supplemental with strict medical supervision for acute episodes or recurrences.

To treat selected connective tissue (collagen) disease (eg, systemic lupus erythematosus).

To treat certain skin diseases (eg, psoriasis, Stevens-Johnson syndrome, hives, dermatitis).

To treat certain allergic conditions not responding to standard treatment (eg, serum sickness, bronchial asthma, allergic rhinitis).

To treat certain eye conditions of an allergic or inflammatory nature (eg, allergic inflammation of the conjunctiva, optic nerve, or eyelids; corneal ulcers; herpes infection of the eye).

To treat certain respiratory disorders (eg, berylliosis, sarcoidosis).

To treat serious blood disorders (eg, various anemias, platelet disorders).

To treat certain cancers (eg, leukemias, lymphomas) (used in combination with other therapy).

To treat certain digestive tract diseases (eg, ulcerative colitis, regional enteritis).

To treat certain edematous states (eg, proteinuria in the nephrotic syndrome).

To treat tuberculosis meningitis when used concurrently with appropriate antituberculosis chemotherapy.

To treat trichinosis with brain or heart involvement.

To treat certain diseases of the nervous system (eg, to assist short term in treating a sudden worsening of multiple sclerosis).

To treat brain swelling associated with brain tumors, brain surgery, or heart injury. (dexamethasone only)

The injectable forms of the various glucocorticoids may be used to treat additional conditions.

Unlabeled Use(s): Occasionally doctors may prescribe glucocorticoids for some types of shock, vomiting, respiratory distress in premature infants, diagnosis of depression, acute mountain sickness, COPD, alcoholic hepatitis, spinal cord injury, and abnormal hair growth.

Precautions:

Do not use in the following situations:

allergy to the medicine or any of its ingredients
fungal infections, systemic
idiopathic thrombocytopenic purpura (intramuscular [IM] injections only)
ileocolostomy during immediate or early postoperative period (enemas only)
live virus vaccines (eg, smallpox)

Use with caution in the following situations:

amebiasis
congestive heart failure

diverticulitis
emotional instability
hepatitis B
herpes simplex in the eye
high blood pressure
infections, active (eg, acute glomerulonephritis, thrombophlebitis)
intestinal anastomosis, recent
kidney disease
liver disease
myasthenia gravis
myocardial infarction, recent
osteoporosis
peptic ulcer
psychotic tendencies
seizure disorders
stress, unusual
Strongyloides (threadworm) infestation, known or suspected
tuberculosis
ulcer, history of
ulcerative colitis, nonspecific
underactive thyroid

Diabetes: Glucocorticoids decrease carbohydrate tolerance. Diabetics may require increased doses of insulin or oral diabetes (hypoglycemic) medications to control blood sugar levels.

Infection: Glucocorticoids may mask signs of infection, and new infections may appear during use. Glucocorticoids may decrease resistance to an infection.

Prolonged use: Prolonged use may produce cataracts, glaucoma, and may enhance the establishment of secondary eye infections due to fungi or viruses.

Immunizations: Immunosuppressive (high) doses of glucocorticoids may reduce the effectiveness of inactivated bacterial and viral vaccines. Use of live virus vaccines is also contraindicated.

Osteoporosis: Corticosteroids increase the risk of osteoporosis. Adequate calcium and vitamin D intake may help reduce this problem.

Pregnancy: Adequate studies have not been done in pregnant women. Use only if clearly needed and potential benefits to the mother outweigh the possible hazards to the fetus.

Breastfeeding: Corticosteroids appear in breast milk. This could cause growth suppression in the infant. Mothers taking these drugs should not breastfeed.

Children: Growth and development of infants and children on prolonged therapy must be closely monitored by a doctor. Some of the injectable medications contain benzyl alcohol, which had been associated with the potentially fatal “gasping syndrome” in premature infants. Consult your doctor.

Elderly: Lower doses may be needed because of body changes caused by aging (such as loss of muscle mass).

Sulfites: Some of these products may contain sulfite preservatives that can cause allergic reactions in certain individuals. Check package label when available or consult your doctor or pharmacist.

Drug Interactions:

Tell your doctor or pharmacist if you are taking or if you are planning to take any over-the-counter or prescription medications or dietary supplements with glucocorticoids. Doses of one or both drugs may need to be modified or a different drug may need to be prescribed. The following drugs and drug classes interact with glucocorticoids.

anticholinesterases (eg, neostigmine)
barbiturates (eg, phenobarbital)
bile acid sequestrants (eg, cholestyramine, colestipol)
contraceptives, oral (eg, *Ortho-Novum*)
estrogens (eg, ethinyl estradiol)
hydantoins (eg, phenytoin)
interferon alfa (eg, *Intron A*)
ketoconazole (eg, *Nizoral*)
macrolide antibiotics (eg, erythromycin)
potassium-depleting diuretics (eg, furosemide)
rifamycins (eg, rifampin)
salicylates (eg, aspirin)
vaccines, live virus (eg, smallpox)

Side Effects:

Every drug is capable of producing side effects. Many glucocorticoid users experience no, or minor, side effects. The frequency and severity of side effects depend on many factors including dose, duration of therapy, and individual susceptibility. Possible side effects include:

Cushing's Syndrome (long-term use) – Appearance of "moonface"; enlargement of some fat pad areas; the appearance of obesity in the midsection; muscle wasting and weakness; abnormal fat deposits; general obesity; high blood pressure; diabetes; osteoporosis; thinning of skin; easy bruising.

Too Rapid Withdrawal of Therapy – Nausea; fatigue; loss of appetite; difficulty breathing; lowered blood pressure; joint and muscle aches; fever; dizziness; fainting; fever; general body discomfort; joint and muscle pain.

Injectables only – Skin pigment changes; abscess; joint damage; injection-site reaction; pain or tenderness at injection site; skin inflammation or hardening; delayed pain or soreness.

Digestive Tract: Nausea; vomiting; increased appetite; weight gain; heartburn; bloating; inflammation of the pancreas; peptic ulcer; stomach pain; rectal bleeding, local pain, or burning with enemas.

Nervous System: Convulsions; increased pressure in the brain; feeling of whirling motion; headache; behavior changes; sleeplessness; hiccups; mood swings; depression; psychotic manifestations; clumsiness; exaggerated sense of well being; seizures.

Circulatory System: Heart failure; high blood pressure; clot formation.

Skin: Impaired wound healing; thin skin and loss of fat under the skin; changes in pigmentation of skin; acne; excessive body hair growth; rash; hives; easy bruising; facial flushing; abnormal skin sensations; increased sweating.

Other: Salt and water retention; general body discomfort; potassium loss; abnormally low calcium; muscle weakness; loss of muscle mass; osteoporosis; bone fractures; menstrual irregularities; growth suppression in children; decreased carbohydrate tolerance; increased blood sugar levels; cataracts; glaucoma; aggravation or masking of an infection; rare instances of blindness; tendon rupture; suppressed reaction to skin tests;

Kaposi's sarcoma; hip or shoulder bone degradation; secondary adrenocortical and pituitary unresponsiveness; increased intraocular pressure; bulging eyes; muscle twitching; rapid eye movement.

Guidelines for Use:

- Dosage will be individualized based on the condition being treated and patient response.
- Injectable glucocorticoids are used when oral therapy is not feasible. They will be prepared and administered by your health care professional.
- Do not change the dose or stop taking unless advised to do so by your doctor.
- May cause stomach upset. Take oral dose forms with meals or snacks. Take single daily or alternate day doses in the morning prior to 9 a.m. Take multiple doses at evenly spaced intervals throughout the day or as advised by your doctor.
- *Alternate day therapy* — Used to retain beneficial drug effects while lowering the risk of side effects. Twice the usual daily dose may be given every other day in the morning before 9 a.m. The benefits of alternate day therapy are obtained when using intermediate-acting agents (eg, prednisone, prednisolone, triamcinolone, methylprednisolone). Alternate day therapy is common if steroid therapy is to be long term. Consult your doctor.
- *Intensol solution* — Mix with liquid or semi-solid food (eg, water, juice, soda-like beverage, applesauce). Use calibrated dropper to measure prescribed dose and then squeeze into liquid or food. Stir until mixed and consume entire amount. Do not store for future use.
- Patients on long-term steroid therapy should wear or carry identification noting that glucocorticoids are being taken.
- Notify your doctor if you experience unusual weight gain; swelling of the lower extremities; muscle weakness; black, tarry stools; vomiting of blood; puffing of the face; prolonged sore throat; fever; cold; or infection.
- *High dose or long-term therapy (longer than 1 month)* — Avoid sudden discontinuation of therapy. Follow a dosage tapering regimen prescribed by your doctor.
- Notify your doctor promptly if these symptoms occur following dosage reduction or withdrawal of therapy: Fatigue, appetite loss, nausea, vomiting, diarrhea, weight loss, weakness, dizziness, low blood sugar, fever, general body discomfort, and joint and muscle pain.
- If you are on immunosuppressant (high) doses of corticosteroids, avoid exposure to chickenpox or measles. If you are exposed, notify your doctor immediately.
- These drugs may cause an elevation in blood pressure and salt and water retention and increased potassium loss. Dietary salt restriction and potassium supplements may be necessary.

Guidelines for Use (cont.):

- Glucocorticoids cause calcium loss and can promote development of osteoporosis. Take adequate calcium and vitamin D supplements.
- Avoid any type of live virus vaccines, especially for smallpox, while taking this medicine.
- Lab tests and doctor visits will be required during therapy. Be sure to keep appointments.

If you have any questions, consult your doctor, pharmacist, or health care provider.

	Generic Name *Brand Name Examples*	Supplied As	Generic Available
Rx	**Alclometasone Dipropionate**		
	Aclovate	**Ointment:** 0.05%	No
	Aclovate	**Cream:** 0.05%	No
Rx	**Amcinonide**		
	Cyclocort	**Ointment:** 0.1%	No
	Cyclocort	**Cream:** 0.1%	No
	Cyclocort	**Lotion:** 0.1%	No
Rx	**Betamethasone Dipropionate**		
	Alphatrex, Diprolene, Diprosone, Maxivate	**Ointment:** 0.05%	Yes
	Alphatrex, Diprolene AF, Diprosone, Maxivate	**Cream:** 0.05%	Yes
	Alphatrex, Diprolene, Diprosone, Maxivate	**Lotion:** 0.05%	Yes
	Diprosone	**Aerosol/Spray:** 0.1%	No
	Diprolene	**Gel**: 0.05%	No
Rx	**Betamethasone Valerate**		Yes
	Beta-Val, Betatrex	**Ointment:** 0.1%	Yes
	Beta-Val, Betatrex	**Cream:** 0.01%, 0.1%	Yes
	Beta-Val, Betatrex	**Lotion:** 0.1%	Yes
Rx	**Clobetasol Propionate**		
	Temovate	**Ointment:** 0.05%	Yes
	Temovate, Temovate E	**Cream:** 0.05%	Yes
	Temovate	**Gel**: 0.05%	Yes
	Temovate	**Scalp application (solution)**: 0.05%	No
Rx	**Clocortolone Pivalate**		
	Cloderm	**Cream:** 0.1%	No
Rx	**Desonide**		
	DesOwen, Tridesilon	**Ointment:** 0.05%	Yes
	DesOwen	**Cream:** 0.05%	Yes
	DesOwen	**Lotion**: 0.05%	No

	Generic Name *Brand Name Examples*	Supplied As	Generic Available
Rx	**Desoximetasone**		
	Topicort	**Ointment:** 0.25%	Yes
	Topicort, *Topicort LP*	**Cream:** 0.05%, 0.25%	Yes
	Topicort	**Gel:** 0.05%	Yes
Rx	**Diflorasone Diacetate**		
	Florone, *Maxiflor*, *Psorcon*	**Ointment:** 0.05%	Yes
	Florone, *Florone E*, *Maxiflor*, *Psorcon E*	**Cream:** 0.05%	Yes
Rx	**Fluocinolone Acetonide**		
	Synalar	**Ointment:** 0.025%	Yes
	Synalar, *Synemol*	**Cream:** 0.025%	Yes
	Fluonid, *Synalar*	**Solution:** 0.01%	Yes
Rx	**Fluocinonide**		
	Lidex	**Ointment:** 0.05%	Yes
	Lidex, *Lidex-E*	**Cream:** 0.05%	Yes
	Lidex	**Solution:** 0.05%	Yes
	Lidex	**Gel:** 0.05%	Yes
Rx	**Flurandrenolide**		
	Cordran	**Ointment:** 0.025%, 0.05%	No
	Cordran SP	**Cream:** 0.025%, 0.05%	No
	Cordran	**Lotion:** 0.05%	Yes
	Cordran	**Tape:** 4 mcg/cm^2	No
Rx	**Fluticasone Propionate**		
	Cutivate	**Ointment:** 0.005%	No
	Cutivate	**Cream:** 0.05%	No
Rx	**Halcinonide**		
	Halog	**Ointment:** 0.1%	No
	Halog, *Halog-E*	**Cream:** 0.025%, 0.1%	No
	Halog	**Solution:** 0.1%	No
Rx	**Halobetasol Propionate**		
	Ultravate	**Ointment:** 0.05%	No
	Ultravate	**Cream:** 0.05%	No

	Generic Name *Brand Name Examples*	Supplied As	Generic Available
Rx/ otc[1]	**Hydrocortisone**		
otc	*Cortizone-5, Cortizone-10, Cortaid Maximum Strength,*	**Ointment:** 0.5%, 1%	Yes
otc	*Cortaid Intensive Therapy, Cortaid Maximum Strength, Cortaid Sensitive Skin with Aloe, Cortizone-5, Cortizone-10, Cortizone-10 External Anal Itch Relief, Cortizone-10 Plus, Cortizone for Kids, KeriCort-10, Preparation H Anti-Itch, Summer's Eve*	**Cream:** 0.5%, 1%	Yes
Rx	*Ala-Cort, Dermacort, Hytone, Penecort, Procto-Cream-HC 2.5%*	**Cream:** 1%, 2.5%	Yes
Rx	*Ala-Scalp, Cetacort, Dermacort, Hytone, Nutracort*	**Lotion:** 1%, 2%, 2.5%	Yes
Rx	*Penecort*	**Solution:** 1%	No
Rx	*Penecort*	**Gel:** 1%	No
otc	*CortaGel, CortiCool*	**Gel:** 1%	No
otc	*Cortizone-10 Quick Shot*	**Aerosol/Spray:** 1%	No
Rx/ otc[1]	**Hydrocortisone Acetate**		
otc	*LanaCort 5*	**Ointment:** 0.5%	No
otc	*Gynecort 5, LanaCort 5*	**Cream:** 0.5%	No
otc	*Caldecort, Gynecort 10, LanaCort 10, LanaCort Cool, Nupercainal*	**Cream**: 1%	No
otc	*Anusol HC-1, LanaCort 10*	**Ointment**: 1%	No
Rx	**Hydrocortisone Probutate**		
	Pandel	**Cream**: 0.1%	No
Rx	**Hydrocortisone Valerate**		
	Westcort	**Ointment:** 0.2%	Yes
	Westcort	**Cream:** 0.2%	Yes

	Generic Name *Brand Name Examples*	Supplied As	Generic Available
Rx	**Mometasone Furoate**		
	Elocon	**Ointment:** 0.1%	No
	Elocon	**Cream:** 0.1%	No
	Elocon	**Lotion:** 0.1%	No
Rx	**Triamcinolone Acetonide**		
	Aristocort A, Kenalog	**Ointment:** 0.025%, 0.1%, 0.5%	Yes
	Aristocort A, Kenalog, Triderm	**Cream:** 0.025%, 0.1%, 0.5%	Yes
	Kenalog	**Lotion:** 0.025%, 0.1%	Yes
	Kenalog	**Aerosol/Spray:** 2 seconds of spray delivers ≈ 0.2 mg	No

[1] Products are available *otc* or *Rx* depending on product labeling.

Type of Drug:

Topical anti-inflammatory, anti-itching agents; anti-inflammatory steroids.

How the Drug Works:

Topical adrenocortical steroids reduce skin inflammation (ie, redness, swelling), itching, and irritation. The exact manner in which the drug works is not fully understood. The effectiveness of the drug depends on many factors, including: The extent of absorption of the drug, the potency of the drug, the size of the area treated, and the doseform (eg, cream, ointment).

Uses:

To treat inflammation and itching caused by corticosteroid-responsive skin disorders.

OTC hydrocortisone: To treat minor skin irritation, itching, and rashes due to eczema; insect bites; poison ivy, oak, or sumac; allergic inflammation from soaps, detergents, cosmetics, or jewelry; itchy genital and anal areas; psoriasis; seborrheic dermatitis; or other minor skin irritations.

Precautions:

Do not use in the following situations:

- acne
- allergy to corticosteroids or any of their ingredients
- bacterial infections of the skin, single therapy for
- cellulitus
- facial, groin, or armpit areas (high potency agents only)
- prolonged use near eyes or eyelids
- rosacea

Use with caution in the following situations:

- blistered, raw, or oozing areas of skin
- diaper dermatosis
- skin infection

Absorption into the body: Absorption into the body of topical corticosteroids has produced manifestations of Cushing's syndrome, reversible hypothalamic-pituitary-adrenal (HPA) axis suppression, and increased blood and urine sugar. This is more likely to occur with application to large body surfaces, use of occlusive dressings, and with the more potent steroids. Patients at higher risk include young children.

Side effects may include growth retardation, delayed weight gain, low plasma cortisol levels and absence of response to ACTH stimulation, including bulging "soft spots," headaches, and bilateral papilledema.

Alcohol-containing preparations: Alcohol-containing preparations may cause drying, burning, or irritation of open lesions.

Formulations: Corticosteroids are specially formulated to maximize their release and potency. Mixing these products with other products is discouraged because it may affect potency and effectiveness.

Occlusive vehicles: A transparent plastic wrap or other vehicles that won't allow air to pass through to the treated area will enhance absorption at least 10 times. These kinds of dressings are not generally recommended (eg, when using clobetasol or halobetasol, when treating children).

Greasy ointment bases are more occlusive and are preferred for dry, scaly lesions. Gels are less occlusive. The aerosols, lotions and solutions are best suited for hairy areas.

Skin atrophy: Skin atrophy may occur in 3 to 4 weeks if the most potent corticosteroids are employed. Skin atrophy occurs most readily at sites where absorption through the skin is highest.

Pregnancy: There are no adequate and well-controlled studies in pregnant women. Use only if clearly needed and the potential benefits to the mother outweigh the possible hazards to the fetus. Do not use large doses or for prolonged periods of time if you are pregnant.

Breastfeeding: It is not known if topical corticosteroids appear in breast milk. Oral corticosteroids appear in breast milk. Consult your doctor before you begin breastfeeding.

Children: Limit therapy to the lowest possible dosage because children may be more susceptible to topical corticosteroid-induced side effects. Safety and effectiveness of alclometasone in children less than 1 year of age have not been established. Clobetasol is not recommended in children less than 12 years of age. Safety and effectiveness of hydrocortisone probutate in children less than 18 years of age have not been established.

Lab tests may be required to monitor therapy. Tests may include urinary-free cortisol, ACTH stimulation, and early morning plasma cortisol tests.

Side Effects:

Every drug is capable of producing side effects. Many topical corticosteroid users experience no, or minor, side effects. The frequency and severity of side effects depend on many factors including dose, duration of therapy, and individual susceptibility. Possible side effects include:

Skin: Burning; itching; irritation; redness; dryness; allergic inflammation; acne; decreased pigmentation in the area being treated; streaks in skin; skin atrophy; infection; stinging; cracking; rash; tingling; scalp pustules (scalp application only); unusual hair growth.

Other: Elevated blood or urine sugar; cataracts and glaucoma (prolonged use near eyes); numbness of fingers; worsening of condition being treated.

Also consider all side effects for oral corticosteroids. See the Glucocorticoids monograph in this chapter.

Guidelines for Use:

- Dosage is individualized.
- Application frequency and duration of therapy are dependent on the condition treated, its location, the potency of the drug, and the vehicle employed. For assistance in product-specific drug selection and dosage guidelines, consult your doctor or pharmacist.
- Wash hands before and after application.
- Wash or soak the affected area before application. This may increase drug penetration.
- Apply sparingly as a thin film. Rub in lightly until the medication disappears.
- For external use only. Avoid contact with the eyes.
- Avoid prolonged use, especially near the eyes, on the face, on genital and rectal areas, and in skin folds.
- The treated area should not be bandaged, covered, or wrapped to be occlusive, unless advised to do so by your doctor.
- Do not use tight-fitting diapers or plastic pants on children treated with topical corticosteroids in the diaper area. Such garments function as occlusive dressings.
- Skin infections may worsen. It may be necessary to stop the corticosteroid and treat the infection.
- Do not use these agents to treat acne, the lesions of rosacea, skin inflammation near the mouth, or for any disorder other than that for which it was prescribed.
- Allergic reactions may occur. Contact your doctor if the condition being treated worsens or irritation, burning, redness, swelling, or stinging persists. Do not reapply the drug.
- If you do not notice improvement within 2 weeks (or 1 week when using OTC hydrocortisone), consult your doctor.
- *Aerosol/Spray* — Take care to cover the eyes while spraying close to the face. Avoid inhalation. Spray the affected area for 3 seconds or less at a time and at a distance of at least 6 inches between the nozzle and skin
- *Scalp application* — Apply to the affected scalp areas twice daily, once in the morning and once at night.
  Do not use more than 50 mL/week.
  Treatment must be limited to 2 consecutive weeks.

Guidelines for Use (cont.):

- *Tape* — Skin should be clean and dry before the tape is applied. Tape should always be cut, never torn.
  Replacement of the tape every 12 hours produces the lowest incidence of side effects, but it may be left in place for 24 hours if it is well-tolerated and adheres well. When replacing the tape, cleanse the skin and allow to dry for 1 hour before applying new tape.
  When necessary, the tape may be used at night only and removed during the day.
  If the ends of the tape loosen prematurely, they may be trimmed off and replaced with fresh tape.
- Lab tests may be required to monitor therapy. Be sure to keep appointments.
- Store at controlled room temperature (59° to 86°F). Protect solutions and lotions from freezing.

If you have any questions, consult your doctor, pharmacist, or health care provider.

	Brand Name Examples	Hydrocortisone %	Other
Rx	Ala-Quin Cream	0.5	3% iodochlorhydroxyquin
Rx	Analpram-HC Cream 2.5%[1], Pramosone Cream 2.5%[1,2]	2.5	1% pramoxine HCl
Rx	Zone-A Forte Lotion	2.5	1% pramoxine HCl
Rx	Analpram-HC Cream, Pramosone Cream[1,2]	1	1% pramoxine HCl
Rx	Epifoam Aerosol Foam, ProctoFoam-HC Aerosol Foam	1	1% pramoxine HCl
Rx	Carmol HC Cream[3]	1	10% urea
otc	HC Derma-Pax Liquid	0.5	0.5% diphenhydramine HCl
Rx	Mantadil Cream	0.5	2% chlorcyclizine HCl
Rx	Vanoxide-HC Lotion	0.5	5% benzoyl peroxide
Rx	Vytone Cream	1	1% iodoquinol

[1] Also available in same strength as a lotion.
[2] Also available in same strength as an ointment.
[3] Contains sodium bisulfite.

Type of Drug:

Topical anti-inflammatory, anti-itching agents.

Uses:

To treat a variety of corticosteroid-responsive skin conditions. Some of these include eczema; insect bites; poison ivy, oak, or sumac; external anal itching; and allergic inflammation from soaps, detergents, cosmetics, or jewelry.

Vanoxide-HC is used to treat acne.

Components of these topical corticosteroid combinations include:

Hydrocortisone is used for its anti-inflammatory, anti-itch, and vasoconstrictive (blood vessel narrowing) effects.

Iodochlorhydroxyquin and *iodoquinol* are used for their antifungal, antibacterial, and antieczematous effects.

Pramoxine HCl is used for its local anesthetic effects.

Urea is a mild keratolytic and hydrates dry skin.

Diphenhydramine and *chlorcyclizine* are antihistamines used to treat itching.

Benzoyl peroxide is used for its peeling and drying effects.

Precautions:

Do not use in the following situations:

- allergy to the medicine or any of its ingredients
- lesions of the eye (*Ala-Quin* only)
- most viral skin lesions (eg, vaccinia, varicella, herpes simplex) (*Ala-Quin* and *Mantadil* only)
- systemic bacterial infection without concomitant antibacterial therapy
- tuberculosis of the skin (*Ala-Quin* and *Mantadil* only)

Use with caution in the following situations:

- use of more potent steroids
- children
- occlusive dressing use
- prolonged use
- use over large surface areas

Pregnancy: There are no adequate and well-controlled studies in pregnant women. Topical corticosteroids should be used during pregnancy only if the potential benefits to the mother outweigh the possible risks to the fetus.

Breastfeeding: It is not known whether topical corticosteroids appear in breast milk. Consult your doctor before you begin breastfeeding.

Children: Pediatric patients may demonstrate greater susceptibility to topical corticosteroid-induced hypothalamic-pituitary-adrenal (HPA) axis suppression and Cushing's syndrome than adult patients because of a larger skin surface area to body weight ratio. Administration of topical corticosteroids to children should be limited to the least amount compatible with an effective therapeutic regimen. Chronic corticosteroid therapy may interfere with the growth and development of children.

Lab tests may be required to monitor long-term or high-dose therapy. Tests may include urinary free cortisol or ACTH stimulation tests.

Sulfites: Some of these products may contain sulfite preservatives that can cause allergic reactions in certain individuals. Check package label when available or consult your doctor or pharmacist.

Drug Interactions:

Tell your doctor or pharmacist if you are taking or if you are planning to take any over-the-counter or prescription medications or dietary supplements with topical corticosteroid combinations. Doses of one or both drugs may need to be modified or a different drug may need to be prescribed.

Side Effects:

Every drug is capable of producing side effects. Many topical corticosteroid combination users experience no, or minor, side effects. The frequency and severity of side effects depend on many factors including dose, duration of therapy, and individual susceptibility. Possible side effects include:

Skin: Burning; itching; rash; irritation; dryness; inflammation of hair follicles; excessive hair growth; acne; hypopigmentation; skin irritation around the mouth; allergic contact dermatitis; tearing of the skin; secondary infection; skin atrophy; stretch marks; plugged or inflamed sweat follicles.

Other: Reversible hypothalamic-pituitary-adrenal (HPA) axis suppression; manifestations of Cushing's syndrome; high blood sugar; sugar in the urine; abnormal thyroid tests (*iodochlorhydroxyquin-containing products only*); false-positive ferric chloride test for phenylketonuria (PKU) (*iodochlorhydroxyquin-containing products only*).

Guidelines for Use:

- For external use only.
- Avoid contact with the eyes.
- *ProctoFoam-HC Aerosol* is for anal or perianal use only.
- Topical corticosteroids are generally applied to the affected area as a thin film and rubbed in gently 3 or 4 times daily depending on the severity of the condition. See individual product information for specific instructions.
- Washing or soaking the affected area and then drying it before application is encouraged, as this may increase drug penetration.
- The treated skin should not be bandaged or otherwise covered or wrapped so as to be occlusive unless directed to do so by your doctor.
- Occlusive dressings may be used for the management of psoriasis or recalcitrant conditions. Discontinue the use of occlusive dressings and notify your doctor if symptoms worsen or an infection develops.
- *HC Derma-Pax* is most effective when used as a wet dressing.
- Avoid prolonged use, especially near the eyes, on the face, on genital and rectal areas, and in skin folds.
- Do not use tight-fitting diapers or plastic pants on children being treated with topical corticosteroids in the diaper area. Such garments function as occlusive dressings.
- Skin infections may worsen. It may be necessary to stop the corticosteroid and treat the infection.
- Allergic reactions may occur. If the condition being treated worsens or irritation, burning, redness, pain, swelling, or stinging persists, discontinue use and contact your doctor.
- Iodochlorhydroxyquin may interfere with thyroid function tests. Tell your doctor if you are using this medicine.
- Benzoyl peroxide may bleach hair or clothing.
- Aerosol containers should never be inserted into the vagina or anus.
- Lab tests may be required to monitor therapy. Be sure to keep appointments.
- Store at room temperature (59° to 86°F) in a tightly closed container.
- Aerosol foams are in pressurized containers. Do not puncture, incinerate, or expose to high heat. Store upright at room temperature (59° to 86°F). Do not refrigerate.

If you have any questions, consult your doctor, pharmacist, or health care provider.

	Generic Name *Brand Name Examples*	Supplied As	Generic Available
Rx	**Fludrocortisone Acetate**		
	Florinef Acetate	**Tablets:** 0.1 mg	No

Type of Drug:

Adrenal cortical steroid.

How the Drug Works:

The mineralocorticoid, fludrocortisone, acts on the kidney to preserve sodium. It increases potassium and hydrogen loss in the urine.

Uses:

To treat insufficient secretion of steroids from the adrenal cortex in Addison's disease. Used in conjunction with glucocorticoid therapy.

To treat excessive salt loss.

Unlabeled Use(s): Occasionally doctors may prescribe fludrocortisone for severe orthostatic hypotension (dizziness or lightheadedness that occurs when rising quickly from a lying or sitting position).

Precautions:

Do not use in the following situations:

allergy to fludrocortisone acetate or any of its ingredients
immunization, concurrent
smallpox vaccination, concurrent
systemic fungal infection

Use with caution in the following situations:

cirrhosis
diverticulitis
heart disease
herpes simplex, ocular
high blood pressure
hypothyroidism
immunosuppression
infection, active
intestinal anastomoses, fresh
kidney disease
liver disease
myasthenia gravis
osteoporosis
patients who have not had chickenpox or measles
peptic ulcer, active or latent
salicylates (eg, aspirin) use in hypoprothombinemic patients
stress (eg, trauma, surgery, severe illness)
tuberculosis, active
ulcerative colitis, non-specific

Pregnancy: Adequate studies have not been done in pregnant women. Use only if clearly needed and potential benefits to the mother outweigh the possible hazards to the fetus.

Breastfeeding: Corticosteroids appear in breast milk. Consult your doctor before you begin breastfeeding.

Children: Safety and effectiveness in children have not been established. Monitor growth and development of infants and children on prolonged therapy.

Lab tests may be required. Tests may include serum electrolyte levels and blood pressure monitoring.

Drug Interactions:

Tell your doctor or pharmacist if you are taking or if you are planning to take any over-the-counter or prescription medications or dietary supplements with fludrocortisone acetate. Doses of one or both drugs may need to be modified or a different drug may need to be prescribed. The following drugs and drug classes interact with fludrocortisone.

amphotericin B (eg, *Fungizone*)
anabolic steroids (eg, oxymetholone, methandrosatenolone, norethandrolone)
anticoagulants, oral (eg, warfarin)
antidiabetics (eg, insulin)
barbiturates (eg, phenobarbital)
cardiac glycosides (eg, digoxin)
cholinesterase inhibitors (eg, neostigmine)
estrogen (eg, *Premarin*)
hydantoins (eg, phenytoin)
immunosuppressive agents (eg, cyclosporine)
potassium-depleting diuretics (eg, benzothiadiazines, furosemide)
rifabutin (*Mycobutin*)
rifampin (eg, *Rifadin*)
salicylates (eg, aspirin)
vaccines (eg, influenza virus vaccine)

Side Effects:

Every drug is capable of producing side effects. Many mineralocorticoid users experience no, or minor, side effects. The frequency and severity of side effects depend on many factors including dose, duration of therapy, and individual susceptibility. Severe side effects may occur if the dose is too high, if the mineralocorticoid is given for a long time, or if it is withdrawn too fast. Fludrocortisone may cause side effects similar to glucocorticoids. Possible side effects include:

Circulatory System: High blood pressure; heart failure; heart enlargement.

Muscular System: Muscle weakness; steroid-induced muscle disease; loss of muscle mass; osteoporosis (brittle bones); compression fractures of the spine; hip bone or shoulder bone degradation; fracture of long bones due to diseases; spontaneous fractures.

Digestive Tract: Peptic ulcer with possible perforation and bleeding; pancreatitis; abdominal distention; inflammation of the esophagus.

Skin: Impaired wound healing; thin, fragile skin; bruising; small red spots under skin; unusual bruising; increased sweating; subcutaneous fat atrophy; red or purple spots or patches under the skin; stretch marks; excessive pigment in the skin and nails; abnormal hairiness or increased hair growth; acne-like eruptions; hives; rash; facial skin redness; itching.

Nervous System: Convulsions; increased intracranial pressure with fluid accumulation at the optic disc (pseudotumor cerebri) usually after treatment; feeling of a whirling motion; headache; severe mental disturbances.

Eyes or Ocular: Posterior subcapsular cataracts; increased intraocular pressure (glaucoma with possible damage to the optic nerve); eye infections.

Other: Fluid retention; unusual weight gain; potassium loss; hypokalemic alkalosis; allergic reaction; high blood sugar; negative nitrogen balance due to protein catabolism; necrotizing angiitis; inflammation of the veins with clot formation; aggravation or masking of infections; sleeplessness; fainting; menstrual irregularities; development of the cushingoid state (eg, buffalo hump obesity, general obesity, high blood pressure, diabetes, osteoporosis); suppression of growth in children; secondary adrenocortical and pituitary unresponsiveness particularly in times of stress (eg, trauma, surgery, illness); decreased carbohydrate tolerance; manifestations of latent diabetes mellitus; increased requirements for insulin or oral hypoglycemic agents in diabetic patients; calcium loss; euphoria; mood swings; personality changes; depression; emotional instability; psychotic tendencies; glucose in the urine.

Guidelines for Use:

- Because of its marked effect on sodium retention, the use of fludrocortisone in the treatment of conditions other than those indicated is not advised.
- Dosage depends on the severity of the disease and the response of the patient.
- *Addison's Disease* — Administer with a glucocorticoid (eg, 10 to 37.5 mg daily of cortisone or 10 to 30 mg daily of hydrocortisone, both in divided doses). The usual dose is 0.1 mg. Doses ranging from 0.1 to 0.2 mg daily have been used. If blood pressure increases, the dose may be decreased to 0.05 mg daily.
- *Salt-Losing Adrenogenital Syndrome* — The recommended dose is 0.1 mg to 0.2 mg daily.
- Carefully monitor salt intake in order to avoid developing high blood pressure, swelling, or weight gain.
- Higher doses may be required in times of stress (eg, trauma, surgery, severe illness) both during and 1 year after treatment with fludrocortisone.
- If a dose is missed, take it as soon as possible. If several hours have passed or it is nearing time for the next dose, do not double the dose in order to catch up, unless advised to do so by your doctor. If more than one dose is missed or if it is necessary to establish a new dosage schedule, contact your doctor or pharmacist.
- Do not stop taking the medicine suddenly.
- Corticosteroids may mask some signs of infection, and new infections may appear during their use. There may be decreased resistance and difficulty in reducing the spread of an infection when used. If an infection occurs during therapy, notify your doctor immediately.
- Dietary salt restriction and potassium supplementation may be necessary. All corticosteroids increase calcium secretion.
- Prolonged use of corticosteroids may produce cataracts, glaucoma with possible damage to optic nerves, and ocular infections.
- *Chickenpox and Measles* — Patients are more susceptible to infections such as chickenpox and measles. These infections can have a more serious or even fatal course in children. Avoid exposure to infections due to fungi or viruses.
- Carry medical identification indicating dependence on steroids and possibly carry an adequate supply of medicine for use in emergencies.
- Notify your doctor if dizziness, severe headaches, joint pain, extreme weakness, swelling of feet or lower legs, or unusual weight gain occurs.
- Lab tests may be needed to determine blood pressure and sodium and potassium levels in the blood. Regular follow-up visits will also be crucial in checking progress. Be sure to keep appointments.
- Store at room temperature (59° to 86°F). Avoid excessive heat.

If you have any questions, consult your doctor, pharmacist, or health care provider.

Generic Name *Brand Name Examples*	Supplied As	Generic Available
Rx **Aminoglutethimide**		
Cytadren	**Tablets:** 250 mg	No

Type of Drug:

Adrenal steroid inhibitor.

How the Drug Works:

Aminoglutethimide inhibits the synthesis of adrenal steroids such as glucocorticoids, mineralocorticoids, estrogens and androgens.

Uses:

To suppress the adrenal gland functions in selected patients with Cushing's syndrome.

Unlabeled Use(s): Occasionally doctors may prescribe aminoglutethimide to treat breast cancer in postmenopausal patients or to treat patients with metastatic prostate cancer.

Precautions:

Do not use in the following situations:
allergy to aminoglutethimide or glutethimide, serious

Use with caution in the following situations:
illness, acute
long-term use (more than 3 months)
low blood pressure
surgery
trauma

Pregnancy: Studies have shown a potential adverse effect on the fetus. Use only if clearly needed and potential benefits outweigh the possible risks.

Breastfeeding: It is not known if aminoglutethimide appears in breast milk. Consult your doctor before you begin breastfeeding.

Children: Safety and effectiveness in children have not been established.

Lab tests will be required to monitor therapy. Be sure to keep appointments. Tests may include:Thyroid function test; adrenal function tests; blood pressure monitoring; serum electrolytes.

Drug Interactions:

Tell your doctor or pharmacist if you are taking or planning to take any over-the-counter or prescription medications or dietary supplements while taking this medicine. Doses of one or both drugs may need to be modified or a different drug may need to be prescribed. The following drugs and drug classes interact with this medicine.

alcohol
anticoagulants, oral (eg, warfarin)
dexamethasone (eg, *Decadron*)
digitoxin
medroxyprogesterone (*Depo-Provera*)
theophylline (eg, *Theo-Dur*)

Side Effects:

Every drug is capable of producing side effects. Most patients experience side effects. The frequency and severity of si'de effects depend on many factors including dose, duration of therapy and individual susceptibility. Possible side effects include:

Digestive Tract: Nausea; appetite loss; vomiting.

Nervous System: Drowsiness; headache; dizziness.

Circulatory System: Low blood pressure (occasionally causing dizziness or lightheadedness when rising from sitting or lying); fast heartbeat.

Skin: Rash; itching.

Other: Muscle pain; fever; reduced adrenal function; underactive thyroid (eg, weight gain); abnormal blood counts.

Guidelines for Use:

- Use exactly as prescribed.
- The usual dose is 250 mg four times daily, every 6 hours.
- If a dose is missed, take it as soon as possible. If several hours have passed or if it is nearing time for the next dose, do not double the dose in order to "catch up" (unless advised to do so by your doctor). If more than one dose is missed or it is necessary to establish a new dosage schedule, contact your doctor or pharmacist.
- May cause dizziness, lightheartedness or fainting, especially when rising quickly from a sitting or lying. If these symptoms should occur, sit or lie down and contact your doctor. Use caution while driving or performing hazardous tasks requiring alertness, coordination or physical dexterity.
- If severe rash, extreme drowsiness, yellowing of skin or eyes, fainting, weakness or headache occur, contact your doctor immediately.
- Nausea and loss of appetite may occur during the first 2 weeks of therapy. Contact you doctor if these do not go away.
- Contraceptive measures (birth control) are recommended during treatment to avoid birth defects. Contact your doctor if pregnancy is suspected.
- Store at room temperature (below 86°F) in a tightly sealed container. Protect from light.

If you have any questions, consult your doctor, pharmacist, or health care provider.

	Generic Name *Brand Name Examples*	Supplied As
otc	**Insulin Injection (Regular Insulin)**	
	Regular Iletin II	**Injection**: 100 units/mL, purified pork
	Novolin R	**Injection**: 100 units/mL, human insulin (rDNA)
	Velosulin BR	**Injection**: 100 units/mL, human insulin (rDNA)
	Novolin R PenFill	**Cartridges**: 100 units/mL, human insulin (rDNA). Use with *NovoPen* and *Novolin Pen*
	Novolin R Prefilled	**Injection**: 100 units/mL, human insulin (rDNA)
	Humulin R	**Injection**: 100 units/mL, regular insulin (rDNA)
Rx	**Insulin Injection Concentrated**	
	Humulin R Regular U-500 (Concentrated)	**Injection**: 500 units/mL, human insulin (rDNA)
otc	**Insulin Zinc Suspension (Lente Insulin)**	
	Lente Iletin I	**Injection** 100 units/mL, beef and pork
	Lente Iletin II	**Injection**: 100 units/mL, purified pork
	Humulin L, Novolin L	**Injection**: 100 units/mL, human insulin (rDNA)
otc	**Insulin Zinc Suspension, Extended (Ultralente Insulin)**	
	Humulin U Ultralente	**Injection**: 100 units/mL, human insulin (rDNA)
otc	**Isophane Insulin Suspension (NPH Insulin)**	
	NPH Iletin I	**Injection**: 100 units/mL, beef and pork
	NPH Iletin II	**Injection**: 100 units/mL, purified pork
	Humulin N, Novolin N	**Injection**: 100 units/mL, human insulin (rDNA)
	Novolin N PenFill	**Cartridges**: 100 units/mL, human insulin-(rDNA). Use with *NovoPen* and *Novolin Pen*
	Novolin N Prefilled	**Injection**: 100 units/mL, human insulin (rDNA)

	Generic Name *Brand Name Examples*	Supplied As
otc	**Isophane Insulin Suspension (NPH) and Regular Insulin Injection Combined**	
	Humulin 50/50	**Injection**: 150 units NPH and 50 units regular insulin/mL, human insulin (rDNA)
	Humulin 70/30, *Novolin 70/30*	**Injection**: 70 units NPH and 30 units regular insulin/mL, human insulin (rDNA)
	Novolin 70/30 PenFill	**Cartridges**: 70 units NPH and 30 units regular insulin/mL, human insulin (rDNA)
	Novolin 70/30 Prefilled	**Injection**: 70 units NPH and 30 units regular insulin/mL, human insulin (rDNA)
Rx	**Insulin Analog Injection**	
	Humalog	**Injection**: 100 units/mL, human insulin lispro (rDNA)
	Humalog Mix 50/50	**Injection**: 50 units insulin lispro protamine and 50 units insulin lispro/mL, human insulin lispro (rDNA)
	Humalog Mix 75/25	**Injection**: 75 units insulin lispro protamine and 25 units insulin lispro/mL, insulin lispro (rDNA)
	NovoLog	**Injection**: 100 units/mL, human insulin aspart (rDNA)
Rx	**Insulin Glargine Injection**	
	Lantus	**Injection**: 100 IU (3.6378 mg)

Beef insulin: Obtained from the pancreas gland of a cow.
Pork insulin: Obtained from the pancreas gland of a pig.
Human insulin (rDNA): Synthesized in a special laboratory.

Type of Drug:

Hormone; antidiabetic agent.

How the Drug Works:

Insulin, normally produced in the pancreas gland, is the major hormone that regulates glucose (sugar) use in the body. Without insulin, sugar is trapped in the bloodstream and cannot enter the cells of the body where it can be utilized for energy, so blood sugar levels increase, resulting in diabetes. In type 1 (insulin-dependent) and advanced type 2 (non-insulin-dependent) diabetes, the pancreas is not able to make enough insulin to control sugar levels.

Insulin must be injected. If taken by mouth, it would be digested by the acids and enzymes in the stomach.

Uses:

To treat type 1 (insulin-dependent) diabetes mellitus.

To treat type 2 (non-insulin-dependent) diabetes mellitus that cannot be properly controlled by diet, exercise, or weight reduction.

Used in a hospital setting to treat dangerously high blood levels of potassium.

Precautions:

Diet and exercise: It is important to follow the diet and exercise regimen prescribed by your doctor in order to effectively control diabetes. Do not change this regimen unless advised to do so by your doctor.

High blood pressure: High blood pressure in combination with diabetes increases the risk for other health problems (eg, eye or kidney problems, heart attack, stroke). Blood pressure should be monitored frequently. Regular checkups and eye examinations are important.

Smoking: Avoid tobacco products. If you are a smoker and stop, your dose of insulin may need to be reduced.

Brand interchange: Do not change from one insulin product to another unless advised to do so by your doctor. Insulins vary by strength, brand, onset, maximum effect, and duration of activity (see the following table). Become familiar with how the products you are using affect your blood sugar levels.

Pharmacokinetics and Compatibility of Various Insulins					
Insulin Preparations		**Onset (hrs)**	**Peak (hrs)**	**Duration (hrs)**	**Compatible mixed with**
Rapid-Acting	Insulin Injection (Regular)	0.5 to 1	variable depending on product	8 to 12	All
	Prompt Insulin Zinc Suspension (semilente)	1 to 1.5	5 to 10	12 to 16	Lente
	Insulin Lispro Solution	0.25	0.5 to 1.5	6 to 8	Ultralente, NPH
	Insulin Aspart Solution	0.25	1 to 3	3 to 5	NPH

Pharmacokinetics and Compatibility of Various Insulins					
Insulin Preparations		Onset (hrs)	Peak (hrs)	Duration (hrs)	Compatible mixed with
Inter-medi-ate-Acting	Isophane Insulin Suspension (NPH)	1 to 1.5	4 to 12	24	Regular
	Insulin Zinc Suspension (Lente)	1 to 2.5	7 to 15	24	Regular, semilente
	Insulin Glargine Solution	1.1	5[1]	24[2]	None
Long-Acting	Protamine Zinc Insulin Suspension (PZI)	4 to 8	14 to 24	36	Regular
	Extended Insulin Zinc Suspension (Ultralente)	4 to 8	10 to 30	28	Regular, semilente

[1] No pronounced peak; small amounts of insulin glargine are slowly released resulting in a relatively constant concentration/time profile over 24 hours.
[2] Studies only conducted up to 24 hours.

Insulin mixtures: Patients stabilized on mixtures should have a consistent response. Unexpected responses are most likely to occur when switching from separate injections to mixtures (or vice versa). When mixing 2 types of insulin, always draw the clear regular insulin into the syringe first. To avoid dosage errors, do not alter the order of mixing insulins or change the model or brand of syringe or needle.

It is recommended to use the self-prepared mixtures within the first 5 minutes after mixing. If this is not possible, clarify with your doctor, pharmacist, or health care provider the instructions on how to store these mixtures.

NPH/regular mixtures of insulin are available in premixed formulations of 70% NPH and 30% regular, and of 50% NPH and 50% regular. Insulin lispro NPH/regular mixtures are available in premixed formulations of 75% NPH and 25% regular and of 50% NPH and 50% regular. These mixtures are stable and are absorbed as if injected separately.

High blood sugar: In patients with type 1 diabetes mellitus, high blood sugar levels (hyperglycemia) that are not treated properly with insulin can develop into diabetic ketoacidosis, a life-threatening condition requiring prompt diagnosis and treatment (see the following table for symptoms). Close monitoring and control of blood sugar levels are required to prevent high blood sugar levels from developing.

Symptoms of Hypoglycemia vs Ketoacidosis		
Reaction	**Onset**	**Symptoms**
Hypoglycemia Too little sugar in the blood (Insulin reaction)	sudden	**Mild to Moderate Hypoglycemia** sweating tremor rapid heart rate pounding in the chest anxiety irritability personality changes slurred speech abnormal behavior inability to concentrate drowsiness headache hunger restlessness tingling in the hands, feet, lips, or tongue vision changes
		Severe Hypoglycemia disorientation unconsciousness seizures death
Ketoacidosis Too much sugar and acid in the blood (Diabetic coma)	slow (hours to days)	drowsiness flushed face thirst fruity breath odor rapid breathing stomach ache appetite loss large amounts of sugar and acetone in the urine

Low blood sugar: Insulin use has the potential to cause hypoglycemia, or low blood sugar (refer to the preceding table for symptoms). Hypoglycemia may be due to taking too much insulin, exercising or working more than usual, not eating enough food, or not eating at the appropriate times. Eating sugar or a sugar-sweetened product will often correct the condition and prevent more serious symptoms. Establish a plan with your doctor on how best to treat hypoglycemic reactions. All diabetic patients should carry a source of rapid-acting sugar (eg, candy mints, glucose tablets) to take if symptoms of low blood sugar develop. Commercial products containing 40% glucose are available, such as *B-D Glucose* tablets. Close self-monitoring of blood glucose is necessary to determine when blood sugar levels are too low. Notify your doctor immediately if you experience ongoing symptoms of low blood sugar.

All patients using insulin should also have a *Glucagon* emergency kit available, so that family members, coworkers, or friends can administer the *Glucagon* to raise blood sugar levels in an unconscious patient with diabetes (see the Glucose Elevating Agents — Glucagon monograph in this chapter). Make sure these people know how to prepare and administer *Glucagon*.

Pregnancy: If you are using insulin and become pregnant, management of your diabetes will require a greater effort and you should self-monitor blood glucose and ketones more often. Rigid control of blood sugar and avoidance of ketones in the blood are desired throughout pregnancy. Insulin requirements may drop immediately following delivery, then increase to pre-pregnancy levels over time.

Breastfeeding: Insulin appears in breast milk, but is destroyed in the stomach of the infant and not absorbed. Breastfeeding women may require adjustments in insulin dose and diet.

Lab tests may be required to monitor therapy. Tests may include blood glucose, urine ketones, and glycohemoglobin tests.

Drug Interactions:

Tell your doctor or pharmacist if you are taking or if you are planning to take any over-the-counter or prescription medications or dietary supplements while taking insulin. Doses of one or both drugs may need to be modified or a different drug may need to be prescribed. The following drugs and drug classes interact with insulin:

Decrease the glucose-lowering effect of insulin —

acetazolamide (eg, *Diamox*)
AIDS antivirals (eg, saquinavir)
albuterol (eg, *Proventil*)
asparaginase (*Elspar*)
calcitonin (eg, *Calcimar*)
clonidine (eg, *Catapres*)
contraceptives, oral (eg, *Ortho-Novum*)
corticosteroids (eg, prednisone)
cyclophosphamide (eg, *Cytoxan*)
danazol (eg, *Danocrine*)
dextrothyroxine (*Choloxin*)
diazoxide (*Proglycem*)
diltiazem (eg, *Cardizem*)
dobutamide (eg, *Dobutrex*)
epinephrine (eg, *Adrenalin Chloride*)
estrogens (eg, *Premarin*)
isoniazid (eg, *Nydrazid*)
lithium carbonate (eg, *Eskalith*)
loop diuretics (eg, furosemide)
morphine sulfate (eg, *MS Contin*)
niacin (vitamin B_3; nicotinic acid)
nicotine
phenothiazines (eg, promethazine)
phenytoin (eg, *Dilantin*)
somatropin (eg, *Genotropin*)
terbutaline (eg, *Brethine*)
thiazide diuretics (eg, hydrochlorothiazide)
thyroid hormone (eg, levothyroxine)

Increase the glucose-lowering effect of insulin —

ACE inhibitors (eg, ramipril)
alcohol
antidiabetic products, oral (eg, glipizide)
beta blockers (eg, propranolol)
clofibrate (*Atromid-S*)
disopyramide (eg, *Norpace*)
fluoxetine (eg, *Prozac*)
lithium carbonate (eg, *Eskalith*)
MAOIs (eg, phenelzine)

propoxyphene (eg, *Darvon-N*)
salicylates (eg, aspirin)
somatostatin analog (eg, octreotide)
sulfonamides (eg, trimethoprim and sulfamethoxazole)
tetracyclines (eg, oxytetracycline)

Side Effects:

Every drug is capable of producing side effects. Many insulin users experience no, or minor, side effects. The frequency and severity of side effects depend on many factors including dose, duration of therapy, and individual susceptibility. Possible side effects include:

Skin: Rash, itching, redness, or other allergic symptoms at injection site; skin puckering at injection site; skin depression at injection site; skin thickening at injection site; fatty lumps at injection site.

For symptoms of high blood sugar and low blood sugar, see Precautions.

Guidelines for Use:

- Read the package inserts of the insulin and understand all aspects of its use.
- Carefully follow the storage, preparation, and injection techniques taught to you by your doctor or diabetes educator.
- Participate in a thorough diabetes education program so that you understand diabetes and all aspects of its treatment, including diet, exercise, personal hygiene, and how to self-monitor blood glucose.
- Become familiar with the specific type of insulin that you are using and how your blood sugar levels are affected by each dose. Do not switch types, brands, strengths, doses, or the order of mixing your insulin without first consulting your doctor or diabetes educator. Overdosage could result in insulin shock.
- Wear an ID tag (eg, Medic Alert) so appropriate treatment can be given if an emergency occurs away from home.
- Always keep an extra supply of insulin, as well as a spare syringe and needle, on hand.
- Visually inspect the solution/suspension before administration.
- Rotate injection sites to prevent scarring and other possible complications.
- Do not switch the model and brand of syringe or needle without first consulting your doctor or diabetes educator.
- Monitor blood glucose and urine for glucose and ketones as prescribed. Keep track of the results so that adjustments in your treatment can be made more easily.
- Contact your doctor if you experience symptoms of hypoglycemia or ketoacidosis (see table in Precautions for symptoms).

Guidelines for Use (cont.):

- Insulin requirements may change when you are ill (eg, vomiting, fever), under stress, or exercising. Stay on your regular diet, if possible. Establish a "sick day" plan with your doctor. A "sick day" plan provides directions for what to do when you are sick and cannot keep food down or are having difficulty eating. The plan should include advice on when to call your doctor or seek emergency care.
- To avoid possible transmission of disease, do not share syringes, needles, or cartridges with anyone else.
- Consult your doctor about your insulin schedule if you will be traveling across 2 or more time zones. You may need to make adjustments in your insulin schedule.
- Be sure to have regular physical and eye examinations. The frequency of these exams will be determined by your regular doctor and your eye doctor.
- Lab tests may be required to monitor therapy. Be sure to keep appointments.
- *Regular insulin* — Do not use if solution is cloudy, colored, thickened, or if particles are seen.
- *Lente and NPH insulins* — Gently mix well before using. Do not use if clumps are seen or if white material (the insulin) remains at the bottom of the insulin bottle.
- Store at room temperature (up to 30 days), away from light and heat. If you buy extra bottles of insulin, store the bottles that you are not using in the door of the refrigerator. Do not freeze insulin. Do not use the bottles after the expiration date stamped on the label or if the insulin has been frozen.

If you have any questions, consult your doctor, pharmacist, or health care provider.

	Generic Name *Brand Name Example*	Supplied As	Generic Available
Rx	**Acarbose**		
	Precose	**Tablets:** 25 mg, 50 mg, 100 mg	No
Rx	**Miglitol**		
	Glyset	**Tablets:** 25 mg, 50 mg, 100 mg	No

Type of Drug:

Oral antidiabetic.

How the Drug Works:

Acarbose and miglitol delay the digestion of ingested carbohydrates; this slows the absorption of glucose and results in a smaller rise in blood sugar levels following meals. May be used alone, as an adjunct to diet, or in combination with a sulfonylurea (eg, glyburide) when diet plus antidiabetic agents or sulfonylureas do not result in adequate blood sugar control. Acarbose may be used in combination with metformin or insulin. Miglitol may also be used in combination with insulin.

Uses:

To help decrease blood sugar levels. Acarbose and miglitol are only prescribed for patients with type 2 diabetes mellitus who are not capable of managing blood sugar levels by diet and exercise alone.

Precautions:

Do not use in the following situations:

- allergy to the drug or any of its ingredients
- cirrhosis (liver disease, severe) (acarbose only)
- colonic ulceration (rectal bleeding)
- conditions that may worsen as a result of increased gas formation in the intestine
- diabetic ketoacidosis
- inflammatory bowel disease
- intestinal disease, chronic
- intestinal obstruction, current or predisposition to

Use with caution in the following situations:

- kidney disease
- insulin or sulfonylurea use (may increase risk of low blood sugar)
- liver disease

Loss of control of blood glucose: When diabetic patients are exposed to stress (eg, fever, trauma, infection, surgery) a temporary loss of control of blood glucose may occur. At such times, temporary insulin therapy may be needed.

Pregnancy: There are no adequate and well-controlled studies in pregnant women. Use only if clearly needed and potential benefits to the mother outweigh the possible hazard to the fetus.

Breastfeeding: It is not known if acarbose appears in breast milk. Miglitol appears in breast milk. Acarbose and miglitol should not be used while breastfeeding. Consult your doctor before you begin breastfeeding.

Children: Safety and effectiveness for use in children have not been established.

Lab tests are required to monitor therapy. Tests include blood glucose or hemoglobin level tests.

Drug Interactions:

Tell your doctor or pharmacist if you are taking or planning to take any over-the-counter or prescription medications or dietary supplements while taking this medicine. Doses of one or both drugs may need to be modified or a different drug may need to be prescribed. The following drugs and drug classes interact with alpha-glucosidase inhibitors:

- calcium channel blockers (eg, diltiazem) (acarbose only)
- corticosteroids (eg, triamcinolone) (acarbose only)
- digestive enzymes (eg, amylase)
- digoxin (eg, *Lanoxin*)
- estrogens (eg, *Premarin*) (acarbose only)
- glyburide (eg, *Micronase*) (miglitol only)
- insulin
- intestinal adsorbents (eg, charcoal)
- phenothiazines (eg, perphenazine) (acarbose only)
- phenytoin (eg, *Dilantin*) (acarbose only)
- propranolol (eg, *Inderal*) (miglitol only)
- ranitidine (eg, *Zantac*) (miglitol only)
- sulfonylureas (eg, glipizide) (miglitol only)
- thiazide diuretics (eg, hydrochlorothiazide) (acarbose only)
- thyroid supplements (acarbose only)

Side Effects:

Every drug is capable of producing side effects. Many patients experience no, or minor, side effects. The frequency and severity of side effects depend on many factors including dose, duration of therapy, and individual susceptibility. Possible side effects include:

Digestive Tract: Stomach pain; diarrhea; gas.

Other: Abnormal blood or liver function tests; rash (miglitol only).

Guidelines for Use:

- Dosage will be individualized on the basis of both effectiveness and tolerance. Take exactly as prescribed. Do not exceed the maximum recommended dosage of 100 mg 3 times daily or stop taking, unless advised by your doctor.
- Start with a low dose and increase gradually to reduce side effects and to identify the minimum dose needed for adequate glycemic control.
- Take 3 times daily at the start (with the first bite) of each main meal.
- Do not take a dose if you are going to skip a meal. If more than one dose is missed, contact your doctor or pharmacist.
- If side effects occur, they usually develop during the first few weeks of therapy. Side effects are commonly mild to moderate gastrointestinal (eg, diarrhea, gas, stomach pain) and generally diminish in frequency and intensity with time.
- Be sure to follow the diet, exercise, urine, and blood glucose testing programs prescribed by your doctor.
- This medicine alone does not cause low blood sugar levels, but it may increase the lowering of blood sugar caused by sulfonylureas or insulin. Because this medicine prevents the breakdown of table (cane) sugar, be sure to use glucose, not table sugar or fruits, to treat symptoms of low blood sugar (eg, fatigue, numbness in arms and legs). Contact your doctor if these symptoms occur.
- Lab tests will be required to monitor therapy. Be sure to keep appointments.
- Store acarbose below 77°F in a tightly closed container. Protect from moisture. Store miglitol between 59° and 86°F.

If you have any questions, consult your doctor, pharmacist, or health care provider.

	Generic Name *Brand Name Example*	Supplied As	Generic Available
Rx	**Pioglitazone HCl**		
	Actos	**Tablets:** 15 mg, 30 mg, 45 mg	No
Rx	**Rosiglitazone Maleate**		
	Avandia	**Tablets:** 2 mg, 4 mg, 8 mg	No

Type of Drug:

Oral antidiabetic (blood sugar lowering) agent used in the management of type 2 diabetes (adult-onset; non-insulin-dependent diabetes mellitus [NIDDM]) not adequately controlled with diet and exercise.

How the Drug Works:

The thiazolidinedione hypoglycemic agents appear to lower blood sugar (glucose) by improving target cell response or sensitivity to insulin. They also decrease glucose output from the liver and increase insulin-dependent glucose disposal in skeletal muscle. They do not stimulate insulin production but lower tissue resistance (ie, increase sensitivity) to insulin.

Uses:

Used alone or as an adjunct to diet and exercise to treat type 2 diabetes or in combination with a sulfonylurea or insulin, or metformin to improve glycemic control when diet, exercise, and a single diabetic drug do not accomplish adequate control of blood glucose levels.

Precautions:

Do not use in the following situations:

allergy to a thiazolidinedione or any of its ingredients
diabetic ketoacidosis
liver disease, active
NYHA class III and IV cardiac status
type 1 diabetes mellitus

Use with caution in the following situations:

congestive heart failure
edema (fluid retention)
liver disease, history of
liver function test abnormalities, history of

Pregnancy: There are no adequate and well-controlled studies in pregnant women. Use only if clearly needed and potential benefits to the mother outweigh the possible hazard to the fetus. Most experts recommend that insulin be used to control diabetes during pregnancy.

Breastfeeding: It is not known if thiazolidinediones appear in breast milk. Do not administer to a nursing woman.

Children: Safety and effectiveness in patients under 18 years of age have not been established.

Lab tests will be required to monitor therapy. Tests may include blood glucose, glycosylated hemoglobin, and liver function.

Drug Interactions:

Tell your doctor or pharmacist if you are taking or planning to take any over-the-counter or prescription medications or dietary supplements while taking thiazolidinediones. Doses of one or both drugs may need to be modified or a different drug may need to be prescribed. Insulin interacts with thiazolidinediones. The following drugs and drug classes interact with pioglitazone only:

- azole antifungals (eg, ketoconazole)
- calcium channel blockers (eg, diltiazem)
- contraceptives, oral (eg, *Ortho-Novum*) (pioglitazone only)
- corticosteroids
- cyclosporine (eg, *Neoral*)
- erythromycin (eg, *E-Mycin*)
- HMG-CoA reductase inhibitors (eg, lovastatin)
- tacrolimus (*Prograf*)
- triazolam (*Halcion*)
- trimetrexate (*Neutrexin*)

Side Effects:

Every drug is capable of producing side effects. Many thiazolidinedione users experience no, or minor, side effects. The frequency and severity of side effects depend on many factors including dose, duration of therapy, and individual susceptibility. Possible side effects include:

Digestive Tract: Nausea; diarrhea; weight gain.

Other: Headache; runny nose; sore throat; muscle or back pain; fluid retention; upper respiratory tract infection; elevated liver enzymes; dark urine; anemia; blood sugar changes; abnormal blood tests.

Guidelines for Use:

- Dosage will be individualized. Take exactly as prescribed.
- Do not change the dose or stop taking unless advised by your doctor. This could have serious consequences.
- Take pioglitazone once daily without regard to meals.
- Take rosiglitazone as a single dose or divided into 2 doses. May be taken without regard to meals.
- Dietary restriction, weight loss (if obese), and exercise are essential to optimal management of diabetes and help improve insulin sensitivity. Follow your prescribed diet and exercise program closely.
- During periods of stress such as fever, trauma, infection, or surgery, medication requirements may change. Consult your doctor.
- Insulin, a sulfonylurea, or a metformin dose may need to be reduced if hypoglycemia occurs when starting a thiazolidinedione.
- Notify your doctor immediately if you experience nausea, vomiting, stomach pain, fatigue, appetite loss, dark urine, yellowing of skin or eyes.
- Talk to your doctor about low blood sugar risks, predisposing conditions, symptoms (eg, numbness, fatigue, hunger, sweating, rapid pulse, confusion) and treatment (administration of sugar-containing beverage or food) associated with combination therapy with insulin or other oral antidiabetic agents.
- Thiazolidinediones may cause ovulation in nonovulating premenopausal women. Talk to your doctor about adequate contraception.
- Pioglitazone may reduce the effectiveness of oral contraceptives (eg, *Ortho-Novum*). Talk to your doctor about an oral contraceptive with higher levels of estrogen and progestin or an alternative method of contraception.
- Lab tests will be required to monitor therapy. Be sure to keep appointments.
- Store at room temperature (59° to 86°F) in a tightly closed container. Protect from light and moisture.

If you have any questions, consult your doctor, pharmacist, or health care provider.

	Generic Name *Brand Name Examples*	Supplied As	Generic Available
Rx	**Acetohexamide**	**Tablets:** 250 mg, 500 mg	Yes
Rx	**Chlorpropamide**		
	Diabinese	**Tablets:** 100 mg, 250 mg	Yes
Rx	**Glimepiride**		
	Amaryl	**Tablets:** 1 mg, 2 mg, 4 mg	No
Rx	**Glipizide**		
	Glucotrol	**Tablets:** 5 mg, 10 mg	Yes
	Glucotrol XL	**Tablets, extended release**: 2.5 mg, 5 mg, 10 mg	No
Rx	**Glyburide (Glibenclamide)**		
	DiaBeta, Micronase	**Tablets:** 1.25 mg, 2.5 mg, 5 mg	Yes
	Glynase PresTab	**Tablets, micronized:** 1.5 mg, 3 mg, 4.5 mg, 6 mg	Yes
Rx	**Tolazamide**		
	Tolinase	**Tablets:** 100 mg, 250 mg, 500 mg	Yes
Rx	**Tolbutamide**		
	Orinase	**Tablets:** 500 mg	Yes

All of the products listed on this table are sulfonylureas; however, they are not interchangeable. For example, glipizide cannot be used for tolazamide. Daily dose may vary depending on individual needs. Do not change the dose without consulting your doctor, pharmacist, or health care provider.

Type of Drug:

Oral antidiabetic agents for use only as an adjunct to diet and exercise in the management of type 2 (non-insulin-dependent) diabetes mellitus.

How the Drug Works:

The sulfonylurea hypoglycemic agents appear to decrease blood sugar by stimulating the release of insulin from the pancreas. Sulfonylureas may also decrease the amount of sugar that is dumped into the blood from the liver and may increase the sensitivity of fat and muscle tissue to the action of insulin. By increasing the amount of insulin or the effectiveness of insulin, blood sugar levels are lowered. Sulfonylureas do not work in type 1 (insulin-dependent) diabetes mellitus in which the pancreas is not capable of manufacturing or releasing insulin.

Uses:

As an adjunct to diet and exercise to lower the blood glucose in patients with type 2 diabetes mellitus whose hyperglycemia cannot be controlled by diet and exercise alone. They may be used alone or combined with other blood sugar lowering medicines (eg, thiazolidinediones, metformin, insulin).

Unlabeled Use(s): Occasionally doctors may prescribe chlorpropamide for the treatment of neurogenic diabetes insipidus.

Precautions:

Do not use in the following situations:

allergy to sulfa drugs
allergy to sulfonylureas or any of their ingredients
diabetes complicated by pregnancy
diabetes complicated by ketoacidosis (with or without coma)
insulin-dependent (type 1) diabetes, sole therapy

Use with caution in the following situations:

debilitation
elderly
gastrointestinal disease (glipizide extended-release only)
kidney disease
liver disease
malnutrition

Alcohol: A reaction may occur, including facial flushing, changes in blood sugar, and breathlessness, when alcohol is ingested. This occurs most often in patients taking chlorpropamide.

Diet and exercise: Diet and exercise are the primary management of type 2 diabetes. Sulfonylureas are used with, not as a substitute for, diet and exercise.

Hyperglycemia (high blood sugar levels): Hyperglycemia is a major risk factor in the development of diabetes complications. Maintaining blood sugar levels as close to normal as possible is important. Symptoms of hyperglycemia include excessive thirst or urination, nausea, and stomach upset.

Hypoglycemia (low blood sugar levels): Patients with kidney or liver problems or patients taking more than 1 blood glucose lowering medicine may be at higher risk for the development of medication-induced hypoglycemia. Symptoms include shaking, dizziness, faintness, headache, irritability, confusion, fatigue, excessive hunger, profuse sweating, numbness of arms or legs, and rapid pulse. May lead to convulsions or coma if extremely severe.

To prevent hypoglycemia:

1. Understand the symptoms of low blood sugar levels.
2. Maintain an adequate diet. Do not miss meals.
3. Frequently monitor blood glucose levels.
4. Keep a source of quick-acting sugar with you at all times.
5. Know how exercise, alcohol, and other drugs affect your blood sugar level.

Hypoglycemia is more of a problem with chlorpropamide than with other medications in this class. Discuss the expected results of your sulfonylurea therapy with your doctor, pharmacist, or diabetes educator. Know the onset of action, peak activity, and total duration of activity.

Heart disease: Long-term use of sulfonylureas has been associated with increased risk for development of heart problems compared with diet alone or diet plus insulin.

Sulfonylureas	Doses/day	Onset (hrs)	Duration (hrs)
Acetohexamide	1 to 2	1	12 to 24
Chlorpropamide	1	1	24 to 60
Glimepiride	1	2 to 3	24
Glipizide	1 to 2	1 to 3	10 to 24
Glyburide, micronized	1 to 2	1	12 to 24
Glyburide, nonmicronized	1 to 2	2 to 4	16 to 24
Tolazamide	1	4 to 6	12 to 24
Tolbutamide	2 to 3	1	6 to 12

Pregnancy: There are no adequate and well-controlled studies in pregnant women. Use only if clearly needed. In general, avoid sulfonylureas in pregnancy. They will not provide good control in patients whose blood glucose levels cannot be controlled by diet alone. Insulin is recommended to treat pregnant patients with diabetes to maintain blood glucose levels as close to normal as possible.

Breastfeeding: Chlorpropamide is excreted in breast milk. It is not known if other sulfonylureas appear in breast milk. Because of the potential for hypoglycemia in nursing infants, decide whether to discontinue nursing or discontinue the drug. Consult your doctor before you begin breastfeeding.

Children: Safety and effectiveness in children have not been established.

Elderly: Elderly, debilitated, or malnourished patients may be particularly sensitive to sulfonylureas. If there is a tendency toward hypoglycemia (low blood sugar levels), dosage will be reduced or therapy discontinued by your doctor. Use with caution.

Lab tests will be required to monitor therapy. Tests may include blood glucose, glycosylated hemoglobin, and kidney and liver function tests.

Drug Interactions:

Tell your doctor or pharmacist if you are taking or if you are planning to take any over-the-counter or prescription medications or dietary supplements while taking sulfonylureas. Doses of one or both drugs may need to be modified or a different drug may need to be prescribed. The following drugs and drug classes interact with sulfonylureas:

Decreased Glucose Lowering Effects	Increased Glucose Lowering Effects
calcium channel blockers (eg, verapamil) charcoal cholestyramine (eg, *Questran*) contraceptives, oral (eg, *Ortho-Novum*) corticosteroids (eg, prednisone) diazoxide (eg, *Proglycem*) estrogens (eg, oral contraceptives, estradiol) glucocorticoids (eg, prednisone) hydantoins (eg, phenytoin) isoniazid (eg, *Laniazid*) nicotinic acid (eg, *Nicobid*) phenothiazines (eg, chlorpromazine) rifampin (eg, *Rifadin*) sympathomimetics (eg, epinephrine) thiazide diuretics (eg, hydrochlorothiazide) thyroid agents (eg, levothyroxine sodium) urinary alkalinizers (eg, sodium bicarbonate)	androgens (eg, testosterone) anticoagulants, oral (eg, warfarin) azole antifungals (eg, ketoconazole) beta adrenergic blockers (eg, propranolol) chloramphenicol (eg, *Chloromycetin*) clofibrate (eg, *Atromid-S*) fenfluramine (*Pondimin*) gemfibrozil (*Lopid*) histamine H_2 antagonists (eg, cimetidine) magnesium salts (eg, *Magonate*) MAOIs (eg, phenelzine) methyldopa (eg, *Aldomet*) probenecid (eg, *Benemid*) salicylates, large doses (eg, aspirin) sulfinpyrazone (eg, *Anturane*) sulfonamides (eg, sulfisoxazole) tricyclic antidepressants (eg, doxepin HCl) urinary acidifiers (eg, ammonium chloride)

Other: Digitalis glycosides (eg, digoxin); ciprofloxacin (eg, *Cipro*); ethanol; barbiturates (eg, phenobarbital).

Side Effects:

Every drug is capable of producing side effects. Many sulfonylurea users experience no, or minor, side effects. The frequency and severity of side effects depend on many factors including dose, duration of therapy, and individual susceptibility. Possible side effects include:

Digestive Tract: Nausea; heartburn; feeling of fullness; diarrhea; vomiting; appetite loss; taste alteration (tolbutamide only); gas; constipation; stomach pain; indigestion; hunger.

Nervous System: Weakness; dizziness; headache; abnormal skin sensations; drowsiness; nervousness; tremor; sleeplessness; anxiety; depression; decreased sensitivity to stimulation; confusion.

Skin: Yellowing of the skin or eyes; rash; hives; dry, red skin; itching; sensitivity to sunlight; sweating.

Other: Abnormal blood counts and blood tests; pain; dark urine; leg cramps; fainting; joint or muscle pain; runny nose; blurred vision; excessive urination; low blood sugar.

Guidelines for Use:

- Dosage is individualized. Do not change dose or stop taking this medicine unless advised to do so by your doctor.
- Follow the diet and exercise program and personal hygiene and infection avoidance regimens exactly as prescribed by your doctor.
- May be taken with food if stomach upset occurs. Always take immediate-release glipizide 30 minutes prior to a meal to increase effectiveness.
- Avoid alcohol. It can cause flushing, breathlessness, and changes in blood sugar.
- Avoid aspirin in large doses.
- Get specific instructions from your doctor on how to examine your feet for complications of diabetes. In addition, obtain equipment for and learn the correct process of home glucose monitoring.
- Monitor blood sugar levels as recommended by your doctor. Notify your doctor if you experience low blood sugar symptoms (eg, fatigue, excessive hunger, profuse sweating, numbness of arms or legs, rapid pulse, confusion) or high blood sugar symptoms (eg, bad breath, excessive thirst or urination).
- Diet and exercise are the primary managements of type 2 diabetes. These medications should be used with, not as a substitute for, diet and exercise.
- *To prevent hypoglycemia* — Understand the symptoms of low blood sugar levels. Maintain an adequate diet. Do not miss meals. Know how exercise, alcohol, and other drugs affect blood sugar levels.
- During periods of stress such as fever, trauma, infection, or surgery, medication requirements may change. Consult your doctor.
- Long-term use of sulfonylureas may be associated with increased heart problems when compared with diet treatment alone, or diet plus insulin. Patients with heart problems or concern about heart problems should consult their doctor.
- *Glipizide, extended-release* — Do not crush, chew, or divide tablets. Do not be alarmed if the tablet shell appears in the stool. This drug is designed to slowly release the medicine and then expel the empty shell from the body.
- May cause sensitivity to sunlight. Avoid prolonged exposure to the sun. Use sunscreens and wear protective clothing until tolerance is determined.
- May cause drowsiness or dizziness. Use caution while driving or performing other tasks requiring alertness, coordination, or physical dexterity.
- Lab tests will be required to monitor therapy. Be sure to keep appointments.
- Store at controlled room temperature. Protect from moisture.

If you have any questions, consult your doctor, pharmacist, or health care provider.

	Generic Name *Brand Name Examples*	Supplied As	Generic Available
Rx	**Nateglinide**		
	Starlix	**Tablets**: 60 mg, 120 mg	No
Rx	**Repaglinide**		
	Prandin	**Tablets:** 0.5 mg, 1 mg, 2 mg	No

Type of Drug:

Oral nonsulfonylurea blood-glucose-lowering drugs for management of type 2 diabetes mellitus (previously known as non-insulin-dependent diabetes mellitus [NIDDM]).

How the Drug Works:

Meglitinides lower blood glucose levels by stimulating the release of insulin from functioning beta cells of the pancreas.

Uses:

To treat high blood glucose, in addition to diet and exercise, in patients with type 2 diabetes mellitus whose blood sugar cannot be controlled by diet and exercise alone.

To treat high blood glucose in combination with metformin (*Glucophage*) when blood sugar cannot be controlled by exercise, diet, and either a meglitinide or metformin alone.

Precautions:

Do not use in the following situations:

- allergy to the meglitinide or any of its ingredients
- diabetic ketoacidosis with or without coma
- type 1 diabetes (previously known as insulin-dependent diabetes)

Use with caution in the following situations:

- adrenal or pituitary insufficiency
- debilitation or malnourishment
- liver disease, moderate to severe
- loss of blood sugar control
- low blood sugar

Diet and exercise: Diet and exercise are the primary managements of type 2 diabetes. Meglitinides are used with, not as a substitute for, diet and exercise.

Heart problems: Meglitinides may increase the risk of heart problems, compared with treatment with diet alone or diet plus insulin.

Pregnancy: There are no adequate and well-controlled studies in pregnant women. Use only if clearly needed and the potential benefits to the mother outweigh the possible hazards to the fetus.

Breastfeeding: It is not known if meglitinides appear in breast milk. Consult your doctor before you begin breastfeeding.

Children: Safety and effectiveness in children have not been established.

Lab tests will be required during treatment. Tests may include blood glucose and glycosylated hemoglobin HbA_{1c} levels.

Drug Interactions:

Tell your doctor or pharmacist if you are taking or planning to take any over-the-counter or prescription medications or dietary supplements while taking a meglitinide. Doses of one or both drugs may need to be modified, or a different drug may need to be prescribed. The following drugs and drug classes interact with meglitinides:

antibacterial agents (eg, chloramphenicol, erythromycin, isoniazid, rifampin, sulfonamides)
antifungal agents (eg, ketoconazole, miconazole)
barbiturates (eg, phenobarbital)
beta-adrenergic blocking agents (eg, atenolol)
calcium channel blockers (eg, verapamil)
carbamazepine (eg, *Tegretol*)
corticosteroids (eg, hydrocortisone, prednisone)
coumarin derivatives (eg, warfarin)
diuretics (eg, thiazides)
estrogens (eg, oral contraceptives, estradiol)
MAO inhibitors (eg, phenelzine)
NSAIDs (eg, ibuprofen)
phenothiazines (eg, *Thorazine*)
phenytoin (eg, *Dilantin*)
probenecid
salicylates (eg, aspirin)
sympathomimetics (eg, pseudoephedrine)
thyroid agents

Side Effects:

Every drug is capable of producing side effects. Many meglitinide users experience no, or minor, side effects. The frequency and severity of side effects depend on many factors including dose, duration of therapy, and individual susceptibility. Possible side effects include:

Digestive Tract: Nausea; diarrhea; constipation; vomiting; indigestion.

Respiratory System: Chest or head congestion; bronchitis; sinus inflammation; upper respiratory tract infection; cough.

Other: Abnormal skin sensations; changes in blood sugar; joint, chest, or back pain; headache; urinary tract infection; flu-like symptoms; dizziness; accidental trauma; heart problems (eg, high blood pressure, abnormal heart rhythm, pounding in the chest).

Guidelines for Use:

- Dosage is individualized. Take exactly as prescribed.
- Do not change the dose or stop taking this medicine unless advised to do so by your doctor.
- Take nateglinide 1 to 30 minutes before a meal. Take repaglinide 15 to 30 minutes before a meal.
- Meglitinides stimulate pancreatic insulin secretion within 20 to 30 minutes of oral administration. Peak insulin levels are attained about 1 hour after dosing and return to baseline within about 4 hours after dosing.
- When a meglitinide is used to replace therapy with another oral hypoglycemic agent, it may be started the day after the final dose is given. Closely monitor for hypoglycemia because of a potential overlapping drug effect (particularly with long-acting sulfonylureas [eg, chlorpropamide]).
- Treatment may need to be adjusted. Your doctor will monitor your treatment for the first few weeks of therapy.
- Patients who skip a meal (or add an extra meal) should skip (or add) a dose for that meal. Contact your doctor or pharmacist if you miss a dose.
- Repaglinide may be taken in combination with metformin. One or both dosages may need to be adjusted.
- Follow the diet and exercise program exactly as prescribed by your doctor.
- Diabetic patients may experience loss of glucose control. Be prepared to monitor blood sugar more often.
- Monitor blood glucose levels daily. Notify your doctor if symptoms of hypoglycemia occur (eg, fatigue, excessive hunger, profuse sweating, numbness of extremities) or if blood glucose is below 60 mg/dL. Notify your doctor if symptoms of hyperglycemia occur (eg, bad breath, excessive thirst or urination) or if blood glucose is consistently above 200 mg/dL.
- Lab tests are required to monitor treatment. Be sure to keep appointments.
- Store below 77°F. Protect from moisture. Keep in tightly closed container.

If you have any questions, consult your doctor, pharmacist, or health care provider.

	Generic Name *Brand Name Examples*	Supplied As	Generic Available
Rx	**Metformin HCl**		
	Glucophage	**Tablets**: 500 mg, 850 mg, 1000 mg	No
	Glucophage XR	**Tablets, extended-release**: 500 mg	No

Type of Drug:

Oral nonsulfoylurea antidiabetic agent used in the treatment of type 2 diabetes mellitus (previously referred to as non-insulin-dependent diabetes mellitus [NIDDM]).

How the Drug Works:

Metformin reduces the amount of glucose produced by the liver and the amount of glucose absorbed by the intestines, and enhances insulin sensitivity by increasing peripheral glucose uptake and utilization.

Uses:

Used as monotherapy along with diet and exercise to treat type 2 diabetes mellitus. May also be prescribed for use with a sulfonylurea, meglitinide, or insulin.

Precautions:

Do not use in the following situations:

- allergy to metformin or any of its ingredients
- congestive heart failure
- diabetic ketoacidosis
- kidney disease or dysfunction
- metabolic acidosis, acute or chronic
- radiologic studies involving "dyes"

Use with caution in the following situations:

- alcohol use
- elderly
- heart disease
- infections
- liver disease
- stroke
- surgery
- vitamin B_{12}, decreased levels

Lactic acidosis: Lactic acidosis is a rare but serious side effect that can occur when taking this medication, particularly if kidney function is impaired. Stop taking this medicine and contact your doctor immediately if you experience general body discomfort, muscle pain, difficulty breathing, drowsiness, stomach pain, chills, dizziness, lightheadedness, or slow heartbeat.

Diet and exercise: Diet and exercise are the primary managements of type 2 diabetes. Metformin is used with, not as a substitute for, diet and exercise.

Heart problems: This medicine may increase the risk of heart problems compared to treatment with diet alone or diet plus insulin.

Pregnancy: There are no adequate and well-controlled studies in pregnant women. Pregnant women with diabetes should be treated with insulin. Metformin is not recommended for control of blood sugar levels in pregnant women.

Breastfeeding: It is not known if metformin appears in breast milk. Consult your doctor before you begin breastfeeding.

Children: Safety and effectiveness for use of metformin tablets in patients under 10 years of age and metformin extended-release tablets in patients under 17 years of age have not been established.

Elderly: Elderly and debilitated patients are more likely to develop hypoglycemia (low blood sugar levels). Use with caution.

Lab tests will be required to monitor therapy. Tests include blood glucose, glycosylated hemoglobin (HbA_{1c}), and kidney function tests.

Drug Interactions:

Tell your doctor or pharmacist if you are taking or planning to take any over-the-counter or prescription medications or dietary supplements while taking metformin. Doses of one or both drugs may need to be modified or a different drug may need to be prescribed. The following drugs and drug classes interact with metformin:

- alcohol (acute or chronic use)
- amiloride (*Midamor*)
- calcium channel blockers (eg, nifedipine)
- cimetidine (eg, *Tagamet*)
- corticosteroids (eg, prednisone)
- digoxin (eg, *Lanoxin*)
- diuretics (eg, thiazides)
- estrogens (eg, oral contraceptives, estradiol)
- furosemide (eg, *Lasix*)
- iodinated contrast material (eg, x-ray dye)
- isoniazid
- morphine (eg, *Duramorph*)
- nicotinic acid (eg, *Niacor*)
- phenothiazines (eg, chlorpromazine)
- phenytoin (eg, *Dilantin*)
- procainamide (eg, *Pronestyl*)
- quinidine (eg, *Quinora*)
- quinine
- ranitidine (eg, *Zantac*)
- sympathomimetics (eg, epinephrine)
- thyroid products
- triamterene (*Dyrenium*)
- trimethorprim (eg, *Trimpex*)
- vancomycin (eg, *Vancocin*)

Side Effects:

Every drug is capable of producing side effects. Many metformin users experience no, or minor, side effects. The frequency or severity of side effects depend on many factors including dose, duration of therapy, and individual susceptibility. Possible side effects include:

Digestive Tract: Diarrhea; nausea; vomiting; stomach bloating or pain; gas; constipation; indigestion; abnormal stools; heartburn.

Nervous System: Light-headedness; headache; weakness; dizziness.

Other: Changes in taste perception; rash; difficulty breathing; increased sweating; low blood pressure; muscle pain; upper respiratory infection; chest discomfort; chills; flu-like symptoms; flushing; palpitations (pounding in the chest).

Guidelines for Use:

- Dosage is individualized. Take exactly as prescribed. May be taken with other antidiabetic medication.
- Tablets are usually taken twice daily with the morning and evening meals. Extended-release tablets are usually taken once daily with the evening meal.
- Follow the diet and exercise program exactly as prescribed by your doctor.
- If a dose is missed, take it as soon as possible. If several hours have passed or it is nearing time for the next dose, do not double the dose to catch up, unless advised to do so by your doctor. If more than one dose is missed or it is necessary to establish a new dosage schedule, contact your doctor or pharmacist.
- Contact your doctor immediately if you experience difficulty breathing, muscle pain, general body discomfort, drowsiness, dizziness, light-headedness, slow heartbeat, stomach pain, or chills.
- Nausea, vomiting, diarrhea, gas, and appetite loss generally stop with continued use. If they continue, contact your doctor immediately.
- Avoid drinking alcohol while undergoing therapy with metformin.
- The effectiveness of this medicine may decrease over time. If you feel that it is losing its effectiveness, contact your doctor.
- Patients switched from metformin tablets to extended-release tablets do not appear to require dosage adjustments, but glycemic control should be closely monitored when switches occur.
- Lab tests will be required to monitor therapy. Be sure to keep appointments.
- Store at room temperature (59° to 86°F).

If you have any questions, consult your doctor, pharmacist, or health care provider.

Generic Name *Brand Name Example*	Supplied As	Generic Available
Rx **Glyburide/Metformin HCl**		
Glucovance	**Tablets**: 1.25 mg/250 mg, 2.5 mg/500 mg, 5 mg/500 mg	No

Type of Drug:

Combination oral antidiabetic agent used in the treatment of type 2 diabetes mellitus (previously referred to as non-insulin-dependent diabetes mellitus [NIDDM]).

How the Drug Works:

Glyburide stimulates the release of insulin from the pancreas acutely and lowers glucose chronically by unknown mechanisms. Metformin reduces the amount of sugar produced by the liver and the amount absorbed by the intestines and enhances insulin sensitivity.

Uses:

Used as initial therapy, along with diet and exercise, to treat type 2 diabetes. Also used as second-line therapy when diet, exercise, and initial treatment with a sulfonylurea or metformin used alone is not sufficient.

Precautions:

Do not use in the following situations:

allergy to glyburide, metformin, or any of their ingredients
congestive heart failure
diabetic ketoacidosis
kidney disease or dysfunction
metabolic acidosis, acute or chronic
radiologic studies involving "dyes"

Use with caution in the following situations:

alcohol use
elderly
heart disease
infections
liver disease
stroke
surgery
vitamin B_{12}, decreased levels

Lactic acidosis: Lactic acidosis is a rare but serious side effect that can occur when taking this medication, particularly if kidney function is impaired. Stop taking this medicine and contact your doctor immediately if you experience general body discomfort, muscle pain, difficulty breathing, drowsiness, stomach pain, chills, dizziness, lightheadedness, or slow heartbeat.

Diet and exercise: Diet and exercise are the primary managements of type 2 diabetes. Glyburide/metformin is used with, not as a substitute for, diet and exercise.

Heart problems: This medicine may increase the risk of heart problems compared to treatment with diet alone or diet plus insulin.

Pregnancy: There are no adequate and well-controlled studies in pregnant women. Pregnant women with diabetes should be treated with insulin. Glyburide/metformin is not recommended for control of blood sugar levels in pregnant women.

Breastfeeding: It is not known if glyburide/metformin appears in breast milk. Consult your doctor before you begin breastfeeding.

Children: Safety and effectiveness in children have not been established.

Elderly: Elderly and debilitated patients are more likely to develop hypoglycemia (low blood sugar levels). Use with caution.

Lab tests will be required to monitor therapy. Tests include blood glucose, glycosylated hemoglobin (HbA_{1c}), and kidney function tests.

Drug Interactions:

Tell your doctor or pharmacist if you are taking or planning to take any over-the-counter or prescription medications or dietary supplements while taking glyburide/metformin. Doses of one or both drugs may need to be modified or a different drug may need to be prescribed. The following drugs and drug classes interact with glyburide/metformin:

alcohol (acute or chronic use)
amiloride (*Midamor*)
beta-adrenergic blocking agents (atenolol)
calcium channel blockers (eg, nifedipine)
chloramphenicol (eg, *Chloromycetin*)
cimetidine (eg, *Tagamet*)
ciprofloxacin (*Cipro*)
clofibrate (eg, *Atromid-S*)
corticosteroids (eg, prednisone)
coumarin derivatives (eg, warfarin)
diazoxide (eg, *Proglycem*)
digoxin (eg, *Lanoxin*)
diuretics (eg, thiazides)
estrogens (eg, oral contraceptives, estradiol)
furosemide (eg, *Lasix*)
iodinated contrast material (eg, x-ray dye)
isoniazid
MAO inhibitors (eg, phenelzine)
miconazole (eg, *Monistat*)
morphine (eg, *Duramorph*)
nicotinic acid (eg, *Niacor*)
NSAIDs (eg, ibuprofen)
phenothiazines (eg, chlorpromazine)
phenylbutazones (eg, oxyphenbutazone)
phenytoin (eg, *Dilantin*)
probenecid
procainamide (eg, *Pronestyl*)
quinidine (eg, *Quinora*)
quinine
ranitidine (eg, *Zantac*)
rifampin (eg, *Rifadin*)
salicylates (eg, aspirin)
sulfonamides (eg, sulfisoxazole)
sympathomimetics (eg, epinephrine)
thyroid products
triamterene (*Dyrenium*)
trimethorprim (eg, *Trimpex*)
vancomycin (eg, *Vancocin*)

Side Effects:

Every drug is capable of producing side effects. Many glyburide/metformin users experience no, or minor, side effects. The frequency or severity of side effects depend on many factors including dose, duration of therapy, and individual susceptibility. Possible side effects include:

Nervous System: Chills; drowsiness; light-headedness; headache; dizziness; shakiness.

Digestive Tract: Diarrhea; nausea; vomiting; stomach pain.

Other: Upper respiratory infection; difficulty breathing; muscle pain; rash; changes in taste perception; low blood pressure; sweating; hunger.

Guidelines for Use:

- Dosage is individualized. Take exactly as prescribed.
- Take with meals.
- Follow the diet and exercise program exactly as prescribed by your doctor.
- If a dose is missed, take it as soon as possible. If several hours have passed or it is nearing time for the next dose, do not double the dose to catch up, unless advised to do so by your doctor. If more than one dose is missed or it is necessary to establish a new dosage schedule, contact your doctor or pharmacist.
- Contact your doctor immediately if you experience difficulty breathing, muscle pain, general body discomfort, drowsiness, dizziness, light-headedness, slow heartbeat, stomach pain, or chills.
- Nausea, vomiting, and diarrhea generally stop with continued use. If they continue, contact your doctor immediately.
- Avoid drinking alcohol while undergoing therapy with glyburide/metformin.
- The effectiveness of this medicine may decrease over time. If you feel that it is losing its effectiveness, contact your doctor.
- Lab tests will be required to monitor therapy. Be sure to keep appointments.
- Store below 77°F. Protect from light.

If you have any questions, consult your doctor, pharmacist, or health care provider.

GLUCOSE ELEVATING AGENTS – GLUCAGON

	Generic Name *Brand Name Examples*	Supplied As	Generic Available
Rx	**Glucagon (rDNA Origin)**		
	Glucagon Diagnostic Kit, Glucagon Emergency Kit	**Injection**: 1 mg (1 unit)	Yes

Type of Drug:

A blood glucose (sugar) elevating agent.

How the Drug Works:

Glucagon is a natural hormone that is released from the pancreas. It elevates blood sugar in a variety of ways (eg, inhibition of glucogen synthesis, enhanced formation of glucose from noncarbohydrates and fat, increased hydrolysis of glucogen to glucose).

Uses:

Used to treat severe hypoglycemia (low blood glucose levels). Because patients with type 1 diabetes may have less of an increase in blood glucose levels compared with a stable type 2 diabetes patient, a supplementary carbohydrate should be given as soon as possible, especially to a pediatric patient.

Used as a diagnostic aid in the x-ray examination of the stomach, duodenum, small intestine, and colon when decreased intestinal motility is desired.

Unlabeled Use(s): Occasionally doctors may prescribe glucagon for treatment of an overdose of propranolol and in cardiovascular emergencies (eg, severely reduced heart rates).

Precautions:

Do not use in the following situations: Allergy to glucagon or any of its ingredients.

Use with caution in the following situations:

pheochromocytoma, active or history of
tumor of the pancreas, history of

Hypoglycemia (low blood sugar levels): Although glucagon may be used for emergency treatment of low blood sugar levels, notify your doctor so that adjustments in insulin dose and dietary factors can be made. In addition, patients should be given food after they become conscious and alert. Frequently self monitor blood glucose so that blood sugar levels are not allowed to get too low.

Pregnancy: There are no adequate and well-controlled studies in pregnant women. Use only if clearly needed and the potential benefits to the mother outweigh the possible hazards to the fetus.

Breastfeeding: It is not known if glucagon appears in breast milk. Consult your doctor before you begin breastfeeding.

Children: Safety and effectiveness for use in the treatment of hypoglycemia in children have been established.

Lab tests will be required to monitor therapy. Tests include blood glucose levels.

Drug Interactions:

Tell your doctor or pharmacist if you are taking or planning to take any over-the-counter or prescription medications or dietary supplements while taking glucagon. Doses of one or both drugs may need to be modified or a different drug may need to be prescribed. Oral anticoagulants (eg, warfarin) interact with glucagon.

Side Effects:

Every drug is capable of producing side effects. Many glucagon users experience no, or minor, side effects. The frequency and severity of side effects depend on many factors including dose, duration of therapy, and individual susceptibility. Possible side effects include: Nausea; vomiting; hives; low blood pressure; difficulty breathing.

Guidelines for Use:

- Carefully read the patient instructions provided with the product.
- All patients with diabetes should have a *Glucagon Emergency Kit.*
- *Low blood sugar (conscious patient)* — Consume fast-acting sugars (eg, *B-D Glucose*, *Glutose*).
- *Low blood sugar (unconscious patient)* — Intravenous (IV; into a vein) glucose use is encouraged, if available and feasible. If not, glucagon is the treatment of choice. Instruct friends, coworkers, and family members of patients with diabetes how to administer glucagon. Prompt treatment is essential.
- The patient will usually awaken within 15 minutes of glucagon use. If not, repeat the dose. Upon awakening, give the patient food (ie, a carbohydrate) as soon as possible and follow the usual dietary regimen.
- The glucagon emergency kit has a diluting fluid in a unit (one) dose syringe. This diluting fluid is injected into a vial of the glucagon crystals. The vial is then shaken and the contents brought back into the syringe. The glucagon crystals now in the diluting fluid are given IV, intramuscularly (IM; into a muscle), or subcutaneously (SC; under the skin).
- Notify your doctor if you experience a hypoglycemic reaction so that your treatment regimen may be adjusted if necessary.
- Lab tests will be required. Be sure to keep appointments.
- Store at controlled room temperature (68° to 77° F) before mixing with the diluting fluid.
- Use glucagon immediately after it has been mixed with the diluting fluid because the drug is stable for only a short time. Discard any unused portion.

If you have any questions, consult your doctor, pharmacist, or health care provider.

THYROID DRUGS — ANTITHYROID AGENTS

	Generic Name *Brand Name Examples*	Supplied As	Generic Available
Rx	**Methimazole**		
	Tapazole	**Tablets**: 5 mg, 10 mg	Yes
Rx	**Propylthiouracil (PTU)**	**Tablets**: 50 mg	Yes
Rx	**Sodium Iodide I 131**	**Capsules**: 0.75 to 100 mCi	Yes
		Solution, oral: 3.5 to 150 mCi	Yes
	Iodotope	**Capsules**: 1 to 130 mCi	No
	Iodotope	**Solution, oral**: 7.05 mCi	No

Type of Drug:

Antithyroid drugs.

How the Drug Works:

The oral antithyroid drugs inhibit the formation of thyroid hormones.

Uses:

To treat hyperthyroidism (overactive thyroid gland). To treat or prepare the overactive thyroid for surgery or radioactive iodine therapy. Sodium iodide I 131 preparations may be used to treat certain forms of thyroid cancer.

Unlabeled Use(s): Occasionally doctors may prescribe propylthiouracil to treat liver disease due to alcoholism.

Precautions:

Do not use in the following situations:

allergy to the antithyroid agent or any of its ingredients
breastfeeding

Pregnancy: Studies have shown a potential adverse effect to the fetus. Use only if clearly needed and the potential benefits to the mother outweigh the possible hazards to the fetus. These agents, if used carefully, are effective in treating hyperthyroidism complicated by pregnancy. Dose must be adequate but not excessive. These drugs cross the placenta and could induce goiter or even cretinism (congenital lack of thyroid secretion which can stop physical and mental development) in the fetus. Propylthiouracil is less likely than methimazole to cross the placenta.

Breastfeeding: Patients receiving antithyroid preparations should not breastfeed.

Children: Safety and effectiveness of sodium iodide I 131 in children have not been established. Sodium iodide I 131 is not usually used for treatment of hyperthyroidism in patients under 30 years of age unless circumstances preclude other methods of treatment.

Lab tests will be required to monitor therapy. Tests include blood counts, bone marrow function, and thyroid function.

Drug Interactions:

Tell your doctor or pharmacist if you are taking or planning to take any over-the-counter or prescription medications or dietary supplements while taking an antithyroid agent. Doses of one or both drugs may need to be modified or a different drug may need to be prescribed. The following drugs or drug classes interact with antithyroid agents:

- anticoagulants (eg, warfarin)
- beta-adrenergic blocking agents (eg, atenolol)
- digoxin (eg, *Lanoxin*)
- theophylline (eg, *Slo-Phyllin*)

Side Effects:

Every drug is capable of producing side effects. Many antithyroid agent users experience no, or minor, side effects. The frequency and severity of side effects depend on many factors including dose, duration of therapy, and individual susceptibility. Possible side effects include:

Digestive Tract: Nausea; vomiting; stomach upset or pain; loss of taste sensation; swelling of salivary glands.

Nervous System: Abnormal skin sensations; headache; drowsiness; depression; feeling of whirling motion; hyperactivity.

Skin: Unusual bleeding or bruising; rash; itching; hives; excessive skin pigmentation; yellowing of skin or eyes; abnormal hair loss.

Other: Joint or muscle pain; fever; fluid retention (edema); swollen lymph glands; abnormal blood counts; kidney disease; lung disease; liver disease; low blood sugar.

Other: Sodium iodide I 131 only: Radiation sickness (eg, nausea, vomiting); anemia; chromosomal abnormalities; tenderness and swelling of the neck; pain on swallowing; sore throat; cough; temporary thinning of hair.

Guidelines for Use:

- Dosage is individualized. Take exactly as prescribed.
- Do not change the dose or stop taking this medicine unless advised to do so by your doctor.
- Take methimazole or propylthiouracil at regular intervals around the clock (usually every 8 hours), unless directed otherwise by your doctor.
- Notify your doctor if fever, sore throat, hay fever, unusual bleeding or bruising, headache, general body discomfort, rash, yellowing of the skin, vomiting, itching, appetite loss, skin surface changes, or pain in the upper right side of your body occurs.
- If a dose of methimazole or propylthiouracil is missed, take it as soon as possible. If several hours have passed or it is nearing time for the next dose, do not double the dose to catch up, unless advised to do so by your doctor. If more than one dose is missed or it is necessary to establish a new dosage schedule, contact your doctor or pharmacist.
- Lab tests will be required to monitor therapy. Be sure to keep appointments.
- Store methimazole or propylthiouracil at room temperature (59° to 86°F). Store sodium iodide I 131 at room temperature controlled in compliance with government regulations.

If you have any questions, consult your doctor, pharmacist, or health care provider.

	Generic Name *Brand Name Examples*	Supplied As	Generic Available
Rx	**Iodine Products**		
	Strong Iodine Solution (Lugol's Solution)	**Solution**: 5% iodine and 10% potassium iodide	No
	Thyro-Block[1]	**Tablets**: 130 mg potassium iodide	No

[1] Available only to state and federal agencies.

Type of Drug:

Iodine drugs.

How the Drug Works:

Iodine intake is necessary for normal thyroid function and the synthesis of thyroid hormones levothyroxine (T_4) and liothyronine (T_3). Adequate iodine is generally consumed with a balanced diet.

Extremely large doses of iodine may, however, decrease the synthesis and release of the thyroid hormones. This effect forms the basis for using large doses of iodine to treat an overactive thyroid gland (hyperthyroidism).

Uses:

For use with an antithyroid drug in hyperthyroid patients prior to thyroid surgery or to treat an overactive thyroid gland.

To block the thyroid gland during a radiation emergency (eg, radioactive fallout).

Unlabeled Use(s): Occasionally, doctors may prescribe potassium iodide with topical steroids to treat Sweet disease (acute febrile neutrophilic dermatosis), to treat lymphocutaneous sporotrichosis (a fungus that infects the skin and lymphatic system), or as an expectorant for cough.

Precautions:

Do not use in the following situations: Allergy to the iodine product or any of its ingredients.

Pregnancy: Studies have shown a potential risk to the fetus. Use only if clearly needed and the potential benefits to the mother outweigh the possible hazards to the fetus.

Breastfeeding: Iodine products appear in breast milk. Consult your doctor before you begin breastfeeding.

Drug Interactions:

Tell your doctor or pharmacist if you are taking or planning to take any over-the-counter or prescription medications or dietary supplements while taking an iodine product. Doses of one or both drugs may need to be modified or a different drug may need to be prescribed. Lithium (eg, *Eskalith*) interacts with iodine products.

Side Effects:

Every drug is capable of producing side effects. Many iodine product users experience no, or minor, side effects. The frequency and severity of side effects depend on many factors including dose, duration of therapy, and individual susceptibility. Possible side effects include:

Digestive Tract: Swelling of the salivary glands; metallic taste; burning mouth and throat; sore teeth and gums; upset stomach; diarrhea.

Respiratory System: Symptoms of a head cold; shortness of breath.

Other: Rash; fever; joint pain; swelling of parts of the face and body.

Guidelines for Use:

- Use exactly as prescribed.
- *Strong iodine solution*— Dilute with water or fruit juice to improve taste.
- *Thyroid surgery*— Oral iodine-containing products are usually given for 10 days prior to surgery.
- Discontinue use and notify your doctor if fever, skin rash, metallic taste, swelling of the throat, burning of the mouth and throat, sore teeth and gums, head cold symptoms, severe stomach distress, diarrhea, shortness of breath or enlargement of the thyroid gland (goiter) occurs.
- If a dose is missed, take it as soon as possible. If several hours have passed or if it is nearing time for the next dose, do not double the dose in order to "catch up" (unless advised to do so by your doctor). If more than one dose is missed or if it is necessary to establish a new dosage schedule, contact your doctor or pharmacist.
- *Recommended Dietary Allowances (RDA)*— Adults: 150 mcg.
- If crystals are present in the solution, dissolve by warming the solution and shaking gently.
- Discard solution if it becomes discolored (eg, brownish yellow).
- Store at room temperature in a tight container. Do not freeze.

If you have any questions, consult your doctor, pharmacist, or health care provider.

	Generic Name *Brand Name Examples*	Supplied As	Generic Available
Rx	**Thyroid Desiccated**		
	Armour Thyroid, Thyrar, Thyroid Strong	**Tablets:** 15 mg, 30 mg, 60 mg, 90 mg, 120 mg, 180 mg, 240 mg, 300 mg	Yes
	Thyroid Strong	**Tablets, sugar coated:** 30 mg, 60 mg, 120 mg, 180 mg	No
	S-P-T	**Capsules:** 60 mg, 120 mg, 180 mg, 300 mg	No
Rx	**Levothyroxine Sodium (T_4; L-thyroxine)**		
	Eltroxin, Levothroid, Levoxyl, Levo-T, Synthroid	**Tablets:** 0.025 mg, 0.05 mg, 0.075 mg, 0.088 mg, 0.1 mg, 0.112 mg, 0.125 mg, 0.137 mg, 0.15 mg, 0.175 mg, 0.2 mg, 0.3 mg	Yes
	Levothroid, Levoxine, Synthroid	**Injection:** 200 mcg/vial, 500 mcg/vial	Yes
Rx	**Liothyronine Sodium (T_3)**		
	Cytomel	**Tablets:** 5 mcg, 25 mcg, 50 mcg	Yes
	Triostat	**Injection:** 10 mcg/vial	No
Rx	**Liotrix**		
	Thyrolar	**Tablets:** 15 mg, 30 mg, 60 mg, 120 mg, 180 mg	No

Note: 16 mg equals $\frac{1}{4}$grain; 32 mg equals grain; 65 mg equals 1 grain.

Type of Drug:

Thyroid hormones.

How the Drug Works:

The natural thyroid hormone products (eg, desiccated thyroid and thyroqlobulin) are obtained from beef and pork. They are economical, but standardization of iodine content is difficult. The synthetic products, including levothyroxine (T_4), liothyronine (T_3) and liotrix (T_3 and T_4), are generally preferred due to more uniform potency.

Thyroid hormones increase the metabolic rate of body tissues. This involves many varied functions such as oxygen use, respiratory rate, body temperature, heart rate, metabolism of foods, enzyme activity and growth and development of the skeletal and nervous system. Thyroid hormones influence every organ system of the body.

Uses:

To treat hypothyroidism (low thyroid hormone production).

To treat thyroid nodules, chronic lymphocytic thyroiditis (Hashimoto's disease), multinodular goiter and thyroid cancer.

To treat thyrotoxicosis (excessive thyroid hormone production). Used with an antithyroid drug to prevent hypothyroidism.

Precautions:

Do not use in the following situations:

allergy to thyroid hormones
heart attack, recent
obesity, treatment
thyroid deficiency (hypothyroidism) and hypoadrenalism (Addison's disease) together
thyroid gland, overactive (thyrotoxicosis)

Use with caution in the following situations:

Addison's disease
angina (chest pain)
diabetes insipidus
diabetes mellitus
elderly
heart disease
infertility
kidney disease
myxedema (swelling due to hypothroidism)

Pregnancy: This drug appears to be safe for use during pregnancy. Do not discontinue thyroid replacement therapy in hypothyroid (decreased thyroid activity) women during pregnancy.

Breastfeeding: Very small amounts of thyroid hormones appear in breast milk. Use with caution during breastfeeding. The mother and nursing infant should be checked periodically.

Children: Thyroid replacement therapy in children may lead to partial hair loss in the first few months of therapy. This is a temporary condition. Normal hair growth and distribution returns.

Lab tests will be required to monitor therapy. Be sure to keep appointments.

Tartrazine: Some of these products may contain the dye tartrazine (FD&C Yellow No. 5) which can cause allergic reactions in certain individuals. Check package label when available or consult your doctor or pharmacist.

Drug Interactions:

Tell your doctor or pharmacist if you are taking or if you are planning to take any over-the-counter or prescription medications or dietary supplements while taking this medicine. Doses of one or both drugs may need to be modified or a different drug may need to be prescribed. The following drugs and drug classes interact with this medicine:

anticoagulants, oral (eg, *Coumadin*)
beta blockers (eg, propranolol)
cholestyramine (eg, *Questran*)
colestipol (*Colestid*)
digoxin (eg, *Lanoxin*)
estrogens (eg, *Premarin*)
theophyllines (eg, *Theo-Dur*)

Side Effects:

Every drug is capable of producing side effects. Many patients experience no, or minor, side effects. The frequency and severity of side effects depend on many factors including dose, duration of therapy and individual susceptibility.

Side effects other than those indicating too much thyroid due to excessive dosage or too rapid dosage increase are rare. Symptoms of too much thyroid include:

Digestive Tract: Diarrhea; vomiting.

Nervous System: Tremors; headache; nervousness; sleeplessness.

Circulatory System: Increased heart rate; palpitations (pounding in the chest); irregular heartbeat; angina (chest pain); cardiac arrest.

Other: Weight loss; menstrual irregularities; sweating; heat intolerance; fever.

Guidelines for Use:

- Use exactly as prescribed.
- Take as a single daily dose on an empty stomach, preferably before breakfast.
- *Brand interchange* — Do not change from one brand of this drug to another without consulting your pharmacist or doctor. Products manufactured by different companies may not be equally effective.
- Replacement therapy is usually taken for life.
- Do not discontinue medication except on advice of your doctor.
- Notify your doctor if headache, nervousness, sleeplessness diarrhea, excessive sweating, heat intolerance, chest pain, increased heart rate, irregular heartbeat or any unusual event occurs.
- Partial loss of hair may be experienced by children in the first few months of thyroid therapy, but this is usually only temporary.
- Do not use this medication to treat obesity. Thyroid hormones are not effective for weight reduction. Large doses of thyroid medications may produce serious or even life-threatening conditions, especially when taken with appetite suppressants.
- If a dose is missed, take it as soon as possible. If several hours have passed or if it is nearing time for the next dose, do not double the dose in order to "catch up" (unless advised to do so by your doctor). If more than one dose is missed or it is necessary to establish a new dosage schedule, contact your doctor or pharmacist.
- Dosage is individualized to approximate the deficit in thyroid secretion. Your response is evaluated by your doctor with lab tests.
- Store at room temperature away from moisture and light.

If you have any questions, consult your doctor, pharmacist, or health care provider.

	Generic Name *Brand Name Examples*	Supplied As	Generic Available
Rx	**Calcitonin-Salmon**		
	Calcimar, *Miacaicin*, *Osteocalcin*	**Injection:** 200 IU/mL	Yes
	Miacalcin	**Nasal spray:** 200 IU/activation	No

Type of Drug:

Hormone.

How the Drug Works:

Calcitonin is a hormone secreted by specialized cells of the thyroid gland. It plays a major role in calcium and bone metabolism and has direct actions on the kidneys and digestive tract.

Uses:

To treat moderate to severe Paget's disease (injection only), a condition of abnormal and accelerated bone formation and calcium uptake.

For early treatment in high calcium emergencies when a rapid decrease in serum calcium is required, until a more specific treatment can be done. It can also be added to existing therapies for high calcium levels (injection only).

To treat postmenopausal osteoporosis. May prevent the progressive loss of bone mass. Use nasal spray only in patients who cannot take estrogen.

Precautions:

Do not use in the following situations:
allergy to calcitonin-salmon

Use with caution in the following situations:
low calcium levels
osteogenic sarcoma (eg, bone cancer)

Pregnancy: Adequate studies have not been done in pregnant women, or animal studies may have shown a risk to the fetus. Use only if clearly needed and potential benefits outweigh the possible hazards to the fetus.

Breastfeeding: It is not known if calcitonin appears in breast milk. Consult your doctor before you begin breastfeeding.

Children: Bone disorders in children (juvenile Paget's disease) have been reported rarely. There are no data to support use in children.

Lab tests or exams may be necessary to monitor treatment. Be sure to keep appointments. Tests may include: Nasal examinations; skin tests for allergy (prior to treatment); blood calcium levels.

Side Effects:

Every drug is capable of producing side effects. Many patients experience no, or minor, side effects. The frequency and severity of side effects depend on many factors including dose, duration of therapy and individual susceptibility. Possible side effects include:

Digestive Tract: Nausea; vomiting; appetite changes; gas; abdominal pain and discomfort; salty taste.

Nervous System: Headache/migraine; sleeplessness; anxiety; vertigo (feeling of a whirling motion); nerve pain; agitation.

Circulatory System: Fast heartbeat; palpitation (pounding in the chest); heart attack or block; anemia; stroke; inflammation of the veins.

Respiratory System: Nasal congestion; nasal symptoms (eg, irritation, redness, sores); difficulty breathing; sore throat; pneumonia; bronchitis; coughing; distorted sense of smell.

Skin: Inflammation at the injection site; flushing of face or hands; itching of ear lobes; swelling of feet; rashes; skin ulcers; eczema; hair loss; sweating.

Senses: Eye pain; blurred vision; eye floaters (black or white spots); ringing in the ears; earache; hearing loss.

Other: Back, muscle or joint pain; nosebleed; increased urination at night; feverish sensation; weight increase; stiffness; taste distortion; overactive thyroid (eg, weight loss); inflammation of kidney or pelvis; blood in urine; gallstone formation; thirst; yellowing of skin or eyes.

Guidelines for Use:

- Patient instructions for use are enclosed in each package.
- Follow the injection procedure taught to you by your healthcare provider.
- Doses vary according to the condition being treated. Do not adjust dose without consulting your doctor.
- If a dose is missed, inject or inhale it as soon as possible. If several hours have passed or if it is nearing time for the next dose, do not double the dose in order to "catch up" (unless advised to do so by your doctor). If more than one dose is missed or it is necessary to establish a new dosage schedule, contact your doctor or pharmacist.
- *Nasal spray* — To activate (prime) the pump, hold the bottle upright and depress the two white side arms toward the bottle six times until a faint spray is emitted. The pump is activated once the first faint spray has been emitted. At this point, firmly place the nozzle into the nostril with the head in the upright position, and depress the pump toward the bottle. It is not necessary to reactivate the pump before each daily dose.
- Nausea, vomiting and flushing tend to decrease with continued use. Administration at bedtime may be helpful.
- Supplemental vitamin D and calcium should be considered in those receiving calcitonin to treat postmenopausal osteoporosis.
- Contact your doctor if any of the following occurs: Allergic reaction to the drug (eg, shortness of breath, difficult breathing, hives, rash), significant nasal irritation or persistent nausea and vomiting.
- *Storage—*

  Injection: Store in the refrigerator between 36° and 43° F.

  Nasal spray: Store unopened bottle in the refrigerator between 36° and 46° F. Once the pump has been activated, store at room temperature.

If you have any questions, consult your doctor, pharmacist, or health care provider.

	Generic Name *Brand Name Examples*	Supplied As	Generic Available
Rx	**Alendronate Sodium**		
	Fosamax	**Tablets**: 5 mg, 10 mg, 35 mg, 40 mg, 70 mg	No
Rx	**Etidronate Disodium**		
	Didronel[1]	**Tablets**: 200 mg, 400 mg	No
Rx	**Pamidronate Disodium**		
	Aredia	**Powder for injection**: 30 mg, 90 mg	No
Rx	**Risedronate**		
	Actonel	**Tablets**: 5 mg, 30 mg	No
Rx	**Tiludronate Disodium**		
	Skelid	**Tablets**: 200 mg	No
Rx	**Zoledronic Acid**		
	Zometa	**Powder for injection**: 4.26 mg zoledronic acid monohydrate (equiv. to 4 mg zoledronic acid anhydrous)	No

[1] Also available as an intravenous injection.

Type of Drug:

Bisphosphonates.

How the Drug Works:

Bisphosphonates help preserve bone mass by inhibiting normal and abnormal bone loss due to resorption (bone tissue loss). Some of these drugs also help control the balance of calcium in bones and blood in certain cancers.

Uses:

To treat Paget disease of bone (alendronate, etidronate, pamidronate, risedronate, tiludronate only).

To treat osteolytic bone metastases of breast cancer and osteolytic bone lesions of multiple myeloma in conjuction with standard antineoplastic therapy (pamidronate only).

To treat high calcium blood levels in combination with adequate hydration (pamidronate, zoledronic acid only) and bone lesions (pamidronate only) caused by cancer.

To treat osteoporosis in men and postmenopausal women; to prevent osteoporosis in postmenopausal women; to treat glucocorticoid-induced osteoporoses in men and women (alendronate, risedronate only).

To prevent and treat heterotopic ossification (unwanted bone calcification) following total hip replacement or due to spinal cord injury (oral etidronate only).

Unlabeled Use(s): To treat osteoporosis in postmenopausal women (etidronate, pamidronate, risedronate only). To prevent osteoporosis in postmenopausal women (risedronate, etidronate only). To treat hyperparathyroidism, high calcium blood levels associated with immobilization; to reduce bone pain in patients with prostatic cancer (pamidronate only). To prevent glucocorticoid-induced osteoporosis (etidronate, pamidronate only).

Precautions:

Do not use in the following situations:

allergy to the bisphosphonate or any of its ingredients
clinically overt bone softening (osteomalacia) (etidronate only)
esophagus abnormalities (alendronate only)
inability to stand or sit upright for at least 30 minutes (alendronate, risedronate only)
kidney disease, severe (alendronate, residronate, tiludronate only)
low blood calcium levels (alendronate, risedronate only)

Use with caution in the following situations:

asthma
bone fractures
digestive system disorders
kidney disease
liver disease (zoledronic acid only)
low calcium blood levels

Pregnancy: There are no adequate or well-controlled studies in pregnant women. Use only if clearly needed and the potential benefits to the mother outweigh the possible hazards to the fetus.

Breastfeeding: It is not known if these drugs appear in breast milk. Consult your doctor before you begin breastfeeding.

Children: Safety and effectiveness in children have not been established.

Lab tests will be required periodically during treatment. Tests may include blood exams and kidney function tests.

Drug Interactions:

Tell your doctor or pharmacist if you are taking or planning to take any over-the-counter or prescription medications or dietary supplements with a bisphosphonate. Doses of one or both drugs may need to be modified or a different drug may need to be prescribed. The following drugs and drug classes interact with bisphosphonates:

aminoglycosides (eg, gentamicin sulfate) (zoledronic acid only)
antacids (alendronate, etidronate, tiludronate only)
aspirin (alendronate, tiludronate only)

calcium supplements (alendronate, etidronate, risedronate, tiludronate only)
food (alendronate, etidronate, risedronate, tiludronate only)
indomethecin (eg, *Indocin*) (tiludronate only)
loop diuretics (eg, furosemide) (zoledronic acid only)
warfarin (eg, *Coumadin*) (etidronate only)

Side Effects:

Every drug is capable of producing side effects. Many bisphosphonate users experience no, or minor, side effects. The frequency or severity of side effects depend on many factors including dose, duration of therapy, and individual susceptibility. Possible side effects include:

Digestive Tract: Inflammation of the stomach, nausea; vomiting; diarrhea; constipation; gas; heartburn; indigestion; ulcers; stomach pain; acid regurgitation; difficulty swallowing; bloating; appetite loss; stomach bleeding; taste changes; dental disorder; mouth sores; inflammation of the colon.

Circulatory System: High blood pressure; fainting; rapid heartbeat; irregular heartbeat; anemia; decreased white blood cell and platelet count; abnormal blood tests.

Nervous System: Headache; fatigue; dizziness; drowsiness; weakness; vertigo (feeling of whirling motion); confusion; anxiety; nervousness; sleep disorders; sleeplessness; hallucinations; amnesia; depression; convulsions.

Respiratory System: Difficulty breathing; runny nose; sore throat; sinus infection; coughing; bronchitis; upper respiratory infections.

Skin: Rash; itching; redness, swelling, hardness, or pain at injection site (pamidronate, zoledronic acid only); fungal infections; sweating; flushing; hair loss.

Other: Urinary tract infection; flu-like symptoms; infection; fracture; vitamin D deficiency; fever; general swelling; joint, muscle, chest, neck, leg, back, or bone pain; involuntary muscle contractions; muscle or leg cramps; abnormal skin sensations (eg, burning, prickling, tingling); cataracts; glaucoma; eye inflammation.

Guidelines for Use:

- Pamidronate and zoledronic acid are prepared and administered by your health care provider in a medical setting.
- Dosage is individualized. Take exactly as prescribed.
- Do not stop taking or change the dose unless directed by your doctor.
- If a dose is missed, take it as soon as possible. If several hours have passed or it is nearing time for the next dose, do not double the dose to catch up, unless advised to do so by your doctor. If more than one dose is missed or it is necessary to establish a new dosage schedule, contact your doctor or pharmacist.
- These medications may cause upset stomach, nausea, or diarrhea.
- Take supplemental calcium and vitamin D as advised by your doctor if dietary intake is inadequate.
- Avoid nicotine and alcohol, which deplete calcium from the bones.
- Consider weight-bearing exercises to increase the calcium density of bones.
- Lab tests will be required to monitor therapy. Be sure to keep appointments.
- Store tablets at controlled room temperature (59° to 86°F) in a tightly sealed container. Do not remove tiludronate tablets from foil strip until they are to be used.
- *Alendronate and risedronate* —
  Take each tablet first thing in morning with a full glass of water (6 to 8 oz) at least 30 minutes before the first food, beverage, or medication of the day.
  Taking with mineral water, fruit juices, or coffee can decrease its effectiveness.
  Do not lie down for at least 30 minutes following administration and until after the first food of the day.
  Discontinue use and notify your physician if you experience new or worsening heartburn or difficult or painful swallowing.
- *Etidronate* —
  Take tablets with a full glass of water (6 to 8 oz) on an empty stomach, at least 2 hours before meals.
  Take tablets as a single dose. If stomach upset occurs, divide the dose.
  Do not eat foods (such as milk or dairy products), vitamins, mineral supplements, or antacids that are high in calcium within 2 hours of taking.
- *Tiludronate* —
  Take with a full glass of water (6 to 8 oz), at least 2 hours before or after meals.
  Do not take calcium supplements, aspirin, or indomethacin 2 hours before or after taking this medication.
  If needed, take aluminum- or magnesium-containing antacids at least 2 hours after taking this medication.

If you have any questions, consult your doctor, pharmacist, or health care provider.

	Generic Name *Brand Name Example*	Supplied As	Generic Available
Rx	**Imiglucerase**		
	Cerezyme	**Injection**: 200 units/vial, 400 units/vial	No

Type of Drug:

Enzyme replacement therapy.

How the Drug Works:

An enzyme used long-term to break down glucocerebroside into glucose and ceramide. This prevents the accumulation of glucocerebroside in Gaucher disease.

Uses:

For long-term enzyme replacement therapy for type I Gaucher disease that results in one or more of the following problems: anemia, low platelet counts, bone disease and deterioration, enlargement of the liver or spleen.

Precautions:

Do not use in the following situations: Allergy to imiglucerase or any of its ingredients.

Use with caution in the following situations: Pulmonary hypertension.

Hypersensitivity: Approximately 15% of patients have developed IgG antibodies reactive with imiglucerase during the first year of therapy. Approximately 46% of those patients experienced allergic reactions.

Pregnancy: There are no adequate and well-controlled studies in pregnant women. Use only if clearly needed and the potential benefits to the mother outweigh the possible hazards to the fetus.

Breastfeeding: It is not known if imiglucerase appears in breast milk. Consult your doctor before you begin breastfeeding.

Side Effects:

Every drug is capable of producing side effects. Many imiglucerase users experience no, or minor, side effects. The frequency and severity of side effects depend on many factors including dose, duration of therapy, and individual susceptibility. Possible side effects include:

Nervous System: Headache; fever; chills; fatigue; dizziness.

Other: Nausea; vomiting; stomach discomfort; diarrhea; back pain; chest discomfort; swelling; difficulty breathing; low blood pressure; rapid heart rate; injection site burning, itching, and swelling; rash; itching; flushing; skin discoloration.

Guidelines for Use:

- This drug is prepared and administered intravenously (IV; into a vein) by your health care provider in a medical setting.
- Dosage is individualized and may be administered as frequently as 3 times per week or as infrequently as once every 2 weeks depending on disease severity.
- Contact your doctor immediately if you experience any symptoms of allergic reaction (eg, rash, difficulty breathing).

If you have any questions, consult your doctor, pharmacist, or health care provider.

Diuretics
- Carbonic Anhydrase Inhibitors, 313
- Loop Diuretics, 317
- Potassium-Sparing Diuretics, 320
- Thiazides and Related Diuretics, 323
- Combinations, 327
- Nonprescription Diuretics, 328

Cardiac Glycosides, 329

Inamrinone Lactate, 333

Milrinone Lactate, 335

Antianginals
- Nitrates, 337

Antiarrhythmics
- Amiodarone, 343
- Disopyramide, 346
- Dofetilide, 349
- Flecainide, 352
- Mexiletine, 354
- Moricizine, 356
- Procainamide, 359
- Propafenone, 361
- Quinidine, 363
- Tocainide, 366

Calcium Channel Blocking Agents, 368

Peripheral Vasodilators
- Isoxsuprine, 375
- Papaverine, 377

Beta-Adrenergic Blocking Agents, 379

Antihypertensives
- Alpha-1-Adrenergic Blockers, 386
- Angiotensin Converting Enzyme Inhibitors, 390
- Angiotensin II Receptor Antagonists, 395
- Clonidine, 398
- Guanabenz Acetate, 401
- Guanadrel Sulfate, 403
- Guanethidine Monosulfate, 405
- Guanafacine, 408
- Hydralazine, 410
- Carvedilol, 413
- Labetalol, 416
- Mecamylamine, 419
- Methyldopa, 421
- Minoxidil, 424
- Reserpine, 427
- Combinations, 430

Salt Substitutes, 434

Antihyperlipidemics
- Bile Acid Sequestrants, 435
- Clofibrate, 439
- Fenofibrate, 442
- Gemfibrozil, 445
- HMG-CoA Reductase Inhibitors, 448

	Generic Name *Brand Name Examples*	Supplied As	Generic Available
Rx	**Acetazolamide**		
	Diamox	**Tablets:** 125 mg, 250 mg	Yes
	Diamox Sequels	**Capsules, sustained release:** 500 mg	No
	Diamox	**Powder for injection:** 500 mg/vial	Yes
Rx	**Dichlorphenamide**		
	Daranide	**Tablets:** 50 mg	No
Rx	**Methazolamide**		
	Neptazane	**Tablets:** 25 mg, 50 mg	No

Type of Drug:

Diuretics (water pills); antiglaucoma agents.

How the Drug Works:

Carbonic anhydrase inhibitors block the activity of the enzyme carbonic anhydrase. This reduces the rate of fluid formation in the inner eye, resulting in reduced pressure within the eye. These drugs also cause increased amounts of electrolytes (sodium, potassium, bicarbonate) and water to be excreted by the kidneys (diuretic effect) and slows abnormal nerve conduction in the brain (anticonvulsant effect).

Uses:

To treat chronic simple (open-angle) glaucoma and secondary glaucoma, and to lower intraocular pressure preoperatively for acute closed-angle glaucoma.

Acetazolamide — To prevent mountain sickness in climbers who are attempting to climb rapidly and in climbers who climb gradually, but who are prone to developing mountain sickness. Also used to treat fluid accumulation and swelling due to congestive heart failure or drugs and to treat some forms of epilepsy (eg, petit mal seizures).

Precautions:

Do not use in the following situations:

- adrenocortical insufficiency (eg, Addison disease)
- allergy to these medicines or any of their ingredients
- cirrhosis
- electrolyte imbalance (eg, low potassium or sodium levels)
- glaucoma, chronic noncongestive angle-closure
- hyperchloremic acidosis
- kidney disease, severe
- liver disease, severe
- lung obstruction, severe

Use with caution in the following situations:

- allergy to sulfa drugs (eg, *Bactrim*)
- aspirin use, high-dose, concurrent
- emphysema
- lung obstruction

Large doses: Taking larger than recommended doses does not increase the diuretic (water pill) activity of the drug. However, it will increase the risk of side effects.

Pregnancy: There are no adequate and well-controlled studies in pregnant women. Use only if potential benefits to the mother outweight potential risks to the fetus.

Breastfeeding: Acetazolamide may appear in breast milk. It is not known if all carbonic anhydrase inhibitors appear in breast milk. Consult your doctor before you begin breastfeeding.

Children: Safety and effectiveness in children have not been established.

Lab tests may be required during treatment. Tests may include electrolyte levels (eg, potassium) and blood counts.

Drug Interactions:

Tell your doctor or pharmacist if you are taking or if you are planning to take any over-the-counter or prescription medications or doetary supplements with carbonic anhydrase inhibitors. Doses of one or both drugs may need to be modified or a different drug may need to be prescribed. The following drugs interact with carbonic anhydrase inhibitors.

- cyclosporine (eg, *Sandimmune*)
- salicylates (eg, aspirin, *Arthropan*, *Doan's*, *Tusal*)
- salsalate (eg, *Disalcid*)
- steroid therapy (eg, prednisone)

Side Effects:

Every drug is capable of producing side effects. Many carbonic anhydrase inhibitor users experience no, or minor, side effects. The frequency and severity of side effects depend on many factors including dose, duration of therapy, and individual susceptibility. Possible side effects include:

Digestive Tract: Appetite loss; nausea; vomiting; diarrhea; sore throat; taste changes.

Nervous System: Drowsiness; confusion; ringing in the ears; impaired coordination; headache; tingling in the hands or feet.

Skin: Rash; itching; unusual bleeding or bruising; sensitivity to light; red or purple spots under the skin.

Urinary and Reproductive Tract: Flank or loin pain; excessive urination; crystals in urine; kidney stones.

Other: Fever; weight loss; nearsightedness when decreasing or discontinuing the drug; abnormal blood counts; hearing dysfunction; severe allergic reaction.

Guidelines for Use:

All:

- If stomach upset occurs, take with food.
- Drink plenty of water and other fluids.
- May cause drowsiness. Use caution while driving or performing other tasks requiring alertness, coordination, or physical dexterity.
- Notify your doctor if sore throat, fever, unusual bleeding or bruising, tingling or tremors in the hands or feet, flank or loin pain, or skin rash occurs.
- May cause sensitivity to sunlight. Avoid prolonged exposure to the sun or ultraviolet (UV) light (eg, tanning beds).
- Store tablets, capsules, and injection at room temperature (59° to 86°F).

Acetazolamide:

- Tablets can be crushed and mixed with sweet foods to mask bitter taste.
- Do not crush or chew sustained release capsules. Capsules can be opened and contents sprinkled on food, if necessary.
- *Acute Mountain Sickness* — Dosage is 500 to 1000 mg daily, in divided doses, using tablets or sustained release capsules as appropiate.
  The higher dose level of 1000 mg is recommended with rapid ascent (eg, rescue or military operations). Dose should be initiated 24 to 48 hours before ascent and continued for 48 hours while at high altitude, or as long as necessary, to control symptoms. Gradual ascent is desirable to avoid acute moutain sickness. If rapid ascent is undertaken and acetazolamide used, prompt descent is still necessary if severe forms of altitude sickness (eg, lung edema or cerebral swelling) occur.
- *Congestive Heart Failure* — Starting dose is usually 250 to 375 mg once daily (5 mg/kg) in the morning. If the initial response fails, do not increase the dose, but allow the kidney to recover by skipping the medicine for a day.
- Acetazolamide yields the best diuretic results when given on alternate days or given for 2 days alternating with a day of rest.
- *Drug-Induced Edema* — Recommended dosage is 250 to 375 mg once a day for 1 to 2 days, alternating with a day of rest.
- *Epilepsy* — Suggested total daily dose is 8 to 30 mg/kg in divided doses. Optimum range appears to be from 375 to 1000 mg daily. When given in combination with other anticonvulsants, starting dose should be 250 mg once daily in addition to existing medicines.

Guidelines for Use (cont.):

- *Glaucoma* — Acetazolamide is used as an adjunct to the usual therapy.
  When using capsules, dosage is 500 mg (1 capsule) 2 times a day, usually given as 1 capsule in the morning and 1 capsule in the evening.
  Dosage for chronic simple (open-angle) glaucoma ranges from 250 to 1000 mg per 24 hours. Daily doses over 250 mg are usually taken in divided doses.
  For secondary glaucoma and in preoperative treatment of acute congestive (closed-angle) glaucoma, the preferred dosage is 250 mg every 4 hours.
- Doses larger than 1000 mg per 24 hours do not increase the effect and may increase drowsiness and other side effects.

Methazolamide:

- Effective therapeutic dose varies from 50 to 100 mg 2 to 3 times daily.
- May be used with miotic (eg, *Pilocarpine*) and osmotic (eg, mannitol) agents.

Dichlorphenamide:

- Usually given in conjunction with topical ocular antiglaucoma agents.
- In acute angle-closure glaucoma, it may be used together with miotic and osmotic agents in an attempt to reduce internal pressure rapidly. If this is not relieved quickly, surgery may be mandatory.
- Dose must be adjusted carefully to each individual.
- A usual initial dose is 100 to 200 mg (2 to 4 tablets), followed by 100 mg (2 tablets) every 12 hours until the desired response has been obtained.
- Recommended maintenance dosage for adults is 25 to 50 mg (½ to 1 tablet) 1 to 3 times daily.

	Generic Name *Brand Name Examples*	Supplied As	Generic Available
Rx	**Bumetanide**		
	Bumex	**Tablets:** 0.5 mg, 1 mg, 2 mg	No
	Bumex	**Injection:** 0.25 mg/mL	Yes
Rx	**Ethacrynic Acid**		
	Edecrin	**Tablets:** 25 mg, 50 mg	No
	Edecrin	**Powder for injection:** 50 mg (as ethacrynate sodium)/vial	No
Rx	**Furosemide**		
	Lasix	**Tablets:** 20 mg, 40 mg, 80 mg	Yes
	Lasix	**Oral solution:** 10 mg/mL, 40 mg/5 mL	Yes
	Lasix	**Injection:** 10 mg/mL	Yes
Rx	**Torsemide**		
	Demadex	**Tablets:** 5 mg, 10 mg, 20 mg, 100 mg	No
	Demadex	**Injection:** 10 mg/mL	No

Type of Drug:

Diuretics or "water pills."

How the Drug Works:

Loop diuretics cause electrolytes (especially sodium and chloride) to be excreted in the urine. Water is excreted with the electrolytes.

Uses:

To treat edema (fluid retention and swelling) due to congestive heart failure, liver disease (eg, cirrhosis), and kidney disease.

Furosemide and torsemide — To treat hypertension (high blood pressure) alone or with other high blood pressure medicine.

Ethacrynic acid — To treat fluid accumulation in the abdomen (ascites) due to cancer, liver failure, and other conditions, and to treat fluid accumulation in children due to congenital heart or kidney disease.

Precautions:

Do not use in the following situations:

allergy to loop diuretics or any of their ingredients
allergy to sulfa drugs
allergy to thiazides
electrolyte loss, severe
inability to urinate
infants (ethacrynic acid only)

Use with caution in the following situations:

diabetes
digoxin therapy
elderly
gout

heart disease
kidney disease
liver disease
systemic lupus erythematosus

Loop diuretics: Loop diuretics are potent diuretics which can lead to profound increase in urine excretion with water and electrolyte depletion when given in large amounts. Careful medical supervision is required. The dose and dose schedule must be adjusted to the individual patient's needs.

Pregnancy: There are no adequate and well-controlled studies in pregnant women. Use only if clearly needed and potential benefits to the mother outweigh the possible hazards to the fetus.

Breastfeeding: Furosemide appears in breast milk. It is not known if other loop diuretics appear in breast milk. Consult your doctor before you begin breastfeeding.

Children: Safety and effectiveness for use of bumetanide in children younger than 18 years of age have not been established. Safety and effectiveness for use of ethacrynic acid in infants have not been established. Furosemide is indicated for use in pediatric patients. Safety and effectiveness for use of torsemide in children have not been established.

Lab tests may be required during therapy. Tests may include electrolytes (eg, sodium, potassium, calcium, magnesium), blood counts, blood glucose (sugar), uric acid, urea nitrogen, creatinine, and cholesterol.

Drug Interactions:

Tell your doctor or pharmacist if you are taking or planning to take any over-the-counter or prescription medications or dietary supplements with loop diuretics. Doses of one or both drugs may need to be modified or a different drug may need to be prescribed. The following drugs and drug classes interact with loop diuretics:

ACE inhibitors (eg, benazepril)
aminoglycosides (eg, gentamicin)
cholestyramine (eg, *Questran*)
cisapride (*Propulsid*)
cisplatin (eg, *Platinol*)
colestipol (*Colestid*)
digitalis glycosides (eg, digoxin)
hydantoins (eg, phenytoin)
lithium (eg, *Eskalith*)
NSAIDs (eg, ibuprofen)
thiazide diuretics (eg, hydrochlorothiazide)

Do not combine furosemide with ethacrynic acid.

Side Effects:

Every drug is capable of producing side effects. Many loop diuretic users experience no, or minor, side effects. The frequency and severity of side effects depend on many factors including dose, duration of therapy, and individual susceptibility. Possible side effects include:

Symptoms of Electrolyte Loss: Weakness; dizziness; confusion; appetite loss; nausea; vomiting; muscle cramps; limb heaviness.

Digestive Tract: Difficulty swallowing; diarrhea (including sudden watery diarrhea); irritation of mouth or stomach; constipation; stomach pain; appetite loss; indigestion; bloating.

Nervous System: Restlessness; tingling or numbness of hands or feet; apprehension; nervousness; headache; insomnia.

Circulatory System: Irregular heartbeat; weak pulse; chest pain; orthostatic hypotension (dizziness or lightheadedness when rising too quickly from a seated or lying position).

Senses: Ringing in the ears; hearing loss (usually reversible).

Skin: Sweating; itching; rash, hives; jaundice (yellowing of skin or eyes); sensitivity to sunlight; unusual bleeding or bruising.

Other: Blood in the urine; dehydration; joint pain; fever; chills; breathing difficulties; yellow vision; blurred vision; premature ejaculation; impotence; difficulty maintaining an erection; dry mouth; excessive urination; rectal bleeding; fluid retention; muscle pain; cold; cough; sore throat; decreased potassium levels; elevated blood sugar.

Guidelines for Use:

- Dosage is individualized.
- If a dose is missed, take it as soon as possible. If several hours have passed or it is nearing time for the next dose, do not double the dose to catch up, unless advised to do so by your doctor. If more than one dose is missed or it is necessary to establish a new dosage schedule, contact your doctor or pharmacist. Use exactly as prescribed.
- Take ethacrynic acid after meals, if necessary.
- Drug will increase urination. Take early in the day to avoid sleep disruption.
- Notify your doctor if muscle weakness, cramps, nausea or dizziness occurs.
- Orthostatic hypotension (dizziness or lightheadedness when arising from a seated or lying position) may occur. Get up slowly.
- *Diabetes mellitus patients* — May increase blood glucose (sugar) levels.
- Photosensitivity (sensitivity to sunlight) may occur. Use sunscreens and wear protective clothing until tolerance is determined.
- Additional potassium may be required while taking loop diuretics.
- Patients with high blood pressure should avoid medications that may increase blood pressure, including nonprescription decongestant products for cold symptoms and stimulant weight-control products.
- Weight should be monitored throughout treatment with loop diuretics. Loss of fluid should not be excessive within a narrow band of time.
- Lab tests will be required. Be sure to keep appointments.
- Store at room temperature (59° to 86°F) in well closed, light-resistant container. Do not freeze.

If you have any questions, consult your doctor, pharmacist, or health care provider.

DIURETICS — POTASSIUM-SPARING DIURETICS

	Generic Name *Brand Name Examples*	Supplied As	Generic Available
Rx	**Amiloride HCl**		
	Midamor	**Tablets:** 5 mg	Yes
Rx	**Spironolactone**		
	Aldactone	**Tablets:** 25 mg, 50 mg, 100 mg	Yes
Rx	**Triamterene**		
	Dyrenium	**Capsules:** 50 mg, 100 mg	No

Type of Drug:

Diuretics or "water pills."

How the Drug Works:

Potassium-sparing diuretics increase the amount of water and sodium being excreted by the kidneys, but reduce the amount of potassium being excreted by the kidneys.

Uses:

To treat edema (fluid accumulation and swelling) due to congestive heart failure, cirrhosis of the liver, and in certain kidney conditions.

To treat high blood pressure, usually in combination with other drugs.

To prevent or treat low potassium levels due to use of other medications (eg, other diuretics).

Spironolactone: To diagnose and treat primary hyperaldosteronism (an abnormality of electrolyte metabolism). To treat edema in children.

Triamterene: To treat edema due to secondary hyperaldosteronism (an abnormality of electrolyte metabolism).

Precautions:

Do not use in the following situations:

allergy to potassium-sparing diuretics
anuria (eg, inability to urinate)
liver disease, severe (triamterene only)
potassium levels, increased
potassium supplement use

Use with caution in the following situations:

diabetes (amiloride and triamterene)
elderly (amiloride and triamterene)
congestive heart failure
kidney disease
kidney stone formation, history (triamterene only)
liver disease

High potassium levels (hyperkalemia): Occasionally hyperkalemia may occur when these agents are used without diuretics. Symptoms include abnormal skin sensations (burning, tingling), muscle weakness, impaired movement and irregular heartbeat.

Pregnancy: Amiloride and *triamterene* — Studies in pregnant women have not shown a risk to the fetus; however, no drug should be used during pregnancy unless clearly needed.

Spironolactone may cross the placenta. Use only if clearly needed and potential benefits outweigh the possible risks.

Breastfeeding: Spironolactone appears in breast milk. However, it is not known if triamterene or amiloride are excreted in breast milk. Safety for use in breastfeeding has not been established. These drugs can cause serious side effects in a nursing infant. Do not breastfeed while taking these drugs.

Children: Safety and effectiveness of triamterene and amiloride in children have not been established.

Lab tests should be performed periodically for serum electrolytes, creatinine, BUN and serum potassium. Periodic blood tests should also be performed.

Drug Interactions:

Tell your doctor or pharmacist if you are taking or planning to take any over-the-counter or prescription medications or dietary supplements with potassium-sparing diuretics. Doses of one or both drugs may need to be modified or a different drug may need to be prescribed. The following drugs and drug classes interact with potassium-sparing diuretics:

- ACE inhibitors (eg, captopril)
- anesthetics (general)
- antihypertensives (spironolactone and triamterene only)
- chlorpropamide (eg, *Diabinese*) (triamterene only)
- digoxin (eg, *Lanoxin*) (spironolactone only)
- indomethacin (eg, *Indocin)* (spironolactone and triamterene only)
- lithium (eg, *Eskalith*) (amiloride and triamterene only)
- nonsteroidal anti-inflammatory agents (eg, aspirin) (amiloride and triamterene only)
- potassium supplements (eg, *Kaon*)
- salt substitutes
- skeletal muscle relaxants (triamterene only)

Side Effects:

Every drug is capable of producing side effects. Many potassium-sparing diuretic users experience no, or minor, side effects. The frequency and severity of side effects depend on many factors including dose, duration of therapy, and individual susceptibility. Possible side effects include:

Digestive Tract: Stomach or intestinal cramps or pain; nausea; vomiting; thirst; diarrhea; constipation; gas; appetite changes (loss of appetite).

Nervous System: Weakness, fatigue; drowsiness; confusion; tingling or numbness of hands or feet; headache; dizziness; lack of coordination.

Circulatory System: Irregular pulse; chest pain.

Respiratory System: Shortness of breath; cough.

Skin: Rash; hives; excessive body hair growth; yellowing of the skin or eyes; sensitivity to sunlight; unusual bleeding or bruising.

Other: Deepening of the voice, breast enlargement in males (spironolactone only); menstrual abnormalities; fever; muscle weakness or cramping; inability to achieve or maintain an erection; difficult urination; dry mouth; allergic reaction.

Guidelines for Use:

- *Amiloride* —
  May cause stomach upset. Take with food.
  Notify your doctor if any of the following occurs: Muscular weakness, irregular heartbeat, shortness of breath, rash, fatigue or muscle cramps.
  May cause dizziness, headache or visual disturbances. Use caution while driving or performing other tasks requiring alertness.
  Avoid large quantities of potassium-rich food.
- *Spironolactone* —
  May cause drowsiness, lack of coordination and mental confusion. Use caution while driving or performing other tasks requiring alertness.
  May cause stomach cramping, diarrhea, lethargy, thirst, headache, skin rash, menstrual abnormalities, deepening of the voice and breast enlargement (in males). Notify your doctor if these effects occur.
- *Triamterene* —
  May cause stomach upset. Take after meals.
  May cause weakness, headache, nausea, vomiting and dry mouth. Notify your doctor if these become severe or persistent.
  Notify your doctor if fever, sore throat, mouth sores, or unusual bleeding or bruising occurs.
  Avoid prolonged exposure to sunlight. Photosensitivity (sensitivity to sunlight) may occur. Take protective measures (eg, sunscreens, protective clothing) against exposure to ultraviolet light or sunlight.
  If single daily dose is prescribed, take in morning to avoid disruption of sleep because of frequent urination.
- Do not use dietary potassium supplements, potassium-containing medications, low-salt milk or salt substitutes.
- If a dose is missed, take it as soon as possible. If several hours have passed or it is nearing time for the next dose, do not double the dose to catch up, unless advised by your doctor. If more than one dose is missed, contact your doctor or pharmacist.
- Occasionally hyperkalemia (high potassium levels) may occur when these agents are used. Symptoms include abnormal skin sensations (burning, tingling), muscle weakness, fatigue, loss of arm and leg movement, irregular heartbeat and shock.
- Patients being treated for high blood pressure often feel tired and rundown for a few weeks after beginning therapy. Continue taking your medication even though you may not feel quite "normal." Contact your doctor or pharmacist about any new symptoms.
- Store below 77°F. Protect from light, moisture, freezing and excessive heat.

If you have any questions, consult your doctor, pharmacist, or health care provider.

	Generic Name *Brand Name Examples*	Supplied As	Generic Available
Rx	**Bendroflumethiazide**		
	Naturetin	**Tablets:** 5 mg, 10 mg	No
Rx	**Benzthiazide**		
	Exna[1]	**Tablets:** 50 mg	No
Rx	**Chlorothiazide**		
	Diurigen, Diuril	**Tablets:** 250 mg, 500 mg	Yes
	Diuril[2]	**Oral suspension:** 250 mg/5 mL	No
Rx	**Chlorthalidone**		
	Hygroton, Thalitone	**Tablets:** 15 mg, 25 mg, 50 mg, 100 mg	Yes
Rx	**Hydrochlorothiazide (HCTZ)**		
	Esidrix, Ezide, HydroDIURIL, Hydro-Par, Oretic	**Tablets:** 25 mg, 50 mg, 100 mg	Yes
	Hydrochlorothiazide	**Solution:** 50 mg/5 mL	No
	Hydrochlorothiazide	**Intensol solution:** 100 mg/mL	No
Rx	**Hydroflumethiazide**		
	Diucardin, Saluron	**Tablets:** 50 mg	Yes
Rx	**Indapamide**		
	Lozol	**Tablets:** 1.25 mg, 2.5 mg	No
Rx	**Methyclothiazide**		
	Aquatensen, Enduron	**Tablets:** 2.5 mg, 5 mg	Yes
Rx	**Metolazone**		
	Mykrox, Zaroxolyn	**Tablets:** 0.5 mg, 2.5 mg, 5 mg, 10 mg	No
Rx	**Polythiazide**		
	Renese	**Tablets:** 1 mg, 2 mg, 4 mg	No
Rx	**Quinethazone**		
	Hydromox	**Tablets:** 50 mg	No
Rx	**Trichlormethiazide**		
	Diurese, Metahydrin[1], *Naqua*	**Tablets:** 2 mg, 4 mg	Yes

[1] Contains the dye tartrazine.
[2] Contains alcohol. *Diuril* is also available as an injection.

All of the products listed in the above table are diuretics; however, they are not interchangeable. For example, metolazone cannot be used for hydroclorothiazide. Daily dose may vary depending on individual needs. Do not adjust the dose without consulting your pharmacist or doctor.

Type of Drug:

Diuretics or "water pills."

How the Drug Works:

Thiazides and related diuretics reduce water in the body and increase urine flow.

Uses:

To treat high blood pressure, either alone or in combination with other high blood pressure medications.

To treat edema (excess fluid accumulation in the tissues) associated with congestive heart failure, kidney problems and during estrogen or corticosteroid therapy.

Unlabeled Use(s): Occasionally doctors may prescribe thiazide diuretics for calcium kidney stones, osteoporosis and diabetes insipidus (not diabetes mellitus).

Precautions:

Do not use in the following situations:

allergy to thiazides, oral diabetic drugs (eg, *Diabinese)* or sulfa drugs (eg, *Gantrisin)*
kidney disease (inability to urinate)

Use with caution in the following situations:

allergy or history of bronchial asthma
diabetes
gout
kidney impairment
liver disease
lupus erythematosus

Diabetes: Thiazide diuretics may increase blood sugar levels. Insulin requirements may need to be adjusted.

Gout attacks may occur in patients with or without a history of gout.

Potassium loss: By increasing urine production, thiazide diuretics may cause an increased loss of electrolytes, especially potassium. (See Side Effects.)

Low potassium levels may be prevented or treated by eating foods and drinking liquids high in potassium content (eg, citrus juice, bananas, dates, raisins, melons and tomatoes). If dietary changes do not increase potassium to a normal level, it may be necessary for your doctor to prescribe a potassium supplement medication to replace lost potassium.

Pregnancy: Thiazides cross the placenta. Use only when clearly needed and when potential benefits outweigh the possible hazards to the fetus.

Breastfeeding: Thiazides appear in breast milk. Stop nursing if thiazide diuretics are necessary. Consult your doctor before you begin breastfeeding.

Children: Metolazone is not currently recommended for use in children. Safety and effectiveness have not been established for hydroflumethiazide or trichlormethiazide.

Tartrazine: Some of these products may contain the dye tartrazine (FD&C Yellow No. 5) which can cause allergic reactions in certain individuals. Check package label when available or consult your pharmacist or doctor if you are sensitive to tartrazine.

Drug Interactions:

Tell your doctor or pharmacist if you are taking or planning to take any over-the-counter or prescription medications with your diuretic. Doses of one or both drugs may need to be modified or a different drug may need to be prescribed. The following drugs and drug classes interact with thiazide diuretics.

- cholestyramine *(Questran)*
- colestipol *(Colestid)*
- corticosteroids (eg, hydrocortisone)
- cough, cold, sinus or hayfever medications
- diazoxide *(Proglycem)*
- digoxin (eg, *Lanoxin)*
- furosemide (eg, *Lasix)*
- lithium (eg, *Eskalith)*
- oral diabetic drugs (eg, *Orinase)*

Side Effects:

Every drug is capable of producing side effects. Many thiazide diuretic users experience no, or minor, side effects. The frequency and severity of side effects depend on many factors including dose, duration of therapy, and individual susceptibility. Possible side effects include:

Potassium loss: Dry mouth; thirst; irregular heartbeat; confusion and mood changes; nausea; vomiting; unusual tiredness; weakness; weak pulse; muscle cramps; joint pain or spasms; heaviness in limbs.

Digestive Tract: Loss of appetite; stomach upset; bloating; diarrhea; constipation.

Nervous System: Dizziness; lightheadedness; headache; tingling of toes and fingers; yellow or blurred vision; depression; nervousness; sleeplessness.

Circulatory System: Orthostatic hypotension (fall in blood pressure upon standing which may cause dizziness, fainting and blurred vision); chest pain.

Skin: Sensitivity to sun; rash; hives; itching; dry skin; flushing; yellowing of skin or eyes; unusual bruising.

Respiratory System: Cough; sinus congestion; sore throat; difficult or painful breathing.

Other: Frequent urination; impotence; reduced sexual drive; electrolyte (eg, potassium) imbalance; blood sugar imbalance; muscle cramps; joint pain; fever; chills; weight loss; bloody nose; gout attack.

Guidelines for Use:

- Take exactly as prescribed.
- If a dose is missed, take it as soon as possible. If several hours have passed or if it is nearing time for the next dose, do not double the dose to catch up, unless advised to do so by your doctor. If more than one dose is missed or it is necessary to establish a new dosage schedule, contact your doctor or pharmacist.
- Increases urination, therefore take early in the day.
- May cause stomach upset. May be taken with food or milk.
- May cause loss of potassium. If signs of potassium loss occur (weakness, cramps, nausea, dizziness, etc), contact your doctor. Ask your doctor about foods containing potassium.
- May increase blood sugar levels in diabetics.
- May cause gout attacks. Contact your doctor if significant sudden joint pain occurs.
- Do not take other medications without your doctor's approval. This includes nonprescription medicines for appetite control, asthma, colds, cough, hayfever or sinus.
- Diuretics are usually given as a single daily dose in the morning. Take as directed by your doctor. The daily dose varies depending on individual needs. Do not adjust the dose without consulting your pharmacist or doctor.

If you have any questions, consult your doctor, pharmacist, or health care provider.

	Generic Name *Brand Name Examples*	Supplied As	Generic Available
Rx	**Amiloride and Hydrochlorothiazide**		
	Moduretic	**Tablets:** 5 mg amiloride HCl and 50 mg hydrochlorothiazide	Yes
Rx	**Spironolactone and Hydrochlorothiazide**		
	Aldactazide, Spirozide	**Tablets:** 25 mg spironolactone and 25 mg hydrochlorothiazide	Yes
	Aldactazide	**Tablets:** 50 mg spironolactone and 50 mg hydrochlorothiazide	No
Rx	**Triamterene and Hydrochlorothiazide**		
	Maxzide-25MG	**Tablets:** 37.5 mg triamterene and 25 mg hydrochlorothiazide	Yes
	Dyazide	**Capsules:** 50 mg triamterene and 25 mg hydrochlorothiazide	Yes
	Maxzide	**Tablets:** 75 mg triamterene and 50 mg hydrochlorothiazide	Yes

Type of Drug:

Diuretic or "water pill"; combination of two diuretics.

How the Drug Works:

Combination diuretics provide additional diuretic activity (increased water excreted by kidneys) and blood-pressure-lowering effects. They minimize the possibility of potassium loss from the body because they contain a potassium-sparing diuretic.

For complete information on hydrochlorothiazide, see the Diuretics-Thiazides and Related Diuretics monograph in this chapter. For complete information on amiloride HCl, spironolactone, and triamterene, see the Diuretics-Potassium-Sparing Diuretics monograph in this chapter.

Guidelines for Use:

- Increases urination, therefore, take early in the day.
- May cause stomach upset. Take with food or milk.
- May cause a sensitivity to sunlight. Take protective measures (eg, sunscreens, protective clothing) until sensitivity is determined.
- If a dose is missed, take it as soon as possible. If several hours have passed or it is nearing time for the next dose, do not double the dose to catch up, unless advised by your doctor. If more than one dose is missed, contact your doctor or pharmacist.
- Patients being treated for low blood pressure often feel tired and run down for a few weeks after beginning therapy. It takes time for the body to adjust to lowered blood pressure. Continue taking your medicine and check with your doctor.
- Diuretics are usually given as a single daily dose in the morning. Take as directed by your doctor. The daily dose varies depending on individual needs. Do not adjust the dose without consulting your pharmacist or doctor.
- May increase blood sugar levels if you are diabetic.

If you have any questions, consult your doctor, pharmacist, or health care provider.

	Brand Name Examples	Supplied As	Generic Available
otc	*Aqua·Ban*	**Tablets, enteric coated:** 325 mg ammonium Cl, 100 mg caffeine	No
otc	*Aqua·Ban Plus*	**Tablets, enteric coated:** 650 mg ammonium, 200 mg caffeine and 6 mg iron	No

Type of Drug:

Over-the-counter (*otc*) diuretics or "water pills."

How the Drug Works:

Ammonium chloride alone has limited value in promoting urine flow. Its use in combination with caffeine is effective since the diuretic actions are additive. Doses up to 3 g/day may be given in divided doses 3 to 4 times daily for up to 6 days. Large doses (4 to 12 g/day) may cause nausea and vomiting, headache, hyperventilation, drowsiness and confusion.

Caffeine increases urination. It may lessen the mental and physical fatigue associated with water retention. Caffeine is effective for relief of premenstrual and menstrual symptoms in doses of 100 to 200 mg every 3 to 4 hours. For more information on caffeine, see page 326.

Uses:

Nonprescription diuretics may lessen menstrual discomfort. When taken 4 to 6 days before onset of a period, they may help relieve symptoms related to water retention, including: Excess water weight, bloating, painful breasts, cramps and tension.

Guidelines for Use:

- *Ammonium chloride* — Do not use if you have impaired kidney or liver function.
- *Caffeine* — May cause sleeplessness when taken within 4 hours of bedtime. Consider this when drinking coffee, tea, or colas, and when taking products containing caffeine. Doses above 100 mg may cause stomach upset.

If you have any questions, consult your doctor, pharmacist, or health care provider.

	Generic Name *Brand Name Examples*	Supplied As	Generic Available
Rx	**Digoxin**		
	Digitek, Lanoxin	**Tablets**: 0.125 mg, 0.25 mg	Yes
	Lanoxicaps[1]	**Capsules**: 0.05 mg, 0.1 mg, 0.2 mg	No
	Lanoxin Pediatric[1]	**Elixir**: 0.05 mg/mL	Yes
	Lanoxin[1]	**Injection**: 0.25 mg/mL, 0.5 mg/2 mL	Yes
	Lanoxin Pediatric[1]	**Injection**: 0.1 mg/mL	No

[1] Contains alcohol.

Type of Drug:

Digitalis; cardiac glycoside; heart medications which act on the heart muscle and heart conduction system.

How the Drug Works:

Cardiac glycosides work on the heart to increase the force with which the heart pumps blood through the body (heart tonic). This increases the amount of blood the heart pumps and improves the blood circulation in patients in whom the heart is not pumping strong enough (eg, congestive heart failure). This may also help reduce fluid retention and swelling due to congestive heart failure. Cardiac glycosides also help slow and steady the heart rhythm in situations in which the heart is beating too fast or in an irregular manner (eg, atrial fibrillation).

Uses:

To treat congestive heart failure.

To treat certain types of abnormal heart rhythms (arrhythmias) in which the heart is beating too fast or too irregularly to function normally (eg, atrial fibrillation).

Precautions:

Do not use in the following situations:

- allergy to the cardiac glycoside or any of its ingredients
- digitalis toxicity, possibility of
- some types of irregular or fast heartbeats (eg, ventricular fibrillation, ventricular tachycardia)

Use with caution in the following situations:

- acute myocardial infarction
- electrolyte disorder (eg, low blood magnesium levels, low blood potassium levels, high blood calcium levels)
- hyperdynamic states (eg, hyperthyroidism, hypoxia, arteriovenous shunt)
- hypermetabolic state (eg, hyperthyroidism)
- hypothyroidism (underactive thyroid)
- idiopathic hypertrophic subaortic stenosis
- incomplete AV block, preexisting
- kidney disease

paroxysmal atrial fibrillation or flutter and a coexisting accessory AV pathway (Wolff-Parkinson-White syndrome)

preserved left ventricular systolic function

sinus node disease, preexisting

Pregnancy: There are no adequate and well-controlled studies in pregnant women. Use only if clearly needed and the potential benefits to the mother outweigh the possible hazards to the fetus.

Breastfeeding: Digoxin appears in breast milk. No adverse effects to the infant have been reported. Consult your doctor before you begin breastfeeding.

Children: Newborns vary considerably in their tolerance and sensitivity to these medications. Premature and immature infants are particularly sensitive to the effects of digoxin, and the dosage of the drug must not only be reduced but must be individualized according to their degree of maturity. Digitalis glycosides are a significant cause of accidental poisoning in children. Use with caution.

Elderly: Elderly patients must be dosed carefully. Changes in weight, kidney function, and other physical changes that occur normally with aging can affect dosing. Frequent electrocardiograph monitoring is important in elderly patients.

Lab tests may be required to monitor therapy. Alterations in potassium, magnesium, calcium, and other electrolyte or mineral levels can affect therapy. Tests may be required to ensure that these levels are normal. It may also be necessary to perform electrocardiograph monitoring, liver and kidney function tests, and digoxin blood level determinations.

Drug Interactions:

Tell your doctor or pharmacist if you are taking or planning to take any over-the-counter or prescription medications or dietary supplements with a cardiac glycoside. Doses of one or both drugs may need to be modified or a different drug may need to be prescribed. The following drugs and drug classes interact with cardiac glycosides:

Increase digoxin blood levels (possibly increasing therapeutic and toxic effects of digoxin) —

aminoglycosides, oral (eg, neomycin)
amiodarone (*Cordarone*)
alprazolam (*Xanax*)
azole antifungal agents (eg, itraconazole)
bepridil (*Vascor*)
cyclosporine (eg, *Sandimmune*)
diphenoxylate (eg, *Lomotil*)
indomethacin (eg, *Indocin*)
macrolide antibiotics (eg, erythromycin)
propafenone (*Rythmol*)
quinidine (eg, *Quinora*)
quinine (eg, *Quinamm*)
spironolactone (eg, *Aldactone*)
tetracyclines (eg, doxycycline)
thioamines (eg, methimazole, propylthiouracil)
tolbutamide (eg, *Orinase*)
verapamil (eg, *Calan*)

Decrease digoxin blood levels (possibly decreasing the therapeutic effects of digoxin) —

acarbose (*Precose*)
aminoglycosides, oral (eg, neomycin)
antacids (eg, *Maalox*)
antineoplastics (eg, bleomycin)
charcoal
cholestyramine (eg, *Questran*)
colestipol (*Colestid*)
diets high in fiber
hydantoins (eg, phenytoin)
metoclopramide (eg, *Reglan*)
penicillamine (eg, *Depen*)
rifampin (eg, *Rifadin*)
sulfasalazine (eg, azulfidine)

Other —

loop diuretics (eg, furosemide)
propantheline (*Pro-Panthine*)
succinylcholine (eg, *Anectine*)
thiazide diuretics (eg, hydrochlorothiazide)
thyroid hormones (eg, *Synthroid)*

Side Effects:

Every drug is capable of producing side effects. Many cardiac glycoside users experience no, or minor, side effects. The frequency and severity of side effects depend on many factors including dose, duration of therapy, and individual susceptibility. Possible side effects include:

Digestive Tract: Loss of appetite; diarrhea; nausea; vomiting.

Circulatory System: Heart block; heart rhythm disturbances (unusually slow or fast pulse); abnormal heartbeats; pounding in chest (palpitations); ECG changes.

Nervous System: Weakness; headache; depression; delirium; restlessness; drowsiness; confusion; hallucinations; dizziness; apathy; anxiety.

Other: Visual disturbances (eg, blurred, yellow vision); rash; itching.

Guidelines for Use:

- *Digoxin* — Dosage is individualized based on age, kidney function, weight, and heart condition. Usual adult maintenance doses range from 0.125 mg to 0.5 mg once daily. A loading dose is sometimes used to achieve a fast response. The loading dose is given in several portions at 6- to 8-hour intervals with careful assessment of the response before each additional portion.
- The injectable doseform will be prepared and administered by your health care provider in a medical setting.
- *Lanoxicaps* have greater bioavailability than standard digoxin tablets. Therefore, the 0.2 mg capsule is equivalent to the 0.25 mg digoxin tablet, the 0.1 mg capsule is equivalent to 0.125 mg tablet, and the 0.05 mg capsule is equivalent to the 0.0625 mg tablet.
- *Pediatric Elixir* — Dosage will be individualized. Divided daily dosing is usually used for infants and children younger than 10 years of age. Use calibrated dropper to carefully withdraw the prescribed dose.
- *Tablets and Capsules* — Individualize dosage for infants and children. Divided daily dosing is recommended for infants and young children under 10 years of age. Children over 10 years of age require adult dosages in proportion to their body weight.
- Do not change the dose or stop taking medication without first consulting your doctor.
- May be taken without regard to meals. Taking with meals high in bran fiber may reduce the amount of medication absorbed.
- If a dose is missed, take it as soon as possible. If several hours have passed or if it is nearing time for the next dose, do not double the dose to catch up, unless advised by your doctor. If more than one dose is missed or it is necessary to establish a new dosage schedule, contact your doctor or pharmacist.
- Avoid nonprescription antacids, cough, cold, allergy, and diet drugs, except on professional advice.
- Notify your doctor if loss of appetite, lower stomach pain, nausea, vomiting, diarrhea, unusual tiredness or weakness, drowsiness, headache, blurred or yellow vision, rash, itching, hives, depression, or a change in heart rate or pulse (eg, slowing, racing) occurs.
- *Brand and doseform interchange* — Do not change from one brand or doseform of this drug to another without consulting your pharmacist or doctor. Products manufactured by different companies may not be equally effective. Different doseforms provide different amounts of medication, requiring dose modification.
- Digitalis glycosides can cause poisoning in children due to accidental ingestion. Keep out of reach of children.
- Lab tests or exams may be required to monitor therapy. Be sure to keep appointments.
- Store tablets and capsules at room temperature (59° to 86°F). Protect from light and moisture.

If you have any questions, consult your doctor, pharmacist, or health care provider.

	Generic Name	Supplied As	Generic Available
Rx	**Inamrinone Lactate**	**Injection**: 5 mg/mL (as lactate)[1]	Yes

[1] Contains metabisulfite.

Type of Drug:

Heart medication that strengthens heart muscle action and improves blood circulation.

How the Drug Works:

Inamrinone works on the heart to increase the force with which the heart pumps blood through the body (heart tonic). This increases the amount of blood the heart pumps and improves blood circulation in patients in whom the heart is not pumping enough blood (eg, congestive heart failure).

Uses:

For the short-term treatment of symptoms of congestive heart failure in patients who have not responded to standard therapy.

Precautions:

Do not use in the following situations:

- allergy to bisulfites
- allergy to inamrinone or any of its ingredients
- heart attack, acute

Use with caution in the following situations:

- decreased platelet counts
- diuretic therapy, vigorous
- heart rhythm disturbances
- hypertrophic subaortic stenosis
- kidney disease
- liver disease
- low blood pressure

Pregnancy: There are no adequate and well-controlled studies in pregnant women. Use only if clearly needed and the potential benefits to the mother outweigh possible hazards to the fetus.

Breastfeeding: It is not known if inamrinone appears in breast milk. Consult your doctor before you begin breastfeeding.

Children: Safety and effectiveness in children have not been established.

Lab tests and exams will be required to monitor therapy. Tests will include kidney and liver function tests, and fluid and electrolyte, blood pressure, blood tests, and heart rate monitoring.

Sulfites: Inamrinone contains sodium metabisulfite, a sulfite preservative that can cause potentially life-threatening allergic reactions in certain individuals. Consult your doctor or pharmacist.

Drug Interactions:

Tell your doctor or pharmacist if you are taking or planning to take any over-the-counter or prescription medications or dietary supplements while taking inamrinone. Doses of one or both drugs may need to be modified or a different drug may need to be prescribed. Disopyramide (eg, *Norpace*) interacts with inamrinone.

Side Effects:

Every drug is capable of producing side effects. Many inamrinone users experience no, or minor, side effects. The frequency and severity of side effects depend on many factors including dose, duration of therapy, and individual susceptibility. Possible side effects include:

Circulatory System: Irregular heartbeat; low blood pressure; decreased blood platelets.

Other: Nausea.

Guidelines for Use:

- Dosage is individualized. Use exactly as prescribed.
- Solutions will be prepared and administered by your health care provider. Dosage will be determined by your doctor. Do not change, adjust, or manipulate the infusion device.
- Visually inspect solution for particles or discoloration before use.
- Duration of therapy will depend on patient responsiveness.
- Because of limited experience and potential for serious side effects, inamrinone should only be used in patients who can be closely monitored and who have not responded adequately to digitalis, diuretics, or vasodilators.
- During intravenous (IV; into a vein) therapy with inamrinone, blood pressure and heart rate should be monitored and the rate of infusion slowed or stopped in patients showing excessive decreases in blood pressure.
- Notify your doctor if you experience an abnormal heartbeat.
- Furosemide should not be administered in IV lines containing inamrinone.
- Lab tests and exams will be required to monitor therapy.

If you have any questions, consult your doctor, pharmacist, or health care provider.

	Generic Name *Brand Name Example*	Supplied As	Generic Available
Rx	**Milrinone Lactate**		
	Primacor	**Injection:** 0.2 mg/mL, 1 mg/mL	No

Type of Drug:

A vasodilator; a heart medication that acts on the heart muscle to increase the strength of contraction.

How the Drug Works:

Milrinone works on the heart to increase the force with which the heart pumps blood through the body (heart tonic). This increases the amount of blood the heart pumps and improves blood circulation in a patient whose heart is not pumping strongly enough (eg, congestive heart failure).

Uses:

For the short-term intravenous (IV; into a vein) treatment of acute decompensated heart failure.

Precautions:

Do not use in the following situations: Allergy to milrinone or any of its ingredients.

Use with caution in the following situations:

arrythmia (irregular heart rhythm)
heart attack, acute
hypokalemia (low potassium levels)
valvular heart disease, untreated

Pregnancy: There are no adequate and well-controlled studies in pregnant women. Use only if clearly needed and the potential benefits to the mother outweigh the possible hazards to the fetus.

Breastfeeding: It is not known if milrinone appears in breast milk. Consult your doctor before you begin breastfeeding.

Children: Safety and effectiveness in children have not been established.

Lab tests will be required to monitor therapy. Tests may include fluid and electrolyte levels and kidney function. Blood pressure, heart rate, and electrocardiogram will also be monitored during treatment.

Drug Interactions:

Tell your doctor or pharmacist if you are taking or planning to take any over-the-counter or prescription medications or dietary supplements while taking milrinone. Doses of one or both drugs may need to be modified or a different drug may need to be prescribed. Furosemide (eg, *Lasix*) interacts with milrinone when given through the same IV line.

Side Effects:

Every drug is capable of producing side effects. Many milrinone users experience no, or minor, side effects. The frequency and severity of side effects depend on many factors including dose, duration of therapy, and individual susceptibility. Possible side effects include:

Nervous System: Headache.

Circulatory System: Irregular heartbeat; chest pain; low blood pressure.

Guidelines for Use:

- This medicine will be prepared and administered IV by your health care provider in a medical setting.
- Lab tests will be required to monitor therapy.

If you have any questions, consult your doctor, pharmacist, or health care provider.

	Generic Name *Brand Name Examples*	Supplied As	Generic Available
Rx	**Isosorbide Dinitrate**		
	Isordil Titradose, Sorbitrate	**Tablets**: 5 mg, 10 mg, 20 mg, 30 mg, 40 mg	Yes
	Sorbitrate	**Tablets, chewable**: 5 mg, 10 mg	No
	Isordil, Sorbitrate	**Tablets, sublingual**: 2.5 mg, 5 mg, 10 mg	Yes
	Dilatrate-SR	**Capsules, sustained release**: 40 mg	Yes
Rx	**Isosorbide Mononitrate**		
	Monoket	**Tablets**: 10 mg	No
	Ismo, Monoket	**Tablets**: 20 mg	Yes
	Imdur	**Tablets, extended release**: 30 mg, 60 mg, 120 mg	Yes
Rx	**Nitroglycerin**[1]		
	NitroQuick, Nitrostat, NitroTab	**Tablets, sublingual**: 0.3 mg, 0.4 mg, 0.6 mg	No
	Nitro-Time	**Capsules, sustained release**: 2.5 mg, 6.5 mg, 9 mg	Yes
	Nitro-Bid	**Ointment, topical**: 2% in a lanolin-petrolatum base	Yes
	Nitrolingual	**Aerosol spray, translingual**: 0.4 mg/metered dose	No
	Nitrogard	**Tablets, buccal, extended release**: 1 mg, 2 mg, 2.5 mg, 3 mg, 5 mg	No

[1] Also available as an intravenous injection.

Rx	Nitroglycerin Transdermal Systems (Patches) *Brand Name Examples*	Release Rate (mg/hr)	Surface Area (cm^2)	Total NTG content (mg)
	Minitran	0.1	3.3	9
	Nitro-Dur	0.1	5	20
	Transderm-Nitro	0.1	5	12.5
	Nitroglycerin Transdermal	0.2	6-10[1]	16-62.5[1]
	Minitran	0.2	6.7	18
	Nitrek	0.2	8	22.4
	Nitrodisc	0.2	8	16
	Nitro-Dur	0.2	10	40
	Transderm-Nitro	0.2	10	25
	Deponit	0.2	16	16
	Nitrodisc	0.3	12	24
	Nitro-Dur	0.3	15	60
	Nitroglycerin Transdermal	0.4	13-20[1]	32-125[1]
	Minitran	0.4	13.3	36
	Nitrek	0.4	16	44.8
	Nitrodisc	0.4	16	32
	Nitro-Dur	0.4	20	80
	Transderm-Nitro	0.4	20	50
	Deponit	0.4	32	32
	Nitroglycerin Transdermal	0.6	20-30[1]	75-187.5[1]
	Minitran	0.6	20	54
	Nitrek	0.6	24	67.2
	Nitro-Dur	0.6	30	120
	Transderm-Nitro	0.6	30	75
	Nitro-Dur	0.8	40	160

[1] Various generic systems have the same release rates but variable surface areas and NTG contents.

Type of Drug:

Angina drugs; nitroglycerin, nitro, NTG.

How the Drug Works:

Nitrates relax blood vessels, allowing them to dilate (widen). This allows more blood to flow through the vessels and reduces the workload of the heart. It also reduces the oxygen demand of the heart and improves blood flow to the heart.

Uses:

To treat and prevent angina attacks. These drugs may be taken before events or activities that are likely to provoke an angina attack.

To treat an acute angina attack.

Unlabeled Use(s): Occasionally doctors may prescribe sublingual and topical nitroglycerin and oral nitrates for reducing the workload on the heart in patients with a history of heart attacks or congestive heart failure. Doctors may also prescribe nitroglycerin ointment with other medications for treatment of Raynaud disease.

Precautions:

Do not use in the following situations:

- allergy to nitrates or any of their ingredients
- anemia, severe
- congestive heart failure
- enlarged heart
- glaucoma, angle closure
- head trauma, bleeding, hemorrhage
- heart attack (isosorbide mononitrate, nitroglycerin only)
- hypotension (low blood pressure)

Excessive dosages: Excessive dosages may produce severe headaches. Lower doses and pain medications can help control this problem. Headaches tend to become less severe or disappear as therapy continues.

Isosorbide mononitrate: Do not avoid headaches by altering the schedule of drug treatment, since headaches are a marker of the activity of the drug. Aspirin or acetaminophen are helpful in relieving headaches without affecting the action of isosorbide.

Tolerance: Tolerance to the effects of nitroglycerin may develop with other nitrates. The effectiveness of nitrate therapy may decrease over time. If this occurs, therapy should be reevaluated by your doctor. Tolerance may be reversed with short periods (8 to 24 hours) of withdrawal. Tolerance may be minimized by using the smallest effective dose, by using intermittent dosing, or by alternating with other vasodilators. Administering isosorbide dinitrate 2 or 3 times daily instead of 4, or using nitroglycerin transdermal patches for only 12 hours during the day, may reduce the possibility of tolerance developing. Nitrates that appear least likely to be associated with tolerance are the short-acting formulations (eg, sublingual, translingual spray). The transmucosal form also appears to be associated with minimal tolerance.

Transient dizziness or weakness: Transient dizziness or weakness (orthostatic hypotension) can occur when arising from a seated or lying position. Alcohol can worsen this side effect. Recovery can be hastened by positions in which the head is lower than the heart, deep breathing, and movements of the arms and legs.

Pregnancy: There are no adequate and well-controlled studies in pregnant women. Use only if clearly needed and the potential benefits to the mother outweigh the possible hazards to the fetus.

Breastfeeding: It is not known if nitrates appear in breast milk. Discontinue nursing during nitrate therapy.

Children: Safety and effectiveness have not been established.

Drug Interactions:

Tell your doctor or pharmacist if you are taking or if you are planning to take any over-the-counter or prescription medications or dietary supplements with nitrates. Doses of one or both drugs may need to be modified or a different drug may need to be prescribed. The following drugs and drug classes interact with nitrates:

alcohol
calcium channel blockers (eg, verapamil)
ergot alkaloids (eg, dihydroergotamine)
heparin (eg, *Liquaemin*)
sildenafil citrate (*Viagra*)
vasodilators (eg, papaverine)

Side Effects:

Every drug is capable of producing side effects. Many nitrate users experience no, or minor, side effects. The frequency and severity of side effects depend on many factors including dose, duration of therapy, and individual susceptibility. Possible side effects include:

Digestive Tract: Nausea; vomiting; diarrhea; stomach pain; appetite loss; dry mouth.

Nervous System: Persistent or severe headache; apprehension; restlessness; agitation; anxiety; flushing; dizziness; muscle twitching; weakness; lightheadedness.

Circulatory System: Abnormally slow or fast pulse; chest pain; palpitations (pounding in the chest); low blood pressure; fainting; irregular heartbeat.

Skin: Rash or itching (nitroglycerin patches); flushing; excessive sweating; cold sweat; local burning or tingling (sublingual or buccal tablets).

Other: Visual disturbances; fever; involuntary passing of urine or feces.

Guidelines for Use:

- *Brand interchange* — Do not change from one brand of this drug to another without consulting your pharmacist or doctor. Products manufactured by different companies may not be equally effective.
- Avoid alcohol while undergoing nitrate therapy.
- May cause headache, dizziness, or flushing. Notify your doctor if blurred vision, dry mouth, or persistent headache occurs.
- Take oral nitrates on an empty stomach with a glass of water.
- Keep tablets and capsules in original container. Keep container closed tightly.
- *Sublingual tablets* —
  Dissolve tablet under tongue. Do not crush or chew. Do not swallow.
  A lack of burning or stinging sensation does not indicate a loss of potency.
  Use when seated. Take at the first sign of an anginal attack (chest pain) before severe pain develops. If angina is not relieved in 5 minutes, dissolve a second tablet under the tongue. If pain is not relieved within another 5 minutes, dissolve a third tablet. If pain continues or intensifies, notify your doctor immediately or report to the nearest hospital emergency room.
  Absorption is dependent on saliva secretion. Dry mouth (including drug-induced dry mouth) decreases absorption.
  Keep in the original container. Store at room temperature. Protect from moisture. Traditionally, unused tablets should be discarded 6 months after the original bottle is opened. Specific manufacturers may have different recommendations.
- *Translingual spray* —
  Do not shake. Spray onto or under tongue. Do not inhale spray.
  At the onset of attack, spray 1 or 2 doses onto oral mucosa. No more than 3 doses are recommended within 15 minutes. If chest pain persists, seek prompt medical attention.
  May be used 5 to 10 minutes prior to engaging in activities that might precipitate an acute attack.
- *Transmucosal tablets* —
  Place tablet between lip and gum above front teeth or between cheek and gum.
  Permit to dissolve slowly over a 3 to 5 hour period.
  Do not chew or swallow tablets. Release of nitroglycerin begins immediately upon contact with the mucosa and will continue until the tablet dissolves. Rate of dissolution is increased by touching tablet with tongue or drinking hot liquids.
- *Sustained-release nitroglycerin* —
  Swallow whole. Do not chew or crush. Not for sublingual use.

Guidelines for Use (cont.):

- *Topical ointment* —
  Patient instructions are available with products.
  Spread a thin layer on skin using applicator or dose-measuring paper. Do not use fingers. Do not rub or massage. Keep tube tightly closed.
  When applying ointment, spread at least a 2¼ × 3½ inch area in a thin, uniform layer. The ointment may be applied to the chest or back.
  Rotate application sites to prevent contact dermatitis.
- *Transdermal nitroglycerin patches* —
  Patient instructions are available with products.
  Patches are not for immediate relief of chest pain. Occasional use of sublingual preparations may be necessary.
  Apply pad once each day to a skin site free of hair and excessive movement. Do not apply to the forearms or below the knees. Avoid cuts or irritations.
  Change the application site slightly each time to avoid undue skin irritation.
  Dispose of used patches carefully. Discarded patches contain significant amounts of nitroglycerin and can be harmful to children or pets.

If you have any questions, consult your doctor, pharmacist, or health care provider.

Generic Name *Brand Name Examples*	Supplied As	Generic Available
Rx **Amiodarone**[1]		
Cordarone, Pacerone	**Tablets**: 200 mg	Yes
Pacerone	**Tablets**: 400 mg	No

[1] This product is also available as an injection.

Type of Drug:

A drug used for specific types of severe irregular heartbeats.

How the Drug Works:

Amiodarone corrects and prevents the occurrence of various types of irregular heart rhythms that may lead to life-threatening situations.

Uses:

To treat certain life-threatening heart rhythm disturbances (ie, recurrent ventricular fibrillation, recurrent hemodynamically unstable ventricular tachycardia) that are not affected by other antiarrhythmics or when other drugs are not tolerated.

Unlabeled Use(s): Sometimes used to treat refractory sustained or paroxysmal atrial fibrillation and paroxysmal supraventricular tachycardia, and symptomatic atrial flutter. May improve left ventricular ejection fraction, exercise tolerance, and ventricular arrhythmias in patients with congestive heart failure.

Precautions:

Do not use in the following situations:

allergy to amiodarone or any of its ingredients
fainting episodes caused by bradycardia (without pacemaker)
heart block, second- and third-degree
sinus-node dysfunction, severe

Use with caution in the following situations:

electrolyte imbalance (eg, potassium)
liver disease
lung disease
thyroid dysfunction

Potentially fatal toxicities: Amiodarone has caused pulmonary toxicity (ie, hypersensitivity pneumonitis or interstitial/alveolar pneumonitis). Overt liver disease has been reported, resulting in a few deaths. Significant heart block or sinus bradycardia has also been reported.

Heart effects: A worsening of heart rhythm irregularities is unusual while under treatment but can occur. Amiodarone can also cause slow heart rates or occasional pauses in the heart rhythm.

Sensitivity to sunlight: Amiodarone has caused sensitivity of the skin to sunlight and to ultraviolet light. During long-term treatment, exposed skin may appear blue-gray. Risk is increased in patients with a fair complexion and in those with excessive exposure to the sun. Use sunscreens and wear protective clothing.

Pregnancy: Amiodarone can cause fetal harm when administered to a pregnant woman. There have been some reports of congenital goiter/hypothyroidism and hyperthyroidism. Use only if clearly needed and potential benefits to the mother outweigh the possible hazards to the fetus.

Breastfeeding: Amiodarone appears in breast milk. Mothers should discontinue breastfeeding during therapy.

Children: Safety and effectiveness have not been established. Benzyl alcohol, contained in some of these products as a preservative, has been associated with a fatal gasping syndrome in premature infants. Amiodarone is not recommended in children.

Lab tests and physical examinations will be required during treatment with amiodarone. Tests may include chest x-rays; blood tests; electrocardiograms; liver, thyroid, and pulmonary function tests; and eye exams.

Drug Interactions:

Tell your doctor or pharmacist if you are taking or if you are planning to take any over-the-counter or prescription medications or dietary supplements with amiodarone. Doses of one or both drugs may need to be modified or a different drug may need to be prescribed. The following drugs and drug classes interact with amiodarone:

antiarrhythmics, other (eg, procainamide)
anticoagulants (eg, warfarin)
calcium channel blockers (eg, verapamil)
cimetidine (eg, *Tagamet*)
cyclosporine (eg, *Neoral*)
digoxin (eg, *Lanoxin*)
disopyramide (eg, *Norpace*)
fentanyl (eg, *Sublimaze*)
flecainide (*Tambocor*)
methotrexate (eg, *Rheumatrex*)
hydantoins (eg, phenytoin)
quinidine (eg, *Quinora*)
quinolones (eg, sparfloxacin)
ritonavir (*Norvir*)

Side Effects:

Every drug is capable of producing side effects. Many amiodarone users experience no, or minor, side effects. The frequency and severity of side effects depend on many factors including dose, duration of therapy, and individual susceptibility. Possible side effects include:

Eyes or Ocular: Appearance of halos around lights; sensitivity to light; blurred or spotty vision; dry eyes; sensitivity to light; permanent blindness; eye discomfort; fluid accumulation at the optic disc; other vision disturbances; eye degeneration; optic nerve disease.

Digestive Tract: Nausea; vomiting; constipation; diarrhea; loss of appetite; stomach pain.

Nervous System: Tremors; twitches; fatigue; loss of coordination; unsteady walking; dizziness; numbness and tingling in hands and feet; difficulty sleeping; headache; general discomfort; abnormal gait.

Circulatory System: Slowing of heartbeat (rhythm); worsening of irregular heart rhythm; decrease in blood pressure; decrease in blood platelets; coagulation abnormalities; heart failure; heart block.

Respiratory System: Difficulty breathing (shortness of breath); coughing; abnormal x-ray or biopsy; fibrosis.

Skin: Sensitivity to sunlight; blue-gray skin color; rash; dermatitis; unexplained bruising; hair loss; flushing; abnormal skin sensations (eg, burning, prickling, tingling).

Other: Disturbances in thyroid, respiratory, kidney and liver function (cirrhosis, hepatitis); abnormal taste and smell; edema (fluid retention); abnormal salivation; loss of sex drive; abnormal blood tests.

Guidelines for Use:

- Dosage is individualized. Take exactly as prescribed.
- Do not change the dose or stop taking unless advised by your doctor.
- High doses of amiodarone are usually required for the first 1 to 3 weeks of treatment.
- Take with meals, especially if stomach upset occurs.
- If a dose is missed, take it as soon as possible. If several hours have passed or it is nearing time for the next dose, do not double the dose to catch up, unless advised by your doctor. If more than one dose is missed, or it is necessary to establish a new dosage schedule, contact your doctor or pharmacist.
- Inform your doctor if you are pregnant, become pregnant, planning to become pregnant, or are breastfeeding before beginning therapy.
- May cause photosensitivity (sensitivity to sunlight). Use sunscreen and wear protective clothing until tolerance is determined.
- Shortness of breath, coughing and abnormal diagnostic tests (eg, chest x-ray, lung biopsy) can occur. Report changes in breathing or vision, or any coughing to your doctor and have a routine chest x-ray.
- Loss of vision can occur. Inform your doctor if your vision changes or your peripheral vision decreases.
- Store at room temperature (59° to 86°F). Keep in a tight container away from light.

If you have any questions, consult your doctor, pharmacist, or health care provider.

	Generic Name *Brand Name Examples*	Supplied As	Generic Available
Rx	**Disopyramide Phosphate**		
	Norpace	**Capsules**: 100 mg, 150 mg	Yes
	Norpace CR	**Capsules, extended release**: 100 mg, 150 mg	Yes

Type of Drug:

A drug used for specific types of irregular heartbeats.

How the Drug Works:

Disopyramide slows the rate at which nerve impulses are conducted through the heart and reduces the tendency of the heart to beat irregularly.

Uses:

To treat documented life-threatening heart rhythm disturbances.

Unlabeled Use(s): Occasionally doctors may prescribe disopyramide for certain types of rapid heart rate.

Precautions:

Do not use in the following situations:

allergy to disopyramide or any of its ingredients
cardiogenic shock
congenital QT prolongation
heart block (without pacemaker), second- or third-degree

Use with caution in the following situations:

abnormal heart conduction
antiarrhythmic therapy, concomitant
arrhythmias, ventricular
asymptomatic ventricular premature contractions
atrial rhythm disturbances
bundle branch block
congestive heart failure
enlarged prostate
glaucoma
heart block, first-degree
kidney disease
liver disease
low blood pressure
myasthenia gravis
potassium imbalance
urinary retention

Low blood sugar: Occasionally low blood glucose (sugar) levels occur with disopyramide therapy. Contact your doctor if symptoms (eg, increased heart rate, sweating, chills, tremor) develop.

Pregnancy: There are no adequate and well-controlled studies in pregnant women. Disopyramide has been found in human fetal blood, and may stimulate contractions of the pregnant uterus. Use only if clearly needed and the potential benefits to the mother outweigh the possible hazards to the fetus.

Breastfeeding: Disopyramide appears in breast milk. A decision should be made whether to discontinue nursing or discontinue the drug, taking into account the importance of the drug to the mother. Consult your doctor.

Lab tests may be required during treatment with disopyramide. Tests may include: blood tests and electrocardiograms.

Drug Interactions:

Tell your doctor or pharmacist if you are taking or planning to take any over-the-counter or prescription medications or dietary supplements with disopyramide. Doses of one or both drugs may need to be modified or a different drug may need to be prescribed. The following drugs and drug classes interact with disopyramide:

antiarrhythmics, other (eg, procainamide, lidocaine)
beta-blockers (eg, propranolol)
clarithromycin (*Biaxin*)
erythromycin (eg, *E-Mycin*)
hydantoins (eg, phenytoin)
quinidine (eg, *Cardioquin*)
rifampin (eg, *Rifadin*)
verapamil (eg, *Calan*)

Side Effects:

Every drug is capable of producing side effects. Many disopyramide users experience no, or minor, side effects. The frequency and severity of side effects depend on many factors including dose, duration of therapy, and individual susceptibility. Possible side effects include:

Digestive Tract: Constipation; nausea; vomiting; stomach pain; bloating and gas; appetite loss; diarrhea.

Nervous System: Headache; nervousness; dizziness; fatigue; difficulty sleeping.

Circulatory System: Chest pain; irregular heartbeat; low blood pressure; heart conduction disturbances; congestive heart failure.

Skin: Rash; itching; hives.

Urinary and Reproductive Tract: Urinary retention, hesitancy, frequency, or urgency; impotence; painful urination.

Other: Shortness of breath; edema (fluid retention); weight gain; blurred vision; dry mouth; dry nose, eyes, and throat; aches and pains; fainting; general body discomfort; muscle weakness; decreased potassium level; increased cholesterol and triglyceride blood levels; decreased blood sugar level.

Guidelines for Use:

- Hospitalization is required when starting this medication.
- Dosage is individualized. Take exactly as prescribed.
- Do not change the dose or stop taking before consulting your doctor. Do not exceed recommended dosage.
- If a dose is missed, take it as soon as possible. If several hours have passed or if it is nearing time for the next dose, do not double the dose to catch up, unless advised by your doctor. If more than one dose is missed, or it is necessary to establish a new dosage schedule, contact your doctor or pharmacist.
- Swallow sustained release capsules whole. Do not break or chew.
- May cause rash, chest pain, dry mouth, dizziness, difficulty breathing, difficult urination, constipation, or blurred vision. Notify your doctor if these symptoms persist.
- Consult your doctor immediately if you experience symptoms of low blood sugar (increased heart rate, sweating, chills, tremors).
- Inform your doctor if you are pregnant, become pregnant, planning to become pregnant, or are breastfeeding before beginning therapy.
- Lab tests may be required to monitor blood counts and heart function. Be sure to keep appointments.
- Store at controlled room temperature (68° to 77°F).

If you have any questions, consult your doctor, pharmacist, or health care provider.

Generic Name *Brand Name Example*	Supplied As	Generic Available
Rx **Dofetilide**		
Tikosyn	**Capsules**: 125 mcg, 250 mcg, 500 mcg	No

Type of Drug:
Antiarrhythmic drug.

How the Drug Works:
Dofetilide delays cardiac cell electrical activity, normalizing cardiac activity and maintaining normal sinus rhythm.

Uses:
For the conversion of atrial fibrillation and atrial flutter to normal sinus rhythm.

For maintaining normal sinus rhythm in patients with atrial fibrillation and atrial flutter.

Unlabeled Use(s): Dofetilide has been used for ventricular arrhythmias.

Precautions:
Do not use in the following situations:
- allergy to dofetilide or any of its ingredients
- concominant use of verapamil, cimetidine, trimethoprim, ketoconazole, prochlorperazine, or megestrol
- congenital or acquired long QT syndromes
- heart rate of less than 50 bpm
- kidney impairment, severe
- QT baseline interval or QTc greater than 440 msec

Use with caution in the following situations:
- hypokalemia
- hypomagnesemia
- kidney disease, mild to moderate
- liver disease
- torsade de pointes type ventricular tachycardia
- QT prolongation

Gender: Dofetilide was associated with a greater risk of torsade de pointes in female patients than in male patients.

Pregnancy: There are no adaquate and well-controlled studies in pregnant women. Use only if clearly needed and the potential benefits to the mother outweigh the possible hazards to the fetus.

Breastfeeding: It is not known if dofetilide appears in breast milk. Consult your doctor before you begin breastfeeding.

Children: The safety and efficacy of use in children younger than 18 years of age have not been established.

Lab tests will be required during treatment. Tests may include ECG monitoring, QTc levels, kidney function, and liver function.

Drug Interactions:

Tell you doctor or pharmacist if you are taking or if you a planning to take any over-the-counter or prescription medications or dietary supplements with dofetilide. Doses of one or both drugs may need to be modified or a different drug may need to be prescribed. The following drugs and drug classes interact with dofetilide:

- amiloride (*Midamor*)
- antiarrhythmic agents (Class I or Class III) (eg, moricizine)
- bepridil (*Vascor*)
- cimetidine (eg, *Tagamet*)
- CYP3A4 isoenzyme inhibitors (eg, ketoconazole)
- digoxin (*Lanoxin*)
- megestrol (*Megace*)
- metformin (*Glucophage*)
- phenothiazines (eg, chlorpromazine)
- potassium-depleting diuretics
- prochlorperazine (eg, *Compazine*)
- tricyclic antidepressants (eg, amitriptyline)
- triamterene (*Dyrenium*)
- trimethoprim (eg, *Proloprim*)
- trimethoprim/sulfamethoxazole (eg, *Bactrim*)
- verapamil (eg, *Calan*)

Side Effects:

Every drug is capable of producing side effects. Many dofetilide users experience no, or minor, side effects. The frequency and severity of side effects depend on many factors including dose, duration of therapy, and individual susceptibility. Possible side effects include:

Circulatory System: Rapid heart beat; slow heart beat; various cardiac rhythm disturbances; pounding in the chest; heart block; heart arrest; stroke.

Nervous System: Headache; chest pain; dizziness; stomach pain; back pain; joint pain; muscle limpness; weakness; anxiety; fainting; muscle dysfunction.

Skin: Rash; hives; sweating; abnormal skin sensations (eg, burning, prickling, tingling).

Other: Respiratory tract infection; difficulty breathing; nausea; vomiting; thirst; appetite loss; flu syndrome; sleeplessness; accidental injury; diarrhea; urinary tract infection; fluid retention; cough; migraine; dizziness; fainting; liver damage.

Guidelines for Use:

- Dosage is individualized. Take exactly as prescribed.
- Do not change the dose or stop taking unless advised by your doctor.
- Dofetilide is only available to hospitals and prescribers who have received appropriate dosing and treatment initiation education.
- Compliance with the dosing schedule and periodic heart and kidney function tests is important for minimizing the risk of developing serious abnormal heart rhythm.
- Notify your health care provider of any change in over-the-counter or prescription medication, or dietary supplement use.
- Inform your health care provider if you are hospitalized or prescribed a new medication for any condition.
- Inform your doctor if you are pregnant, become pregnant, planning to become pregnant, or are breastfeeding before beginning therapy.
- Notify your doctor immediately of symptoms associated with altered electrolyte balance, such as excessive or prolonged diarrhea, sweating, vomiting, appetite loss, thirst, or diuretic use.
- If a dose is missed, take it as soon as possible. If several hours have passed or if it is nearing time for the next dose, do not double the dose to catch up, unless advised by your doctor. If more than one dose is missed or it is necessary to establish a new dosage schedule, contact your doctor or pharmacist.
- Store at controlled room temperature (59° to 86°F) in a tight container. Protect from moisture and humidity.

If you have any questions, consult your doctor, pharmacist, or health care provider.

	Generic Name *Brand Name Example*	Supplied As	Generic Available
	Flecainide Acetate		
Rx	*Tambocor*	**Tablets:** 50 mg, 100 mg, 150 mg	No

Type of Drug:

Drug used for specific types of irregular heartbeats.

How the Drug Works:

Flecainide corrects and prevents the occurrence of various types of irregular heartbeats that lead to serious life-threatening situations.

Uses:

To treat life-threatening heart rhythm disturbances.

Precautions:

Do not use in the following situations:

allergy to flecainide
cardiogenic shock
heart block (without a pacemaker)
specific types of irregular heartbeats

Use with caution in the following situations:

heart attack, recent
heart disease (eg, congestive heart failure, sick sinus syndrome)
heart rate, occasional slowing or pausing
kidney disease
liver disease
pacemaker, permanent
potassium imbalance

Heart rhythm disturbances: New or worsened heart rhythm disturbances can result. The likelihood of heart rhythm disturbances occurring as a result of using flecainide is greater at high doses or in patients with heart disease. Therefore, the dose of flecainide should not be changed unsupervised.

Pregnancy: Adequate studies have not been done in pregnant women. Use only if clearly needed and potential benefits outweigh the possible hazards to the fetus.

Breastfeeding: Flecainide appears in breast milk. Because of the potential for serious side effects in nursing infants, decide whether to discontinue nursing or the drug, taking into account the importance of the drug to the mother. Consult your doctor.

Children: Safety and effectiveness in children younger than 18 years of age have not been established.

Lab tests may be required during treatment with flecainide. Tests may include monitoring of blood levels.

Drug Interactions:

Tell your doctor or pharmacist if you are taking or planning to take any over-the-counter or prescription medications or dietary supplements with flecainide. Doses of one or both drugs may need to be modified or a different drug may need to be prescribed. The following drugs and drug classes interact with flecainide:

amiodarone *(Cordarone)*
cimetidine (eg, *Tagamet)*
digoxin (eg, *Lanoxin)*
disopyramide (eg, *Norpace*)
propranolol (eg, *Inderal)*
urinary acidifiers (eg, ammonium chloride)
urinary alkalinizers (eg, sodium bicarbonate)
verapamil (eg, *Calan*)

Side Effects:

Every drug is capable of producing side effects. Many flecainide users experience no, or minor, side effects. The frequency and severity of side effects depend on many factors including dose, duration of therapy, and individual susceptibility. Possible side effects include:

Digestive Tract: Nausea; vomiting; constipation; indigestion; appetite loss; diarrhea; stomach pain.

Nervous System: Dizziness; numbness and tingling of toes and fingers; tremor; headache; depression; sleeplessness; paralysis; fatigue; weakness; incoordination; vertigo (feeling of whirling motion); anxiety.

Circulatory System: New or worsened heart rhythm disturbances; heart rate changes; chest pain; palpitations (pounding in the chest).

Skin: Rash; flushing; sweating.

Other: Edema (fluid retention); blurred vision; difficulty focusing eyes; spots in front of eyes; double vision; ringing in the ears; difficulty breathing; fever; general body discomfort; fainting.

Guidelines for Use:

- Take as prescribed by your doctor. Serious heartbeat disturbances can result from missing any doses and serious side effects can result from increasing or decreasing doses without supervision.
- Blood tests for flecainide levels may be required to monitor your therapy.

If you have any questions, consult your doctor, pharmacist, or health care provider.

Generic Name *Brand Name Example*	Supplied As	Generic Available
Rx **Mexiletine** *Mexitil*	**Capsules:** 150 mg, 200 mg, 250 mg	No

Type of Drug:

A drug used for specific types of irregular heartbeats.

How the Drug Works:

Mexiletine reduces the tendency of the heart to beat irregularly.

Uses:

To treat documented life-threatening heart rhythm disturbances.

Unlabeled Use(s): Occasionally doctors may prescribe mexiletine to reduce the incidence of irregular heartbeats during heart attacks. It may also be used to reduce pain, impaired sense of touch and abnormal sensations associated with diabetic neuropathy.

Precautions:

Do not use in the following situations:

- cardiogenic shock
- heart block (without pacemaker)

Use with caution in the following situations:

- certain heart disorders
- congestive heart failure, severe
- heart block (with pacemaker)
- liver disease
- low blood pressure
- seizures, history

Heart rhythm disturbances: Worsened heart rhythm disturbances can result from taking mexiletine. Close monitoring and careful dosage adjustment will be required.

Pregnancy: Mexiletine crosses the placenta. Adequate studies have not been done in pregnant women. Use only if clearly needed and potential benefits outweigh the possible hazards to the fetus.

Breastfeeding: Mexiletine appears in breast milk. Discontinue nursing if mexiletine therapy is needed.

Children: Safety and effectiveness have not been established.

Drug Interactions:

Tell your doctor or pharmacist if you are taking or planning to take any over-the-counter or prescription medications or dietary supplements with mexiletine. Doses of one or both drugs may need to be modified or a different drug may need to be prescribed. The following drugs and drug classes interact with mexiletine:

- aluminum-magnesium hydroxide (eg, *Maalox)*
- atropine
- caffeine
- cimetidine *(Tagamet)*
- hydantoins (eg, phenytoin)
- metoclopramide (eg, *Reglan)*
- narcotics (eg, codeine)
- rifampin (eg, *Rifadin)*
- theophylline (eg, *Theo-Dur)*
- urinary acidifiers (eg, potassium acid phosphate)
- urinary alkalinizers (eg, potassium citrate)

Side Effects:

Every drug is capable of producing side effects. Many mexiletine users experience no, or minor, side effects. The frequency and severity of side effects depend on many factors including dose, duration of therapy, and individual susceptibility. Possible side effects include:

Digestive Tract: Nausea; vomiting; heartburn; stomach pain, cramps or discomfort; constipation; diarrhea; changes in appetite.

Nervous System: Dizziness; tremor; lightheadedness; nervousness; confusion; incoordination;headache; numbness; abnormal sensations; changes in sleep habits; weakness; fatigue; depression.

Circulatory System: Palpitations (pounding in the chest); chest pain; increased irregular heartbeats.

Other: Joint pain; blurred vision; vision problems; ringing in the ears; speech difficulties; rash; dry mouth; difficulty breathing; edema (fluid retention); fever.

Guidelines for Use:

- Take medication with food or an antacid.
- Notify your doctor if unexplained general tiredness, yellowing of the skin, fever or sore throat occurs.
- Side effects such as nausea, vomiting, heartburn, diarrhea, constipation, dizziness, tremor, nervousness, in-coordination, changes in sleep habits, headache, visual disturbances, tingling/numbness, weakness, ringing in the ears and palpitations/chest pain may occur. Notify your doctor if they become bothersome.
- Avoid changes in diet that could drastically acidify or alkalinize the urine.
- Hospitalization is required when starting this medication.

If you have any questions, consult your doctor, pharmacist, or health care provider.

Generic Name / *Brand Name Example*	Supplied As	Generic Available
Rx **Moricizine**		
Ethmozine	**Tablets:** 200 mg, 250 mg, 300 mg	No

Type of Drug:

A drug used for specific types of irregular heartbeats.

How the Drug Works:

Moricizine prevents the occurrence of certain types of heart disturbances involving the ventricle of the heart that lead to serious life-threatening situations.

Uses:

To treat life-threatening heart rhythm disturbances. Because of certain effects of this drug, moricizine use should be reserved for patients in whom the benefits of treatment outweigh the risks.

Unlabeled Use(s): Occasionally doctors may prescribe moricizine for certain other heart rhythm disturbances.

Precautions:

Do not use in the following situations:

allergy to moricizine
cardiogenic shock
heart block

Use with caution in the following situations:

congestive heart failure
electrolyte imbalances (eg, potassium, magnesium)
heart conduction abnormalities, preexisting
kidney disease
liver disease
sick sinus syndrome

Heart Rhythm Disturbances: New or worsened heart rhythm disturbances can result from taking moricizine, especially in patients with serious or advanced heart disease. Close monitoring and careful dosage adjustment will be required.

Pregnancy: Adequate studies have not been done in pregnant women. Use only if clearly needed and potential benefits outweigh the possible hazards to the fetus.

Breastfeeding: Moricizine appears in breast milk. Because of the potential for serious adverse effects, a decision should be made whether to discontinue nursing or the drug, taking into account the importance of the drug to the mother. Consult your doctor.

Children: Safety and effectiveness in children under 18 have not been established.

Lab tests may be required during treatment with moricizine. Tests may include: Electrocardiograms; kidney and liver function tests.

Drug Interactions:

Tell your doctor or pharmacist if you are taking or planning to take any over-the-counter or prescription medications or dietary supplements with moricizine. Doses of one or both drugs may need to be modified or a different drug may need to be prescribed. The following drugs and drug classes interact with moricizine:

cimetidine (eg, *Tagamet*)
digoxin (eg, *Lanoxin*)
propranolol (eg, *Inderal*)
theophylline (eg, *Theo-Dur*)

Side Effects:

Every drug is capable of producing side effects. Many moricizine users experience no, or minor, side effects. The frequency and severity of side effects depend on many factors including dose, duration of therapy, and individual susceptibility. Possible side effects include:

Digestive Tract: Nausea; vomiting; diarrhea; stomach pain; indigestion; appetite loss; gas; bitter taste; intestinal blockage.

Nervous System: Dizziness; drowsinesss; headache; fatigue; nervousness; restlessness; sleep disturbances; vertigo (feeling of whirling motion); abnormal coordination or movement; tremor; anxiety; depression; confusion; seizures; coma; hallucinations; memory loss; euphoria (exaggerated sense of well being); agitation; abnormal gait; weakness.

Circulatory System: Palpitations (pounding in the chest); chest pain; changes in heart rate and blood pressure; heart rhythm disturbances; heart failure; heart attack or stroke.

Respiratory System: Difficult, accelerated or cessation of breathing; asthma; cough; sore throat; inflamed sinuses.

Urinary and Reproductive Tract: Urinary retention, frequency or incontinence; kidney pain; difficult or painful urination.

Skin: Rash; dry skin; itching; hives; abnormal or decreased sensation; sweating. *Senses:* Blurred vision; double vision; involuntary eye movements; eye pain; ringing in the ears; difficulty speaking.

Other: Dry mouth; difficulty swallowing; swollen lips and tongue; decreased sex drive; impotence; abnormally low body temperature or fever; edema (fluid retention) around the eye socket; muscle and bone pain; fainting; temperature intolerance.

Guidelines for Use:

- Take exactly as prescribed by your doctor. Serious heartbeat disturbances can result from taking too much or too little of this drug. Dosage changes must be supervised by your doctor.
- Contact your doctor immediately if you develop chest pain or discomfort, palpitations (pounding in the chest), irregular heartbeat or fever.
- Unless instructed otherwise by your doctor, if a dose is missed, take it as soon as possible. If several hours have passed or it is nearing time for the next dose, do not double the dose to catch up, unless advised to do so by your doctor. If more than one dose is missed or it is necessary to establish a new dosage schedule, contact your doctor or pharmacist. Use exactly as prescribed.
- Hospitalization is required when starting on this medication.

If you have any questions, consult your doctor, pharmacist, or health care provider.

	Generic Name *Brand Name Examples*	Supplied As	Generic Available
Rx	**Procainamide**[1]		
	Pronestyl	**Capsules:** 250 mg, 375 mg, 500 mg	Yes
	Pronestyl[2]	**Tablets:** 250 mg, 375 mg, 500 mg	Yes
	Procan SR, Pronestyl-SR	**Tablets, sustained release:** 250 mg, 500 mg, 750 mg, 1000 mg	Yes

[1] Some of these products are also available as an injection.
[2] Contains the dye tartrazine.

Type of Drug:

A drug used for specific types of irregular heartbeats.

How the Drug Works:

Procainamide slows the rate at which nerve impulses are conducted through the heart and reduces the tendency of the heart to beat irregularly.

Uses:

To treat documented life-threatening heart rhythm disturbances.

Precautions:

Do not use in the following situations:

- allergies to procainamide, procaine or procaine-like anesthetics
- heart block
- lupus erythematosus
- torsade de pointes

Use with caution in the following situations:

- bone marrow failure, preexisting
- congestive heart failure
- cytopenia
- digitalis intoxication
- heart disease
- kidney disease
- myasthenia gravis

Lupus erythematosus-like syndrome: A syndrome similar to systemic lupus erythematosus may occur (see Side Effects). Contact your doctor if symptoms develop.

Pregnancy: Procainamide crosses the placenta. Adequate studies have not been done in pregnant women. Use only if clearly needed and potential benefits outweigh the possible hazards to the fetus.

Breastfeeding: Procainamide is excreted in breast milk. Because of the potential for adverse effects, a decision should be made whether to discontinue nursing or the drug, taking into account the importance of the drug to the mother. Contact your doctor.

Children: Safety and effectiveness have not been established.

Lab tests may be required during treatment with procainamide. Tests may include: Electrocardiograms, procainamide blood levels and blood counts.

Tartrazine: Some of these products may contain the dye tartrazine (FD&C Yellow No. 5) which can cause allergic reactions in certain individuals. Check package label when available or consult your doctor or pharmacist.

Drug Interactions:

Tell your doctor or pharmacist if you are taking or if you are planning to take any over-the-counter or prescription medications with procainamide. Doses of one or both drugs may need to be modified or a different drug may need to be prescribed. The following drugs and drug classes interact with procainamide.

alcohol
beta-blockers (eg, propranolol)
histamine H_2 antagonists (eg, cimetidine)
lidocaine (eg, *Xylocaine*)
quinidine (eg, *Quinora*)
succinylcholine (eg, *Sucostrin*)
trimethoprim (eg, *Proloprim*)

Side Effects:

Every drug is capable of producing side effects. Many procainamide users experience no, or minor, side effects. The frequency and severity of side effects depend on many factors including dose, duration of therapy and individual susceptibility. Possible side effects include:

Lupus Erythematosus-like Syndrome: Joint pain or stiffness; skin lesions; muscle aches; chest pain with breathing; fever; chills; abdominal pain.

Digestive Tract: Appetite loss; nausea; vomiting; diarrhea; abdominal pain.

Nervous System: Depression; dizziness; weakness; giddiness; hallucinations.

Skin: Rash; itching; hives; flushing.

Other: Irregular heartbeat; fibrillation; bitter taste.

Guidelines for Use:

- Notify your doctor of any drug allergies, especially to procaine, other local anesthetic agents or aspirin, and report any history of kidney disease, congestive heart failure, myasthenia gravis, liver disease or lupus erythematosus.
- Notify your doctor promptly of the following symptoms: joint or muscle pain, fever, chills, rash, easy bruising, sore throat or mouth, infections, dark urine, yellowing of skin or eyes, wheezing, muscular weakness, chest or abdominal pain, palpitations, nausea, vomiting, appetite loss, diarrhea, hallucinations, dizziness or depression.
- Do not break or chew sustained-release tablets.

If you have any questions, consult your doctor, pharmacist, or health care provider.

Generic Name *Brand Name Example*	Supplied As	Generic Available
Rx **Propafenone HCl**		
Rythmol	**Tablets:** 150 mg, 300 mg	No

Type of Drug:

Drug used for specific types of irregular heartbeats.

How the Drug Works:

Propafenone reduces the tendency of the heart to beat irregularly. It stabilizes the activity of the heart muscle under certain conditions.

Uses:

To treat documented life-threatening heart rhythm disturbances. Because of certain effects of this drug, propafenone use should be reserved for patients in whom the benefits of treatment outweigh the risks.

Unlabeled Use(s): Occasionally doctors may prescribe propafenone for heart rhythm disturbances associated with Wolff-Parkinson-White syndrome.

Precautions:

Do not use in the following situations:

- allergy to propafenone
- cardiogenic shock
- congestive heart failure (uncontrolled)
- decreased blood pressure, marked
- decreased heart rate
- electrolyte imbalance
- heart disorders, certain (without pacemaker)
- lung disorders

Use with caution in the following situations:

- bronchospasm, nonallergic
- kidney disease
- liver disease
- pacemakers

Heart rhythm disturbances: New or worsened heart rhythm disturbances can result. Therefore, periodic electrocardiograms (EKGs) will be required prior to, and during, treatment with propafenone.

Pregnancy: Adequate studies have not been done in pregnant women. Use only if clearly needed and potential benefits outweigh the possible hazards to the fetus.

Breastfeeding: It is not known if propafenone appears in breast milk. A decision should be made whether to discontinue nursing or the drug, taking into account the importance of the drug to the mother. Consult your doctor.

Children: Safety and effectiveness have not been established.

Elderly: Use with caution. The usual adult dose may need to be lowered in these patients.

Lab tests may be required during treatment with propafenone. These tests may include electrocardiograms (EKGs); blood counts; liver and kidney function tests.

Drug Interactions:

Tell your doctor or pharmacist if you are taking or planning to take any over-the-counter or prescription medications or dietary supplements with propafenone. Doses of one or both drugs may need to be modified or a different drug may need to be prescribed. The following drugs and drug classes interact with propafenone:

anesthetics, local (eg, benzocaine)
anticoagulants (eg, warfarin)
beta-blockers (eg, propranolol)
cimetidine (eg, *Tagamet*)
cyclosporine (eg, *Sandimmune*)
digoxin (eg,*Lanoxin*)
quinidine (eg,*Quinora*)
rifampin (eg,*Rifadin*)

Side Effects:

Every drug is capable of producing side effects. Many propafenone users experience no, or minor, side effects. The frequency and severity of side effects depend on many factors including dose, duration of therapy, and individual susceptibility. Possible side effects include:

Digestive Tract: Nausea; vomiting; constipation; diarrhea; gas; appetite loss; indigestion; stomach pain; abdominal cramping; dry mouth; unusual taste.

Nervous System: Dizziness; headache; fatigue; anxiety; sleeplessness; drowsiness; incoordination; tremor.

Circulatory System: Congestive heart failure; chest pain; palpitations (pounding in the chest); irregular heartbeats (rhythm); decrease in blood pressure.

Other: Blurred vision; rash; difficulty breathing; edema (fluid retention); joint pain; sweating; weakness; fainting.

Guidelines for Use:

- Unless instructed otherwise by your doctor, if a dose is missed, take it as soon as possible. If several hours have passed or it is nearing time for the next dose, do not double the dose to catch up, unless advised to do so by your doctor. If more than one dose is missed, or it is necessary to establish a new dosage schedule, contact your doctor or pharmacist. Take this medication at evenly spaced intervals around the clock.
- Palpitations (pounding in the chest), chest pain, blurred or abnormal vision, or difficulty breathing may occur. Notify your doctor if these symptoms become bothersome.
- Notify your doctor if you develop any signs of infection such as fever, sore throat, chills or unusual bleeding or bruising.
- Watch for signs of overdose or toxicity, such as lowered blood pressure, excessive drowsiness, slowed heart rate or abnormal heartbeat.

If you have any questions, consult your doctor, pharmacist, or health care provider.

	Generic Name *Brand Name Examples*	Supplied As	Generic Available
Rx	**Quinidine Gluconate**[1]		
	Quinaglute Dura-Tabs, Quinalan	**Tablets, sustained release:** 324 mg	Yes
Rx	**Quinidine Polygalact-uronate**		
	Cardioquin	**Tablets:** 275 mg (equiv. to 200 mg sulfate)	No
Rx	**Quinidine Sulfate**		
	Quinora	**Tablets:** 200 mg, 300 mg	Yes
	Quinidex Extentabs	**Tablets, sustained release:** 300 mg	No

[1] Some of these products are also available as an injection.

Type of Drug:

Drugs used to treat irregular heartbeats.

How the Drug Works:

Quinidine reduces excitability of the heart muscle, slows the rate at which nerve impulses are conducted through the heart and reduces the ability of the heart to contract.

Uses:

To treat abnormal heart rhythms.

Injection: To treat *Plasmodium falciparum* malaria when oral therapy is not feasible or when a rapid effect is required.

Precautions:

Do not use in the following situations:

- allergy to quinidine
- certain heart rate or rhythm disturbances
- digitalis intoxication
- discoloration or "bruising" associated with quinidine, history
- heart block
- myasthenia gravis

Use with caution in the following situations:

- heart disease
- heart flutters or fibrillations
- kidney disease
- liver disease

Pregnancy: Adequate studies have not been done in pregnant women. Quinidine crosses the placenta and is found in fetal blood. Use only if clearly needed and potential benefits outweigh the possible hazards to the fetus.

Breastfeeding: Quinidine appears in breast milk. Consult your doctor before you begin breastfeeding.

Children: Safety and effectiveness have not been established.

Lab tests may be required during treatment with quinidine. Tests may include: Electrocardiograms; potassium and quinidine blood levels; kidney and liver function tests.

Drug Interactions:

Tell your doctor or pharmacist if you are taking or planning to take any over-the-counter or prescription medications or dietary supplements with quinidine. Doses of one or both drugs may need to be modified or a different drug may need to be prescribed. The following drugs and drug classes interact with quinidine:

- acetazolamide (eg, *Diamox*)
- amiodarone (*Cordarone*)
- antacids (eg, *Tums*)
- anticholinergics (eg, diphenhydramine)
- anticoagulants, oral (eg, warfarin)
- barbiturates (eg, phenobarbital)
- beta-blockers (eg, propranolol)
- cholinergic drugs (eg, pilocarpine)
- cimetidine (eg, *Tagamet*)
- dichlorphenamide (*Daranide*)
- digitoxin (eg, *Crystodigin*)
- digoxin (eg, *Lanoxin*)
- disopyramide (*Norpace*)
- hydantoins (eg, phenytoin)
- methazolamide (*Neptazane*)
- nifedipine (eg, *Procardia*)
- procainamide (*Pronestyl*)
- propafenone (*Rythmol*)
- rifampin (eg, *Rifadin*)
- sucralfate (*Carafate*)
- succinylcholine (eg, *Quelicin*)
- tricyclic antidepressants (eg, amitriptyline)
- urinary alkalinizers (eg, potassium citrate)
- verapamil (eg, *Calan*)

Side Effects:

Every drug is capable of producing side effects. Many quinidine users experience no, or minor, side effects. The frequency and severity of side effects depend on many factors including dose, duration of therapy, and individual susceptibility. Possible side effects include:

Quinidine Overdose: Ringing in the ears; hearing loss; headache; nausea; dizziness; vertigo (feeling of whirling motion); lightheadedness; disturbed vision. These may appear after a single dose.

Digestive Tract: Nausea; vomiting; stomach pain; diarrhea; appetite loss.

Nervous System: Headache; confusion; excitement; apprehension; vertigo (feeling of whirling motion); incoordination, depression; dementia; delirium.

Circulatory System: Low blood pressure; changes in heart rate or rhythm; heart flutter.

Respiratory System: Respiratory distress; asthma (allergic reaction).

Skin: Rash; itching; hives; sensitivity to sunlight; flushing; eczema; psoriasis; abnormal pigmentation.

Eyes or Ocular: Blurred vision; disturbed color perception; decreased visual field; double vision; night blindness; blind or dark spot in visual field; sensitivity to light.

Other: Hepatitis; lupus erythematosus; hearing disturbances; abnormal blood counts; fainting; fever; joint or muscle pain.

Guidelines for Use:

- Do not discontinue medication unless instructed by your doctor.
- May cause stomach upset. Take with food.
- Notify your doctor if ringing in the ears, visual disturbances, dizziness, headache, nausea, rash, or difficulty breathing occurs.
- Do not crush or chew sustained release tablets.
- Hospitalization is sometimes required when starting on this medication.

If you have any questions, consult your doctor, pharmacist, or health care provider.

Generic Name *Brand Name Example*	Supplied As	Generic Available
Rx **Tocainide** *Tonocard*	**Tablets:** 400 mg, 600 mg	No

Type of Drug:

A drug for specific types of irregular heartbeats.

How the Drug Works:

Tocainide reduces the tendency of the heart to beat irregularly.

Uses:

To treat life-threatening heart rhythm disturbances.

Unlabeled Use(s): Occasionally doctors may prescribe tocainide for the treatment of myotonic dystrophy and trigeminal neuralgia.

Precautions:

Do not use in the following situations:

allergy to tocainide or to amide-type local anesthetics
heart block (without ventricular pacemaker)

Use with caution in the following situations:

bone marrow failure, preexisting
cytopenia
heart disease, certain types (eg, heart failure)
kidney disease, severe
liver disease, severe

Heart rhythm disturbances: Worsened heart rhythm disturbances can result from taking tocainide. Close monitoring and careful dosage adjustment will be required.

Pregnancy: Adequate studies have not been done in pregnant women. Use only if clearly needed and potential benefits outweigh the possible hazards to the fetus.

Breastfeeding: Tocainide appears in breast milk. Because of the potential for adverse effects, a decision should be made whether to discontinue nursing or the drug, taking into account the importance of the drug to the mother. Consult your doctor.

Children: Safety and effectiveness have not been established.

Lab tests may be required during treatment with tocainide. Tests may include: Electrocardiograms; potassium levels; blood counts and chest x-rays, especially during the first 3 months of therapy. Report any unusual bruising or bleeding, signs of infection (fever, sore throat, chills) painful or difficult breathing, coughing or wheezing to your doctor.

Drug Interactions:

Tell your doctor or pharmacist if you are taking or planning to take any over-the-counter or prescription medications or dietary supplements with tocainide. Doses of one or both drugs may need to be modified or a different drug may need to be prescribed. The following drugs and drug classes interact with tocainide:

cimetidine (eg, *Tagamet*)
metoprolol (*Lopressor*)
rifampin (*eg, Rifadin*)

Side Effects:

Every drug is capable of producing side effects. Many tocainide users experience no, or minor, side effects. The frequency and severity of side effects depend on many factors including dose, duration of therapy, and individual susceptibility. Possible side effects include:

Digestive Tract: Appetite loss; nausea; vomiting; diarrhea; loose stools.

Nervous System: Dizziness; vertigo (feeling of whirling motion); drowsiness; tremor; confusion; disorientation; hallucinations; change in mood or awareness; incoordination; unsteadiness; walking disturbances; anxiety; headache; abnormal sensations.

Circulatory System: Irregular heartbeats; palpitations (pounding in the chest); decreased blood pressure; chest pain; congestive heart failure.

Other: Blurred vision; visual disturbances; ringing in the ears; hearing loss; sweating; hot/cold feelings; rash; skin lesion/disorder; joint or muscle pain.

Guidelines for Use:

- Notify your doctor if any of the following occurs: painful or difficult breathing; cough; wheezing; tremor; palpitations; rash; easy bruising or bleeding; fever; sore throat; soreness and ulcers in the mouth; or chills.
- May cause drowsiness or dizziness. Observe caution while driving or performing other tasks requiring alertness.
- May cause nausea, vomiting or diarrhea. Notify your doctor if these persist or become severe.

If you have any questions, consult your doctor, pharmacist, or health care provider.

	Generic Name *Brand Name Examples*	Supplied As	Generic Available
Rx	**Amlodipine**		
	Norvasc	**Tablets**: 2.5 mg, 5 mg, 10 mg	No
Rx	**Bepridil HCl**[1]		
	Vascor	**Tablets**: 200 mg, 300 mg, 400 mg	No
Rx	**Diltiazem HCl**[2]	**Capsules, extended-release**: 60 mg, 90 mg	Yes
	Tiamate	**Tablets, extended-release**: 120 mg, 180 mg, 240 mg	No
	Cardizem[1]	**Tablets**: 30 mg, 60 mg, 90 mg, 120 mg	Yes
	Cardizem SR	**Capsules, sustained-release**: 60 mg, 90 mg	Yes
	Cardizem CD, Cardizem SR, Dilacor XR, Tiazac	**Capsules, sustained-release**: 120 mg	Yes
	Cardizem CD, Dilacor XR, Tiazac	**Capsules, sustained-release**: 180 mg, 240 mg	No
	Cardizem CD, Tiazac	**Capsules, sustained-release**: 300 mg	No
	Cartia XT, Diltia XT, Tiazac	**Capsules, extended-release**: 120 mg, 180 mg, 240 mg	Yes
	Cartia XT	**Capsules, extended-release**: 300 mg	No
	Cardizem CD, Tiazac	**Capsules, extended-release**: 360 mg	No
	Tiazac	**Capsules, extended-release**: 420 mg	No
Rx	**Felodipine**		
	Plendil[1]	**Tablets, sustained-release**: 2.5 mg, 5 mg, 10 mg	No
Rx	**Isradipine**		
	DynaCirc CR	**Tablets, controlled-release**: 5 mg, 10 mg	No
	DynaCirc[1]	**Capsules**: 2.5 mg, 5 mg	No
Rx	**Nicardipine HCl**[2]		
	Cardene	**Capsules**: 20 mg, 30 mg	Yes
	Cardene SR[1]	**Capsules, sustained-release**: 30 mg, 45 mg, 60 mg	No

	Generic Name *Brand Name Examples*	Supplied As	Generic Available
Rx	**Nifedipine**		
	Nifedical XL	**Tablets, extended-release**: 30 mg, 60 mg	No
	Adalat CC[1], *Procardia XL*	**Tablets, sustained-release**: 30 mg, 60 mg, 90 mg	Yes
	Adalat, Procardia	**Capsules**: 10 mg[3], 20 mg	Yes
Rx	**Nimodipine**		
	Nimotop[1]	**Capsules**: 30 mg	No
Rx	**Nisoldipine**		
	Sular	**Tablets, extended-release**: 10 mg, 20 mg, 30 mg, 40 mg	No
Rx	**Verapamil HCl**[2]	**Capsules, extended-release**: 120 mg, 180 mg, 240 mg	Yes
	Calan[1]	**Tablets**: 40 mg, 80 mg, 120 mg	Yes
	Calan SR, Isoptin SR	**Tablets, sustained-release**: 120 mg, 180 mg, 240 mg	Yes
	Covera-HS	**Tablets, extended-release**: 180 mg, 240 mg	No
	Verelan	**Capsules, sustained-release**: 120 mg, 180 mg, 240 mg, 360 mg	Yes
	Verelan PM	**Capsules, sustained-release**: 100 mg, 200 mg, 300 mg	No

[1] Contains lactose.
[2] Also available as an injection.
[3] Contains saccharin.

Type of Drug:

Calcium channel blockers (ie, slow channel blockers, calcium ion antagonists); drugs that inhibit the movement of calcium across the cell membrane of cardiac muscle and vascular smooth muscle.

How the Drug Works:

Calcium is involved in blood vessel and heart muscle contraction, nerve impulse transmission and energy storage, and energy use in the heart. Calcium channel blocking agents dilate arteries of the heart and other arteries, may increase or decrease heart rate, may decrease heart contraction, slow ability of the heart to contract, and slow the rate at which nerve impulses are conducted through the heart.

Uses:

To treat angina due to coronary artery spasm (Prinzmetal angina) (amlodipine, nifedipine, nifedipine sustained-release, verapamil).

To treat chronic stable (stress-associated) angina in patients who cannot tolerate or are unresponsive to beta-adrenergic blockers or nitrates (amlodipine, bepridil, diltiazem, nicardipine, nifedipine, nifedipine sustained-release, verapamil only).

To treat unstable angina (verapamil only).

To treat arrhythmias (irregular heartbeats) at rest and during stress in association with digitalis (verapamil only).

To treat high blood pressure (amlodipine, diltiazem sustained-release, felodipine, isradipine, nicardipine, nifedipine sustained-release, nisoldipine, verapamil only).

To improve neurological deficiencies caused by spasms following subarachnoid hemorrhage (SAH) (ruptured vessels in the brain). Therapy must begin within 96 hours and continue for 21 days (nimodipine only).

Unlabeled Use(s): Occasionally doctors may prescribe diltiazem to treat unstable angina, Raynaud syndrome, and tardive dyskinesia, and to prevent certain types of heart attack. Isradipine may be useful in the treatment of chronic stable angina. Nicardipine may be useful in the treatment of congestive heart failure and in combination with aminocaproic acid for SAH. Occasionally doctors may prescribe nifedipine to lower blood pressure in hypertensive emergencies; to prevent or treat migraine headaches; and to treat primary pulmonary (lung) and pregnancy-associated hypertension, asthma, preterm labor, disorders of the esophagus, certain types of heart disorders, coronary artery disease, congestive heart failure, Raynaud syndrome, biliary and renal colic, and cardiomyopathy. Nimodipine appears to be beneficial in some patients with common and classic migraine and chronic cluster headache. Occasionally doctors may prescribe verapamil to prevent migraine headache, cluster headache, and exercise-induced asthma; to treat manic-depressive states, night leg cramps, and hypertrophic cardiomyopathy. Verapamil has also been used for paroxysmal supraventricular tachycardia.

Precautions:

Do not use in the following situations:

- allergy to calcium channel blocking agents or their ingredients
- aortic stenosis, advanced (nicardipine only)
- arrhythmias, serious, history of (bepridil only)
- atrial flutter or atrial fibrillation and an accessory bypass tract (eg, Wolff-Parkinson-White, Lown-Ganong-Levine syndromes) (verapamil only)
- AV block, second or third degree, except with functioning pacemaker (bepridil, diltiazem, verapamil only)
- cardiac insufficiency, uncompensated (bepridil only)
- cardiogenic shock (verapamil only)
- congenital QT interval prolongation (bepridil only)
- drugs that prolong QT interval, (eg, antiarrhythmics), concurrent use (bepridil only)
- low blood pressure (bepridil, diltiazem, verapamil only)
- myocardial infarction, acute (diltiazem only)
- severe left ventricular dysfunction (verapamil only)
- sick sinus syndrome, without pacemaker (bepridil, diltiazem, verapamil only)

Use with caution in the following situations:

- agranulocytosis
- beta-blocker withdrawal (nifedipine, nicardipine only)
- bradycardia, transient (verapamil only)
- chest pain (nicardipine, nifedipine only)
- congestive heart failure
- coronary artery disease (nisoldipine only)
- Duchenne muscular dystrophy (verapamil only)
- edema (felodipine, nifedipine only)
- heart attack
- heart conduction problems
- hypertrophic cardiomyopathy (enlarged heart) (verapamil only)
- hypokalemia (bepridil only)
- kidney disease
- left bundle branch block (bepridil only)
- liver disease
- low blood pressure
- sinus bradycardia (bepridil only)

New serious arrhythmias: Bepridil has been associated with the occurrence of new serious arrhythmias. Use should be limited to patients in whom other antianginal drugs have failed.

Pregnancy: There are no adaquate and well-controlled studies in pregnant women. Use only if clearly needed and the potential benefits to the mother outweigh the possible hazards to the fetus.

Breastfeeding: Bepridil, diltiazem, nifedipine, and verapamil appear in breast milk. It is not known if amlodipine, felodipine, isradipine, nicardipine, nimodipine, or nisoldipine appear in breast milk. Decide whether to discontinue nursing or the drug, taking into account the importance of the drug to the mother. Consult your doctor.

Children: Safety and effectiveness have not been established in children.

Elderly: Felodipine, nifedipine, and verapamil may result in a greater lowering of blood pressure than in younger patients.

Lab tests may be required periodically during treatment. Tests may include electrocardiograms, serum potassium levels, liver and kidney function tests, blood pressure, and blood and platelet counts.

Drug Interactions:

Tell your doctor or pharmacist if you are taking or planning to take any over-the-counter or prescription medications or dietary supplements with calcium channel blocking agents. Doses of one or both drugs may need to be modified or a different drug may need to be prescribed.The following drugs and drug classes interact with calcium channel blocking agents:

- alcohol (verapamil only)
- anesthetics
- antiarrhythmics (eg, flecainide) (verapamil only)
- antihistamines, nonsedating (eg, loratadine) (bepridil only)
- antihypertensives (eg, diuretics) (verapamil only)
- azole antifungals (eg, ketoconazole, itraconazole) (felodipine, nisoldipine only)
- barbiturates (eg, phenobarbital) (felodipine, nifedipine only)
- benzodiapines (eg, midazolam) (diltiazem only)
- beta-blockers (eg, propranolol)
- calcium salts (verapamil only)

carbamazepine (eg, *Tegretol*) (diltiazem, felodipine, verapamil only)
cardiac glycosides (eg, digoxin) (bepridil only)
cimetidine (eg, *Tagamet*)
cyclosporine (eg, *Neoral*) (diltiazem, nicardipine, verapamil only)
digoxin (eg, *Lanoxin*)
diltiazem (eg, *Cardizem*) (nifedipine only)
encainide (*Enkaid*) (diltiazem only)
erythromycin (eg, *E-Mycin*) (felodipine only)
fentanyl (eg, *Duragesic*)
grapefruit juice (felodipine, nifedipine, nisoldipine only)
HMG-CoA reductase inhibitors (eg, lovastatin) (diltiazem, verapamil only)
lithium (eg, *Eskalith*) (verapamil only)
neuromuscular blockers (eg, atracurium) (verapamil only)
nifedipine (eg, *Procardia*) (diltiazem only)
nondepolarizing muscle relaxants (eg, pancuronium) (verapamil only)
phenytoin (eg, *Dilantin*) (felodipine, nisoldipine only)
prazosin (eg, *Minipress*) (verapamil only)
primidone (eg, *Mysoline*) (nifedipine only)
procainamide (eg, *Pronestyl*) (bepridil only)
quinidine (eg, *Quinora*) (bepridil, nisoldipine, verapamil only)
rifampin (eg, *Rifadin*) (diltiazem, isradipine, nifedipine, verapamil only)
tacrolimus (*Prograf*) (diltiazem only)
theophyllines (eg, aminophylline) (diltiazem, verapamil only)
tricyclic antidepressants (eg, amitriptyline) (bepridil only)

Side Effects:

Every drug is capable of producing side effects. Many calcium channel blocking agent users experience no, or minor, side effects. The frequency and severity of side effects depend on many factors including dose, duration of therapy, and individual susceptibility. Possible side effects include:

Nervous System: Headache; dizziness; giddiness (felodipine only); lightheadedness; fainting; weakness; fatigue; nervousness; anxiety; tremor; general body discomfort; impaired movement; excessive movement (nicardipine only); confusion; irritability; drowsiness; sleep disturbances; difficulty sleeping; abnormal dreams; psychiatric disturbances (eg, depression, amnesia, paranoia, psychosis).

Digestive Tract: Nausea; vomiting; diarrhea; constipation; gas; stomach pain or cramps; indigestion; changes in taste perception; dry mouth; swollen gums (felodipine only); appetite changes (bepridil only).

Respiratory System: Congestion; runny nose; sinus infection; cough; shortness of breath; wheezing; sore throat; sneezing; bronchitis; fluid retention in lungs.

Circulatory System: Fluid retention; low blood pressure; high blood pressure; anemia; pounding in the chest; chest pain; decreased heart rate; increased heart rate; abnormal heart rhythm; abnormal electrocardiogram readings; myocardial infarction; AV block; congestive heart failure.

Skin: Rash; skin irritation; flushing; sweating; acne (nimodipine only); itching; hives; abnormal skin sensations (eg, burning, prickling, tingling); hair loss.

Other: Fever; chills; flu-like symptoms; muscle cramps or pain; joint stiffness or pain; back pain (felodipine only); weight loss; weight gain; nosebleed; ringing in ears; pain; blurred vision; difficult urination; painful urination; frequent urination; sexual difficulties; infection (nicardipine only).

Guidelines for Use:

- Dosage is individualized. Take exactly as prescribed.
- Do not change the dose or stop taking this medicine unless advised to do so by your doctor. Abrupt withdrawal may result in increased angina attacks.
- All of the products listed are calcium channel blockers; however, they are not interchangeable. For example, diltiazem cannot be used for nimodipine.
- *Extended- or sustained-release* — Swallow whole; do not chew, crush, or divide. An empty tablet may appear in stool; this is no cause for concern.
- *Amlodipine, felodipine, isradipine, nicardipine* — May be taken with or without food. Do not take felodipine with grapefruit juice.
- *Verapamil* — Verapamil extended-release is usually taken at bedtime with or without food. Take verapamil sustained-release with food in the morning. If heart failure is not severe or rate-related, use digitalis and diuretics before verapamil.
- *Diltiazem sustained-release* — The usual dose is taken in the morning on an empty stomach.
- *Bepridil* — If stomach upset occurs, take with meals or at bedtime. Notify any doctor who treats that you are taking bepridil, as well as any other medications you may be taking. Bepridil use has been associated with the occurrence of new arrhythmias. Use should be limited to patients in whom other antianginal drugs have failed.
- *Nimodipine* — Take preferably less than 1 hour before or 2 hours after meals. Therapy to improve neurological deficiencies caused by spasms following SAH must begin within 96 hours and continue for 21 days. If capsule cannot be swallowed (eg, time of surgery, unconsciousness), a hole can be made in both ends of the capsule with an 18 gauge needle, and the contents extracted into a syringe for oral administration.
- *Nisoldipine* — Do not take with grapefruit juice or with high-fat meals.
- *Adalat CC* — Take once daily on an empty stomach.

Guidelines for Use (cont.):

- *Felodipine* — May cause swollen or bleeding gums. Good dental hygiene decreases incidence and severity of this condition.
- Calcium channel blockers may interfere with normal blood-clotting mechanisms. Contact your doctor if unusual bleeding or bruising of the skin occurs.
- Low blood pressure may occur, but is usually well tolerated. It is more likely to occur in patients who are also taking beta-blockers (eg, propranolol).
- Beta-blockers should be tapered slowly rather than stopped abruptly before starting nicardipine or nifedipine therapy. When starting nicardipine therapy, taper beta-blockers over 8 to 10 days with coadministration.
- Maintain use of potassium supplementation or potassium-sparing diuretics.
- If a dose is missed, take it as soon as possible. If several hours have passed or it is nearing time for the next dose, do not double the dose to catch up, unless advised to do so by your doctor. If more than one dose is missed or it is necessary to establish a new dosage schedule, contact your doctor or pharmacist.
- Notify your doctor if you experience irregular heartbeat, increased frequency or severity of angina, shortness of breath, swelling of hands and feet, dizziness, constipation, nausea, or low blood pressure (eg, light-headedness).
- Notify your doctor if you experience symptoms of an allergic reaction (eg, itching, rash, hives, difficulty breathing).
- Inform your doctor if you are pregnant, become pregnant, plan on becoming pregnant, or are breastfeeding.
- Lab tests may be required to monitor therapy. Be sure to keep appointments.
- Store at controlled room temperature (59° to 77°F) in a tightly sealed container. Keep away from light and moisture. Protect nimodipine from freezing.

If you have any questions, consult your doctor, pharmacist, or health care provider.

Generic Name *Brand Name Example*	Supplied As	Generic Available
Rx **Isoxsuprine HCl**		
Vasodilan	**Tablets:** 10 mg, 20 mg	Yes

Type of Drug:

Peripheral vasodilator (relaxes blood vessels in skeletal muscles).

How the Drug Works:

Isoxsuprine increases blood flow in skeletal muscle by relaxing and dilating (widening) blood vessels in these muscles.

Uses:

"Possibly effective" to relieve symptoms of disorders related to inadequate blood flow or blood supply to the brain and extremities (arms and legs). These disorders include: Vascular disease, Buerger disease, and Raynaud disease.

Unlabeled Use(s): Occasionally doctors may provide isoxsuprine for painful menstrual periods and premature labor.

Precautions:

Do not use in the following situations:

- arterial bleeding
- immediately after childbirth

Pregnancy: Safety in pregnancy has not been established. Risks of fluid accumulation in lungs in pregnant women is increased. Lower amounts of calcium and glucose in the blood, lower blood pressure and poorly functioning intestines in newborns have resulted. Consult your doctor.

Drug Interactions:

Tell your doctor or pharmacist if you are taking or planning to take any over-the-counter or prescription medications or dietary supplements with isoxsuprine. Doses of one or both drugs may need to be modified or a different drug may need to be prescribed.

Side Effects:

Every drug is capable of producing side effects. Many isoxsuprine users experience no, or minor, side effects. The frequency and severity of side effects depend on many factors including dosage, duration of therapy, and individual susceptibility. Possible side effects include:

Circulatory System: Decreased blood pressure; orthostatic hypotension (dizziness or lightheadedness when arising from a seated or lying position); rapid heartbeat; pounding in the chest (palpitations); chest pain.

Other: Severe rash; dizziness; nausea; vomiting; stomach pain.

Guidelines for Use:

- Take exactly as prescribed.
- Do not stop taking this medicine or change the dosage without checking with your doctor; this could have serious adverse effects.
- Pounding sensation in chest (palpitations) and skin rash can occur. Notify your doctor if these symptoms persist.
- Dizziness or weakness may occur after sudden changes in posture (eg, when rising from a lying position). This can usually be avoided by rising slowly or sitting upright for a few minutes before standing.
- Store at controlled room temperature (59° to 86°F). Protect from moisture.

If you have any questions, consult your doctor, pharmacist, or health care provider.

	Generic Name *Brand Name Examples*	Supplied As	Generic Available
Rx	**Papaverine HCl**		
	Pavabid Plateau Caps	**Capsules, timed release:** 150 mg	Yes

Type of Drug:

Peripheral vasodilator (relaxes blood vessels in skeletal muscles).

How the Drug Works:

Papaverine relaxes and dilates (widens) blood vessels to increase blood flow.

Uses:

To treat problems associated with blood vessel constriction or spasm in the brain, heart, arms and legs.

Precautions:

Do not use in the following situations:

allergy to papaverine
irregular heartbeats, history of

Use with caution in the following situations:

glaucoma
heart attack, history of
heart beat irregularities
liver disease

Heart: Large doses can produce serious arrhythmias (irregular heartbeats).

Liver sensitivity has been reported with intestinal symptoms, yellowing of the skin and eyes and altered liver function tests. Discontinue medication if these symptoms occur.

Pregnancy: Adequate studies have not been done in pregnant women or animal studies may have shown a risk to the fetus. Use only if clearly needed and potential benefits outweigh the possible hazards to the fetus.

Breastfeeding: It is not known if papaverine appears in breast milk. Consult your doctor before you begin breastfeeding.

Children: Safety and effectiveness have not been established.

Drug Interactions:

Tell your doctor or pharmacist if you are taking or planning to take any over-the-counter or prescription medications or dietary supplements with papaverine. Doses of one or both drugs may need to be modified or a different drug may need to be prescribed. Levodopa (eg, *Larodopa*) interacts with papaverine.

Side Effects:

Every drug is capable of producing side effects. Many papaverine users experience no, or minor, side effects. The frequency and severity of side effects depend on many factors including dosage, duration of therapy, and individual susceptibility. Possible side effects include:

Digestive Tract: Nausea; stomachache; appetite loss; constipation; diarrhea.

Nervous System: Headache; dizziness; drowsiness; feeling of whirling motion.

Circulatory System: Increased heart rate; increased blood pressure.

Skin: Yellowing of skin or eyes; sweating; flushing of face; rash.

Other: Fatigue and general body aches; increase in depth of respirations; abnormal liver tests.

Guidelines for Use:

- May cause drowsiness or dizziness. Use caution when driving or performing tasks requiring alertness. Alcohol may intensify these effects.
- May cause flushing, sweating, headache, tiredness, jaundice, rash, nausea, appetite loss, abdominal distress, constipation or diarrhea. Notify your doctor if these effects become pronounced.
- Take at evenly spaced intervals throughout the day.
- Store at controlled room temperature (59° to 86°F). Protect from moisture.

If you have any questions, consult your doctor, pharmacist, or health care provider.

	Generic Name *Brand Name Examples*	Supplied As	Generic Available
Rx	**Acebutolol HCl**		
	Sectral	**Capsules**: 200 mg, 400 mg	Yes
Rx	**Atenolol**[1]		
	Tenormin	**Tablets**: 25 mg, 50 mg, 100 mg	Yes
Rx	**Betaxolol HCl**		
	Kerlone	**Tablets**: 10 mg, 20 mg	No
Rx	**Bisoprolol Fumarate**		
	Zebeta	**Tablets**: 5 mg, 10 mg	Yes
Rx	**Carteolol HCl**		
	Cartrol	**Tablets**: 2.5 mg, 5 mg	No
Rx	**Metoprolol**[1]		
	Toprol XL	**Tablets, extended release**: 25 mg, 50 mg, 100 mg, 200 mg	No
	Lopressor	**Tablets**: 50 mg, 100 mg	No
Rx	**Nadolol**		
	Corgard	**Tablets**: 20 mg, 40 mg, 80 mg, 120 mg, 160 mg	Yes
Rx	**Penbutolol Sulfate**		
	Levatol	**Tablets**: 20 mg	No
Rx	**Pindolol**		
	Visken	**Tablets**: 5 mg, 10 mg	Yes
Rx	**Propranolol HCl**[1]	**Tablets**: 90 mg	Yes
		Solution, oral:[2] 4 mg/mL 8 mg/mL	Yes
	Inderal	**Tablets**: 10 mg, 20 mg, 40 mg, 60 mg, 80 mg	Yes
	Inderal LA	**Capsules, sustained release**: 60 mg, 80 mg, 120 mg, 160 mg	Yes
	Propranolol Intensol[2]	**Solution, concentrated oral**: 80 mg/mL	No
Rx	**Sotalol HCl**		
	Betapace, Sorine	**Tablets**: 80 mg, 120 mg, 160 mg, 240 mg	Yes
	Betapace AF	**Tablets**: 80 mg, 120 mg, 160 mg	No
Rx	**Timolol Maleate**		
	Blocadren	**Tablets**: 5 mg, 10 mg, 20 mg	Yes

[1] Also available as an injection.
[2] Sugar free.

All of the products listed in the above table are beta-blockers; however, they are not interchangeable. For example, atenolol cannot be used for nadolol.

Type of Drug:

Beta-blockers; antihypertensives; drugs used to lower high blood pressure; antianginal drugs; antiarrhythmic drugs.

How the Drug Works:

Beta-adrenergic blocking agents interfere with the action of adrenalin and similar chemicals on heart muscle contraction (heart may beat with less force and pump out less blood) and nerve conduction in the heart (heart may beat more slowly and regularly). Beta-adrenergic blocking agents reduce the amount of work the heart has to do (reduces angina chest pain) and the amount of blood the heart pumps out (lowers elevated blood pressure) and stabilize heart rhythm in conditions in which the heart is beating too fast or irregularly (antiarrhythmic effects).

Uses:

Beta-Adrenergic Blocking Agents

Indications ✓ = labeled x = unlabeled	Acebutolol	Atenolol	Betaxolol	Bisoprolol	Carteolol	Metoprolol[1]	Nadolol	Penbutolol	Pindolol	Propranolol[1]	Sotalol	Timolol
Hypertension	✓	✓	✓	✓	✓	✓	✓	✓	✓	✓		✓
Angina pectoris	x	✓		x		✓	✓			✓		
Cardiac arrhythmias												
Supraventricular arrhythmias/tachycardias										✓		
Ventricular arrhythmias/tachycardias										✓	✓[2]	
Premature ventricular contractions (PVCs)	✓									✓		
Digitalis-induced tachyarrhythmias										✓		
Resistant tachyarrhythmias (during anesthesia)										✓		
Atrial ectopy						x						
Maintenance of normal sinus rhythm											✓[3]	
Myocardial Infarction		✓				✓[4]						✓
CHF (stable)[5]				x		✓[6]						
Pheochromocytoma										✓		
Migraine prophylaxis		x				x	x			✓		✓

Beta-Adrenergic Blocking Agents												
Indications ✓= labeled x = unlabeled	Acebutolol	Atenolol	Betaxolol	Bisoprolol	Carteolol	Metoprolol[1]	Nadolol	Penbutolol	Pindolol	Propranolol[1]	Sotalol	Timolol
Hypertrophic subaortic stenosis										✓		
Parkinsonian tremors							x			x[7]		
Akathisia, antipsychotic-induced						x				x		
Variceal bleeding in portal hyper-tension, prevention of		x				x	x			x		x
Atrial fibrillation												
Rapid heart rate control						x						
Maintenance heart rate control						x						
Generalized anxiety disor-der										x		
Angina, unstable		x				x						
Stable	x			x								
Unstable		x				x						
Essential Tremor										✓		

[1] Includes long-acting formulation.
[2] Not *Betapace AF*.
[3] Not *Betapace*.
[4] Immediate-release tablets only.
[5] See Precautions.
[6] *Toprol-XL* only.
[7] Sustained-release only.

Precautions:

Do not use in the following situations:

- allergy to beta-blockers or any of their ingredients
- bronchial asthma, bronchospasm, or severe chronic obstructive pulmonary diseases (eg, emphysema, bronchitis)
- cardiac failure, moderate to severe (metoprolol only)
- cardiac failure, uncontrolled
- cardiac shock
- heart block, greater than first degree
- long QT syndromes, congenital or acquired (sotalol only)
- low blood pressure, less than 100 mmHg (metoprolol only)
- renal impairment, severe (sotalol only)
- slow heart rate, severe

Use with caution in the following situations:

- acute myocardial infarction, recent
- adrenal gland tumor
- anesthesia for major surgery
- AV block, first block
- bronchospastic diseases
- calcium channel blocker therapy, concurrent
- congestive heart failure, controlled
- diabetes

electrolyte disturbances (eg, potassium, magnesium)
kidney disease
liver disease
low blood pressure
low blood sugar
low heart rate
overactive thyroid
peripheral vascular disease
sick sinus syndrome
Wolff-Parkinson-White syndrome

Discontinuing therapy: When discontinuing these medications, slowly reduce the dose over 1 to 2 weeks. Sudden discontinuation of these drugs has caused worsening of angina (chest pain), heart attacks, irregular heartbeats, and death. Other serious withdrawal symptoms include: sweating, palpitations (pounding in the chest), headache, tremulousness, discomfort, and allergy to catecholamines. If discontinued suddenly, beta-blockers may mask the signs of hyperthyroidism (overactive thyroid). If thyroid patients stop taking these medications too suddenly, symptoms of hyperthyroidism (eg, a rapid pulse) may occur.

Diabetes: These products can mask some of the signs of hypoglycemia (low blood sugar) such as rapid heart rate and tremors, and alter blood sugar levels. It may be necessary for your doctor to alter your dose of diabetic medications while taking beta-blockers.

Proarrhythmia: Betapace AF can cause or worsen ventricular arrhythmias, a different type of heartbeat that can be dangerous and even cause death. To minimize the risk of this heartbeat, patients should be placed in a medical facility that can provide cardiac resuscitation, continuous ECG monitoring, and calculations of creatinine clearance for a minimum of 3 days when starting or restarting therapy.

Allergic reaction: Patients with a history of allergic reactions to various allergens may be unresponsive to the usual doses of epinephrine used to treat the allergic reaction.

Pregnancy: There are no adequate or well-controlled studies in pregnant women. Use only if clearly needed and the potential benefits to the mother outweigh the possible hazards to the fetus.

Atenolol, acebutolol, and sotalol – Acebutolol crosses the placenta; reduced birth weight and decreased blood pressure and heart rate have occurred.

Breastfeeding: Acebutolol, atenolol, betaxolol, metoprolol, nadolol, pindolol, propranolol, sotalol, and timolol appear in breast milk. It is not known if carteolol, bisoprolol, or penbutolol appear in breast milk. Discontinue nursing when taking any beta-blockers.

Children: Safety and effectiveness have not been established.

Drug Interactions:

Tell your doctor or pharmacist if you are taking or planning to take any over-the-counter or prescription medications or dietary supplements with beta-blockers. Doses of one or both drugs may need to be modified or a different drug may need to be prescribed. The following drugs and drug classes interact with beta-blockers:

antacids (eg, aluminum carbonate)
antiarrhythmics (eg, quinidine)
antidiabetic drugs, oral (eg, glipizide)
barbiturates (eg, phenobarbital)
calcium channel blockers (eg, verapamil)
cimetidine (eg, *Tagamet*)
clonidine (eg, *Catapres*)
colestipol (eg, *Colestid*)
contraceptives, oral (eg, *Ortho-Novum*)
cyclosporine (eg, *Neoral*)
epinephrine (eg, *Adrenalin*)
ergot alkaloids (eg, ergotamine)
hydantoins (eg, phenytoin)
hydralazine (eg, *Apresoline*)
insulin
lidocaine (eg, *Xylocaine*)
NSAIDs (eg, ibuprofen)
penicillins (eg, ampicillin)
phenothiazines (eg, chlorpromazine)
prazosin (eg, *Minipress*)
propafenone (eg, *Rythmol*)
rifamycins (eg, rifampin)
selective serotonin reuptake inhibitors (eg, paroxetine)
theophyllines (eg, aminophylline)
thioamines (eg, methimazole)

Side Effects:

Every drug is capable of producing side effects. Many beta-blocker users experience no, or minor, side effects. The frequency and severity of side effects depend on many factors including dose, duration of therapy, and individual susceptibility. Possible side effects include:

Digestive Tract: Nausea; vomiting; stomach pain; gas; bloating; diarrhea; constipation; heartburn; indigestion; stomach cramping; appetite changes; dry mouth; colon or rectal problems.

Nervous System: Depression; anxiety; nervousness; disorientation; confusion; fainting; weakness; dizziness; catatonia; vertigo (feeling of whirling motion); lightheadedness; fatigue; sleeplessness; drowsiness; lethargy; sleep disturbances; nightmares; abnormal, vivid dreams; hallucinations; short-term memory loss; decreased concentration; sedation; headache; emotional lability; mood changes; behavior changes; slurred speech.

Circulatory System: Changes in heart rate; decreased heart rate; irregular heart rate; heart rhythm abnormalities; chest pain; palpitations (pounding in the chest); cold extremities; changes in blood pressure; heart arrest; heart block; congestive heart failure; abnormal ECG; decreased blood platelets; decreased white blood cells; blood clot; vein inflammation; stroke.

Respiratory System: Shortness of breath or difficulty breathing; cough; nasal congestion; wheezing; upper respiratory infection; sinus infection; fluid in the lungs; bronchitis; asthma; bronchospasm; sore or inflamed throat; throat spasms.

Skin: Rash; swelling; flushing or paleness; abnormal skin sensations (eg, burning, prickling, tingling); increased or decreased skin sensitivity to stimulation; itching and irritation; hair loss; sweating; dry skin; numbness of the hands.

Muscular System: Aching or painful joints and muscles; back pain; limb pain; shoulder pain; muscle weakness; muscle cramps or twitching; tremor.

Urinary and Reproductive Tract: Painful urination; inability to urinate; frequent urination; urinary tract infection; excessive urination at night; sexual problems; decreased sex drive; impotence.

Senses: Blurred vision; dry, burning, or irritated eyes; eye inflammation; visual disturbances; ringing in the ears; earache; taste changes; eye pain; abnormal tearing.

Other: Fever; weight changes; changes in blood sugar levels; infection; swelling of arms and legs; general body discomfort; decreased exercise tolerance; gout; cold- or flu-like symptoms.

Guidelines for Use:

- Dosage is individualized. Take exactly as prescribed.
- Do not stop taking or change the dose unless directed by your doctor. Abrupt withrawal has resulted in worsening of angina and ventricular arrhythmias and can cause myocardial infarction and death.
- If a dose is missed, take it as soon as possible. If several hours have passed or it is nearing time for the next dose, do not double the dose to catch up, unless advised to do so by your doctor. If more than one dose is missed or it is necessary to establish a new dosage schedule, contact your doctor or pharmacist.
- Do not chew or crush sustained-release or extended-release products.
- *Diabetes* — May mask some signs of low blood sugar (eg, rapid heart rate, tremors) or alter blood glucose levels.
- *Glaucoma* — May reduce intraocular pressure and interfere with the glaucoma screening test.
- Consult your pharmacist or doctor before using dietary supplements or other prescription or nonprescription products including nasal decongestants, diet aids, and nonprescription cold preparations.
- May cause drowsiness, dizziness, lightheadedness, or blurred vision. Use caution while driving or performing other tasks requiring alertness, coordination, or physical dexterity.
- Notify your doctor if you experience difficulty breathing (especially on exertion or when lying down), night cough, swelling of the extremities, slow pulse rate, dizziness, light-headedness, fainting, confusion, depression, rash, fever, sore throat, unusual bleeding or bruising, fatigue with exertion, cough, fast heartbeat, severe diarrhea, or unusual bleeding.
- Inform your doctor or dentist of therapy before any type of surgery.
- Inform your doctor if you are pregnant, become pregnant, plan on becoming pregnant, or are breastfeeding.
- *Brand interchange* — Do not change from one brand of this drug to another without consulting your pharmacist or doctor. For example, *Betapace* and *Betapace AF* are not interchangeable.

Guidelines for Use (cont.):

- *Nadolol, pindolol, acebutolol, atenolol, carteolol, bisoprolol, betaxolol, and penbutolol* — May be taken without regard to meals.
- *Metoprolol and propranolol* — Take consistently with or without food at the same time each day.
- *Propranolol Intensol* — Mix prescribed dose with liquid or semi-solid food such as water, juices, soda or soda-like beverages, applesauce, or pudding. Use calibrated dropper to measure dose. Administer entire amount of mixture immediately after mixing. Do not store mixture after mixing.
- *Sotalol* — Food may reduce absorption. Take on an empty stomach.
- *Sotalol* — To reduce the risk of induced arrhythmias, patients should be placed in a medical facility that can provide cardiac resuscitation, continuous ECG monitoring, and calculations of creatine clearance for a minimum of 3 days when starting or restarting therapy.
- Store at room temperature (59° to 86°F). Avoid excessive heat. Protect from light, moisture, and freezing.

If you have any questions, consult your doctor, pharmacist, or health care provider.

	Generic Name *Brand Name Examples*	Supplied As	Generic Available
Rx	**Doxazosin Mesylate**		
	Cardura	**Tablets:** 1 mg, 2 mg, 4 mg, 8 mg	No
Rx	**Prazosin**		
	Minipress	**Capsules:** 1 mg, 2 mg, 5 mg	Yes
Rx	**Tamsulosin HCl**		
	Flomax	**Capsules:** 0.4 mg	No
Rx	**Terazosin**		
	Hytrin	**Capsules:** 1 mg, 2 mg, 5 mg, 10 mg	No

Type of Drug:

Drugs used to lower high blood pressure.

How the Drug Works:

Alpha-1-adrenergic blockers dilate both veins and arteries to reduce resistance against which the blood must flow. This lowers blood pressure.

Alpha-1-adrenergic blockers relax the muscles around the urethra and improve symptoms of benign prostatic hyperplasia.

Prazosin also helps to increase output of the heart.

Uses:

To treat high blood pressure alone or in combination with other blood pressure lowering medications (eg, diuretics) (except tamsulosin, which is not used to treat high blood pressure).

Doxazosin, terazosin and tamsulosin are also used for the symptomatic treatment of benign prostatic hyperplasia (BPH).

Unlabeled Use(s): Occasionally doctors may prescribe prazosin for treatment of congestive heart failure, Raynaud's syndrome and benign prostatic hypertrophy. Doxazosin occasionally may be prescribed for the treatment of CHF with concurrent digoxin and diuretics.

Precautions:

Do not use in the following situations: Allergy to these alpha-1-adrenergic blockers.

Use with caution in the following situations:

liver disease
prostate cancer

"First dose" effect: Dizziness, fainting and falling are possible because of lowered blood pressure, especially early in therapy. These symptoms are more likely to occur when rising quickly from a seated or lying position, if the dose is increased, if the therapy is stopped and then started again, or if more than one antihypertensive drug is being taken. To lessen the chances of problems, the first dose should be given at bedtime. Sit or lie down if you feel lightheaded.

Priapism: Painful penile erection, sustained for hours, occurs rarely. Contact your physician if condition occurs.

Tamsulosin: Tamsulosin is not indicated for use in women or children.

Pregnancy: Adequate studies have not been done in pregnant women, or animal studies may have shown a risk to the fetus. Use only if clearly needed and potential benefits outweigh the possible hazards to the fetus.

Breastfeeding: Prazosin appears in breast milk. It is not known if doxazosin or terazosin appear in breast milk. Consult your doctor before you begin breastfeeding.

Children: Safety and effectiveness in children have not been established.

Lab tests may be required to monitor treatment. Be sure to keep appointments.

Drug Interactions:

Tell your doctor or pharmacist if you are taking or planning to take any over-the-counter or prescription medications or dietary supplements while taking this medicine. Doses of one or both drugs may need to be modified or a different drug may need to be prescribed. The following drugs and drug classes interact with this medicine:

cimetidine (eg, *Tagamet*) (tamsulosin only)
clonidine (eg, *Catapres*) (prazosin only)
verapamil (eg, *Calan*) (terazosin only)

Side Effects:

Every drug is capable of producing side effects. Many patients experience no, or minor, side effects. The frequency and severity of side effects depend on many factors including dose, duration of therapy, and individual susceptibility. Possible side effects include:

Digestive Tract: Nausea; vomiting; stomachache; indigestion; diarrhea; constipation; gas.

Nervous System: Depression; dizziness; incoordination; vertigo (feeling of whirling motion); nervousness; anxiety; drowsiness; fatigue; sleeplessness; headache; abnormal skin sensations; lightheadedness; lack of energy; fainting.

Circulatory System: Palpitations (pounding in the chest); orthostatic hypotension (dizziness or lightheadedness when rising quickly from a sitting or lying position); rapid or irregular pulse; low blood pressure.

Respiratory System: Difficulty breathing; nasal congestion; sore throat; runny nose; inflamed sinuses; cold symptoms; bronchitis; increased cough; nosebleed; flu symptoms.

Skin: Rash; itching; sweating; flushing.

Other: Painful erections; sexual problems; fainting; swelling of arms and legs (edema); facial swelling; dry mouth; ringing in the ears; weight gain; loss of bladder control; frequent urination; abnormal or blurred vision; eye pain or irritation; fever; urinary tract infections; gout; muscle cramps/spasms; neck, shoulder, back, chest, joint, muscle or general body pain/discomfort; red eyes; infection; weakness; tooth disorder.

Guidelines for Use:

- Dosage is individualized. Take exactly as prescribed.
- Do not stop taking or change dose unless advised by your doctor.
- If a dose is missed, take it as soon as possible. If several hours have passed or if it is nearing time for the next dose, do not double the dose to catch up, unless advised by your doctor. If more than one dose is missed or it is necessary to establish a new dosage schedule, contact your doctor or pharmacist.
- Patients being treated for high blood pressure often feel tired and run down for a few weeks after beginning therapy. It takes time for the body to adjust to lowered blood pressure. Continue taking your medication even though you may not feel quite normal. Check with your doctor or pharmacist during this time regarding any new symptoms that occur to ensure that these new feelings are a normal consequence of changes in blood pressure.
- Take the first dose at bedtime in order to reduce the risk of dizziness and lightheadedness which may occur early in therapy. Take without regard to food. Take tamsulosin about 30 minutes after the same meal each day.
- Do not crush, chew, or open tamsulosin capsules.
- May cause drowsiness, dizziness, lightheadedness, or blurred vision. Use caution when driving or performing other tasks requiring alertness, coordination, or physical dexterity. Avoid engaging in any hazardous tasks for at least 12 to 24 hours after taking the first dose of these medications, missing several doses, increasing the dose or taking other high blood pressure medications with these products. Sit or lie down if you feel lightheaded.
- Dizziness or lightheadedness may also occur following alcohol ingestion, standing for long periods of time, exercise, or during exposure to extreme heat.
- Use caution when rising from a sitting or lying position. If dizziness, lightheadedness, or palpitations become bothersome, notify your doctor.
- Do not take nonprescription decongestants; weight loss products; or cold, sinus, or allergy medications without first consulting your pharmacist or doctor.
- These agents may cause sodium and water retention when used alone to treat high blood pressure.
- Lab and blood pressure testing may be required to monitor therapy. Be sure to keep appointments.
- Store at room temperature (68° to 77°F). Protect from light and moisture.

	Generic Name *Brand Name Examples*	Supplied As	Generic Available
Rx	**Benazepril HCl** *Lotensin*	**Tablets:** 5 mg, 10 mg, 20 mg, 40 mg	No
Rx	**Benazepril HCl and Hydrochlorothiazide** *Lotensin HCT*	**Tablets:** 5 mg/6.25 mg, 10 mg/12.5 mg, 20 mg/12.5 mg, 20 mg/25 mg	No
Rx	**Captopril** *Capoten*	**Tablets:** 12.5 mg, 25 mg, 50 mg, 100 mg	Yes
Rx	**Enalapril Maleate** *Vasotec*	**Tablets:** 2.5 mg, 5 mg, 10 mg, 20 mg	Yes
	Vasotec I.V.	**Injection:** 1.25 mg enalaprilat/mL	Yes
Rx	**Fosinopril Sodium** *Monopril*	**Tablets:** 10 mg, 20 mg, 30 mg, 40 mg	No
Rx	**Lisinopril** *Prinivil*, *Zestril*	**Tablets:** 2.5 mg, 5 mg, 10 mg, 20 mg, 40 mg	No
Rx	**Moexipril HCl** *Univasc*	**Tablets:** 7.5 mg, 15 mg	No
Rx	**Perindopril Erbumine** *Aceon*	**Tablets:** 2 mg, 4 mg, 8 mg	No
Rx	**Quinapril HCl** *Accupril*	**Tablets:** 5 mg, 10 mg, 20 mg, 40 mg	No
Rx	**Ramipril** *Altace*	**Capsules:** 1.25 mg, 2.5 mg, 5 mg, 10 mg	No
Rx	**Trandolapril** *Mavik*	**Tablets:** 1 mg, 2 mg, 4 mg	No

Type of Drug:

Angiotensin converting enzyme inhibitors (ACEIs); drugs used to lower blood pressure.

How the Drug Works:

ACE is involved in certain chemical reactions that constrict (narrow) blood vessels and cause sodium and fluid retention by the kidney. This can cause an increase in blood pressure. ACE inhibitors lower blood pressure by interferring with ACE, which causes blood vessels to relax (widen). Blow flows more freely and at a lower pressure.

ACEIs also increase the heart's ability to pump blood in some types of heart failure.

Uses:

To treat high blood pressure alone or in combination with other blood pressure-lowering medications.

Captopril, enalapril, fosinopril, lisinopril, quinapril, ramipril — To treat certain types congestive of heart failure, usually with other medications (eg, diuretics, digitalis).

Captopril — To treat diabetic nephropathy (kidney damage) in patients with Type I (insulin-dependent) diabetes mellitus and retinopathy.

Lisinopril — To improve survival in patients who have had a heart attack within 24 hours.

Unlabeled Use(s): Occasionally, doctors may prescribe some of these medications for the management of specific types of hypertensive crises or neonatal and childhood hypertension; treatment of rheumatoid arthritis; certain types of edema; diabetic nephropathy; Bartter and Raynaud syndromes; and diagnosis of primary aldosteronism and certain kidney disorders.

Precautions:

Do not use in the following situations:

allergy to angiotensin converting enzyme inhibitors
ACEIs angioedema (difficulty breathing), history of
pregnancy, second and third trimester

Use with caution in the following situations:

agranulocytosis
anesthesia, surgical
angioedema, history of
aortic stenosis
diabetes mellitus
heart disease
low blood pressure
hemodialysis
high potassium levels
kidney disease
liver disease (fosinopril, ramipril, trandolapril only)
lupus erythematosus, systemic
neutropenia (low white blood cell count)
pregnancy, first trimester
protein in the urine (captopril only)

Low blood pressure: Dizziness and fainting due to lowered blood pressure may occur early in therapy. This effect is more likely to occur with diuretic treatment and when arising from a seated or lying position, but can occur at any time early in therapy. This effect can also occur if several doses are missed and then the medicine is restarted, if the dosage is increased rapidly, or if other blood pressure medications are added.

Potassium: Elevated serum potassium levels have occurred. Use with caution in the presence of kidney disease, diabetes, and with potassium-containing products (eg, salt substitutes, potassium supplements).

Photosensitivity: Sensitivity to light may occur; therefore, caution patients to take protective measures (eg, sunscreens, protective clothing) against exposure to ultraviolet (UV) light or sunlight until tolerance is determined.

Cough: A persistent, dry, nonproductive cough can be caused by ACEIs. The cough is more likely to occur in women and at low doses. Recovery is rapid and complete in 1 to 4 days when the drug has been discontinued.

Race: ACEIs may not be as effective in black patients.

Pregnancy: Report pregnancy or suspected pregnancy to your doctor immediately.

First trimester – Mothers whose embryos and fetuses are exposed to ACEIs only during the first trimester should be informed and the drug discontinued as soon as possible. Continue use only if clearly needed and potential benefits outweigh the possible hazards to the fetus.

Second and third trimesters – Studies have shown a potential adverse effect on the fetus. When used during the second and third trimesters, ACEIs can cause fetal harm or even death. Discontinue the drug as soon as possible.

Breastfeeding: Benazepril, captopril, enalapril, and fosinopril appear in breast milk. It is not known if lisinopril, moexipril, quinapril, perindopril, ramipril, or trandolapril appear in breast milk. Consult your doctor before you begin breastfeeding.

Children: Safety and effectiveness in children have not been established. There is limited experience with the use of captopril in children. Unpredictable decreases in blood pressure and associated complications have occurred. Use catopril in children only when other measures for controlling blood pressure have not been effective.

Elderly: Older patients tend to develop higher blood levels of these drugs than younger patients. Do not adjust dose without consulting with your doctor.

Lab tests will be required periodically during treatment. Tests may include urine protein, liver function, kidney function, electrolyte and white blood cell counts, and potassium levels.

Drug Interactions:

Tell your doctor or pharmacist if you are taking or planning to take any over-the-counter or prescription medications or dietary supplements with an ACEI. Doses of one or both drugs may need to be modified, or a different drug may need to be prescribed. The following drugs and drug classes interact with an ACEI:

- antacids (eg, *Maalox*)
- digoxin (eg, *Lanoxin*)
- diuretics (eg, furosemide)
- food (captopril, moexepril, and quinapril only)
- indomethacin (eg, *Indocin*)
- lithium (eg, *Eskalith*)
- potassium-containing salt substitutes (eg, *Nu-Salt*)

potassium-sparing diuretics (eg, triamterene)
potassium supplements
tetracyclines (eg, oxytetracyline) (quinapril only)

Side Effects:

Every drug is capable of producing side effects. Many ACEI users experience no, or minor, side effects. The frequency and severity of side effects depend on many factors including dose, duration of therapy, and individual susceptibility. Possible side effects include:

Digestive Tract: Stomach pain or ache; nausea; vomiting; diarrhea; constipation; indigestion; ulcers; appetite changes; gas; tongue swelling; difficulty swallowing; taste changes; mouth ulcer.

Nervous System: Depression; headache; dizziness; nervousness; sleeping difficulties; drowsiness; sleeplessness; fatigue; vertigo (feeling of whirling motion); abnormal skin sensations; weakness; taste changes.

Circulatory System: Chest pain; pounding of the chest; rapid or irregular heart beat; lowered blood pressure; orthostatic hypotention (dizziness or lightheadedness when rising quickly from a sitting or lying position); fainting; heart attack; stroke.

Respiratory System: Difficulty breathing or shortness of breath; cough; sore throat; runny nose; sinus irritation; pneumonia; upper respiratory infection.

Skin: Rash; itching; hives; flushing; hair loss; jaundice (yellowing of skin or eyes).

Other: Fluid retention; pain in arms or legs; weight changes; back, joint, muscle or shoulder pain; menstrual disorder; decreased or increased urination; protein in urine; fever; general body discomfort; flu syndrome; cold symptoms; ringing in the ears; ear infection; urinary tract infection; sexual problems; impotence; low serum sodium levels; elevated serum uric acid; elevated serum potassium levels; low serum calcium levels.

Guidelines for Use:

- Dosage is individualized. Take exactly as prescribed.
- Do not stop taking or change the dose unless advised by your doctor.
- All of these drugs *except* captopril, moexipril, and quinapril may be taken without regard to food. Take captopril, moexipril, and quinapril 1 hour before meals or 2 hours after meals if possible.
- *Ramipril* — R amipril capsules are usually swallowed whole. However, the capsules may be opened and the contents sprinkled on approximately 4 oz of applesauce or mixed in apple juice or water. Consume the entire mixture. Pre-prepared mixtures can be stored for up to 24 hours at room temperature or for up to 48 hours under refrigeration.

Guidelines for Use (cont.):

- *Ramipril* (cont.)—
- If a dose is missed, take it as soon as possible. If several hours have passed or if it is nearing time for the next dose, do not double the dose to catch up, unless advised by your doctor. If more than one dose is missed, or it is necessary to establish a new dosage schedule, contact your doctor or pharmacist.
- Inform your doctor if you are pregnant, become pregnant, or are planning to become pregnant. ACEIs can cause injury to and even death to a developing fetus.
- Inform your doctor if you are intending to breastfeed or are breastfeeding.
- Notify your doctor if you experience any of the following: sore throat, fever, swelling of hands or feet, irregular heartbeat, chest pains, hoarseness, or yellowing of the skin or eyes.
- Stop taking and notify your doctor immediately if swelling of the face, eyes, lips, or tongue occur, or if you experience difficulty in swallowing or breathing.
- Excessive perspiration, inadequate fluid intake, dehydration, vomiting, and diarrhea may lead to a fall in blood pressure while taking this medicine.
- May cause dizziness, fainting, or lightheadedness, especially after the first dose or during the first days of therapy; avoid sudden changes in posture. If actual fainting occurs, stop taking your medicine until you talk to your doctor. Heart failure patients should avoid rapid increases in physical activity. Sit or lie down if you feel lightheaded.
- May cause skin rash or impaired taste perception. Notify your doctor if these persist.
- A persistent dry cough may occur and usually does not go away unless the medication is stopped. Notify your doctor if this effect becomes bothersome.
- Do not use potassium supplements or salt substitutes containing potassium without consulting your doctor.
- May cause photosensitivity (sensitivity to sunlight). Avoid prolonged exposure to the sun or other forms of ultraviolet light (UV) light (eg, tanning beds). Use sunscreens and wear protective clothing until tolerance is determined.
- Lab tests may be required to monitor therapy. Be sure to keep appointments.
- Store in a tight, light-resistant container at room temperature (59° to 86°F). Protect from moisture.

If you have any questions, consult your doctor, pharmacist, or health care provider.

	Generic Name *Brand Name Examples*	Supplied As	Generic Available
Rx	**Candesartan Cilexetil**		
	Atacand	**Tablets:** 4 mg, 8 mg, 16 mg, 32 mg	No
Rx	**Eprosartan Mesylate**		
	Teveten	**Tablets:** 400 mg, 600 mg	No
Rx	**Irbesartan**		
	Avapro	**Tablets:** 75 mg, 150 mg, 300 mg	No
Rx	**Losartan Potassium**		
	Cozaar	**Tablets:** 25 mg, 50 mg, 100 mg	No
Rx	**Telmisartan**		
	Micardis	**Tablets:** 40 mg, 80 mg	No
Rx	**Valsartan**		
	Diovan	**Capsules:** 80 mg, 160 mg	No

Type of Drug:

Antihypertensive; blood pressure lowering agent.

How the Drug Works:

Angiotensin II is a chemical transmitter (key) that combines with chemical receptors (key holes) in blood vessels and other tissues and causes blood vessels to constrict (narrow) and the kidneys to retain sodium and fluids. Angiotensin II receptor antagonists inhibit the action of angiotensin II (plug up the keyholes) and allow the blood vessels to dilate (widen) and the kidneys to eliminate extra sodium and fluids. These actions combine to help lower elevated blood pressure.

Uses:

To lower blood pressure in patients older than 18 years of age. It may be used alone or in combination with other antihypertensive agents.

Unlabeled Use(s): These agents may be beneficial in the treatment of heart failure; however, further studies are needed. Irbesartan may reduce progression of kidney disease and its complications in patients with high blood pressure and diabetic kidney damage caused by type 2 diabetes.

Precautions:

Do not use in the following situations:

allergy to an angiotensin II receptor antagonist or any of its ingredients
pregnancy (second and third trimesters)

Use with caution in the following situations:

diuretic use, concurrent
kidney disease
liver disease
volume or salt-depletion (eg, dehydration) from diarrhea, vomiting, or sweating

Race: Angiotensin II may not be as effective in black patients.

Pregnancy:

First trimester – When pregnancy is detected, the patient should discontinue use as soon as possible. Use only if clearly needed and potential benefits to the mother outweigh the possible hazards to the fetus.

Second and third trimesters – Studies have shown a potential adverse effect on the fetus.

Breastfeeding: It is not known if angiotensin II receptor antagonists are excreted in breast milk. Because of the potential for adverse effects, a decision should be made whether to discontinue nursing or discontinue the drug, taking into account the importance of the drug to the mother. Consult your doctor before you begin breastfeeding.

Children: Safety and effectiveness in children younger than 18 years of age have not been established.

Elderly: Older patients may be more sensitive to the blood pressure-lowering effects of these agents.

Lab tests may be required to monitor therapy. Tests may include blood pressure readings, kidney function tests, liver function tests, and blood tests for electrolytes (eg, potassium).

Drug Interactions:

Tell your doctor or pharmacist if you are taking or planning to take any over-the-counter or prescription medications or dietary supplements while taking an angiotensin II receptor antagonist. Doses of one or both drugs may need to be modified or a different drug may need to be prescribed. The following drugs and drug classes interact with angiotensin II receptor antagonists:

digoxin (eg, *Lanoxin*) (telmisartan only)
potassium-containing salt substitutes
potassium-sparing diuretics (eg, spironolactone)
potassium supplements

Side Effects:

Every drug is capable of producing side effects. Many angiotensin II receptor antagonist users experience no, or minor, side effects. The frequency and severity of side effects depend on many factors including dose, duration of therapy, and individual susceptibility. Possible side effects include:

Digestive Tract: Indigestion; diarrhea; nausea; heartburn; stomach pain; vomiting; nausea.

Nervous System: Anxiety; dizziness; headache; fatigue; nervousness; sleeplessness; depression.

Respiratory System: Upper respiratory tract infection; cough; nasal congestion; sinus irritation; runny nose; sore throat; bronchitis.

Other: Rapid heartbeat; high blood pressure; chest, muscle, back, leg, or joint pain; muscle cramps; viral infection; fluid retention (swelling); trauma; weakness; flu; urinary tract infection; rash; protein in the urine.

Guidelines for Use:

- Dosage is individualized. Take exactly as prescribed.
- Do not change the dose or stop taking unless advised to do so by your doctor.
- May be taken without regard to food.
- *Telmisartan* — Do not remove tablets from blister pack until just before taking.
- May be taken with other blood pressure-lowering agents prescribed by your doctor.
- Maximum effect is generally attained after 2 to 4 weeks.
- If a dose is missed, take it as soon as possible. If several hours have passed or if it is nearing time for the next dose, do not double the dose to catch up, unless advised by your doctor. If more than one dose is missed or it is necessary to establish a new dosage schedule, contact your doctor or pharmacist.
- May cause dizziness or drowsiness. Use caution while driving or performing other tasks requiring alertness, coordination, or physical dexterity until tolerance is determined.
- Dehydration (eg, excess sweating, vomiting, diarrhea) may increase the blood pressure-lowering effect, causing dizziness or fainting. Notify your doctor if dizziness develops.
- A low dose of a diuretic may be added if blood pressure is not controlled.
- Inform your doctor immediately if you are pregnant, become pregnant, are planning to become pregnant, or are breastfeeding.
- Lifestyle changes (eg, stop smoking, lose weight, exercise, limit salt in diet) also help to reduce blood pressure.
- Lab tests may be required to monitor therapy. Be sure to keep appointments.
- Store at room temperature (59° to 86°F) in a tightly closed container. Protect from light and moisture.

If you have any questions, consult your doctor, pharmacist, or health care provider.

Generic Name *Brand Name Examples*	Supplied As	Generic Available
Rx **Clonidine HCl**		
Catapres	**Tablets:** 0.1 mg, 0.2 mg, 0.3 mg	Yes
Catapres-TTS-1, Catapres-TTS-2, Catapres-TTS-3	**Transdermal patches:** 0.1 mg/day, 0.2 mg/day, 0.3 mg/day	No

Type of Drug:

Drug used to lower blood pressure.

How the Drug Works:

Clonidine lowers blood pressure primarily by relaxing and dilating (widening) blood vessels.

Uses:

To treat high blood pressure. Used either alone or in combination with other blood pressure-lowering drugs.

Unlabeled Use(s): Occasionally, doctors may prescribe clonidine for atrial fibrillation, attention deficit hyperactivity disorder, kidney damage from cyclosporine, excessive sweating, mania, restless legs syndrome, psychosis, alcohol withdrawal, growth delay in children, diabetic diarrhea, Tourette's syndrome, hypertensive "urgencies," menopausal flushing, methadone/opiate detoxification, postherpetic neuralgia, reduction of inflammatory reactions in patients with asthma, smoking cessation, ulcerative colitis, and diagnosing pheochromocytoma.

Precautions:

Do not use in the following situations: Allergy to clonidine or any of its ingredients, including adhesive on patch.

Use with caution in the following situations:

- coronary artery disease
- depression, history of
- heart attack, recent
- heart disease, severe
- heart rhythm disturbances
- kidney disease, chronic
- stroke, history of

Withdrawal reaction: Abrupt discontinuation of clonidine, particularly the tablets, can cause a sudden, intense increase in blood pressure. Symptoms may include nervousness, agitation, headache, and tremors. Do not stop taking clonidine without consulting your doctor.

Tolerance: Tolerance may develop. Clonidine's effectiveness may decrease over time. If this occurs, therapy will have to be reevaluated by your doctor.

Pregnancy: There are no adequate or well-controlled studies in pregnant women. Use only if clearly needed and the potential benefits to the mother outweigh the possible hazards to the fetus.

Breastfeeding: Clonidine appears in breast milk. Consult your doctor before you begin breastfeeding.

Children: Safety and effectiveness in children have not been established.

Lab tests may be required to monitor therapy. Tests may include eye examinations and blood pressure monitoring.

Drug Interactions:

Tell your doctor or pharmacist if you are taking or planning to take any over-the-counter or prescription medications or dietary supplements with clonidine. Doses of one or both drugs may need to be modified or a different drug may need to be prescribed. The following drugs and drug classes interact with clonidine:

- alcohol
- barbiturates (eg, phenobarbital)
- beta blockers (eg, propranolol)
- digitalis (eg, digoxin)
- levodopa (eg, *Dopar*)
- prazosin (eg, *Minipress*)
- sedative drugs (eg, tranquilizers, sleeping pills, antihistamines)
- tricyclic antidepressants (eg, amitriptyline)
- verapamil (eg, *Calan*)

Side Effects:

Every drug is capable of producing side effects. Many clonidine users experience no, or minor, side effects. The frequency and severity of side effects depend on many factors including dose, duration of therapy, and individual susceptibility. Possible side effects include:

Digestive Tract: Constipation; nausea; vomiting; decreased appetite; weight gain; dry mouth.

Nervous System: Drowsiness; depression; headache; nervousness; weakness; sedation; dizziness; agitation; fatigue; sleeplessness; vivid dreams or nightmares.

Skin: Rash; flushing; facial hives; localized blisters; hives; itching; skin inflammation; discoloration; swelling; burning; pain; bruising; redness (patches); pale skin.

Other: Impotence; loss of sex drive; general body discomfort; excessive urination at night; fainting after rising from a lying or sitting position; breast growth in males; pounding in chest; abnormal heart rate; increased sensitivity to alcohol; fever.

Guidelines for Use:

- *Tablets* — Usual adult tablet dose is 0.2 to 0.6 mg in 2 divided doses (morning and bedtime).
  If a dose is missed, take it as soon as possible. If several hours have passed or if it is nearing time for the next dose, do not double the dose in order to catch up (unless advised to do so by your doctor). If more than one dose is missed or it is necessary to establish a new dosage schedule, contact your doctor or pharmacist.
  Do not stop taking this medicine suddenly. If your doctor discontinues this drug, the dose must be gradually reduced over 2 to 4 days in order to avoid a rapid increase in blood pressure, nervousness, agitation, or headache.
  Store tablets below 86°F, in a tight, light-resistant container.
- *Patches* — Patient instructions are included with each box of patches.
  Apply to hairless area on upper outer arm or chest once every 7 days.
  Do not apply over any abnormal or damaged skin. Do not shave skin before applying.
  Use a different skin site from the previous application. If the patch loosens during the 7–day wearing, apply the white adhesive overlay directly over the patch to ensure good adhesion.
  Tell your doctor if an allergic reaction or skin irritation extends beyond the local patch area.
  It may take 2 to 3 days after first application of patch before blood pressure is reduced.
  Doctors will occasionally have patients wear more than 1 patch at a time to adjust the dose. Apply patches at different locations.
  If mild skin irritation occurs during the 7-day wearing, remove and discard the patch and apply a new patch in another area.
  Usual exposure to water (eg, showering, bathing, swimming) should not affect the patch.
  After removal, fold used patch in half with sticky sides together and dispose of carefully.
- Take this medication exactly as directed, have your blood pressure checked regularly, and keep your appointments with your doctor even if you feel well. Most patients with high blood pressure do not feel sick.
- Patients being treated for high blood pressure often feel tired or rundown for a few weeks after beginning therapy. Continue taking your medication even though you may not feel quite normal. Contact your doctor or pharmacist about any new symptoms.
- This medicine may cause drowsiness or dizziness. Use caution while driving or performing other tasks requiring alertness, coordination, or physical dexterity.
- Avoid alcohol and other mental depressants (eg, tranquilizers) while you are taking this medicine. They may cause excessive drowsiness.
- *Unlabeled administration route* — Sublingual (under the tongue) clonidine may be effective for high blood pressure in patients who are unable to take oral medication.

If you have any questions, consult your doctor, pharmacist, or health care provider.

	Generic Name *Brand Name Example*	Supplied As	Generic Available
Rx	**Guanabenz Acetate**		
	Wytensin	**Tablets:** 4 mg, 8 mg	Yes

Type of Drug:

Drug used to lower high blood pressure.

How the Drug Works:

Guanabenz acetate lowers blood pressure primarily by relaxing and dilating (widening) blood vessels. Blood flows more freely at a lower pressure.

Uses:

To treat high blood pressure alone or in conjunction with a diuretic (water pill).

Precautions:

Do not use in the following situations: Allergy to guanabenz acetate or any of its ingredients.

Use with caution in the following situations:

coronary insufficiency
heart attack, recent
kidney disease, severe
liver disease, severe
stroke, history of

Discontinuing treatment: Do not stop taking this medicine without consulting your doctor. Abrupt withdrawal of treatment may result in high blood pressure.

Pregnancy: Adequate studies have not been done in pregnant women, or animal studies may have shown a risk to the fetus. Use only if clearly needed and potential benefits outweigh the possible hazards to the fetus.

Breastfeeding: It is not known if guanabenz appears in breast milk. Consult your doctor before you begin breastfeeding.

Children: Safety and effectiveness in children under 12 years of age have not been established.

Drug Interactions:

Tell your doctor or pharmacist if you are taking or planning to take any over-the-counter or prescription medications or dietary supplements while taking guanabenz acetate. Doses of one or both drugs may need to be modified or a different drug may need to be prescribed.

Side Effects:

Every drug is capable of producing side effects. Many patients experience no, or minor, side effects. The frequency and severity of side effects depend on many factors including dose, duration of therapy, and individual susceptibility. Possible side effects include:

Digestive Tract: Nausea; vomiting; stomach pain; diarrhea; constipation; dry mouth.

Nervous System: Depression; sleep disturbances; dizziness; drowsiness; headache; anxiety; taste disturbances; blurred vision; weakness.

Circulatory System: Irregular heartbeat; chest pain; pounding in the chest.

Respiratory System: Difficulty breathing; nasal congestion.

Other: Edema (fluid retention); muscle pain in arms and legs; breast growth in males; impotence, decreased sex drive; urinary frequency; rash; itching.

Guidelines for Use:

- Use exactly as prescribed.
- Take twice a day. Do not exceed 32 mg twice daily.
- If a dose is missed, take it as soon as possible. If several hours have passed or it is nearing time for the next dose, do not double the dose to catch up, unless advised to do so by your doctor. If more than one dose is missed or it is necessary to establish a new dosage schedule, contact your doctor or pharmacist.
- Take this medication daily as directed, have your blood pressure checked regularly and keep your appointments with your doctor even if you feel well. Most patients with high blood pressure do not feel sick.
- Do not stop taking this medicine suddenly or without consulting your doctor. Abrupt withdrawal of treatment may result in high blood pressure.
- Patients being treated for high blood pressure often feel tired or rundown for a few weeks after beginning therapy. Continue taking your medication even though you may not feel quite "normal." Contact your doctor or pharmacist about any new symptoms.
- This medicine may cause drowsiness or dizziness. Use caution while driving or performing other tasks requiring alertness, coordination, or physical dexterity.
- Avoid alcohol and other mental depressants (eg, tranquilizers) while you are taking this medicine. They may cause excessive drowsiness.
- Lab tests may be required to monitor therapy. Keep appointments.
- Store at room temperature (approximately 77°F) in a tightly closed container. Protect from light.

If you have any questions, consult your doctor, pharmacist, or health care provider.

	Generic Name *Brand Name Example*	Supplied As	Generic Available
Rx	**Guanadrel Sulfate**		
	Hylorel	**Tablets:** 10 mg, 25 mg	No

Type of Drug:

Drug used to lower high blood pressure.

How the Drug Works:

Guanadrel allows blood vessels to relax and dilate (widen), decreasing the resistance of the blood vessels to blood flow and resulting in lower blood pressure.

Uses:

To treat high blood pressure in conjunction with a diuretic ("water pill").

Precautions:

Do not use in the following situations:

allergy to this medication
congestive heart failure
MAO inhibitor antidepressant use (eg, phenelzine), within 1 week
pheochromocytoma (tumor of the adrenal gland)

Use with caution in the following situations:

asthma
kidney disease
peptic ulcer
surgery
tricyclic antidepressant use
vascular disease

Pregnancy: Studies in pregnant women or in animals have been judged not to show a risk to the fetus. However, no drug should be used during pregnancy unless clearly needed.

Breastfeeding: It is not known if guarandrel appears in breast milk. Consult your doctor before you begin breastfeeding.

Children: Safety and effectiveness have not been established.

Drug Interactions:

Tell your doctor or pharmacist if you are taking or planning to take any over-the-counter or prescription medications or dietary supplements while taking this medicine. Doses of one or both drugs may need to be modified or a different drug may need to be prescribed. The following drugs and drug classes interact with this medicine:

alpha-blocking agents (eg, prazosin)
beta blockers (eg, propanolol)
ephedrine
MAOIs (eg, phenelzine)
norepinephrine
phenothiazines (eg, promethazine)
phenylpropanolamine (eg, *Propagest*)
reserpine
tricyclic antidepressants (eg, amitriptyline)
vasodilators (eg, hydralazine)

Side Effects:

Every drug is capable of producing side effects. Many patients experience no, or minor, side effects. The frequency and severity of side effects depend on many factors including dose, duration of therapy, and individual susceptibility. Possible side effects include:

Digestive Tract: Nausea; vomiting; increased bowel movements; stomach pain; constipation; gas; indigestion; appetite loss; weight changes; dry mouth or throat; swollen tongue.

Nervous System: Headache; sleep disturbances; confusion; drowsiness; fatigue; fainting; depression; psychological problems; tingling or numbness.

Circulatory System: Chest pain; pounding in the chest.

Respiratory System: Shortness of breath; cough.

Other: Vision problems; swelling in hands and feet; impotence; back or neck ache; leg cramps and aches; joint pain or inflammation; urination frequency; urine retention; increased urination at night; blood in urine; ejaculation disturbances.

Guidelines for Use:

- Use exactly as prescribed.
- Usual adult daily dose is 20 to 75 mg, taken in two divided doses.
- If a dose is missed, take it as soon as possible. If several hours have passed or it is nearing time for the next dose, do not double the dose to catch up, unless advised to do so by your doctor. If more than one dose is missed or it is necessary to establish a new dosage schedule, contact your doctor or pharmacist.
- Take this medicine daily as directed, have your blood pressure checked regularly and keep your appointments with your doctor even if you feel well. Most patients do not feel sick.
- Do not stop taking this medicine suddenly or without consulting your doctor.
- Patients being treated for high blood pressure often feel tired or rundown for a few weeks after beginning therapy. Continue taking your medication even though you may not feel quite "normal." Contact your doctor or pharmacist about any new symptoms.
- This medicine may cause dizziness, lightheadedness, blurred vision or fainting, especially when rising or standing. This condition is worsened by alcohol use, fever, hot weather, prolonged standing or excersise. If these symptoms should occur, sit or lie down and contact your doctor.
- This medicine may cause drowsiness. Use caution while driving or performing other tasks requiring alertness, coordination or physical dexterity.
- Do not take any prescription or over-the-counter medications, especially for colds, allergy or asthma, without the advice of your doctor or pharmacist.
- Store at controlled room temperature (59° to 86°F).

If you have any questions, consult your doctor, pharmacist, or health care provider.

	Generic Name *Brand Name Example*	Supplied As	Generic Available
Rx	**Guanethidine Monosulfate**		
	Ismelin	**Tablets:** 10 mg, 25 mg	No

Type of Drug:

Drug used to lower high blood pressure.

How the Drug Works:

Guanethidine lowers blood pressure by relaxing and dilating (widening) blood vessels. Blood flows more freely at a lower pressure.

Uses:

To treat moderate and severe high blood pressure, either alone or in conjuction with a diuretic ("water pill").

To treat high blood pressure caused by certain kidney diseases.

Precautions:

Do not use in the following situations:

allergy to this medicine
congestive heart failure, not due to hypertension
MAOI (eg, phenelzine), use
pheochromocytoma (adrenal gland tumor)

Use with caution in the following situations:

asthma
cerebral vascular disease (stroke)
coronary insufficiency
fever
heart attack, recent
heart failure
kidney disease
nitrogen retention
peptic ulcers
surgery

Pregnancy: Adequate studies have not been done in pregnant women, or animal studies may have shown a risk to the fetus. Use only if clearly needed and potential benefits outweigh the possible hazards to the fetus.

Breastfeeding: Guanethidine appears in breast milk. Contact your doctor before you begin breastfeeding.

Children: Safety and effectiveness in children have not been established.

Drug Interactions:

Tell your doctor or pharmacist if you are taking or planning to take any over-the-counter or prescription medications or dietary supplements while taking this medicine. Doses of one or both drugs may need to be modified or a different drug may need to be prescribed. The following drugs and drug classes interact with this medicine:

- alcohol
- appetite suppressants (eg, amphetamines)
- barbiturates (eg, phenobarbital)
- blood sugar lowering medications (eg, insulin)
- contraceptives, oral (eg, *Ortho-Novum*)
- digoxin (eg, *Lanoxin*)
- haloperidol (eg, *Haldol*)
- MAO inhibitor antidepressants (eg, phenelzine)
- maprotiline (*Ludiomil*)
- methylphenidate (eg, *Ritalin*)
- minoxidil (eg, *Loniten*)
- phenylthiazine (eg, *Compazine*)
- rauwolfia derivatives (eg, reserpine)
- sympathomimetics (eg, ephedrine)
- thioxanthenes (eg, thiothixene)
- tricyclic antidepressants (eg, amitriptyline)

Side Effects:

Every drug is capable of producing side effects. Many patients experience no, or minor, side effects. The frequency and severity of side effects depend on many factors including dose, duration of therapy, and individual susceptibility. Possible side effects include:

Digestive Tract: Diarrhea; nausea; vomiting; increased bowel movements; dry mouth.

Nervous System: Dizziness; weakness; depression; fainting; drowsiness; blurred vision; tiredness.

Circulatory System: Slowed heart rate; chest pain or numbness.

Respiratory System: Nasal congestion; difficulty breathing; asthma.

Other: Hair loss; impotence; muscle tremors or aches; edema (fluid retention); increased urination at night; loss of bladder control; drooping eyelids; skin inflammation; ejaculation problems; scalp hair loss.

Guidelines for Use:

- Use exactly as prescribed.
- Usual adult dose is 25 to 50 mg taken once daily.
- If a dose is missed, take it as soon as possible. If several hours have passed or it is nearing time for the next dose, do not double the dose to catch up, unless advised to do so by your doctor. If more than one dose is missed or it is necessary to establish a new dosage schedule, contact your doctor or pharmacist.
- Take this medication daily as directed, have your blood pressure checked regularly and keep your appointments with your doctor even if you feel well. Most patients with high blood pressure do not feel sick.
- Do not stop taking this medicine suddenly or abruptly.
- Patients being treated for high blood pressure often feel tired or run-down for a few weeks after beginning therapy. Continue taking your medication even though you may not feel quite "normal." Contact your doctor or pharmacist about any new symptoms.
- Dizziness or lightheadedness may occur if you stand up too fast from a lying or sitting position. If this occurs, get up slowly and avoid sudden changes in posture.
- This medicine can cause dizziness. Use caution while driving or performing other tasks requiring alertness, coordination or physical dexterity.
- Contact your doctor if severe diarrhea, nausea, vomiting, frequent dizziness or fainting occurs.
- This medicine may interfere with ejaculation.
- Avoid alcohol while you are taking this medicine, as it aggravates the orthostatic hypotensive effects (dizziness or lightheadedness when rising quickly from a sitting or lying position) of this medicine.
- Do not take any prescription or over-the-counter medications, especially for colds, allergy or asthma, without consulting with your doctor or pharmacist.
- Store below 86°F in a tightly closed container.

If you have any questions, consult your doctor, pharmacist, or health care provider.

	Generic Name *Brand Name Example*	Supplied As	Generic Available
Rx	**Guanfacine HCl** *Tenex*	**Tablets:** 1 mg, 2 mg	No

Type of Drug:

Drug used to lower high blood pressure.

How the Drug Works:

Guanfacine lowers blood pressure by relaxing and dilating (widening) blood vessels. Blood flows more freely at a lower pressure.

Uses:

To treat high blood pressure. May be used alone or in conjunction with other blood pressure lowering drugs, especially a thiazide diuretic ("water pill").

Unlabeled Use(s): Occasionally doctors may prescribe guanfacine for heroin withdrawal, to reduce the frequency of migraine headaches or to reduce nausea and vomiting.

Precautions:

Do not use in the following situations: Allergy to guanfacine or any of its ingredients.

Use with caution in the following situations:

cerebrovascular disease (stroke)
coronary insufficiency, severe
heart attack, recent
kidney disease, chronic
liver disease, chronic

Drug withdrawal reaction: Do not stop taking this medicine without consulting with your doctor. Abrupt withdrawal may result in high blood pressure.

Pregnancy: Studies in pregnant women or in animals have been judged not to show a risk to the fetus. However, no drug should be used during pregnancy unless clearly needed.

Breastfeeding: It is not known if guanfacine appears in breast milk. Consult your doctor before you begin breastfeeding.

Children: Safety and effectiveness in children under 12 years of age have not been established.

Drug Interactions:

Tell your doctor or pharmacist if you are taking or planning to take any over-the-counter or prescription medications or dietary supplements while taking this medicine. Doses of one or both drugs may need to be modified or a different drug may need to be prescribed. The following drugs and drug classes interact with this medicine:

barbiturates (eg, phenobarbital)
phenytoin (eg, *Dilantin*)
tricyclic antidepressants (eg, amitriptyline)

Side Effects:

Every drug is capable of producing side effects. Many patients experience no, or minor, side effects. The frequency and severity of side effects depend on many factors including dose, duration of therapy, and individual susceptibility. Possible side effects include:

Digestive Tract: Nausea; constipation; dry mouth; stomach pain; diarrhea; indigestion; difficulty swallowing.

Nervous System: Dizziness; headache; drowsiness; weakness; sleeplessness; memory loss; confusion; depression; numbness or tingling; paralysis.

Circulatory System: Slow heartbeat; pounding in the chest; chest pain.

Respiratory System: Nasal congestion; difficulty breathing.

Skin: Inflammation; itching; hives; sweating.

Other: Impotence; decrease in sexual desire; problems with testicles; changes in taste or vision; ringing in the ears; eye inflammation or infection; leg cramps, tremors; loss of bladder control; general body discomfort; decreased mobility or activity; unusual bleeding.

Guidelines for Use:

- Use exactly as prescribed.
- Usual adult dose is 1 mg daily. Take at bedtime to decrease daytime drowsiness.
- If a dose is missed, take it as soon as possible. If several hours have passed or it is nearing time for the next dose, do not double the dose to catch up, unless advised to do so by your doctor. If more than one dose is missed or it is necessary to establish a new dosage schedule, contact your doctor or pharmacist.
- Take this medication daily as directed, have your blood pressure checked regularly and keep your appointments with your doctor even if you feel well. Most patients with high blood pressure do not feel sick.
- Do not stop taking this medicine suddenly. If your doctor discontinues this drug, the dose must be gradually reduced in order to avoid a rapid increase in blood pressure, nervousness or agitation.
- Patients being treated for high blood pressure often feel tired or rundown for a few weeks after beginning therapy. Continue taking your medication even though you may not feel quite "normal." Contact your doctor or pharmacist about any new symptoms.
- This medicine may cause drowsiness or dizziness. Use caution while driving or performing other tasks requiring alertness, coordination or physical dexterity.
- Avoid alcohol and other mental depressants (eg, tranquilizers) while you are taking this medicine. They may cause excessive drowsiness.
- Store at controlled room temperature (59° to 86°F) in a tight, light-resistant container.

If you have any questions, consult your doctor, pharmacist, or health care provider.

	Generic Name *Brand Name Example*	Supplied As	Generic Available
Rx	**Hydralazine HCl**		
	Apresoline[1]	**Tablets:** 10 mg, 25 mg, 50 mg, 100 mg	Yes
	Apresoline	**Injection:** 20 mg/mL	Yes

[1] 100 mg tablet contains the dye tartrazine.

Type of Drug:

Drug used to lower high blood pressure.

How the Drug Works:

Hydralazine lowers blood pressure by relaxing and dilating (widening) the blood vessels. Blood flows more freely at a lower pressure.

Uses:

To treat high blood pressure alone or in conjunction with other blood pressure lowering medications.

Unlabeled Use(s): Occasionally doctors may prescribe hydralazine for the treatment of congestive heart failure, severe aortic insufficiency and after heart valve replacement.

Precautions:

Do not use in the following situations:

allergy to this medicine
coronary artery disease
mitral valvular rheumatic heart disease

Use with caution in the following situations:

kidney disease, advanced
stroke

Systemic lupus erythematosus: Hydralazine may produce symptoms similar to lupus (joint pain, fever, chest pain, continued general body discomfort, enlarged spleen, skin problems). Symptoms usually go away when the drug is discontinued.

Pregnancy: Adequate studies have not been done in pregnant women, or animal studies may have shown a risk to the fetus. Use only if clearly needed and potential benefits outweigh the possible hazards to the fetus.

Breastfeeding: Hydralazine appears in breast milk. Consult your doctor before you begin breastfeeding.

Children: Safety and effectiveness have not been established.

Lab tests may be required to monitor therapy. Tests may include blood tests. Be sure to keep appointments.

Tartrazine: Some of these products may contain the dye tartrazine (FD&C yellow No. 5) which can cause allergic reactions in certain individuals. Check package label when available or consult your doctor or pharmacist.

Drug Interactions:

Tell your doctor or pharmacist if you are taking or planning to take any over-the-counter or prescription medications or dietary supplements while taking this medicine. Doses of one or both drugs may need to be modified or a different drug may need to be prescribed. The following drugs and drug classes interact with this medicine:

beta blockers (eg, propranolol)
diazoxide (*Hyperstat IV*)
indomethacin (eg, *Indocin*)
MAO inhibitor antidepressants (eg, phenelzine)

Side Effects:

Every drug is capable of producing side effects. Many patients experience no, or minor, side effects. The frequency and severity of side effects depend on many factors including dose, duration of therapy, and individual susceptibility. Possible side effects include:

Digestive Tract: Nausea; vomiting; diarrhea; appetite loss; constipation.

Nervous System: Headache; dizziness; tremors; depression; anxiety; disorientation; drowsiness.

Circulatory System: Chest pain; palpitations (pounding in the chest); increased heart beat; fainting.

Respiratory System: Difficulty breathing; nasal congestion.

Skin: Rash; itching; flushing; hives.

Other: Muscle pain or cramps; joint pain; difficult urination; red, swollen, puffy, infected, watery eyes; numbness or tingling in the hands or feet; fever; chills; fluid retention (edema); flushing.

Guidelines for Use:

- Use exactly as prescribed.
- Usual adult tablet dose is 50 mg taken four times daily.
- Take with meals.
- If a dose is missed, take it as soon as possible. If several hours have passed or it is nearing time for the next dose, do not double the dose to catch up, unless advised to do so by your doctor. If more than one dose is missed or it is necessary to establish a new dosage schedule, contact your doctor or pharmacist.
- Take this medication daily as directed. Have your blood pressure checked regularly and keep your appointments with your doctor even if you feel well. Most patients with high blood pressure do not feel sick.
- Patients being treated for high blood pressure often feel tired or rundown for a few weeks after beginning therapy. Continue taking your medication even though you may not feel quite "normal." Contact your doctor or pharmacist about any new symptoms.
- This medicine may cause dizziness or drowsiness. Use caution while driving or performing other tasks requiring alertness, coordination or physical dexterity.
- Contact your doctor if rash, joint pain, fever, chest pain or prolonged tiredness or general body discomfort occurs.
- Lab tests may be required to monitor therapy. Be sure to keep appointments.
- *Injection* — Follow the injection procedure taught to you by your healthcare provider.
  Visually inspect solution for particles or discoloration before use.
- Store tablets below 86°F in a tight, light-resistant container.

If you have any questions, consult your doctor, pharmacist, or health care provider.

	Generic Name *Brand Name Example*	Supplied As	Generic Available
Rx	**Carvedilol**		
	Coreg	**Tablets:** 6.25 mg, 12.5 mg, 25 mg	No

Type of Drug:

Drug used to lower high blood pressure; antihypertensive; alpha/beta-adrenergic blocking agent.

How the Drug Works:

Carvedilol lowers blood pressure by dilating blood vessels, thereby decreasing blood pressure and pulse rate.

Uses:

For the management of high blood pressure. It can be used alone or in combination with other antihypertensive drugs such as thiazide diuretics ("water pills").

Unlabeled Use(s): Occasionally doctors may prescribe carvedilol for congestive heart failure, chest pain (angina pectoris) or idiopathic cardiomyopathy.

Precautions:

Do not use in the following situations:

- allergy to this medicine
- bronchial asthma (or related bronchial conditions)
- heart problems, severe (eg, slow heartbeat or shock)
- liver disease, severe

Use with caution in the following situations:

- anesthesia/surgery
- heart failure
- hyperthyroidism (overactive thyroid)
- hypoglycemia (low blood sugar)
- peripheral vascular disease (hardening of the arteries)

Diabetes: These products can mask signs of hypoglycemia (low blood sugar) and alter blood sugar levels. It may be necessary for your doctor to alter your dose of diabetic medications while you are taking this medicine.

Bronchospasm, nonallergic (eg, chronic bronchitis, emphysema): In general, patients with bronchospastic disease should not take carvedilol. However, carvedilol may be used with caution in patients who do not respond to or cannot tolerate other high blood pressure drugs. Use the lowest possible dose in these cases.

Pregnancy: Adequate studies have not been done in pregnant women, or animal studies may have shown a risk to the fetus. Use only if clearly needed and potential benefits outweigh the possible hazards to the fetus.

Breastfeeding: It is not known if carvedilol appears in breast milk. Consult your doctor before you begin breastfeeding.

Children: Safety and effectiveness in children under 18 years of age have not been established.

Drug Interactions:

Tell your doctor or pharmacist if you are taking or planning to take any over-the-counter or prescription medications while taking this medicine. Doses of one or both drugs may need to be modified or a different drug may need to be prescribed. The following drugs and drug classes interact with this medicine:

calcium channel blockers (eg, nifedipine)
catecholamine-depleting agents (eg, reserpine, MAOIs)
cimetidine (eg, *Tagamet*)
clonidine (eg, *Catapres*)
digoxin (eg, *Lanoxin*)
insulin
oral hypoglycemics (eg, sulfonylureas)
rifampin (eg, *Rifadin*)

Side Effects:

Every drug is capable of producing side effects. Many patients experience no, or minor, side effects. The frequency and severity of side effects depend upon many factors including dose, duration of therapy, and individual susceptibility. Possible side effects include:

Digestive Tract: Stomach pain; diarrhea.

Nervous System: Dizziness; sleeplessness; drowsiness; fatigue.

Circulatory System: Slow heart rate; postural hypotension (dizziness or lightheadedness when rising from a sitting or lying position); swelling of the lower legs.

Other: Runny nose; sore throat; difficulty breathing; back pain; infections; unusual bleeding or bruising.

Guidelines for Use:

- Use exactly as prescribed.
- Take with food to reduce lightheadedness when rising or standing.
- If a dose is missed, take it as soon as possible. If several hours have passed or it is nearing time for the next dose, do not double the dose to catch up, unless advised to do so by your doctor. If more than one dose is missed or it is necessary to establish a new dosage schedule, contact your doctor or pharmacist.
- Do not stop taking this medicine or change the dose without checking with your doctor; this could cause serious adverse effects.
- May cause drowsiness, dizziness, lightheadedness or fainting (especially when rising or standing). If these symptoms should occur, sit or lie down and contact your doctor. Use caution when driving or performing other tasks requiring alertness, coordination or physical dexterity.
- Patients being treated for high blood pressure often feel tired and run down for a few weeks after beginning therapy. It takes time for the body to adjust to lowered blood pressure. The full effect may take 7 to 14 days. Continue taking your medication even though you may not feel quick "normal." Check with your doctor or pharmacist during this time regarding any new symptoms that occur to assure that these new feelings are a normal consequence of changes in blood pressure.
- If itching, dark urine, appetite loss, yellowing of skin or eyes, pain in the upper right side or flu-like symptoms occur, contact your doctor immediately.
- Dose adjustments may be required after checking blood pressure. Be sure to keep appointments.
- Contact lens wearers may notice decreased tearing (dry eyes).
- Store at room temperature (59° to 86°F) away from moisture and light.

If you have any questions, consult your doctor, pharmacist, or health care provider.

	Generic Name *Brand Name Examples*	Supplied As	Generic Available
Rx	**Labetalol HCl**		
	Normodyne, Trandate	**Tablets:** 100 mg, 200 mg, 300 mg	No
	Normodyne, Trandate	**Injections:** 5 mg/mL	No

Type of Drug:

Drug used to lower high blood pressure; antihypertensive; alpha/beta blocker.

How the Drug Works:

Labetalol lowers blood pressure alone and prevents blood pressure and pulse rate from increasing during exercise.

Uses:

To treat high blood pressure alone or with other blood pressure lowering drugs, such as thiazide diuretics (water pills).

Unlabeled Use(s): Occasionally doctors may prescribe labetalol for pheochromocytoma and for clonidine withdrawal.

Precautions:

Do not use in the following situations:

allergy to this medicine
bronchial asthma
heart problems, severe (eg, slow heartbeat or shock)

Use with caution in the following situations:

anesthesia/surgery
bronchitis, chronic
congestive heart failure, history
emphysema
hypoglycemia (low blood sugar
liver disease
pheochromocytoma (tumor)

Diabetes: These products can mask signs of hypoglycemia (low blood sugar) and alter blood sugar levels. It may be necessary for your doctor to alter your dose of diabetic medications while you are taking labetalol.

Discontinuing therapy: Do not suddenly discontinue labetalol without consulting your doctor. Angina (chest pain) or blood pressure may worsen.

Pregnancy: Adequate studies have not been done in pregnant women, or animal studies may have shown a risk to the fetus. Use only if clearly needed and potential benefits outweigh the possible hazards to the fetus.

Breastfeeding: Labetalol appears in breast milk. Consult your doctor before you begin breastfeeding.

Children: Safety and effectiveness have not been established.

Lab tests may be required to monitor therapy. Be sure to keep appointments.

Drug Interactions:

Tell your doctor or pharmacist if you are taking or planning to take any over-the-counter or prescription medications or dietary supplements while taking this medicine. Doses of one or both drugs may need to be modified or a different drug may need to be prescribed. The following drugs and drug classes interact with this medicine:

- alkalines (eg, furosemide) (*Normodyne* injection only)
- beta-adrenergic agonists (eg, albuterol)
- cimetidine (eg, *Tagamet*)
- halothane anesthesia
- nitroglycerin (eg, *Nitro-Bid*)
- tricyclic antidepressants (eg, imipramine)
- verapamil (eg, *Isoptin*)

Side Effects:

Every drug is capable of producing side effects. Many patients experience no, or minor, side effects. The frequency and severity of side effects depend on many factors including dose, duration of therapy, and individual susceptibility. Possible side effects include:

Digestive Tract: Nausea; vomiting; indigestion.

Nervous System: Dizziness; headache; fatigue; drowsiness; abnormal skin sensations; tingling of scalp or skin; weakness; yawning; numbness; feeling of whirling motion.

Circulatory System: Postural hypotension (dizziness or lightheadedness when rising from a sitting or lying position); slow heartbeat.

Skin: Itching; rash; yellowing of skin or eyes; hair loss.

Other: Difficulty breathing; wheezing; nasal congestion; swelling of lower legs; visual disturbances; taste changes; muscle cramps; sexual difficulty; urinary problems.

Guidelines for Use:

- Use exactly as prescribed.
- Usually taken twice a day. Tablets may be taken with or without food, but should be taken the same way each time.
- Do not stop taking this medicine without contacting your doctor; this could cause serious adverse effects.
- If a dose is missed, take it as soon as possible. If several hours have passed or it is nearing time for the next dose, do not double the dose to catch up, unless advised to do so by your doctor. If more than one dose is missed or it is necessary to establish a new dosage schedule, contact your doctor or pharmacist.
- Patients being treated for high blood pressure often feel tired and run down for a few weeks after beginning therapy. It takes time for the body to adjust to lowered blood pressure. Continue taking your medication even though you may not feel quite "normal." Check with your doctor or pharmacist during this time regarding any new symptoms that occur to assure that these new feelings are a normal consequence of changes in blood pressure.
- May cause dizziness or fainting, especially when rising or standing. If these symptoms should occur, sit or lie down and contact your doctor. Use caution when driving or performing other tasks requiring alertness, coordination or physical dexterity.
- Temporary scalp tinging may occur, especially at the start of treatment.
- Contact your doctor if any of the following occurs: Difficulty breathing; chest pain; slowed heartbeat; swelling of the lower legs; itching; dark urine; appetite loss; stomach pain; flu-like symptoms; yellowing of skin or eyes; upper right side pain.
- Diabetics may require adjustments in the dose of their antidiabetic medicine.
- Lab tests/exams will be required. Be sure to keep appointments.
- Store at room temperature (36° to 86°F) away from light and moisture. Do not freeze.

If you have any questions, consult your doctor, pharmacist, or health care provider.

Generic Name *Brand Name Example*	Supplied As	Generic Available
Rx **Mecamylamine HCl**		
Inversine	**Tablets:** 2.5 mg	No

Type of Drug:

Drug used to lower high blood pressure.

How the Drug Works:

Mecamylamine lowers blood pressure primarily by relaxing and dilating (widening) blood vessels. Blood flows more freely at a lower pressure.

Uses:

To treat moderately severe to severe high blood pressure or uncomplicated malignant hypertension.

Precautions:

Do not use in the following situations:

allergy to this medicine
antibiotic use
coronary insufficiency
glaucoma
heart attack, recent
high blood pressure, mild, moderate or labile
kidney disease
pyloric stenosis
sulfonamide use
noncompliant patients
uremia

Use with caution in the following situations:

arteriosclerosis (hardening of the arteries)
urination difficulties
prostate enlargement
stroke, recent

Discontinuing treatment: Do not discontinue this medicine without consulting your doctor. Abrupt withdrawal may result in a sudden return of high blood pressure and may result in a stroke or heart failure.

Action of mecamylamine may be increased by: Excessive heat; fever; infection; hemorrhage; pregnancy; anesthesia; surgery; vigorous exercise; other high blood pressure drugs; alcohol; salt depletion from diminished intake or increased excretion due to diarrhea, vomiting, excessive sweating or diuretics. Do not restrict sodium ingestion during therapy.

Pregnancy: Adequate studies have not been done in pregnant women, or animal studies may have shown a risk to the fetus. Use only if clearly needed and potential benefits outweigh the possible hazards to the fetus.

Breastfeeding: Because of the potential for serious adverse reactions in nursing infants, either discontinue nursing or discontinue the drug. Consult your doctor before you begin breastfeeding.

Side Effects:

Every drug is capable of producing side effects. Many patients experience no, or minor, side effects. The frequency and severity of side effects depend on many factors including dose, duration of therapy, and individual susceptibility. Possible side effects include:

Digestive Tract: Nausea; vomiting; constipation; appetite loss; tongue inflammation; dry mouth; intestinal obstruction.

Nervous System: Convulsions; lightheadedness; weakness; drowsiness; fainting and dizziness when rising from a sitting or lying position; low blood pressure when standing; tremors; abnormal involuntary movements; abnormal mental state.

Other: Dilated pupils; blurred vision; shortness of breath; urinary retention; impotence; decreased sexual desire; tingling or numbness.

Guidelines for Use:

- Use exactly as required.
- Usual adult dose is 25 mg, taken in three divided daily doses. Take after meals.
- The timing of doses in relation to meals should be consistent. Take the largest dose at noontime or in the evening. The smallest dose should be in the morning.
- Do not restrict dietary salt. Depleted salt states may increase the action of this medicine. Loss of salt can occur through sweating, vomiting, diarrhea or dehydration.
- If a dose is missed, take it as soon as possible. If several hours have passed or it is nearing time for the next dose, do not double the dose to catch up, unless advised to do so by your doctor. If more than one dose is missed or it is necessary to establish a new dosage schedule, contact your doctor or pharmacist.
- May cause dizziness, lightheadedness or fainting, especially when rising from a lying or sitting position. This effect may be increased by alcoholic beverages, exercise or during hot weather.
- Take this medication daily as directed, have your blood pressure checked regularly and keep your appointments with your doctor even if you feel well. Most patients with high blood pressure do not feel sick.
- Do not stop taking this medicine suddenly. If your doctor discontinues this drug, the dose must be gradually reduced in order to avoid a rapid increase in blood pressure and may result in a stroke or heart failure.
- Patients being treated for high blood pressure often feel tired or rundown for a few weeks after beginning therapy. Continue taking your medication even though you may not feel quite "normal." Contact your doctor or pharmacist about any new symptoms.
- Stop taking this medicine and contact your doctor immediately if tremors, diarrhea, bloating, decreased stomach rumbling or signs of bowel obstruction occur.
- This medicine may cause drowsiness. Use caution while driving or performing other tasks requiring alertness, coordination or physical dexterity.
- Avoid alcohol while you are taking this medicine. It may cause excessive drowsiness.
- Store at room temperature in a tight, light-resistant container.

If you have any questions, consult your doctor, pharmacist, or health care provider.

	Generic Name *Brand Name Example*	Supplied As	Generic Available
Rx	**Methyldopa HCl**		
	Aldomet	**Tablets:** 125 mg, 250 mg, 500 mg	Yes
	Aldomet[1]	**Oral Suspension:** 250 mg/5 mL	Yes
	Aldomet[2]	**Injection:** 250 mg/5 mL	Yes

[1] Contains sulfites and alcohol.
[2] Contains sulfites.

Type of Drug:

Drug used to lower high blood pressure.

How the Drug Works:

Methyldopa lowers blood pressure by relaxing and dilating (widening) blood vessels. Blood flows more freely at a lower pressure.

Uses:

To treat high blood pressure alone or in conjunction with other blood pressure lowering drugs.

Precautions:

Do not use in the following situations:

allergy to any component of this medicine
blood vessel disease
cirrhosis, active
hepatitis, active
MAOI (eg, phenelzine), use

Use with caution in the following situations:

anemia or other blood disorders
anesthetics
kidney disease
liver disease, history

Pregnancy:

Tablets, oral suspension - Studies in pregnant women have not shown a risk to the fetus. However, no drug should be used during pregnant unless clearly needed.

Injection – Adequate studies have not been done in pregnant women or animal studies may have shown a risk to the fetus. Use only if clearly needed and potential benefits outweigh the possible hazards to the fetus.

Breastfeeding: Methyldopa appears in breast milk. Contact your doctor before you begin breastfeeding.

Elderly: Dizziness and lightheadedness in older patients may be related to an increased sensitivity and to the patient's physical condition. Lower doses may need to be prescribed.

Lab tests may be required to monitor treatment. Tests may include Coombs test, liver function tests, hemoglobin, hematocrit, white and red cell counts. Be sure to keep appointments.

Sulfites: The oral suspension and injection contain sulfite preservatives which can cause allergic reactions in certain individuals (eg, asthmatics).

Drug Interactions:

Tell your doctor or pharmacist if you are taking or planning to take any over-the-counter or prescription medications or dietary supplements while taking this medicine. Doses of one or both drugs may need to be modified or a different drug may need to be prescribed. The following drugs and drug classes interact with this medicine:

barbiturates (eg, phenobarbital)
beta blockers (eg, propranolol)
haloperidol (eg, *Haldol*)
levodopa (eg, *Larodopa*)
lithium (eg, *Eskalith*)
MAOIs (eg, phenelzine)
phenothiazines (eg, trifluoperazine)
sulfonylureas (eg, tolbutamide)
sympathomimetics (eg, ephedrine)
tricyclic antidepressants (eg, amitriptyline)

Side Effects:

Every drug is capable of producing side effects. Many patients experience no, or minor, side effects. The frequency and severity of side effects depend on many factors including dose, duration of therapy, and individual susceptibility. Possible side effects include:

Digestive Tract: Nausea; vomiting; diarrhea; constipation; gas; colitis; bloating; dry mouth; inflammation of salivary glands; sore or black tongue; weight gain; mouth sores; stomach pain.

Nervous System: Dizziness; weakness; lightheadedness; drowsiness; headache; depression; decreased concentration; nightmares; tingling or numbness; unusual body movements; fainting.

Circulatory System: Slow heart rate; chest pain; congestive heart failure.

Respiratory System: Nasal congestion; sore throat; difficulty breathing.

Skin: Rash; yellowing of skin or eyes; easy bruising or bleeding.

Other: Joint or muscle pain; edema (fluid retention); fever; absence of menstruation; impotence; decrease sexual desire; breast swelling; breast secretions; anemia; dark or amber urine; breast growth in males; pancreatitis; liver or blood disorders; abnormal liver functions tests; Parkinsonism; Bell palsy.

Guidelines for Use:

- Take exactly as prescribed.
- Usual adult dose of tablets and suspension is 500 mg to 2 g in two to four divided daily doses.
- If a dose is missed, take it as soon as possible. If several hours have passed or it is nearing time for the next dose, do not double the dose to catch up, unless advised to do so by your doctor. If more than one dose is missed or it is necessary to establish a new dosage schedule, contact your doctor or pharmacist.
- Take this medication daily as directed, have your blood pressure checked regularly and keep your appointments with your doctor even if you feel well. Most patients with high blood pressure do not feel sick.
- Do not stop taking this medicine suddenly. If your doctor discontinues this drug, the dose must be gradually reduced over 2 to 4 days in order to avoid a rapid increase in blood pressure.
- Patients being treated for high blood pressure often feel tired or rundown for a few weeks after beginning therapy. Continue taking your medication even though you may not feel quite "normal." Contact your doctor or pharmacist about any new symptoms.
- Dizziness or lightheadedness may occur if you stand up too fast from a lying or sitting position. If this occurs, get up slowly and avoid sudden changes in posture.
- This medicine may cause drowsiness. Use caution while driving or performing other tasks requiring alertness, coordination or physical dexterity.
- Avoid alcohol and other mental depressants (eg, tranquilizers) while you are taking this medicine. They may cause excessive drowsiness.
- Notify your doctor if prolonged general tiredness, edema (fluid retention), shortness of breath, involuntary movements, fever, mouth sores, sore throat or yellowing of skin or eyes occurs.
- Tolerance may occur, usually between the second or third month of therapy. Your doctor may increase the dosage of methyldopa or add a diuretic (water pill).
- When urine is exposed to air, it may darken. This is not a problem.
- *Injection* — Usual adult dose is 250 to 500 mg every 6 hours. Follow the injection procedure taught to you by a healthcare provider.
  Visually inspect solution for particles or discoloration before use.
- Lab tests may be required to monitor treatment. Be sure to keep appointments.
- *Storage* — Store tablets at room temperature in a tight, light-resistant container.
  Store suspension below 78°F in a light, light-resistant container. Do not freeze.

If you have any questions, consult your doctor, pharmacist, or health care provider.

	Generic Name *Brand Name Example*	Supplied As	Generic Available
Rx	**Minoxidil**		
	Loniten	**Tablets:** 2.5 mg, 10 mg	Yes

Type of Drug:

Drug used to lower high blood pressure.

How the Drug Works:

Minoxidil lowers blood pressure by relaxing and dilating (widening) the arteries. Blood flows more freely at a lower pressure.

Uses:

To treat severe elevations of blood pressure. It is always used in combination with other blood pressure lowering agents (eg, beta blockers, diuretics).

Unlabeled Use(s): Occasionally doctors may prescribe topical minoxidil to treat male pattern baldness. See the Miscellaneous-Minoxidil monograph in the Topical Products chapter.

Precautions:

Do not use in the following situations:

allergy to any component of this medicine
aortic aneurysm, dissecting
heart attack, acute
pheochromocytoma (tumor of the adrenal gland)

Use with caution in the following situations:

angina
circulation, compromised
cryoglobulinemia
guanethidine use (*Ismelin*)
heart attack, recent
hypertension, severe
kidney dialysis
kidney failure

Doctor supervision: Minoxidil may produce serious side effects. Use of this drug must be closely supervised by your doctor. Minoxidil is given with other blood pressure medications. Take all medications exactly as prescribed. Notify your doctor if any of the following occur: Increased heart rate; rapid weight gain (over 5 pounds); unusual swelling of face, hands, ankles or abdomen; breathing difficulty; chest pain; severe indigestion; dizziness; lightheadedness or fainting.

Fluid and electrolyte balance and body weight must be monitored. Diuretics alone, or with restricted salt intake, usually minimize fluid retention. Fluid retention rarely may require discontinuation of minoxidil. Under close medical supervision, it may be possible to discontinue the drug for 1 or 2 days and then resume treatment in conjunction with diuretic therapy.

Increased hair growth: 80% of patients who are taking this medicine develop elongation, thickening and enhanced pigmentation of fine body hair within 3 to 6 weeks after starting therapy. It is usually first noticed on the temples, between the eyebrows, between the hairline and eyebrows or in the sideburn area of the upper cheek, later extending to the back, arms, legs and scalp. Upon discontinuation of the drug, new hair growth stops, but 1 to 6 months may be required for restoration to pretreatment appearance. Unwanted hair can be controlled by a hair remover or by shaving. For further information on minoxidil as a treatment for male pattern baldness, see the Miscellaneous-Minoxidil monograph in the Topicals chapter.

Lab tests: Your doctor may require lab tests at 1 to 3 month intervals in the beginning of minoxidil therapy, and at 6 to 12 month intervals later. Some of the tests that may be required include: Urine tests, kidney function tests, echocardiograms, electrocardiograms and chest x-rays.

Pregnancy: Adequate studies have not been done in pregnant women, or animal studies may have shown a risk to the fetus. Use only if clearly needed and potential benefits outweigh the possible hazards to the fetus.

Breastfeeding: Minoxidil appears in breast milk. It should not be given to nursing women. Contact your doctor before beginning breastfeeding.

Children: Experience in children is limited. Doses must be adjusted very carefully. Consult your doctor.

Drug Interactions:

Tell your doctor or pharmacist if you are taking or planning to take any over-the-counter or prescription medications or dietary supplements while take this medicine. Doses of one or both drugs may need to be modified or a different drug may need to be prescribed. Guanethidine (eg, *Ismelin*) interacts with this medicine.

Side Effects:

Many patients experience side effects. The frequency and severity of side effects depend on many factors including dose, duration of therapy and individual susceptibility. Possible side effects include:

Digestive Tract: Nausea; vomiting; severe indigestion.

Circulatory System: Chest pain; rapid pulse.

Respiratory System: Shortness of breath; difficulty breathing.

Skin: Rash; increased hair growth and darkening of fine body hair.

Other: Weight gain or swelling of arms, legs, face or abdomen; dizziness.

Guidelines for Use:

- Use exactly as prescribed.
- Usual adult dose (patients over 12 years of age) is 10 to 40 mg as a single daily dose. Do not exceed 100 mg per day.
- Minoxidil is usually taken with at least two other antihypertensive drugs (a beta blocker and a diuretic). Take all medications as prescribed.
- If a dose is missed, take it as soon as possible. If several hours have passed or it is nearing time for the next dose, do not double the dose to catch up, unless advised to do so by your doctor. If more than one dose is missed or it is necessary to establish a new dosage schedule, contact your doctor or pharmacist.
- A low salt diet should be closely followed.
- Take this medication daily as directed, have your blood pressure checked regularly and keep your appointments with your doctor even if you feel well. Most patients with high blood pressure do not feel sick.
- Do not stop taking this medicine suddenly. If your doctor discontinues this drug, the dose must be gradually reduced in order to avoid a rapid increase in blood pressure, nervousness, agitation or headache.
- Patients being treated for high blood pressure often feel tired or run-down for a few weeks after beginning therapy. Continue taking your medication even though you may not feel quite "normal." Contact your doctor or pharmacist about any new symptoms.
- This medicine may cause dizziness or drowsiness. Use caution while driving or performing other tasks requiring alertness, coordination or physical dexterity.
- Notify your doctor if any of the following occurs: Increased heart rate; rapid weight gain of more than 5 pounds; unusual swelling of hands, feet, face or abdomen; breathing difficulty, especially when lying down; new or aggravated angina symptoms (chest, arm or shoulder pain); severe indigestion; dizziness; lightheadedness or fainting.
- Enhanced growth and darkening of fine body hair occurs in most patients. This may become bothersome. However, do not discontinue medication without consulting your doctor. Unwanted hair can be controlled by a hair remover or by shaving.
- Lab tests may be required to monitor treatment. Be sure to keep appointments.
- Store at controlled room temperature (59° to 86°F).

If you have any questions, consult your doctor, pharmacist, or health care provider.

	Generic Name	Supplied As	Generic Available
Rx	**Reserpine**	**Tablets:** 0.1 mg, 0.25 mg	Yes

Type of Drug:

Antihypertensive; drug used to lower high blood pressure.

How the Drug Works:

Reserpine (a rauwolfia alkaloid) lowers blood pressure by altering nerve function and decreasing the heart rate. It also has sedative and tranquilizing properties.

Uses:

To treat mild high blood pressure. May be used with other blood pressure lowering drugs to treat serious high blood pressure.

To relieve symptoms in agitated mental states (eg, schizophrenia).

Precautions:

Do not use in the following situations:

- allergy to rauwolfia derivatives
- depression, history of
- electroshock therapy
- peptic ulcer, active
- ulcerative colitis

Use with caution in the following situations:

- anesthetics, surgical
- gallstones
- kidney disease
- peptic ulcer, history
- ulcerative colitis, history

Depression: Reserpine may cause mental depression. Contact your doctor at the first sign of extreme sadness, early morning sleeplessness, loss of appetite, impotence, or low self-esteem.

Pregnancy: Adequate studies have not been done in pregnant women, or animal studies may have shown a potential hazard to the fetus. Use only if clearly needed and potential benefits outweigh the possible hazards to the fetus.

Breastfeeding: Reserpine appears in breast milk. Consult your doctor before you begin breastfeeding.

Children: Safety and effectiveness have not been established.

Lab tests may be required to monitor therapy. Be sure to keep appointments.

Drug Interactions:

Tell your doctor or pharmacist if you are taking or planning to take any over-the-counter or prescription medications or dietary supplements while taking this medicine. Doses of one or both drugs may need to be modified or a different drug may need to be prescribed. The following drugs and drug classes interact with this medicine:

amphetamines
anesthesia, general
digoxin (eg, *Lanoxin*)
isoproterenol (eg, *Isuprel*)
MAO inhibitor antidepressant use (eg, phenelzine)
quinidine (eg, *Quinidex*)
sympathomimetics (eg, ephedrine)
tricyclic antidepressants (eg, amitriptyline)

Side Effects:

Every drug is capable of producing side effects. Many patients experience no, or minor, side effects. The frequency and severity of side effects depend on many factors including dose, duration of therapy, and individual susceptibility. Possible side effects include:

Digestive Tract: Nausea; vomiting; diarrhea; loss of appetite; increased stomach acid; dry mouth; black/bloody stools.

Nervous System: Depression; dizziness; headache; nervousness; anxiety; nightmares; drowsiness; tremors; involuntary movements.

Circulatory System: Irregular pulse; chest pain (angina); slow pulse; edema (swelling of the lower legs).

Respiratory System: Shortness of breath; difficult or painful breathing; congestion.

Skin: Rash; itching.

Other: Dulling of the senses; deafness; breast secretions; breast swelling in men; changes in sex drive; muscle aches; weight gain; glaucoma, inflammation and redness of eyes, blurred vision and other eye problems; difficulty urinating; fainting; nosebleeds.

Guidelines for Use:

- Use exactly as prescribed.
- May cause stomach upset. Take with food or milk.
- Do not take this medication for any disorder other than for which it was prescribed.
- If a dose is missed, take it as soon as possible. If several hours have passed or it is nearing time for the next dose, do not double the dose to catch up, unless advised by your doctor. If more than one dose is missed or it is necessary to establish a new dosage schedule, contact your doctor or pharmacist.
- Do not discontinue medication without consulting your doctor.
- Patients being treated for high blood pressure often feel tired and run down for a few weeks after beginning therapy. It takes time for the body to adjust to lowered blood pressure. Continue taking your medication even though you may not feel quite "normal." Check with your doctor or pharmacist during this time regarding any new symptoms that occur to assure that these new feelings are a normal consequence of changes in blood pressure.
- This medicine may cause drowsiness, dizziness or blurred vision. Use caution when driving or performing other tasks requiring alertness, coordination or physical dexterity.
- Notify your doctor of continued or severe stomach pain, mental depression, early-morning insomnia, loss of appetite, impotence, nausea, vomiting, chest pain, nervousness, dizziness, breast enlargement or changes in mood or sleep habits.
- Avoid tyramine-containing foods (eg, yogurt, cheddar cheese, raisins).
- Check with your doctor before using a nonprescription cold, flu or weight loss medication.
- Store at room temperature (59° to 86° F). Protect from heat and light.

If you have any questions, consult your doctor, pharmacist, or health care provider.

	Generic Name *Brand Name Examples*	Diuretic	Other
Rx	**Thiazide Diuretics and Reserpine Derivatives**		
	Renese-R Tablets	2 mg polythiazide	0.25 mg reserpine
	Regroton Tablets	50 mg chlorthali-done	0.25 mg reserpine
	Hydropres-50 Tablets, Hydro-Serp Tablets, Hydroserpine #2 Tablets	50 mg hydrochlorothiazide	0.125 mg reserpine
	Hydroserpine #1 Tablets	25 mg hydrochlorothiazide	0.125 mg reserpine
	Salutensin Tablets	50 mg hydro-flumethiazide	0.125 mg reserpine
	Demi-Regroton Tablets	25 mg chlorthali-done	0.125 mg reserpine
	Diutensen-R Tablets	2.5 mg methyclo-thiazide	0.1 mg reserpine
	Metatensin #4 Tablets	4 mg trichlor-methiazide	0.1 mg reserpine
	Metatensin #2 Tablets[1]	2 mg trichlor-methiazide	0.1 mg reserpine
	Rauzide Tablets	4 mg bendroflumethiazide	50 mg powdered rauwolfia serpentina
	Enduronyl Forte Tablets	5 mg methyclo-thiazide	0.5 mg deserpidine
	Enduronyl Tablets	5 mg methyclo-thiazide	0.25 mg deserpidine
Rx	**Thiazide Diuretic, Reserpine and Hydralazine**		
	Hydrap-ES Tablets, Marpres Tablets, Ser-Ap-Es Tablets, Tri-Hydroserpine Tablets	15 mg hydrochlorothiazide	0.1 mg reserpine, 25 mg hydralazine
Rx	**Thiazide Diuretic and Hydralazine**		
	Apresazide 100/50 Capsules	50 mg hydrochlorothiazide	100 mg hydralazine
	Apresazide 50/50 Capsules	50 mg hydrochlorothiazide	50 mg hydralazine
	Apresazide 25/25 Capsules	25 mg hydrochlorothiazide	25 mg hydralazine
Rx	**Thiazide Diuretic and Beta-Blockers**		
	Tenoretic 100 Tablets	25 mg chlorthali-done	100 mg atenolol
	Tenoretic 50 Tablets	25 mg chlorthali-done	50 mg atenolol
	Corzide Tablets 80/5	5 mg bendroflumethiazide	80 mg nadolol

	Generic Name *Brand Name Examples*	Diuretic	Other
	Corzide Tablets 40/5	5 mg bendroflumethiazide	40 mg nadolol
	Timolide 10-25 Tablets	25 mg hydrochloro-thiazide	10 mg timolol maleate
	Inderide LA 160/50 Capsules	50 mg hydrochlorothiazide	160 mg propranolol HCl
	Inderide LA 120/50 Capsules	50 mg hydrochlorothiazide	120 mg propranolol HCl
	Inderide LA 80/50 Capsules	50 mg hydrochlorothiazide	80 mg propranolol HCl
	Inderide 80/25 Capsules	25 mg hydrochlorothiazide	80 mg propranolol HCl
	Inderide 40/25 Capsules	25 mg hydrochlorothiazide	40 mg propranolol HCl
	Lopressor HCT 100/50 Tablets	50 mg hydrochlorothiazide	100 mg metoprolol tartrate
	Lopressor HCT 100/25 Tablets	25 mg hydrochlorothiazide	100 mg metoprolol tartrate
	Lopressor HCT 50/25 Tablets	25 mg hydrochlorothiazide	50 mg metoprolol tartrate
	Ziac Tablets	6.25 mg hydrochlorothiazide 6.25 mg hydrochlorothiazide 6.25 mg hydrochlorothiazide	2.5 mg bisoprolol fumarate 5 mg bisoprolol fumarate 10 mg bisoprolol fumarate
Rx	**Thiazide Diuretics and Methyldopa**		
	Aldoril D50 Tablets	50 mg hydrochlorothiazide	500 mg methyldopa
	Aldoril D30 Tablets	30 mg hydrochlorothiazide	500 mg methyldopa
	Aldoril-25 Tablets	25 mg hydrochloro-thiazide	250 mg methyldopa
	Aldoril-15 Tablets	15 mg hydrochloro-thiazide	250 mg methyldopa
	Aldoclor-250 Tablets	250 mg chloro-thiazide	250 mg methyldopa
	Aldoclor-150 Tablets	150 mg chloro-thiazide	250 mg methyldopa
Rx	**Thiazide Diuretic and ACEIs**		
	Lotensin HCT Tablets 20/25	25 mg hydrochlorothiazide	20 mg benazepril
	Lotensin HCT Tablets 20/12.5	12.5 mg hydrochlorothiazide	20 mg benazepril

	Generic Name *Brand Name Examples*	Diuretic	Other
	Lotensin HCT Tablets 10/12.5	12.5 mg hydrochlorothiazide	10 mg benazepril
	Lotensin HCT Tablets 5/6.25	6.25 mg hydrochlorothiazide	5 mg benazepril
	Capozide 50/25	25 mg hydrochlorothiazide	50 mg captopril
	Capozide 25/25	25 mg hydrochlorothiazide	25 mg captopril
	Capozide 50/15	15 mg hydrochlorothiazide	50 mg captopril
	Capozide 25/15	15 mg hydrochlorothiazide	25 mg captopril
	Vaseretic 10-25 Tablets	25 mg hydrochlorothiazide	10 mg enalapril maleate
	Prinzide 12.5 Tablets, Zestoretic Tablets	12.5 mg hydrochlorothiazide	20 mg lisinopril
	Prinzide 25 Tablets, Zestoretic Tablets	25 mg hydrochlorothiazide	20 mg lisinopril
Rx	**Thiazide Diuretic and Clonidine**		
	Combipres 0.3 Tablets	15 mg chlorthalidone	0.3 mg clonidine HCl
	Combipres 0.2 Tablets	15 mg chlorthalidone	0.2 mg clonidine HCl
	Combipres 0.1 Tablets	15 mg chlorthalidone	0.1 mg clonidine HCl
Rx	**Thiazide Diuretic and Prazosin**		
	Minizide 5 Capsules	0.5 mg polythiazide	5 mg prazosin
	Minizide 2 Capsules	0.5 mg polythiazide	2 mg prazosin
	Minizide 1 Capsules	0.5 mg polythiazide	1 mg prazosin
Rx	**Thiazide Diuretics and Miscellaneous Antihypertensives**		
	Esimil Tablets	25 mg hydrochlorothiazide	10 mg guanethidine monosulfate
	Hyzaar Tablets	12.5 mg hydrochlorothiazide	50 mg losartan potassium, 4.24 mg potassium
Rx	**Miscellaneous Antihypertensives**		
	Lotrel Capsules	†	2.5 mg amlodipine, 10 mg benazepril
	Lotrel Capsules	†	5 mg amlodipine, 10 mg benazepril
	Lotrel Capsules	†	5 mg amlodipine, 20 mg benazepril

[1] Contains the dye tartrazine.
† Products do not contain a diuretic.

For more information on the ingredients in these combinations, see the individual drug monographs in this chapter.

Type of Drug:

Antihypertensive; drugs used to lower high blood pressure.

Uses:

To treat high blood pressure. Used with other drugs when adequate control is not achieved by a single drug.

Guidelines for Use:

- Use exactly as prescribed.
- May cause stomach upset. May be taken with food or milk.
- Take as directed by your doctor. The daily dose varies depending on individual needs. Do not adjust the dose without consulting your pharmacist or doctor.
- May increase urination. Therefore, take early in the day.
- If a dose is missed, take it as soon as possible. If several hours have passed or it is nearing time for the next dose, do not double the dose to catch up, unless advised to do so by your doctor. If more than one dose is missed or it is necessary to establish a new dosage schedule, contact your doctor or pharmacist.
- Do not interrupt or stop medication without consulting your doctor.
- Do not use salt substitutes without consulting your doctor or pharmacist.
- May cause a persistent dry cough. Tell your doctor or pharmacist. Recovery is rapid when the medicine is stopped.
- Dizziness, fainting or lightheadedness is most likely to occur after the first dose or in the first days of therapy. Avoid sudden changes in posture. If dizziness persists, contact your doctor.
- Do not take other medications without your doctor's approval. This includes nonprescription medicines for appetite control, asthma, colds, cough, hay fever or sinus.
- May cause sensitivity to sunlight. Avoid prolonged exposure to the sun. Use sunscreens and wear protective clothing until tolerance is determined.
- May increase blood sugar levels in diabetics.
- Contact your doctor if significant, sudden joint pain occurs.
- Lab tests may be required. Be sure to keep appointments.
- Inform your doctor if you are pregnant, become pregnant, are planning to become pregnant or if you are breastfeeding.
- Store at room temperature in a tightly sealed container away from light.

If you have any questions, consult your doctor, pharmacist, or health care provider.

	Product	Contents
otc	**Adolph's Salt Substitute**	Potassium chloride, silicon dioxide and tartaric acid. Also available seasoned with sugar, paprika, garlic and onion powder, cottonseed and soybean oil.
otc	**Morton Salt Substitute**	Potassium chloride, fumaric acid, tricalcium phosphate and monocalcium phosphate. Also available seasoned with spices and sugar.
otc	**NoSalt**	Potassium chloride, potassium bitartrate, adipic acid, mineral oil and fumaric acid. Also available seasoned with dextrose, onion, garlic, spices, lactose, cream of tartar, paprika, silica, disodium inosinate, disodium guanylate, turmeric and paprika.
otc	**Nu-Salt**	Potassium chloride, potassium bitartrate, calcium silicate, natural flavor derived from yeast.

Uses:

Food seasoning to be used as a substitute for salt or sodium chloride (NaCl) at the table or in cooking to help regulate dietary sodium intake. Appropriate for persons on low sodium diets (ie, persons whose sodium intake has been restricted for medical reasons).

Persons with diabetes, heart (taking diuretics) or kidney disease, or receiving medical treatment should consult a doctor before using a salt substitute.

Precautions:

Do not use in the following situations:

high potassium level
kidney disease, severe

Use with caution in the following situations:

diabetes
heart disease
kidney disease

Drug Interactions:

Tell your doctor or pharmacist if you are taking or if you are planning to take any over-the-counter or prescription medications or dietary supplements with this medicine. Doses may need to be modified or a different drug may need to be prescribed. The following drugs and drug classes interact this medicine:

ACE inhibitors (eg, *Vasotec)*
amiloride *(Midamor)*
potassium supplements (eg, *K-Dur)*
spironolactone *(Aldactone)*
triamterene *(Dyrenium)*

Side Effects:

Every drug is capable of producing side effects. Many patients experience no side effects. However, excessive sodium depletion may lead to weakness, nausea and muscle weakness/cramps, vomiting, diarrhea, or stomach upset.

If you have any questions, consult your doctor, pharmacist, or health care provider.

	Generic Name / *Brand Name Examples*	Supplied As	Generic Available
Rx	**Cholestyramine**		
	LoCHOLEST	**Powder:** 4 g cholestyramine resin/9 g powder	No
	Questran	**Powder:** 4 g cholestyramine resin/9 g powder	Yes
	Questran Light	**Powder:** 4 g cholestyramine resin/6.4 g powder	Yes
	LoCHOLEST Light[1]	**Powder:** 4 g cholestyramine resin/5.7 g powder	No
	Prevalite	**Powder:** 4 g cholestyramine resin/5.5 g powder	No
Rx	**Colesevelam HCl**		
	Welchol	**Tablets:** 625 mg	No
Rx	**Colestipol HCl**		
	Colestid	**Tablets:** 1 g colestipol HCl	No
	Colestid	**Granules:** 5 g packets, 300 g bottle, 500 g bottle	No
	Flavored Colestid[1]	**Granules:** 7.5 g packets, 450 g bottle	No

[1] Contains phenylalanine.

Type of Drug:

Drugs used as adjunctive therapy to diet and exercise to lower the level of LDL cholesterol and total cholesterol in the blood.

How the Drug Works:

Bile acid sequestrants increase the removal of bile acids from the body. As the body loses bile acids, it replaces them by converting cholesterol from the blood to bile acids. This causes the blood level of cholesterol to decrease.

High blood levels of cholesterol may increase the risk of developing heart, coronary artery, or other vascular disease.

Uses:

To lower high levels of cholesterol in the blood alone or in conjunction with proper diet, exercise, and possibly other lipid-lowering drugs.

Cholestyramine: To relieve itching associated with partial biliary obstruction.

Unlabeled Use(s): Occasionally doctors may prescribe cholestyramine to bind the toxins produced by *Clostridium difficile,* the organism which causes antibiotic-induced pseudomembranous colitis. Cholestyramine has also been used for treatment of chlordecone *(Kepone)* pesticide poisoning, bile salt-mediated and postvagotomy diarrhea, and thyroid hormone overdose. Cholestyramine and colestipol have both been used to treat digitalis toxicity.

Precautions:

Do not use in the following situations:

allergy to a bile acid sequestrant or any of its ingredients
bowel obstruction
complete biliary obstruction
gallstones or other obstructive gallbladder diseases
phenylketonuria (*Questran Light* only)

Use with caution in the following situations:

constipation
dysphagia
gastrointestinal motility disorder (*Questran Light* only)
gastrointestinal surgery, recent
swallowing disorder

Before treatment: Before treatment with a bile acid sequestrant, a vigorous attempt should be made to control cholesterol with appropriate diet, exercise, and weight reduction (in obese people).

Diseases that may increase cholesterol and must be treated before beginning treatment with bile acid sequestrants include:

diabetes mellitus
hypothyroidism
nephrotic syndrome (kidney)
obstructive liver disease
protein in the blood

Phenylketonuria: Some of these products contain phenylalanine. Consult your doctor or pharmacist.

Supplementation: Treatment with bile acid sequestrants may require supplementation with vitamins A , E, and D, oral vitamin K, or folic acid.

Pregnancy: Safety for use during pregnancy has not been established. These agents are not absorbed systemically, and are not expected to cause fetal harm when administered during pregnancy in recommended doses. Use only when clearly needed the potential benefits to the mother outweigh the possible hazards to the fetus.

Breastfeeding: Use caution when breastfeeding. The possible lack of proper vitamin absorption may have an effect on nursing infants. Consult your doctor.

Children: Dosage schedules have not been established. The effects of long-term use and effectiveness in maintaining lowered cholesterol levels are unknown.

Lab tests will be required periodically during treatment with bile acid sequestrants. Tests may include blood counts, triglycerides, and cholesterol levels.

Drug Interactions:

Tell your doctor or pharmacist if you are taking or planning to take any over-the-counter or prescription medications or dietary supplements while taking bile acid sequestrants. Doses of one or both drugs may need to be modified or a different drug may need to be prescribed. The following drugs and drug classes interact with bile acid sequestrants:

diclofenac (eg, *Cataflam*)
dicumarol
digoxin (eg, *Lanoxin*)
divalproex sodium (eg, *Depakote*)
furosemide (eg, *Lasix*)
hydrocortisone (eg, *Cortef*)
piroxicam (eg, *Feldene*)
sulindac (eg, *Clinoril*)
thiazide diuretics (eg, hydrochlorothiazide)
thyroid hormones (eg, levothyroxine sodium)
valproic acid (eg, *Depakene*)
warfarin (eg, *Coumadin*)

Side Effects:

Every drug is capable of producing side effects. Many bile acid sequestrant users experience no, or minor, side effects. The frequency and severity of side effects depend on many factors including dose, duration of therapy, and individual susceptibility. Possible side effects include:

Digestive Tract: Severe constipation or other persistent stomach problems; gastrointestinal bleeding or irritation; fatty or black stools; loose stools; occasional stomach pain or gas; indigestion; ulcer attack; bloating; belching; nausea; vomiting; heartburn; aggravated hemorrhoids; appetite loss; difficulty swallowing; diarrhea.

Nervous System: Headache; leg pain; anxiety; vertigo; dizziness; fatigue; insomnia; drowsiness; fainting.

Respiratory System: Asthma; wheezing; shortness of breath.

Skin: Rash; itching; hives; abnormal skin sensations.

Other: Unusual bruising or bleeding (eg, gums, rectum); hiccups; sour taste; weight loss or gain; difficulty swallowing; muscle pain; anemia, backache; chest pain; arthritis; ringing in the ears; blood in urine; painful urination; increased urination; burnt urine odor; fluid retention; tingling or numbness in legs and arms; swelling of hands or feet; inflammation of the uveal tract; inflammation of the pancreas or gall bladder; gall stones; increased libido; deficiencies of fat-soluble vitamins (eg, A and D).

Guidelines for Use:

- Dosage is individualized. Take exactly as prescribed.
- Do not stop taking or change the dose unless advised by your doctor.
- *Granules or powder* — Mix with liquid (water or noncarbonated drinks), very liquid soups or cereals, or with pulpy fruits (applesauce or crushed pineapple). Do not take the dry powder or granules.
- *Tablets* — Take with food and liquids.
- *Cholestyramine tablets* — May be taken with meals. Swallowing tablets is easier if you drink plenty of fluid as you swallow each tablet.
- *Cholestyramine powder* — Mix the contents of one powder packet or one level scoopful with 2 to 6 fl oz water or noncarbonated beverage. Avoid accidental inhalation. Do not take dry.
- *Colestipol preparation* — Add the prescribed amount to a glassful (3 oz or more) of liquid. Stir until completely mixed. Colestipol will not dissolve. May also mix with carbonated beverages, slowly stirred in a large glass. Rinse glass with a small amount of additional beverage to ensure that all the medication is taken.
- If a dose is missed, take it as soon as possible. If several hours have passed or if it is nearing time for the next dose, do not double the dose to catch up, unless advised by your doctor. If more than one dose is missed or it is necessary to establish a new dosage schedule, contact your doctor or pharmacist.
- May interfere with the effects of other drugs taken at the same time. Take other drugs either 1 hour before or 4 to 6 hours after bile acid sequestrants.
- Contact your doctor if you experience unusual bleeding (eg, gums, rectum).
- May cause constipation, gas, nausea, or heartburn. These effects usually disappear with continued use, but contact your doctor if these effects continue and are bothersome.
- Most effective when used with a diet which decreases the intake of cholesterol and saturated fats.
- Lab tests may be required to monitor therapy. Be sure to keep appointments.
- Store at room temperature (59° to 86°F) in a dry place.

If you have any questions, consult your doctor, pharmacist, or health care provider.

	Generic Name *Brand Name Example*	Supplied As	Generic Available
Rx	**Clofibrate**		
	Atromid-S	**Capsules:** 500 mg	Yes

Type of Drug:

Drug used to lower high levels of cholesterol and triglycerides (fat-like substances) in the blood.

How the Drug Works:

Clofibrate increases the rate of removal of cholesterol and triglycerides from the blood. High levels of cholesterol and triglycerides may block blood vessels, increasing the risk of heart or blood vessel disease.

Uses:

To lower high levels of triglycerides and cholesterol. Used alone or in conjunction with other drugs and proper diet.

Precautions:

Do not use in the following situations:

- allergy to clofibrate or any of its ingredients
- breastfeeding
- gallbladder disease or gallstones
- kidney disease
- liver disease
- pregnancy

Use with caution in the following situations:

- heart disease
- peptic ulcer

Before treatment: Before treatment with clofibrate, an attempt should be made to control high cholesterol and triglycerides with appropriate diet, exercise, and weight reduction (in obese people).

Pregnancy: Clofibrate should not be used during pregnancy. Contact your doctor if you become pregnant or plan to become pregnant while taking clofibrate.

Breastfeeding: Do not breastfeed if clofibrate therapy is necessary. Consult your doctor.

Children: Safety and effectiveness have not been established. Use is not recommended.

Lab tests will be required periodically during treatment with clofibrate. Tests may include blood counts, cholesterol, triglycerides, and liver function tests.

Drug Interactions:

Tell your doctor or pharmacist if you are taking or planning to take any over-the-counter or prescription medications or dietary supplements with clofibrate. Doses of one or both drugs may need to be modified or a different drug may need to be prescribed. The following drugs and drug classes interact with clofibrate:

- anisindione (*Miradon*)
- dicumarol
- insulin
- sulfonylureas (eg, *Glipizide*)
- warfarin (eg, *Coumadin*)

Side Effects:

Every drug is capable of producing side effects. Many clofibrate users experience no, or minor, side effects. The frequency and severity of side effects depend on many factors including dose, duration of therapy, and individual susceptibility. Possible side effects include:

Digestive Tract: Nausea; vomiting; diarrhea; loose stools; indigestion; gas; bloating; stomach pain; upset stomach or heartburn; increased appetite.

Nervous System: Fatigue; weakness; drowsiness; dizziness; headache.

Circulatory System: Chest pain; irregular heart rate.

Skin: Rash; itching; dry skin; hair loss; dry, brittle hair; hives; redness.

Other: Weight gain; decreased urination; painful urination; blood in urine; decreased sexual function; flu-like symptoms (eg, muscle aches, soreness, weakness or cramps); joint pain; skin lesions; gallstones; mouth sores; unusual blood counts (eg, anemia); increased liver function tests; decreased kidney function.

Guidelines for Use:

- Usual dosage is 2 g (4 capsules) daily in divided doses.
- If upset stomach occurs, take with food.
- This medicine does not reduce the importance of adhering to a diet that will lower intake of cholesterol and saturated fats.
- If a dose is missed, take it as soon as possible. If several hours have passed or it nearing time for the next dose, do not double the dose to catch up, unless advised to do so by your doctor. If more than one dose is missed, or if it is necessary to establish a new dosage schedule, contact your doctor or pharmacist. Use exactly as prescribed.
- Strict birth control procedures must be exercised by women of child-bearing potential. This medicine should be withdrawn several months prior to conception. However, talk to your doctor prior to changing your dosing regimen.
- Avoid alcohol while taking this medicine.
- Dosage adjustment may be required for oral anticoagulants (eg, warfarin sodium) when given with clofibrate.
- Do not take this medicine with HMG-CoA reductase inhibitors (eg, lovastatin).
- May cause photosensitivity (sensitivity to sunlight). Avoid prolonged exposure to the sun or other forms of ultraviolet (UV) light (eg, tanning beds). Use sunscreens and wear protective clothing until tolerance is determined.
- Notify your doctor if any of the following occurs: Chest pain; shortness of breath; irregular heartbeat; severe stomach pain with nausea and vomiting; fever and chills or sore throat; blood in the urine; unusually low urine output; swelling of feet or ankles; weight gain; muscle tenderness or weakness.
- Lab tests may be required. Be sure to keep appointments.
- Store at room temperature in a tightly closed container. Protect from light, freezing, and excessive heat.

If you have any questions, consult your doctor, pharmacist, or health care provider.

	Generic Name *Brand Name Example*	Supplied As	Generic Available
Rx	**Fenofibrate**		
	Tricor	**Capsules:** 67 mg	No

Type of Drug:

Triglyceride (fat-like substances) lowering agent. Fenofibrate does not affect cholesterol levels significantly.

How the Drug Works:

Fenofibrate decreases triglyceride blood levels by reducing triglyceride production by the liver and increasing its breakdown.

Uses:

Used in addition to diet to lower high triglyceride levels (Types IV and V hyperlipidemia) in patients at risk of pancreatitis who are not responding adequately to diet alone. Fenofibrate does not replace the need for diet and exercise.

Precautions:

Do not use in the following situations:

allergy to fenofibrate
breastfeeding
cirrhosis of the liver
gallbladder disease, preexisting
liver disease
liver function abnormalities
kidney disease, severe

Use with caution in the following situations:

anticoagulant (eg, warfarin) therapy
HMG-CoA reductase inhibitor (eg, atorvastatin, cerivastatin, fluvastatin, lovastatin, pravastatin, simvastatin) therapy
medicines which increase triglyceride levels (eg, beta blockers, thiazides, estrogens)

Pregnancy: Adequate studies have not been done in pregnant women. Use only if clearly needed and potential benefits outweigh the possible hazards to the fetus.

Breastfeeding: Fenofibrate should not be used in nursing mothers. A decision should be made whether to discontinue nursing or discontinue use of fenofibrate. Consult your doctor before you begin breastfeeding.

Children: Safety and efficacy in children have not been established.

Lab tests will be required to monitor therapy. Be sure to keep appointments. Tests may include: Kidney and liver function tests, blood counts, and triglyceride and cholesterol levels.

Drug Interactions:

Tell your doctor or pharmacist if you are taking or planning to take any over-the-counter or prescription medications or dietary supplements while taking fenofibrate. Doses of one or both drugs may need to be modified or a different drug may need to be prescribed. The following drugs and drug classes may interact with fenofibrate:

anticoagulants, oral (eg, warfarin)
bile acid binding resins (eg, cholestyramine)
HMG-CoA reductase inhibitors (eg, lovastatin)
immunosuppressants (eg, azathioprine)
nephrotoxic agents (eg, cyclosporine)

Side Effects:

Every drug is capable of producing side effects. Many fenofibrate users experience no, or minor, side effects. The frequency and severity of side effects depend on many factors including dose, duration of therapy, and individual susceptibility. Possible side effects include:

Digestive Tract: Belching; gas; nausea; vomiting; constipation.

Nervous System: Dizziness; fatigue; headache.

Skin: Itching; rash.

Other: Muscle aches, tenderness, or weakness with or without fever or malaise (general feeling of discomfort); infections; flu-like symptoms; pain; joint pain; eye floaters; eye irritation; decreased sex drive; runny nose.

Guidelines for Use:

- Usual daily dose is 67 mg (1 capsule) per day. Dosage will be individualized. This medicine may be increased by your doctor up to 201 mg (3 capsules) per day.
- Take with meals to increase effectiveness.
- Continue the diet regimen prescribed by your doctor while taking fenofibrate.
- If a dose is missed, take it as soon as possible. If several hours have passed or it is nearing time for the next dose, do not double the dose to catch up, unless advised to do so by your doctor. If more than one dose is missed, contact your doctor or pharmacist.
- Fenofibrate is not a replacement for diet and exercise. Every effort should be made to control triglyceride levels with diet, exercise, weight loss (if appropriate), and control of any medical problems such as diabetes mellitus or hypothyroidism.
- Notify your doctor immediately if you experience muscle pain, tenderness, or weakness, especially if accompanied by fever or general body discomfort. This could be a sign of a serious medical condition.
- Notify your doctor if you develop abdominal pain, which may vary from mild to very severe and may be felt in back, chest, or sides. This could be a sign of a serious medical condition.
- Discontinue use at first appearance of rash or other signs of an allergic reaction (eg, difficulty breathing).
- Take fenofibrate at least 1 hour before or 4 to 6 hours after taking a bile acid binding resin (eg, cholestyramine).
- If fenofibrate is not effective after 2 months of treatment, your doctor may discontinue therapy with fenofibrate.
- Do not take fenofibrate while breastfeeding.
- Lab tests will be required. Be sure to keep appointments.
- Store at room temperature. Protect from moisture.

If you have any questions, consult your doctor, pharmacist, or health care provider.

	Generic Name *Brand Name Example*	Supplied As	Generic Available
Rx	**Gemfibrozil**		
	Lopid	**Tablets:** 600 mg	Yes

Type of Drug:

Drug that lowers elevated blood levels of triglycerides (fat-like substances), raises HDL (good) cholesterol, and has variable effects on LDL (bad) cholesterol.

How the Drug Works:

Gemfibrozil decreases the blood level of triglycerides and some types of cholesterol (LDL) by reducing the production of these items by the liver. It also increases blood levels of HDL cholesterol. High levels of LDL cholesterol and triglycerides may block blood vessels, increasing the risk of heart or blood vessel disease (arteriosclerosis).

Uses:

As an adjunct to diet to lower elevated triglyceride levels (Types IV and V hyperlipidemia) in adult patients at risk for pancreatitis and who are unable to control triglyceride levels by diet and exercise alone.

To reduce risk of developing coronary artery disease in adult patients with low HDL cholesterol levels and elevated LDL cholesterol and triglycerides (Type IIb hyperlipidemia) and who have not responded to weight loss, diet, exercise, and other lipid-lowering drugs.

Precautions:

Do not use in the following situations:

- allergy to gemfibrozil
- cirrhosis
- gallbladder disease
- kidney disease
- liver disease

Use with caution in the following situations:

- alcohol use, chronic or excessive
- anticoagulants, oral (eg, warfarin)
- diabetes
- estrogen therapy
- HMG-CoA reductase inhibitors (eg, lovastatin)
- hypothyroidism (underactive thyroid)

Before treatment with gemfibrozil, an attempt should be made to control high LDL cholesterol and triglycerides with appropriate diet, exercise, and weight reduction (in obese people), and to control any medical problems such as diabetes mellitus or hypothyroidism that are contributing to the lipid abnormalities.

Pregnancy: Adequate studies have not been done in pregnant women. Use only if clearly needed and potential benefits outweigh the possible hazards to the fetus.

Breastfeeding: It is not known if gemfibrozil appears in breast milk. Consult your doctor before you begin breastfeeding.

Children: Safety and efficacy in children have not been established.

Lab tests may be required during treatment with gemfibrozil. Tests may include: Blood counts, cholesterol and triglycerides, liver and kidney function tests. Be sure to keep appointments.

Drug Interactions:

Tell your doctor or pharmacist if you are taking or planning to take any over-the-counter or prescription medications or dietary supplements with gemfibrozil. Doses of one or both drugs may need to be modified or a different drug may need to be prescribed. The following drugs and drug classes interact with gemfibrozil:

anticoagulants (eg, warfarin)
HMG-CoA reductase inhibitors (eg, lovastatin)

Side Effects:

Every drug is capable of producing side effects. Many gemfibrozil users experience no, or minor, side effects. The frequency and severity of side effects depend on many factors including dose, duration of therapy, and individual susceptibility. Possible side effects include:

Digestive Tract: Indigestion; stomach pain; vomiting; nausea; diarrhea; constipation; acute appendicitis.

Nervous System: Headache; dizziness; vertigo (feeling of whirling motion); fatigue.

Skin: Rash; itching; hives; inflamed or irritated skin; abnormal skin sensations (eg, burning, prickling, tingling); abnormal sensitivity to touch, pain, or other stimuli.

Other: Muscle pain or weakness; changes in taste perception; blurred vision.

Guidelines for Use:

- Dosage is individualized. Take exactly as prescribed.
- Do not change the dose or stop taking this medicine unless advised to do so by your doctor.
- Take this drug 30 minutes before the morning and evening meal.
- Most effective when used with a diet that reduces the intake of cholesterol and saturated fats, and an exercise program.
- If a dose is missed, take it as soon as possible. If several hours have passed or it nearing time for the next dose, do not double the dose to catch up, unless advised to do so by your doctor. If more than one dose is missed or it is necessary to establish a new dosage schedule contact your doctor or pharmacist.
- Avoid alcohol while taking this medicine.
- Inform your doctor if you are pregnant, become pregnant, plan on becoming pregnant, or are breastfeeding.
- May cause dizziness or blurred vision. Use caution when driving or performing other tasks requiring alertness, coordination, or physical dexterity.
- Notify your doctor immediately if you experience muscle pain, tenderness, or weakness.
- May cause stomach pain, diarrhea, nausea, or vomiting. Contact your doctor if these effects become particularly bothersome or severe.
- Lab tests may be required to monitor therapy. Be sure to keep appointments.
- Store below 86°F in a tightly sealed container.

If you have any questions, consult your doctor, pharmacist, or health care provider.

	Generic Name *Brand Name Examples*	Supplied As	Generic Available
Rx	**Atorvastatin Calcium**		
	Lipitor	**Tablets**: 10 mg, 20 mg, 40 mg, 80 mg	No
Rx	**Fluvastatin Sodium**		
	Lescol	**Capsules**: 20 mg, 40 mg	No
	Lescol XL	**Tablets, extended-release**: 80 mg	No
Rx	**Lovastatin**		
	Mevacor	**Tablets**: 10 mg, 20 mg, 40 mg	No
Rx	**Pravastatin Sodium**		
	Pravachol	**Tablets**: 10 mg, 20 mg, 40 mg	No
Rx	**Simvastatin**		
	Zocor	**Tablets**: 5 mg, 10 mg, 20 mg, 40 mg, 80 mg	No

Type of Drug:

Drugs used to lower high blood levels of certain types of lipids or fats (eg, LDL cholesterol, triglycerides) in the blood.

How the Drug Works:

HMG-CoA reductase inhibitors lower the blood levels of triglycerides and LDL ("bad") cholesterol by reducing their production by the liver. They also increase blood levels of HDL ("good") cholesterol.

Uses:

As an adjunct to diet for reducing elevated total and LDL cholesterol, apo-B, and triglyceride levels; and to increase HDL cholesterol in patients with primary hypercholesterolemia and mixed dyslipidemia (Fredrickson IIa and IIb).

Atorvastatin: As an adjunct to other lipid-lowering treatments to reduce total and LDL cholesterol in patients with homozygous familial hypercholesterolemia; to treat primary dysbetalipoproteinemia (Fredrickson type III); and to lower elevated serum triglyceride levels (Fredrickson type IV).

Fluvastatin: To slow the progression of coronary atherosclerosis in patients with coronary heart disease.

Lovastatin: To slow the progression of coronary atherosclerosis in patients with coronary heart disease; to reduce the risk of heart attack, unstable angina, or the chance of coronary revascularization procedures (eg, angioplasty) in patients without symptomatic cardiovascular disease, average to moderately elevated total and LDL cholesterol, and below average HDL cholesterol.

Pravastatin: To reduce the risk of myocardial infarction, stroke and stroke/transient ischemic attack, cardiovascular mortality, or the chance of coronary revascularization procedures (eg, angioplasty) in patients with clinically evident coronary heart disease; to slow the progression of coronary atheroclerosis; to treat primary dysbetalipoproteinemia (Fredrickson type III); to lower elevated serum triglyceride levels (Fredrickson type IV).

Simvastatin: To reduce the risk of heart attack, stroke or transient ischemic attack, cardiovascular mortality, or the chance of coronary revascularization procedures (eg, angioplasty) in patients with clinically evident coronary heart disease; as an adjunct to other lipid-lowering treatments to reduce total and LDL cholesterol; to lower elevated serum triglyceride levels (Fredrickson type IV); to treat primary dysbetalipoproteinemia (Fredrickson type III).

Unlabeled Use(s): Occasionally doctors may prescribe atorvastatin or fluvastatin to lower elevated total cholesterol levels in patients with heterozygous familial hypercholesterolemia and diabetic dyslipidemia in type 2 diabetic patients. Lovastatin may be useful to treat diabetic dyslipidemia, nephrotic hyperlipidemia, neck artery disease, familial dysbetalipoproteinemia, and familial combined hyperlipidemia. Pravastatin and Simvastatin can lower elevated cholesterol levels in patients with heterozygous familial hypercholesterolemia, familial combined hyperlipidemia, diabetic dyslipidemia in type 2 diabetic patients, hyperlipidemia secondary to the nephrotic syndrome, and homozygous familial hypercholesterolemia in patients with reduced LDL receptors.

Precautions:

Do not use in the following situations:

allergy to HMG-CoA reductase inhibitors or any of their ingredients
breastfeeding
elevated liver function tests, unexplained and persistent
liver disease, active
pregnancy

Use with caution in the following situations:

alcohol use, concurrent
electrolyte, hormone, or metabolic disorders
endocrine dysfunction
high creatine phosphokinase levels
immunosuppressant therapy, concurrent
infection, severe and acute
kidney disease
lipid-lowering therapy, concurrent
liver disease, history of
low blood pressure
ophthalmic disorders
seizures, uncontrolled
surgery, major
trauma

Pregnancy: Do not use during pregnancy. The risk to the fetus clearly outweighs any possible benefit to the mother. Women of childbearing age should use only if it is highly unlikely that they will become pregnant and they have been informed of the potential hazards. If you become pregnant while taking one of these drugs, discontinue use immediately and consult your doctor.

Breastfeeding: Fluvastatin and pravastatin appear in breast milk. It is not known if atorvastatin, lovastatin, or simvastatin appear in breast milk. Do not breastfeed while taking these drugs.

Children: Safety and effectiveness in children younger than 18 years of age have not been established. Treatment is not recommended.

Elderly: Lower starting doses of lovastatin and pravastatin may be considered in patients older than 70 years of age.

Lab tests will be required to monitor therapy. Tests may include cholesterol levels, eye exams, liver and kidney function tests, and liver (transaminase) and muscle (creatine phosphokinase) enzymes.

Drug Interactions:

Tell your doctor or pharmacist if you are taking or planning to take any over-the-counter or prescription medications or dietary supplements with HMG-CoA reductase inhibitors. Doses of one or both drugs may need to be modified or a different drug may need to be prescribed. The following drugs and drug classes interact with HMG-CoA reductase inhibitors:

- antacids (atorvastatin only)
- azole antifungals (eg, ketoconazole, itraconazole)
- bile acid sequestrants (eg, cholestyramine)
- cimetidine (eg, *Tagamet*) (fluvastatin only)
- cyclosporine (eg, *Sandimmune*)
- diltiazem (eg, *Cardizem*)
- gemfibrozil (eg, *Lopid*)
- grapefruit juice
- isradipine (*DynaCirc*)
- macrolide antibiotics (eg, erythromycin)
- nefazodone (*Serzone*)
- niacin (eg, *Nicobid*)
- omeprazole (*Prilosec*) (fluvastatin only)
- protease inhibitors (eg, ritonavir)
- ranitidine (eg, *Zantac*) (fluvastatin only)
- rifampin (eg, *Rifadin*) (fluvastatin only)
- verapamil (eg, *Calan*)
- warfarin (eg, *Coumadin*)

Side Effects:

Every drug is capable of producing side effects. Many HMG-CoA reductase inhibitor users experience no, or minor, side effects. The frequency and severity of side effects depend on many factors including dose, duration of therapy, and individual susceptibility. Possible side effects include:

Digestive Tract: Nausea; vomiting; diarrhea; stomach pain; constipation; gas; indigestion; heartburn.

Nervous System: Headache; dizziness; weakness; fatigue; sleeplessness.

Respiratory System: Cold or flu-like symptoms; cough; congestion; upper respiratory tract infection; sore throat; sinus infection; runny nose.

Other: Muscle pain or cramps; urinary abnormality; abnormal blood tests; blurred vision; accidental trauma; tooth disorders; localized pain; urinary tract infection; chest, leg, back, or joint pain; joint inflammation; swelling of arms and legs; infection; rash.

Guidelines for Use:

- Exercise and a diet that reduces the intake of cholesterol and saturated fats should accompany HMG-CoA reductase inhibitor treatment.
- Dosage is individualized. Take exactly as prescribed.
- Do not change the dose or stop taking this medicine unless advised to do so by your doctor.
- *Atorvastatin, fluvastatin, simvastatin* — Take once daily in the evening with or without food.
- *Lovastatin* — Take with evening meals.
- *Pravastatin* — Take once daily with or without food.
- If a dose is missed, take it as soon as possible. If several hours have passed or it is nearing time for the next dose, do not double the dose to catch up, unless advised to do so by your doctor. If more than one dose is missed or it is necessary to establish a new dosage schedule, contact your doctor or pharmacist.
- If taken in conjunction with cholestyramine or colestipol, take HMG-CoA reductase inhibitors either 1 hour before or at least 4 hours after the cholestyramine or colestipol.
- Inform your doctor if you are pregnant, become pregnant, plan on becoming pregnant, or are breastfeeding.
- Notify your doctor immediately if you experience unexplained headache, muscle pain, tenderness or weakness, nausea, vomiting, or diarrhea, particularly if accompanied by fever or general body discomfort.
- Lab tests will be required to monitor therapy. Be sure to keep appointments.
- Store between 41° and 86°F. Protect from light and moisture.

If you have any questions, consult your doctor, pharmacist, or health care provider.

Bronchodilators
- Sympathomimetics, 455
- Xanthine Derivatives, 462

Leukotriene Receptor Antagonists/Formation Inhibitors, 468

Inhalants
- Corticosteroids, 471
- Cromolyn Sodium, 476
- Ipratropium Bromide, 479
- Ipratropium Bromide/Albuterol Sulfate, 482
- Mucolytics, 485
- Nedocromil Sodium, 488

Intranasal Steroids, 490

Antihistamines, 494

Decongestants, 501

Antitussives
- Narcotic, 506
- Nonnarcotic, 509

Expectorants, 513

Miscellaneous Nasal Products, 517

Upper Respiratory Combinations, 518

	Generic Name *Brand Name Examples*	Supplied As	Generic Available
Rx	**Albuterol Sulfate**		
	Proventil, Proventil HFA, Ventolin	**Aerosol:** 90 mcg/actuation	Yes
	Proventil	**Tablets:** 2 mg, 4 mg	Yes
	Proventil Repetabs, Volmax	**Tablets, extended release:** 4 mg, 8 mg	No
	Proventil, Ventolin	**Syrup:** 2 mg/5 mL	Yes
	Airet, Proventil, Ventolin Nebules	**Solution for inhalation:** 0.083% (in unit dose containers)	Yes
	Proventil, Ventolin	**Solution for inhalation:** 0.5%	Yes
	Ventolin Rotocaps	**Capsules for inhalation:** 200 mcg microfine (as sulfate)	No
Rx	**Bitolterol Mesylate**		
	Tornalate	**Solution for inhalation:** 0.2%	No
	Tornalate	**Aerosol:** 0.8% (0.37 mg/actuation)	No
	Ephedrine Sulfate		
otc	*Ephedrine Sulfate*	**Capsules:** 25 mg	Yes
Rx	*Ephedrine Sulfate*	**Injection:** 50 mg/mL	Yes
	Epinephrine		
Rx	*Adrenalin Chloride*[1]	**Solution for inhalation:** 1:100 epinephrine solution	No
otc	*microNefron*[1], *Nephron*[1], *S-2*[1]	**Solution for inhalation:** 2.25% racepinephrine (1.125% epinephrine base)	No
otc	*AsthmaHaler Mist, Primatene Mist*	**Aerosol:** 0.22 mg epinephrine/spray	No
Rx	*Adrenalin Chloride*[1], *Ana-Guard*[1]	**Injection:**1:1000 (1 mg/mL as HCl) solution	Yes
Rx	**Isoetharine HCl**[1]	**Solution for inhalation:** 1%	Yes
Rx	**Isoproterenol**[1]	**Injection:** 1:50,000 (0.02 mg/mL)	Yes
	Isuprel[1]	**Injection:** 1:5000 (0.2 mg/mL)	Yes
Rx	**Levalbuterol HCl**		
	Xopenex	**Solution for inhalation:** 0.063 mg/3 mL, 1.25 mg/3 mL	No

	Generic Name *Brand Name Examples*	Supplied As	Generic Available
Rx	**Metaproterenol Sulfate**	**Tablets:** 10 mg, 20 mg	Yes
		Syrup: 10 mg/5 mL	Yes
	Alupent	**Solution for inhalation:** 0.4% (in unit dose containers), 0.6%, 5% (in unit dose containers)	Yes
	Alupent	**Aerosol:** 75 mg as micronized powder (0.65 mg/dose; 100 inhalations)	No
	Alupent	**Aerosol:** 150 mg as micronized powder (0.65 mg/dose; 200 inhalations)	No
Rx	**Pirbuterol Acetate**		
	Maxair Autohaler, Maxair Inhaler	**Aerosol:** 0.2 mg/actuation	No
Rx	**Salmeterol Xinafoate**		
	Serevent	**Aerosol:** 25 mcg base/actuation	No
	Serevent Diskus	**Powder for inhalation:** 50 mcg	No
Rx	**Terbutaline Sulfate**		
	Brethine	**Tablets:** 2.5 mg, 5 mg	No
	Brethine	**Injection:** 1 mg/mL	No

[1] Contains sulfites.

All of the products listed in this table are bronchodilators; however, they are not interchangeable. For example, albuterol cannot be used for epinephrine, and salmeterol cannot be used for albuterol. Daily dose may vary depending on individual needs. Do not adjust the dose or change products without consulting your pharmacist or doctor.

Type of Drug:

Bronchodilators; "rescue" medicines. Drugs that make breathing easier by opening breathing tubes (bronchial tubes) of the lung.

How the Drug Works:

Sympathomimetics dilate (open) the bronchioles (air tubes) of the lung by relaxing the smooth muscle around the bronchioles. They are also used to prevent spasms or contractions of the smooth muscles around the bronchioles. This allows easier airflow into and out of the lungs. This may also assist in removing (expectorating) mucus and other debris causing congestion in the lungs.

Uses:

To treat and prevent reversible bronchospasm associated with bronchial and nocturnal (nighttime) asthma, chronic bronchitis, emphysema, exercise-induced bronchospasm, and other obstructive airway diseases of the lungs.

To treat serious allergic reactions (epinephrine injection only).

Precautions:

Do not use in the following situations:

allergy to a sympathomimetic or any of its ingredients
asthma (acute, significantly worsening, or deteriorating) (salmeterol only)
asthma, manageable with occasional short use of short-acting, inhaled
beta$_2$-agonists (bronchodilators) (salmeterol only)
asthma attack, once it has begun (salmeterol only)
glaucoma, narrow angle (ephedrine and epinephrine injection only)
heart rhythm disturbances associated with a rapid heart rate (metaproterenol only)
substitute for inhaled or oral corticosteroids (salmeterol only)

Use with caution in the following situations:

abnormal heart rhythm
bronchospasm, life threatening (salmeterol only)
diabetes mellitus
elderly (epinephrine only)
heart disease
high blood pressure
hyperthyroidism
pregnancy, labor, and delivery
prostate enlargement (ephedrine and epinephrine only)
psychoneurosis (eg, obsessions, phobias) (epinephrine only)
seizures, history of
sensitivity to sympathomimetics

Pregnancy: There are no adequate and well-controlled studies in pregnant women. Use only if clearly needed and the potential benefits to the mother outweigh the possible risks to the fetus.

Breastfeeding: It is not known if these drugs appear in breast milk. Consult your doctor before you begin breastfeeding.

Children:

Aerosol – Safety and effectiveness for use of albuterol, bitolterol, metaproterenol, pirbuterol, salmeterol, and terbutaline in children younger than 12 years of age (younger than 4 years of age for *Ventolin*) have not been established. Consult a doctor about the use of epinephrine in children younger than 4 years of age.

Oral doseforms – Safety and effectiveness of albuterol have not been established for children younger than 2 years (syrup) and younger than 6 years (tablets and extended-release tablets) of age. Ephedrine is rarely used alone in children. Metaproterenol is not recommended for use in children younger than 6 years of age. Terbutaline is not recommended for use in children younger than 12 years of age.

Powder for inhalation – Safety and effectiveness of albuterol and salmeterol have not been established in children younger than 4 years of age.

Solution for inhalation – Safety and effectiveness of albuterol, bitolterol, epinephrine, isoetharine, and levalbuterol have not been established in children younger than 12 years of age (younger than 2 years of age for *Ventolin*). Safety and effectiveness of metaproterenol have not been established in children younger than 6 years of age.

Sulfites: Some of these products may contain sulfite preservatives, which can cause allergic reactions in certain individuals. Check package label when available or consult your doctor or pharmacist.

Drug Interactions:

Tell your doctor or pharmacist if you are taking or planning to take any over-the-counter or prescription medications or dietary supplements while taking sympathomimetics. Doses of one or both drugs may need to be modified or a different drug may need to be prescribed. The following drugs and drug classes interact with sympathomimetics:

- beta blocking agents (eg, propranolol)
- digoxin (eg, *Lanoxin)*
- diuretics, non-potassium sparing (eg, loop diuretics, thiazide)
- ergot alkaloids (eg, *Hydergine)* (epinephrine only)
- furazolidone *(Furoxone)* (ephedrine only)
- guanethidine (eg, *Ismelin)* (ephedrine and epinephrine only)
- methyldopa (eg, *Aldomet)* (ephedrine and epinephrine only)
- MAO inhibitors (eg, phenelzine)
- phenothiazines (eg, chlorpromazine) (epinephrine only)
- rauwolfia alkaloids (eg, reserpine) (ephedrine and epinephrine only)
- tricyclic antidepressants (eg, amitriptyline)
- urinary acidifiers (eg, ammonium chloride) (ephedrine only)
- urinary alkalinizers (eg, sodium bicarbonate) (ephedrine only)

Side Effects:

Every drug is capable of producing side effects. Many sympathomimetic bronchodilator users experience no, or minor, side effects. The frequency and severity of side effects depend on many factors including dose, duration of therapy, and individual susceptibility. Possible side effects include:

Digestive Tract: Nausea; vomiting; appetite changes; heartburn; diarrhea; stomach pain; dry mouth; indigestion; constipation; mouth fungal infection; mouth or throat irritation; gastrointestinal distress; belching; gas.

Nervous System: Vertigo (feeling of whirling motion); dizziness; lightheadedness; headache; anxiety; tension; tremor; drowsiness; weakness; fatigue; nervousness; unstable emotions; aggressive behavior; restlessness; excitement; hyperactivity; sleeplessness; agitation; nightmares; irritability; shakiness.

Circulatory System: Changes in heart rate or rhythm; changes in blood pressure; chest pain or discomfort; pounding in the chest; irregular pulse.

Respiratory System: Breathing problems; bronchospasm; respiratory infections; nasal congestion; lower respiratory infections; bronchitis; increased mucous or phlegm discharge; cough; wheezing; nosebleed; sinus headache; hoarseness (especially in children); worsening of asthma; chest discomfort; runny nose; viral infection; sneezing.

Skin: Flushing; pallor; sweating; hives; rash; pain at the injection site (injections only); eczema; skin inflammation.

Other: Muscle cramps, stiffness, or soreness; unusual or bad taste; tooth pain or discoloration; painful menstruation; general body discomfort; joint, arm, neck, chest, shoulder, or back pain; low potassium levels; localized aches and pains; urinary tract infection; flu-like symptoms; allergic reaction; fever; decreased sensitivity to stimulation; accidental injury; pain; migraine; leg cramps; chills; abnormal lab tests; fainting; abnormal skin sensations; eye itch; sweating; eye inflammation.

Guidelines for Use:

- Read and follow the patient instructions provided with the products.
- Dosage will be individualized. Do not use more frequently or at higher doses than recommended by your doctor.
- Do not crush or chew extended-release tablets. Swallow whole with liquids. The outer coating of the tablet may not be absorbed and may be noticeable in the stool.
- *Brand interchange* — Do not change from one brand of these drugs to another without consulting your pharmacist or doctor.
- While you are using a sympathomimetic bronchodilator, take other inhaled drugs and asthma medications only as directed by your doctor.
- If asthma attack continues or worsens, discontinue use and contact your doctor.
- *Salmeterol* — Do not use once an asthma attack begins. Use a quick-acting bronchodilator (eg, albuterol) instead. This medicine is not a substitute for inhaled or oral corticosteroids.
- If a dose is missed, take it as soon as possible. If several hours have passed or it is nearing time for the next dose, do not double the dose to catch up, unless advised to do so by your doctor. If several doses are missed, contact your doctor or pharmacist.
- May cause dizziness or drowsiness. Use caution while driving or performing other tasks requiring alertness, coordination, or physical dexterity.
- May cause nervousness, restlessness, or sleeplessness. Notify your doctor if the effects continue.
- Notify your doctor if palpitations, fast heartbeat, chest pain, muscle tremors, dizziness, headache, flushing, or difficulty in urination occurs, or if difficulty breathing persists.
- *Oral doseforms* — Do not exceed recommended dosage. If stomach upset occurs, take with food.
- *Nebulizer* — Mix medication as directed. Do not use if solution is brown or cloudy. Dilute concentrated solution (0.5%) before use. Do not mix different types of medication, unless advised to do so by your doctor.

  Assemble mask or mouthpiece. Administer treatment while sitting in a comfortable, upright position. Take slow, deep breaths until medication canister is empty. Wash mask or mouthpiece and medication container with hot water. Allow to air dry.

Guidelines for Use (cont.):

- *Pressurized aerosol* — Follow administration, storage, and disposal instructions exactly.
  Shake aerosol canister before each use.
  Use of a spacing device (eg, *Aerochamber*) will enhance effectiveness and decrease side effects.
  Protect from heat and light.
  Do not stop or adjust the dose unless directed by your doctor. Overuse may result in the drug losing its effectiveness.
  Breathe out fully through the mouth, expelling as much air from the lungs as possible. Place the mouthpiece of the inhaler (or spacer) into your mouth and, while breathing deeply and slowly through the mouth, activate the medication canister. Hold your breath for 3 to 5 seconds and then breathe out.
  If more than 1 inhalation per dose is necessary, wait at least 1 full minute between doses. (Administer second inhalation at 3 to 5 minutes for albuterol and epinephrine; 10 minutes for metaproterenol).
  If a previously effective dosage regimen fails to provide the usual relief, consult your doctor immediately. This may be a sign of seriously worsening asthma, which requires reassessment of therapy. Consult your doctor.
  If any of the following occurs with the use of a short-acting $beta_2$-agonist (eg, albuterol, bitolterol, pirbuterol, terbutaline), contact your doctor: Use of 4 or more inhalations daily for more than 2 consecutive days; use of more than 1 canister in an 8-week period (ie, canister with 200 inhalations); sudden need for increased inhalations.
  Do not interchange medication canisters and adapters (plastic colored sleeves) from different aerosol products.

If you have any questions, consult your doctor, pharmacist, or health care provider.

	Generic Name *Brand Name Examples*	Supplied As	Generic Available
Rx	**Aminophylline (Theophylline Ethylenediamine)**	**Tablets:** 100 mg, 200 mg	Yes
		Liquid: 105 mg/5 mL	Yes
		Suppositories: 250 mg, 500 mg	Yes
		Injection: 250 mg/10 mL	Yes
Rx	**Dyphylline (Dihydroxypropyl Theophylline)**		
	Dilor, Dilor-400, Lufyllin, Lufyllin-400	**Tablets:** 200 mg, 400 mg	Yes
	Dilor, Lufyllin	**Elixir:** 100 mg/15 mL, 160 mg/15 mL	No
	Dilor	**Injection:** 250 mg/mL	No
Rx	**Oxtriphylline (Choline Theophyllinate)**		
	Choledyl SA	**Tablets, extended release (8 to 12 hours):** 400 mg, 600 mg	No
Rx	**Theophylline**	**Oral solution:** 80 mg/15 mL	Yes
	Quibron-T Accudose, Slo-Phyllin, Theolair	**Tablets:** 100 mg, 125 mg, 200 mg, 250 mg, 300 mg	Yes
	Theochron	**Tablets, extended release:** 100 mg, 200 mg, 300 mg	No
	Quibron-T/SR Accudose, Respbid, Theolair-SR, T-Phyl	**Tablets, sustained release (8 to 12 hours):** 200 mg, 250 mg, 300 mg, 500 mg	No
	Theo-Dur	**Tablets, extended release (8 to 24 hours):** 100 mg, 200 mg, 300 mg, 450 mg	No
	Theo-X	**Tablets, extended release (12 to 24 hours):** 100 mg, 200 mg, 300 mg	No
	Uniphyl, Uni-Dur	**Tablets, extended release (24 hours):** 400 mg, 600 mg	No
	Theo-24	**Capsules, extended release (24 hours):** 100 mg, 200 mg, 300 mg, 400 mg	No
	Elixophyllin	**Elixir:** 80 mg/15 mL	Yes
	Slo-Phyllin	**Syrup:** 80 mg/15 mL	No

All of the products listed in the table are bronchodilators; however, they are not all equivalent on a weight basis and cannot be interchanged without adjusting the dose. For example, oxtriphylline cannot be used for theophylline without adjusting the dose. Daily dose may vary depending on individual needs. Do not adjust the dose or change products without consulting your pharmacist or doctor.

Theophylline Content and Equivalent Dose of Various Theophylline Salts		
Theophylline salts	Theophylline %	Equivalent dose
Theophylline anhydrous	100	100 mg
Aminophylline anhydrous	86	116 mg
Aminophylline dihydrate	79	127 mg
Oxtriphylline	64	156 mg

Type of Drug:

Bronchodilators; theophylline products; drugs that make breathing easier by relaxing and widening certain breathing passages (bronchial tubes) of the lung.

How the Drug Works:

The xanthine derivatives directly relax the smooth muscle surrounding the bronchial tubes (air passages) of the lungs, allowing the tubes to widen, making breathing easier. These drugs may improve contraction of the diaphragm (the major breathing muscle) in patients with chronic obstructive airway disease.

Uses:

To prevent and relieve symptoms of bronchial asthma. Not for use by themselves in an acute attack (status asthmaticus).

To treat bronchospasm (spasm in breathing tubes) associated with chronic bronchitis and emphysema.

Unlabeled Use(s): Occasionally doctors may prescribe xanthine bronchodilators for other breathing problems and slow heart rates in premature infants.

Precautions:

Do not use in the following situations:

- allergy to any xanthine compounds (eg, caffeine, chocolate) or any of their ingredients
- allergy to ethylenediamine (aminophylline only)
- irritation or infection of the rectum or lower colon (aminophylline suppositories only)
- peptic ulcer disease, active
- seizure disorder, underlying (unless receiving anticonvulsants)
- xanthine use, concurrent

Use with caution in the following situations:

- abnormal heart rhythm
- alcoholism (some liquid forms)
- congestive heart failure
- dehydration
- elderly (particularly males with chronic lung disease)
- heart disease, severe
- high blood pressure
- high fever, sustained
- hyperthyroidism
- hypothyroidism
- hypoxemia (deficient oxygenation of the blood)
- influenza vaccine
- kidney function, impaired (infants younger than 3 months old)
- liver function, impaired (except dyphylline)
- low blood pressure
- myocardial injury, acute
- newborns and infants younger than 1 year of age
- peptic ulcer disease, history
- pregnancy, third trimester
- pulmonary edema, acute
- sepsis with multiple organ failure
- smoking (decreases theophylline levels)
- status asthmaticus (oral products act too slowly)
- viral infection

Acute asthma attacks (status asthmaticus) are a medical emergency and are not rapidly responsive to usual doses of conventional bronchodilators. Therapy frequently requires IV medication and close monitoring. These products alone are not appropriate treatment for an acute asthma attack.

Pregnancy: There are no adequate and well-controlled studies in pregnant women. Use only if clearly needed and potential benefits outweigh the possible hazards to the fetus.

Breastfeeding: Xanthines appear in breast milk. Because of the potential for serious adverse reactions in nursing infants, decide whether to discontinue nursing or to discontinue the drug, taking into account the importance of the drug to the mother. Consult your doctor before you begin breastfeeding.

Children: Safety and effectiveness of aminophylline and theophylline for use in children younger than 1 year of age have not been established. Caution should be exercised for younger children who cannot complain of side effects. If used in children younger than 1 year of age, strict attention should be directed at dosing and monitoring of serum levels. However, some dosage forms of theophylline are not recommended for certain age groups. Please check individual dosing and administration in package inserts. Oxtriphylline is not recommended for children younger than 6 years of age. Dyphylline is not recommended for children.

Elderly: Reduced theophylline elimination has been documented in patients older than 55 years of age, particularly in males with chronic lung disease, congestive heart failure, or liver disease. It is important to consider reduction of dosage and frequent measurement of serum theophylline levels in these individuals, as they may experience toxicity more easily.

Lab tests may be necessary. High blood levels of xanthine bronchodilators may cause severe side effects. Therapy is monitored with lab tests to maintain nontoxic levels of medication, as serious toxicity is not reliably preceded by less severe side effects. Lung function measurements before and after a period of treatment may also be necessary to determine therapy effectiveness. Note that dyphylline is not converted to theophylline; thus, theophylline blood levels cannot be used to monitor it use.

Drug Interactions:

Tell your doctor or pharmacist if you are taking or planning to take any over-the-counter or prescription medications or dietary supplements while taking xanthine bronchodilators. Doses of one or both drugs may need to be modified or a different drug may need to be prescribed. The following drugs and drug classes interact with xanthine bronchodilators:

These drugs *decrease* the effectiveness of xanthine bronchodilators:

aminoglutethimide (*Cytadren*)
barbiturates (eg, phenobarbital)
carbamazepine (eg, *Tegretol*)[1]
charcoal
hydantoins (eg, phenytoin)
moricizine (*Ethmozine*)
rifampin (eg, *Rifadin*)
ritonavir (*Norvir*)
smoking (cigarettes and marijuana)
sucralfate (*Carafate*)
sulfinpyrazone (eg, *Anturane*)

These drugs *increase* the effects of xanthine bronchodilators (increasing side effects):

alcohol
allopurinol (eg, *Zyloprim*)
beta blockers (nonselective) (eg, propranolol)
carbamazepine (eg, *Tegretol*)[1]
cimetidine (eg, *Tagamet*)
clarithromycin (*Biaxin*)
contraceptives, oral estrogen-containing (eg, *Ortho-Novum*)
corticosteroids (eg, hydrocortisone)
disulfiram (*Antabuse*)
ephedrine (eg, *Sudafed*)
erythromycin (eg, *Eryc*)
fluoroquinolones (eg, ciprofloxacin, enoxacin, norfloxacin, ofloxacin)
fluvoxamine (*Luvox*)
influenza vaccine (eg, *Fluzone*)
interferon, human recombinant alpha-A
isoniazid (eg, *Laniazid*)[1]
methotrexate (eg, *Rheumatrex*)
mexiletine (*Mexitil*)
pentoxifylline (*Trental*)
propafenone (*Rythmol*)
propranolol (eg, *Inderal*)
tacrine (*Cognex*)
thiabendazole (*Mintezol*)[1]
thyroid hormones (eg, levothyroxine)
ticlopidine (*Ticlid*)
troleandomycin (*Tao*)
verapamil (eg, *Verelan*)

Other drugs which xanthine bronchodilators affect:

adenosine (*Adenocard*)
benzodiazepines (eg, diazepam)
beta agonists
halothane (eg, *Fluothane*)
ketamine (*Ketalar*)
lithium (eg, *Eskalith*)
nondepolarizing muscle relaxants (eg, metocurine iodide)
probenecid (dyphylline only)
tetracyclines (eg, *Sumycin*)

[1]May increase or decrease effects.

Side Effects:

Every drug is capable of producing side effects. Many xanthine bronchodilator users experience no, or minor, side effects, particularly if serum theophylline levels are less than 20 mcg/mL. The frequency and severity of side effects depend on many factors including dose, duration of therapy, and individual susceptibility. High blood levels (generally higher than 30 mcg/mL) of these medications will cause serious side effects, although high blood levels and serious toxicity are not always preceded by side effects. Possible side effects include:

Digestive Tract: Stomach pain; nausea; vomiting; vomiting of blood; diarrhea; gastroesophageal reflux (nocturnal).

Nervous System: Seizures; headache; sleeplessness; irritability; restlessness; muscle twitching; reflex hyperexcitability; agitation.

Circulatory System: Decreased blood pressure; abnormal heart beat; pounding in the chest (palpitations); fast heartbeat.

Skin: Flushing; rash; hair loss.

Other: Increased urination; high blood sugar; rectal irritation or bleeding (suppository only); muscle tremors or twitching.

Guidelines for Use:

- Take exactly as prescribed. Individual doses are determined by response (decrease in symptoms) and blood levels (except with dyphylline). Do not take a different dose, take the drug more often, or for a longer time than prescribed.
- *Immediate Release Tablets and Liquids:*
  Take at regular intervals around the clock.
  If a dose is missed, take it as soon as possible. If several hours have passed or if it is nearing time for the next dose, do not double the dose in order to catch up, unless advised to do so by your doctor. If more than one dose is missed or it is necessary to establish a new dosage schedule, contact your doctor or pharmacist.
- *Sustained, Extended, or Controlled Release Products:*
  Take 8- to 12-hour release products at regular intervals (8 or 12 hours) around the clock. Try to take at the same time each day.
  Take 12- to 24-hour release products generally every 12 hours. However, a few patients may be able to take once a day.
  Take 24-hour release products once daily, preferably in the morning. Try to take at the same time each day.
  Although normally given once daily, patients who require very large doses may be asked to split the dose and take 2 doses per day. In this event, the second dose should be taken 10 to 12 hours after the first dose and before the evening meal.
  If a dose is missed, take the next dose at the usually scheduled time. Do not make up the missed dose.

Guidelines for Use (cont.):

- *Brand interchange* — Do not change from one brand of this drug to another without consulting your pharmacist or doctor. Products are not equivalent on a weight basis and cannot be interchanged without adjusting the dose.
- If stomach upset occurs with liquid preparations or non-sustained release forms, take with food.
- Do not crush or chew enteric coated or sustained, extended, or controlled release tablets or capsules.
- Taking theophylline immediately after a high-fat meal or a fasting period may alter its rate of absorption.
- Do not use for an acute episode of bronchospasm.
- If rash, nausea, vomiting, restlessness, irregular heartbeat, or convulsions occur, contact your doctor immediately
- Inform your doctor of bothersome side effects such as headache, stomach pain, sleeplessness, or jitteriness.
- Notify your doctor if respiratory symptoms return repeatedly near the end of the dosing interval.
- Avoid large amounts of caffeine-containing beverages, such as tea, coffee, cocoa, and cola drinks, or eating large amounts of chocolate. These products may increase side effects.
- Tell your doctor if you are a smoker. Smoking increases the clearance rate of theophylline and may decrease overall effect. Nicotine replacement therapy (NRT) used in smoking cessation programs does not adversely affect theophylline clearance.
- *Uniphyl, Theolair SR* — Take this drug consistently with respect to food, either with meals or fasting (at least 2 hours pre- or 2 hours post-meals).
- *Theo-24* — In patients receiving once-daily doses of 900 mg or more, avoid eating a high-fat morning meal or take at least 1 hour before eating. If you cannot comply with this regimen, talk to your doctor about alternative therapy.
- Lab tests will be required. Be sure to keep appointments. Blood levels must be checked regularly to avoid underdosing and overdosing.
- Store oral dosage forms at room temperature (59° to 86°F) in a tightly closed container. Store suppositories between 36° to 46°F (refrigerated).

If you have any questions, consult your doctor, pharmacist, or health care provider.

	Generic Name *Brand Name Examples*	How Supplied	Generic Available
Rx	**Montelukast Sodium**		
	Singulair	**Tablets**: 10 mg	No
	Singulair[1]	**Tablets, chewable**: 4 mg, 5 mg	No
Rx	**Zafirlukast**		
	Accolate	**Tablets**: 10 mg, 20 mg	No
Rx	**Zileuton**		
	Zyflo Filmtabs	**Tablets**: 600 mg	No

[1] Contains phenylalanine.

Type of Drug:

Anti-asthma drug.

How the Drug Works:

Zileuton inhibits the formation of certain chemicals (leukotrienes) that are responsible for causing some forms of asthma. Montelukast and zafirlukast block the action of certain chemicals (leukotrienes) that are responsible for causing some forms of asthma.

These drugs are useful for controlling or preventing some forms of asthma but do not help during an acute asthma attack.

Uses:

For the prevention and chronic treatment of asthma in adult and children 2 years of age and older (montelukast), 7 years of age and older (zafirlukast), and 12 years of age and older (zileuton).

Precautions:

Do not use in the following situations:

allergy to the leukotriene receptor antagonist or any of its ingredients
liver disease, active (zileuton only)
to treat bronchospasm in acute asthmatic attacks

Use with caution in the following situations:

alcohol use (zileuton only)
elderly (zafirlukast only)
liver disease, history of (zileuton only)

Phenylketonuria: Montelukast chewable tablets contain phenylalanine. Consult your doctor or pharmacist.

Pregnancy: There are no adequate and well-controlled studies in pregnant women. Use only if clearly needed and potential benefits to the mother outweigh the possible hazards to the fetus.

Breastfeeding: Zafirlukast appears in breast milk. Do not breastfeed while taking zafirlukast. It is not known if zileuton or montelukast appear in breast milk. Consult your doctor before you begin breastfeeding.

Children: Safety and effectiveness for use in children younger than 12 years of age (zileuton), younger than 5 years of age (zafirlukast), and younger than 2 years of age (montelukast) are not established.

Elderly: Patients older than 65 years of age are more likely to experience infections while taking zafirlukast. These infections are usually mild to moderate and mostly affect the respiratory tract.

Lab tests may be required to monitor therapy. Tests may include breathing tests. Liver enzymes will be monitored with zileuton therapy.

Drug Interactions:

Tell your doctor or pharmacist if you are taking or planning to take any over-the-counter or prescription medications or dietary supplements while taking a leukotriene receptor antagonist or formation inhibitor. Doses of one or both drugs may need to be modified or a different drug may need to be prescribed. The following drugs and drug classes may interact with leukotriene receptor antagonists or formation inhibitors:

aspirin (zafirlukast only)
calcium channel blockers (eg, nifidipine) (zafirlukast and zileuton only)
cyclosporine (eg, *Sandimmune*) (zafirlukast and zileuton only)
erythromycin (eg, *E-Mycin*) (zafirlukast only)
propranolol (eg, *Inderal*) (zileuton only)
theophylline (eg, *Theo-Dur*) (zafirlukast and zileuton only)
warfarin (eg, *Coumadin*) (zafirlukast and zileuton only)

Side Effects:

Every drug is capable of producing side effects. Many leukotriene receptor antagonist or formation inhibitor users experience no, or minor, side effects. The frequency or severity of side effects depend on many factors including dose, duration of therapy, and individual susceptibility. Possible side effects include:

Nervous System: Headache; weakness; dizziness; sleeplessness; nervousness; drowsiness; fatigue.

Digestive Tract: Nausea; vomiting; diarrhea; stomach pain; indigestion; gas; constipation.

Other: Infection; accidental injury; generalized pain; muscle, chest, joint, leg, or back pain; fever; eye inflammation; stiffness; swollen lymph nodes; general body discomfort; neck pain; itching; urinary tract infection; inflammation of the vagina; flu; cough; nasal congestion; dental pain; rash; laryngitis; sore throat; ear pain or inflammation; sinus inflammation; viral infection; thirst; sneezing; hives; pus in the urine.

Guidelines for Use:

- Dosage is individualized. Take exactly as prescribed.
- These medicines are used for long-term control or prevention of asthma and should be taken regularly as prescribed, even during symptom-free periods. They should also be continued during acute exacerbations of asthma.
- Do not decrease the dose or stop taking any other asthma medications unless instructed by your doctor.
- Take zafirlukast 2 times a day on an empty stomach, at least 1 hour before or 2 hours after meals.
- Take zileuton 4 times a day with meals and at bedtime.
- Take montelukast once a day in the evening without regard to meals. Take with food if stomach upset occurs.
- If a dose is missed, take it as soon as possible. If several hours have passed or it is nearing time for the next dose, do not double the dose to catch up, unless advised by your doctor. If more than one dose is missed or it is necessary to establish a new dosage schedule, contact your doctor or pharmacist.
- May cause dizziness. Use caution when driving or performing other tasks requiring alertness, coordination or physical dexterity.
- These medicines are not bronchodilators and should not be used as "rescue medicines" to treat acute episodes of asthma.
- Do not breastfeed while taking zafirlukast.
- Contact your doctor if you need your short-acting bronchodilators ("rescue medicines") more often than usual.
- Contact your doctor if you are taking zileuton and experience right upper quadrant pain, nausea, tiredness, unconsciousness, itchiness, yellowing of the skin or the whites of the eyes, "flu-like" symptoms, or unusually dark urine.
- Lab tests may be required to monitor therapy. Be sure to keep appointments.
- Store at controlled room temperature (68° to 77°F). Protect from light and moisture.

If you have any questions, consult your doctor, pharmacist, or health care provider.

	Generic Name *Brand Name Examples*	Supplied As	Generic Available
Rx	**Beclomethasone Dipropionate**		
	Vanceril	**Aerosol**: 42 mcg/actuation	No
	Vanceril Double Strength	**Aerosol**: 84 mcg/actuation	
	QVAR	**Aerosol**: 40 mcg/actuation, 80 mcg/actuation	No
Rx	**Budesonide**		
	Pulmicort Turbuhaler	**Inhalation powder**: ≈ 160 mcg/actuation	No
	Pulmicort Respules	**Inhalation suspension**: 0.25 mg/2 mL, 0.5 mg/2 mL	No
Rx	**Flunisolide**		
	AeroBid, AeroBid-M[1]	**Aerosol:** ≈ 250 mcg/actuation	No
Rx	**Fluticasone Propionate**		
	Flovent	**Aerosol:** 44 mcg/actuation, 110 mcg/actuation, 220 mcg/actuation	No
	Flovent Rotadisk	**Inhalation powder:** 44 mcg/actuation, 88 mcg/actuation, 220 mcg/actuation	No
Rx	**Fluticasone Propionate/Salmeterol**		
	Advair Diskus	**Inhalation powder**: 93 mcg/45 mcg/actuation, 233 mcg/45 mcg/actuation, 465 mcg/45 mcg/actuation	No
Rx	**Triamcinolone Acetonide**		
	Azmacort[2]	**Aerosol:** 100 mcg/actuation	No

[1] Contains menthol
[2] Contains alcohol

Type of Drug:

Respiratory inhalants; drugs that produce an anti-inflammatory effect in lungs of stable asthma patients; asthma controllers; asthma preventatives.

How the Drug Works:

Irritation and inflammation (swelling) of the bronchial tubes (air tubes) of the lung is frequently a cause of persistent or recurrent asthma symptoms. These synthetic "anti-inflammatory steroids" decrease the irritation and swelling (inflammation) of the air tubes of the lungs and control or prevent asthma symptoms. These drugs do not directly open the bronchial tubes and do not provide rapid relief. They are useful for controlling or preventing asthma symptoms but do not help during an acute asthma attack. When inhaled into the bronchial tubes, the effect is local and the incidence of side effects is very low when compared to side effects when these medications are given by mouth.

Uses:

To prevent or reduce the frequency and severity of bronchial asthma attacks in patients requiring chronic (long-term) treatment.

Corticosteroid inhalants are *not* to be used to treat an acute asthma attack or in the treatment of nonasthmatic bronchitis.

Flovent Rotadisk — For treatment of chronic asthma attacks in patients 4 years of age and older or for asthma requiring long-term corticosteroid therapy.

Patients using corticosteroid inhalants may also take oral corticosteroid therapy or specific bronchodilator therapy.

Precautions:

Do not use in the following situations:

acute bronchospasm, treatment of
allergy to any ingredient of the formulation
asthma that can be controlled by bronchodilators and other nonsteroidal medicine (beclomethasone aerosol only)
nonasthmatic bronchitis (beclomethasone aerosol only)
systemic corticosteroid treatment, infrequently required (beclomethasone aerosol only)

Use with caution in the following situations:

adrenal insufficiency
chicken pox, exposure
herpes infection in the eye
measles, exposure
oral corticosteroid use, chronic
respiratory infections (fungal, bacterial, or viral)
systemic fungal, bacterial, parasitic, or viral infection, untreated
tuberculosis, active or inactive

Changing from other dosage forms: Patients who have been on long-term oral corticosteroids may lose their body's natural ability to produce corticosteroid hormones. Switching or lessening current oral doses may cause symptoms of withdrawal (eg, joint or muscle pain, tiredness, depression). Therefore, taper dosage of oral steroid gradually and only with the instruction of a doctor.

Pregnancy: There are no adequate and well-controlled studies in pregnant women. Use only if clearly needed and the potential benefits to the mother outweigh the possible hazards to the fetus.

Breastfeeding: It is not known if inhaled corticosteroids appear in breast milk. Consult your doctor before you begin breastfeeding.

Children: There is insufficient information available to warrant use in children younger than 12 months of age (budesonide suspension), younger than 6 years of age (beclomethasone, budesonide inhalation powder, flunisolide, and triamcinolone), or younger than 12 years of age (fluticasone aerosol). Extended regular use may suppress growth in children and teenagers.

Drug Interactions:

Tell your doctor or pharmacist if you are taking or planning to take any over-the-counter or prescription medications or dietary supplements with inhaled corticosteroids. Doses of one or both drugs may need to be modified or a different drug may need to be prescribed. Ketoconazole (eg, *Nizoral)* interacts with inhaled corticosteroids.

Side Effects:

Every drug is capable of producing side effects. Many inhaled corticosteroid users experience no, or minor, side effects. The frequency and severity of side effects depend on many factors including dose, duration of therapy, and individual susceptibility. Possible side effects include:

Digestive Tract: Diarrhea; toothache; nausea; vomiting; stomach pain or upset; constipation; gas; oral thrush (white patches in mouth); heartburn; indigestion; changes in appetite.

Nervous System: Headache; migraine; fatigue; dizziness; irritability; sleeplessness; fainting; shakiness; nervousness; mental disturbances; depression; agitation; lightheadedness; anxiety; changes in energy level; moodiness; numbness; vertigo (feeling of whirling motion); emotional lability.

Respiratory System: Sore throat; flu-like symptoms; head, nasal, or chest congestion; dry or irritated mouth, nose, or throat; hoarseness; voice changes; mouth infections; coughing; wheezing; difficulty breathing; runny nose; sneezing; throat infection; upper respiratory tract infection; loss of voice; nosebleed; sinus inflammation; chest tightness; phlegm; chest tightness; worsening of asthma.

Skin: Acne; red, itchy skin; rash; itching; hives; bruising; skin discoloration; sensitivity to sunlight.

Other: Fever; urinary tract or vaginal infections; neck pain; back problems; pain; weight gain; unpleasant taste and smell; blurred vision; eye discomfort; speech problems; high blood pressure; rapid heartbeat; ear or eye infection; loss of sense of taste and smell; menstrual problems; bone fracture; palpitations (pounding in the chest); chest pain; suppression of HPA function; weakness; pain; back pain; enlarged lymph nodes; general body discomfort; sweating; swelling of the arms or legs; muscle or joint pain; chills; fever.

Guidelines for Use:

- Read and follow patient instructions provided with the product.
- Use exactly as prescribed. Do not increase recommended dose. Benefits are not immediate and effectiveness requires regular use. Contact your doctor if symptoms do not improve or condition worsens.
- *Aerosol* — Using the inhaler beyond the labeled number of actuations (puffs) will result in ineffective doses of medication and loss of control of asthma.
  Canisters should only be used with their actuator (plastic holder). Administering with a spacing device (eg, *OptiHaler*, *Aerochamber*) will enhance medication delivery and effectiveness.
- *QVAR* — Prime the aerosol canister before using the first time or if it has not been used for 10 or more days. Activating the aerosol into the air 2 times will prime the canister.
- *Inhalation suspension* — Must be administered by air-driven jet nebulizer. Shake gently before adding to nebulizer canister.
- Do not stop using when you feel better, unless advised by your doctor. These medicines are designed to prevent asthma symptoms and must be used on a daily basis, even when you feel well.
- Rinse mouth thoroughly, without swallowing, after completing inhalations. This reduces the risk of mouth infection.
- Do not use for an acute asthma attack requiring rapid relief. Inhaled corticosteroids are not bronchodilators.
- Avoid spraying in eyes.
- *Bronchodilator inhaler use* — Use the bronchodilator (eg, isoproterenol, albuterol, epinephrine) several minutes before the corticosteroid aerosol. This opens the air tubes and increases penetration of the steroid into the passageways.
- Notify your doctor if you experience oral thrush (white patches in mouth or throat), voice changes, sore throat, sore mouth, mental disturbances, increased bruising, weight gain, cushingoid features, acne, or cataracts.
- Contact your doctor when asthma attacks do not adequately respond to bronchodilators or if you notice a sudden increase in the need for your bronchodilator. Oral or injectable steroids may be required.
- May cause dizziness or lightheadedness. Use caution while driving or performing other tasks requiring alertness, coordination, or physical dexterity.
- May cause photosensitivity (sensitivity to sunlight). Avoid prolonged exposure to the sun and other ultraviolet (UV) light (eg, tanning beds). Use sunscreens and wear protective clothing until tolerance is determined.
- Supplementary oral steroids may be necessary during periods of high stress such as surgery, trauma, infection, or severe asthma attack. Carry a warning card indicating this potential need.

Guidelines for Use (cont.):

- Notify your doctor immediately if symptoms of steroid withdrawal occur when changing from oral to inhalant therapy (eg, joint or muscle pain, lack of energy, depression, more problems breathing, wheezing, dizziness). Your doctor may increase your oral steroid dose temporarily and then begin decreasing the oral steroid dose more slowly.
- Allergic reactions (eg, rash, hives, difficulty breathing) have occurred following beclomethasone use. These may be immediate or delayed. Contact your doctor if you suspect a reaction.
- Avoid exposure to chicken pox, measles, or other infections involving the respiratory tract. If exposed, consult your doctor immediately.
- Store at room temperature. Use inhalation suspension within 2 weeks of opening foil pouch. Use fluticasone powder within 2 months of opening foil pouch. Use fluticasone/salmeterol powder within 1 month of opening foil pouch.

If you have any questions, consult your doctor, pharmacist, or health care provider.

	Generic Name *Brand Name Examples*	Supplied As	Generic Available
	Cromolyn Sodium	**Inhalation (for nebulizer only)**: 20 mg/2 mL	Yes
Rx	*Intal Inhaler*	**Aerosol**: 800 mcg/spray	No
Rx	*Intal Nebulizer Solution*	**Solution (for nebulizer only)**: 20 mg/2 mL amp	No
otc	*Nasalcrom*[1]	**Nasal solution**: 5.2 mg/spray	No
otc	*Children's Nasalcrom*[1]	**Nasal solution**: 5.2 mg/spray	No

[1] Contains 0.01% benzalkonium chloride and 0.01% EDTA.

Type of Drug:

Respiratory inhalant.

How the Drug Works:

Cromolyn sodium is an antiasthmatic, antiallergic stabilizer of mast cells, which release histamine and slow-reacting substances of anaphylaxis. The decreased release of these and other chemicals assist in preventing constriction (narrowing) of the breathing airways in asthma and allergy attacks.

Uses:

Cromolyn Sodium and Intal: To prevent symptoms in the management of bronchial asthma, exercise-induced bronchospasm (spasm of breathing airways in the lungs), and acute bronchospasm due to environmental pollution and known allergens (chemicals that may produce an asthmatic or allergic reaction).

Nasalcrom: To prevent or treat symptoms of allergic rhinitis (eg, runny, itchy, stuffy nose; sneezing).

Unlabeled Use(s): Oral use of cromolyn is being evaluated in patients with food allergies, eczema, ulcers, hives (chronic), and postexercise-induced bronchospasms.

Precautions:

Do not use in the following situations:

- allergy to cromolyn or any of its ingredients
- asthma attack, prolonged and severe
- eosinophilic pneumonia (bacterial lung infection)
- sinus infection (nasal solution only)
- cold symptoms

Use with caution in the following situations:

- coronary artery disease (aerosol only)
- coughing or wheezing
- irregular heartbeat (aerosol only)
- kidney disease
- liver disease

Pregnancy: Safety for use during pregnancy has not been established. Use only if clearly needed and potential benefits to the mother outweigh the possible hazards to the fetus.

Breastfeeding: It is not known if cromolyn appears in breast milk. Consult your doctor before you begin breastfeeding.

Children: Safety and effectiveness for use in children under 6 (nasal solution), 5 (aerosol), or 2 (nebulizer) years of age have not been established.

Drug Interactions:

Tell your doctor or pharmacist if you are taking or if you are planning to take any over-the-counter or prescription medications or dietary supplements while taking cromolyn. Doses of one or both drugs may need to be modified or a different drug may need to be prescribed. Isoproterenol interacts with this medicine.

Side Effects:

Every drug is capable of producinq side effects. Many patients experience no, or minor, side effects. The frequency and severity of side effects depend on many factors including dose, duration of therapy, and individual susceptibility. Possible side effects include:

Aerosol: Dizziness; dry or irritated throat; joint swelling and pain; painful or difficult urination; urinary frequency; hives; skin infammation; excessive eye tearing; swollen parotid gland.

Nasal Solution: Nasal stinging; nasal burning; postnasal drip.

Nebulizer Solution: Drowsiness; serum sickness; stomach ache.

Other: Headache; nausea; cough; wheezing; nasal irritation; sneezing; nosebleed; bad taste in mouth; rash.

Guidelines for Use:

- Use exactly as prescribed.
- Not for the treatment of an existing asthma attack. Only use when an asthma attack is under control and you can breathe well.
- Notify your doctor if coughing, wheezing, or other unusual symptoms occur.
- Blow your nose before administering the nasal solution. If congested, use a shortacting topical decongestant before the solution. Nasal solution may cause mild stinging or sneezing, but this rarely requires stopping therapy.
- Instructions for use of inhalation devices accompany each product.
- Use continuously. Effectiveness depends on regularity of use. Do not stop therapy suddenly. Consult your doctor before stopping the drug.
- *To prevent exercise-induced bronchospasm* — Administer no longer than 1 hour before beginning exercise.
- If a dose is missed, inhale it as soon as possible. If several hours have passed or it is nearing time for the next dose, do not double the dose to catch up, unless advised to do so by your doctor. If more than one dose is missed or it is necessary to establish a new dosage schedule, contact your doctor or pharmacist.
- Improvement ordinarily occurs within the first 4 weeks of use. Improvement should be apparent by a decrease in the severity of symptoms and the need for other therapy (eg, oral steroids, inhaled bronchodilators).
- Long-term use is justified if cromolyn produces a significant reduction in frequency or severity of symptoms, permits reduction of doses or elimination of oral steroids, or improves management of patients experiencing intolerable side effects from other asthma drugs.
- If allergic rhinitis (eg, runny nose) is seasonal, continue treatment throughout exposure period. If it is year-round, continuous use may be necessary. Cromolyn use may decrease or eliminate the need for antihistamines or decongestants.
- Store nebulizer solution, aerosol, and nasal solution at room temperature, away from light. Do not use nebulizer solution if it is discolored or contains particles. Do not puncture the aerosol container or store near heat, cold, or open flame. Keep away from children.

If you have any questions, consult your doctor, pharmacist, or health care provider.

	Generic Name *Brand Name Example*	Supplied As	Generic Available
Rx	**Ipratropium Bromide**		
	Atrovent	**Aerosol**: Delivers 18 mcg/ actuation (200 actuations/ canister)	No
	Atrovent	**Solution**: 0.02%	Yes

Type of Drug:

Respiratory inhalant; bronchodilator.

How the Drug Works:

Ipratropium bromido blocks the action of the chemical transmitter acetylcholine when inhaled orally. Acetylcholine stimulates the muscles around the bronchial tubes (air passages in the lung) to spasm or constrict. This closes the bronchial tubes and makes it harder to breath. By blocking acetylcholine, ipratropium allows the muscles around the bronchial tubes to relax. This allow the bronchial tubes to open wider (bronchodilation) and makes it easier to breath.

Uses:

To treat bronchospasms (spasms of air passages) occurring in chronic obstructive pulmonary disease (COPD), including chronic bronchitis, and emphysema.

Precautions:

Do not use in the following situations:

allergy to ipratropium bromide, atropine, or any of its anticholinergic derivatives
allergy to soya lecithin or related food products (eg, soybeans, peanuts) (aerosol only)

Use with caution in the following situations:

acute bronchospasm attacks (eg, asthma attacks)
enlarged prostate
glaucoma, narrow-angle
obstruction of the neck of the urinary bladder

Pregnancy: There are no adequate and well-controlled studies in pregnant women. Use only if clearly needed and benefits outweigh the possible hazards to the fetus.

Breastfeeding: It is not known if ipratropium bromide appears in breast milk. Consult your doctor before you begin breastfeeding.

Children: Safety and effectiveness in children younger than 12 years of age have not been established.

Side Effects:

Every drug is capable of producing side effects. Many patients experience no, or minor, side effects. The frequency and severity of side effects depend on many factors including dose, duration of therapy, and individual susceptibility. Possible side effects include:

Digestive Tract: Nausea; stomach ache.

Nervous System: Headache; nervousness; dizziness; sleeplessness.

Circulatory System: Increased heart rate or irregular heartbeat; palpitations (pounding in the chest); low blood pressure; increased blood pressure.

Skin: Rash; itching; hives; flushing; hair loss.

Respiratory System: Cough; difficulty breathing; bronchitis; bronchospasm; increased sputum; upper respiratory tract infection; respiratory disorder; sore throat; dry mouth or throat; hoarseness; sinus infection; nasal irritation or congestion; runny nose; blood-tinged mucus.

Other: Worsening of narrow-angle glaucoma with acute eye pain; blurred vision; eye irritation; eye inflammation; ear ringing; tremors; pain; flu-like symptoms; joint, back, or chest pain; general pain; difficult urination; thirst.

Guidelines for Use:

- Dosage is individualized. Use exactly as prescribed.
- Do not stop taking or change the dose unless directed by your doctor.
- If a dose is missed, inhale it as soon as possible. If several hours have passed or it is nearing time for the next dose, do not double the dose to catch up, unless advised to do so by your doctor. If more than one dose is missed or it is necessary to establish a new dosage schedule, contact your doctor or pharmacist.
- Shake the aerosol canister well before using.
- The pump requires 7 actuations to initiate first dose. If not used for more than 24 hours, the pump will require 2 actuations; if not used for more than 7 days, the pump will require 7 actuations to reprime.
- Use of a spacer (eg, *OptiHaler*) with the aerosol may increase the amount of medicine that gets into the bronchial tubes and its effectiveness.
- The aerosol contains enough medication for 200 inhalations. Discard the canister after you have used 200 inhalations. Use of the aerosol after 200 inhalations will not provide the correct amount of medication.
- The aerosol total daily dose should not exceed 12 inhalations in 24 hours. If the recommended dosage does not provide relief or symptoms become worse, contact your doctor immediately.
- Do not use the aerosol with other inhaled drugs unless directed by your doctor.
- Do not use for the treatment of acute episodes of bronchospasm in which rapid response is required. This medicine is considered maintenance therapy. Drugs with faster action may be preferred for initial therapy in this situation.
- Temporary blurring of vision, causing or worsening of narrow-angle glaucoma, or eye pain may occur if the drug comes into contact with the eye. For the solution form, use of a nebulizer with a mouthpiece (rather than a face mask) may be preferable to reduce the chance of getting the solution in the eyes.
- The solution can be mixed in the nebulizer with albuterol. The combination should then be used within 1 hour.
- Inform your doctor if you are pregnant, become pregnant, are planning to become pregnant, or are breastfeeding.
- *Aerosol* — Store at room temperature (59° to 86°F). Avoid excessive humidity.
- *Solution* — Store at room temperature (59° to 86°F) away from light. Store unused vials in the foil pouch.

If you have any questions, consult your doctor, pharmacist, or health care provider.

	Generic Name *Brand Name Example*	Supplied As	Generic Available
Rx	**Ipratropium Bromide/ Albuterol Sulfate**		
	Combivent	**Aerosol**: 18 mcg ipratropium bromide/103 mcg albuterol sulfate per actuation	No

Type of Drug:

Respiratory inhalant; anticholinergic bronchodilator (ipratropium), $beta_2$-adrenergic bronchodilator (albuterol).

How the Drug Works:

Ipratropium blocks the action of the chemical transmitter acetylcholine. Acetylcholine causes the muscles around the bronchial (air) tubes to spasm and constrict, which makes it harder to breathe. By blocking acetylcholine, ipratropium allows these muscles to relax, thus widening the bronchial tubes (bronchodilation) and allowing more air into the lungs.

Albuterol dilates (opens) the bronchial (air) tubes of the lungs by relaxing the muscles around the bronchial tubes. This allows for easier air flow into and out of the lungs. It also assists in removing (expectorating) mucus and other debris causing congestion in the lungs.

Uses:

To treat bronchospasm in patients with chronic obstructive pulmonary disease (COPD) who are on a regular inhalant but require an additional bronchodilator.

Precautions:

Do not use in the following situations:

- allergy to ipratropium bromide, albuterol sulfate, atropine, sympathomimetic amines, or any other ingredients within the inhalant
- allergy to soya lecithin or related food products (eg, soybeans, peanuts)

Use with caution in the following situations:

- abnormal heart rhythm
- acute bronchospasm attacks (eg, asthma attacks)
- cardiovascular disorders (eg, coronary insufficiency)
- convulsive disorders
- diabetes mellitus
- enlarged prostate
- glaucoma, narrow-angle
- high blood pressure
- hyperthyroidism (overactive thyroid)
- hypokalemia (low blood potassium)
- kidney disease
- liver disease
- obstruction of the neck of the urinary bladder

Do not exceed recommended dose: Fatalities have been reported in association with excessive use of inhaled sympathomimetic drugs in patients with asthma.

Pregnancy: There are no adequate and well-controlled studies in pregnant women. Use only if clearly needed and the potential benefits to the mother outweigh the possible hazards to the fetus. Restrict use during labor because of the potential for albuterol interference with uterine contractility.

Breastfeeding: It is not known whether ipratropium/albuterol appears in breast milk. Consult your doctor before you begin breastfeeding.

Children: Safety and effectiveness in children have not been established.

Drug Interactions:

Tell your doctor or pharmacist if you are taking or planning to take any over-the-counter or prescription medications or dietary supplements with ipratropium/albuterol. Doses of one or both drugs may need to be modified or a different drug may need to be prescribed. The following drugs and drug classes interact with ipratropium/albuterol:

- anticholinergic agents (eg, flavoxate)
- beta-adrenergic agents (eg, epinephrine)
- beta-receptor blocking agents (eg, propranolol)
- diuretics (eg, thiazides)
- MAOIs (eg, phenelzine)
- tricyclic antidepressants (eg, maprotiline)

Side Effects:

Every drug is capable of producing side effects. Many ipratropium/albuterol users experience no, or minor, side effects. The frequency and severity of side effects depend on many factors including dose, duration of therapy, and individual susceptibility. Possible side effects include:

Digestive Tract: Nausea; vomiting; heartburn; indigestion; taste changes; dry mouth; diarrhea.

Nervous System: Headache; fatigue; sleeplessness; dizziness; nervousness; tremor.

Respiratory System: Runny nose; sore throat; coughing; difficulty breathing; bronchospasm; bronchitis; pneumonia; sinus infection; upper respiratory tract infection; flu-like symptoms; increased mucus.

Circulatory System: Abnormal heart rhythm; pounding in the chest; rapid heartbeat; high blood pressure.

Other: Chest, joint, or general body pain; edema; difficulty speaking; abnormal skin sensations (eg, burning, prickling, tingling); urinary tract infection.

Guidelines for Use:

- Read and follow the patient instructions provided.
- Dosage is individualized. Do not exceed recommended dosage. Take exactly as prescribed.
- Do not stop taking or change the dose unless directed by your doctor.
- Use of a spacing device (eg, *Aerochamber*) will enhance effectiveness and decrease side effects.
- The recommended dose is 2 inhalations 4 times daily, which should last 4 to 5 hours or longer. Do not exceed 12 inhalations in 24 hours.
- Breathe out fully through the mouth, expelling as much air from the lungs as possible. Place the mouthpiece of the inhaler (or spacer) into your mouth and, while breathing deeply and slowly through the mouth, activate the medication canister. Hold your breath for 3 to 5 seconds and then breathe out.
- Wait at least 5 minutes between doses (puffs).
- Contact your doctor immediately if your aerosol becomes less effective, your breathing symptoms become worse, or if you need to use the aerosol more frequently than usual.
- If a dose is missed, inhale it as soon as possible. If several hours have passed or it is nearing time for the next dose, do not double the dose to catch up, unless advised to do so by your doctor. If more than one dose is missed or it is necessary to establish a new dosage schedule, contact your doctor or pharmacist.
- Shake aerosol canister well before each use.
- Test spray 3 times before using the first time or if the aerosol has not been used for longer than 24 hours.
- Contact your doctor if symptoms continue or occur suddenly during therapy.
- Avoid spraying the aerosol into the eyes. Thoroughly wash eyes immediately should this occur. Contact your doctor if you experience blurring vision, eye pain or discomfort, visual halos, or colored images.
- Inform your doctor if you are pregnant, become pregnant, plan on becoming pregnant, or are breastfeeding.
- Do not use actuator with other aerosol medications. Use aerosol canister with the included actuator only.
- Do not take other inhaled drugs during therapy unless advised to do so by your doctor.
- Discard canister after labeled number of actuations have been used. Each canister contains 200 actuations.
- Keep out of the reach of children.
- Aerosol contents are under pressure. Do not puncture canister. Do not use or store near heat or open flame. Exposure to temperatures higher than 120°F may cause bursting. Do not throw canister into a fire or incinerator.
- Store at room temperature (59° to 86°F). Avoid excessive humidity.

If you have any questions, consult your doctor, pharmacist, or health care provider.

Generic Name *Brand Name Examples*	Supplied As	Generic Available
Rx **Acetylcysteine**		
Mucomyst, Mucosil-10	**Solution**: 10%	Yes
Mucomyst, Mucosil-20	**Solution**: 20%	Yes
Rx **Dornase Alfa**		
Pulmozyme	**Solution**: 1 mg/mL	No

Type of Drug:

Respiratory inhalant; drug that thins mucus.

How the Drug Works:

Acetylcysteine decreases the thickness and stickiness of mucus secretions of the lung, making them easier to cough up, and therefore promoting removal (expectoration) of this fluid.

Dornase alfa decreases the thickness and stickiness of mucus secretions of cystic fibrosis patients.

Uses:

Acetylcysteine: To treat abnormally thick mucus secretions in chronic emphysema, emphysema with bronchitis, chronic asthmatic bronchitis, tuberculosis, bronchiectasis (chronic dilation of the airways), pneumonia, bronchitis, tacheobronchitis, cystic fibrosis, and other conditions involving excess mucus accumulation in the lung that is significant enough to affect breathing.

To reduce abnormally thick mucus secretion during tracheostomy care and diagnostic bronchial tests (eg, bronchograms, bronchospirometry, bronchial wedge catheterization).

To reduce abnormally thick mucus secretions during anesthesia in or after surgery or chest injuries.

As an emergency oral antidote drug to decrease liver damage after acetaminophen (eg, *Tylenol)* poisoning.

Dornase alfa: To reduce frequency of respiratory infections requiring parenteral (injectable) antibiotics and to improve pulmonary function in conjunction with standard therapies for patients with cystic fibrosis.

Unlabeled Use(s): Occasionally, doctors may prescribe acetylcysteine as an eye solution to treat severe dry eyes or as an enema to treat bowel obstruction.

Precautions:

Do not use in the following situations: Allergy to acetylcysteine, dornase alfa, Chinese hamster ovary cell products (dornase alfa only), or any other ingredients within the mucolytic.

Use with caution in the following situations:

asthma (eg, bronchospasm) (acetylcysteine only)
inadequate cough reflex (acetylcysteine only)
liver failure (acetylcysteine only)

Prolonged use: Safety and effectiveness of daily administration of dornase alfa for longer than 12 months have not been established.

Pregnancy: There are no adequate or well-controlled studies in pregnant women. Use only if clearly needed and the potential benefits to the mother outweigh the possible hazards to the fetus.

Breastfeeding: It is not known if acetylcysteine or dornase alfa appear in breast milk. Consult your doctor before you begin breastfeeding.

Children: Safety and effectiveness of dornase alfa in children younger than 5 years of age have not been established.

Side Effects:

Every drug is capable of producing side effects. Many mucolytic users experience no, or minor, side effects. The frequency and severity of side effects depend on many factors including dose, duration of therapy, and individual susceptibility. Possible side effects include:

Respiratory System: Increased mucus; runny nose; sore throat; voice changes; voice loss; cough; difficulty breathing; bronchitis; bronchspasm (spasm of the air tubes); chest tightness.

Digestive Tract: Nausea; vomiting; stomach pain; mouth inflammation.

Other: Fever; rash; drowsiness; eye inflammation; clamminess.

Guidelines for Use:

- Dosage is individualized. Take exactly as prescribed.
- Do not stop taking or change the dose unless directed by your doctor.
- If a dose is missed, inhale it as soon as possible. If several hours have passed or it is nearing time for the next dose, do not double the dose to catch up, unless advised to do so by your doctor. If more than one dose is missed or it is necessary to establish a new dosage schedule, contact your doctor or pharmacist.
- Discontinue therapy if symptoms of allergy appear, unless symptoms can be controlled with other drugs and therapy is considered essential.
- Inform your doctor if you are pregnant, become pregnant, plan on becoming pregnant, or are breastfeeding.
- Do not mix other drugs in tho nebulizer unless advised to do so by your doctor.
- Only administer with equipment provided by, or recommended by, your doctor.
- *Acetylcysteine* — Follow dilution and administration techniques taught by your doctor.
  When used to treat acetaminophen poisoning, it will be prepared and administered by a health care professional in a medical setting.
  May produce an increased volume of liquified secretions that must be coughed up. Notify your doctor if you have difficulty coughing up these secretions.
  May initially produce a slight disagreeable odor which soon disappears.
  May cause a stickiness on the face after nebulization with a face mask. This can be easily removed by washing with water.
  Color of the solution may change in the opened bottle, but the light purple color does not significantly reduce the drug's safety or effectiveness if used within 96 hours after opening.
  The 20% solution may be diluted with either Normal Saline, Water for Injection, or Sterile Water for inhalation. The 10% solution may be used undiluted.
  Continued nebulization of acetylcysteine with a dry gas results in concentration of the drug in the nebulizer due to evaporation. This may reduce nebulization and drug delivery. Dilute with Sterile Water for Injection as concentration occurs.
  Store unopened vial at controlled room temperature (59° to 86°F). Store unused portion in refrigerator once opened and use within 96 hours.
- *Dornase alfa* — The recommended dose is one 2.5 mg single-use ampule inhaled once daily using a recommended nebulizer. Some patients may benefit from twice daily administration. Use in conjunction with standard therapies for cystic fibrosis.
  Discard solution if it is cloudy or discolored. Dornase alfa contains no preservatives; therefore, once opened, the entire ampule must be used or discarded.
  Do not dilute or mix dornase with other drugs in the nebulizer.
  Store in protective foil pouch under refrigeration (36° to 46°F). Protect from light. Do not use beyond the expiration date.

If you have any questions, consult your doctor, pharmacist, or health care provider.

Generic Name *Brand Name Example*	Supplied As	Generic Available
Rx **Nedocromil Sodium**		
Tilade	**Aerosol:** 1.75 mg/actuation	No

Type of Drug:

Respiratory inhalant.

How the Drug Works:

Nedocromil sodium inhibits the activity of inflammatory cells associated with asthma.

Uses:

As maintenance therapy in the management of mild to moderate bronchial asthma. Nedocromil sodium is not used to reverse acute bronchospasm.

Precautions:

Do not use in the following situations: Allergy to nedocromil sodium or any ingredient in the product.

Pregnancy: Adequate studies have not been done in pregnant women. Use only if clearly needed and potential benefits outweigh the possible hazards to the fetus.

Breastfeeding: It is not known if nedocromil sodium appears in breast milk. Consult your doctor before you begin breastfeeding.

Children: Safety and effectiveness in children under 12 have not been established.

Side Effects:

Every drug is capable of producing side effects. Many nedocromil sodium users experience no, or minor, side effects. The frequency and severity of side effects depend on many factors including dose, duration of therapy and individual susceptibility. Possible side effects include:

Digestive Tract: Nausea; vomiting; indigestion; diarrhea; stomach pain.

Nervous System: Dizziness; headache; fatigue; difficulty speaking.

Respiratory System: Coughing; sore throat; congestion; upper respiratory tract infection; increased sputum; bronchitis; difficulty breathing; wheezing.

Other: Dry mouth; chest pain; viral infection; unpleasant taste.

Guidelines for Use:

- Proper inhalation technique is very important. Follow the directions that are in the patient information leaflet that is included with the medicine.
- Use continuously. Effectiveness depends on regularity of use, even during symptom-free periods.
- Notify your doctor if coughing or wheezing occurs.
- Not for the treatment of an existing asthma attack. Nedocromil sodium should generally be continued during an asthma attack though, unless intolerance develops.
- This medicine should be added to your existing treatment therapy. Once a positive response is made to the inhaler, and the asthma is undor good control, your doctor may gradually reduce your other medicine usage.

If you have any questions, consult your doctor, pharmacist, or health care provider.

	Generic Name *Brand Name Examples*	Supplied As	Generic Available
Rx	**Beclomethasone Dipropionate**		
	Beconase Inhalation, Vancenase Nasal Inhaler	**Aerosol**: 42 mcg/actuation	No
	Beconase AQ Nasal Vancenase AQ Nasal	**Spray**: 42 mcg/actuation	No
	Vancenase AQ 84 Nasal	**Spray**: 84 mcg/actuation	No
Rx	**Budesonide**		
	Rhinocort	**Aerosol**: 32 mcg/actuation	No
Rx	**Flunisolide**		
	Nasalide	**Spray**: 25 mcg/actuation	No
Rx	**Fluticasone Propionate**		
	Flonase	**Spray**: 50 mcg/actuation	No
Rx	**Mometasone Furoate**		
	Nasonex[1]	**Spray**: 50 mcg/actuation (monohydrate)	No
Rx	**Triamcinolone Acetonide**		
	Nasacort[1]	**Aerosol**: 55 mcg/actuation	No
	Nasacort AQ	**Spray**: 55 mcg/actuation	No

[1] Contains alcohol.

Type of Drug:

Nasal corticosteroids; anti-inflammatory agents.

How the Drug Works:

Intranasal steroids for inhalation shrink swollen and irritated nasal tissue by reducing inflammation.

Uses:

To relieve nasal symptoms of seasonal or perennial allergic rhinitis (eg, hay fever) which involves inflammation of the mucous membranes of the nasal passages. Symptoms of allergic rhinitis include itching, runny nose, postnasal drip, nasal congestion and sneezing.

Budesonide and beclomethasone (spray): Also used to treat nonallergic perennial rhinitis in adults.

Beclomethasone: Also used to prevent the recurrence of nasal polyps after surgical removal.

Precautions:

Do not use in the following situations:

allergy to the drug or any ingredient in the formulation
untreated infection of the nasal mucous membranes

Use with caution in the following situations:

children (growth suppression), extended use
chickenpox, exposure
herpes infection, in the eye
immunosuppressant therapy (eg, prednisone, methotrexate)
infections (fungal, bacterial or viral), untreated
inhaled glucocorticoids, use
lesions (sores, injuries) in nasal tissue (eg, nasal surgery, frequent nosebleed)
measles, exposure
stress, related to adrenal insufficiency
tuberculosis, active or inactive

Changing from other dosage forms: Patients on long-term oral corticosteroids may lose their body's natural ability to produce corticosteroid hormones. Switching or lessening current doses may cause symptoms of withdrawal (eg, joint or muscle pain, tiredness, depression). Therefore, taper dosage of oral steroid gradually and only with the instruction of a doctor.

Nasal decongestants: In the presence of excessive nasal congestion, the drug may fail to reach the site of intended action. In such cases, use a nasal decongestant spray just before use during the first 2 to 3 days of therapy. Do not use a nasal decongestant spray for more than 3 consecutive days.

Intranasal Steroids are absorbed into the circulation system. Using higher than recommended doses may interfere with normal adrenal functions.

Pregnancy: Adequate studies have not been done in pregnant women. Use only if clearly needed and potential benefits outweigh the possible hazards to the fetus.

Breastfeeding: It is not known whether these drugs are excreted in breast milk. Other corticosteroids do appear in breast milk. Consult your doctor before you begin breastfeeding.

Children: Safety and effectiveness in children under 12 years of age *(mometasone)* under 6 years of age *(beclomethasone, budesonide, flunisolide, triamcinolone)* or under 4 years of age *(fluticasone)* have not been established. Use is not recommended. May suppress growth in children and teenagers with extended use.

Side Effects:

Every drug is capable of producing side effects. Many intranasal steroid users experience no, or minor, side effects. The frequency and severity of side effects depend on many factors including dose, duration of therapy and individual susceptibility. Possible side effects include:

Respiratory System: Nasal or throat irritation; stinging; burning; dryness; nosebleed; runny nose; sneezing (especially in children); blood in nasal mucus; congestion; asthma; increased cough; sore throat; thrush or sores in nose or throat.

Other: Headache; lightheadedness; dizziness; hives; nausea; vomiting; dry mouth; indigestion; joint or muscle pain; weakness; depression; watery eyes; eye disorders; taste changes; earache; ringing in ears; diarrhea; painful menstruation; fever.

Guidelines for Use:

- Dosage is individualized. Take exactly as prescribed.
- Do not change the dose or stop taking before consulting your doctor. Do not exceed recommended dosage.
- Read and follow patient instructions provided with these products.
- If a dose is missed, take it as soon as possible. If several hours have passed or it is nearing time for the next dose, do not double the dose to catch up, unless advised by your doctor. If more than one dose is missed, or it is necessary to establish a new dosage schedule, contact your doctor or pharmacist.
- Effects are not immediate. Product requires daily use, and improvement usually occurs in a few days. Improvement time varies with each patient. Consult your doctor if condition does not improve or worsens after 3 weeks of daily use.
- May cause irritation and drying of nasal mucosa. Contact physician if symptoms do not improve or the condition worsens.
- Report any unusual fever, muscle/joint pain, weakness, sneezing, dizziness, nasal irritation, depression, or fluid retention to your doctor.
- Use with caution in patients with infections (fungal, bacterial, or viral), lesions/sores in the nasal tissues (eg, nasal surgery, frequent nosebleeds), herpes infections near the eye, or tuberculosis (active or inactive).

Guidelines for Use (cont.):

- Clear nasal passages prior to use by blowing the nose. If nasal passages are congested or blocked, use a decongestant nasal spray just before use to ensure adequate penetration of the spray. Do not use the decongestant nasal spray for more than 3 consecutive days.
- Clean outer portion of the nose with a damp tissue and wash hands with soap and water after drug administration.
- Infection of the nose and throat by a fungus *(Candida albicans)* has been associated with chronic use. Such infection (thrush) may require stopping the intranasal steroid to treat the infection.
- Avoid exposure to chickenpox, measles, or other infections. Consult your doctor immediately if exposed.
- *Nasal polyps* — Treatment may have to be continued for several weeks or more before results can be fully assessed. Recurrence of symptoms due to polyps can occur after stopping treatment, depending on the severity of the disease.
- Inform your doctor if you are pregnant, become pregnant, planning to become pregnant, or are breastfeeding before beginning therapy.
- Lab tests may be necessary if using this medicine for several months. Be sure to keep appointments.
- *Beclomethasone* — Shake well before using. Beneficial effects may decrease when the aerosol canister is cold. This medicine comes in different strengths and dosage forms. Products and use may not be interchangeable.
- *Budesonide* — Store with valve upward. Shake well before use. After opening aluminum pouch, use within 6 months. Avoid storage in areas of high humidity.
- *Flunisolide* — After the desired effect is obtained, reduce the maintenance dose to the smallest amount necessary to control the symptoms.
- *Fluticasone* — Shake gently before use. Do not exceed more than 2 sprays per nostril per day. Adolescents/children should start at one spray per nostril per day.
- *Mometasone* — Shake well before using. In patients with known seasonal allergies, preventive use is recommended 2 to 4 weeks prior to the start of pollen season. Store at a temperature of 36° to 77°F. Keep away from light and moisture.
- Store at room temperature (59° to 86°F) in a dry place (except mometasone).

If you have any questions, consult your doctor, pharmacist, or health care provider.

	Generic Name *Brand Name Examples*	Supplied As	Generic Available
Rx	**Azatadine Maleate**		
	Optimine[1]	**Tablets**: 1 mg	No
Rx	**Azelastine**		
	Astelin	**Nasal spray**: 137 mcg/spray	No
Rx	**Cetirizine HCl**		
	Zyrtec	**Tablets**: 5 mg, 10 mg	No
	Zyrtec	**Syrup**: 5 mg/5 mL	No
	Chlorpheniramine Maleate		
otc	*Chlo-Amine*	**Tablets, chewable**: 2 mg	No
otc	*Allergy*[1]	**Tablets**: 4 mg	Yes
otc	*Chlor-Trimeton Allergy 8-Hour, Chlor-Trimeton Allergy 12-Hour, Efidac 24*	**Tablets, extended release**: 8 mg, 12 mg, 16 mg	Yes
	Clemastine Fumarate		
otc	*Antihist-1*[1], *Dayhist-1*[1], *Tavist Allergy*[1]	**Tablets**: 1.34 mg	Yes
Rx	*Tavist*[1]	**Tablets**: 2.68 mg	Yes
otc	*Aller-Chlor, Chlor-Trimeton*	**Syrup**: 0.5mg/5 mL	Yes
Rx	**Cyproheptadine HCl**		
	Periactin[1]	**Tablets**: 4 mg	Yes
	Periactin[2]	**Syrup**: 2 mg/5 mL	Yes
Rx	**Dexchlorpheniramine Maleate**		
	Polaramine[1]	**Tablets**: 2 mg	No
	Polaramine Repetabs	**Tablets, timed release**: 4 mg, 6 mg	Yes
	Polaramine[2]	**Syrup**: 2 mg/5 mL	Yes

	Generic Name *Brand Name Examples*	Supplied As	Generic Available
	Diphenhydramine HCl		
otc	*Banophen*[1], *Banophen Softgels, Benadryl Dye Free Allergy Liqui-Gels, Complete Allergy Relief, Diphen, Diphenhist*[1], *Genahist*[1]	**Capsules**: 25 mg, 50 mg	Yes
Rx	*Diphenhydramine HCl*	**Capsules**: 25 mg, 50 mg	Yes
otc	*AllerMax*[1], *Banophen, Benadryl Allergy Ultratab, Diphenhist Caplabs*[1]	**Tablets**: 25 mg, 50 mg	Yes
otc	*Benadryl Allergy*[3]	**Tablets, chewable**: 12.5 mg	No
otc	*AllerMax Allergy and Cough Formula*[2], *Banophen Allergy, Benadryl Allergy*, Benadryl Dye-Free Allergy, *Diphen AF, Genahist, Scot-Tussin Allergy*	**Liquid**: 6.25 mg/5 mL, 12.5 mg/5 mL	No
otc	*Diphen Cough*[2], *Diphenhist*[2], *Hydramine Cough*[2]	**Syrup**: 12.5 mg/5 mL	Yes
Rx	*Benadryl, Hyrexin-50*	**Injection**: 50 mg/mL	Yes
Rx	**Fexofenadine HCl**		
	Allegra	**Tablets**: 30 mg, 60 mg, 180 mg	No
	Allegra[1]	**Capsules**: 60 mg	No
Rx	**Hydroxyzine**		
	Atarax[1]	**Tablets**: 10 mg, 25 mg, 50 mg (as HCl)	Yes
	Atarax 100[1]	**Tablets**: 100 mg (as HCl)	No
	Atarax[1]	**Syrup**: 10 mg/5 mL (as HCl)	Yes
	Vistaril	**Capsules**: 25 mg, 50 mg, 100 mg (as pamoate)	Yes
	Vistaril	**Suspension, oral**: 25 mg/5 mL (as pamoate)	No
	Vistaril	**Injection**: 25 mg/mL, 50 mg/mL (as HCl)	No

	Generic Name *Brand Name Examples*	Supplied As	Generic Available
Rx	**Loratadine**		
	Claritin[1]	**Tablets**: 10 mg	No
	Claritin	**Syrup**: 1 mg/mL	No
	Claritin Reditabs	**Tablets, rapidly disintegrating**: 10 mg	No
otc	**Phenindamine Tartrate**		
	Nolahist	**Tablets**: 25 mg	No
Rx	**Promethazine HCl**		
	Phenergan[1]	**Tablets**: 12.5 mg, 25 mg, 50 mg	Yes
	Phenergan Plain,[2] *Phenergan Fortis*[2]	**Syrup**: 6.25 mg/5 mL, 25 mg/5 mL	Yes
	Phenergan	**Suppositories**: 12.5 mg, 25 mg, 50 mg	Yes
	Phenergan[4]	**Injection**: 25 mg/mL, 50 mg/mL	Yes

[1] Contains lactose.
[2] Contains alcohol.
[3] Contains aspartame.
[4] Contains sulfites.

Type of Drug:

Antihistamine; allergy medications.

How the Drug Works:

Antihistamines block the effects of histamine at H_1 receptors in the body. Histamine is one of the chemicals released in the body during an allergic reaction. It causes redness, itching, and irritation of respiratory mucosal tissues, and can cause watery eyes, runny nose, sneezing, itchy nose, eyes, palate, and throat, and hives.

Uses:

To provide relief of symptoms associated with seasonal and year-round allergies causing runny nose, sneezing, itching of the nose or throat, or watery, itchy eyes; hives; and rash, insect bites, and stings where there is mild to moderate itching and no complications.

Certizine and fexofenadine: To treat chronic idiopathic urticaria (hives).

Diphenhydramine: To treat or prevent motion sickness, sleeplessness, and parkinsonism. Also used as a suppressant for coughs caused by colds or allergies.

Promethazine: To treat or prevent motion sickness, nausea, and vomiting associated with anesthesia and surgery, apprehension, and sleeplessness. Used with pain medication (eg, meperidine) to help control pain following surgery.

Unlabeled Use(s): Occasionally doctors may prescribe cyproheptadine to stimulate appetite in underweight people (eg, anorexia nervosa) and to treat cluster headaches.

Precautions:

Do not use in the following situations:

alcohol and other depressants (eg, tranquilizers)
allergy to antihistamines
anesthesia, local
bone marrow depression
breastfeeding
digestive tract obstruction
enlarged prostate
glaucoma, narrow angle
liver disease
MAOI use, concurrent
newborns or premature infants
peptic ulcer
ulcers (promethazine only)
urinary bladder obstruction

Use with caution in the following situations:

asthma
hypertension (high blood pressure)
hyperthyroidism (overactive thyroid)
increased pressure in the eye
kidney disease
liver disease
pregnancy
seizures (promethazine only)

Pregnancy: Safety for use during pregnancy has not been established. Several possible associations with malformations have been found, but significance is unknown. Use only when clearly needed and the potential benefits outweigh the possible hazards to the fetus. Do not use during the third trimester; newborns and premature infants may have severe reactions (eg, convulsions) to some antihistamines.

Breastfeeding: Antihistamines appear in breast milk. Breastfeeding should be discouraged while taking these medications, or antihistamines should be avoided during the breastfeeding months.

Children: Antihistamine overdosage in children may cause hallucinations, convulsions, or death. Antihistamines may decrease mental alertness or produce hyperactivity in young children. Consult your pharmacist or product label to determine the appropriate dose of nonprescription drugs to be given to children younger than 12 years of age. Do not give prescription antihistamines to children younger than 12 years of age unless advised by your doctor or approved in the package labeling.

Elderly: Elderly patients may require lower doses. Antihistamines are more likely to cause dizziness, sedation, confusion, disorientation, fainting, excitation, and decreased blood pressure.

Drug Interactions:

Tell your doctor or pharmacist if you are taking or planning to take any over-the-counter or prescription medications or dietary supplements while taking antihistamines. Doses of one or both drugs may need to be modified or a different drug may need to be prescribed. Alcohol, sedatives (sleeping pills), tranquilizers, antianxiety medications, and narcotic pain relievers all are known to interact with antihistamines. The following drugs and drug classes also interact antihistamines:

aluminum- and magnesium-containing antacids (eg, *Maalox*)
anesthesia (promethazine only)
barbiturates (promethazine only)
cimetidine (azelastine only)
epinephrine (eg, *Adrenalin)*
erythromycin (eg, *E-Mycin*) (fexofenadine only)
ketoconazole (eg, *Nizoral*)
MAOIs (eg, phenelzine)
tricyclic antidepressants (eg, *Elavil*)

Side Effects:

Every drug is capable of producing side effects. Many antihistamine users experience no, or minor, side effects. The frequency and severity of side effects depend on many factors including dose, duration of therapy, and individual susceptibility. Possible side effects include:

Digestive Tract: Stomachache; constipation; appetite changes; nausea; vomiting; diarrhea; indigestion; decreased salivation; gas; altered sense of taste; dry mouth.

Nervous System: Drowsiness; dizziness; confusion; disorientation; nervousness; restlessness; excitation; tremor; decreased coordination; fatigue; headache; sleeplessness; sedation; irritability; exaggerated sense of well being; fainting; migraine; abnormal skin sensations; feeling of whirling motion; impaired concentration; hallucination; hysteria; amnesia; abnormal thinking; agitation; anxiety; depersonalization; depression; convulsions.

Circulatory System: Changes in blood pressure; irregular heartbeat; fast heartbeat; shock; palpitations (pounding in the chest); chest pain.

Respiratory System: Dry nose and throat; cough; sore throat; thickening of mucus in respiratory tract; chest tightness; wheezing; nasal stuffiness; hyperventilation; upper respiratory tract infection; laryngitis; bronchospasm; nasal and throat burning; nosebleed; difficulty breathing; sneezing.

Skin: Rash; hives; sweating; itching; flushing; dry skin; excessively oily skin; skin inflammation; red or purple patches under the skin; acne; excessive sweating; hair loss.

Other: Weight gain; joint pain; muscle pain; sensitivity to light; frequent, abnormal, or difficult urination; urine retention; ringing in the ears; blurred or double vision; itchy, watery eyes; yellowing of skin or eyes; chills; painful menstruation (loratadine and fexofenadine only); thirst; earache; fever; leg cramps; weakness; decreased sensitivity to stimulation; eye pain or abnormality; altered tearing; twitching eyes; tight muscles; breast pain; heavy menstruation; allergic reaction; back pain; "flu-like" symptoms; general body discomfort; pain in extremities; twitching; decreased sex drive; excessive movement; inflammation of the vagina with itching or abnormal discharge; urinary discoloration; distorted sense of smell; hot flashes; anemia.

Guidelines for Use:

- Dosage is individualized. Use exacty as prescribed.
- If a dose is missed, take it as soon as possible. If several hours have passed or it is nearing time for the next dose, do not double the dose to catch up, unless advised by your doctor. If more than one dose is missed or it is necessary to establish a new dosage schedule, contact your doctor or pharmacist.
- Loratadine tablets and syrup should be taken once daily on an empty stomach (1 hour before or 2 hours after a meal). Loratadine rapidly-disintegrating tablets break down quickly after being placed on the tongue; they may be given with or without water.
- Do not crush or chew sustained-release preparations.
- May cause drowsiness or dizziness. Avoid alcohol and other sedatives (eg, tranquilizers). Chlorpheniramine, loratadine, cetirizine, and fexofenadine cause the least amount of drowsiness; promethazine and diphenhydramine cause the most. Use caution while driving or performing tasks requiring alertness, coordination, or physical dexterity.
- *Promethazine* — Report any involuntary muscle movements or unusual sensitivity to sunlight.
- Use alone when sneezing and runny nose exist, but nasal congestion is slight. When nasal congestion accompanies sneezing and runny nose, an oral decongestant (eg, pseudoephedrine) may be added.
- Avoid therapy with combination products containing antihistamines, decongestants, anticholinergics, expectorants, pain medication, cough suppressants, caffeine, and vitamins. Deal with symptoms as specifically as possible. Combination products frequently contain some ingredients in ineffective amounts. They also increase risk for side effects and drug interactions. They usually cost more than products with fewer ingredients.
- A persistent cough may be a sign of a serious condition. Contact your doctor if cough persists for more than 1 week, tends to recur, or is accompanied by a high fever, rash, or persistent headache.
- Do not take antihistamines for persistent or chronic cough, such as occurs with smoking, asthma, or emphysema or if cough is accompanied by excessive phlegm, unless directed by a doctor. Cough is a protective reflex that helps clear the respiratory tract of mucus and other debris.
- Do not take for 7 days before allergy skin testing.
- If fainting, dizziness, unusual heartbeats, stomach pain, chest pain, vomiting, or any other unusual symptoms occur, contact your doctor immediately.
- If sleeplessness persists continuously for more than 2 weeks, consult your doctor.
- If the medication loses effectiveness with continued use, make sure you are taking it according to directions. Sometimes, loss of effectiveness indicates that your condition has gotten worse. Treatment may require a different medication or dose.

Guidelines for Use (cont.):

- May rarely cause photosensitivity (sensitivity to sunlight). Avoid prolonged exposure to the sun or other forms of ultraviolet (UV) light (eg, tanning beds). Use sunscreens and wear protective clothing until tolerance is determined.
- *Azelastine* — Prime the nasal spray delivery system before initial use and after storage for 3 or more days. Avoid spraying in the eyes.
- Store at room temperature (59° to 77°F) in a tightly closed container. Protect from heat, light, and moisture. Keep away from children.
- *Suppositories and some syrups* — Store in the refrigerator (36° to 46°F) in a tightly closed container. See individual labels for specific storage information.

If you have any questions, consult your doctor, pharmacist, or health care provider.

	Generic Name / *Brand Name Examples*	Supplied As	Generic Available
otc	**Ephedrine Sulfate**		
	Pretz-D	**Solution (nasal spray)**: 0.25%	No
Rx	**Epinephrine HCl**		
	Adrenalin Chloride[1]	**Solution**: 0.1%	No
otc	**Naphazoline HCl**		
	Privine	**Solution (nasal spray and drops)**: 0.05%	No
otc	**Oxymetazoline HCl**		
	Afrin, Dristan 12-hr, Duramist Plus 12 Hour, Genasal, Neo-Synephrine 12-Hour, Nōstrilla 12 Hour, Twice-A-Day 12 Hour, Vicks Sinex 12 Hour	**Solution (nasal spray)**: 0.05%	Yes
	Phenylephrine HCl		
Rx	*AH-chew D*	**Tablets, chewable**: 10 mg	No
otc	*Neo-Synephrine Extra Strength, Neo-Synephrine Mild Formula, Neo-Synephrine Regular Strength, Vicks Sinex*	**Solution (nasal spray)**: 0.25%, 0.5%, 1%	Yes
otc	*Neo-Synephrine Extra Strength, Neo-Synephrine Regular Strength, Rhinall*[1]*, Tur-bi-kal*	**Solution (nasal drops)**: 0.17%, 0.5%, 1%	No
	Pseudoephedrine HCl	**Syrup**: 30 mg/5 mL	Yes
otc	*Genaphed, Sudafed, SudoGest*	**Tablets**: 30 mg, 60 mg	Yes
otc	*Sudafed 12 Hour*	**Tablets, extended release:** 120 mg	No
otc	*Efidac 24*	**Tablets, extended release**: 240 mg	No
otc	*Sinustop*	**Capsules**: 60 mg	No
otc	*Children's Sudafed, Triaminic AM Decongestant*	**Liquid**: 15 mg/5 mL	Yes
otc	*PediaCare Infants' Decongestant, Triaminic Infant Decongestant*	**Drops, oral**: 7.5 mg/0.8 mL	No

	Generic Name *Brand Name Examples*	Supplied As	Generic Available
otc	**Pseudoephedrine Sulfate**		
	Drixoral	**Tablets, extended release**: 120 mg	No
Rx	**Tetrahydrozoline HCl**		
	Tyzine Pediatric	**Solution (nasal drops)**: 0.05%	No
	Tyzine	**Solution (nasal drops and spray)**: 0.1%	No
otc	**Xylometazoline HCl**		
	Otrivin Pediatric	**Solution (nasal drops)**: 0.05%	No
	Otrivin	**Solution (nasal spray)**: 0.1%	No

[1] Contains sulfites.

Type of Drug:

Nasal decongestants.

How the Drug Works:

Nasal decongestants shrink swollen and congested nasal tissues (mucous membranes) by constricting blood vessels. This should relieve congestion (stuffy feeling), promote drainage of mucus, relieve the stuffy feeling, and improve breathing. Local application (eg, nasal drops, sprays) causes more intense rapid nasal vasoconstriction than oral drugs (eg, tablets, syrup).

Uses:

To treat nasal congestion due to the common cold, hay fever, sinusitis, and other upper respiratory allergies.

To treat eustachian tube congestion (plugged ears).

To promote nasal or sinus drainage.

To relieve air block and pressure pain in air travel.

Precautions:

Do not use in the following situations:

allergy to the decongestant or any of its ingredients
breastfeeding (oral agents only)
coronary artery disease (oral agents only)
glaucoma (topical naphazoline only)
high blood pressure, severe (oral agents only)
MAOI (eg, phenelzine) use, current or within the previous 14 days
pregnancy (phenylephrine chewable tablets)

Use with caution in the following situations:

angina (chest pain)
bowel obstruction or narrowing (pseudoephedrine extended-release only)
diabetes mellitus
dizziness with previous use
elderly
glaucoma (increase in intraocular pressure)
heart disease
high blood pressure
hyperthyroidism (overactive thyroid)
insomnia (sleeplessness) with previous use
irregular heartbeat with previous use
prostatic hypertrophy (enlarged prostate)
weakness with previous use

Excessive use: Excessive use of topical decongestants may cause side effects (eg, nervousness, dizziness, sleeplessness) that are more likely in infants and in the elderly. Long-term high-dose therapy may be habit forming (ie, rebound congestion).

Hypertension (high blood pressure): Use these products only with medical advice. You may experience a change in blood pressure because of the increased narrowing of the blood vessels.

Rebound congestion: Rebound congestion (rhinitis medicamentosa) following several days of regular topical application may occur. Rebound congestion, which is worse than the original symptoms, occurs when the dose wears off. Increasing the amount of drug or frequency of use only perpetuates rebound congestion and increases the risks of medication toxicity. Talk to your doctor or pharmacist if congestion continues to return when the drug effect wears off.

Treatment for rebound congestion: A simple but uncomfortable solution is to completely withdraw the topical medication. A more acceptable method is to gradually withdraw therapy by discontinuing the medication in one nostril, followed by total withdrawal. Substituting an oral decongestant for a topical one also may be useful.

Sulfite sensitivity: Some of these products contains sulfites that may cause allergic-type reactions in certain individuals. Check package label when available or consult your doctor or pharmacist.

Pregnancy: There are no adequate and well-controlled studies in pregnant women. Use only if clearly needed and the potential benefits to the mother outweigh the possible hazards to the fetus.

Breastfeeding: Consult your doctor before taking an oral decongestant while breastfeeding. It is not known if topical decongestants appear in breast milk. Use caution when administering to a nursing woman.

Children: Dosage restrictions may vary according to product instructions; refer to individual product information for dosage and administration.

Elderly: Patients 60 years and older are more likely to experience side effects. Overdosage may cause hallucinations, convulsions, depression, and death.

Drug Interactions:

Tell your doctor or pharmacist if you are taking or planning to take any over-the-counter or prescription medications or dietary supplements with decongestants. Doses of one or both drugs may need to be modified or a different drug may need to be prescribed. The following drugs and drug classes interact with decongestants:

- furazolidone *(Furoxone)*
- guanethidine (eg, *Ismelin*)
- MAOIs (eg, phenelzine)
- methyldopa (eg, *Aldomet*)
- rauwolfia alkaloids (eg, reserpine)
- tricyclic antidepressants (eg, amitriptyline)

Side Effects:

Every drug is capable of producing side effects. Many nasal decongestant users experience no, or minor, side effects. The frequency and severity of side effects depend on many factors including dose, duration of therapy, individual susceptibility, and method of administration. Side effects are more likely to occur with oral nasal decongestants. Oral agents, however, cause less local irritation and are not associated with rebound congestion (rhinitis medicamentosa). Possible side effects include:

Digestive Tract: Nausea; vomiting; appetite loss; stomachache.

Nervous System: Anxiety; restlessness; tremor; CNS depression; weakness; tenseness; headache; dizziness; drowsiness; sleeplessness; lightheadedness; nervousness.

Circulatory System: Irregular heartbeat; changes in blood pressure; palpitations (pounding in the chest).

Other: Sweating; pallor; chest pain; eye sensitivity to light; painful or difficult urination. *Topical Use:* Burning; stinging; sneezing; dryness; local irritation; rebound congestion; nasal discharge; rash; hives; weakness.

Guidelines for Use:

- Dosage is individualized. Take exactly as prescribed.
- Do not exceed recommended dosage.
- Patients with high blood pressure or other cardiovascular diseases, thyroid disease, glaucoma, diabetes mellitus, or enlarged prostate should use these products only with medical advice.
- To prevent pressure pain in air travel or other situations where there is a rapid change in altitude, nose drops and nasal sprays act quickly. Take oral dosage forms 1 to 2 hours prior to a major altitude change.
- Side effects are most likely in the elderly and children. Excessive use (misuse) increases risk for side effects.
- Contact your doctor if you experience persistent stomach pain or vomiting.
- *Oral* — If symptoms do not improve within 7 days or are accompanied by a high fever, consult your doctor before continuing use. Do not exceed recommended dosage. Higher doses may cause nervousness, irregular heartbeat, dizziness, or sleeplessness. If these occur, stop use and contact your doctor. Do not divide, dissolve, crush, or chew extended-release preparations.
- *Topical* — Notify your doctor if you experience sleeplessness, dizziness, weakness, tremor, or irregular heartbeat. Do not exceed recommended dosage and do not use longer than 3 to 5 days. Stinging or burning sensations or drying of the nose may occur. This often disappears after a few applications. If rebound congestion occurs from excessive doses and frequent use, withdraw the topical drug gradually. Stop using the medication in one nostril, then both nostrils. An oral decongestant may be used. Notify your doctor if symptoms persist.
- *Nasal spray* — Inhale through each nostril while blocking off other nostril. Use only as needed. Avoid excessive use. Hold head upright, insert nozzle into nostril, spray quickly and firmly and sniff deeply. Wipe nozzle clean after use.
- *Nasal drops* — Recline on a bed and hang your head over the edge. Remain in this position for several minutes after using the drops, turning your head from side to side.
- Use of nasal spray or drops by more than 1 person may spread infection.

If you have any questions, consult your doctor, pharmacist, or health care provider.

	Generic Name	Supplied As	Generic Available
C-II	**Codeine Sulfate**	**Tablets**: 15 mg, 30 mg, 60 mg	Yes
C-II	**Codeine Phosphate**	**Tablets, soluble**: 30 mg, 60 mg	Yes
		Oral solution: 15 mg	Yes
		Injection: 30 mg/mL, 60 mg/mL	Yes

Cough is a normal, protective reflex. It helps clear mucus, irritants, and other foreign matter from the throat, trachea, and lungs. Caution is advised in attempting to suppress a productive cough (mucus is coughed up). If mucus is not removed from the lungs, it may support growth of bacteria and make breathing more difficult. Moderate cough suppression may be used to reduce discomfort and allow sleep, but do not attempt to completely suppress a productive cough.

The dry, nonproductive cough is a good candidate for therapeutic cough suppression, although increased fluid intake is also appropriate to help produce a productive cough. If such coughs are persistent, bothersome, or sleep disrupting, they may respond well to treatment with codeine.

Type of Drug:

Cough medicine; cough suppressant; narcotic analgesic (pain reliever).

How the Drug Works:

Codeine suppresses the "cough center" in the brain. The dose required to suppress coughing is lower than the dose required for pain relief. The risk of dependence is slight if taken as directed.

Uses:

To suppress cough induced by irritation of the respiratory tract. To relieve mild to moderate pain.

Precautions:

Do not use in the following situations:

allergy to codeine or any of its ingredients
during labor, premature
premature infants

Use with caution in the following situations:

abdominal conditions, acute (undiagnosed)
Addison disease
asthma attack
bronchitis, chronic
convulsive disorders
cough, persistent (10 days)
emphysema
enlarged prostate
fever
gastrointestinal or urinary tract surgery, recent
head injury
hypothyroidism (underactive thyroid)
kidney disease
liver disease
respiratory tract diseases
urethra, abnormally narrow
ulcers

Pregnancy: There are no adequate and well-controlled studies in pregnant women. Use only if clearly needed and the potential benefits to the mother outweigh the possible hazards to the fetus. Dependence has been reported in newborns whose mothers took narcotics regularly during pregnancy.

Breastfeeding: Codeine appears in breast milk. Consult your doctor before you begin breastfeeding.

Children: Give to infants and small children only with great caution and carefully monitor dosage. Safety and effectiveness in newborn infants have not been established.

Elderly: Use with caution in elderly patients.

Drug Interactions:

Tell your doctor or pharmacist if you are taking or planning to take any over-the-counter or prescription medications or dietary supplements with codeine. Doses of one or both drugs may need to be modified or a different drug may need to be prescribed. Drugs which have central nervous system depressant activity have additive effects when given with codeine. The following drugs are examples of such agents.

alcohol
anesthetics, general (eg, methohexital)
benzodiazepines (eg, diazepam)
phenothiazines (eg, chlorpromazine)
tricyclic antidepressants (eg, amitriptyline)

Consider all drug interactions reported for narcotic pain relievers (see Analgesics - Narcotic Pain Relievers in the CNS Drugs chapter) when using codeine.

Side Effects:

Every drug is capable of producing side effects. Many codeine users experience no, or minor, side effects. The frequency and severity of side effects depend on many factors including dose, duration of therapy, and individual susceptibility. Possible side effects include:

Nervous System: Sedation; hallucinations; headache; convulsions; euphoria; dizziness; weakness; disorientation; lightheadedness; nervous system depression; shock; restlessness.

Circulatory System: Irregular heartbeat; palpitations (pounding heart); circulatory depression; cardiac arrest.

Other: Dependency; urine retention; infrequent urination; allergic reaction (eg, itching, hives, rash); respiratory arrest; fainting; visual disturbances; nausea; vomiting; constipation; biliary tract spasm. Consider all side effects reported for narcotic pain relievers (see Analgesics - Narcotic Pain Relievers in the CNS Drugs chapter) when using codeine.

Guidelines for Use:

- May cause stomach upset. Take with food or milk.
- Do not exceed recommended daily dose.
- May impair mental or physical ability. Use caution when driving or performing other tasks requiring alertness. Use of alcohol, sedatives, hypnotics, tranquilizers, promethazine, and antihistamines may have an additive effect.
- *Injection* — Visually inspect for particulate matter and discoloration prior to administration. Do not use if solution is discolored or contains precipitate.
- May produce orthostatic hypotension (dizziness or lightheadedness when rising from a standing or lying position), dry mouth, and constipation in some patients.
- Do not take for persistent or chronic cough, such as occurs with smoking, asthma, or emphysema, or where cough is accompanied by mucus (productive cough) except under supervision of your doctor. Consult your doctor regarding use of a cough suppressant.
- If a cough continues beyond 7 to 10 days or is accompanied by a fever, consult your doctor.

If you have any questions, consult your doctor, pharmacist, or health care provider.

	Generic Name *Brand Name Examples*	Supplied As	Generic Available
Rx	**Benzonatate**		
	Tessalon Perles	**Capsules:** 100 mg	No
otc	**Dextromethorphan HBr**		
	Hold DM, Scot-Tussin DM Cough Chasers, Sucrets 4-hour Cough Suppressant	**Lozenges:** 2.5 mg, 5 mg	No
	Benylin, Benylin Pediatric, Pertussin CS, Pertussin DM[1]*, Silphen–DM*	**Syrup:** 3.5 mg/5 mL, 7.5 mg/5 mL, 10 mg/5 mL, 15 mg/5 mL	No
	Delsym	**Suspension, extended release:** 30 mg/5 mL	No
	Diphenhydramine HCl		
otc	*Beldin*[1]*, Bydramine Cough*[1]*, Diphen AF, Diphen Cough*[1]*, Hydramine Cough*[1]	**Syrup:** 12.5 mg/5 mL	Yes
Rx	*Tusstat*[1]	**Syrup:** 12.5 mg/5 mL	Yes
	Nonnarcotic Antitussive Combinations		
otc	*Spec-T Cough Suppressant*[2]	**Lozenges:** 10 mg dextromethorphan HBr and 10 mg benzocaine	No

[1] Contains alcohol.
[2] Contains the dye tartrazine.

Cough is a normal protective reflex. It helps clear mucus, irritants, and other foreign matter from the throat, trachea, and lungs. Caution is advised in attempting to suppress a productive cough (mucus is coughed up). The productive cough is essential to the removal of foreign debris. If mucus is not removed from the lungs, it may support growth of bacteria and make breathing more difficult. Moderate cough suppression may be used to reduce discomfort and allow sleep, but do not attempt to completely suppress a productive cough.

The dry, nonproductive cough is a good candidate for therapeutic cough suppression. If such coughs are persistent, bothersome, or sleep-disrupting, they may respond well to treatment with antitussives.

Type of Drug:

Cough medicine; cough suppressant.

How the Drug Works:

Nonnarcotic antitussives depress the cough center in the brain.

Benzonatate: Reduces the cough reflex by anesthetizing the nerve receptors in the breathing passages and lungs.

Uses:

To relieve or suppress nonproductive cough (no mucus production) or cough due to colds or allergy.

Precautions:

Do not use in the following situations:

allergy to the drug or any of its ingredients
newborn or premature infants (diphenhydramine)

Use with caution in the following situations:

asthma
bladder obstruction (diphenhydramine)
bronchitis, chronic
chronic cough (smoker, etc)
cough with mucus
CNS stimulants
difficulty urinating (diphenhydramine)
difficulty breathing
emphysema
fever
glaucoma (diphenhydramine)
headache, persistent
MAO inhibitor use (dextromethorphan, diphenhydramine)
nausea or vomiting
prostate gland enlargement (diphenhydramine)
pulmonary disease, chronic (diphenhydramine)
pyloroduodenal obstruction (diphenhydramine)
rash
shortness of breath (diphenhydramine)

Pregnancy: Adequate studies have not been done in pregnant women. Use only if clearly needed and potential benefits outweigh the possible hazards to the fetus.

Breastfeeding: It is not known if nonnarcotic antitussives appear in breast milk. Consult your doctor before you begin breastfeeding. Nursing women should not use *Tusstat* syrup.

Children: Use only as directed by your doctor or pharmacist. Most of these products are not recommended for children under 2 to 12 years of age. Consult individual product information for pediatric dosing.

Elderly: Products containing an antihistamine are more likely to cause dizziness, sedation, and hypotension in the elderly.

Tartrazine: Some of these products may contain the dye tartrazine (FD&C Yellow No. 5) which can cause allergic reactions in certain individuals. Check package label when available or consult your doctor or pharmacist.

Drug Interactions:

Tell your doctor or pharmacist if you are taking or planning to take any over-the-counter or prescription medications or dietary supplements with nonnarcotic antitussives. Doses of one or both drugs may need to be modified or a different drug may need to be prescribed. The following drugs and drug classes may interact with nonnarcotic antitussives:

alcohol
MAOIs (eg, isocarboxazid)
sedatives (eg, benzodiazepines)
tranquilizers (eg, perphenazine, phenobarbital)

Side Effects:

Every drug is capable of producing side effects. Many nonnarcotic antitussive users experience no, or minor, side effects. The frequency and severity of side effects depend on many factors including dose, duration of therapy, and individual susceptibility. Possible side effects include:

Circulatory System: Pounding in chest; rapid heartbeat; low blood pressure; extrasystoles.

Digestive Tract: Constipation; nausea; stomach upset; loss of appetite; vomiting.

Eyes or Ocular: Burning sensation in eyes; blurred vision; vision problems.

Nervous System: Headache; mental confusion; visual hallucinations; sedation; dizziness; excitability in children; neuritis.

Respiratory System: Tightness in chest; wheezing; chest numbness; nasal congestion; thick bronchial secretions.

Skin: Itching; skin eruptions; abnormal skin sensations.

Urinary and Reproductive Tract: Urinary frequency; difficult urination; urinary retention; early menstruation.

Other: A vague "chilly" sensation; allergy; shock; sensitivity to light; excessive perspiration; dryness of mouth, nose, and throat; decreased blood platelets; agranulocytosis; incoordination; feeling of whirling motion; ringing in ears; acute labyrinthritis; hysteria; convulsions.

Guidelines for Use:

- Take only as directed. Do not exceed recommended dose.
- See individual package instructions for dosing information.
- *Pertussin CS, Pertussin DM, and Delsym* — Shake well before use.
- Do not take for persistent or chronic cough, such as occurs with smoking, asthma, chronic bronchitis, emphysema, or where cough is accompanied by excessive phelgm, except under supervision of your doctor.
- Do not use *Spec-T* lozenges for more than 2 days unless directed by your doctor.
- Some products may cause drowsiness, whether they contain alcohol or not. Alcohol, sedatives, and tranquilizers may increase the drowsiness effect. Avoid alcoholic beverages while taking this product and do not take sedatives or tranquilizers without consulting your doctor.
- May cause drowsiness, dizziness, or blurred vision. Use caution while driving or performing other tasks requiring mental alertness, coordination, or physical dexterity.
- A persistent cough may be a sign of a serious condition. If cough persists for more than 1 week, tends to recur, or is accompanied by fever, rash, or persistent headache, notify your doctor.
- Do not use dextromethorphan or diphenhydramine if you are taking an MAO inhibitor or for 2 weeks after stopping MAO inhibitor therapy.
- *Benzonatate* — Do not chew or suck *Tessalon Perles*. Severe hypersensitivity reactions (eg, bronchospasm, laryngospasm, and cardiovascular collapse) have occurred.
- Store at room temperature (59° to 86°F).

If you have any questions, consult your doctor, pharmacist, or health care provider.

	Generic Name *Brand Name Examples*	Supplied As	Generic Available
	Guaifenesin (Glyceryl Guaiacolate)		
otc	*Gee-Gee, Glytuss, Hytuss*	**Tablets:** 100 mg, 200 mg	Yes
Rx	*Fenesin, Humibid L.A., Sinumist-SR*	**Tablets, sustained release:** 600 mg	No
otc	*Breonesin*[1]*, Hytuss 2X*	**Capsules:** 200 mg	No
Rx	*Humibid Sprinkle*	**Capsules, sustained release:** 300 mg	No
otc	*Anti-Tuss*[2]*, Genatuss, Guiatuss*[1,2,3]*, Mytussin*[2]*, Robitussin, Scot-tussin*[1,3]	**Syrup:** 100 mg/5 mL	Yes
otc	*Naldecon Senior EX*[1]	**Liquid:** 200 mg/5 mL	No
	Iodine Products		
Rx	*Potassium Iodide, SSKI*	**Solution:** 1 g potassium iodide/mL	Yes
Rx	*Pima*	**Syrup:** 325 mg potassium iodide/5 mL	No

[1] Sugar free.
[2] Contains alcohol.
[3] Dye free.

Only one expectorant, guaifenesin, is safe and effective for use in nonprescription cough and cold medications to help loosen excessive respiratory secretions, mucus, and other foreign debris, according to a recent standard published by the Food and Drug Administration. No other nonprescription expectorant is considered both safe and effective by the FDA.

Type of Drug:

Loosens excessive respiratory secretions, mucus, and other foreign debris.

How the Drug Works:

Expectorants thin mucous secretions in the lungs and make the phlegm less sticky. The mucus is easier to cough up. This reduces chest congestion and makes coughs more productive. The exact mechanism by which expectorants thin mucous secretions in the lung is not known.

Uses:

Guaifenesin: For symptomatic relief of respiratory conditions characterized by dry, nonproductive cough and in the presence of mucus in the respiratory tract.

Iodine Products: For symptomatic treatment of lung disease where mucus complicates the condition (eg, emphysema, bronchial asthma, chronic bronchitis, bronchiectasis). Also used as adjunctive treatment in respiratory conditions such as cystic fibrosis, chronic sinusitis, and after surgery to help prevent lung collapse.

Precautions:

Do not use in the following situations:

Guaifenesin —
allergy to guaifenesin or any of its ingredients

Potassium iodide —
Addison disease, untreated
allergy to iodides
bronchitis, acute
dehydration, acute
heat cramps
hyperkalemia
iodine poisoning
kidney disease

Use with caution in the following situations:

Guaifenesin —
cough with excessive secretions
cough (7 to 10 days in duration)
cough, recurring (eg, asthma, chronic bronchitis, emphysema, smoking)
cough with fever, rash, or persistent headache
diabetes
heart disease
high blood pressure
prostate enlargement
thyroid disease

Potassium iodide —
cough (7 to 10 days duration)
cystic fibrosis in children
heart disease
hyperthyroidism
iodine-induced goiters
kidney function impairment
myotonia congenita (hereditary muscle disease)
tuberculosis

Pregnancy: Guaifenesin — Adequate studies have not been done in pregnant women. Use only if clearly needed and the benefits outweigh the possible risks.

Potassium iodide – Studies have shown a potential risk to the fetus, including abnormal thyroid function and goiter development. Use only if clearly needed and potential benefits outweigh the possible risks.

Breastfeeding: It is not known if guaifenesin appears in breast milk. Potassium iodide appears in breast milk and may cause skin rash and thyroid suppression in the infant. Decide whether to discontinue nursing or the drug. Consult your doctor.

Children: Safety and effectiveness in children under 2 years of age have not been established for guaifenesin. Safety and effectiveness in children have not been established for potassium iodide.

Drug Interactions:

Tell your doctor or pharmacist if you are taking, have recently discontinued, or are planning to take any over-the-counter or prescription medications with these expectorants. Doses of one or both drugs may need to be modified or a different drug may need to be prescribed. The following drugs and drug classes may interact with guaifenesin or potassium iodide expectorants.

- angiotensin-converting enzyme (ACE) inhibitors (eg, captopril)
- antithyroid agents (eg, propylthiouracil (PTU), methimazole)
- lithium (eg, *Eskalith)*
- monoamine oxidase inhibitors (MAOIs) (eg, phenelzine sulfate)
- potassium products (eg, *Slow-K)*
- potassium-sparing diuretics (eg, spironolactone, triamterene, amiloride)

Side Effects:

Every drug is capable of producing side effects. Many expectorant users experience no, or minor, side effects. The frequency and severity of side effects depend on many factors including dose, duration of therapy, and individual susceptibility. Possible side effects include:

Guaifenesin — Nausea; vomiting; diarrhea; gas; abnormal urine tests.

Potassium iodide —

Iodism or chronic iodine poisoning: Sore or burning mouth or throat; severe headache; productive cough; metallic taste; sneezing; eyelid swelling; increased salivation; acneiform skin lesions in oily skin areas; severe skin eruptions.

Allergic Reactions: Nerve swelling; skin and mucous membrane bleeding; serum sickness-like symptoms (eg, fever, bloating, lymph node enlargement, joint pain, blood disorder, fluid in lungs).

Digestive Tract: Nausea; vomiting; diarrhea; stomach upset or pain; bleeding.

Nervous System: Mental confusion; numbness.

Skin: Acne; rash; minor skin eruptions.

Other: Benign thyroid tumor; goiter; myxedema (hypothyroidism); irregular heartbeat; swelling of salivary glands, neck, or throat; tingling, pain, or weakness in hands or feet; weakness or heaviness of legs; fever; abnormal thyroid tests; unusual tiredness; metallic aftertaste.

Guidelines for Use:

- Use as directed. Do not exceed recommended dosage.
- Do not take these products for persistent or chronic cough such as occurs with smoking, asthma, chronic bronchitis, or emphysema, or when cough is accompanied by excessive phlegm, unless directed by your doctor.
- A persistent cough may be a sign of a serious condition. If cough persists for more than 1 week, tends to recur, or is accompanied by fever, rash, or persistent headache, consult a doctor.
- Guaifenesin is the only expectorant approved by the FDA as safe and effective. It is well tolerated. Iodine-containing products have the potential to produce many adverse effects.
- Drink a glass of water or other fluid with each dose of expectorant. Most authorities believe a well hydrated body (due to fluid intake) is responsible for thinning respiratory tract mucus and may be as valuable as or more so than the expectorant itself.
- Do not cut, crush, or chew sustained release tablets or capsules.
- *Iodine-containing expectorants* — Stop taking if stomach pain, rash, nausea, vomiting, bloating, gastrointestinal bleeding, or a metallic taste develops.

If you have any questions, consult your doctor, pharmacist, or health care provider.

	Brand Name Examples	Supplied As
otc	*Ayr Saline Nasal Drops*[1], *Ayr Saline Mist*[1], *Ayr Baby Saline Nose Spray/ Drops*[1], *HuMist Moisturizing Nasal Mist*[1], *NaSal Saline*[1], *Ocean Nasal Mist*[2]	**Solution:** 0.65% sodium chloride
otc	*Salinex Nasal Mist, Salinex Nasal Drops*	**Solution:** 0.4% sodium chloride
otc	*Benzedrex*	**Inhaler:** 250 mg propylhexedrine
otc	*Dristan Nasal Spray*[2]	**Solution:** 0.5% phenylephrine HCl and 0.2% pheniramine maleate
otc	*4-Way Long Lasting Nasal Spray*	**Solution:** 0.05% oxymetazoline HCl
otc	*Pretz-D*	**Solution:** 0.025% ephedrine sulfate

[1] Alcohol free [2] Contains benzyl alcohol.

For more information, see topical antihistamines and decongestants monographs.

Type of Drug:

Nasal decongestants; antihistamines; moisturizing agents.

Uses:

Sodium chloride: A saline moisturizing solution to restore moisture, thin nasal secretions, and relieve dry, crusted, and inflamed nasal membranes due to colds, low humidity, nasal decongestant overuse, allergies, nosebleeds, sinus infection, and other irritations.

Phenylephrine, oxymetazoline HCl, ephedrine sulfate, and propylhexedrine: Decongestants for relief of nasal congestion (swelling).

Pheniramine maleate: Antihistamine for relief of nasal symptoms (eg, itching, runny nose, congestion) due to allergies.

Guidelines for Use:

- Follow directions for use provided on each package.
- Do not use in eyes or ears.
- Moisturizing drops or sprays can be used every 2 hours if needed.
- Use of dispenser by more than 1 person may spread infection.
- *Inhalers* — Inhale through each nostril while blocking the other. Keep inhalers tightly closed between doses.
- If symptoms persist, contact your doctor or pharmacist.
- Avoid excessive or prolonged use (eg, more than 3 days) of products containing decongestants to prevent rebound congestion.

If you have any questions, consult your doctor, pharmacist, or health care provider.

Combination products are frequently used in the therapy of respiratory conditions. These fixed-dose combination products may present two problems: (1) The patient may not need all the components in the product; (2) the patient may need the components, but in different strengths or at different dosing intervals.

Product Selection Guidelines: The following guidelines should be employed when choosing a respiratory combination product.

Symptoms – Pain, fever, congestion, runny nose, cough (productive or nonproductive).

Medical history and health – Age, allergy history, pregnancy, heart disease, high blood pressure, asthma, bronchitis, glaucoma, hyperthyroidism (overactive thyroid), diabetes, depression.

Drugs you are currently taking – Other cold or allergy medications; medications for high blood pressure, diabetes, etc.

Do not exceed the recommended dosage – Do not take a nonprescription *(otc)* respiratory product for more than 7 days. If symptoms do not improve or are accompanied by fever, consult a doctor.

Humidification – Humidification of room air and adequate fluid intake (6 to 8 glasses/day) are important in treating cold symptoms.

Sulfites and Tartrazine – Some of these products contain sulfites or tartrazine, which may cause allergic-type reactions (eg, rash, hives, itching, wheezing) in certain susceptible persons. Although the overall prevalence of sensitivity in the general population is probably low, it is seen more frequently in asthmatics or in atopic nonasthmatic persons (sulfites) or in patients who have aspirin allergy (tartrazine).

Sugar free liquid products – The small amount of sugar in usual doses of medication is probably insignificant to the well-controlled diabetic. However, consider the effects of alcohol and sympathomimetics in addition to the sugar content of these formulations.

Sustained release formulations – Products with identical active ingredients are listed together. Due to formulation differences, do not consider them bioequivalent.

Groups: These combination products are presented in groups based on their formulations. Products with identical or similar ingredients are listed next to each other, regardless of therapeutic claims, which may differ even for identical formulas. Pediatric preparations (those products intended mainly or exclusively for children) are grouped together at the end of the main sections.

Antiasthmatic Combinations contain xanthine derivatives and sympathomimetics for bronchodilation (widening of air passages). Many products also contain expectorants to facilitate break up and removal of mucus.

Xanthine Combinations
Xanthine-Sympathomimetic Combinations

Upper Respiratory Combinations are used primarily for relief of symptoms associated with colds, upper respiratory infections and allergies (eg, inflammation of nose and sinuses, etc). Cough preparations include an antitussive (cough suppressant) or expectorant, but may also contain ingredients for relief of other symptoms.

- Decongestant and Analgesic Combinations
- Pediatric Decongestant and Analgesic Combinations
- Decongestant and Expectorant Combinations
- Pediatric Decongestant and Expectorant Combinations
- Antihistamine and Analgesic Combinations
- Decongestant, Antihistamine, and Expectorant Combinations
- Pediatric Decongestant, Antihistamine, and Expectorant Combinations
- Decongestants and Antihistamines
- Pediatric Decongestants and Antihistamines
- Decongestant, Antihistamine, and Analgesic Combinations
- Decongestant, Antihistamine, and Anticholinergic Combinations
- Pediatric Decongestant, Antihistamine, and Anticholinergic Combinations
- Antitussive Combinations
- Pediatric Antitussive Combinations
- Antitussive and Expectorant Combinations
- Pediatric Antitussive and Expectorant Combinations
- Antitussives with Expectorants
- Pediatric Antitussives with Expectorants
- Topical Combinations

Ingredients:

Antihistamines are used for relief from allergic symptoms (hay fever) including runny nose, sneezing, itching of the nose or throat and itchy, watery eyes. The anticholinergic (drying) effects of antihistamines may cause a thickening of lung secretions; therefore, these agents may not be helpful in respiratory conditions characterized by congestion. Antihistamines may cause drowsiness. Antihistamines can also cause drying of the eyes. This can be a problem for people who wear contact lenses. Appropriate lubricating drops may be indicated.

Xanthines primarily theophylline, relieve spasms of the air passages by direct action on the bronchial smooth muscle in asthma and chronic bronchitis. Some xanthine-containing combination products are available over-the-counter, but asthmatic patients should use them only under supervision of a doctor.

Sympathomimetics are used for their decongestant or bronchodilator (widening of air passages) effects. Side effects may include nervousness, heart stimulation and high blood pressure if taken orally.

Decongestants – Used for temporary relief of nasal congestion due to colds or allergy. Given orally, they are less effective than topical nasal decongestants, and they have a potential for side effects. Frequent or prolonged topical use may lead to local irritation and rebound congestion. Topical decongestants (sprays and drops) should not be used for more than 3 to 5 days in a row. After that, switch to an oral product, or avoid use of decongestants altogether.

Bronchodilators – Ephedrine is common in these combinations; however, it may stimulate the heart. Bronchodilation effects may decrease congestion of mucous membranes. Pseudoephedrine is not an effective bronchodilator.

Narcotic Antitussives – The antitussive dose is lower than that required for pain relief. Consider general precautions for the use of narcotics, including the potential for abuse, when using these products.

Nonnarcotic Antitussives decrease the cough reflex without inducing many of the common characteristics of narcotic preparations. Examples include: Dextromethorphan, diphenhydramine, carbetapentane and caramiphen edisylate.

Expectorants may be of limited value in loosening and liquifying respiratory mucus, in soothing the irritated lining of the lungs (bronchial mucosa) and in making coughs more productive. Guaifenesin is the only FDA-recognized safe and effective ingredient for use in *otc* cough and cold medicines to loosen phlegm. Humidification of room air and adequate fluid intake (6 to 8 glasses/day) are important measures as well.

Analgesics (eg, pain relievers, acetaminophen, aspirin, ibuprofen) are frequently included for symptoms of headache, fever, muscle aches and pain.

Anticholinergics are included for their drying effects on mucus secretions. This action may be beneficial in acute runny nose; however, drying of respiratory secretions may lead to obstruction. Traditionally, anticholinergics have been avoided in patients with asthma or chronic obstructive pulmonary disease (COPD); however, some patients respond well to these agents. Caution is still advised, particularly among patients with heart disease.
An anticholinergic for oral inhalation is available as a bronchodilator for maintenance of air passage spasms (bronchospasms) associated with COPD, including chronic bronchitis and emphysema.

Papaverine relaxes the smooth muscle of the air passageways tree.

Barbiturates are included for their sedative effects in combination with xanthines or sympathomimetics which may cause CNS stimulation. The sedative effectiveness of low doses (eg, 8 mg phenobarbital) is questionable. OTC availability of phenobarbital-containing products may be limited according to state laws.

Caffeine is included in some combinations for CNS stimulation to counteract antihistamine depression and to enhance the effects of pain relievers.

Xanthine Combinations

Content given per capsule, tablet, or 15 mL.

	Brand Name Examples	Xanthine	Expectorant
Rx	*Quibron-300 Capsules*	300 mg theophylline	180 mg guaifenesin
Rx	*Quibron Capsules*	150 mg theophylline	90 mg guaifenesin
Rx	*Slo-Phyllin GG Syrup*		
Rx	*Theolate Liquid*		
Rx	*Elixophyllin-GG Liquid*	100 mg theophylline	100 mg guaifenesin
Rx	*Elixophyllin-KI Elixir*	80 mg theophylline	130 mg potassium iodide
Rx	*Dilor-G Liquid*	300 mg dyphylline	300 mg guaifenesin
Rx	*Dy-G Liquid*		
Rx	*Panfil-G Syrup*	300 mg dyphylline	150 mg guaifenesin
Rx	*Dilor-G Tablets*	200 mg dyphylline	200 mg guaifenesin
Rx	*Dyflex-G Tablets*		
Rx	*Lufyllin-GG Tablets*		
Rx	*Panfil-G Capsules*	200 mg dyphylline	100 mg guaifenesin
Rx	*Dyphylline-GG Elixir*	100 mg dyphylline	100 mg guaifenesin
Rx	*Lufyllin-GG Elixir*		
Rx	*Brondelate Elixir*	300 mg oxtriphylline	150 mg guaifenesin

Xanthine-Sympathomimetic Combinations

Content given per tablet.

	Brand Name Examples	Xanthine	Bronchodilator	Expectorant	Other
Rx	*Lufyllin-EPG Tablets*	100 mg dyphylline	16 mg ephedrine HCl	200 mg guaifenesin	16 mg phenobarbital

Decongestant and Analgesic Combinations

Content given per capsule, tablet, or 5 mL.

	Brand Name Examples	Deconges-tant	Analgesic
otc	*Alka-Seltzer Plus Cold & Sinus Tablets*[1]	5 mg phenylephrine HCl	250 mg acetaminophen
otc	*Cepacol Sore Throat Liquid*[2,3]	10 mg pseudoephedrine HCl	106.7 mg acetaminophen
otc	*Alka-Seltzer Plus Cold & Sinus Liqui-Gels*[3]	30 mg pseudoephedrine HCl	325 mg acetaminophen
otc	*Ornex No Drowsiness Tablets*[3]		
otc	*Phenapap Tablets*[3]		
otc	*Sinutab Sinus Without Drowsiness Regular Strength Tablets*		
otc	*Sudafed Cold & Sinus Non-Drowsy Liqui-Caps*		
otc	*Dristan Cold Non-Drowsy Maximum Strength Tablets*	30 mg pseudoephedrine HCl	500 mg acetaminophen
otc	*Mapap Sinus Maximum Strength Geltabs*		
otc	*Nasal Decongestant Sinus Non-Drowsy Tablets*		
otc	*Ornex No Drowsiness Maximum Strength Tablets*		
otc	*Sine-Off No-Drowsiness Formula Tablets*		
otc	*Sinus-Relief Maximum Strength Tablets*		
otc	*Sinutab Sinus Without Drowsiness Maximum Strength Tablets*		

	Brand Name Examples	Deconges-tant	Analgesic
otc	*Sudafed Sinus Headache Non-Drowsy Tablets*	30 mg pseudo-ephedrine HCl	500 mg acetaminophen
otc	*SudoGest Sinus Maximum Strength Tablets*		
otc	*Tavist Sinus Maximum Strength Tablets*		
otc	*Tylenol Sinus Non-Drowsy Maximum Strength Geltabs, Tablets, and Gel-caps*		
otc	*Advil Cold & Sinus Tablets*	30 mg pseudo-ephedrine HCl	200 mg ibuprofen
otc	*Advil Flu & Body Ache Tablets*		
otc	*Dristan Sinus Tablets*		
otc	*Motrin Sinus Headache Tablets*		
otc	*Aleve Cold & Sinus Tablets*	120 mg pseudo-ephedrine HCl	220 mg naproxen sodium (200 mg naproxen)
otc	*Aleve Sinus & Headache Tablets*[4]		

[1] Contains phenylalanine.
[2] Alcohol free.
[3] This product may also be used in children; refer to package labeling.
[4] Extended release.

Pediatric Decongestant and Analgesic Combinations

Content given per tablet, 5 mL (liquid), or 1 mL (drops).

	Brand Name Examples	Deconges-tant	Analgesic
otc	*Tylenol Infant's Cold Con-centrated Drops*[1]	9.375 mg/mL pseudo-ephedrine HCl	100 mg/mL acetamino-phen
otc	*Tylenol Children's Sinus Suspension*	15 mg pseudo-ephedrine HCl	160 mg acetaminophen
otc	*Triaminic Softchews Allergy Sinus & Headache Tablets*[2]		

	Brand Name Examples	Deconges-tant	Analgesic
otc	*Motrin Children's Cold Suspension*	15 mg pseudo-ephedrine HCl	100 mg ibuprofen

[1] Alcohol free.
[2] Contains phenylalanine.

Decongestant and Expectorant Combinations

Content given per capsule, tablet, or 5 mL.

	Brand Name Examples	Deconges-tant	Expectorant
Rx	*Broncholate Syrup*	6.25 mg ephedrine HCl	600 mg guaifenesin
Rx	*KIE Syrup*[1]	8 mg ephed-rine HCl	150 mg potassium iodide
otc	*Mini Two-Way Action Tablets*	12.5 mg ephedrine HCl	200 mg guaifenesin
otc	*Primatene Tablets*		
otc	*Dynafed Asthma Relief Tablets*	25 mg ephedrine HCl	200 mg guaifenesin
otc	*Mini Two-Way Action Tablets*		
otc	*Bronkaid Dual Action Tablets*	25 mg ephedrine sulfate	400 mg guaifenesin
otc	*Rescon-GG Liquid*[1,2,5]	5 mg phenyl-ephrine HCl	100 mg guaifenesin
Rx	*Entex Liquid*[1,2,3,5]	7.5 mg phenyl-ephrine HCl	100 mg guaifenesin
Rx	*Endal Tablets*[4]	20 mg phenyl-ephrine HCl	300 mg guaifenesin
Rx	*GFN 600/Phenylephrine 20 Tablets*[1,5]	20 mg phenyl-ephrine HCl	600 mg guaifenesin

	Brand Name Examples	Deconges-tant	Expectorant
Rx	*Entex LA Tablets*[1,5,6]	30 mg phenyl-ephrine HCl	600 mg guaifenesin
Rx	*Liquibid-D Tablets*[1]	40 mg phenyl-ephrine HCl	600 mg guaifenesin
otc	*Guiatuss PE Liquid*[2]	30 mg pseudo-ephedrine HCl	100 mg guaifenesin
otc	*Robafen PE Liquid*[1,2]		
otc	*Robitussin PE Liquid*[1]		
otc	*Sudafed Non-Drowsy Non-Drying Sinus Liquid Caps*	30 mg pseudo-ephedrine HCl	120 mg guaifenesin
otc	*Guaifed Syrup*[1,2]	30 mg pseudo-ephedrine HCl	200 mg guaifenesin
otc	*Robitussin Severe Con-gestion Liqui-Gels*[1]		
otc	*Severe Congestion Tussin Softgels*[1]		
otc	*Sinutab Non-Drying Liquid Caps*		
otc	*Robitussin Cold Sinus & Congestion Tablets*[1,7]	30 mg pseudo-ephedrine HCl	200 mg guaifenesin
Rx	*PanMist-S Syrup*[1]	45 mg pseudo-ephedrine HCl	200 mg guaifenesin
Rx	*Coldmist JR Tablets*[1,6]	45 mg pseudo-ephedrine HCl	600 mg guaifenesin
Rx	*PanMist JR Tablets*[1,8]		
Rx	*Profen II Tablets*[1,8]	45 mg pseudo-ephedrine HCl	800 mg guaifenesin

	Brand Name Examples	Deconges-tant	Expectorant
Rx	*Respa-1st Tablets*[1,6]	58 mg pseudo-ephedrine HCl	600 mg guaifenesin
Rx	*Respaire-60 SR Capsules*[1,8]	60 mg pseudo-ephedrine HCl	200 mg guaifenesin
Rx	*Guaifed-PD Capsules*[1,6]	60 mg pseudo-ephedrine HCl	300 mg guaifenesin
Rx	*Versacaps Capsules*[1,6]		
otc	*Congestac Tablets*[1]	60 mg pseudo-ephedrine HCl	400 mg guaifenesin
otc	*Refenesen Plus Severe Strength Cough & Cold Medicine Tablets*		
Rx	*Sudal 60/500 Tablets*[1,6]	60 mg pseudo-ephedrine HCl	500 mg guaifenesin
Rx	*Maxifed-G Tablets*[1,6]	60 mg pseudo-ephedrine HCl	550 mg guaifenesin
Rx	*Guaifenesin/Pseudo-ephedrine HCl Tablets*[1,6]	60 mg pseudo-ephedrine HCl	600 mg guaifenesin
Rx	*AquatabD Dose Pack Tablets*[1,6]		
Rx	*Deconsal II Tablets*[1,6]		
Rx	*Defen-LA Tablets*[1,6]		
Rx	*Guaifenex PSE 60 Tablets*[1,8]		
Rx	*Iosal II Tablets*[1,6]		
Rx	*Guaifenex-Rx Tablets*[8]	*Day:* 60 mg pseudo-ephedrine HCl	600 mg guaifenesin
		Night:	600 mg guaifenesin

	Brand Name Examples	Deconges-tant	Expectorant
Rx	*AquatabD Tablets*	60 mg pseudo-ephedrine HCl	1200 mg guaifenesin
Rx	*G/P 1200/60 Tablets*[1,6]		
Rx	*Maxifed Tablets*[1]	80 mg pseudo-ephedrine HCl	700 mg guaifenesin
Rx	*Coldmist LA Tablets*[1,8]	80 mg pseu-dopehedrine HCl	800 mg guaifenesin
Rx	*PanMist LA Tablets*[1,8]		
Rx	*H 9600 SR Tablets*[1,5,6]	90 mg pseudo-ephedrine HCl	600 mg guaifenesin
Rx	*Profen Forte Tablets*[1,8]	90 mg pseudo-ephedrine HCl	800 mg guaifenesin
Rx	*Dynex Tablets*[1,5,6]	90 mg pseudo-ephedrine HCl	1200 mg guaifenesin
Rx	*Guaifed Capsules*[6]	120 mg pseudo-ephedrine HCl	250 mg guaifenesin
Rx	*Pseudovent Capsules*[6]		
Rx	*Respaire-120 SR Capsules*[8]		
Rx	*GP-500 Tablets*[1,3,5,6]	120 mg pseudo-ephedrine HCl	500 mg guaifenesin
Rx	*Nasatab LA Tablets*[1,6]		
Rx	*Stamoist E Tablets*[1,6]		
Rx	*V-Dec-M Tablets*[1,6]		
Rx	*Touro LA Tablets*[6]	120 mg pseudo-ephedrine HCl	525 mg guaifenesin

	Brand Name Examples	Deconges-tant	Expectorant
Rx	*Duratuss Tablets*[5,6]	120 mg pseudo-ephedrine HCl	600 mg guaifenesin
Rx	*Entex PSE Tablets*[1,6]		
Rx	*Guaifenex PSE 120 Tablets*[1,5,8]		
Rx	*GuaiMAX-D Tablets*[1,8]		
Rx	*Guaipax PSE Tablets*[1,6]		
Rx	*Guai-Vent/PSE Tablets*[1,6]		
Rx	*Miraphen PSE Tablets*[1,8]		
Rx	*Duratuss GP Tablets*[5,6]	120 mg pseudo-ephedrine HCl	1200 mg guaifenesin
Rx	*GFN/PSE Tablets*[1,6]		
Rx	*Guaifenex GP Tablets*[5,8]		

[1] This product may also be used in children; refer to package labeling.
[2] Alcohol free.
[3] Sugar free.
[4] Timed release.
[5] Dye free.
[6] Sustained release.
[7] Also contains 325 mg acetaminophen.
[8] Extended release.

Pediatric Decongestant and Expectorant Combinations

Content given per capsule or 5 mL.

	Brand Name Examples	Deconges-tant	Expectorant
otc	*Thera-Hist Expectorant Chest Congestion Liquid*	15 mg pseudo-ephedrine HCl	50 mg guaifenesin
otc	*Triacting Liquid*		
otc	*Triaminic Chest Congestion Liquid*		
Rx	*Pseudovent-PED Capsules*[1]	60 mg pseudo-ephedrine HCl	300 mg guaifenesin

[1] Sustained release.

Anthistamine and Analgesic Combinations

Content given per capsule or tablet.

	Brand Name Examples	Antihista-mine	Analgesic
otc	*Coricidin HBP Cold & Flu Tablets*[1]	2 mg chlor-pheniramine maleate	325 mg acetaminophen
otc	*Percogesic Extra Strength Tablets*	12.5 mg diphenhydra-mine HCl	500 mg acetaminophen
otc	*Tylenol Severe Allergy Tablets*		
otc	*Tylenol PM Extra Strength Tablets, Gelcaps, and Geltabs*	25 mg diphenhydra-mine HCl	500 mg acetaminophon
Rx	*Ed-Flex Capsules*[1]	20 mg phenyltolox-amine citrate	300 mg acetaminophen, 200 mg salicylamide
otc	*Aceta-Gesic Tablets*[1]	30 mg phenyltolox-amine citrate	325 mg acetaminophen
otc	*Major-gesic Tablets*[1]		
otc	*Percogesic Tablets*[1]		
otc	*Phenylgesic Tablets*[1]		

[1] This product may also be used in children; refer to package labeling.

Decongestant, Antihistamine, and Expectorant Combinations

Content given per tablet or 5 mL.

	Brand Name Examples	Decongestant	Antihistamine	Expectorant
Rx	*Decolate Tablets*	5 mg phenyl-ephrine HCl	4 mg chlor-pheniramine maleate	100 mg guai-fenesin
Rx	*Polaramine Expectorant Liquid*[1,2]	20 mg pseudo-ephedrine sul-fate	2 mg dexchlor-pheniramine maleate	100 mg guai-fenesin

[1] This product may also be used in children; refer to package labeling.
[2] Contains alcohol.

Pediatric Decongestant, Antihistamine, and Expectorant Combinations

Content given per 1 mL.

	Brand Name Examples	Decongestant	Antihistamine	Expectorant
Rx	*Donatussin Drops*	2 mg/mL phenylephrine HCl	1 mg/mL chlorpheniramine maleate	20 mg/mL guaifenesin

Decongestants and Antihistamines

Content given per capsule, tablet, or 5 mL.

	Brand Name Examples	Decongestant	Antihistamine
otc	*Histatab Plus Tablets*[1]	5 mg phenylephrine HCl	2 mg chlorpheniramine maleate
Rx	*Ed A-Hist Liquid*[1,2]	10 mg phenylephrine HCl	4 mg chlorpheniramine maleate
Rx	*Ed A-Hist Tablets*[3]	20 mg phenylephrine HCl	8 mg chlorpheniramine maleate
Rx	*Promethazine HCl and Phenylephrine HCl Syrup*[1,2]	5 mg phenylephrine HCl	6.25 mg promethazine HCl
Rx	*Phenergan VC Syrup*[1,2]		
Rx	*Prometh VC Plain Syrup*[1,2]		
Rx	*Rynatan Tablets*	25 mg phenylephrine HCl	9 mg chlorpheniramine tannate
Rx	*Semprex-D Capsules*	60 mg pseudoephedrine HCl	8 mg acrivastine
otc	*Bromfed Syrup*	30 mg pseudoephedrine HCl	2 mg brompheniramine maleate
Rx	*Brofed Liquid*[1]	30 mg pseudoephedrine HCl	4 mg brompheniramine maleate

	Brand Name Examples	Deconges-tant	Antihistamine
Rx	*Rondec Syrup*[1]	45 mg pseudo-ephedrine HCl	4 mg brompheniramine maleate
Rx	*Brompheniramine Maleate/Pseudoephedrine HCl Syrup*[1]	60 mg pseudo-ephedrine HCl	4 mg brompheniramine maleate
Rx	*Andehist Syrup*[1,4,5]		
Rx	*Bromfed Tablets*[1]		
Rx	*Lodrane Liquid*[1,4-6]		
Rx	*Touro Allergy Capsules*[1,3]	60 mg pseudo-ephedrine HCl	5.75 mg brompheniramine maleate
Rx	*Lodrane LD Capsules*[1,6]	60 mg pseudo-ephedrine HCl	6 mg brompheniramine maleate
Rx	*Respahist Capsules*[1,3]		
Rx	*Histex SR Capsules*[7]	120 mg pseudo-ephedrine HCl	10 mg brompheniramine maleate
Rx	*Bromfed Capsules*[7]	120 mg pseudo-ephedrine HCl	12 mg brompheniramine maleate
Rx	*Bromfenex Capsules*[7]		
Rx	*ULTRAbrom Capsules*[7]		
Rx	*Cardec-S Liquid*[1]	60 mg pseudo-ephedrine HCl	4 mg carbinoxamine maleate
Rx	*Rondec Tablets*[1]		
Rx	*Coldec D Tablets*[1]	90 mg pseudo-ephedrine HCl	8 mg carbinoxamine maleate
Rx	*Palgic-D Tablets*[1]		
Rx	*Rondec-TR Tablets*[8]	120 mg pseudo-ephedrine HCl	8 mg carbinoxamine maleate

	Brand Name Examples	Decongestant	Antihistamine
Rx	*Zyrtec-D 12 Hour Tablets*[7]	120 mg pseudoephedrine HCl	5 mg cetirizine HCl
otc	*Allerest Maximum Strength Tablets*	30 mg pseudoephedrine HCl	2 mg chlorpheniramine maleate
Rx	*Deconamine Syrup*[1,5,6]		
otc	*Scot-Tussin Hayfebrol Liquid*[1,4-6]		
Rx	*Histex Liquid*[1]		
otc	*Ryna Liquid*[1,4-6]		
Rx	*Deconamine Tablets*	60 mg pseudoephedrine HCl	4 mg chlorpheniramine maleate
Rx	*Kronofed-A Jr. Capsules*[3]		
otc	*Sudafed Cold & Allergy Maximum Strength Tablets*[1]		
Rx	*Chlorpheniramine Maleate/Pseudoephedrine HCl ER Capsules*[7]	120 mg pseudoephedrine HCl	8 mg chlorpheniramine maleate
Rx	*Brexin-L.A. Capsules*		
Rx	*Colfed-A Capsules*[7]		
Rx	*Deconamine SR Capsules*[3]		
Rx	*Deconomed SR Capsules*[3]		
Rx	*Kronofed-A Capsules*[3]		
Rx	*N D Clear Capsules*[3]		
Rx	*Rinade B.I.D. Capsules*[6,7]		
Rx	*Time-Hist Capsules*[3]		
Rx	*Biohist-LA Tablets*[1,3]	120 mg pseudoephedrine HCl	12 mg chlorpheniramine maleate
Rx	*Histade Capsules*[3]		
Rx	*Rescon 12 Hour Capsules*[3]		

	Brand Name Examples	Deconges-tant	Antihistamine
otc	*Benadryl Allergy & Sinus Fastmelt Dissolving Tablets*[9]	30 mg pseudo-ephedrine HCl	19 mg diphenhydramine citrate (12.5 mg diphen-hydramine HCl)
otc	*Benadryl Allergy & Sinus Liquid*[1]	30 mg pseudo-ephedrine HCl	12.5 mg diphenhydramine HCl
otc	*Benadryl Allergy & Sinus Tablets*	60 mg pseudo-ephedrine HCl	25 mg diphenhydramine HCl
Rx	*Allegra-D Tablets*[7]	120 mg pseudo-ephedrine HCl	60 mg fexofenadine HCl
Rx	*Quadra-Hist D Capsules*[7]	80 mg pseudo-ephedrine HCl	16 mg phenyltoloxamine citrate, 16 mg pyrilamine maleate, 16 mg pheni-ramine maleate
otc	*Triprolidine HCl w/Pseudo-ephedrine HCl Syrup*[1]	30 mg pseudo-ephedrine HCl	1.25 mg triprolidine HCl
otc	*Allerfrim Syrup*[1]		
otc	*Aprodine Syrup*[1]		
otc	*Silafed Syrup*[1]		
otc	*Actifed Cold & Allergy Tablets*[1]	60 mg pseudo-ephedrine HCl	2.5 mg triprolidine HCl
otc	*Allerfrim Tablets*[1]		
otc	*Aprodine Tablets*[1]		
otc	*Cenafed Plus Tablets*[1]		
otc	*Genac Tablets*[1]		
otc	*Sudafed Sinus Nighttime Maximum Strength Tablets*[1]		

	Brand Name Examples	Deconges-tant	Antihistamine
Rx	*Trinalin Repetabs Tablets*[3]	120 mg pseudo-ephedrine sulfate	1 mg azatadine maleate
otc	*Chlor-Trimeton Allergy-D 4 Hour Tablets*[1]	60 mg pseudo-ephedrine sulfate	4 mg chlorpheniramine maleate
otc	*Chlor-Trimeton Allergy-D 12 Hour Tablets*	120 mg pseudo-ephedrine sulfate	8 mg chlorpheniramine maleate
Rx	*Drixomed Tablets*[3]	120 mg pseudo-ephedrine sulfate	6 mg dexbrompheniramine maleate
otc	*Drixoral Cold & Allergy Tablets*		
Rx	*Claritin-D 12 Hour Tablets*[7]	120 mg pseudo-ephedrine sulfate	5 mg loratadine
Rx	*Claritin-D 24 Hour Tablets*[7]	240 mg pseudo-ephedrine sulfate	10 mg loratadine
Rx	*C-PHED Tannate Suspension*[1]	75 mg pseudo-ephedrine tannate	4.5 mg chlorpheniramine tannate
Rx	*CP-TANNIC Suspension*[1]		
Rx	*Tanafed Suspension*		

[1] This product may also be used in children; refer to package labeling.
[2] Contains alcohol.
[3] Sustained release.
[4] Sugar free.
[5] Alcohol free.
[6] Dye free.
[7] Extended release.
[8] Timed release.
[9] Contains phenylalanine.

Pediatric Decongestants and Antihistamines

Content given per tablet, capsule, 5 mL (liquid), or 1 mL (drops).

	Brand Name Examples	Decongestant	Antihistamine
Rx	*Rhinatate-NF Pediatric Suspension*	5 mg phenylephrine tannate	4.5 mg chlorpheniramine tannate
Rx	*Rynatan Pediatric Suspension*[1]		
Rx	*Phenylephrine Tannate/Chlorpheniramine Tannate/Pyrilamine Tannate Pediatric Suspension*	5 mg phenylephrine tannate	2 mg chlorpheniramine tannate, 12.5 mg pyrilamine tannate
Rx	*Rhinatate Pediatric Suspension*		
Rx	*Triotann Pediatric Suspension*		
Rx	*Triotann-S Pediatric Suspension*		
Rx	*Duonate-12 Suspension*	5 mg phenylephrine tannate	30 mg pyrilamine tannate
Rx	*R-Tanna 12 Suspension*		
Rx	*R-Tannic-S A/D Suspension*		
Rx	*Ryna-12 S Suspension*		
otc	*Bromanate Elixir*[2]	15 mg pseudoephedrine HCl	1 mg brompheniramine maleate
otc	*Dimaphen Elixir*[2,3]		
otc	*Dimetapp Cold & Allergy Elixir*[2,3]		
Rx	*Brompheniramine Maleate/Pseudoephedrine HCl Syrup*	60 mg pseudoephedrine HCl	4 mg brompheniramine maleate

	Brand Name Examples	Decongestant	Antihistamine
Rx	*Bromfed-PD Capsules*[3,4]	60 mg pseudoephedrine HCl	6 mg brompheniramine maleate
Rx	*Bromfenex PD Capsules*[3,4]		
Rx	*DALLERGY-JR Capsules*[3,4]		
Rx	*ULTRAbrom PD Capsules*[3,4]		
Rx	*Rondec Oral Drops*	15 mg pseudoephedrine HCl	1 mg carbinoxamine maleate
Rx	*Andehist Drops*[2,5]	15 mg pseudoephedrine HCl	2 mg carbinoxamine maleate
Rx	*Palgic DS Syrup*		
Rx	*Pediatex-D Liquid*[2,5,6]		
Rx	*Carbinoxamine Oral Drops*[2,5]	25 mg pseudoephedrine HCl	2 mg carbinoxamine maleate
Rx	*Cydec Oral Drops*		
Rx	*Carbinoxamine Syrup*[2,3,5]	60 mg pseudoephedrine HCl	4 mg carbinoxamine maleate
otc	*PediaCare Children's Cold & Allergy Liquid*[2]	15 mg pseudoephedrine HCl	1 mg chlorpheniramine maleate
otc	*Thera-Hist Cold & Allergy Syrup*		
otc	*Tri-Acting Cold & Allergy Syrup*[2]		
otc	*Triacting Cold & Allergy Liquid*[2]		
otc	*Triaminic Cold & Allergy Liquid*[2]		
otc	*Triaminic Softchews Tablets*[7]		

	Brand Name Examples	Deconges-tant	Antihistamine
Rx	*Rescon-Jr. Capsules*[3,8]	60 mg pseudo-ephedrine HCl	4 mg chlorpheniramine maleate
otc	*Benadryl Children's Allergy & Cold Fastmelt Tablets*[3,7]	30 mg pseudo-ephedrine HCl	19 mg diphenhydramine citrate (12.5 mg diphen-hydramine HCl)
otc	*Benadryl Children's Allergy & Sinus Liquid*[2,3,5]	30 mg pseudo-ephedrine HCl	12.5 mg diphenhydramine HCl
Rx	*Quadra-Hist D PED Capsules*[4]	40 mg pseudo-ephedrine HCl	8 mg phenyltoloxamine citrate, 8 mg pyrilamine maleate, 8 mg pheni-ramine maleate
Rx	*Chlorpheniramine Tan-nate/Pseudoephedrine Tannate Suspension*[2,5]	75 mg pseudo-ephedrine tannate	4.5 mg chlorpheniramine tannate

[1] Contains tartrazine dye.
[2] Alcohol free.
[3] This product may also be used in adults; refer to package labeling.
[4] Extended release.
[5] Sugar free.
[6] Dye free.
[7] Contains phenylalanine.
[8] Sustained release.

Decongestant, Antihistamine, and Analgesic Combinations

Content given per capsule, tablet, packet, or 5 mL.

	Brand Name Examples	Decongestant	Antihistamine	Analgesic/ Other
otc	*Alka-Seltzer Plus Cold Medicine Effervescent Tablets*[1]	5 mg phenyl-ephrine HCl	2 mg chlor-pheniramine maleate	250 mg aceta-minophen
otc	*Decodult Tablets*	5 mg phenyl-ephrine HCl	2 mg chlor-pheniramine maleate	300 mg aceta-minophen

	Brand Name Examples	Decongestant	Antihistamine	Analgesic/ Other
otc	*Dristan Cold Multi-Symptom Formula Tablets*	5 mg phenylephrine HCl	2 mg chlorpheniramine maleate	325 mg acetaminophen
otc	*Dryphen Multi-Symptom Formula Tablets*			
otc	*Scot-Tussin Original Clear 5-Action Cold and Allergy Formula Liquid*[2,3-5]	4.2 mg phenylephrine HCl	13.3 mg pheniramine maleate	83.3 mg Na citrate, 83.3 mg Na salicylate, 25 mg caffeine citrate
otc	*Scot-Tussin Original 5-Action Cold and Allergy Formula Syrup*[2,4]			
otc	*Comtrex Acute Head Cold & Sinus Pressure Relief, Multi-Symptom Maximum Strength Tablets*	30 mg pseudoephedrine HCl	2 mg brompheniramine maleate	500 mg acetaminophen
otc	*Alka-Seltzer Plus Cold Medicine Liqui-Gels*[2]	30 mg pseudoephedrine HCl	2 mg chlorpheniramine maleate	325 mg acetaminophen
otc	*Kolephrin Tablets*[2]			
otc	*Actifed Cold & Sinus Maximum Strength Tablets*	30 mg pseudoephedrine HCl	2 mg chlorpheniramine maleate	500 mg acetaminophen
otc	*Comtrex Allergy-Sinus Treatment, Maximum Strength Tablets*			
otc	*Good Sense Maximum Strength Dose Sinus Tablets*			

	Brand Name Examples	Decongestant	Antihistamine	Analgesic/ Other
otc	*Good Sense Maximum Strength Pain Relief Allergy Sinus Gelcaps*	30 mg pseudoephedrine HCl	2 mg chlorpheniramine maleate	500 mg acetaminophen
otc	*Sine-Off Sinus Medicine Tablets*			
otc	*Sinutab Sinus Allergy, Maximum Strength*			
otc	*Tylenol Allergy Sinus, Maximum Strength Tablets, Gelcaps, and Geltabs*			
otc	*Comtrex Flu Therapy & Fever Relief Day & Night, Multi-Symptom Maximum Strength Tablets*	*Day:* 30 mg pseudoephedrine HCl		500 mg acetaminophen
		Night: 30 mg pseudoephedrine HCl	2 mg chlorpheniramine maleate	500 mg acetaminophen
Rx	*Simplet Tablets*	60 mg pseudoephedrine HCl	4 mg chlorpheniramine maleate	650 mg acetaminophen
otc	*Singlet for Adults Tablets*			
otc	*TheraFlu Flu and Cold Medicine Original Formula Powder*			
otc	*Triaminicin Cold, Allergy, Sinus Medicine Tablets*			
otc	*TheraFlu Flu & Cold Medicine for SoraeThroat, Maximum Strength Powder*[1]	60 mg pseudoephedrine HCl	4 mg chlorpheniramine maleate	1000 mg acetaminophen

	Brand Name Examples	Decongestant	Antihistamine	Analgesic/ Other
otc	*TheraFlu Flu & Sore Throat, Maximum Strength Powder*	60 mg pseudo-ephedrine HCl	4 mg chlor-pheniramine maleate	1000 mg aceta-minophen
otc	*TheraFlu Flu & Sore Throat Night Time, Maximum Strength Powder*[A]			
otc	*Tavist Allergy/ Sinus/Headache Tablets*	30 mg pseudo-ephedrine HCl	0.335 mg clemastine fumarate	500 mg aceta-minophen
otc	*Benadryl Allergy & Cold Tablets*	30 mg pseudo-ephedrine HCl	12.5 mg diphenhydra-mine HCl	500 mg aceta-minophen
otc	*Benadryl Allergy & Sinus Head-ache Tablets and Gelcaps*			
otc	*Benadryl Maxi-mum Strength Severe Allergy & Sinus Headache Tablets*	30 mg pseudo-ephedrine HCl	25 mg diphen-hydramine HCl	500 mg aceta-minophen
otc	*Sine-Off Night Time Formula Sinus, Cold, & Flu Medicine Geltabs*			
otc	*Sudafed Maxi-mum Strength Sinus Nighttime Plus Pain Relief Tablets*			
otc	*Tylenol Allergy Sinus NightTime, Maximum Strength Tablets*			
otc	*Tylenol Flu NightTime, Maxi-mum Strength Gelcaps*			

	Brand Name Examples	Decongestant	Antihistamine	Analgesic/ Other
otc	*Contac Day & Night Allergy/ Sinus Relief Tablets*	*Day:* 60 mg pseudoephedrine HCl		650 mg acetaminophen
		Night: 60 mg pseudoephedrine HCl	50 mg diphenhydramine HCl	650 mg acetaminophen
otc	*Tylenol Sinus NightTime, Maximum Strength Tablets*	30 mg pseudoephedrine HCl	6.25 mg doxylamine succinate	500 mg acetaminophen
otc	*Coricidin 'D' Cold, Flu, & Sinus Tablets*[2]	30 mg pseudoephedrine sulfate	2 mg chlorpheniramine maleate	325 mg acetaminophen
otc	*Drixoral Allergy Sinus Tablets*[6]	60 mg pseudoephedrine sulfate	3 mg dexbrompheniramine maleate	500 mg acetaminophen

[1] Contains phenylalanine.
[2] This product may also be used in children; refer to package labeling.
[3] Sugar free.
[4] Alcohol free.
[5] Dye free.
[6] Extended release.

Pediatric Decongestant, Antihistamine, and Analgesic Combinations

Content given per tablet or 5 mL.

	Brand Name Examples	Decongestant	Antihistamine	Analgesic
otc	*Tylenol Children's Cold Chewable Tablets*[1]	7.5 mg pseudoephedrine HCl	0.5 mg chlorpheniramine maleate	80 mg acetaminophen
otc	*Tylenol Children's Cold Liquid*	15 mg pseudoephedrine HCl	1 mg chlorpheniramine maleate	160 mg acetaminophen

[1] Contains phenylalanine.
[2] Alcohol free.

Decongestant, Antihistamine, and Anticholinergic Combinations

Content given per tablet or 5 mL.

	Brand Name Examples	Decongestant	Antihistamine	Anticholinergic
Rx	*Dallergy Syrup*[1]	10 mg phenylephrine HCl	2 mg chlorpheniramine maleate	0.625 mg methscopolamine nitrate
Rx	*AH-chew Tablets*[1,2]	10 mg phenylephrine HCl	2 mg chlorpheniramine maleate	1.25 mg methscopolamine nitrate
Rx	*D.A. Chewable Tablets*[1]			
Rx	*Dehistine Syrup*[1,3]			
Rx	*Duradryl Syrup*[1]			
Rx	*Extendryl Chewable Tablets*[1]			
Rx	*Extendryl Syrup*[1]			
Rx	*Ex-Histine Syrup*[1]			
Rx	*D.A. II Tablets*[1,4]	10 mg phenylephrine HCl	4 mg chlorpheniramine maleate	1.25 mg methscopolamine nitrate
Rx	*Dallergy Tablets*[1]			
Rx	*Dallergy Extended Release Tablets*[1]	20 mg phenylephrine HCl	8 mg chlorpheniramine maleate	2.5 mg methscopolamine nitrate
Rx	*Dura-Vent/DA Tablets*[1,4]			
Rx	*Extendryl SR Capsules*			
otc	*Hista-Vent DA Tablets*[1,4]			
Rx	*OMNIhist L.A. Tablets*[4]			
Rx	*Pre-Hist-D Tablets*[1,4]			

	Brand Name Examples	Decongestant	Antihistamine	Anticholinergic
Rx	*Stahist Tablets*[4,5]	25 mg phenylephrine HCl, 40 mg pseudoephedrine	8 mg chlorpheniramine maleate	0.19 mg hyoscyamine sulfate, 0.04 mg atropine sulfate, 0.01 mg scopolamine HBr
Rx	*AlleRx-D Tablets*[6]	120 mg pseudoephedrine HCl		2.5 mg methscopolamine nitrate
Rx	*PSE 120/MSC 2.5 Tablets*[1]			
Rx	*Pannaz S Syrup*[1]	15 mg pseudoephedrine HCl	2 mg carbinoxamine maleate	1.25 mg methscopolamine nitrate
Rx	*Respa A.R. Tablets*[5,7]	90 mg pseudoephedrine HCl	8 mg chlorpheniramine maleate	0.024 mg belladonna alkaloids (atropine, hyoscyamine, scopolamine)
Rx	*CPM 8/PSE 90/MSC 2.5 Tablets*[1,4]	90 mg pseudoephedrine HCl	8 mg chlorpheniramine maleate	2.5 mg methscopolamine nitrate
Rx	*Pannaz Tablets*[1,4]			
Rx	*Mescolor Tablets*[1,4,5]	120 mg pseudoephedrine HCl	8 mg chlorpheniramine maleate	2.5 mg methscopolamine nitrate
Rx	*Rescon-MX Tablets*[1,4]			
Rx	*Xiral Tablets*[1,4,5]			
Rx	*AlleRx Dose Pack Tablets*[6]	*Day:* 120 mg pseudoephedrine HCl		2.5 mg methscopolamine nitrate
		Night:	8 mg chlorpheniramine maleate	2.5 mg methscopolamine nitrate

[1] This product may also be used in children; refer to package labeling.
[2] Chewable.
[3] Alcohol free.
[4] Sustained release.
[5] Dye free.
[6] Controlled release.
[7] Sugar free.

Pediatric Decongestant, Antihistamine, and Anticholinergic Combinations

Content given per capsule.

	Brand Name Examples	Decongestant	Antihistamine	Anticholinergic
Rx	*Duradryl JR Capsules*	10 mg phenylephrine HCl	4 mg chlorpheniramine maleate	1.25 mg methscopolamine nitrate
Rx	*Extendryl JR Capsules*			

Antitussive Combinations

Content given per tablet, capsule, packet, pouch, or 5 mL.

	Brand Name Examples	Antitussive	Antihistamine	Decongestant	Other
Rx	*Tannic-12 Tablets*[1]	60 mg carbetapentane tannate	5 mg chlorpheniramine tannate		
Rx	*Trionate Tablets*				
Rx	*Tussi-12 Tablets*				
Rx	*Quad Tann Tablets*	60 mg carbetapentane tannate	5 mg chlorpheniramine tannate	10 mg phenylephrine tannate, 10 mg ephedrine tannate	
Rx	*Rynatuss Tablets*				
c-III	*Cycofed Syrup*[2]	20 mg codeine phosphate		60 mg pseudoephedrine HCl	
c-III	*Nucofed Syrup*[2,3]				
c-III	*Nucofed Capsules*				
c-V	*Dihistine DH Elixir*[2,4]	10 mg codeine phosphate	2 mg chlorpheniramine maleate	30 mg pseudoephedrine HCl	
c-V	*Decohistine DH Liquid*[4]				
c-V	*Ryna-C Liquid*[1,2,3,5]				
c-V	*Prometh w/Codeine Cough Syrup*[2,4]	10 mg codeine phosphate	6.25 mg promethazine HCl		
c-V	*Promethazine HCl w/Codeine Syrup*[2]				

	Brand Name Examples	Antitussive	Antihistamine	Decongestant	Other
c-v	*Promethazone VC w/Codeine Cough Syrup*[2,4]	10 mg codeine phosphate	6.25 mg promethazine HCl	5 mg phenylephrine HCl	
c-v	*Prometh VC w/Codeine Cough Syrup*[2,4]				
c-v	*Tricodene Cough & Cold Liquid*[2]	8.2 mg codeine phosphate	12.5 mg pyrilamine maleate		
c-v	*Codimal PH Syrup*[2,3]	10 mg codeine phosphate	8.33 mg pyrilamine maleate	5 mg phenylephrine HCl	
c-v	*Triacin-C Cough Syrup*[2,4]	10 mg codeine phosphate	1.25 mg triprolidine HCl	30 mg pseudoephedrine HCl	
otc	*Robitussin Honey Cough & Cold Liquid*	10 mg dextromethorphan HBr		20 mg pseudoephedrine HCl	
otc	*Top Care Maximum Strength Soothing Cough & Head Congestion Relief D Liquid*[2,4]				
otc	*Vicks 44D Cough & Head Congestion Relief Liquid*[2,4]				
otc	*Robitussin Maximum Strength Cough & Cold Syrup*[4]	15 mg dextromethorphan HBr		30 mg pseudoephedrine HCl	
otc	*666 Cold Preparation, Maximum Strength Liquid*[2]	3.3 mg dextromethorphan HBr		10 mg pseudoephedrine HCl	108.3 mg acetaminophen
otc	*Vicks DayQuil Multi-Symptom Cold/Flu Relief Liquid*[2]				

	Brand Name Examples	Antitussive	Antihistamine	Decongestant	Other
otc	*Robitussin Honey Flu Multi-Symptom Liquid*	6.6 mg dextromethorphan HBr		20 mg pseudoephedrine HCl	166.6 mg acetaminophen
otc	*Vicks DayQuil LiquiCaps Multi-Symptom Cold/Flu Relief Capsules*[2]	10 mg dextromethorphan HBr		30 mg pseudoephedrine HCl	250 mg acetaminophen
otc	*Alka-Seltzer Plus Cold & Flu Liqui-Gels*[2]	10 mg dextromethorphan HBr		30 mg pseudoephedrine HCl	325 mg acetaminophen
otc	*Alka-Seltzer Plus Liqui-Gels Flu Medicine*[2]				
otc	*Tylenol Cold Non-Drowsy Formula Gelcaps and Tablets*[2]	15 mg dextromethorphan HBr		30 mg pseudoephedrine HCl	325 mg acetaminophen
otc	*Top Care Multi-Symptom Pain Relief Cold Tablets*[2]				
otc	*Comtrex Multi-Symptom Maximum Strength Non-Drowsy Cold & Cough Relief Tablets*	15 mg dextromethorphan HBr		30 mg pseudoephedrine	500 mg acetaminophen
otc	*TheraFlu Non-Drowsy Formula Maximum Strength Tablets*				
otc	*Tylenol Flu Maximum Strength Non-Drowsy Gelcaps*				
otc	*Sudafed Non-Drowsy Severe Cold Formula Maximum Strength Tablets*				

	Brand Name Examples	Antitussive	Antihistamine	Decongestant	Other
otc	*Robitussin Honey Flu Non-Drowsy Syrup*	20 mg dextromethorphan HBr		60 mg pseudoephedrine HCl	500 mg acetaminophen
otc	*TheraFlu Non-Drowsy Flu, Cold & Cough Maximum Strength Powder*	30 mg dextromethorphan HBr		60 mg pseudoephedrine HCl	1000 mg acetaminophen
otc	*TheraFlu Severe Cold & Congestion Non-Drowsy, Maximum Strength Powder*				
Rx	*Bromatane DX Syrup*[2,4,5]	10 mg dextromethorphan HBr	2 mg brompheniramine maleate	30 mg pseudoephedrine HCl	
Rx	*Bromfed DM Cough Syrup*[2]				
Rx	*Dimetane-DX Cough Syrup*[2,4,5]				
otc	*Robitussin Allergy & Cough Liquid*[1,2,3]				
Rx	*Alacol DM Syrup*[3,5]	10 mg dextromethorphan HBr	2 mg brompheniramine maleate	5 mg phenylephrine HCl	
Rx	*Carbodex DM Syrup*	15 mg dextromethorphan HBr	4 mg brompheniramine maleate	45 mg pseudoephedrine HCl	
Rx	*Carbofed DM Syrup*[2]				
Rx	*Rondec-DM Syrup*[2]				

	Brand Name Examples	Antitussive	Antihistamine	Decongestant	Other
Rx	*Andehist-DM Syrup*[2,3]	15 mg dextromethorphan HBr	4 mg brompheniramine maleate	60 mg pseudoephedrine HCl	
Rx	*Coldec DM Syrup*[2,3,5]				
Rx	*Rondamine DM Syrup*				
Rx	*Sildec-DM Syrup*[2,3,5]				
Rx	*Anaplex-DM Liquid*[1,2,3,5]	30 mg dextromethorphan HBr	4 mg brompheniremine maleate	60 mg pseudoephedrine HCl	
Rx	*Balamine DM Syrup*[2]	12.5 mg dextromethorphan HBr	4 mg carbinoxamine maleate	60 mg pseudoephedrine HCl	
Rx	*Carbinoxamine Compound Syrup*[4]	15 mg dextromethorphan HBr	4 mg carbinoxamine maleate	60 mg pseudoephedrine HCl	
Rx	*Cardec DM Syrup*[2,4]				
Rx	*Cydec-DM Syrup*[2]				
Rx	*Tussafed Syrup*[2,3,5]				
otc	*Tricodene Sugar Free Liquid*[2,3,5]	10 mg dextromethorphan HBr	2 mg chlorpheniramine maleate		
otc	*Scot-Tussin DM Liquid*[1,2,3,5]	15 mg dextromethorphan HBr	2 mg chlorpheniramine maleate		
otc	*Coricidin HBP Cough & Cold Tablets*	30 mg dextromethorphan HBr	4 mg chlorpheniramine maleate		

	Brand Name Examples	Antitussive	Antihistamine	Decongestant	Other
otc	*Coricidin HBP Maximum Strength Flu Tablets*	15 mg dextromethorphan HBr	2 mg chlorpheniramine maleate		500 mg acetaminophen
otc	*Alka-Seltzer Plus Flu Medicine Effervescent Tablets*[6]	15 mg dextromethorphan HBr	2 mg chlorpheniramine maleate		500 mg aspirin
otc	*Father John's Medicine Plus Liquid*[8]	1.66 mg dextromethorphan HBr	0.66 mg chlorpheniramine maleate	1.66 mg phenylephrine HCl	
otc	*Alka-Seltzer Plus Cold & Cough Medicine Effervescent Tablets*[6]	10 mg dextromethorphan HBr	2 mg chlorpheniramine maleate	5 mg phenylephrine HCl	
Rx	*Atuss DM Syrup*[2,3]	15 mg dextromethorphan HBr	2 mg chlorpheniramine maleate	10 mg phenylephrine HCl	
otc	*Rescon-DM Liquid*[1,2,3,5]	10 mg dextromethorphan HBr	2 mg chlorpheniramine maleate	30 mg pseudoephedrine HCl	
otc	*Robitussin Flu Liquid*[2,3]	5 mg dextromethorphan HBr	1 mg chlorpheniramine maleate	15 mg pseudoephedrine HCl	160 mg acetaminophen
otc	*Vicks 44M Cough, Cold, & Flu Relief Liquid*[4]	7.5 mg dextromethorphan HBr	1 mg chlorpheniramine maleate	15 mg pseudoephedrine HCl	162.5 mg acetaminophen

	Brand Name Examples	Antitussive	Antihistamine	Decongestant	Other
otc	*Alka-Seltzer Plus Cold & Cough Liqui-Gels*[2]	10 mg dextromethorphan HBr	2 mg chlorpheniramine maleate	30 mg pseudoephedrine HCl	325 mg acetaminophen
otc	*Kolephrin/DM Tablets*[2]				
otc	*Top Care Multi-Symptom Pain Relief Cold Tablets*[2]	15 mg dextromethorphan HBr	2 mg chlorpheniramine maleate	30 mg pseudoephedrine HCl	325 mg acetaminophen
otc	*Tylenol Cold Complete Formula Tablets*[2]				
otc	*Mapap Cold Formula Tablets*[2]				
otc	*Contac Severe Cold & Flu Maximum Strength Tablets*	15 mg dextromethorphan HBr	2 mg chlorpheniramine maleate	30 mg pseudoephedrine HCl	500 mg acetaminophen
otc	*Comtrex Day & Night Cold & Cough Relief, Multi-Symptom Maximum Strength Tablets*				
otc	*Genacol Maximum Strength Cold & Flu Relief Tablets*				
otc	*Comtrex Cough and Cold Relief, Multi-Symptom Maximum Strength Tablets*[2]				
otc	*Cold Symptoms Relief Maximum Strength Tablets*				
otc	*TheraFlu Maximum Strength NightTime Formula Flu, Cold, & Cough Medicine Tablets*				

	Brand Name Examples	Antitussive	Antihistamine	Decongestant	Other
otc	*Robitussin Honey Flu Nighttime Syrup*	20 mg dextromethorphan HBr	4 mg chlorpheniramine maleate	60 mg pseudoephedrine HCl	500 mg acetaminophen
otc	*TheraFlu Flu, Cold & Cough Powder*	20 mg dextromethorphan HBr	4 mg chlorpheniramine maleate	60 mg pseudoephedrine HCl	650 mg acetaminophen
otc	*TheraFlu Cold & Cough Night Time Powder*				
otc	*TheraFlu Flu, Cold, & Cough and Sore Throat, Maximum Strength Powder*[6]	30 mg dextromethorphan HBr	4 mg chlorpheniramine maleate	60 mg pseudoephedrine HCl	1000 mg acetaminophen
otc	*TheraFlu Flu & Cough Night Time, Maximum Strength Powder*[6]				
otc	*TheraFlu Flu, Cold, & Cough Night Time, Maximum Strength Powder*				
otc	*TheraFlu Severe Cold & Congestion Night Time, Maximum Strength Powder*				
otc	*Top Care Maximum Strength Flu, Cold, & Cough Medicine Night Time Powder*				

	Brand Name Examples	Antitussive	Antihistamine	Decongestant	Other
otc	*Contac Day & Night Cold & Flu Tablets*	*Day:* 30 mg dextromethorphan HBr		60 mg pseudoephedrine HCl	650 mg acetaminophen
		Night:	50 mg diphenhydramine HCl	60 mg pseudoephedrine HCl	650 mg acetaminophen
otc	*Vicks NyQuil Cough Syrup*[2,4]	5 mg dextromethorphan HBr	2.1 mg doxylamine succinate		
otc	*Alka-Seltzer Plus Night-Time Cold Medicine Effervescent Tablets*[6]	10 mg dextromethorphan HBr	6.25 mg doxylamine succinate	5 mg phenylephrine HCl	
otc	*All-Nite Liquid*[4]	5 mg dextromethorphan HBr	2.1 mg doxylamine succinate	10 mg pseudoephedrine HCl	167 mg acetaminophen
otc	*Nite Time Cold Formula for Adults Liquid*[4]				
otc	*Tylenol Flu Night-Time, Maximum Strength Liquid*[2]				
otc	*Vicks NyQuil Multi-Symptom Cold/Flu Relief Liquid*[4]				
otc	*Top Care LiquiCaps Nite Time Multi-Symptom Cold/Flu Relief Capsules*	10 mg dextromethorphan HBr	6.25 mg doxylamine succinate	30 mg pseudoephedrine HCl	250 mg acetaminophen
otc	*Vicks NyQuil Multi-Symptom Cold & Flu Relief LiquiCaps Capsules*				

	Brand Name Examples	Antitussive	Antihistamine	Decongestant	Other
otc	*Alka-Seltzer Plus NightTime Cold Liqui-Gels*[3]	10 mg dextromethorphan HBr	6.25 mg doxylamine succinate	30 mg pseudoephedrine HCl	325 mg acetaminophen
Rx	*Prometh w/Dextromethorphan Syrup*[2,4]	15 mg dextromethorphan HBr	6.25 mg promethazine		
Rx	*Promethazine w/Dextromethorphan Cough Syrup*[2,4]				
otc	*Codal-DM Syrup*[1,2,3,5]	10 mg dextromethorphan HBr	8.33 mg pyrilamine maleate	5 mg phenylephrine HCl	
otc	*Codimal DM Syrup*[1,2,3,5]				
otc	*Dicomal-DM Syrup*[1,2,3,5]				
otc	*Robitussin Night Relief Liquid*[3]	5 mg dextromethorphan HBr	8.3 mg pyrilamine maleate	10 mg pseudoephedrine HCl	108.3 mg acetaminophen
c-III	*Hycodan Tablets*[2]	5 mg hydrocodone bitartrate			1.5 mg homatropine MBr
c-III	*Hycodan Syrup*[2]				
c-III	*Hydromet Syrup*[2]				
c-III	*Hydromide Syrup*[2,1]				
c-III	*Hydropane Syrup*[2]				
c-III	*Tussigon Tablets*[2]				
c-III	*Detussin Liquid*[2,4]	5 mg hydrocodone bitartrate		60 mg pseudoephedrine HCl	
c-III	*Histussin D Liquid*[2]				
c-III	*P-V-Tussin Tablets*				

Brand Name Examples	Antitussive	Antihistamine	Decongestant	Other
c-III *Anaplex HD Liquid*[1,2,3,5]	1.7 mg hydrocodone bitartrate	2 mg brompheniramine maleate	30 mg pseudoephedrine HCl	
c-III *S-T Forte 2 Liquid*[1,2,3,5]	2.5 mg hydrocodone bitartrate	2 mg chlorpheniramine maleate		
c-III *ED-TLC Liquid*[2]	1.67 mg hydrocodone bitartrate	2 mg chlorpheniramine maleate	5 mg phenylephrine HCl	
c-III *Hydrocodone HD Liquid*[2,3]				
c-III *Endagen-HD Liquid*[2]	1.7 mg hydrocodone bitartrate	2 mg chlorpheniramine maleate	5 mg phenylephrine HCl	
c-III *Vanex HD Liquid*[1]				
c-III *Hydro-PC Liquid*[2]	2 mg hydrocodone bitartrate	2 mg chlorpheniramine maleate	5 mg phenylephrine HCl	
c-III *Hydro-PC II Liquid*[2]	2 mg hydrocodone bitartrate	2 mg chlorpheniramine maleate	7.5 mg phenylephrine HCl	
c-III *Comtussin HC Syrup*[1,5]	2.5 mg hydrocodone bitartrate	2 mg chlorpheniramine maleate	5 mg phenylephrine HCl	
c-III *Cytuss HC Liquid*[2]				
c-III *Histussin HC Syrup*[3,5]				
c-III *Hydrocodone CP Syrup*[2,3,5]				
c-III *Histinex HC Syrup*[2,3,5]				

	Brand Name Examples	Antitussive	Antihistamine	Decongestant	Other
c-III c-III c-III	Atuss HD Liquid[2] ED Tuss HC Syrup[2,4] Maxi-Tuss HC Liquid[2]	2.5 mg hydrocodone bitartrate	4 mg chlorpheniramine maleate	10 mg phenylephrine HCl	
c-III	Atuss MS Liquid[2]	5 mg hydrocodone bitartrate	2 mg chlorpheniramine maleate	10 mg phenylephrine HCl	
c-III c-III c-III c-III	Histinex PV Syrup[2,3,5] Hyphed Liquid[2,4] P-V-Tussin Syrup[2,4] Tussend Syrup[2,4]	2.5 mg hydrocodone bitartrate	2 mg chlorpheniramine maleate	30 mg pseudoephedrine HCl	
c-III c-III	Hydro-Tussin HC Syrup[1,2,3,5] Pancof-HC Liquid[1,2,3,5]	3 mg hydrocodone bitartrate	2 mg chlorpheniramine maleate	15 mg pseudoephedrine HCl	
c-III	Tussend Tablets[2]	5 mg hydrocodone bitartrate	4 mg chlorpheniramine maleate	60 mg pseudoephedrine HCl	
c-III	Statuss Green Liquid[2,3,5]	2.5 mg hydrocodone bitartrate	2 mg chlorpheniramine maleate, 3.3 mg pyrilamine maleate	5 mg phenylephrine HCl, 3.3 mg pseudoephedrine HCl	
c-III	Tussionex Pennkinetic Suspension[2,3,7]	10 mg hydrodone (as polistirex)	8 mg chlorpheniramine (as polistirex)		

	Brand Name Examples	Antitussive	Antihistamine	Decongestant	Other
c-III	*Hydrocodone Bitartrate 5 mg/ Pseudoephedrine HCl 30 mg/Carbinoxamine Maleate 2 mg* Liquid	5 mg hydrocodone bitartrate	2 mgcarbinoxamine maleate	30 mg pseudoephedrine HCl	
c-III	*Codal-DH Syrup*[2]	1.66 mg hydrocodone bitartrate	8.33 mg pyrilamine maleate	5 mg phenylephrine HCl	
c-III	*Codimal DH Syrup*[2,3]				
c-III	*Dicomal-DH Syrup*[2]	1.66 mg hydrocodone bitartrate	8.33 mg pyrilamine maleate	5 mg phenylephrine HCl	

[1] Dye free.
[2] This product may also be used in children; refer to package labeling.
[3] Alcohol free.
[4] Contains alcohol.
[5] Sugar free.
[6] Contains phenylalanine.
[7] Extended release.

Pediatric Antitussive Combinations

Content given per tablet, 5 mL (liquid), or 1 mL (drops).

	Brand Name Examples	Decongestant	Antihistamine	Antitussive	Other
Rx	*Tussi-12 S Suspension*[1]		4 mg chlorpheniramine tannate	30 mg carbetapentane tannate	
Rx	*Tannic-12 Suspension*	5 mg phenylephrine tannate	4 mg chlorpheniramine tannate	30 mg carbetapentane tannate	
Rx	*Rynatuss Pediatric Suspension*[1]	5 mg phenylephrine tannate, 5 mg ephedrine tannate	4 mg chlorpheniramine tannate	30 mg carbetapantane tannate	

	Brand Name Examples	**Decongestant**	**Antihistamine**	**Antitussive**	**Other**
otc	*Dimetapp Decongestant Plus Cough Infant Drops*[2]	9.375 mg/mL pseudoephedrine HCl		3.125 mg/mL dextromethorphan HBr	
otc	*Pedia Care Infants' Decongestant & Cough Drops*[2]				
otc	*Pedia Relief Decongestant Plus Cough Infants' Drops*[2]	9.375 mg/mL pseudoephedrine HCl		3.125 mg/mL dextromethorphan HBr	
otc	*Tylenol Infants' Cold Decongestant & Fever Reducer Plus Cough Concentrated Drops*[2]	9.375 mg/mL pseudoephedrine HCl		3.125 mg/mL dextromethorphan HBr	100 mg/mL acetaminophen
otc	*Sudafed Children's Non-Drowsy Cold & Cough Liquid*[2-4]	15 mg pseudoephedrine HCl		5 mg dextromethorphan HBr	
otc	*Dimetapp Children's Non-Drowsy Flu Syrup*[2,3]	15 mg pseudoephedrine HCl		5 mg dextromethorphan HBr	160 mg acetaminophen
otc	*Triaminic Throat Pain & Cough Softchews Tablets*[1,3]				

	Brand Name Examples	**Decongestant**	**Antihistamine**	**Antitussive**	**Other**
otc	*Pedia Care Children's Long-Lasting Cough Plus Cold Liquid*[2]	15 mg pseudoephedrine HCl		7.5 mg dextromethorphan HBr	
otc	*Robitussin Pediatric Cough & Cold Formula Liquid*[2,3]				
otc	*Triaminic AM Non-Drowsy Cough & Decongestant Liquid*[3]				
otc	*Triaminic Cough & Congestion Liquid*[2]				
otc	*Triaminic Cough & Sore Throat Liquid*[2]	15 mg pseudoephedrine HCl		7.5 mg dextromethorphan HBr	160 mg acetaminophen
otc	*Bromanate DM Cold & Cough Elixir*[2,3]	15 mg pseudoephedrine HCl	1 mg brompheniramine maleate	5 mg dextromethorphan HBr	
otc	*Children's Elixir DM Cough & Cold Elixir*[2,3]				
otc	*Dimaphen DM Cold & Cough Elixir*[2,3]				
otc	*Dimetapp DM Children's Cold & Cough Elixir*[2,3]				
otc	*Dimetapp Children's Nighttime Flu Syrup*[2,3]	15 mg pseudoephedrine HCl	1 mg brompheniramine maleate	5 mg dextromethorphan HBr	160 mg acetaminophen
Rx	*C.P.-DM Drops*	15 mg/mL pseudoephedrine HCl	1 mg/mL carbinoxamine maleate	4 mg/mL dextromethorphan HBr	
Rx	*Carbofed DM Oral Drops*[2,4]				
Rx	*Rondec-DM Oral Drops*				

	Brand Name Examples	Decongestant	Antihistamine	Antitussive	Other
Rx	*Andehist DM Oral Drops*	15 mg/mL pseudoephedrine HCl	2 mg/mL carbinoxamine maleate	4 mg/mL dextromethorphan HBr	
Rx	*Carbodex DM Drops*				
Rx	*Sildec-DM Oral Drops*[2,4]				
Rx	*Pediatex-DM Liquid*[3]	15 mg pseudoephedrine HCl	2 mg carbinoxamine maleate	15 mg dextromethorphan HBr	
Rx	*Balamine DM Oral Drops*	25 mg/mL pseudoephedrine HCl	2 mg/mL carbinoxamine maleate	3.5 mg/mL dextromethorphan HBr	
Rx	*Carbinoxamine Compound Drops*	25 mg/mL pseudoephedrine HCl	2 mg/mL carbinoxamine maleate	4 mg/mL dextromethorphan HBr	
Rx	*Cydec-DM Drops*				
Rx	*Balamine DM Syrup*[3]	60 mg pseudoephedrine HCl	4 mg carbinoxamine maleate	12.5 mg dextromethorphan HBr	
Rx	*Cydec-DM Syrup*[3]	60 mg pseudoephedrine HCl	4 mg carbinoxamine maleate	15 mg dextromethorphan HBr	
otc	*Tylenol Children's Cold Plus Cough Chewable Tablets*	7.5 mg pseudoephedrine HCl	0.5 mg chlorpheniramine maleate	2.5 mg dextromethorphan HBr	80 mg acetaminophen

	Brand Name Examples	Decongestant	Antihistamine	Antitussive	Other
otc	*All-Nite Children's Cold/Cough Relief Liquid*[2,3]	10 mg pseudoephedrine HCl	0.67 mg chlorpheniramine maleate	5 mg dextromethorphan HBr	
otc	*Nite Time Children's Liquid*[2,3]				
otc	*Vicks Children's NyQuil Cold/Cough Relief Liquid*[2,3]				
otc	*Vicks Pediatric 44M Cough & Cold Relief Liquid*[2,3]				
otc	*Kid Kare Children's Cough/Cold Liquid*[2]	15 mg pseudoephedrine HCl	1 mg chlorpheniramine maleate	5 mg dextromethorphan HBr	
otc	*Pedia Care Cough-Cold Liquid*[2]				
otc	*Pedia Care Multi-Symptom Cold Liquid*[2]				
otc	*Thera-Hist Cold & Cough Syrup*[3]	15 mg pseudoephedrine HCl	1 mg chlorpheniramine maleate	5 mg dextromethorphan HBr	
otc	*Tri-Acting Cold & Cough Syrup*[2]				
otc	*Triaminic Cold & Cough Liquid*[2]				
otc	*Triaminic Cold & Cough Softchews Tablets*[5]				
otc	*Triaminic Cough Softchews Tablets*[3,5]				
otc	*Tylenol Children's Cold Plus Cough Suspension*[2]	15 mg pseudoephedrine HCl	1 mg chlorpheniramine maleate	5 mg dextromethorphan HBr	160 mg acetaminophen

	Brand Name Examples	Decongestant	Antihistamine	Antitussive	Other
otc	*Pedia Care Night-Rest Cough & Cold Liquid*[2]	15 mg pseudoephedrine HCl	1 mg chlorpheniramine maleate	7.5 mg dextromethorphan HBr	
otc	*Robitussin Pediatric Night Relief Cough & Cold Liquid*[2]				
otc	*Triaminic Cold & Night Time Cough Liquid*[2]				
otc	*Triaminic Cold, Cough & Fever Liquid*	15 mg pseudoephedrine HCl	1 mg chlorpheniramine maleate	7.5 mg dextromethorphan HBr	160 mg acetaminophen
otc	*Tylenol Children's Flu Suspension*[2]				

[1] Contains tartrazine.
[2] Alcohol free.
[3] This product may also be used in adults; refer to package labeling.
[4] Sugar free.
[5] Contains phenylalanine.

Antitussive and Expectorant Combinations

Content given per tablet, 5 mL, or packet.

	Brand Name Examples	Antitussive	Expectorant	Decongestant	Antihistamine/ Other
Rx	*Levall Liquid*[1,2]	20 mg carbetapantane citrate	100 mg guaifenesin	15 mg phenylephrine HCl	
c-v	*Dihistine Expectorant Liquid*	10 mg codeine phosphate	100 mg guaifenesin	30 mg pseudoephedrine HCl	
c-v	*Guiatuss DAC Liquid*[1,3]				
c-v	*Halotussin DAC Syrup*[1,3,4]				
c-v	*Mytussin DAC Liquid*[1,3,4]				
c-v	*Novagest Expectorant with Codeine Liquid*[1,3]				
c-III	*Nucofed Expectorant Syrup*[1,3]	20 mg codeine phosphate	200 mg guaifenesin	60 mg pseudoephedrine HCl	
c-III	*Nucotuss Expectorant Syrup*[1,3]				
c-v	*Tussirex Syrup*[2,5]	10 mg codeine phosphate	83.3 mg sodium citrate	4.17 mg phenylephrine HCl	13.33 mg pheniramine maleate, 83.33 mg sodium salicylate, 25 mg caffeine citrate
c-v	*Tussirex Sugar Free Liquid*[2,4,5]				
Rx	*Donatussin Syrup*[1,2]	7.5 mg dextromethorphan HBr	100 mg guaifenesin	10 mg phenylephrine HCl	2 mg chlorpheniramine maleate

	Brand Name Examples	Antitussive	Expectorant	Decongestant	Antihistamine/ Other
otc	*Tussex Cough Syrup*[1,2,4]	10 mg dextromethorphan HBr	100 mg guaifenesin	5 mg phenylephrine HCl	
otc	*Tussafed Ex Syrup*[1,2]	30 mg dextromethorphan HBr	200 mg guaifenesin	10 mg phenylephrine HCl	
otc	*Guiatuss CF Syrup*[1,2]	10 mg dextromethorphan HBr	100 mg guaifenesin	30 mg pseudoephedrinc HCl	
otc	*Robafen CF Syrup*[1,2]				
otc	*Robitussin CF Syrup*[1,2]				
otc	*Comtrex Multi-Symptom Deep Chest Cold & Congestion Relief Softgels*	10 mg dextromethorphan HBr	100 mg guaifenesin	30 mg pseudoephedrine HCl	250 mg acetaminophen
otc	*Robitussin Cold, Multi-Symptom Cold & Flu Softgels*				
otc	*Sudafed Multi-Symptom Cold & Cough Liquid Caps*				
Rx	*Profen II DM Liquid*[1,2,4,5]	10 mg dextromethorphan HBr	200 mg guaifenesin	15 mg pseudoephedrine HCl	
otc	*Cold & Cough Tussin Softgels*[1]	10 mg dextromethorphan HBr	200 mg guaifenesin	30 mg pseudoephedrine HCl	
otc	*Robitussin Cold, Cold & Cough Softgels*[1]				

	Brand Name Examples	Antitussive	Expectorant	Decongestant	Antihistamine/ Other
otc	*Robitussin Cold, Cold & Congestion Softgels and Tablets*[1]	10 mg dextromethorphan HBr	200 mg guaifenesin	30 mg pseudoephedrine HCl	
otc	*Robitussin Cold, Multi-Symptom Cold & Flu Tablets*[1]	10 mg dextromethorphan HBr	200 mg guaifenesin	30 mg pseudoephedrine HCl	325 mg acetaminophen
Rx	*PanMist-DM Syrup*[1,2,4,5]	15 mg dextromethorphan HBr	100 mg guaifenesin	45 mg pseudoephedrine HCl	
otc	*Tylenol Multi-Symptom Cold Severe Congestion Tablets*[1]	15 mg dextromethorphan HBr	200 mg guaifenesin	30 mg pseudoephedrine HCl	325 mg acetaminophen
Rx	*Z-Cof DM Syrup*[1,2,4]	15 mg dextromethorphan HBr	200 mg guaifenesin	40 mg pseudoephedrine HCl	
otc	*TheraFlu Maximum Strength Flu & Congestion Non-Drowsy Powder*[6]	30 mg dextromethorphan HBr	400 mg guaifenesin	60 mg pseudoephedrine HCl	1000 mg acetaminophen
otc	*TheraFlu Maximum Strength Flu, Cold & Cough Powder*[2,6]				
Rx	*Maxifed DM Tablets*[1,5,7]	30 mg dextromethorphan HBr	550 mg guaifenesin	60 mg pseudoephedrine HCl	
Rx	*Touro CC Tablets*[1,5,7]	30 mg dextromethorphan HBr	575 mg guaifenesin	60 mg pseudoephedrine HCl	
Rx	*PanMist-DM Tablets*[1,8]	30 mg dextromethorphan HBr	600 mg guaifenesin	45 mg pseudoephedrine HCl	

	Brand Name Examples	Antitussive	Expectorant	Decongestant	Antihistamine/ Other
Rx	*Protuss DM Tablets*[1,5,7]	30 mg dextromethorphan HBr	600 mg guaifenesin	60 mg pseudoephedrine HCl	
Rx	*Tussafed-LA Tablets*[1,5,7]	30 mg dextromethorphan HBr	600 mg guaifenesin	60 mg pseudoephedrine HCl	
Rx	*Guaifenex-Rx DM Tablets*[8]	*Day:*	600 mg guaifenesin	60 mg pseudoephedrine HCl	
		Night: 30 mg dextromethorphan HBr	600 mg guaifenesin		
Rx	*MED-Rx DM Tablets*[9]	*Day:*	600 mg guaifenesin	60 mg pseudoephedrine HCl	
		Night: 30 mg dextromethorphan HBr	600 mg guaifenesin		
Rx	*Profen II DM Tablets*[1,8]	30 mg dextromethorphan HBr	800 mg guaifenesin	45 mg pseudoephedrine HCl	
Rx	*Medent-DM Tablets*[1,5,7]	30 mg dextromethorphan HBr	800 mg guaifenesin	60 mg pseudoephedrine HCl	
Rx	*Profen Forte DM Tablets*[1,7]	60 mg dextromethorphan HBr	800 mg guaifenesin	90 mg pseudoephedrine HCl	
Rx	*Aquatab C Tablets*	60 mg dextromethorphan HBr	1200 mg guaifenesin	120 mg pseudoephedrine HCl	
Rx	*GFN 1200/DM 60/PSE 120 Tablets*[5,7]	60 mg dextromethorphan HBr	1200 mg guaifenesin	120 mg pseudoephedrine HCl	

	Brand Name Examples	Antitussive	Expectorant	Decongestant	Antihistamine/ Other
C-III	*Atuss-G Syrup*[1]	2 mg hydrocodone bitartrate	100 mg guaifenesin	10 mg phenylephrine HCl	
C-III	*Donatussin DC Syrup*[1,2]	2.5 mg hydrocodone bitartrate	50 mg guaifenesin	7.5 mg phenylephrine HCl	
C-III	*Tussafed HC Syrup*[1,2]				
C-III	*Entex HC Liquid*[1,2,4,5]	5 mg hydrocodone bitartrate	100 mg guaifenesin	7.5 mg phenylephrine HCl	
C-III	*Levall 5.0 Liquid*[1,2,4]	5 mg hydrocodone bitartrate	100 mg guaifenesin	15 mg phenylephrine HCl	
C-III	*ZTuss Expectorant Liquid*[1,6]	2.5 mg hydrocodone bitartrate	100 mg guaifenesin	15 mg pseudoephedrine HCl	2 mg chlorpheniramine maleate
C-III	*Duratuss HD Elixir*[1,3]	2.5 mg hydrocodone bitartrate	100 mg guaifenesin	30 mg pseudoephedrine HCl	
C-III	*Hydro-Tussin HD Liquid*[1,2]				
C-III	*Su-Tuss HD Elixir*[1,3]				
C-III	*Pancof-XP Liquid*[1,2,4,5]	3 mg hydrocodone bitartrate	100 mg guaifenesin	15 mg pseudoephedrine HCl	
C-III	*Protuss-D Liquid*[1,2,4,5]	5 mg hydrocodone bitartrate	300 mg potassium guaiacolsulfonate	30 mg pseudoephedrine HCl	

[1] This product may also be used in children; refer to package labeling.
[2] Alcohol free.
[3] Contains alcohol.
[4] Sugar free.
[5] Dye free.
[6] Contains phenylalanine.
[7] Sustained release.
[8] Extended release.
[9] Controlled release.

Pediatric Antitussive and Expectorant Combinations

Content given per 5 mL.

	Brand Name Examples	Decongestant	Antitussive	Expectorant
c-v	*Nucofed Pediatric Expectorant Syrup*[1,2]	30 mg pseudoephedrine HCl	10 mg codeine phosphate	100 mg guaifenesin
c-v	*Nucotuss Pediatric Expectorant Syrup*[1,2]			
otc	*Robitussin Cough & Cold Infant Drops*[1]	6 mg/mL pseudoephedrine HCl	2 mg/mL dextromethorphan HBr	40 mg/mL guaifenesin

[1] This product may also be used in adults; refer to package labeling.
[2] Contains alcohol.

Antitussives with Expectorants

Content given per tablet or 5 mL.

	Brand Name Examples	Antitussive	Expectorant
c-v	*Chreracol Cough Syrup*[1,2]	10 mg codeine phosphate	100 mg guaifenesin
c-v	*Gani-Tuss NR Liquid*[1,3,4]		
c-v	*Guiatuss AC Syrup*[1,2,3]		
c-v	*Halotussin AC Liquid*[1,3,4]		
c-v	*Mytussin AC Cough Syrup*[1,2,3]		
c-v	*Romilar AC Liquid*[1,3-6]		
c-v	*Tussi-Organidin NR Liquid*[1]		
c-v	*Tussi-Organidin-S NR Liquid*[1]		
c-III	*Codeine Phosphate and Guaifenesin Tablets*	10 mg codeine phosphate	300 mg guaifenesin
otc	*Benylin Expectorant Liquid*[1,3,4]	5 mg dextromethorphan HBr	100 mg guaifenesin

	Brand Name Examples	Antitussive	Expectorant
otc	*Vicks 44E Cough & Chest Congestion Relief Liquid*[1,2]	6.67 mg dextromethorphan HBr	66.7 mg guaifenesin
otc	*Cheracol D Cough Formula Syrup*[1,2]	10 mg dextromethorphan HBr	100 mg guaifenesin
otc	*Cheracol Plus Liquid*[1,2]		
otc	*Diabetic Tussin DM Liquid*[1,3-6]		
otc	*Extra Action Cough Syrup*[1]		
Rx	*Gani-Tuss-DM NR Liquid*[1,3,4]		
otc	*Genatuss DM Syrup*[1,4]		
otc	*Guaifenesin DM Syrup*[1,4]		
Rx	*Guaifenesin-DM NR Liquid*[1,3,4]		
otc	*Guiatuss-DM Syrup*[1,4]		
otc	*Mytussin DM Syrup*[1,4]		
otc	*Phanatuss DM Cough Syrup*[1,3,4]		
otc	*Robitussin-DM Liquid*[1]		
otc	*Robitussin Sugar Free Cough Liquid*[1,3-5]		
otc	*Siltussin DM Cough Syrup*[1,4]		
otc	*Tolu-Sed DM Liquid*[1-3]		
Rx	*Tussi-Organidin-DM NR Liquid*[1]		
otc	*Kolephrin GG/DM Liquid*[1,4]	10 mg dextromethorphan HBr	150 mg guaifenesin

	Brand Name Examples	Antitussive	Expectorant
otc	*Diabetic Tussin Maximum Strength DM Liquid*[β-6]	10 mg dextromethorphan HBr	200 mg guaifenesin
otc	*Naldecon Senior DX Liquid*[β,4]		
otc	*Robitussin Cough & Congestion Formula Liquid*[1,4]		
otc	*Tuss-DM Tablets*[1]		
otc	*Safe Tussin Liquid*[1,3-5]	15 mg dextromethorphan HBr	100 mg guaifenesin
otc	*Scot-Tussin Senior Clear Liquid*[β,4,6]	15 mg dextromethorphan HBr	200 mg guaifenesin
Rx	*Duratuss DM Elixir*[1,2]	20 mg dextromethorphan HBr	200 mg guaifenesin
Rx	*Hydro-Tussin DM Liquid*[1]		
Rx	*Maxi-tuss DM Liquid*[1]		
Rx	*SU-TUSS DM Liquid*[1,2]		
Rx	*Respa-DM Tablets*[1,5,7]	28 mg dextromethorphan HBr	600 mg guaifenesin
Rx	*Sudal-DM Tablets*[1,5,7]	30 mg dextromethorphan HBr	500 mg guaifenesin
Rx	*Touro DM Tablets*[1,7]	30 mg dextromethorphan HBr	575 mg guaifenesin
Rx	*Fenesin DM Tablets*[1,7]	30 mg dextromethorphan HBr	600 mg guaifenesin
Rx	*Guaifenex DM Tablets*[1,8]		
Rx	*Guiadrine DM Tablets*[1,7]		
Rx	*Humibid DM Tablets*[1,7]		
Rx	*Iobid DM Tablets*[1,7]		
Rx	*Muco-Fen-DM Tablets*[1,7]		
Rx	*Allfen-DM Tablets*[1,5,7]	50 mg dextromethorphan HBr	1000 mg guaifenesin

	Brand Name Examples	Antitussive	Expectorant
Rx	*Dex GG TR Tablets*[1,8]	60 mg dextromethorphan HBr	1000 mg guaifenesin
Rx	*GFN 1000/DM 60 Tablets*[7]		
Rx	*Guaifenesin 1000 mg and Dextromethorhan HBr 60 mg LA Tablets*[1]		
Rx	*Aquatab DM Tablets*	60 mg dextromethorphan HBr	1200 mg guaifenesin
Rx	*GFN 1200/DM 60 Tablets*[1,7]		
Rx	*TUSSI-bid Tablets*[1,7]		
C-III	*Pneumotussin 2.5 Cough Syrup*[1,3-5]	2.5 mg hydrocodone bitartrate	200 mg guaifenesin
C-III	*Pneumotussin Tablets*[1,5]	2.5 mg hydrocodone bitartrate	300 mg guaifenesin
C-III	*Hydrocodone Bitartrate and Guaifenesin Liquid*[1,3-5]	5 mg hydrocodone bitartrate	100 mg guaifenesin
C-III	*Codiclear DH Syrup*[1,3-5]		
C-III	*Hycosin Expectorant Syrup*[1,2]		
C-III	*Hycotuss Expectorant Syrup*[1,2]		
C-III	*Hydrocodone GF Syrup*[1,3-5]		
C-III	*Kwelcof Liquid*[1,3-5]		
C-III	*Vicodin Tuss Syrup*[1,3-5]		
C-III	*Vitussin Syrup*[1,3-5]		
C-III	*Atuss EX Syrup*[1,3-5]	2.5 mg hydrocodone bitartrate	120 mg potassium guaiacolsulfonate
C-III	*Prolex DH Liquid*[1,3,4]	4.5 mg hydrocodone bitartrate	300 mg potassium guaiacolsulfonate

	Brand Name Examples	Antitussive	Expectorant
C-III	*Hydron KGS Liquid*[1,3,4]	5 mg hydrocodone bitartrate	300 mg potassium guaiacolsulfonate
C-III	*Protuss Liquid*[1,3,4]		
C-III	*Marcof Expectorant Syrup*[1,3-5]	5 mg hydrocodone bitartrate	350 mg potassium guaiacolsulfonate
C-II	*Dilaudid Cough Syrup*[2]	1 mg hydromorphone HCl	100 mg guaifenesin

[1] This product may also be used in children; refer to package labeling.
[2] Contains alcohol.
[3] Sugar free.
[4] Alcohol free.
[5] Dye free.
[6] Contains phenylalanine.
[7] Sustained release.
[8] Extended release.

Pediatric Antitussives with Expectorants

Content given per 5 mL (liquid) or 1 mL (drops).

	Brand Name Examples	Antitussive	Expectorant
otc	*Robitussin DM Infant Drops*[1]	2 mg/mL dextromethorphan HBr	40 mg/mL guaifenesin
otc	*Vicks Pediatric 44E Cough & Chest Congestion Relief Liquid*[2]	3.3 mg dextromethorphan HBr	33.3 mg guaifenesin

[1] Alcohol free.
[2] This product may also be used in adults; refer to package labeling.

Topical Combinations

	Brand Name Examples	Ingredients
otc	*Nose Better Gel*	0.5% allantoin, 0.75% camphor, 0.5% menthol
otc	*TheraPatch Vapor Patch for Kids Cough Suppressant*	4.7% camphor, 2.6% menthol
otc	*Triaminic Vapor Patch for Cough*	
otc	*Mentholatum Cherry Chest Rub for Kids*	4.7% camphor, 2.6% menthol, 1.2% eucalyptus oil
otc	*Tom's of Maine Natural Cough & Cold Rub Cough Suppressant*	4.8% camphor, 2.6% menthol
otc	*Vicks VapoRub Cream*	5.2% camphor, 2.8% menthol, 1.2% eucalyptus oil
otc	*Mentholatum Ointment*	9% camphor, 1.3% menthol
otc	*Breathe Right Children's Colds Nasal Strips*	Menthol
otc	*Breathe Right Colds Nasal Strips*	

If you have any questions, consult your doctor, pharmacist, or health care provider.

CNS Stimulants
- Amphetamines, 575
- Appetite Suppressants (Non-Amphetamine), 579
- Appetite Suppressants - Sibutramine, 584
- Caffeine, 587
- Methylphenidate, 590
- Pemoline, 594

Analgesics
- Acetaminophen, 597
- Aspirin and Salicylates, 601
- Buffered Aspirin, 606
- Nonnarcotic Combinations, 608
- Diflunisal, 613
- Narcotic Pain Relievers, 615
- Narcotic Pain Reliever Combinations, 623
- Butorphanol Tartrate, 631
- Pentazocine, 633
- Tramadol, 636

Nonsteroidal Anti-Inflammatory Agents, 638

Antirheumatic Agents
- Gold Compounds, 646
- Hydroxychloroquine, 649
- Methotrexate, 651

Agents for Gout
- Allopurinol, 655
- Colchicine, 658
- Probenecid, 662
- Sulfinpyrazone, 666

Agents for Migraine
- Migraine Combinations, 668
- Methysergide, 671
- Almotriptan, 674
- Naratriptan, 676
- Rizatriptan, 679
- Sumatriptan Succinate, 683
- Zolmitriptan, 687

Antiemetic/Antivertigo Agents
- Anticholinergic Agents, 689
- Cannabinoids, 693
- 5-HT_3 Receptor Antagonists, 696
- Phenothiazines, 699
- Phosphorated Carbohydrate Solution, 705

Vasopressor/Antihypotensive Agents
- Midodrine, 707

Antianxiety Agents
- Benzodiazepines, 710
- Buspirone, 716
- Hydroxyzine, 719
- Meprobamate, 721

Antidepressant Agents
- Bupropion, 724
- Nefazodone, 727
- Fluoxetine, 730
- Fluvoxamine, 734
- Citalopram Hydrobromide, 737
- Tetracyclic Compounds, 740
- Monoamine Oxidase Inhibitors, 743
- Paroxetine, 749
- Sertraline, 752
- Trazodone, 754
- Venlafaxine, 757
- Tricyclic Antidepressants, 760

Antipsychotic Agents
- Antipsychotic Agents, 770
- Quetiapine Fumarate, 781
- Risperidone, 784
- Olanzapine, 787
- Clozapine, 791

Psychotherapeutic Agents
- Pimozide, 794
- Ergoloid Mesylates, 797
- Lithium, 799
- Cholinesterase Inhibitors, 803
- Psychotherapeutic Combinations, 807

Sedatives
- Barbiturates, 812
- Hypnotics, 817

Nonprescription Sleep Aids, 822

Anticonvulsants
- Acetazolamide, 825
- Carbamazepine, 828
- Clonazepam, 832
- Felbamate, 836
- Gabapentin, 839
- Hydantoins, 842
- Oxazolidinediones, 847
- Oxcarbazepine, 849
- Zonisamide, 852
- Primidone, 855
- Topiramate, 858
- Succinimides, 861
- Lamotrigine, 864
- Tiagabine, 867
- Levetiracetam, 870
- Valproic Acid, 872

Muscle Relaxants
- Baclofen, 876
- Dantrolene Sodium, 879
- Tizanidine, 882
- Skeletal Muscle Relaxants, 885
- Skeletal Muscle Relaxant Combinations, 889

Antiparkinson Agents
- Anticholinergics, 891
- Dopaminergics, 895
- Pramipexole Dihydrochloride, 900
- Ropinirole, 903
- Pergolide Mesylate, 906
- Selegiline, 909
- Entacapone, 912

	Generic Name *Brand Name Examples*	Supplied As	Generic Available
c-II	**Methamphetamine HCl**		
	Desoxyn	**Tablets:** 5 mg	No
	Desoxyn Gradumets	**Tablets, long-acting:** 5 mg, 10 mg, 15 mg[1]	No
c-II	**Amphetamine Mixtures**		
	Adderall	**Tablets:** 5 mg, 10 mg, 20 mg, 30 mg containing a mixture of dextroamphetamine saccharate, amphetamine aspartate, dextroamphetamine sulfate, amphetamine sulfate	No

[1] Contains the dye tartrazine.

Type of Drug:

Central nervous system stimulants: "Bennies," "dexies," "speed" or "crystal."

How the Drug Works:

These synthetic drugs are a stronger form of the natural body stimulant adrenaline. They work by altering natural chemicals (neurotransmitters) in the brain and can affect other body systems in high doses.

Uses:

To treat attention deficit disorder with hyperactivity in children older than 6 years of age. The total treatment program includes psychological, educational and social guidance along with the drug.

For short-term (eg, a few weeks) use as part of an overall diet plan to reduce weight (methamphetamine only).

For narcolepsy, a rare sleep disorder which causes people to uncontrollably fall asleep (amphetamine mixtures).

Precautions:

Do not use in the following situations:

- agitated states
- allergy to stimulant drugs
- arteriosclerosis (hardening of the arteries)
- drug abuse tendencies
- glaucoma
- heart disease, symptomatic
- high blood pressure, moderate to severe
- monoamine oxidase inhibitor use
- overactive thyroid gland

Do not use to combat fatigue or to replace rest.

Use with caution in the following situations:

- high blood pressure, mild
- Tourette's syndrome

Diabetes: Insulin requirements may be altered with the use of amphetamines and diet restriction.

Abuse: Amphetamines have a high potential for abuse. Use in weight reduction programs only when alternative therapy (diets, group programs, other drugs) has been ineffective. Use for prolonged periods may lead to drug dependence.

Drug dependence: Tolerance, extreme dependence and severe social disability have occurred with amphetamine abuse. Patients may gradually increase the dosage to many times that recommended. Abrupt discontinuation following a long period of using high doses results in extreme fatigue, mental depression, and changes in sleep habits.

Chronic intoxication: Severe skin rash, marked sleeplessness, irritability, hyperactivity, personality changes, disorganization of thoughts, poor concentration, hallucinations, and compulsive behavior often occur. The most severe side effect of chronic intoxication is psychosis, often indistinguishable from paranoid schizophrenia.

Attention deficit disorders: Drug treatment is not indicated in all cases. Amphetamine prescriptions depend on the chronicity and severity of the child's symptoms and appropriateness for his/her age. When symptoms are associated with acute stress reactions, treatment with amphetamines is usually not indicated.

Pregnancy: Adequate studies have not been done in pregnant women, or animal studies may have shown a risk to the fetus. Birth defects have been reported with amphetamine use in pregnancy. Use only if clearly needed and potential benefits outweigh the possible hazards to the fetus. Infants born to mothers dependent on amphetamines have an increased risk of premature delivery and low birth weight. These infants may experience symptoms of withdrawal demonstrated by restlessness including agitation and weakness.

Breastfeeding: Amphetamines appear in breast milk. Consult your doctor before you begin breastfeeding.

Children: Long-term effects in children have not been well established. Do not use as weight loss medications in children younger than 12 years old. Amphetamines are not recommended in children younger than 3 years old. In psychotic children, amphetamines may worsen symptoms of behavior disturbance and thought disorder. Amphetamines may precipitate or worsen Tourette's disorder.

Tartrazine: Some of these products may contain the dye tartrazine (FD&C Yellow No. 5) which can cause allergic reactions in certain individuals. Check package labeling when available or consult your doctor or pharmacist.

Drug Interactions:

Tell your doctor or pharmacist if you are taking or if you are planning to take any over-the-counter or prescription medications or dietary supplements while taking this medicine. Doses of one or both drugs may need to be modified or a different drug may need to be prescribed. The following drugs and drug classes interact with amphetamines.

antihistamines (eg, diphenhydramine)
chlorpromazine (*Thorazine*)
ethosuximide (*Zarontin*)
gastrointestinal acidifying agents (eg, ascorbic acid, fruit juice, glutamic acid)
gastrointestinal alkalinizing agents (eg, sodium bicarbonate)
guanethidine (eg, *Ismelin*)
haloperidol (*Haldol*)
lithium carbonate (*Eskalith*)
MAO Inhibitor antidepressants (eg, phenelzine)
meperidine (*Demerol*)
methenamine therapy (eg, methenamine mandelate)
norepinephrine (*Levophed*)
phenobarbitol (*Sofoton*)
phenothiazines (eg, promazine)
phenytoin (*Dilantin*)
propoxyphene (eg, *Dolene*)
reserpine
tricyclic antidepressants (eg, amitriptyline)
urinary acidifiers (eg, ammonium chloride)
urinary alkalinizers (eg, acetazolamide)
veratrum alkyloids

Side Effects:

Every drug is capable of producing side effects. Many patients experience no, or minor, side effects. The frequency and severity of side effects depend on many factors including dosage, duration of therapy, and individual susceptibility. Possible side effects include:

Digestive Tract: Diarrhea; constipation; appetite loss; dry mouth; bad taste.

Nervous System: Dizziness; sleeplessness; depression; irritability; restlessness; nervousness; headache; muscle tremor; exacerbation of motor and phonic tics and Tourette's syndrome; exaggerated sense of well-being; overstimulation; difficulty moving; unpleasant feelings.

Circulatory System: Pounding in the chest (palpitations); rapid or irregular heartbeat; high blood pressure.

Skin: Hives.

Other: Impotence; changes in sex drive; drowsiness between doses or after stopping medicine; weight loss.

Guidelines for Use:

- Use exactly as prescribed.
- Do not chew or crush sustained-release or long-acting tablets.
- Do not take more frequently than prescribed. These drugs can be addicting.
- May cause insomnia. Avoid taking these medications late in the day.
- Do not increase dosage without consulting with your doctor.
- Take methamphetamine 30 minutes before each meal.
- This medicine may cause dizziness. Use caution while driving or performing other tasks requiring mental alertness, coordination, or physical dexterity.
- May cause nervousness, restlessness, sleeplessness, dizziness, appetite loss, dry mouth, and digestive tract disturbances. Contact your doctor if these become pronounced.
- If a dose is missed, take it as soon as possible. If several hours have passed or if it is nearing time for the next dose, do not double the dose in order to "catch up" (unless advised to do so by your doctor). If more than one dose is missed or it is necessary to establish a new dosage schedule, contact your doctor or pharmacist.
- Inform your doctor if you are pregnant, become pregnant, are planning to become pregnant, or if you are breastfeeding.
- Use of many of these drugs to improve athletic skills, mental alertness, or to stay awake is dangerous and illegal. Never share drugs with others.
- Monitor growth during treatment.
- *Attention deficit disorder in children* – Your doctor may occasionally interrupt drug therapy to determine if there is a recurrence of symptoms.
- *Weight control* – Appropriate lifestyle changes (eg, diet and exercise) should be made while on therapy in order to avoid continued use of the drug.
- Store at room temperature (59° to 86°F).

If you have any questions, consult your doctor, pharmacist, or health care provider.

Generic Name *Brand Name Examples*	Supplied As	Generic Available
c-*III* **Benzphetamine HCl**		
Didrex	**Tablets:** 50 mg	No
c-*IV* **Diethylpropion HCl**		
Tenuate	**Tablets:** 25 mg	Yes
Tenuate Dospan	**Tablets, controlled-release:** 75 mg	Yes
c-*IV* **Mazindol**		
Mazanor, *Sanorex*	**Tablets:** 1 mg, 2 mg	No
c-*III* **Phendimetrazine Tartrate**		
Bontril PDM, *Plegine*	**Tablets:** 35 mg	Yes
Adipost, *Bontril Slow-Release*, *Melfiat-105*, *Prelu-2*	**Capsules, sustained-release:** 105 mg	Yes
c-*IV* **Phentermine HCl**		
Adipex-P, *Fastin*, *Obenix*,[1] *Oby-Cap*, *Oby-Trim*, *Zantryl*	**Capsules:** 30 mg, 37.5 mg	Yes
Adipex-P	**Tablets:** 37.5 mg	Yes
c-*IV* **Phentermine Resin**		
Ionamin	**Capsules:** 15 mg, 30 mg	Yes

[1] Contains the dye tartrazine.

Type of Drug:

Non-amphetamine appetite suppressants. Anorexiants, anorectics, anorexigenics, diet pills.

How the Drug Works:

Appetite suppressants appear to temporarily stimulate the appetite center of the brain, which reduces hunger or craving of food. Although most of these drugs are related to amphetamines, they are less likely to stimulate other systems and are slightly less habit-forming.

Uses:

For short-term (8 to 12 weeks) use to reduce weight as part of an overall diet plan that includes dietary calorie restriction, exercise, and behavioral modification.

Precautions:

Do not use in the following situations:

- agitated states
- allergy to these drugs or any of their ingredients
- arteriosclerosis (hardening of the arteries), advanced
- cardiovascular disease, symptomatic (eg, heart failure, heart rhythm disturbance, coronary artery disease)
- CNS stimulants, use
- drug or alcohol abuse, history
- glaucoma
- high blood pressure, moderate to severe
- MAO inhibitor antidepressants (eg, phenelzine) use, within 14 days
- pregnancy (benzphetamine only)
- thyroid, overactive (untreated)

Use with caution in the following situations:

- abnormal heart rhythm (diethylpropion)
- anesthesia (diethylpropion)
- diabetes
- eating disorders, history
- epilepsy (diethylpropion)
- high blood pressure, mild
- primary pulmonary hypertension
- valvular heart disease

To avoid dependency, use these drugs only for a short period of time (not to exceed 12 weeks) and discontinue use at the first sign of ineffectiveness.

Tolerance (loss of effectiveness) to appetite suppressants may develop within a few weeks. Discontinue the drug rather than increase the dosage.

Drug dependence: These drugs have abuse potential. Intense dependence and severe social dysfunction may be associated with long-term therapy or abuse. Abrupt cessation after long-term, high-dose therapy results in extreme fatigue and mental depression. Gradually reducing the dose in this situation may minimize withdrawal symptoms.

Chronic intoxication: Chronic intoxication is manifested by severe rash, marked sleep loss, irritability, hyperactivity, and personality changes. Psychosis, often indistinguishable from schizophrenia, is the most severe side effect.

Primary pulmonary hypertension: Pulmonary hypertension (elevated blood pressure in blood vessels in lungs) has been reported in some patients taking appetite suppressants for longer than 3 months. Symptoms of this serious condition include: Difficulty breathing; decreased exercise tolerance; chest pain; fainting; swelling of ankles or feet.

Diabetes: These drugs may lower blood sugar (glucose) levels independent of appetite suppressant effects. Carefully monitor blood sugar levels and watch for symptoms of low blood sugar.

Pregnancy: Adequate studies have not been done in pregnant women or animal studies may have shown a risk to the fetus. Use only if clearly needed and potential benefits outweigh the possible hazards to the fetus.

Benzphetamine – Do not use during pregnancy. The risk of use in a pregnant woman clearly outweighs any possible benefit.

Diethylpropion – Studies in pregnant women or in animals have been judged not to show a risk to the fetus. However, no drug should be used during pregnancy unless clearly needed.

Breastfeeding: Safety for use of these drugs in the nursing mother has not been established. Diethylpropion appears in breast milk. Consult your doctor before you begin breastfeeding.

Children: Use of these drugs as appetite suppressants in children younger than 12 years of age is not recommended.

Phentermine resin – Use in children younger than 16 years of age is not recommended.

Tartrazine: Some of these products may contian the dye tartrazine (FD&C Yellow No. 5), which can cause allergic reactions in certain individuals. Check package label when available or consult your doctor or pharmacist.

Drug Interactions:

Tell your doctor or pharmacist if you are taking or if you are planning to take any over-the-counter or prescription medications or dietary supplements while taking these medicines. Doses of one or both drugs may need to be modified or a different drug may need to be prescribed. The following drugs and drug classes interact with these medicines.

- alcohol
- adrenergic neural blocking agents (eg, propranolol) (phentermine resin only)
- anesthetics
- antihypertensives (eg, guanethidine)
- catecholamines (eg, levarterenol, norepinephrine) (mazindol, diethylpropion only)
- fluoxetine *(Prozac)*
- fluvoxamine *(Luvox)*
- insulin
- MAO inhibitor antidepressants (eg, phenelzine)
- paroxetine *(Paxil)*
- phenothiazines (eg, chlorpromazine)
- sertraline (*Zoloft*)
- sulfonylureas (eg, glipizide)
- tricyclic antidepressants (eg, amitriptyline)
- urinary acidifiers (eg, ammonium chloride) (benzphetamine only)
- urinary alkalinizers (eg, sodium bicarbonate) (benzphetamine only)

Side Effects:

Every drug is capable of producing side effects. Many patients experience no, or minor, side effects. The frequency and severity of side effects depend on many factors including dose, duration of therapy and individual susceptibility. Possible side effects include:

Digestive Tract: Nausea; vomiting; constipation; stomach pain; diarrhea; thirst; dry mouth; unpleasant taste.

Nervous System: Restlessness; nervousness; anxiety; tension; mental confusion; depression; sleeplessness; fainting; overstimulation; weakness;

headache; drowsiness; dizziness; clumsiness; convulsions; involuntary movements; euphoria (exaggerated sense of well-being); moodiness; jitteriness; difficulty moving; agitation; psychotic states.

Circulatory System: Pounding in the chest (palpitations); rapid pulse; irregular heartbeat; chest pain; changes in blood pressure; primary pulmonary hypertension; ECG changes; regurgitant cardiac valvular disease.

Skin: Hair loss; sweating; hives; rash; flushing; burning sensation; clamminess; bruising.

Other: Difficulty breathing; fever; muscle aches; tremors; menstrual changes; changes in sexual desire; impotence; double vision; blurred vision; eye irritation; frequent urination; painful or difficult urination; breast swelling in males; pupil dilation; general body discomfort; chills.

Guidelines for Use:

- Use exactly as prescribed.
- Take phendimetrazine, mazindol, and phentermine resin 30 to 60 minutes before meals.
- Take phentermine before or 1 to 2 hours after breakfast.
- Appetite suppressants are not a substitute for proper dieting. Lifestyle changes (eg, diet and exercise) are necesary to initially lose weight and then maintain weight loss.
- Do not exceed prescribed dose or take more frequently than prescribed. These drugs can be addicting.
- Do not crush or chew sustained-release products.
- *Phentermine resin* — Swallow capsules whole.
- May cause insomnia. Avoid taking these medications late in the day.
- If a dose is missed, take it as soon as possible. If several hours have passed or if it is nearing time for the next dose, do not double the dose in order to "catch up" (unless advised to do so by your doctor). If more than one dose is missed or it is necessary to establish a new dosage schedule, contact your doctor or pharmacist.
- Do not stop taking this medicine suddenly. It may result in extreme tiredness and depression.
- Avoid alcohol and other mental depressants (eg, narcotics, tranquilizers, antihistamines) while you are taking this medicine.
- May cause dizziness or blurred vision. Use caution while driving or performing other tasks requiring alertness, coordination, or physical dexterity.
- May cause dry mouth and constipation. Notify your doctor if these become pronounced.
- Contact your doctor if deterioration in exercise tolerance, difficulty breathing, chest pain, fainting, swelling, palpitations (heart pounding), nervousness, or dizziness occurs.
- *Diabetic patients* may experience loss of glucose control. Be prepared to monitor blood sugar more often.
- *Epilepsy patients* — Diethylpropion may increase the incidence of convulsions.
- Inform your doctor if you are pregnant, become pregnant, are planning to become pregnant, or are breastfeeding.
- Lab tests, including blood pressure tests, may be required to monitor therapy. Be sure to keep appointments.
- Never share your medication with others.
- Store at room temperature (59° to 86°F) in a tightly sealed container. Protect from light and moisture.

If you have any questions, consult your doctor, pharmacist, or health care provider.

	Generic Name *Brand Name Example*	Supplied As	Generic Available
c-IV	**Sibutramine HCl Monohydrate**		
	Meridia	**Capsules:** 5 mg, 10 mg, 15 mg	No

Type of Drug:

Weight loss drug, appetite suppressant.

How the Drug Works:

Sibutramine reduces appetite by preventing the reuptake of neurotransmitters in the brain involved with hunger.

Uses:

For the management of obesity, including weight loss and maintenance of weight loss, in conjunction with a reduced-calorie diet, exercise (if possible), and behavioral modification. This drug should be reserved for use in obese patients with an initial body mass index (BMI) of at least 30 kg/m^2 in the presence of other risk factors (eg, hypertension, diabetes, hyperlipidemia).

Precautions:

Do not use in the following situations:

abnormal heartbeat, history
allergy to sibutramine or any of its ingredients
anorexia nervosa
appetite suppressant drugs, use with other
congestive heart failure, history
coronary artery disease, history
kidney disease, severe
liver disease, severe
MAO inhibitor antidepressant (eg, phenelzine) use, within 14 days
stroke, history

Use with caution in the following situations:

drug abuse, history
gall stones
glaucoma, narrow-angle
high blood pressure
kidney disease
liver disease
obesity, organic causes (eg, underactive thyroid)
pulmonary hypertension, history
seizures, history

Pregnancy: Adequate studies have not been done in pregnant women. Use in pregnancy is not recommended.

Breastfeeding: It is not known if sibutramine appears in breast milk. Consult your doctor before you begin breastfeeding.

Children: Safety and effectiveness in children younger than 16 years of age have not been established.

Lab tests or exams may be required to monitor treatment. Be sure to keep appointments. Tests may include: blood pressure, pulse rate, heart rhythm.

Drug Interactions:

Tell your doctor or pharmacist if you are taking or if you are planning to take any over-the-counter or prescription medications or dietary supplements with sibutramine. Doses of one or both drugs may need to be modified or a different drug may need to be prescribed. The following drugs and drug classes interact with sibutramine:

alcohol
antidepressants (tricyclics)
centrally acting weight-reducing agents, other
cimetidine (eg, *Tagamet*)
decongestants (eg, pseudoephedrine, phenylpropanolamine)
dihydroergotamine *(D.H.E. 45)*
erythromycin (eg, *E-Mycin*)
dextromethorphan (eg, *Vicks 44*)
fentanyl *(Duragesic)*
ketoconazole *(Nizoral)*
lithium (eg, *Eskalith*)
MAO inhibitor antidepressants (eg, phenelzine)
meperidine (eg, *Demerol*)
pentazocine (*Talwin NX*)
serotonin reuptake inhibitors (eg, fluoxetine, fluvoxamine, paroxetine, sertraline, venlafaxine)
sumatriptan *(Imitrex)*
tryptophan

Side Effects:

Every drug is capable of producing side effects. Many sibutramine users experience no, or minor, side effects. The frequency and severity of side effects depend on many factors including dose, duration of therapy and individual susceptibility. Possible side effects include:

Digestive Tract: Dry mouth; constipation; stomach pain; increased appetite; nausea; indigestion; stomach inflammation; vomiting; rectal problems; thirst; diarrhea; gas.

Nervous System: Headache; migraine; sleeplessness; dizziness; nervousness; anxiety; depression; abnormal skin sensations; drowsiness; stimulation; unstable emotions; agitation; abnormal thinking.

Circulatory System: Rapid heartbeat; high/increased blood pressure; pounding in the chest (palpitations).

Respiratory System: Runny nose; sinus infection; sore throat; increased cough; laryngitis; bronchitis; difficulty breathing.

Skin: Flushing; rash; sweating; herpes simplex; acne; itching.

Other: Back pain; weakness; stomach pain; chest pain; neck pain; allergic reaction; general swelling; joint pain/problems/inflammation; muscle pain; tendon pain; changes in taste; ear problems/pain; painful menstruation; urinary tract infection; vaginal bleeding; vaginal yeast infection; fever; swelling of arms and legs; leg cramps; tight muscles or muscle tension; vision problems; menstrual problems.

Guidelines for Use:

- Usual dose is 10 mg once daily.
- May be taken with or without food.
- If a dose is missed, take it as soon as possible. If several hours have passed or if it is nearing time for the next dose, do not double the dose in order to "catch up" (unless advised to do so by your doctor). If more than one dose is missed or it is necessary to establish a new dosage schedule, contact your doctor or pharmacist. Use exactly as prescribed.
- Wait at least 2 weeks before starting treatment with sibutramine after stopping MAOIs and before starting MAOIs after stopping sibutramine.
- Read the package insert before starting therapy.
- If rash, hives or other allergic reactions occur, contact your doctor immediately.
- Discontinue this medicine and contact your doctor if seizures occur.
- Do not exceed prescribed dose or take more frequently than prescribed. These drugs can be addicting.
- This medicine may cause drowsiness or dizziness. Use caution while driving or performing other tasks requiring mental alertness, coordination, or physical dexterity.
- Do not take other medicaton without your doctor's approval. This includes nonprescription medicines for appetite control, asthma, colds, cough, hay fever, or sinus problems.
- Avoid alcohol and other mental depressants (eg, narcotics, tranquilizers, antidepressants, hypnotics, antihistamines) while you are taking this medicine unless approved by your doctor.
- Inform you doctor if you are pregnant, become pregnant, are planning to become pregnant, or if you are breastfeeding.
- Appetite suppressants are not a substitute for proper dieting. Lifestyle changes (eg, diet and exercise) are necessary to initially lose weight and then maintain weight loss.
- May cause insomnia (sleeplessness). Avoid taking late in the day.
- The long-term effects of this medicine are unknown.
- Lab tests or exams may be required to monitor treatment. Be sure to keep appointments. Tests may include: blood pressure, pulse rate, heart rhythm.
- Store at controlled room temperature. Protect from heat and moisture.

If you have any questions, consult your doctor, pharmacist, or health care provider.

	Generic Name *Brand Name Examples*	Supplied As	Generic Available
	Caffeine		
otc	*20-20, 357 HR Magnum, Caffedrine, Keep Alert, Keep Going, Maximum Strength NoDoz, Overtime, Stay Awake, Valentine, Vivarin*	**Tablets:** 200 mg	Yes
otc	*.44 Magnum, Fastlene, Molie*	**Capsules**: 200 mg	No
otc	*Enerjets*	**Lozenges**: 75 mg	No
Rx	*Cafcit*	**Oral solution**: 20 mg/mL	No
Rx	*Cafcit*	**Injection**: 20 mg/mL	No
Rx	**Caffeine and sodium benzoate**	**Injection**: 250 mg/mL (121 mg caffeine and 129 mg sodium benzoate or 125 mg caffeine and 125 mg sodium benzoate)	Yes

Type of Drug:

Central nervous system stimulant.

How the Drug Works:

Caffeine stimulates the brain. It also stimulates the heart, dilates (widens) blood vessels in the body, constricts (narrows) blood vessels in the brain, increases acid secretion in the stomach, and acts as a mild or weak diuretic (water pill).

Uses:

To aid in staying awake or restoring alertness. Caffeine is also used as an ingredient in various pain medications (eg, aspirin, acetaminophen) to increase the pain-relieving effects; to treat respiratory depression associated with overdosage with CNS depressants (eg, narcotic analgesics, alcohol) in conjunction with other supportive measures; and to treat breathing problems in premature infants.

Unlabeled Use(s): Occasionally doctors may prescribe caffeine for the treatment of atopic dermatitis (topical cream), headaches, excited or comatose alcoholic patients, postprandial hypotension (low blood pressure in elderly following meal high in carbohydrates), obesity (combined with ephedrine), or as an appetite suppressant.

Precautions:

Do not use in the following situations: Allergy to caffeine or any of its ingredients.

Use with caution in the following situations:

- depression
- esophagitis, reflux
- heart disease
- irritable intestinal disease
- kidney function impairment (infants)

liver function impairment (infants)
osteoporosis
seizure disorder (infants)
ulcers, duodenal

Diabetes: Higher blood sugar (glucose) levels may result from caffeine use. Closely monitor your sugar level. Use with caution in patients with pre-existing diabetes.

Pregnancy: There are no adequate and well-controlled studies in pregnant women. Use only if clearly needed and the potential benefits to the mother outweigh the possible hazards to the fetus.

Breastfeeding: Caffeine appears in breast milk. Consult your doctor before you begin breastfeeding.

Children: Do not give to children younger than 12 years of age unless recommended by a doctor.

Caffeine in the diet:

DIETARY CAFFEINE[1]		
Dietary Source	**Range of Caffeine Content**	
Coffee - Regular	Espresso Brewed Instant	120 mg/2 oz 40-180 mg/5 to 8 oz 30-120 mg/5 to 8 oz
Coffee - Decaffeinated	Brewed Instant	2-5 mg/5 to 8 oz 1-5 mg/5 to 8 oz
Tea	Brewed Instant Iced	20-110 mg/5 to 8 oz 25-50 mg/5 to 8 oz ≈ 70 mg/12 oz
Other	Soft drinks Cocoa Chocolate milk Milk chocolate Bakers chocolate	0-72 mg/12 oz 2-50 mg/5 to 8 oz 2-7 mg/5 oz 1-15 mg/1 oz 25-58 mg/1 oz

[1] Depending on strength of brew and product.

Drug Interactions:

Tell your doctor or pharmacist if you are taking or if you are planning to take any over-the-counter or prescription medications or dietary supplements with caffeine. Doses of one or both drugs may need to be modified or a different drug may need to be prescribed. The following drugs and drug classes interact with caffeine.

allopurinol (eg, *Lopurin*)
aspirin
beta-blockers (eg, acebutolol)
cimetidine (eg, *Tagamet*)
clozapine (*Clozaril*)
contraceptives, oral (eg, *Ortho-Novum*)
disulfiram (eg, *Antabuse*)
fluoroquinolones (eg, ciprofloxacin, norfloxacin, enoxacin)
iron
mexiletine (*Mexitil*)

nicotine (eg, smoking, nicotine replacement therapy)
phenobarbital (eg, *Solfoton*)
phenylpropanolamine (eg, *Dexatrim*)
phenytoin (eg, *Dilantin*)
terbinafine (*Lamisil*)
theophylline (eg, *TheoDur)*

Side Effects:

Every drug is capable of producing side effects. Many caffeine users experience no, or minor, side effects. The frequency and severity of side effects depend on many factors including dose, duration of therapy and individual susceptibility. Possible side effects include:

Withdrawal: Headache, anxiety, depression, sleeplessness, difficulty sleeping, fatigue, and muscle tension may occur following abrupt stopping of the drug after regular consumption of as little as 100 mg/day. Symptoms usually start between 12 to 18 hours after the last caffeine ingestion.

Digestive Tract: Nausea; vomiting; diarrhea; stomach pain.

Nervous System: Headache; inability to sleep; anxiety; nervousness; restlessness; excitement; lightheadedness; irritability.

Circulatory System: Rapid heartbeat; pounding in the chest (palpitations); abnormal heartbeat.

Other: Increased urination; ringing in the ears; muscle tremor; visual problems; rash; itching; increased blood sugar.

Guidelines for Use:

- Stop taking this drug if an increased or abnormal heart rate or rhythm, dizziness, or palpitations occurs.
- Do not take more than the recommended dose.
- If you continue to be tired or drowsy, call your doctor.
- This drug is intended for occasional use and is not intended to replace normal sleep.
- If you stop taking this medicine after regular daily doses, you may develop a headache, anxiety, fatigue, depression, difficulty sleeping, or muscle tightness. These feelings will usually begin 12 to 24 hours after your last dose of caffeine. The feelings will go away after your body readjusts.
- Store at controlled room temperature (59° to 86°F).

If you have any questions, consult your doctor, pharmacist, or health care provider.

Generic Name *Brand Name Examples*	Supplied As	Generic Available
C-II **Methylphenidate HCl**		
Methylin, Ritalin	**Tablets:** 5 mg, 10 mg, 20 mg	Yes
Concerta	**Tablets, extended-release:** 18 mg, 36 mg, 54 mg	No
Metadate ER, Methylin ER	**Tablets, extended-release:** 10 mg, 20 mg	Yes
Ritalin-SR[1]	**Tablets, sustained-release:** 20 mg	Yes
Metadate CD	**Capsules, extended-release:** 20 mg	No

[1] Dye free.

Type of Drug:

Central nervous system stimulant.

How the Drug Works:

Methylphenidate mildly stimulates the central nervous system.

Uses:

To aid in treatment of children with behavior problems (attention deficit disorder) characterized by hyperactivity, moderate-to-severe distractibility, short attention span, impulsive behavior, and extreme mood changes that are not stress induced. Stimulants are not for a child who exhibits symptoms due to living conditions or psychiatric disorders, or when symptoms are caused by acute stress reactions.

To treat narcolepsy (sudden or irresistable periods of spontaneous sleep lasting less than 15 minutes that occur during any type of activity).

Do not use methylphenidate for the prevention or treatment of normal fatigue states.

Unlabeled Use(s): Occasionally doctors may prescribe methylphenidate to treat depression in elderly patients, poststroke patients, or patients with cancer, brain injury, or HIV infection, or to treat anesthesia-related hiccups.

Precautions:

Do not use in the following situations:

- allergy to methylphenidate or any of its ingredients
- anxiety, agitation, or tension, moderate to severe
- GI obstruction (*Concerta* only)
- glaucoma
- MAOI therapy, concurrent or within 14 days
- motor tics
- Tourette syndrome, diagnosed or family history of

Use with caution in the following situations:

- alcoholism, history of
- children with psychosis
- drug dependence, history of
- emotional instability
- high blood pressure
- seizure disorders

Drug dependence: Chronic abuse of methylphenidate can lead to marked tolerance and psychic dependence with varying degrees of abnormal behavior. Methylphenidate should be given with caution to emotionally unstable patients who may increase the dosage on their own.

Neuroleptic malignant syndrome: Neuroleptic malignant syndrome (NMS) is a potentially fatal syndrome which has been rarely associated with methylphenidate use. Symptoms include increased body heat; muscle rigidity; altered mental abilities, including catatonia; irregular pulse and blood pressure; increased heart rate; sweating; and irregular heart rhythm.

Total treatment program: Methylphenidate therapy should be a part of a total treatment program that includes psychological, educational, and social measures.

Pregnancy: There are no adequate and well-controlled studies in pregnant women. Use only if clearly needed and the potential benefits to the mother outweigh the possible hazards to the fetus.

Breastfeeding: Safety for use in the nursing mother has not been established. Consult your doctor before you begin breastfeeding.

Children: Do not use in children younger than 6 years of age, since safety and effectiveness have not been established. In psychotic children, the drug may worsen symptoms of behavior disturbance and thought disorder. Aggravation of Tourette syndrome has been reported. Safety and effectiveness of long-term use in children have not been established. Suppression of growth (eg, not gaining height or weight) has been reported with long-term use of stimulants in children. Carefully monitor patients on long-term therapy.

Lab tests may be required during therapy. Tests include blood counts, platelet counts, and blood pressure measurements.

Drug Interactions:

Tell your doctor or pharmacist if you are taking or planning to take any over-the-counter or prescription medications or dietary supplements with methylphenidate. Doses of one or both drugs may need to be modified or a different drug may need to be prescribed. The following drugs and drug classes interact with methylphenidate:

- anticoagulants, oral (eg, warfarin)
- anticonvulsants (eg, phenobarbital, primidone, phenytoin)
- guanethidine (eg, *Ismelin)*
- MAOIs (eg, phenelzine)
- pressor agents (eg, norepinephrine)
- selective serotonin reuptake inhibitors (eg, paroxetine)
- tricyclic antidepressants (eg, imipramine, clomipramine, desipramine)

Side Effects:

Every drug is capable of producing side effects. Many methylphenidate users experience no, or minor, side effects. The frequency and severity of side effects depend on many factors including dose, duration of therapy, and individual susceptibility. Possible side effects include:

Children: Appetite loss; stomach pain; weight loss during prolonged therapy; sleeplessness; and fast heartbeat occur more frequently in children; however, any of the following side effects may also occur.

Allergic Reactions: Rash; hives; fever; joint pain; peeling skin; skin redness; itching.

Digestive Tract: Appetite loss; nausea; stomach pain.

Nervous System: Nervousness; dizziness; sleeplessness; difficulty moving; drowsiness; Tourette syndrome; headache.

Circulatory System: Palpitations (pounding in chest); pulse rate changes; chest pain; fast heartbeat; abnormal heart rhythm; blood pressure changes (usually increased).

Other: Weight loss; depression; visual disturbances.

Guidelines for Use:

- Dosage will be individualized. Take exactly as prescribed.
- Do not stop taking or change the dose, unless directed by your doctor.
- Take regular tablets 30 to 45 minutes before taking other medication, if possible.
- *Children older than 6 years of age:* Methylphenidate will be initiated in small doses, with gradual weekly incremental adjustments.
- *Adults:* Administer regular tablets in divided doses 2 to 3 times daily.
- Patients who are unable to sleep if medication is taken late in the day should take the last dose before 6 PM.
- Sustained-release tablets have a duration of action of approximately 8 hours (12 hours for *Concerta* and *Metadate CD*).
- Do not crush or chew sustained-release tablets.
- If a dose is missed, take it as soon as possible. If several hours have passed or it is nearing time for the next dose, do not double the dose to catch up, unless advised by your doctor. If more than one dose is missed or it is necessary to establish a new dosage schedule, contact your doctor or pharmacist.
- May disguise tiredness, impair physical coordination, or cause dizziness, drowsiness, or blurred vision. Use caution when driving or performing other tasks requiring alertness, coordination, or physical dexterity.
- Notify your doctor if you experience nervousness, sleeplessness, chest pain, palpitations, vomiting, fever, rash, or other unusual, unexplained effects.
- Drug treatment for attention deficit disorders is not indefinite and is usually discontinued after puberty.
- Prolonged use may cause tolerance to the drug. Dose may need to be adjusted. Your doctor may recommend "drug-free days" to evaluate the need for continued use and to re-establish drug potency. Consult your doctor before withdrawing the drug.
- Very rare reports of neuroleptic malignant syndrome have been reported. It is uncertain whether these cases were caused by methylphenidate alone or by some other combination of factors. Notify your doctor if you experience fever, excessive sweating, shortness of breath, urinary incontinence, muscle rigidity, tremors, or unusual muscle movements.
- Inform your doctor if you are pregnant, become pregnant, are planning to become pregnant, or are breastfeeding.
- Lab tests may be required during therapy. Be sure to keep appointments.
- Store at room temperature (59° to 86°F). Protect from moisture and light.

If you have any questions, consult your doctor, pharmacist, or health care provider.

Generic Name *Brand Name Examples*	Supplied As	Generic Available
C-IV **Pemoline**		
Cylert, PemADD	**Tablets**: 18.75 mg, 37.5 mg, 75 mg	Yes
Cylert, PemADD CT	**Tablets, chewable**: 37.5 mg	No

Type of Drug:

Central nervous system stimulant.

How the Drug Works:

Pemoline stimulates the central nervous system. How it does this is not fully understood.

Uses:

To aid in treatment of children with behavior problems (attention deficit disorder) characterized by hyperactivity, moderate to severe distractibility, short attention span, impulsive behavior, and extreme mood changes.

Unlabeled Use(s): Occasionally doctors may prescribe pemoline for narcolepsy (irresistible periods of sleep lasting less than 15 minutes during normal waking hours) and excessive daytime sleepiness.

Precautions:

Do not use in the following situations:

allergy to pemoline or any of its ingredients
liver disease, active or history of

Use with caution in the following situations:

children with psychosis
drug dependence, history of
emotional instability
kidney disease
seizure disorders
Tourette syndrome

Drug dependence: The similarity of pemoline to other brain stimulants with known dependence liability suggests that psychological and physical dependence might also occur. There have been isolated reports of temporary psychotic symptoms occurring in adults following the long-term misuse of excessive doses. Pemoline should be given with caution to emotionally unstable patients who may increase the dosage on their own initiative.

CNS stimulants: CNS stimulants, including pemoline, have been reported to precipitate motor and phonic tics, and Tourette syndrome. Therefore, clinical evaluation for tics and Tourette syndrome in children and their families should precede use of stimulant medications.

Potential liver toxicity: Report any unexplained appetite loss, nausea, vomiting, general body discomfort, weakness, or yellowing of the skin or eyes to your doctor.

Total treatment program: Pemoline therapy should be a part of a total treatment program that includes psychological, educational, and social measures.

Pregnancy: There are no adequate and well-controlled studies in pregnant women. Use only if clearly needed and the potential benefits to the mother outweigh the possible hazards to the fetus.

Breastfeeding: It is not known if pemoline appears in breast milk. Consult your doctor before you begin breastfeeding.

Children: Safety and effectiveness in children less than 6 years of age have not been established. Pemoline use may worsen symptoms of behavior disturbance and thought disorder in psychotic children. Aggravation of Tourette syndrome and seizure disorders have been reported after starting pemoline therapy. Chronic administration of stimulants to children may be associated with growth inihibition. Therefore, growth must be monitored during treatment. Long-term effects in children have not been well established. Treatment is not indicated in all cases of attention deficit disorder with hyperactivity. The decision to prescribe pemoline should depend on the assessment of the severity of the child's symptoms for his or her age, and not depend solely on the presence of one or more of the behavioral characteristics.

Lab tests will be required before and during pemoline therapy. Tests may include periodic liver function evaluation.

Drug Interactions:

Tell your doctor or pharmacist if you are taking or planning to take any over-the-counter or prescription medications or dietary supplements while taking pemoline. Doses of one or both drugs may need to be modified or a different drug may need to be prescribed. Decreased seizure threshold has been reported in patients also taking antiepileptic medications (eg, phenytoin).

Side Effects:

Every drug is capable of producing side effects. Many pemoline users experience no, or minor, side effects. The frequency and severity of side effects depend on many factors including dose, duration of therapy, and individual susceptibility. Possible side effects include:

Digestive Tract: Nausea; stomachache; loss of appetite.

Nervous System: Sleeplessness; seizures; hallucinations; dizziness; drowsiness; increased irritability; involuntary movements of tongue, lips, face, arms, and legs; Tourette syndrome; depression; headache; abnormal eye movements.

Other: Rash; yellowing of skin or eyes; dark urine; abnormal liver function tests; weight loss; liver dysfunction.

Guidelines for Use:

- Do not use pemoline until you have discussed with your doctor the risks and benefits of treatment. A written informed consent is required before beginning therapy.
- Dosage is individualized. Take exactly as prescribed. Administer as a single dose each morning.
- Do not stop taking or change the dose unless directed your doctor.
- If a dose is missed, take it as soon as possible. If several hours have passed or it is nearing time for the next dose, do not double the dose to catch up, unless advised by your doctor. If more than one dose is missed or it is necessary to establish a new dosage schedule, contact your doctor or pharmacist.
- Clinical improvement with pemoline is gradual. Significant benefit may not be evident until after 3 to 4 weeks of therapy.
- Because of its association with life-threatening liver failure, pemoline should not ordinarily be considered as first-line drug therapy for attention deficit hyperactivity disorder (ADHD).
- May cause drowsiness or dizziness. Use caution while driving or performing other tasks requiring alertness, coordination, or physical dexterity until tolerance is determined.
- Inform your doctor if you are pregnant, become pregnant, are planning to become pregnant, or are breastfeeding.
- Notify your doctor immediately if you experience darkening of urine, appetite loss, general body discomfort, nausea, vomiting, yellowing of the skin or eyes, or uncontrolled movement.
- Notify your doctor if sleeplessness occurs and is bothersome.
- Chronic use may suppress growth in children.
- Your doctor may interrupt treatment occasionally to determine if there is a recurrence of behavioral symptoms sufficient to require continued therapy.
- Pemoline therapy should be stopped if no benefit is noted after 3 weeks of taking the maximum dose.
- Lab tests will be required to monitor therapy. Be sure to keep appointments.
- Store at room temperature (59° to 86°F).

If you have any questions, consult your doctor, pharmacist, or health care provider.

Generic Name *Brand Name Examples*	Supplied As	Generic Available
otc **Acetaminophen**		
Aceta, Arthritis Pain Formula Aspirin Free, Aspirin Free Anacin Maximum Strength, Aspirin Free Pain Relief, Dapa, Genapap Extra Strength, Genebs, Genebs Extra Strength, Mapap Extra Strength, Mapap Regular Strength, Maranox, Moda Tab, Panadol, Panex, Redutemp, Tapanol Extra Strength, Tylenol Caplets, Tylenol Extra Strength, Tylenol Junior Strength, Tylenol Regular Strength	**Tablets:** 160 mg, 325 mg, 500 mg, 650 mg	Yes
Apacet, Children's Genapap, Children's Panadol[1]*, Children's Tylenol, St. Joseph Aspirin-Free for Children, Tylenol Junior Strength*	**Tablets, chewable:** 80 mg, 160 mg	Yes
Dapa Extra Strength, Feverall Sprinkle Caps, Meda Cap	**Capsules:** 80 mg, 160 mg, 500 mg	Yes
Tylenol Extended Relief	**Caplets, extended release:** 650 mg	No
Arthritis Foundation Pain Reliever Aspirin Free, Aspirin Free Anacin Maximum Strength, Panadol Junior Strength[1]	**Caplets:** 160 mg, 500 mg	No
Aspirin Free Anacin Maximum Strength	**Gel caplets:** 500 mg	No
Snaplets-FR	**Granules:** 80 mg	No
Aceta[2]*, Children's Genapap,*[3] *Children's Mapap*[3]*, Children's Silapap*[1,3]*, Children's Tylenol*[3]*, Dolanex*[1,2]*, Liquiprin, Oraphen-PD*[2]*, Ridenol*	**Elixir:** 80 mg/tsp, 120 mg/tsp, 130 mg/tsp, 160 mg/tsp, 325 mg/tsp	Yes

	Generic Name *Brand Name Examples*	Supplied As	Generic Available
	Children's Halenol[3], Children's Panadol[1,3], St. Joseph Aspirin-Free Fever Reducer for Children[1,3], Tylenol Extra Strength[2]	**Liquid:** 160 mg/tsp, 500 mg/tbsp	Yes
	Genapap Infants' Drops[3], Liquiprin Infants' Drops[3], Mapap Infants' Drops[3], Myapap Drops[1,3], Panadol Infants' Drops[1,3], Silapap Infants' Drops[3], St. Joseph Aspirin-Free Infants' Drops[1,3], Tempra Drops[3], Tylenol Infants' Drops[3], Uni-Ace[3]	**Solution:** 80 mg/0.8 mL, 100 mg/mL, 120 mg/2.5 mL	Yes
	Children's Tylenol[3], Tylenol Infants' Drops[3]	**Suspension:** 80 mg/tsp, 160 mg/tsp	No
	Acetaminophen Uniserts, Acephen, Children's Feverall, Infants' Feverall, Neopap, Suppap	**Suppositories:** 80 mg, 120 mg, 125 mg, 325 mg, 650 mg	Yes
otc	**Acetaminophen, Buffered**		
	Bromo Seltzer	**Effervescent granules:** 325 mg with 2.781 g sodium bicarbonate and 2.224 g citric acid/¾ capful	No

[1] Sugar free.
[2] Contains alcohol.
[3] Alcohol free.

Type of Drug:

Non-aspirin pain reliever and fever reducer. "Tylenol," APAP.

How the Drug Works:

Acetaminophen reduces fever by increasing the removal of body heat through increased sweating and dilating of the blood vessels. It changes the body's thermostat. It is unclear how it relieves pain. The pain relieving and fever reducing qualities of acetaminophen are similar to aspirin.

Uses:

To relieve pain.

To reduce fever.

Unlabeled Use(s): Occasionally, doctors may use acetaminophen in children receiving DTP vaccination to reduce the chances for fever and injection site pain. A dose given immediately after the vaccination and every 4 to 6 hours for 2 to 3 days is suggested.

Precautions:

Do not use in the following situations: Allergy to acetaminophen.

Use with caution in the following situations:

kidney disease
liver disease

Alcohol use: Liver toxicity and liver failure have occurred in chronic alcoholics taking normal doses of acetaminophen. Chronic alcoholics should take no more than 2 g of acetaminophen per day.

Overdosage: Do not exceed recommended dosage. Even a small amount over the maximum daily dose can cause liver or kidney damage. Maintain adequate food and fluid intake while taking this medicine.

Pregnancy: This drug appears to be safe for short-term use during pregnancy. However, no drug should be used during pregnancy unless clearly needed. Long-term use during pregnancy should be avoided.

Breastfeeding: Acetaminophen appears in breast milk. Consult your doctor before you begin breastfeeding.

Children: Safety and effectiveness in children younger than 3 years of age have not been established.

Drug Interactions:

Tell your doctor or pharmacist if you are taking or will be taking any over-the-counter or prescription medication or dietary supplements while taking this medicine. Doses of one or both drugs may need to be modified or a different drug may need to be prescribed. The following drugs and drug classes interact with this medicine:

alcohol
barbiturates (eg, phenobarbital)
carbamazepine (eg, *Tegretol*)
charcoal
hydantoins (eg, phenytoin)
rifampin (eg, *Rifadin*)
sulfinpyrazone (*Anturane*)

Side Effects:

Every drug is capable of producing side effects. Many patients experience no, or minor, side effects. The frequency and severity of side effects include many factors including dose, duration of therapy, and individual susceptibility. Possible side effects include:

Allergic reactions: Difficulty breathing; rash; fever; skin eruptions; hives.

Other: Low blood sugar; abnormal blood counts and liver function tests; yellowing of skin or eyes.

Guidelines for Use:

- Severe or recurrent pain or high or continued fever may indicate serious illness. If pain persists for more than 5 days, if redness is present or in arthritic and rheumatic conditions affecting children younger than 12 years of age, consult your doctor immediately.
- Do not exceed the recommended dosage. Consult your doctor for use in children younger than 3 years of age or for oral use longer than 5 days (children), 10 days (adults) or 3 days for fever.
- If fever, difficulty breathing, rash, or hives occur, discontinue use and contact your doctor immediately.
- Poisoning or overdose may cause few early symptoms (eg, nausea, vomiting, drowsiness, confusion, liver pain, yellowing of skin or eyes), but requires immediate medical treatment.
- Avoid alcohol while taking this medicine.
- Keep out of reach of children.
- Store at room temperature. Store suppositories at room temperature (59° to 86°F) or in the refrigerator (36° to 46°F).

If you have any questions, consult your doctor, pharmacist, or health care provider.

	Generic Name *Brand Name Examples*	Supplied As	Generic Available
otc	**Aspirin, Children's**		
	Bayer Children's	**Chewable tablets:** 81 mg	No
	Aspirin		
otc	*Aspergum*	**Gum tablets:** 227.5 mg	No
otc	*St. Joseph Adult Chewable Aspirin*	**Chewable tablets:** 81 mg	No
otc	*Arthritis Foundation Pain Reliever,Empirin, Genprin, Genuine Bayer Aspirin Tablets and Caplets, Maximum Bayer Aspirin Tablets and Caplets, Norwich, Norwich Extra Strength*	**Tablets:** 325 mg, 500 mg	Yes
otc	*Ecotrin Tablets and Caplets, Ecotrin Maximum Strength Tablets and Caplets, Extra Strength Bayer Enteric 500, Halfprin, Halfprin 81, Regular Strength Bayer Enteric Coated Caplets*	**Tablets, enteric coated:** 165 mg, 325 mg, 500 mg, 650 mg	Yes
otc	*Bayer Low Adult Strength*	**Tablets, delayed release:** 81 mg	No
otc	*8-Hour Bayer Caplets*	**Tablets, timed release:** 650 mg	No
otc	*Adprin-B, Asprimox Extra Protection for Arthritis Pain, Bayer Buffered, Extra Strength Adprin-B, Extra Strength Bayer Plus*	**Tablets, buffered:** 325 mg, 500 mg	No
Rx	*Eastprin*	**Tablets, enteric coated:** 975 mg	Yes
Rx	*ZORprin*	**Tablets, controlled release:** 800 mg	No
otc	*Aspirin*	**Suppositories[1]:** 120 mg, 200 mg, 300 mg, 600 mg	Yes
otc	**Choline Salicylate**		
	Arthropan	**Liquid:** 870 mg/tsp	No

	Generic Name *Brand Name Examples*	Supplied As	Generic Available
	Magnesium Salicylate		
otc	*Backache Maximum Strength Relief, Bayer Select Maximum Strength Backache, Extra Strength Doan's PM, Momentum Muscular Backache Formula, Original Doan's*	**Caplets:** 325 mg, 467 mg, 500 mg, 580 mg	No
Rx	*Magan, Mobidin*	**Tablets:** 545 mg, 600 mg	No
Rx	**Salsalate**		
	Amigesic, Disalcid	**Capsules:** 500 mg	No
	Amigesic, Disalcid Amigesic, Argesic-SA, Artha-G, Disalcid, Marthritic, Mono-Gesic, Salflex, Salsitab	**Tablets:** 500 mg, 750 mg	Yes
otc	**Sodium Salicylate**	**Tablets, enteric coated:** 325 mg, 650 mg	Yes
Rx	**Salicylate Combinations**		
	Trilisate	**Tablets:**500 mg salicylate (as 293 mg choline salicylate and 362 mg magnesium salicylate); 750 mg salicylate (as 440 mg choline salicylate and 544 mg magnesium salicylate); 1000 mg salicylate (as 587 mg choline salicylate and 725 mg magnesium salicylate)	No
	Trilisate	**Liquid:** 500 mg salicylate (as 293 mg choline salicylate and 362 mg magnesium salicylate)/tsp	No

[1] Refrigerate.

Type of Drug:

Aspirin pain reliever, fever reducer and anti-inflammatory agent. ASA.

How the Drug Works:

Salicylates relieve pain by inhibiting pain perception by pain receptors and by inhibiting the formation of chemicals called prostaglandins. Prostaglandins cause pain receptors to be more sensitive to pain-producing stimuli.

They reduce fever by direct action on the heat regulating center of the brain (the body's "thermostat"). This increases the removal of heat through increased sweating and dilation (widening) of blood vessels in the skin.

Salicylates also help in preventing blood platelets from clumping together to form clots.

Uses:

To relieve mild to moderate pain.

To reduce fever.

To reduce inflammation, redness, swelling (eg, in arthritis).

Aspirin: To reduce the risk of recurrent transient ischemic attacks (TIAs) or stroke in men.

To reduce risk of death or nonfatal heart attacks (myocardial infarction) in people with previous heart attack or unstable angina.

Unlabeled Use(s): Occasionally doctors may prescribe aspirin-like pain relievers for the possible protective effect against cataract formation and to prevent toxemia of pregnancy. It may also be of benefit in pregnant women with inadequate uteroplacental blood flow.

Precautions:

Do not use in the following situations:

- allergy to salicylates
- allergy to nonsteroidal anti-inflammatory drugs (NSAIDs)
- bleeding disorder
- bleeding ulcers
- children younger than 18 with chicken-pox or flu symptoms
- hemophilia
- kidney disease (magnesium salicylate only)
- tartrazine sensitivity

Use with caution in the following situations:

- anemia
- anticoagulant therapy
- bleeding disorders, history
- diabetes, mild
- gout
- kidney disease
- liver disease
- surgery (within 1 week)
- ulcers
- vitamin K deficiency

Ears: Discontinue use if dizziness, ringing in the ears, or any hearing difficulty occurs. These symptoms are indications that salicylate blood level may be too high. Temporary hearing loss disappears gradually after the drug is stopped.

Controlled release aspirin Because of its relatively long onset of action, controlled-released aspirin is not recommended for fevers or short-term pain relief. It is not recommended in children younger than 12 or children with fever accompanied by dehydration.

Aspirin intolerance: Symptoms (spasms in bronchioles, hives, swelling, inflammation of the nose) occur within 3 hours after ingestion. Aspirin intolerance is more common in patients with a history of asthma and nasal polyps.

Foods containing salicylate may contribute to a reaction. Some foods with salicylate include curry powder, paprika, licorice, Benedictine liqueur, prunes, raisins, tea, and gherkins. A typical American diet contains 10 to 200 mg/day salicylate.

Desensitization has been successful. It should be done in a hospital. It is generally maintained with 1 aspirin/day. Any NSAID can maintain desensitization. However, if maintenance is interrupted, sensitivity will reappear (2 to 5 days).

Pregnancy: Salicylates cross the placenta. Avoid use during pregnancy, especially the third trimester. Aspirin studies have shown a potential effect to the fetus. Adequate studies have not been done in pregnant women. Use only if clearly needed and potential benefits outweigh the possible hazards to the fetus.

Breastfeeding: Salicylates appear in breast milk. Consult your doctor before you begin breastfeeding.

Children: Administration of aspirin to children (including teenagers) with fever-causing illnesses (eg, chickenpox, flu) has been associated with the development of Reye syndrome. Reye is a rare illness characterized by vomiting, lethargy, and belligerence that may progress to delirium and coma. Safety and effectiveness of magnesium salicylate or salsalate in children have not been established.

Drug Interactions:

Tell your doctor or pharmacist if you are taking or if you are planning to take any over-the-counter or prescription medications or dietary supplements with salicylates. Doses of one or both drugs may need to be modified or a different drug may need to be prescribed. The following drugs and drug classes interact with salicylates.

Drugs affecting aspirin —

acetazolamide (eg, *Diamox)*
antacids (eg, *Tums)*
charcoal, activated
contraceptives, oral (eg, *Ortho-Novum)*
corticosteroids (eg, prednisone)
dichlorphenamide (*Daranide)*
methazolamide (eg, *Neptazane)*
nizatidine (eg, *Axid)*
ticlopidine (eg, *Ticlid)*
urinary acidifiers (eg, vitamin C)
urinary alkalinizers (eg, sodium bicarbonate)

Drugs affected by aspirin —

ACE inhibitors (eg, captopril)
alcohol
anticoagulants, oral (eg, warfarin)
beta-blockers (eg, propranolol)
heparin
hydantoins (eg, phenytoin)
insulin
loop diuretics (eg, furosemide)
methotrexate (eg, *Rheumatrex*)
nitroglycerin (eg, *Nitrostat)*
nonsteroidal anti-inflammatory agents (eg, ibuprofen)
probenecid
spironolactone (eg, *Aldactone)*
sulfinpyrazone (eg, *Anturane)*
sulfonylureas (eg, chlorpropamide)
valproic acid (eg, *Depakene)*

Side Effects:

Every drug is capable of producing side effects. Many salicylate users experience no, or minor, side effects. The frequency and severity of side effects depend on many factors including dose, duration of therapy, and individual susceptibility. Possible side effects include:

Allergic Reactions: Difficulty breathing and inflammation in nose may occur in people with a history of nasal polyps or asthma.

Digestive Tract: Stomach upset; nausea; vomiting; appetite loss; indigestion; heartburn; diarrhea; ulcers; GI bleeding.

Nervous System: Dizziness; weakness; confusion; headache.

Other: Ringing in the ears; difficulty hearing; thirst; sweating; liver problems; prolonged bleeding; abnormal blood counts; black or bloody stools; rapid breathing; iron deficiency anemia (chronic use); dim vision; rash; fever; hives.

Guidelines for Use:

- Dosage is individualized. Take exactly as prescribed.
- Do not stop taking or change the dose unless directed by your doctor.
- May cause stomach upset. Take with food or after meals.
- Do not crush or chew sustained-release preparations.
- Take with a full glass of water (8 oz) to reduce the risk of medication lodging in the throat.
- Patients allergic to tartrazine dye should avoid aspirin; use caution with asthma or nasal polyps.
- Avoid use during pregnancy.
- Avoid use in children with a fever-causing illness.
- Notify your doctor if ringing in ears or persistent stomach pain occurs.
- Do not use aspirin if it has a strong vinegar-like odor.
- Do not place or dissolve on an oral lesion (eg, canker sore, cold sore) or directly on an aching tooth. A serious local inflammatory reaction could occur.

If you have any questions, consult your doctor, pharmacist, or health care provider.

	Brand Name Examples	Aspirin	Buffering Agents
otc	*Alka-Seltzer Extra Strength Antacid and Pain Relief Effervescent Tablets*[1]	500 mg	1000 mg citric acid, 1985 mg sodium bicarbonate
otc	*Bufferin Arthritis Strength Pain Reliever Caplets, Bufferin Extra Strength Coated Caplets*	500 mg	Calcium carbonate, magnesium carbonate, magnesium oxide
otc	*Maximum Strength Ascriptin Coated Caplets*	500 mg	Alumina-magnesia, calcium carbonate
otc	*Alka-Seltzer Original Antacid and Pain Relief Effervescent Tablets*[1]	325 mg	1000 mg citric acid, 1916 mg sodium bicarbonate
otc	*Alka-Seltzer Flavored Antacid and Pain Relief Effervescent Tablets*[1,2]	325 mg	1000 mg citric acid, 1700 mg sodium bicarbonate
otc	*Magnaprin Film Coated Tablets*	325 mg	50 mg aluminum hydroxide, 50 mg magnesium hydroxide, calcium carbonate
otc	*Adprin-B Coated Caplets, Bufferin Coated Tablets*	325 mg	Calcium carbonate, magnesium carbonate, magnesium oxide
otc	*Arthritis Pain Ascriptin Coated Caplets, Ascriptin Regular Strength Coated Tablets*	325 mg	Alumina-magnesia, calcium carbonate
otc	*Buffered Aspirin Enteric Coated Tablets*	325 mg	
otc	*Aspirin Regimen Bayer Adult Low Strength with Calcium Caplets*	81 mg	250 mg calcium carbonate

[1] Contains sodium.
[2] Contains phenylalanine.

For more information on aspirin, see the Analgesics-Aspirin and Salicylates monograph in this chapter.

Type of Drug:

Aspirin pain reliever (analgesic); fever reducer (antipyretic); anti-inflammatory agent.

Guidelines for Use:

- Dosage is individualized. Take exactly as advised.
- May cause stomach upset. Take with food or after meals.
- Take with a full glass of water (8 oz) to reduce the risk of medication sticking in the throat.
- Do not use for pain for more than 10 days or for fever for more than 3 days unless directed by your health care provider.
- Patients allergic to tartrazine dye (FD&C Yellow No. 5) should avoid aspirin.
- Use with caution if you havo asthma or nasal polyps.
- Consult your health care provider if pain or fever persists or gets worse, if new symptoms occur, or if redness or swelling is present. These could be signs of a serious condition.
- Discontinue use and notify your doctor if you experience ringing in ears or persistent stomach pain.
- Limit alcohol intake while taking these products.
- Do not use aspirin if it has a strong vinegar-like odor.
- Avoid use during pregnancy unless advised by your health care provider.
- Avoid use in children with fever-causing illness.
- Store at room temperature (59° to 86°F). Protect from moisture.

If you have any questions, consult your doctor, pharmacist, or health care provider.

Content given per capsule, tablet, or powder packet.

	Brand Name Examples	**APAP†**	**Aspirin**	**Other Analgesics**	**Other**
Rx	*Axocet Capsules, Bupap Tablets, Phrenilin Forte Capsules, Repan CF Tablets, Sedapap Tablets*	650 mg			50 mg butalbital
Rx	*Esgic-Plus Tablets*	500 mg			50 mg butalbital, 40 mg caffeine
otc	*Maximum Strength Midol PMS Caplets and Gelcaps, Maximum Strength Multi-Symptom Pamprin Caplets and Tablets, Premsyn PMS Caplets*	500 mg			25 mg pamabrom, 15 mg pyrilamine maleate
otc	*Maximum Strength Midol Menstrual Caplets and Gelcaps*	500 mg			60 mg caffeine, 15 mg pyrilamine maleate
otc	*Vitelle Lurline PMS Tablets*	500 mg			25 mg pamabrom, 50 mg pyridoxine HCl
otc	*Anacin P.M. Caplets*	500 mg			25 mg diphenhydramine HCl
otc	*Excedrin PM Tablets*	500 mg			38 mg diphenhydramine citrate
Rx	*Flextra-DS Tablets*	500 mg			50 mg phenyltoloxamine citrate
otc	*Aspirin Free Excedrin Caplets*	500 mg			65 mg caffeine

Content given per capsule, tablet, or powder packet.

	Brand Name Examples	APAP†	Aspirin	Other Analgesics	Other
otc	*Fem-1 Tablets, Maximum Strength Midol Teen Caplets, Women's Tylenol Multi-Symptom Menstrual Relief Caplets*	500 mg			25 mg pamabrom
otc	*Goody's Body Pain Powder*	325 mg	500 mg		
otc	*Aceta-Gesic Tablets*	325 mg			30 mg phenyltoloxamine citrate
c-III	*Fiortal Capsules*	325 mg			50 mg butalbital, 40 mg caffeine
Rx	*Butalbital, Acetaminophen and Caffeine Tablets, Esgic Tablets, Fioricet Tablets, Margesic Capsules, Medigesic Capsules, Repan Tablets, Triad Capsules*	325 mg			50 mg butalbital, 40 mg caffeine
Rx	*Phrenilin Tablets*	325 mg			50 mg butalbital
otc	*Goody's Extra Strength Headache Powder*	260 mg	520 mg		32.5 mg caffeine
otc	*Excedrin Extra Strength Caplets, Geltabs, and Tablets, Summit Extra Strength Coated Tablets*	250 mg	250 mg		65 mg caffeine
otc	*Maximum Cramp Relief Pamprin Caplets*	250 mg		250 mg magnesium salicylate	25 mg pamabrom

Content given per capsule, tablet, or powder packet.

	Brand Name Examples	**APAP†**	**Aspirin**	**Other Analgesics**	**Other**
otc	*Vanquish Caplets*	194 mg	227 mg		25 mg aluminum hydroxide, 33 mg caffeine, 50 mg magnesium hydroxide
otc	*Extra Strength Goody's Tablets*	130 mg	260 mg		16.25 mg caffeine
otc	*Saleto Tablets*	115 mg	210 mg	65 mg salicylamide	16 mg caffeine
otc	*BC Powder Original Formula*		650 mg	195 mg salicylamide	38 mg caffeine
otc	*Maximum Strength Anacin Tablets*		500 mg		32 mg caffeine
otc	*Extra Strength Bayer PM Aspirin Plus Sleep Aid Caplets*		500 mg		25 mg diphenhydramine HCl
otc	*Cope Analgesic Tablets*		421 mg		32 mg caffeine
otc	*Anacin Caplets and Tablets, P-A-C Analgesic Tablets*		400 mg		32 mg caffeine
c-III	*Butalbital Compound Capsules and Tablets, Fiorinal Capsules*		325 mg		50 mg butalbital, 40 mg caffeine
c-IV	*Equagesic Tablets, Micrainin Tablets*		325 mg		200 mg meprobamate
Rx	*Magsal Tablets*			600 mg magnesium salicylate tetrahydrate	25 mg phenyltoloxamine dihydrogen citrate

Content given per capsule, tablet, or powder packet.

	Brand Name Examples	**APAP†**	**Aspirin**	**Other Analgesics**	**Other**
otc	*Mobigesic Backache Pain Reliever Tablets*			404 mg magnesium salicylate tetrahydrate	30 mg phenyltoloxamine citrate
Rx	*Arthrotec Tablets*			75 mg diclofenac sodium	200 mcg misoprostol
Rx	*Arthrotec Tablets*			50 mg diclofenac sodium	200 mcg misoprostol

† APAP = Acetaminophen.

Type of Drug:

Nonnarcotic pain reliever combinations.

Uses:

Components of these combinations include:

Nonnarcotic analgesics: Acetaminophen (APAP); aspirin (ASA) and salicylates (eg, salsalate, salicylamide). For more information, see the individual monographs in this chapter.

Antacids (eg, magnesium hydroxide, aluminum hydroxide): Used to minimize gastric upset from salicylates. For more information, see the monograph in the Gastrointestinals chapter.

Barbiturates (eg, butalbital), meprobamate, and antihistamines (eg, diphenhydramine, pyrilamine, phenyltoloxamine): Used for their sedative effects. For more information on barbiturates or meprobamate, see the individual monographs in this chapter. For more information on antihistamines, see the monograph in the Respiratory Drugs chapter.

Caffeine: A traditional component of many analgesic formulations, may be beneficial in certain vascular headaches. For more information, see the monograph in this chapter.

Misoprostol: Prevents nonsteroidal anti-inflammatory-induced gastric ulcers in patients at high risk for complications from a gastric ulcer or at high risk of developing gastric ulceration. For more information, see the Anti-Ulcer-Misoprostol monograph in the Gastrointestinals chapter.

Pamabrom: Used as a diuretic.

Guidelines for Use:

- Dosage is individualized. Take exactly as prescribed.
- Do not stop taking or change the dose, unless directed by your doctor.
- May cause stomach upset. Take with food or after meals.
- Do not crush or chew sustained-release preparations.
- Take with a full glass (8 oz) of water or other fluid to reduce the risk of lodging medication in the throat.
- Patients allergic to tartrazine dye should avoid aspirin.
- Notify your doctor if you experience ringing in ears, skin rash, difficulty breathing, easy bruising, or persistent stomach pain.
- Do not use an aspirin-containing product if it has a strong vinegar-like odor.
- Severe or recurrent pain or high or continued fever may indicate serious illness. If pain persists for more than 10 days or if redness is present, consult your doctor immediately.
- Consult your doctor before using in arthritic and rheumatic conditions affecting children less than of age.
- Avoid aspirin-containing products in patients suspected of having chickenpox or the flu because of the risk of Reye syndrome.
- Do not exceed the recommended dosage. Consult your doctor for use in children younger than 3 years of age, or for oral use more than 10 days.
- Poisoning or overdose may cause few early symptoms but requires immediate medical treatment.

If you have any questions, consult your doctor, pharmacist, or health care provider.

	Generic Name *Brand Name Example*	Supplied As	Generic Available
Rx	**Diflunisal**		
	Dolobid	**Tablets**: 250 mg, 500 mg	Yes

Type of Drug:

Anti-inflammatory; analgesic (pain reliever).

How the Drug Works:

Diflunisal decreases inflammation and relieves pain by inhibiting prostaglandin synthesis. It is not a steroid or a narcotic.

Uses:

To relieve mild to moderate pain, inflammation, and rheumatoid arthritis and osteoarthritis pain.

Precautions:

Do not use in the following situations:

- allergy to aspirin or nonsteroidal anti-inflammatory drugs
- allergy to diflunisal or any of its ingredients
- pregnancy, third trimester

Use with caution in the following situations:

- heart disease
- high blood pressure
- kidney disease
- peptic ulcer

Pregnancy: Safety for use during pregnancy has not been established. Use with caution during the first and second trimesters. Do not use during the third trimester.

Breastfeeding: Diflunisal appears in breast milk. Consult your doctor before you begin breastfeeding.

Children: Safety and effectiveness have not been established. Use in children younger than 12 years of age is not recommended. Acetylsalicylic acid has been associated with Reye syndrome. Since diflunisal is a salicylic acid derivative, the possibility of its association with Reye syndrome cannot be excluded. Consult your doctor.

Drug Interactions:

Tell your doctor or pharmacist if you are taking or if you are planning to take any over-the-counter or prescription medications or dietary supplements with diflunisal. Doses of one or both drugs may need to be modified or a different drug may need to be prescribed. The following drugs and drug classes interact with diflunisal:

- acetaminophen (eg, *Tylenol*)
- antacids (eg, *Tums*)
- anticoagulants, oral (eg, warfarin)
- cyclosporine (eg, *Sandimmune*)
- hydrochlorothiazide (eg, *HydroDIURIL*)
- indomethacin (eg, *Indocin*)
- methotrexate (eg, *Rheumatrex*)
- sulindac (*Clinoril*)

Side Effects:

Every drug is capable of producing side effects. Many diflunisal users experience no, or minor, side effects. The frequency and severity of side effects depend on many factors including dose, duration of therapy, and individual susceptibility. Possible side effects include:

Digestive Tract: Stomach pain; gas; diarrhea; nausea; constipation; ulcers; indigestion; vomiting.

Nervous System: Headache; dizziness; nervousness; sleeplessness; confusion; fatigue or tiredness.

Skin: Rash; itching; sweating; sensitivity to light.

Other: Ringing in the ears or difficulty hearing; edema (fluid retention); swelling.

Guidelines for Use:

- May cause stomach upset. Take with water, milk, or meals.
- Chronic gastrointestinal upset or any signs of bleeding should be reported to your doctor.
- Swallow tablets whole. Do not crush or chew.
- Do not take aspirin or acetaminophen with diflunisal. Consult your doctor.
- If a dose is missed, take it as soon as possible. If several hours have passed or if it is nearing time for the next dose, do not double the dose to catch up, unless advised by your doctor. If more than 1 dose is missed, contact your doctor or pharmacist.
- May cause sensitivity to sunlight. Avoid prolonged exposure to the sun. Use sunscreens and wear protective clothing until tolerance is determined.

If you have any questions, consult your doctor, pharmacist, or health care provider.

	Generic Name *Brand Name Examples*	Supplied As	Generic Available
C-II	**Codeine**		
	Codeine Sulfate	**Tablets:** 15 mg, 30 mg, 60 mg	Yes
	Codeine Phosphate	**Solution, oral**: 15 mg/5 mL	Yes
C-II	**Fentanyl**		
	Actiq[1]	**Lozenge on a stick (transmucosal system)**: 200 mcg, 400 mcg, 600 mcg, 800 mcg, 1200 mcg, 1600 mcg	No
	Duragesic	**Transdermal system**: 2.5 mg/hr, 5 mg/hr[1], 7.5 mg/hr[1], 10 mg/hr[1]	No
C-II	**Hydromorphone**	**Solution, oral**: 1 mg/mL	Yes
	Dilaudid	**Tablets:** 2 mg, 4 mg, 8 mg[2]	Yes
	Dilaudid	**Liquid**: 5 mg/5 mL[2]	Yes
	Dilaudid	**Suppositories:** 3 mg	Yes
C-II	**Levomethadyl Acetate HCl**		
	ORLAAM	**Solution, oral**: 10 mg/mL	No
C-II	**Levorphanol Tartrate**		
	Levo-Dromoran	**Tablets:** 2 mg	Yes
C-II	**Meperidine HCl**		
	Demerol	**Tablets:** 50 mg, 100 mg	Yes
	Demerol	**Syrup:** 50 mg/5 mL	Yes
	Demerol	**Injection**: 10 mg/mL, 25 mg/mL, 50 mg/mL, 75 mg/mL, 100 mg/mL	Yes
C-II	**Methadone HCl**	**Solution, oral**: 5 mg/5 mL, 10 mg/5 mL	Yes
	Dolophine HCl, Methadose	**Tablets:** 5 mg, 10 mg	Yes
	Methadone HCl Diskets	**Tablets, dispersible**: 40 mg	Yes
	Methadone HCl Intensol, Methadose	**Liquid, oral concentrate:** 10 mg/mL	Yes

	Generic Name *Brand Name Examples*	Supplied As	Generic Available
C-II	**Morphine Sulfate**	**Tablets, soluble**: 10 mg, 15 mg, 30 mg	Yes
	MSIR	**Tablets:** 15 mg, 30 mg	No
	MS Contin, Oramorph SR	**Tablets, sustained-release:** 15 mg, 30 mg, 60 mg, 100 mg, 200 mg[1]	Yes
	MSIR	**Capsules**: 15 mg, 30 mg	No
	Kadian	**Capsules, sustained-release**: 20 mg, 50 mg, 100 mg	No
	MSIR	**Solution, oral**: 10 mg/5 mL, 20 mg/5 mL,	Yes
	MSIR, OMS Concentrate, Roxanol, Roxanol 100, Roxanol T	**Solution, oral concentrate:** 20 mg/mL, 100 mg/5 mL	Yes
	RMS	**Suppositories**: 5 mg, 10 mg, 20 mg, 30 mg	Yes
	Astramorph PF, Duramorph, Infumorph	**Injection**: 0.5 mg/mL, 1 mg/mL, 2 mg/mL, 4 mg/mL, 5 mg/mL, 8 mg/mL, 10 mg/mL, 15 mg/mL, 25 mg/mL, 50 mg/mL	
C-II	**Oxycodone HCl**		
	Percolone, Roxicodone	**Tablets:** 5 mg	No
	Oxycontin	**Tablets, controlled-release**: 10 mg, 20 mg, 40 mg, 80 mg[1], 160 mg[1]	No
	OxyIR	**Capsules**: 5 mg	No
	Roxicodone	**Solution, oral:** 5 mg/5 mL	No
	OxyFast, Roxicodone Intensol	**Solution, oral concentrate**: 20 mg/mL	No
C-II	**Oxymorphone HCl**		
	Numorphan	**Suppositories:** 5 mg	No
C-IV	**Propoxyphene (Detropropoxyphene)**		
	Darvon-N	**Tablets:** 100 mg (as napsylate)	No
	Darvon Pulvules	**Capsules:** 65 mg (as HCl)	Yes

[1] For use only in opioid-tolerant patients.
[2] Contains sulfites.

Type of Drug:

Narcotic analgesics (pain relievers).

How the Drug Works:

Narcotic pain relievers relieve pain by dulling the pain perception center of the brain. They may also affect other systems in the body at higher doses. Natural narcotics include opium, codeine, and morphine. Other narcotics are synthetic (opioids) and vary in potency, addictive ability, and side effects.

Uses:

For relief of mild-to-moderate pain and for coughing induced by viral, bacterial, chemical, or mechanical irritation of the respiratory system (codeine only).

For the management of chronic pain in patients requiring continuous opioid analgesia for pain that cannot be managed by lesser means such as acetaminophen-opioid combinations, nonsteroidal analgesics, or PRN (as-needed) dosing with short-acting opioids (fentanyl only).

For the management of breakthrough cancer pain in patients with malignancies who are already receiving and are tolerant to opioid therapy for their underlying persistent cancer pain (fentanyl lozenge only).

For relief of moderate-to-severe pain (hydromorphone, meperidine, methadone, morphine, oxycodone, and oxymorphone only).

For the management of opiate dependence (levomethadyl acetate only).

For the management of moderate-to-severe pain or as a preoperative medication where an opioid analgesic is appropriate (levorphanol only).

For relief of severe pain, and for detoxification and temporary maintenance treatment of narcotic addiction (methadone only).

For relief of moderate-to-severe acute and chronic pain; for the management of pain not responsive to nonnarcotic analgesics; dyspnea (shortness of breath) associated with acute left ventricle failure and pulmonary edema; used preoperatively for patient sedation; to decrease apprehension; effective in the control of postoperative pain (morphine only).

For relief of pain in patients who require opioid analgesics for more than a few days (morphine sustained-release only).

For relief of mild-to-moderate pain (propoxyphene only).

Unlabeled Use(s): Occasionally doctors may prescribe injectable morphine for difficult breathing associated with acute left ventricular failure and pulmonary edema.

Precautions:

Do not use in the following situations:

- alcoholism, acute (levorphanol only)
- allergy to the narcotic or any of its ingredients
- bronchial asthma, acute or severe
- diarrhea caused by poisoning until the toxic material has been eliminated (opium only)
- hypercarbia (oxycodone only)
- MAOI use, concurrent or within the last 14 days (fentanyl and meperidine only)

paralytic ileus (oxycodone and oxymorphone sustained-release only)
respiratory depression
upper airway obstruction

fentanyl lozenge only —
management of acute pain
management of postoperative pain
opioid nontolerant patients

fentanyl transdermal system only —
allergy to adhesives
management of acute pain
management of mild or intermittent pain responsive to
as-needed narcotics or nonnarcotic analgesics
management of postoperative pain

hydromorphone only —
intracranial lesions associated with increased intracranial pressure
parenteral narcotic therapy, concurrent
respiratory depression in the absence of resuscitative equipment
status asthmaticus
ventilatory function, severely depressed (eg, chronic obstructive pulmonary disease, cor pulmonale)

Use with caution in the following situations:
abdominal condition, acute
abnormal heart rhythm
Addison's disease
alcoholism, acute
arteriosclerosis (hardening of the arteries)
asthma
brain tumor
bronchitis, chronic
chronic obstructive pulmonary disease
circulatory shock
CNS depressant drug therapy (eg, barbiturates, tranquilizers, narcotics, general anesthetics)
coma
curvature of the spine
debilitation
delirium tremens (DTs)
diarrhea
drug abuse, history
elderly
emphysema
fever (fentanyl transdermal system only)
gallbladder disease
gallstones
gastrointestinal bleeding
gastrointestinal surgery, recent
genitourinary surgery, recent
head injury
heart disease
hypercapnia (excess of carbon dioxide in the blood)
hypoxia (low blood oxygen levels)
inflammatory bowel disease
intracranial pressure, increased
kidney disease
kyphoscoliosis
liver disease
low blood pressure
lung disease
MAOI use, concurrent or within the last 14 days
myxedema
obesity, severe
ocular pressure, increased
prostate, enlarged
respiratory depression, preexisting
respiratory reserve, decreased
seizure disorder
suicidal or addiction-prone individuals
supraventricular tachycardias
toxic psychosis
underactive thyroid
urethra, narrowing

Labor and Delivery: Fentanyl transdermal system is not recommended for use.

Drug dependence: Narcotic pain relievers have high abuse potential. Dependence and physical tolerance may develop upon repeated use. However, most patients who receive these agents for medical reasons and do not take more than prescribed do not develop dependence.

Tolerance: Some patients may develop tolerance to narcotic pain relievers. This may develop after days or months of continuous therapy. Consult your doctor if tolerance is suspected.

Withdrawal syndrome: Severity is related to the degree of dependence, the abruptness of withdrawal and the drug used. Generally, withdrawal symptoms begin to develop at the time the next dose would ordinarily be given. For heroin and morphine, symptoms gradually increase in intensity, reach a maximum in 36 to 72 hours and subside over 5 to 10 days. In contrast, methadone withdrawal is slower in onset and the patient may not recover for 6 to 7 weeks. Meperidine withdrawal often runs its course within 4 to 5 days. Hydrocodone withdrawal symptoms peak at 48 to 72 hours. Withdrawal precipitated by narcotic antagonists (antidotes) is manifested by onset of symptoms within minutes and maximum intensity within 30 minutes. Symptoms of withdrawal include:

Early — Yawning; tearing; runny nose; restless sleep; sweating.

Intermediate — Flushing; increased heart rate; twitching; tremor; restlessness; anxiety; irritability; goosebumps; appetite loss; dilated pupils.

Late — Muscle spasm; fever; nausea; diarrhea; vomiting; spontaneous orgasm; severe backache; stomach and leg pains; stomach and muscle cramps; hot and cold flashes; sleeplessness; intestinal spasm; repetitive sneezing; excessively runny nose; increased body temperature, blood pressure, respiratory rate and heart rate; chills; bone and muscle pain.

Pregnancy: There are no adequate and well-controlled studies in pregnant women. Regular narcotic use late in pregnancy may cause withdrawal reactions in newborns. Use only if clearly needed and the potential benefits outweigh the possible risks to the fetus.

Breastfeeding: Many of these narcotics appear in breast milk, but the effects on the infant may not be significant. Consult your doctor before you begin or continue breastfeeding if narcotic therapy is required.

Children: Safety and effectiveness of fentanyl transmucosal in children younger than 16 years of age are not established. Safety and effectiveness of codeine in children younger than 3 years of age have not been established. Do not administer fentanyl transdermal systems to children younger than 12 years of age or patients less than 18 years of age who weigh less than 50 kg except in an authorized investigational research setting. Use of levomethadyl or levorphanol is not recommended in those less than 18 years of age. Safety and effectiveness of oxymorphone in children younger than 18 years of age have not been established. Methadone is not recommended as an analgesic in children; documented clinical experience is insufficient to establish suitable dosage regimens. Safety of propoxyphene, morphine, opium, oxycodone, and hydromorphone are not established in children.

Elderly: Appropriately reduce the initial dose in elderly and debilitated patients. Consider the effect of the initial dose in determining supplemental doses. Use caution because opioids have the ability to depress breathing.

Sulfites: Some of these products may contain sulfite preservatives which can cause allergic reactions in certain individuals (eg, asthmatics). Check package label when available or consult your doctor or pharmacist.

Drug Interactions:

Tell your doctor or pharmacist if you are taking or if you are planning to take any over-the-counter or prescription medications or dietary supplements with narcotic pain relievers. Doses of one or both drugs may need to be modified or a different drug may need to be prescribed. The following drugs and drug classes interact with narcotic pain relievers:

agonist/antagonist analgesics
alcohol
amitriptyline (eg, *Elavil*)
anticoagulants (eg, warfarin)
antihistamines (eg, diphenhydramine)
barbiturate anesthetics (eg, thiopental)
carbamazepine (eg, *Tegretol)*
charcoal
chloral hydrate (eg, *Aquachloral*)
chlorpromazine (eg, *Thorazine*)
clomipramine (eg, *Anafranil*)
desipramine (eg, *Norpramin*)
diazepam (eg, *Valium)*
droperidol (*Inapsine)*
fluvoxamine (*Luvox*)
furazolidone (*Furoxone)*
glutethimide (not available in the US)
hydantoins (eg, phenytoin)
hypnotics (eg, zolpidem)
MAOIs (eg, phenelzine)
methocarbamol (eg, *Robaxin*)
nitrous oxide
nortriptyline (eg, *Pamelor*)
protease inhibitors (eg, saquinavir)
rifampin (eg, *Rifadin)*
thioridazine (eg, *Mellaril*)

Side Effects:

Every drug is capable of producing side effects. Many narcotic analgesic users experience no, or minor, side effects. The frequency and severity of side effects depend on many factors including dose, duration of therapy, and individual susceptibility. Possible side effects include:

Most Serious – Respiratory depression; skeletal muscle rigidity; difficulty breathing; slow heartbeat.

Most Frequent – Lightheadedness; dizziness; sedation; nausea; vomiting; sweating.

Digestive Tract: Nausea; vomiting; diarrhea; stomach cramps or pain; taste alterations; dry mouth; appetite loss; constipation; biliary tract spasm; ileus (obstruction of the bowels); paralytic ileus; toxic megacolon in patients with inflammatory bowel disease; gas; indigestion; difficulty swallowing.

Nervous System: Exaggerated sense of well being; restless mood; delirium; sleeplessness; agitation; anxiety; hallucinations; disorientation; drowsiness; sedation; lethargy; mental and physical impairment; uncoordinated movements; coma; mood changes; weakness; headache; mental cloudiness; blurred vision; double vision; pupil constriction; tremor; convulsions; psychic dependence; toxic psychoses; depression; increased intracranial pressure; headache; abnormal skin sensations; confusion; abnormal dreams; continual rapid eye movement; muscle twitching; amnesia; paranoid reaction; drug withdrawal; suicide attempt; decreased mobility; difficulty moving; excessive movement; speech disorder; abnormal gait; abnormal skin sensations; stupor; apathy.

Circulatory System: Flushing; faintness; peripheral circulatory collapse; change in heart rate; abnormal heart rhythm; heart pounding in the chest; chest wall rigidity; change in blood pressure; dizziness or lightheadedness when rising from a seated or lying position; fainting; cardiac arrest; shock.

Urinary and Reproductive Tract: Urinary retention or hesitancy; infrequent urination; antidiuretic effect; reduced libido; difficult urination; impotence; difficult ejaculation; urinary incontinence.

Other: Depression of cough reflex; chills; asthma exacerbation; vision changes; itching; rash; hives; muscle weakness; sweating; runny nose; tearing; yawning; joint pain; general body discomfort; flu syndrome; hot flashes; hiccups; coughing up blood; sore throat; back pain; runny nose; reversible jaundice, including cholestatic jaundice (propoxyphene).

Guidelines for Use:

- Dosage is individualized.
- Do not change the dose or stop taking unless advised to do so by your doctor.
- May cause drowsiness, dizziness, or blurred vision. Use caution while driving or performing other tasks requiring alertness, coordination, or physical dexterity.
- May cause dizziness or lightheadedness when rising from a seated or lying position.
- Avoid alcohol and drowsiness-causing drugs while taking a narcotic pain reliever.
- May cause nausea, vomiting, or constipation. Notify your doctor if these occur and become a problem.
- Long-term use may lead to addiction. Early signs include drug ineffectiveness. Dependence is not an issue in terminal illness where patient comfort is more important.
- If stomach upset occurs, take with food.
- May cause constipation (long-term use). Stool softeners or fiber laxatives may be required if use is prolonged.
- These drugs work best if taken on a routine basis. Narcotics are more effective in preventing pain than in treating pain after it occurs.
- Give the drug ample time to work before determining if more is needed (at least 30 minutes to 1 hour for oral agents).

Guidelines for Use (cont.):

- If a dose is missed, take it as soon as possible. If several hours have passed or if it is nearing time for the next dose, do not double the dose to catch up, unless advised to do so by your doctor. If more than one dose is missed or it is necessary to establish a new dosage schedule, contact your doctor or pharmacist.
- Sometimes these drugs are given in combination with other nonnarcotic pain relievers such as aspirin or acetaminophen (eg, *Tylenol*). Make sure your doctor knows if you have had problems taking aspirin or acetaminophen in the past.
- Notify your doctor if shortness of breath or difficulty breathing occurs.
- Do not crush or chew controlled- or sustained-release medications.
- *Fentanyl transdermal system* — Keep both used and unused systems out of the reach of children. Used systems should be flushed down the toilet immediately upon removal.
  If the application site needs to be cleansed before application, the area should be washed with clear water and allowed to dry. Do not use soaps, alcohol, or other products to cleanse skin.
  Do not cut the patch.
  Remove the old patch before applying a new one.
  Avoid exposing the application site to a direct external heart source, such as an electric blanket.
- *Fentanyl transmucosal system* — This product is extremely toxic to children. Carefully follow the storage, administration, and disposal techniques included in the patient package insert and instructional video.
  Remove from the foil pouch just before use.
  The lozenge should be sucked. Do not chew.
  Store in foil pouch at room temperature (59° to 86°F). Do not freeze. Protect from moisture.
- Refrigerate suppositories.
- It is illegal to share these potent, addictive drugs with others.

If you have any questions, consult your doctor, pharmacist, or health care provider.

Content given per capsule, tablet, suppository, or 1 ml or 5 ml liquid.

	Brand Name Examples	Narcotic	APAP†	Aspirin	Other
	Codeine Phosphate Containing				
c-v	*Acetaminophen w/Codeine Elixir*[2] *Capital w/Codeine Suspension* *Tylenol w/Codeine Elixir*[2]	12 mg codeine phosphate	120 mg		
c-III	*Acetaminophen w/Codeine Tablets* *Tylenol w/Codeine No. 2 Tablets*[1]	15 mg codeine phosphate	300 mg		
c-III	*Aspirin w/Codeine Tablets No. 2*	15 mg codeine phosphate		325 mg	
c-III	*Acetaminophen w/Codeine Tablets* *Tylenol w/Codeine No. 3 Capsules and Tablets*	30 mg codeine phosphate	300 mg		
c-III	*Phenaphen w/ Codeine No. 3 Capsules*	30 mg codeine phosphate	325 mg		
c-III	*Margesic No. 3 Tablets* *Phenaphen-650 w/Codeine Tablets*[1]	30 mg codeine phosphate	650 mg		
c-III	*Aspirin w/Codeine Tablets No. 3* *Empirin w/Codeine No. 3 Tablets*	30 mg codeine phosphate		325 mg	

	Brand Name Examples	Narcotic	APAP†	Aspirin	Other
	Codeine Phosphate (cont.)				
c-III	*Amaphen w/Codeine No. 3 Capsules* *Fioricet w/Codeine Capsules*	30 mg codeine phosphate	325 mg		40 mg caffeine, 50 mg butalbital
c-III	*Fiorinal w/Codeine No. 3 Capsules*	30 mg codeine phosphate		325 mg	40 mg caffeine, 50 mg butalbital
c-III	*Acetaminophen w/Codeine Tablets* *Tylenol w/Codeine No. 4 Tablets*	60 mg codeine phosphate	300 mg		
c-III	*Phenaphen w/Codeine No. 4 Capsules*	60 mg codeine phosphate	325 mg		
c-III	*Aspirin w/Codeine Tablets No.4* *Empirin w/Codeine No. 4 Tablets*	60 mg codeine phosphate		325 mg	
	Hydrocodone Bitartrate Containing				
c-III	*Lortab Liquid*[2]	2.5 mg hydrocodone bitartrate	120 mg		
c-III	*Lortab Tablets*	2.5 mg hydrocodone bitartrate	500 mg		

	Brand Name Examples	Narcotic	APAP†	Aspirin	Other
	Hydrocodone Bitartrate (cont.)				
c-III	*Amacodone Tablets* *Anexsia 5/500 Tablets* *Anodynos DHC Tablets* *Bancap HC Capsules* *Dolacet Capsules* *Hydrocet Capsules* *Hydrocodone Bitartrate and Acetaminophen Capsules and Tablets* *Hy-Phen Tablets* *Lorcet-HD Capsules* *Lorcet Tablets* *Lortab 5/500 Tablets* *Margesic H Capsules* *Vicodin Tablets* *Zydone Capsules*	5 mg hydro-codone bitartrate	500 mg		
c-III	*Azdone Tablets* *Damason-P Tablets* *Lortab ASA Tablets*	5 mg hydro-codone bitartrate		500 mg	

	Brand Name Examples	Narcotic	APAP†	Aspirin	Other
	Hydrocodone Bitartrate (cont.)				
C-III	*Lortab 7.5/500 Tablets*	7.5 mg hydrocodone bitartrate	500 mg		
C-III	*Vicodin ES Tablets*	7.5 mg hydrocodone bitartrate	750 mg		
C-III	*Anexsia 7.5/650 Tablets* *Lorcet Plus Tablets*	7.5 mg hydrocodone bitartrate	650 mg		
C-III	*Lorcet 10/650 Tablets*	10 mg hydrocodone bitartrate	650 mg		
	Dihydrocodeine Bitartrate Containing				
C-III	*Synalgos-DC Capsules*	16 mg dihydrocodeine bitartrate		356.4 mg	30 mg caffeine
	Opium Containing				
C-II	*B & O Supprettes No. 15A Suppositories*	30 mg powdered opium			16.2 mg powdered belladonna extract
C-II	*Opium and Belladonna Suppositories*	60 mg powdered opium			15 mg belladonna extract

	Brand Name Examples	Narcotic	APAP†	Aspirin	Other
	Opium Containing (cont.)				
c-II	*B & O Supprettes No. 16A Suppositories*	60 mg powdered opium			16.2 mg powdered bella-donna extract
	Oxycodone Containing				
c-II	*Oxycodone HCl and Acetamino-phen Tablets* *Oxycet Tablets* *Percocet Tablets* *Roxicet Tablets and Solution*[1]	5 mg oxy-codone HCl	325 mg		
	Oxycodone with Acetaminophen Capsules *Roxicet 5/500 Caplets* *Roxilox Capsules* *Tylox Capsules*[1]	5 mg oxy-codone HCl	500 mg		
c-II	*Oxycodone 2 Aspirin Tablets* *Percodan Tablets* *Roxiprin Tablets*	4.5 mg oxy-codone HCl and 0.38 mg oxy-codone terephtha-late		325 mg	

	Brand Name Examples	Narcotic	APAP†	Aspirin	Other
	Oxycodone Containing (cont.)				
C-II	*Percodan-Demi Tablets*	2.25 mg oxycodone HCl and 0.19 mg oxycodone terephthalate		325 mg	
	Meperiding Containing				
C-II	*Mepergan Fortis Capsules*	50 mg meperidine HCl			25 mg promethazine HCl
	Propoxyphene Nepsylate Containing				
C-IV	*Darvocet-N 50 Tablets* *Propoxyphene Napsylate and Acetaminophen Tablets*	50 mg propoxyphene napsylate	325 mg		
	Darvocet-N 100 Tablets *Propacet 100 Tablets* *Propoxyphene Napsylate and Acetaminophen Tablets*	100 mg propoxyphene napsylate	650 mg		

	Brand Name Examples	Narcotic	APAP†	Aspirin	Other
	Propoxyphene HCl Containing				
C-IV	*E-LOR Tablets* *Genagesic Tablets* *Propoxyphene HCl w/Acetaminophen Tablets* *Wygesic Tablets*	65 mg propoxyphene HCl	650 mg		
C-IV	*Propoxyphene HCl Compound Capsules* *Darvon Compound-65 Pulvules*	65 mg propoxyphene HCl		389 mg	32.4 mg caffeine

† APAP=Acetaminophen.

Type of Drug:

Narcotic pain reliever combinations.

Uses:

To relieve moderate to severe pain.

Components of these combinations include:

Narcotic analgesics: Codeine, hydrocodone bitartrate, dihydrocodeine bitartrate, opium, oxycodone HCl, oxycodone terephthalate, meperidine HCl, propoxyphene HCl and propoxyphene napsylate, used as a pain reliever.

Nonnarcotic analgesics: Acetaminophen; salicylates, salicylamide, used as a pain reliever.

Caffeine, a traditional component of many analgesic formulations, may be beneficial in certain vascular headaches and may enhance the analgesic effect of selected narcotics.

Magnesium-aluminum hydroxides and calcium carbonate, used as buffers.

Barbiturates, acetylcarbromal, carbromal and bromisovalum, are used for their sedative effects.

Promethazine HCl (a phenothiazine derivative with antihistaminic properties), is used for its sedative effect. It may enhance the analgesic effect of selected narcotics.

Belladonna alkaloids, used as antispasmodics.

Guidelines for Use:

- May cause drowsiness, dizziness or blurred vision. Use caution while driving or performing other tasks requiring alertness, coordination and/or physical dexterity.
- Avoid alcohol and drowsiness-causing drugs.
- May cause nausea, vomiting or constipation. Notify your doctor if these become prominent.
- Notify your doctor if shortness of breath or difficulty in breathing occurs.
- Long-term use may lead to addiction. The early sign of this is drug ineffectiveness. Dependence is not an issue in terminal illness pain where patient comfort is more important.
- May cause nausea; take with food.
- May cause constipation with long-term use. Stool softeners or fiber laxatives may be required if use is prolonged.
- Narcotics are more effective in preventing pain, than in treating pain after it occurs.
- Sometimes these drugs are given in combination with other nonnarcotic pain relievers. Make sure your doctor knows if you have had problems taking aspirin or acetaminophen (eg, *Tylenol*) in the past.
- It is illegal to share these potent, addictive drugs with others.

If you have any questions, consultyour doctor, pharmacist or health care provider.

	Generic Name *Brand Name Example*	Supplied As	Generic Available
Rx	**Butorphanol Tartrate**[1] *Stadol NS*	**Nasal Spray:** 10 mg/mL	No

[1] This product is also available as an injection.

Type of Drug:

Pain reliever; analgesic.

How the Drug Works:

Butorphanol is a potent pain reliever similar to the opioid (narcotic) analgesics.

Uses:

To relieve pain (including postoperative and migraine headache pain).

Precautions:

Do not use in the following situations: Allergy to butorphanol tartrate or benzethonium chloride.

Use with caution in the following situations:

- drug addiction or misuse, history
- elderly
- emotional instability
- head injury
- heart disease
- kidney disease
- labor
- liver disease
- lung disease
- nervous system diseases

Drug dependence: Butorphanol has abuse potential. Dependence may develop upon repeated use. However, most patients who receive these agents for medical reasons do not develop dependence.

Pregnancy: Adequate studies have not been done in pregnant women. Use only if clearly needed and potential benefits outweigh the possible hazards to the fetus.

Breastfeeding: Butorphanol appears in breast milk. Consult your doctor before you begin breastfeeding.

Children: Safety and effectiveness have not been established. Use is not recommended.

Elderly: Elderly patients may be more sensitive to side effects.

Drug Interactions:

Tell your doctor or pharmacist if you are taking or if you are planning to take any over-the-counter or prescription medications or dietary supplements with butorphanol. Doses of one or both drugs may need to be modified or a different drug may need to be prescribed. Barbiturates (eg, phenobarbital) interact with butorphanol.

Side Effects:

Every drug is capable of producing side effects. Many butorphanol users experience no, or minor, side effects. The frequency and severity of side effects depend on many factors including dose, duration of therapy, and individual susceptibility. Possible side effects include:

Digestive Tract: Nausea; vomiting; appetite loss; constipation; stomach pain.

Nervous System: Dizziness; drowsiness; sleeplessness; weakness; headache; anxiety; confusion; euphoria (exaggerated sense of well being); floating feeling; nervousness; abnormal sensation; tremor.

Circulatory System: Palpitations (pounding in the chest).

Respiratory System: Cough; difficulty breathing; nasal congestion/irritation; runny nose; sinus/upper respiratory infection.

Skin: Sweating; clamminess; itching.

Other: Sensation of heat; dry mouth; sore throat; nosebleed; blurred vision; ear pain; ringing in ears; unpleasant taste.

Guidelines for Use:

- Patient package insert available with product.
- The pharmacist will assemble product before dispensing to patients.
- May cause drowsiness or dizziness. Use caution while driving or performing other tasks requiring alertness.
- Avoid alcohol and other drowsiness-causing drugs.
- Give the drug ample time to work before determining if more is needed (approximately 1 to 1 hours).

If you have any questions, consult your doctor, pharmacist, or health care provider.

Generic Name *Brand Name Examples*	Supplied As	Generic Available
C-IV **Pentazocine**[1]		
Talwin Nx	**Tablets:** 50 mg with 0.5 mg naloxone HCl	No
C-IV **Pentazocine Combinations**		
Talwin Compound Caplets	**Tablets:** 12.5 mg with 325 mg aspirin	No
Talacen Caplets	**Tablets:** 25 mg with 650 mg acetaminophen	No

[1] This product is also available as an injection.

Type of Drug:

Pain reliever; analgesic.

How the Drug Works:

Pentazocine is a potent pain reliever similar to selected opioid (narcotic) analgesics.

Uses:

To relieve moderate to severe pain (oral and injection).

To supplement surgical anesthesia (injection only).

Precautions:

Do not use in the following situations: Allergy to pentazocine, naloxone (in Talwin Nx) or any component of the products.

Use with caution in the following situations:

- asthma
- drug abuse, history
- emotional instability
- head injury
- heart attack with high blood pressure, nausea and vomiting
- kidney disease
- liver disease
- lung disease
- pregnancy, premature delivery
- seizures, history
- ulcers (Talwin compound only)

Patients receiving narcotics: Pentazocine is a mild narcotic antagonist. Some patients previously given narcotics, including drugs for narcotic dependence, have experienced withdrawal symptoms after receiving pentazocine.

Drug dependence: Emotionally unstable patients and those with a history of drug abuse must be closely supervised when therapy exceeds 4 or 5 days. Dependence has occurred in such patients. Abrupt discontinuation following extended use of pentazocine has resulted in withdrawal symptoms. Pentazocine must be withdrawn gradually following long-term therapy.

Talwin Nx is intended for oral use only. Severe, potentially lethal reactions (eg, clots in the lungs, blood vessel blockage, ulcers and abscesses, withdrawal symptoms in narcotic-dependent individuals) may result from misuse of this drug by injection or in combination with other substances.

Drug abuse: Injection of oral preparations of pentazocine (Talwin, "Ts") and tripelennamine (PBZ, "Blues") has become a common form of drug abuse. The combination is used as a "substitute" for heroin.

The most frequent and serious complication of "Ts and Blues" addiction is pulmonary (lung) disease, caused by the blocking of arteries and arterioles in the lungs with unsterile particles of cellulose and talc used as tablet binders. Nervous system complications from IV injection of "Ts and Blues" include seizures, strokes, and infections.

Pregnancy:

Pentazocine and pentazocine with acetaminophen – Adequate studies have not been done in pregnant women, and animal studies may have shown a risk to the fetus. Use only if clearly needed and potential benefits outweigh the possible hazards to the fetus.

Pentazocine with aspirin – Safe use of pentazocine during pregnancy has not been established. Studies of aspirin have shown a potential effect to the fetus. Use only if clearly needed and potential benefits outweigh the possible risks.

Breastfeeding: It is not known if pentazocine appears in breast milk. Acetaminophen is excreted in breast milk in low concentrations. No side effects in nursing infants were reported. Salicylates (eg, aspirin) are excreted in breast milk in low concentrations. Effects on platelet function in the nursing infant have not been reported, but are a potential risk. Consult your doctor before you begin breastfeeding.

Children: Safety and effectiveness have not been established in children younger than 12 years of age.

Sulfites: Some of these products may contain sulfite preservatives which can cause allergic reactions in certain individuals. Check package labels when available or consult your doctor or pharmacist.

Drug Interactions:

Tell your doctor or pharmacist if you are taking or if you are planning to take any over-the-counter or prescription medications or dietary supplements while taking this medicine. Doses of one or both drugs may need to be modified or a different drug may need to be prescribed. Alcohol, barbiturate anesthetics and anticoagulants (Talwin compound only) interact with this medicine. The effect of this medicine may decrease if you are a smoker.

Side Effects:

Every drug is capable of producing side effects. Many patients experience no, or minor, side effects. The frequency and severity of side effects depend on many factors including dose, duration of therapy and individual susceptibility. Possible side effects include:

Digestive Tract: Nausea; vomiting; constipation; cramps; appetite loss; stomach ache; diarrhea.

Nervous System: Dizziness; lightheadedness; euphoria (exaggerated sense of well being); sleepiness; sleeplessness; disturbed dreams; depression; irritability; excitement; hallucinations; tremor; headache; weakness; fainting; confusion.

Circulatory System: Changes in blood pressure; rapid heart rate; shock.

Skin: Swelling of the face; rash; hives; stinging on injection; sweating; hardening of skin, sloughing or small lumps at injection site; flushing; itching; abnormal skin sensations; discoloration.

Other: Dry mouth; taste changes; ringing in the ears; blurred vision; difficulty focusing; rapid eye movement; pinpoint pupils; double vision; difficulty breathing; urine retention; temporary absence of breathing in newborns whose mothers took this medicine; chills.

Guidelines for Use:

- Take exactly as prescribed.
- May be taken without regard to food.
- After prolonged use, do not discontinue medication without first checking with your doctor or pharmacist.
- If a dose is missed, take it as soon as possible. If several hours have passed, or if it is nearing time for the next dose, do not double the dose to "catch up" (unless directed to do so by your doctor). If more than one dose is missed, or if it is necessary to establish a new dosing schedule, contact your doctor or pharmacist.
- *Talwin Nx* and combination products are intended for oral use only.
- May cause drowsiness, dizziness, or euphoria. Use caution while driving or performing other tasks requiring alertness, coordination, or physical dexterity.
- Avoid alcohol and other depressants (or drowsiness-causing medications).
- Notify your doctor if skin rash, difficulty breathing, confusion, or disorientation occurs.
- Do not use in anticipation of pain, but only for existing pain.
- Store in tight container at room temperature (59° to 86°F). Protect from light.

If you have any questions, consult your doctor, pharmacist, or health care provider.

	Generic Name *Brand Name Example*	Supplied As	Generic Available
Rx	**Tramadol HCl** *Ultram*	**Tablets:** 50 mg	No

Type of Drug:
Pain reliever; analgesic.

How the Drug Works:
Tramadol is a centrally acting, synthetic analgesic compound that acts in the brain to relieve pain. It is not chemically related to opiates, but its actions are similar to those of opioid (narcotic) analgesics.

Uses:
To relieve moderate to moderately severe pain in patients older than 16 years of age.

Precautions:

Do not use in the following situations:
alcohol use, acute
allergy to this medicine
centrally acting analgesic use, acute
hypnotics use, acute
opioid use, acute
psychotropic drug use, acute

Use with caution in the following situations:
abdominal conditions, acute
CNS depressant use (eg, alcohol, opioids, sedatives, tranquilizers)
drug addiction
epilepsy
head injuries
kidney disease
liver disease
monoamine oxidase inhibitor use
narcotic agonist analgesic use (eg, codeine)
promethazine (eg, *Phenergan*)
seizures, history

Respiratory depression: When tramadol is taken with anesthetic medications or alcohol, respiratory depression (slow, shallow, or absent breathing) may occur.

Pregnancy: Adequate studies have not been done in pregnant women, or animal studies may have shown a risk to the fetus. Use only if clearly needed and potential benefits outweigh the possible hazards to the fetus.

Breastfeeding: Tramadol appears in breast milk. Use in nursing mothers is not recommended. Consult your doctor before you begin breastfeeding.

Children: Safety and effectiveness in children younger than 16 years of age have not been established.

Elderly: Daily doses of more than 300 mg are not recommended in patients older than 75 years of age.

Drug Interactions:

Tell your doctor or pharmacist if you are taking or if you are planning to take any over-the-counter or prescription medications or dietary supplements while taking this medicine. Doses of one or both drugs may need to be modified or a different drug may need to be prescribed. The following drugs or drug classes interact with this medicine:

carbamazepine (eg, *Tegretol)*
MAO inhibitors (eg, *phenelzine)*
quinidine (eg, *Quinalan)*

Side Effects:

Every drug is capable of producing side effects. Many patients experience no, or minor, side effects. The frequency and severity of side effects depend on many factors including dose, duration of therapy, and individual susceptibility. Possible side effects include:

Digestive Tract: Nausea; constipation; vomiting; stomach ache; appetite loss; gas; indigestion; diarrhea.

Nervous System: Dizziness; feeling of whirling motion; headache; drowsiness; nervousness; confusion; agitation; tremor; exaggerated sense of well-being; unstable emotions; weakness; incoordination; sleep disorders; anxiety; hallucinations; spasticity.

Skin: Itching; sweating; rash; flushing; redness; warmness of the skin.

Urinary and Reproductive Tract: Urinary frequency; urinary retention; menopausal symptoms.

Other: Dry mouth; general body discomfort; muscle stiffness; visual problems.

Guidelines for Use:

- Use exactly as prescribed.
- For the treatment of a painful condition, take 50 to 100 mg every 4 to 6 hours, not exceeding 400 mg per day. In patients older than 75 years of age, no more than 300 mg/day in divided doses (every 4 to 6 hours) is recommended.
- May be taken without regard to food.
- Do not take this medicine more frequently or in larger doses than prescribed. This drug may be addicting and can cause breathing difficulties if taken in large doses.
- Withdrawal symptoms may occur if this medicine is discontinued abruptly. Tapering the medication should relieve symptoms.
- May cause drowsiness, dizziness, or confusion. Use caution while driving or performing other tasks requiring alertness, coordination, or physical dexterity.
- Do not use alcohol or other mental depressants (eg, hypnotics, tranquilizers) as they may cause increased drowsiness, dizziness, confusion, or breathing problems.
- Store at room temperature (from 59° up to 77°F) in a tight container.

If you have any questions, consult your doctor, pharmacist, or health care provider.

	Generic Name *Brand Name Example*	Supplied As	Generic Available
Rx	**Celecoxib**		
	Celebrex	**Capsules:** 100 mg, 200 mg	No
Rx	**Diclofenac Potassium**		
	Cataflam	**Tablets:** 50 mg	Yes
Rx	**Diclofenac Sodium**		
	Voltaren	**Tablets, delayed-release:** 25 mg, 50 mg, 75 mg	Yes
	Voltaren-XR	**Tablets, extended-release:** 100 mg	No
Rx	**Etodolac**		
	Lodine	**Capsules:** 200 mg, 300 mg	Yes
	Lodine	**Tablets:** 400 mg, 500 mg	Yes
	Lodine XL	**Tablets, extended-release:** 400 mg, 500 mg, 600 mg	No
Rx	**Fenoprofen Calcium**	**Tablets:** 600 mg	Yes
	Nalfon Pulvules	**Capsules:** 200 mg, 300 mg	Yes
Rx	**Flurbiprofen**		
	Ansaid	**Tablets:** 50 mg, 100 mg	Yes
	Ibuprofen		
Rx	*Motrin*	**Tablets:** 400 mg, 600 mg, 800 mg	Yes
otc	*Genpril, Junior Strength Motrin*	**Tablets:** 100 mg	Yes
otc	*Advil, Genpril, Haltran, Menadol, Maximum Strength Midol, Motrin IB, Nuprin*	**Tablets:** 200 mg	Yes
otc	*Advil Liqui-Gels, Motrin IB*	**Capsules:** 200 mg	No
otc	*Children's Advil[1], Children's Motrin[1]*	**Tablets, chewable:** 50 mg	No
otc	*Junior Strength Advil[1], Junior Strength Motrin[1]*	**Tablets, chewable:** 100 mg	No
otc	*Children's Advil, Children's Motrin, PediaCare Fever*	**Oral suspension:** 100 mg/5 mL	Yes
otc	*Infant's Motrin, PediaCare Fever, Pediatric Advil*	**Oral drops:** 50 mg/1.25 mL	No

	Generic Name *Brand Name Example*	Supplied As	Generic Available
Rx	**Indomethacin**		
	Indocin	**Capsules:** 25 mg, 50 mg	Yes
	Indocin SR, Indochron E-R	**Capsules, extended-release:** 75 mg	Yes
	Indocin	**Oral suspension:** 25 mg/5 mL	No
	Indocin	**Suppositories:** 50 mg	No
	Ketoprofen		
Rx	*Orudis*	**Capsules:** 25 mg, 50 mg, 75 mg	Yes
Rx	*Oruvail*	**Capsules, extended-release:** 100 mg, 150 mg, 200 mg	No
otc	*Orudis KT*	**Tablets:** 12.5 mg	No
Rx	**Ketorolac Tromethamine**		
	Toradol	**Tablets:** 10 mg	Yes
	Toradol	**Injection:** 15 mg/mL, 30 mg/mL	No
Rx	**Meclofenamate Sodium**	**Capsules:** 50 mg, 100 mg	Yes
Rx	**Mefenamic Acid**		
	Ponstel	**Capsules:** 250 mg	No
Rx	**Nabumetone**		
	Relafen	**Tablets:** 500 mg, 750 mg	No
Rx	**Naproxen**		
	Naprosyn	**Tablets:** 250 mg, 375 mg, 500 mg	Yes
	EC-Naprosyn	**Tablets, delayed-release:** 375 mg, 500 mg	Yes
	Naprosyn	**Oral suspension:** 125 mg/5 mL	Yes
	Naproxen Sodium		
Rx	*Anaprox, Anaprox DS*	**Tablets:** 275 mg, 550 mg	Yes
Rx	*Naprelan*	**Tablets, controlled-release:** 412.5 mg, 550 mg	No
otc	*Aleve*	**Tablets:** 220 mg	Yes
Rx	**Oxaprozin**		
	Daypro	**Caplets:** 600 mg	No

	Generic Name / *Brand Name Example*	Supplied As	Generic Available
Rx	**Piroxicam**		
	Feldene	**Capsules:** 10 mg, 20 mg	Yes
Rx	**Rofecoxib**		
	Vioxx	**Tablets:** 12.5 mg, 25 mg	No
	Vioxx	**Oral suspension:** 12.5 mg/5 mL, 25 mg/5 mL	No
Rx	**Sulindac**		
	Clinoril	**Tablets:** 150 mg, 200 mg	Yes
Rx	**Tolmetin Sodium**		
	Tolectin 200, Tolectin 600	**Tablets:** 200 mg, 600 mg	No
	Tolectin DS	**Capsules:** 400 mg	Yes

[1] Contains phenylalanine.

Type of Drug:

Nonsteroidal anti-inflammatory drugs (NSAIDs); mild-to-moderate pain relievers; fever reducers; anti-inflammatory agents; arthritis (eg, osteoarthritis, rheumatoid arthritis) pain relievers.

How the Drug Works:

Inflammation (pain, redness, swelling, warmth) occurs when chemicals are released from injured tissues. NSAIDs reduce inflammation by inhibiting those chemicals causing the inflammation. It may take several days before maximum relief is noticed. These agents relieve symptoms but do not alter the course of the underlying disease.

Uses:

To relieve mild-to-moderate pain in conditions such as headache, post-extraction dental pain, athletic injury, menstrual cramps, colds, flu, or sore throat.

Some of these drugs may also be used to treat long-term (chronic) pain of rheumatoid arthritis, acute gout, ankylosing spondylitis, acute painful shoulder, bursitis, tendinitis, osteoarthritis, juvenile rheumatoid arthritis, and migraine; to reduce fever; and to treat heavy menstrual blood loss of unknown cause and primary dysmenorrhea.

Unlabeled Use(s): Occasionally doctors may prescribe certain NSAIDs for juvenile rheumatoid arthritis, sunburn, migraine or cluster headaches, closure of persistent patent ductus arteriosus, polyhydramnios, premenstrual syndrome (PMS), acne treatment, or as eye drops for cystoid macular edema.

Precautions:

Do not use in the following situations:

- allergy to any NSAID
- allergy to aspirin
- allergy to sulfonamides (celecoxib only)
- aspirin or other NSAID use

gastritis, colitis, or ulcer (ketorolac, mefenamic acid only)
gastrointestinal bleeding
gastrointestinal bleeding, history of (ketorolac only)
kidney disease, preexisting
labor and delivery (ketorolac only)
peptic ulcer, active or history of (ketorolac only)
rectal bleeding or inflammation of the rectum (indomethacin suppositories only)
surgery, prior to (ketorolac only)

Use with caution in the following situations:
alcoholism
anticoagulant use, concomitant
asthma
bleeding disorders
corticosteriod use, concomitant
dehydration
diuretic use
edema (fluid retention)
elderly
epilepsy (indomethacin only)
gastrointestinal bleeding, history of
gastrointestinal disease, history of
gastrointestinal lesions (eg, ulcers), active or history of
heart disease or failure
high blood pressure
infection
kidney disease
liver disease
low platelet count (thrombocytopenia)
Parkinson disease (indomethacin only)
peptic ulcer, history of
poor general health
psychic disturbances (indomethacin only)
smoking (oxaprozin only)

Allergy: Asthma, breathing distress, and rapid fall in blood pressure resembling shock are signs of an allergic reaction. A potentially fatal apparent allergy syndrome has occurred with sulindac. Severe allergy reactions with fever, rashes, abdominal pain, headache, nausea, vomiting, signs of liver damage, and meningitis have occurred in patients receiving ibuprofen, especially those with systemic lupus erythematosus.

Severe allergic reactions have also occurred in patients with aspirin allergy and in patients who discontinued tolmetin, then restarted the drug.

Digestive Tract: Serious effects such as bleeding, ulceration, and perforation of the stomach or small or large intestine can occur at any time, with or without warning symptoms, in patients treated chronically with NSAIDs. Although minor upper GI problems are common, report any ulceration or bleeding, even in the absence of previous symptoms.

Eyes: Effects include blurred or diminished vision, spots in vision, changes in color vision, corneal deposits, and retinal disturbances. Discontinue therapy if eye side effects are noted. Blurred vision may be significant and warrants a thorough examination.

Headaches: Some of these agents may cause headaches (most common with fenoprofen, indomethacin, and ketorolac). Dosage reduction or discontinuation may be necessary. Consult your doctor or pharmacist.

Indomethacin: May aggravate depression or other psychiatric problems, epilepsy, and Parkinson's disease. Use with caution. If severe CNS adverse reactions develop, discontinue use. Consult your doctor or pharmacist.

Phenylketonuria: Some of these products contain phenylalanine. Consult your doctor or pharmacist.

Pregnancy: For most NSAIDs, there are no adequate and well-controlled studies in pregnant women. Use only if clearly needed and potential benefits outweigh the possible hazards to the fetus. Digestive tract side effects are increased in pregnant women in the third trimester of pregnancy. Some of these agents may prolong pregnancy if given before the onset of labor. Avoid use during pregnancy, especially in the third trimester.

Breastfeeding: Most NSAIDs appear in breast milk. Consult your doctor before you begin breastfeeding.

Children: The safety and effectiveness of most NSAIDs in children have not been established. Consult your doctor or pharmacist. Indomethacin, meclofenamate, and mefenamic acid are not recommended in children 14 years of age and younger. Over-the-counter ibuprofen suspensions may be used in children 2 to 11 years of age. Carefully follow dosing recommendations provided in package label, or consult your doctor or pharmacist. Naproxen and tolmetin are the only agents labeled for the treatment of juvenile rheumatoid arthritis. Safety and effectiveness of naproxen and tolmetin in infants younger than 2 years of age have not been established.

Elderly: Age appears to increase the possibility of side effects, particularly stomach and intestinal irritation, ulcers, and bleeding. Elderly patients should use NSAIDs with great care, begin with reduced dosages, and use for the shortest period possible.

Lab tests may be required during treatment. Tests may include eye exams, hearing exams, liver and kidney function tests, blood chemistry, and complete blood counts.

Drug Interactions:

Tell your doctor or pharmacist if you are taking or if you are planning to take any over-the-counter or prescription medications or dietary supplements while taking NSAIDs. Doses of one or both drugs may need to be modified or a different drug may need to be prescribed. The following drugs and drug classes interact with NSAIDs:

- aminoglycosides (eg, neomycin sulfate)
- angiotensin converting enzyme (ACE) inhibitors (eg, captopril)
- anticoagulants (eg, warfarin)
- beta-blockers (eg, propranolol)
- cholestyramine *(Questran)*
- cimetidine (eg, *Tagamet*)
- colestipol (*Colestid*)
- cyclosporine (eg, *Neoral*)
- diflunisal (*Dolobid*) (indomethacin only)
- digoxin (eg, *Lanoxin)* (ibuprofen and indomethacin only)
- dimethyl sulfoxide (DMSO) (sulindac only)
- dipyridamole (eg, *Persantine)* (indomethacin only)
- fluconazole (*Diflucan*) (celecoxib only)
- hydantoins (eg, phenytoin)
- lithium (eg, *Eskalith*)
- loop diuretics (eg, furosemide)
- methotrexate (eg, *Rheumatrex)*
- penicillamine *(Cuprimine)* (indomethacin only)
- phenobarbital (eg, *Solfoton*) (fenoprofen only)
- potassium-sparing diuretics (eg, amiloride) (indomethacin and diclofenac only)
- probenecid

rifampin (eg, *Rifadin*) (rofecoxib only)
ritonavir (*Norvir*) (piroxicam only)
salicylates (eg, aspirin)
sodium bicarbonate
sucralfate *(Carafate)* (diclofenac only)
sympathomimetics (eg, phenylpropanolamine) (indomethacin only)
thiazide diuretics (eg, hydrochlorothiazide)

Side Effects:

Every drug is capable of producing side effects. Many NSAID users experience no, or minor, side effects. The frequency and severity of side effects depend on many factors including dose, duration of therapy, and individual susceptibility. Possible side effects include:

Digestive Tract: Nausea; vomiting; indigestion; stomach upset, cramps, or pain; heartburn; diarrhea; constipation; ulcer; bloating; belching; gas; appetite changes; mouth sores; dry mouth; dark, bloody stools; bloody diarrhea; vomiting of blood; salivation; tongue inflammation; feeling of fullness.

Nervous System: Headache; drowsiness; fatigue; dizziness; feeling of whirling motion; clumsiness; lightheadedness; nervousness; depression; sleeplessness; abnormal dreams; sleepiness; tremor; involuntary muscle movements; weakness; confusion; difficulty concentrating; mental disturbances; migraine; amnesia; anxiety; coma; aggravation of epilepsy and Parkinson's disease; hallucinations; mood changes; depersonalization; convulsions; stupor; irritability; memory disturbances.

Circulatory System: Changes in blood pressure; pounding in the chest; chest pain; irregular heart rhythm or heart rate; congestive heart failure.

Urinary and Reproductive Tract: Blood, glucose, or protein in urine; kidney disease; painful, difficult, or increased urination; interstitial nephritis; nephrotic syndrome; pelvic pain; urinary tract infection; vaginal infection; vaginal bleeding; impotence; menstrual problems.

Skin: Rash; hives; itching; redness; irritation; peeling; discoloration; hair loss; dry skin; abnormal skin sensations; inflammation; flushing; paleness.

Senses: Visual disturbances; swollen, dry, or irritated eyes; blurred, diminished, or double vision; cataracts; reversible loss of color vision; ringing in the ears; hearing disturbances or loss; ear pain; change in taste (metallic or bitter); change in sense of smell; blind spot; deafness; night blindness; eye pain; corneal deposits; retinal disturbances; eye infection.

Other: Rectal irritation, swelling, or bleeding (indomethacin suppository only); unexplained bleeding/bruising; general body discomfort; abnormal blood cell and platelet counts; abnormal lab tests; liver disease; yellowing of skin or eyes; difficulty breathing; runny nose; shortness of breath; coughing up blood; fainting; weight changes; fluid retention; fever; chills; sweating; thirst; sore throat; sore or dry mucous membranes; meningitis; diabetes mellitus; breast changes or pain; dry throat; back, arm, hip, or muscle pain; hemorrhoids; swelling of the arms or legs;

asthma; injection-site reaction (ketorolac injection only); pneumonia; muscle twitching; changes in blood sugar; hiatal hernia; upper respiratory tract infection; bronchitis; changes in sensitivity to stimulation; exaggerated sense of well-being; flu-like symptoms; fungal infection; joint swelling; sensitivity to sunlight; sinus infection.

Guidelines for Use:

- Dosage will be individualized. Take exactly as prescribed. Do not change the dose or discontinue use unless advised to do so by your doctor.
- If a dose is missed, take it as soon as possible. If several hours have passed or if it is nearing time for the next dose, do not double the dose to catch up, unless advised to do so by your doctor.
- Avoid aspirin and alcoholic beverages while taking medication.
- Take with food, milk, or antacids if stomach upset occurs. Take tolmetin on an empty stomach or with milk only. For stomach upset with tolmetin, use antacids other than sodium bicarbonate. If symptoms persist, notify your doctor.
- Do not crush, chew, or break extended- or delayed-release products.
- Shake suspensions well before use.
- *Digestive tract* — Long-term treatment with NSAIDs may cause serious effects such as bleeding, ulceration, and perforation. Notify your doctor immediately of signs of ulceration and bleeding (eg, bloody vomit, black or bloody stools, dizziness).
- May cause drowsiness, dizziness, or blurred vision. Use caution while driving or performing other tasks requiring alertness, coordination, or physical dexterity.
- May cause sensitivity to sunlight. Avoid prolonged exposure to the sun. Use sunscreens and wear protective clothing until tolerance is determined.
- Notify your doctor immediately if skin rash, itching, visual disturbances, weight gain, swelling, stomach pain, black stools, bloody vomit, fatigue, lethargy, flu-like symptoms, yellowing of the skin or eyes, nausea, or persistent headache occurs.
- *Diclofenac* – Do not use immediate-, extended-, or delayed-release diclofenac concomitantly with other diclofenac-containing products.
- *Ibuprofen (chewable tablets)* — May cause burning sensation in the mouth or throat. Take with water or food.
- *Ibuprofen (OTC products)* – Do not take for more than 3 days for fever, or more than 10 days for pain. If these symptoms persist or worsen, or if new symptoms develop, contact your doctor.
- *Ketorolac* – Do not use for more than 5 days.

Guidelines for Use (cont.):

- *Meclofenamate* – Women taking meclofenamate for heavy menstrual flow should notify their doctor if they have spotting or bleeding between cycles or worsening of their menstrual flow. These symptoms may be signs of the development of a more serious condition.
- *Sulindac* – If unexplained fever, rash, or other signs of allergic reaction occur, discontinue use and consult your doctor.
- Lab tests may be required to monitor therapy. Be sure to keep appointments.
- Store at room temperature (59° to 86°F).

If you have any questions, consult your doctor, pharmacist, or health care provider.

	Generic Name *Brand Name Examples*	Supplied As	Generic Available
Rx	**Auranofin**		
	Ridaura	**Capsules:** 3 mg	No
Rx	**Aurothioglucose**		
	Solganal	**Injection:** 50 mg/mL suspension	No
Rx	**Gold Sodium Thiomalate**		
	Aurolate	**Injection:** 50 mg/mL	Yes

Type of Drug:

Antirheumatic agents.

How the Drug Works:

The exact mechanism of action of gold compounds is unknown. They suppress or prevent joint swelling and retard cartilage and bone destruction, but do not cure rheumatoid arthritis.

Therapeutic effects from gold compounds occur slowly. Early improvement, often limited to reduction in morning stiffness, may begin after 6 to 8 weeks of treatment, but other beneficial effects may not be observed until after months of therapy.

Uses:

To treat early active adult or juvenile rheumatoid arthritis not adequately controlled by other therapies (eg, NSAIDs).

Unlabeled Use(s): Occasionally doctors may prescribe gold compounds for pemphigus and psoriatic arthritis.

Precautions:

Do not use in the following situations:

allergy to gold compounds or any of their ingredients
blood/bleeding disorders
bone marrow, lack of development (auranofin only)
colitis
congestive heart failure, uncontrolled
debilitation, severe
diabetes mellitus, uncontrolled
eczema
exfoliative dermatitis (auranofin only)
hematologic disorders, severe (auranofin only)
hepatitis, history of
high blood pressure, severe
hives
kidney disease (injectable gold compounds only)
liver disease (injectable gold compounds only)
necrotizing enterocolitis (auranofin only)
pregnancy
pulmonary fibrosis (auranofin only)
radiation therapy, recent (injectable gold compounds only)
systemic lupus erythematosus
toxicity from previous exposure to gold or other heavy metals, severe

Use with caution in the following situations:

blood circulation disorders
blood dyscrasis (eg, granulocytopenia, anemia) caused by drug sensitivity, history of (injectable gold only)
bone marrow depression, history of
congestive heart failure
diabetes mellitus
high blood pressure
inflammatory bowel disease
kidney disease, history of
kidney disease, progressive (auranofin only)
liver disease, active (auranofin only)
liver disease, history of
rash

Injection reaction: Increased joint pain may occur for 1 or 2 days after injection. They usually subside after the first few injections. These reactions are usually mild, but occasionally may be so severe that treatment is stopped prematurely.

Use of other antirheumatic drugs: Use of salicylates, aspirin, NSAIDs, and systemic corticosteroids may be continued when gold injection therapy is started. After improvement begins, slowly discontinue pain relievers and NSAIDs as symptoms permit. Safety of auranofin with injectable gold or high doses of corticosteroids has not been established. Gold salts should not be used concomitantly with penicillamine or hydroxychloroquine. See Drug Interactions.

Pregnancy: There are no adequate and well-controlled studies in pregnant women. Gold therapy is generally contraindicated in pregnant patients. Use only if clearly needed and potential benefits to the mother outweigh the possible hazards to the fetus.

Breastfeeding: Gold appears in breast milk. A decision should be made whether to discontinue nursing or discontinue the drug, taking into account the importance of the drug to the mother. Consult your doctor before you begin breastfeeding.

Children: Safety and effectiveness of auranofin and gold sodium have not been established. Safety and effectiveness of aurothioglucose in children younger than 6 years of age have not been established.

Elderly: Tolerance to gold usually decreases with advancing age.

Lab tests will be required during treatment. Tests include complete blood cell and platelet counts, urinalysis, and kidney and liver function tests. All women of child-bearing potential must have a pregnancy test before treatment begins to rule out the possibility of pregnancy.

Drug Interactions:

Tell your doctor or pharmacist if you are taking or if you are planning to take any over-the-counter or prescription medications or dietary supplements with gold compounds. Doses of one or both drugs may need to be modified or a different drug may need to be prescribed. The following drugs and drug classes interact with gold compounds:

antimalarials (eg, hydroxychloroquine)
immunosuppressive agents (eg, azathioprine, cyclophosphamide, methotrexate)
penicillamine (eg, *Depen)*
phenytoin (eg, *Dilantin)* (auranofin only)

Side Effects:

Every drug is capable of producing side effects. Many gold compound users experience no, or minor, side effects. The frequency and severity of side effects depend on many factors including dose, duration of therapy, and individual susceptibility. Possible side effects include:

Digestive Tract: Indigestion; nausea; vomiting; diarrhea; constipation; stomach cramps; appetite loss; gas; dark or loose stools; mouth inflammation or ulcers.

Skin: Rash; itching; hives; redness; unusual bruising.

Other: Blood in the urine; skin inflammation; metallic taste; abnormal blood cell counts; abnormal liver or kidney function tests; anemia; yellowing of the skin or eyes.

Guidelines for Use:

- Dosage will be individualized. Do not exceed the recommended dosage.
- *Injectable gold products* — The appropriate dose will be prepared and administered by your health care provider.
- Notify your doctor immediately if any of the following occurs: Rash, mouth inflammation, persistent diarrhea, sore mouth, indigestion, metallic taste, unusual bleeding or bruising, itching, blood in the urine, fainting, slow heartbeat, thickening of the tongue, difficulty swallowing or breathing, yellowing of the skin or eyes.
- Notify your doctor immediately if you suspect you have become pregnant during therapy. All women of child-bearing potential must have a pregnancy test before treatment begins to rule out the possibility of pregnancy.
- Increased joint pain may occur for 1 or 2 days after injection. This usually subsides after the first few injections.
- Observe good oral hygiene during therapy.
- Improvement of symptoms is not immediate. Improvement may be seen after 6 to 8 weeks of treatment, although it has not been seen in some patients for up to several months.
- Lab tests and exams will be required to monitor therapy. Be sure to keep appointments.
- Store at room temperature (59° to 86°F). Protect from light.

If you have any questions, consult your doctor, pharmacist, or health care provider.

	Generic Name *Brand Name Example*	Supplied As	Generic Available
Rx	**Hydroxychloroquine**		
	Plaquenil Sulfate	**Tablets:** 200 mg	No

Type of Drug:

Antirheumatic agent; antimalarial drug.

How the Drug Works:

Although the mechanism by which hydroxychloroquine works is not completely understood, it is believed that it inhibits the actions of various enzymes and results in the reduction of joint inflammation due to chronic rheumatoid arthritis. There now is evidence that early use of this agent will preserve joint function and may prevent progression of disease.

Full benefit of the drug may not be fully realized for 6 to 12 months. Hydroxychloroquine may have serious side effects and is usually prescribed after other drugs have failed.

Uses:

To treat acute or chronic rheumatoid arthritis. Hydroxychloroquine also is prescribed for treatment of acute attacks of malaria and lupus erythematosus.

Precautions:

Do not use in the following situations:

- allergy to 4-aminoquinoline compounds
- long-term therapy in children
- retinal or visual field changes due to any 4-aminoquinoline compound

Use with caution in the following situations:

- alcoholism
- in conjunction with known hepatotoxic drugs
- liver disease
- porphyria
- psoriasis

Pregnancy: Avoid use during pregnancy.

Breastfeeding: Hydroxychloroquine appears in breast milk. Consult your doctor before you begin breastfeeding.

Children: Do not use as long-term therapy in children. A number of fatalities have been reported following ingestion of hydroxychloroquine in very young children. Safe use in the treatment of juvenile rheumatoid arthritis has not been established.

Lab tests may be required during treatment with hydroxychloroquine. Tests may include eye exams, blood counts, and knee and ankle reflex testing.

Drug Interactions:

Tell your doctor or pharmacist if you are taking or if you are planning to take any over-the-counter or prescription medications or dietary supplements with hydroxychloroquine. Doses of one or both drugs may need to be modified or a different drug may need to be prescribed. The following drugs and drug classes interact with hydroxychloroquine.

digoxin (eg, *Lanoxin)*
hepatotoxic drugs
phenylbutazone, gold compounds

Side Effects:

Every drug is capable of producing side effects. Many hydroxychloroquine users experience no, or minor, side effects. The frequency and severity of side effects depend on many factors including dose, duration of therapy, and individual susceptibility. Possible side effects include:

Digestive Tract: Appetite loss; nausea; vomiting; diarrhea; abdominal cramps.

Nervous System: Irritability; nervousness; emotional changes; nightmares; psychosis; headache; weakness; dizziness; vertigo (feeling of whirling motion); convulsions; incoordination.

Eyes or Ocular: Visual difficulties/disturbances; blurred vision; missing or blacked-out areas in the central or peripheral visual field; light flashes and streaks; sensitivity to light.

Skin: Hives; bleaching of hair; hair loss; itching; changes in pigmentation.

Other: Muscle weakness; absent or sluggish deep tendon reflexes; ringing in ears; nerve deafness; blood disorders; weight loss.

Guidelines for Use:

- Do not exceed prescribed dosage. Retinal toxicity may occur if dosage is exceeded.
- May cause stomach upset. Take with food or milk.
- Notify your doctor if any of the following occurs: Vision problems; hearing loss; ringing in ears; fever, sore throat; unusual bleeding or bruising; unusual pigmentation of skin or inside of mouth (blue-black); skin rash; itching; unusual muscle weakness; bleaching/loss of hair; mood/mental changes.
- Periodic blood counts should be taken if therapy is prolonged.
- Avoid long-term therapy in children.
- If favorable results do not occur within 6 months, consult your doctor about discontinuing use.

If you have any questions, consult your doctor, pharmacist, or health care provider.

Generic Name *Brand Name Examples*	Supplied As	Generic Available
Rx **Methotrexate (MTX)**		
Rheumatrex Dose Pack[1]	**Tablets:** 2.5 mg	Yes

[1] Contains lactose.

Type of Drug:

Agent for rheumatoid arthritis, psoriasis, and certain types of cancer.

How the Drug Works:

Methotrexate (MTX) is an antimetabolite which interferes with folic acid production, DNA production, and cellular reproduction.

Uses:

To treat severe, disabling rheumatoid arthritis when other therapy fails.

To treat severe, disabling psoriasis when other therapy fails (see Agent for Psoriasis - Methotrexate in the Topicals chapter).

To treat certain types of cancer, alone or with other anticancer agents (see Antimetabolites in the Antineoplastics chapter).

Unlabeled Use(s): Occasionally doctors may prescribe methotrexate for Reiter's disease.

Precautions:

Do not use in the following situations:

- alcoholism
- allergy to methotrexate or any of its ingredients
- blood disorders before MTX therapy (eg, anemia, bone marrow hypoplasia, low platelet and white-cell count)
- breastfeeding
- immunodeficiency syndrome
- liver disease
- pregnancy

Use with caution in the following situations:

- bone marrow depression
- infection, active
- kidney disease
- liver damage
- peptic ulcer, active
- poor health and debility
- ulcerative colitis
- women of childbearing potential

Liver: Methotrexate may be highly toxic to the liver, particularly at high doses or with prolonged therapy. Liver atrophy, necrosis, cirrhosis, fatty liver, and liver fibrosis may occur. Liver function should be determined before methotrexate therapy begins and monitored regularly.

Pregnancy: Methotrexate has caused fetal death and severe birth defects. Defective egg (ovum) or sperm formation caused by methotrexate has been reported. Do not administer to pregnant women and women of childbearing potential unless the benefits outweigh the risks. Not recommended for pregnant patients with psoriasis or rheumatoid arthritis.

Breastfeeding: Methotrexate appears in breast milk. Since the drug may accumulate in newborns and cause serious adverse effects, breastfeeding is not recommended. Decide whether to discontinue nursing or discontinue the drug, taking into account the importance of the drug to the mother.

Children: Safety and effectiveness in children have not been established other than in cancer chemotherapy.

Elderly: Due to diminished liver and kidney function and folate deficiency, consider low doses for elderly patients and closely monitor for early signs of toxicity.

Lab tests will be required before and during treatment with methotrexate. Tests will include: Blood counts; urine tests; kidney, liver, and pulmonary function tests; and chest x-rays. Perform a liver biopsy if there are persistent abnormal liver function tests or a decrease in serum albumin below the normal range in patients with well controlled rheumatoid arthritis.

Drug Interactions:

Tell your doctor or pharmacist if you are taking or if you are planning to take any over-the-counter or prescription medications or dietary supplements with methotrexate. Doses of one or both drugs may need to be modified or a different drug may need to be prescribed. The following drugs or drug classes interact with methotrexate.

- aminoglycosides, oral (eg, neomycin sulfate)
- broad-spectrum antibiotics, nonabsorbable (eg, polymyxin B, neomycin)
- charcoal
- chemotherapeutic agents, nephrotoxic (eg, cisplatin)
- chloramphenicol (eg, *Chloromycetin Palmitate*)
- folic acid (eg, *Folvite*)
- leucovorin calcium (*Wellcovorin*)
- nonsteroidal anti-inflammatory agents (eg, indomethacin)
- penicillins (eg, penicillin G)
- phenylbutazone (eg, *Azolid*)
- phenytoin (eg, *Dilantin*)
- probenecid
- retinoids (eg, etretinate)
- salicylates (eg, aspirin)
- sulfonamides (eg, trimethoprim, sulfamethoxazole)
- tetracycline (eg, *Sumycin*)
- theophylline (eg, *Slo-Phyllin*)

Side Effects:

Every drug is capable of producing side effects. Many methotrexate users experience no, or minor, side effects. The frequency and severity of side effects depend on many factors including dose, duration of therapy, and individual susceptibility. Possible side effects include:

Digestive Tract: Nausea; vomiting; appetite loss; diarrhea; mouth sores; sore throat; dark, bloody stools; black vomit; stomach pain; stomach bleeding.

Hematologic: Decreased platelet count; decreased white blood cell count; excess urea in blood.

Nervous System: Dizziness; headache; general body discomfort; ringing in the ears; unusual tiredness; chills; fever; drowsiness; convulsions; partial or incomplete paralysis; mood changes; strange head sensations; mental disease.

Respiratory System: Interstitial pneumonitis; cough; nosebleed; upper respiratory tract infection.

Skin: Rash; itching; sensitivity to ultraviolet (UV) light; sweating; boils; toxic epidermal necrolysis (blistering, skin sloughing); Stevens-Johnson syndrome; acne; flushing; redness; pigment changes; dilated vessels.

Urinary and Reproductive Tract: Vaginal discharge; painful urination; blood in the urine; menstrual problems; kidney disease; infertility.

Other: Fever; joint pain; decreased resistance to infection (eg, *Pneumocystis carinii* pneumonia); liver disease; chest pain; hair loss; blurred vision; unusual bleeding or bruising; abnormal liver function tests; low blood pressure; eye discomfort; blood clots; visual changes; eye infection.

Guidelines for Use:

- For the treatment of rheumatoid arthritis, the usual starting dose of methotrexate is 7.5 mg once weekly, or a divided dose of 2.5 mg at 12-hour intervals for 3 doses given as a course once weekly.
- Taking methotrexate incorrectly can result in serious side effects. If doses are taken too often, notify your doctor immediately.
- Deaths have been reported from methotrexate use. Patients given methotrexate must receive close medical supervision. Risks of therapy must be fully understood.
- Avoid alcohol, antibiotics, aspirin, other salicylates, and NSAIDs.
- May cause sensitivity to sunlight. Avoid prolonged exposure to the sun or other forms of ultraviolet (UV) light (eg, tanning beds). Use sunscreens and wear protective clothing until tolerance is determined.
- May cause dizziness, drowsiness, or blurred vision. Use caution while driving or performing other tasks requiring mental alertness, coordination, or physical dexterity.
- Contact your doctor immediately if nausea, vomiting, appetite loss, infection, hair loss, skin rash, boils, or acne occurs or persists.
- Discontinue the drug and contact your doctor if any of the following symptoms occur: Diarrhea; abdominal pain; fever; signs of infection; unusual bleeding or bruising; cough; shortness of breath; skin rash. Most adverse reactions are reversible if detected early.
- Do not use methotrexate if you are pregnant.
- Avoid pregnancy if either partner is using methotrexate.
- *Conception* — Men should wait at least 3 months and women should wait at least 1 ovulatory cycle after stopping use of methotrexate before attempting to conceive.
- Unrelated conditions, especially dehydration, can increase the risk of toxicity. Upset stomach, especially when accompanied by significant vomiting, diarrhea, or decreased fluid intake can lead to dehydration. Notify your doctor immediately if these symptoms develop.
- For rheumatoid arthritis treatment, stop methotrexate immediately if there is a significant drop in blood counts or if liver function test abnormalities occur.
- Prior to therapy, a complete blood workup, urinalysis, chest x-ray, and kidney and liver function tests are required. Follow-up tests will also be required.
- Store at 77°F. Excursions are permitted between 59° to 86°F.

If you have any questions, consult your doctor, pharmacist, or health care provider.

Generic Name *Brand Name Examples*	Supplied As	Generic Available
Rx **Allopurinol**		
Zyloprim	**Tablets:** 100 mg, 300 mg	Yes

Type of Drug:

Agent for gout; xanthine oxidase inhibitor.

How the Drug Works:

Gout is a hereditary form of arthritis caused by increased uric acid levels in the blood. Allopurinol prevents the formation of uric acid in the body by inhibiting an enzyme (xanthine oxidase) involved in the production of uric acid.

Uses:

To prevent the signs and symptoms of primary or secondary gout (eg, acute attacks, tophi, joint destruction, uric acid kidney stones, kidney damage).

To manage uric acid elevations in serum (hyperuricemia) and urine (uricosuria) in patients treated for leukemia, lymphoma, and other malignancies.

To manage some types of kidney stones (calcium oxalate).

Precautions:

Do not use in the following situations: Allergy or severe reaction to allopurinol.

Use with caution in the following situations:

- blood or bone marrow disorders
- kidney disease
- liver disease
- thiazide diuretic use, concurrent

Acute attacks of gout may increase during the early stages of allopurinol use. The attacks usually become shorter and less severe after several months of therapy. Even with adequate therapy, it may require several months to deplete the uric acid pool sufficiently to control acute episodes.

Fluid intake: Drink a sufficient amount of fluid to yield a urinary output of at least 2 quarts a day and to maintain a neutral or slightly alkaline urine. This will help prevent the formation of kidney stones while taking allopurinol.

Allergy: Discontinue at the first appearance of rash or other signs of an allergic reaction. In some instances, rash may be followed by more severe reactions such as itching; hives; red lesions; and loss of hair, skin, or fingernails.

Pregnancy: There are no adequate and well-controlled studies in pregnant women. Use only if clearly needed and potential benefits to the mother outweigh the possible hazards to the fetus.

Breastfeeding: Allopurinol appears in breast milk. Consult your doctor before you begin breastfeeding.

Children: Allopurinol is rarely used in children with the exception of those with hyperuricemia secondary to malignancy or to certain rare inborn errors of purine metabolism.

Lab tests will be required during treatment with allopurinol. Tests may include uric acid level, blood counts, and kidney and liver function tests.

Drug Interactions:

Tell your doctor or pharmacist if you are taking or if you are planning to take any over-the-counter or prescription medications or dietary supplements with allopurinol. Doses of one or both drugs may need to be modified or a different drug may need to be prescribed. The following drugs and drug classes interact with allopurinol.

- amoxicillin (eg, *Amoxil*)
- ampicillin (eg, *Principen*)
- anticoagulants (eg, dicumarol)
- azathioprine (eg, *Imuran*)
- chlorpropamide (eg, *Diabinese*)
- cyclosporine (eg, *Sandimmune*)
- cytotoxic agents (eg, cyclophosphamide)
- mercaptopurine (*Purinethol*)
- theophylline (eg, *Theo-Dur*)
- thiazide diuretics (eg, hydrochlorothiazide)
- tolbutamide (eg, *Orinase*)
- uricosuric agents (eg, sulfinpyrazone)

Side Effects:

Every drug is capable of producing side effects. Many allopurinol users experience no, or minor, side effects. The frequency and severity of side effects depend on many factors including dose, duration of therapy, and individual susceptibility. Possible side effects include:

Digestive Tract: Stomach upset; diarrhea; nausea.

Skin: Chills; rash; scaling or sloughing of skin.

Other: Acute gout attacks; joint pain; drowsiness.

Guidelines for Use:

- *Gout and secondary hyperuricemia (maintenance)* — The average dose of allopurinol is 200 to 300 mg/day for patients with mild gout and 400 to 600 mg/day for those with moderate-to-severe gout. The dose may be administered in divided doses or as a single equivalent dose with the 300 mg tablet. Daily doses more than 300 mg should be administered in divided doses. The minimum effective dose is 100 to 200 mg/day, and the maximum recommended dose is 800 mg/day. It is recommended that the patient be started with a low dose (100 mg) and increased at weekly intervals by 100 mg until a serum uric acid level of 6 mg/dL or less is attained, not exceeding the maximum recommended dose.
- *Prevention of uric acid kidney disease during the vigorous chemotherapy of tumors* — 600 to 800 mg/day for 2 or 3 days along with a high fluid intake.
- *Recurrent kidney stones in patients with high levels of uric acid in the urine* — 200 to 300 mg/day in single or divided doses.
- *Secondary hyperuricemia in children* — Children 6 to 10 years of age with secondary hyperuricemia (increased uric acid in the blood) associated with severe diseases may be given 300 mg/day, while those less than 6 years of age are generally given 150 mg/day.
- To minimize stomach upset, take after meals.
- If a dose is missed, simply take your next dose at the regularly scheduled time. Do not attempt to make up for the missed dose.
- May take 2 to 6 weeks to become effective. Do not skip doses or stop taking this drug prematurely.
- Drink plenty of fluids while taking allopurinol, at least 10 to 12 full (8 oz) glasses a day, to prevent kidney stones.
- May cause drowsiness. Use caution while driving or performing other tasks requiring alertness, coordination, or physical dexterity.
- Discontinue allopurinol and notify your doctor immediately at the first sign of appetite loss, weight loss, rash, painful urination, blood in the urine, irritation of the eyes, or swelling of the lips or mouth.
- Avoid large doses of vitamin C as this may increase the possibility of kidney stone formation.
- Allopurinol does not treat acute gout attacks. Other medications (eg, colchicine, indomethacin) are used to treat the acute attack.
- Lab tests will be required to monitor therapy. Be sure to keep appointments.
- Store at 59° to 77°F in a dry place. Protect from light.

If you have any questions, consult your doctor, pharmacist, or health care provider.

	Generic Name *Brand Name Examples*	Supplied As	Generic Available
Rx	**Colchicine**	**Tablets:** 0.5 mg, 0.6 mg **Injection:** 0.5 mg/mL	Yes
Rx	**Probenecid[1] and Colchicine Combinations**		
	Col-Probenecid	**Tablets:** 500 mg probenecid and 0.5 mg colchicine	Yes

[1] For further information on probenecid, see the Probenecid monograph.

Type of Drug:

Agent for treating acute gout attacks and preventing or delaying a recurrence of symptoms.

How the Drug Works:

Gout is a hereditary form of arthritis characterized by increased blood levels of uric acid. Colchicine decreases the inflammatory response to uric acid crystals that occurs in gout. However, it does not lower uric acid levels and thus does not treat the underlying cause of gout. Colchicine relieves pain but it is not an analgesic. Its suppressive effect helps reduce the incidence of gout attacks.

Uses:

Colchicine —

To relieve pain of acute gout attacks. Works most effectively if administered early in the attack.

To prevent or delay acute attacks of gout (prophylaxis).

Probenecid and colchicine combination —

For the treatment of chronic gouty arthritis when complicated by frequent, recurrent acute attacks of gout.

Unlabeled Use(s): Occasionally doctors may prescribe colchicine for treatment of certain types of cirrhosis, familial Mediterranean fever, primary amyloidosis, Behcet's disease, pseudogout, skin manifestations of scleroderma, refractory idiopathic thrombocytopenic purpura, and chronic progressive multiple sclerosis.

Precautions:

Do not use in the following situations:

allergy to colchicine
allergy to probenecid (probenecid and colchicine combination only)
blood dyscrasias (probenecid and colchicine combination only)
children younger than 2 years of age (probenecid and colchicine combination only)
gastrointestinal disorders, severe
heart disease, severe
kidney disease, severe
uric acid kidney stones (probenecid and colchicine combination only)

Use with caution in the following situations:

- elderly (especially those with kidney, gastrointestinal, or heart disease)
- gastrointestinal disorders
- heart disease
- kidney disease
- peptic ulcer, history (probenecid and colchicine combination only)

Men: May adversely affect spermatogenesis.

Pregnancy: Colchicine can cause fetal harm when administered to a pregnant woman. If this drug is used during pregnancy, or if the patient becomes pregnant while taking it, notify the woman of the potential hazard to the fetus.

Breastfeeding: It is not known if colchicine appears in breast milk. Consult your doctor before you begin breastfeeding.

Children: Safety and effectiveness for use in children have not been established. Do not use the probenecid and colchicine combination in children younger than 2 years of age.

Elderly: Administer colchicine with great caution to elderly and debilitated patients, especially those with kidney, digestive tract, or heart disease. Reduce dosage if weakness, appetite loss, nausea, vomiting, or diarrhea appears.

Lab tests may be required during treatment with colchicine. Tests may include blood counts and uric acid levels.

Drug Interactions:

Tell your doctor or pharmacist if you are taking or if you are planning to take any over-the-counter or prescription medications or dietary supplements with colchicine or the probenecid and colchicine combination. Doses of one or both drugs may need to be modified or a different drug may need to be prescribed. The following drugs and drug classes interact with colchicine.

Colchicine:

- CNS depressants (eg, diazepam)
- immunomodulatory agents (eg, cyclosporine)
- sympathomimetic agents (eg, ephedrine)
- vitamin B_{12}

Probenecid and colchicine combination:

- acetaminophen (eg, *Tylenol*)
- barbituate anesthetics (eg, midazolam)
- beta-lactams (eg, penicillin)
- ketamine (*Ketalar*)
- lorazepam (eg, *Ativan*)
- methotrexate (eg, *Rheumatrex*)
- nonsteroidal anti-inflammatory agents (NSAIDs) (eg, indomethacin, sulindac, ketoprofen, meclofenamate, naproxen)
- pyrazinamide
- rifampin (eg, *Rifadin*)
- salicylates (eg, aspirin)
- sulfonamide (eg, sulfamethoxazole)
- sulfonylureas, oral (eg, tolbutamide)
- theophylline (eg, *Theo-Dur*)
- thiopental (eg, *Pentothal*)
- zidovudine (*Retrovir*)

Side Effects:

Every drug is capable of producing side effects. Many colchicine users experience no, or minor, side effects. The frequency and severity of side effects depend on many factors including dose, duration of therapy, and individual susceptibility. Possible side effects include:

Colchicine: Vomiting; nausea; diarrhea; stomach pain; muscle weakness; hair loss; sore throat; unusual bleeding or bruising; tingling in hands or feet; abnormal blood counts; bone marrow depression; rash; agranulocytosis; decreased blood platelets; red or purple spots under the skin; aplastic anemia.

Probenecid and colchicine combination: Headache; dizziness; hepatic necrosis; vomiting; nausea; appetite loss; sore gums; nephrotic syndrome; uric acid stones with or without blood in the urine; renal colic; rib and vertebra pain; frequent urination; precipitation of acute gouty arthritis; allergic reaction; fever; rash; hives; itching; aplastic anemia; decreased white blood counts; hemolytic anemia; anemia; skin inflammation; hair loss; flushing; diarrhea; stomach pain; muscle weakness; sore throat; unusual bleeding or bruising; tingling in hands or feet; agranulocytosis; red or purple spots under the skin; abnormal blood counts; bone marrow depression.

Guidelines for Use:

- *Colchicine* — Take medicine at the first warning of an acute gout attack. A delay of a few hours reduces the drug's effectiveness. The usual adult dose is 1 or 2 tablets initially, followed by 1 tablet every 1 or 2 hours until pain is relieved or nausea, vomiting, or diarrhea develops. Some doctors prescribe 2 tablets every 2 hours. Since the number of doses may range from 6 to 16, the total dose is variable. As prophylaxis, 1 tablet may be taken 1 to 4 times a week for mild or moderate cases, and once or twice daily for severe cases.
- The colchicine dose that relieves gout pain is very close to the dose that causes side effects. Stop taking colchicine once your pain is relieved or at the first sign of side effects (eg, stomach pain, nausea, vomiting, diarrhoa). Continuing to take colchicine is of no benefit and will only worsen the side effects.
- *Probenecid and colchicine* — Do not start therapy until an acute gout attack has subsided. If an acute attack occurs during therapy, use additional colchicine or other appropriate therapy to control the attack. The recommended adult dose is 1 tablet daily for 1 week, followed by 1 tablet twice daily thereafter. In patients with varying degrees of kidney impairment, a daily dose of 2 tablets may be adequate. However, the daily dose may be increased by 1 tablet every 4 weeks within tolerance (and usually not above 4 tablets per day) if symptoms of gouty arthritis are not controlled.
- To reduce the chance of forming uric acid crystals or stones in the kidney, your doctor may want you to take sodium bicarbonate or potassium citrate as well as have you take extra fluid. Follow instructions carefully.
- Notify your doctor if you experience appetite loss, nausea, vomiting, or diarrhea. Dosage may need to be reduced.
- Discontinue use and notify your doctor if rash, sore throat, fever, unusual bleeding or bruising, tiredness, weakness, numbness, or tingling occurs.
- Colchicine does not relieve pain or inflammation from causes other than gout. It is of no value in other (non-gouty) types of arthritis.
- Lab tests will be required to monitor therapy. Be sure to keep appointments.
- Store at room temperature (59° to 86°F). Protect from light and moisture.

If you have any questions, consult your doctor, pharmacist, or health care provider.

	Generic Name *Brand Name Examples*	Supplied As	Generic Available
Rx	**Probenecid**	**Tablets:** 500 mg	Yes
Rx	**Probenecid and Colchicine[1] Combinations**		
	Col-Probenecid	**Tablets:** 500 mg probenecid and 0.5 mg colchicine	Yes

[1] For further information on colchicine, see the colchicine monograph.

Type of Drug:

Uricosuric; agent for treating gout.

How the Drug Works:

Gout is a hereditary form of arthritis characterized by increased blood levels of uric acid. Probenecid decreases the amount of uric acid in the body by increasing the excretion of uric acid into the urine. Probenecid also inhibits secretion of many penicillin and cephalosporin antibiotics by the kidneys. This increases the blood levels of the antibiotics, thereby increasing their effectiveness.

Uses:

To treat increased uric acid blood levels seen with gout and gouty arthritis.

For use with some antibiotics to make them more effective in treating infections.

Precautions:

Do not use in the following situations:

- allergy to probenecid or colchicine or any of their ingredients
- blood disorders (eg, acute intermittent porphyria, G-6-PD deficiency)
- children younger than 2 years of age
- gout attack, acute
- salicylates use, concurrent
- uric acid kidney stones

Use with caution in the following situations:

- allergy to sulfa drugs
- kidney disease
- methotrexate use, concurrent
- peptic ulcer, history
- pregnancy

Pregnancy: Routine use during normal pregnancy is not appropriate. Probenecid crosses the placenta. Use only when clearly needed and when the potential benefits to the mother outweigh the potential hazards to the fetus.

Breastfeeding: It is not known if probenecid appears in breast milk. Consult your doctor before you begin breastfeeding.

Children: Do not use in children younger than 2 years of age.

Drug Interactions:

Tell your doctor or pharmacist if you are taking or if you are planning to take any over-the-counter or prescription medications or dietary supplements with probenecid or colchicine. Doses of one or both drugs may need to be modified or a different drug may need to be prescribed. The following drugs and drug classes interact with probenecid.

- β-lactam antibiotics (eg, penicillin, cephalosporins)
- barbiturate anesthetics (eg, thiopental)
- cyclosporine (eg, *Sandimmune*)
- diflunisal (eg, *Dolobid)*
- dyphylline (eg, *Lufyllin)*
- ketamine (*Ketalar*)
- ketorolac (*Toradol*)
- methotrexate (eg, *Rheumatrex)*
- salicylates (eg, aspirin)
- zidovudine (AZT; *Retrovir*)

Probenecid may give a false-positive result to copper sulfate tests *(Clinitest)* for urine glucose (sugar) but not to enzyme urine glucose tests *(Clinistix)*.

Side Effects:

Every drug is capable of producing side effects. Many probenecid and probenecid and colchicine users experience no, or minor, side effects. The frequency and severity of side effects depend on many factors including dose, duration of therapy, and individual susceptibility. Possible side effects include:

Probenecid —

Digestive Tract: Nausea; vomiting; loss of appetite.

Nervous System: Headache; dizziness.

Skin: Rash; redness of face; itching; hives; skin inflammation.

Other: Fever, blood in the urine; increased urination; sore gums; anemia; abnormal blood cell counts; hair loss; precipitation of acute gouty arthritis; liver damage; kidney disease; uric acid kidney stones; colicky pain due to kidney stones; flank pain; allergic reaction.

Colchicine —

Digestive Tract: Nausea; vomiting; stomach pain; diarrhea.

Skin: Rash; hives; skin inflammation.

Other: Peripheral neuritis; muscular weakness; abnormal blood counts; hair loss; red or purple spots or patches under the skin.

Guidelines for Use:

- Do not begin therapy until an acute gout attack has subsided. However, if an acute attack is precipitated during therapy, the medicine may be continued without changing the dosage. Take additional appropriate therapy (eg, colchicine) to control the attack.
- Avoid taking aspirin or aspirin-like products since they can block the effect of probenecid. If you require a mild analgesic agent, the use of acetaminophen (eg, *Tylenol*) rather than salicylates (eg, aspirin) is preferred.
- May cause stomach upset. Take with food or antacids.
- If nausea, vomiting, or loss of appetite persist, call your doctor. Stomach problems may be an indication of overdosage.
- Drink plenty of fluids, at least 6 to 8 full (8 oz) glasses daily, to prevent development of kidney stones.
- Your doctor may also want you to "alkalinize" your urine by taking sodium bicarbonate or potassium citrate. Follow directions carefully.
- A gout attack may occur when you first begin taking probenecid. You may need other medications for the gout attack. Continue taking probenecid.
- Probenecid may not be effective in chronic kidney insufficiency.
- Store at room temperature (59° to 86°F).

Probenecid —

- *Gout* — Recommended adult dosage is 250 mg (½ tablet) twice a day for 1 week, followed by 500 mg (1 tablet) twice a day thereafter.
- In children between 2 and 14 years of age, initial dose is 25 mg/kg body weight per day. Maintenance dose is 40 mg/kg, divided into 4 doses. For children weighing more than 110 lbs (50 kg), the adult dosage is recommended.
- *Kidney impairment with gout* — Some degree of kidney impairment may be present in patients with gout and this may decrease the effectiveness of probenecid. A daily dosage of 1000 mg may be adequate. However, if necessary, the daily dosage may be increased by 500 mg increments every 4 weeks within tolerance (and usually not above 2000 mg per day) if symptoms of gouty arthritis are not controlled or the 24-hour uric acid excretion is not more than 700 mg.
- Continue therapy at the dose that will maintain normal serum urate levels. When acute attacks have been absent for 6 months or more and serum urate levels remain within normal limits, decrease the daily dose by 1 tablet every 6 months. Do not reduce the maintenance dose to the point at which serum urate levels tend to rise.
- *Probenecid and penicillin therapy (general)* — Recommended dosage is 2000 mg (4 tablets) in divided doses. Reduce the dose in older patients in whom kidney impairment may be present.
- *Neurosyphilis aqueous procaine* — Administer penicillin G 2.4 million units/day IM plus probenecid 500 mg orally 4 times a day for 10 to 14 days.

Guidelines for Use (cont.):

Probenecid and Colchicine —

- Recommended dosage is 1 tablet daily for 1 week, followed by 1 tablet twice a day thereafter.
- Some degree of kidney impairment may be present in patients with gout. A daily dose of 2 tablets may be adequate. However, if necessary, the daily dosage may be increased by 1 tablet every 4 weeks within tolerance (and usually not above 4 tablets per day) if symptoms of gouty arthritis are not controlled or the 24-hour uric acid excretion is not above 700 mg.
- Continue therapy at the dosage that will maintain normal serum urate levels. When acute attacks have been absent for 6 months or more and serum urate levels remain within normal limits, decrease the daily dose by 1 tablet every 6 months. Do not reduce the maintenance dose to the point at which serum urate levels tend to rise.

If you have any questions, consult your doctor, pharmacist, or health care provider.

	Generic Name *Brand Name Examples*	Supplied As	Generic Available
Rx	**Sulfinpyrazone**		
	Anturane	**Tablets:** 100 mg	Yes
	Anturane	**Capsules:** 200 mg	Yes

Type of Drug:

Uricosuric; agent for treating gout.

How the Drug Works:

Gout is a metabolic form of arthritis caused by increased blood levels of uric acid. Sulfinpyrazone decreases the amount of uric acid in the body by increasing the elimination of uric acid into the urine.

Uses:

To treat chronic gouty arthritis and intermittent gouty arthritis. Sulfinpyrazone has a minimal anti-inflammatory effect and is not intended for relief of an acute attack of gout.

Unlabeled Use(s): Occasionally doctors may prescribe sulfinpyrazone to decrease the risk of blood clots in some patients with a heart valve disorder.

Precautions:

Do not use in the following situations:

- allergy to phenylbutazone
- allergy to sulfinpyrazone
- blood cell disorders
- digestive tract inflammation or ulceration
- peptic ulcer, active
- salicylate use, concomitant

Use with caution in the following situations:

- anticoagulants (eg, warfarin), concurrent use of
- hypoglycemic agents (eg, tolbutamide), concurrent use
- insulin, concurrent use
- kidney disease
- peptic ulcer, history
- pregnancy
- sulfa drugs (eg, sulfisoxazole), concurrent use
- urolithiasis

Pregnancy: Adequate studies have not been done in pregnant women. Use only if clearly needed and potential benefits to the mother outweigh the possible hazards to the fetus.

Breastfeeding: It is not known if sulfinpyrazone appears in breast milk. Consult your doctor before you begin breastfeeding.

Children: Safety and effectiveness in children have not been established.

Lab tests may be required to monitor therapy. Tests may include blood uric acid, blood cell counts, kidney function, and urine tests.

Drug Interactions:

Tell your doctor or pharmacist if you are taking or if you are planning to take any over-the-counter or prescription medications or dietary supplements with sulfinpyrazone. Doses of one or both drugs may need to be modified or a different drug may need to be prescribed. The following drugs and drug classes interact with sulfinpyrazone:

acetaminophen (eg, *Tylenol*)
anticoagulants, oral (eg, warfarin)
insulin
niacin (eg, *Nicobid*)
salicylates (eg, aspirin)
sulfonamides (eg, sulfisoxazole)
sulfonylureas (eg, tolbutamide)
theophylline (eg, *Theo-Dur*)
verapamil (eg, *Isoptin*)

Side Effects:

Every drug is capable of producing side effects. Many sulfinpyrazone users experience no, or minor, side effects. The frequency and severity of side effects depend on many factors including dose, duration of therapy, and individual susceptibility. Possible side effects include: Stomach upset; nausea; aggravation of peptic ulcers; rash; blood cell disorders.

Guidelines for Use:

- Initial dosage is 200 to 400 mg daily in 2 divided doses. Maintenance dosage is 400 mg daily given in 2 divided doses. Dose may be increased to 800 mg daily. After blood urate levels are controlled, dose may be reduced to 200 mg daily for long-term control.
- Take sulfinpyrazone regularly as prescribed by your doctor. Do not stop taking or change the dose unless directed by your doctor.
- May cause stomach upset. Take with food, milk, or antacids.
- Initiation of therapy may initially cause acute attacks of gouty arthritis. These initial attacks can be treated with colchicine or other agents used to treat gouty attacks. These attacks subside with continued use of sulfinpyrazone. Do not stop taking sulfinpyrazone during these attacks.
- Continue treatment without interruption, even during acute gouty attacks.
- If a dose is missed, take it as soon as possible. If several hours have passed or if it is nearing time for the next dose, do not double the dose to catch up unless advised to do so by your doctor. If more than 1 dose is missed, or if it is necessary to establish a new dosage schedule, contact your doctor or pharmacist.
- Do not take with aspirin or other products that contain aspirin since they can decrease the effect of sulfinpyrazone.
- Drink plenty of fluids while taking sulfinpyrazone.
- Notify your doctor if you experience nausea, vomiting, severe stomach pain, rash, lethargy, blood in vomit or stool, or unusual bleeding or bruising.
- Inform your doctor if you are pregnant, become pregnant, are planning to become pregnant, or are breastfeeding.
- Lab tests may be required. Be sure to keep appointments.
- Store at room temperature (59° to 86°F). Keep in a tightly closed container.

If you have any questions, consult your doctor, pharmacist, or health care provider.

	Brand Name Examples	Supplied As	Generic Available
Rx	*Duradrin, Midrin, Migratine*	**Capsules**: 65 mg isometheptene mucate/100 mg dichloralphenazone/325 mg acetaminophen	Yes
Rx	*Wigraine*	**Tablets**: 1 mg ergotamine tartrate/100 mg caffeine	No
Rx	*Cafatine-PB*	**Tablets**: 1 mg ergotamine tartrate/100 mg caffeine/30 mg pentobarbital sodium/0.125 mg l-alkaloids of belladonna	No
Rx	*Cafergot*	**Suppositories**: 2 mg ergotamine tartrate/100 mg caffeine	No
otc	*Excedrin Migraine*	**Tablets, coated**: 250 mg acetaminophen/250 mg aspirin/65 mg caffeine	No
otc	*Excedrin Migraine*	**Caplets**: 250 mg acetaminophen/250 mg aspirin/65 mg caffeine	No
otc	*Excedrin Migraine*	**Geltabs**: 250 mg acetaminophen/250 mg aspirin/65 mg caffeine	No

Type of Drug:

Combinations of drugs used to treat migraine attacks.

How the Drug Works:

Ergotamine tartrate, caffeine, and isometheptene constrict blood vessels in the brain, an action that may be related to the relief of migraines. For more information on caffeine, see the CNS Stimulants-Caffeine monograph in this chapter.

Acetaminophen and aspirin are used for their pain-relieving effect. For more information, see the Analgesics-Acetaminophen and Analgesics-Aspirin and Salicylates monographs in this chapter.

Belladonna alkaloids are used to treat nausea and vomiting during migraine attacks.

Barbiturates and dichloralphenazone are used for sedation to reduce the emotional reaction to migraine pain. For more information on barbiturates, see the Sedatives-Barbiturates monograph in this chapter.

Uses:

To stop or prevent vascular (migraine) headaches.

Isometheptene: For relief of tension and vascular (migraine) headaches.

Precautions:

Do not use in the following situations:

- allergy to the migraine combination or any of its ingredients
- chest pain
- coronary artery disease (ergotamine and isometheptene only)
- glaucoma (isometheptene only)
- high blood pressure, severe (ergotamine and isometheptene only)
- kidney disease (ergotamine and isometheptene only)
- liver disease (ergotamine and isometheptene only)
- MAOI therapy, concurrent (isometheptene only)
- peripheral vascular disease (ergotamine only)
- pregnancy (ergotamine only)
- sepsis (blood poisoning) (ergotamine only)

Use with caution in the following situations:

- heart attack, recent
- high blood pressure
- kidney problems
- liver problems
- peripheral vascular disease

Pregnancy: Do not use ergotamine/caffeine products if you are pregnant or planning to become pregnant. Use isometheptene, dichloralphenazone, or acetaminophen products only if clearly needed and the potential benefits to the mother outweigh the possible hazards to the fetus.

Breastfeeding: It is not known if ergotamine is excreted in breast milk.

Children: Safety and effectiveness of use of ergotamine in children have not been established.

Drug Interactions:

Tell your doctor or pharmacist if you are taking or if you are planning to take any over-the-counter or prescription medications or dietary supplements while taking a migraine combination. Doses of one or both drugs may need to be modified or a different drug may need to be prescribed. The following drugs and drug classes interact with migraine combinations containing belladonna alkaloids or ergotamine. For more information on other agents, see the individual monographs in this chapter:

- beta-blockers (eg, propranolol) (ergotamine only)
- haloperidol (eg, *Haldol*) (belladonna only)
- macrolide antibiotics (eg, erythromycin) (ergotamine only)
- MAOIs (eg, phenelzine) (isometheptene only)
- NNRT inhibitors (eg, delavirdine) (ergotamine only)
- phenothiazines (eg, perphenazine) (belladonna only)
- protease inhibitors (eg, ritonavir) (ergotamine only)
- selective 5-HT_1 receptor agonists (eg, sumatriptan) (ergotamine only)
- sibutramine (*Meridia*) (ergotamine only)

Side Effects:

Every drug is capable of producing side effects. Many migraine combination users experience no, or minor, side effects. The frequency and severity of side effects depend on many factors including dose, duration of therapy, and individual susceptibility. Possible side effects include:

Ergotamine — Chest pain; muscle pain in the arms and legs; numbness and tingling in fingers and toes; cold or pale fingers or toes; abnormal heart rhythm; vomiting; nausea; weakness in the legs; diarrhea; localized swelling and itching; vertigo (feeling of whirling motion); rectal or anal ulcer (due to overuse of suppositories).

Isometheptene — Dizziness; rash.

Guidelines for Use:

- Dosage is individualized. Take exactly as prescribed.
- Do not stop taking or change the dose, unless directed by your doctor.
- Take at the first sign or "hint" of a migraine attack.
- Suppositories are used when tablets and capsules cannot be taken because the migraine attack caused nausea or vomiting.
- *Ergotamine products* — Stop taking and notify your doctor if you experience numbness, tingling, coldness, or paleness in fingers or toes; muscle pain in arms or legs; weakness in legs; chest pain; heart rate changes; sudden worsening of headache; swelling; or itching.
- Store tablets and capsules at room temperature. Protect from moisture.
- Store suppositories below 77°F in the foil wrapper. If suppository is soft, chill in the refrigerator before opening.

If you have any questions, consult your doctor, pharmacist, or health care provider.

	Generic Name *Brand Name Example*	Supplied As	Generic Available
Rx	**Methysergide Maleate**		
	Sansert[1]	**Tablets**: 2 mg	No

[1] Contains lactose, tartrazine.

Type of Drug:

Synthetic ergotamine derivative; agent for prevention of vascular headaches (migraine headaches).

How the Drug Works:

The mechanism by which methysergide prevents vascular headaches (migraines) or reduces their frequency or severity is not completely understood. It is believed that it blocks a chemical indicator (serotonin) in the brain which may be the cause of the migraine.

Uses:

To prevent or reduce the intensity and frequency of vascular (migraine) headaches in patients suffering from 1 or more severe vascular headaches per week and for patients whose headaches are so severe that preventive therapy is indicated, regardless of the frequency of the attack. It is not for the management of acute attacks.

Precautions:

Do not use in the following situations:

- allergy to methysergide or any of its ingredients (eg, tartrazine)
- arteriosclerosis (hardening of the arteries), severe
- blood flow problems, extremities
- breastfeeding
- connective tissue disease
- debilitation
- heart disease
- high blood pressure, severe
- infection, serious
- kidney disease
- liver disease
- lung disease
- pregnancy
- vein or tissue inflammation, especially of lower limbs

Nonspecific fibroid formation: Nonspecific fibroid formation in the connective tissue of the pelvic area may occur. Symptoms include fatigue, weight loss, backache, low grade fever, urinary obstruction, stomach or back pain, painful urination, increased urination, and leg pain and swelling. Fibroid formation may also occur in the tissues surrounding the lungs and valves of the heart. Symptoms include difficulty breathing, chest tightness and pain, and heart murmur.

Prolonged therapy: Long-term, uninterrupted administration should not exceed 6 months. There must be a drug-free interval of 3 to 4 weeks after each 6-month treatment course. Gradually reduce the dosage during the last 2 to 3 weeks of each treatment course to avoid "headache rebound."

Weight gain: Methysergide use may promote weight gain. Patients should watch their caloric intake.

Pregnancy: Do not use during pregnancy. The risk of use in a pregnant woman clearly outweighs any possible benefit. Methysergide may induce contractions of the uterus.

Breastfeeding: Methysergide may appear in breast milk. Ergot derivatives in the milk of nursing mothers have caused symptoms of ergotism (eg, vomiting, diarrhea, seizures) in the infant. Due to the potential for serious side effects, a decision should be made whether to discontinue breastfeeding or to discontinue the drug, taking into consideration the importance of the drug to the mother.

Children: Safety and effectiveness for use in children have not been established. Not recommended for use in children.

Tartrazine: This product contains tartrazine dye (FD&C Yellow No. 5), which can cause allergic reactions in certain individuals.

Drug Interactions:

Tell your doctor or pharmacist if you are taking or planning to take any over-the-counter or prescription medications or dietary supplements while taking methysergide. Doses of one or both drugs may need to be modified or a different drug may need to be prescribed. The following drugs or drug classes interact with methysergide:

- beta-blockers (eg, propranolol)
- narcotic analgesics (eg, morphine, codeine)
- selective 5-HT_1 receptor antagonists (eg, sumatriptan)
- sibutramine (*Meridia*)
- vasoconstrictors (eg, ergot alkaloids, sumatriptan, nicotine)

Side Effects:

Every drug is capable of producing side effects. Many methysergide users experience no, or minor, side effects. The frequency and severity of side effects depend on many factors including dose, duration of therapy, and individual susceptibility. Possible side effects include:

Digestive Tract: Nausea; vomiting; diarrhea; stomach pain; heartburn; constipation.

Nervous System: Seizures; sleeplessness; drowsiness; euphoria; weakness; dizziness; light-headedness; hallucinations; incoordination; increased sensitivity (eg, to touch, pain); disassociation.

Other: Fatigue; general body discomfort; weight loss; backache; fever; difficult or painful urination; increased urination; blood clots; leg pain and swelling; difficulty breathing; chest tightness and pain; heart murmur; irregular heartbeat; facial flush; rash; hair loss; bruising; swelling of feet and hands; weight gain; cold, numb, or painful hands or feet; joint and muscle pain; abnormal blood counts; dilated pupils; pain in the side.

Guidelines for Use:

- Methysergide is used on a daily basis to prevent migraine headaches. It does not work if not taken every day. It should not be used to treat a migraine once it has started.
- Dosage is individualized. Take exactly as prescribed.
- Do not stop taking or change the dose, unless directed by your doctor.
- Take with meals to avoid stomach upset.
- If a dose is missed, take it as soon as possible. If several hours have passed or it is nearing time for the next dose, do not double the dose to catch up, unless advised to do so by your doctor. If more than one dose is missed, contact your doctor or pharmacist.
- May cause drowsiness or dizziness. Use caution while driving or performing other tasks that require alertness, coordination, or physical dexterity.
- Use caution regarding caloric intake. Methysergide could promote weight gain.
- Allow 1 to 2 days for protective effects to develop. The protective effects will subside 1 to 2 days after stopping drug therapy.
- Discontinue use and notify your doctor immediately if you experience cold, numb, or painful hands and feet; leg cramps when walking; stomach, back, or chest pain; or shortness of breath.
- Notify your doctor if improvement has not taken place after 3 weeks of therapy.
- Inform your doctor if you are pregnant, become pregnant, are planning to become pregnant, or are breastfeeding. Do not use methysergide if you are pregnant or breastfeeding.
- Follow-up visits and exams will be necessary to monitor therapy. Be sure to keep appointments.
- Store below 86°F in a tightly closed container.

If you have any questions, consult your doctor, pharmacist, or health care provider.

	Generic Name *Brand Name Example*	Supplied As	Generic Available
Rx	**Almotriptan Malate**		
	Axert	**Tablets**: 6.25 mg, 12.5 mg	No

Type of Drug:

Agent for treating migraine headaches.

How the Drug Works:

Almotriptan constricts blood vessels in the brain, an action that provides relief from migraine headaches.

Uses:

For the acute management of migraine with or without aura in adults. It is not intended for the prevention of migraine or for use in the management of hemiplegic or basilar migraine. Safety and efficacy have not been established for the treatment of cluster headache, which is present in an older, predominantly male population.

Precautions:

Do not use in the following situations:

- 5-HT$_1$ agonist (eg, naratriptan) therapy, within 24 hours
- allergy to almotriptan or any of its ingredients
- certain types of migraine (eg, basilar, hemiplegic)
- ergot-containing drug (eg, methysergide) therapy, within 24 hours
- heart disease or symptoms of heart disease
- high blood pressure, uncontrolled
- MAOI (eg, phenelzine) therapy, within the last 14 days

Use with caution in the following situations:

- kidney disease
- liver disease
- risk factors for heart disease (eg, smoking, diabetes, high blood pressure)

Pregnancy: There are no adequate and well-controlled studies in pregnant women. Use only if clearly needed and the potential benefits to the mother outweigh the possible hazards to the fetus.

Breastfeeding: It is not known if almotriptan appears in breast milk. Consult your doctor before you begin breastfeeding.

Children: Safety and effectiveness in children have not been established. Not recommended for use in patients younger than 18 years of age.

Lab tests may be required prior to or during therapy. Tests include cardiovascular system evaluations.

Drug Interactions:

Tell your doctor or pharmacist if you are taking or planning to take any over-the-counter or prescription medications or dietary supplements while taking almotriptan. Doses of one or both drugs may need to be modified or a different drug may need to be prescribed. The following drugs or drug classes interact with almotriptan:

5-HT_1 agonists (eg, naratriptan)
ergot-containing drugs (eg, methysergide)
erythromycin (eg, *E-Mycin*)
itraconazole (*Sporanox*)
ketoconazole (eg, *Nizoral*)
MAOI antidepressants (eg, phenelzine)
ritonavir (*Norvir*)
sibutramine (*Meridia*)

Side Effects:

Every drug is capable of producing side effects. Many almotriptan users experience no, or minor, side effects. The frequency and severity of side effects depend on many factors including dose, duration of therapy, and individual susceptibility. Possible side effects include:

Digestive Tract: Stomach pain; bloody diarrhea; nausea; dry mouth.

Nervous System: Drowsiness; headache; abnormal skin sensations; dizziness.

Other: Increase in blood pressure.

Guidelines for Use:

- Almotriptan is only used to treat migraine headaches. It should not be used to prevent a migraine.
- Review patient information leaflet before use.
- Your doctor may want you to take the first dose of almotriptan in the office if you have any risk factors for coronary artery disease.
- Dosage is individualized. Take exactly as prescribed.
- Do not stop taking or change the dose, unless directed by your doctor.
- If the headache returns after the first dose, you may take a second dose 2 hours or more after the first dose. If pain continues after the first dose, do not take a second dose without first checking with your doctor.
- Do not take more than 2 tablets within a 24-hour period.
- May be taken without regard to food.
- Do not take any other drug in the same class within 24 hours of taking almotriptan. These include sumatriptan (*Imitrex*), naratriptan (*Amerge*), zolmitriptan (*Zomig*), rizatriptan (*Maxalt*), or frovatriptan (*Frova*).
- May cause drowsiness or dizziness. Use caution while driving or performing other tasks requiring alertness, coordination, or physical dexterity.
- Notify your doctor immediately if you experience tightness, pain, pressure, or heaviness in your chest, throat, neck, or jaw.
- The safety of treating more than 4 headaches in a 30-day period is unknown.
- Inform your doctor if you are pregnant, become pregnant, are planning to become pregnant, or are breastfeeding.
- Lab tests may be required prior to or during therapy. Be sure to keep appointments. Long-term users who have or develop risk factors for coronary artery disease will need periodic heart tests.
- Store at controlled room temperature (59° to 86°F).

If you have any questions, consult your doctor, pharmacist, or health care provider.

	Generic Name *Brand Name Example*	Supplied As	Generic Available
Rx	**Naratriptan HCl**		
	Amerge	**Tablets:** 1 mg, 2.5 mg	No

Type of Drug:

Agent for treating acute migraine attacks (with or without aura) in adults.

How the Drug Works:

Naratriptan constricts blood vessels in the brain, an action that provides relief from migraine headaches.

Uses:

For the acute treatment of migraine attacks with or without aura (pre-attack symptoms).

Precautions:

Do not use in the following situations:

- $5\text{-}HT_1$ agonist (eg, almotriptan) therapy, within 24 hours
- allergy to naratriptan or any of its ingredients
- angina (chest pain)
- blood vessel disease, ischemic
- bowel disease, ischemic
- certain types of migraines (hemiplegic or basilar)
- cluster headaches
- ergot-containing drug (eg, methysergide) therapy, within 24 hours
- hardening of the arteries
- heart attack, history of
- heart disease, ischemic
- high blood pressure, uncontrolled
- kidney disease, severe
- liver disease, severe
- poor peripheral circulation
- Prinzmetal angina
- stroke
- vascular diseases of the brain, heart, or peripheral vessels

Use with caution in the following situations:

- cardiac rhythm disturbance
- chest discomfort (eg, pain)
- heart artery disease, risk of or family history of diabetes
- high blood pressure
- high cholesterol
- kidney function, reduced
- liver disease
- males older than 40 years of age
- obesity
- smokers
- women, postmenopausal

Medical evaluation: A cardiovascular evaluation may be required in some patients before being given naratriptan or during long-term use. This evaluation can identify patients with unrecognized coronary artery disease.

First dose: Your physician may want you to take the first dose of naratriptan in the office, particularly if there is a concern about unrecognized coronary artery disease.

Pregnancy: There are no adequate and well-controlled studies in pregnant women. Use only if clearly needed and the potential benefits to the mother outweigh the possible hazards to the fetus.

Breastfeeding: Naratriptan may appear in breast milk. Caution should be exercised when naratriptan is given to breastfeeding women.

Children: Safety and effectiveness have not been established in children younger than 18 years of age.

Elderly: The use of naratriptan in elderly patients is not recommmended due to the increased risk of adverse reactions.

Drug Interactions:

Tell your doctor or pharmacist if you are taking or if you are planning to take any over-the-counter or prescription medications or dietary supplements while taking naratriptan. Doses of one or both drugs may need to be modified or a different drug may need to be prescribed.

ergotamine-containing or ergot-type medications (eg, *Ergomar, Sansert*)
$5\text{–}HT_1$ agonists (sumatriptan, zolmitriptan, rizatriptan)
oral contraceptives
SSRIs (eg, fluoxetine, fluvoxamine, paroxetine, sertraline)

Side Effects:

Every drug is capable of producing side effects. Many naratriptan users experience no, or minor, side effects. The frequency and severity of side effects depend on many factors including dose, duration of therapy, and individual susceptibility. Possible side effects include:

Digestive Tract: Dry mouth; vomiting; nausea.

Nervous System: Dizziness; drowsiness; fatigue; feeling of a whirling motion (veritgo).

Other: Abnormal skin sensations (tingling); cold and warm sensations; flushing; pain or tightness in neck and throat; ear, nose, and throat infections; light sensitivity; abnormal chest sensations (eg, pressure, tightness, and heaviness); irregular heartbeat; general body discomfort.

Guidelines for Use:

- Naratriptan is only intended for the treatment of acute migraine attacks (with or without aura) in adults. It does not prevent or reduce the number of attacks. It should not be used for other types of headaches or for the prevention of a headache or migraine.
- Take a single dose with fluids as soon as migraine symptoms appear; a second dose may be taken if there is only a partial response or if symptoms return, but no sooner than 4 hours following the first dose. Although the 2.5 mg dose may provide a greater effect than the 1 mg dose, talk with your doctor about the increased side effects. Do not take more than 5 mg in any 24-hour period.
- For a given attack, if you have no reponse to the first tablet, do not take a second tablet without first consulting with your doctor.
- *Kidney disease patients* — In patients with mild-to-moderate kidney disease, the maximum dose should not exceed 2.5 mg over a 24–hour period. Patients with severe kidney disease should not use naratriptan.
- *Liver disease patients* — In patients with mild-to-moderate liver disease, the maximum dose should not exceed 2.5 mg over a 24–hour period. Patients with severe liver disease should not use naratriptan.
- Contact your doctor immediately if any of the following occurs: Sudden or severe abdominal pain; pain or tightness in chest or throat; shortness of breath; wheezing; heart throbbing; irregular heartbeat; swelling of eyelids, face, or lips; skin rash, lumps, or hives.
- Some people may experience warm, cold, or abnormal skin sensations involving flushing, heaviness, or pressure. Discuss these and any other symptoms with your doctor.
- May cause drowsiness or dizziness. Use caution while driving or performing other tasks that require alertness, coordination, or physical dexterity. Sit or lie down if you feel dizzy.
- Do not use this medicine if you are pregnant, think you might be pregnant or are not using adequate contraception, unless you have contacted your doctor.
- Do not use any other drug in the same class within 24 hours such as sumatriptan *(Imitrex)*, rizatriptan *(Maxalt)* or zolmitriptan *(Zomig)*.
- Do not use within 24 hours of ergotamine/ergot-containing drugs (eg, *Ergomar*, *Sansert)*.
- Safety of treating more than 4 headaches in a 30-day period is not known.
- Intermittent long-term users who have or develop risk factors for coronary artery disease will need periodic heart tests.
- If your medicine has expired, throw it away. If your doctor stops your treatment, throw away any leftover medicine unless otherwise instructed by your doctor.
- Lab tests or examinations may be required before or during naratriptan therapy. Be sure to keep appointments.
- Store medicine at controlled room temperature (68° to 77°F), away from heat and light. Keep out of the reach of children.

If you have any questions, consult your doctor, pharmacist, or health care provider.

	Generic Name *Brand Name Example*	Supplied As	Generic Available
Rx	**Rizatriptan Benzoate**	**Tablets:** 5 mg, 10 mg	No
	Maxalt	**Tablets, oral disintegrating:**	No
	Maxalt-MLT[1]	5 mg, 10 mg	

[1] Contains phenylalanine (component of aspartame).

Type of Drug:

Agent for treating migraine headaches.

How the Drug Works:

RIzatriptan constricts blood vessels in the brain, an action that provides relief from migraine headaches.

Uses:

For the acute treatment of migraine attacks in adults with or without aura (pre-attack symptoms).

Precautions:

Do not use in the following situations:

allergy to rizatriptan
blood vessel disease, ischemic
bowel disease, ischemic
brain blood vessel disease
certain types of migraines (hemiplegic or basilar)
cluster headaches
ergotamine-containing preparation, use
5–HT_1 agonists, use (within 24 hours)
heart attack, history of
heart disease, ischemic (angina)
high blood pressure, uncontrolled
MAOI antidepressant, use (current or recent)
Prinzmetal's angina

Use with caution in the following situations:

coronary artery disease, risk of or family history of
diabetes
high blood pressure
high cholesterol
kidney disease
kidney function, reduced
liver disease
males older than 40 years old
obesity
smokers
women, postmenopausal

First Dose: Your physician may want you to take your first dose of rizatriptan in his or her office, particularly if there is any concern about unrecognized coronary artery disease.

Medical evaluation: A cardiovascular evaluation may be required in some patients before being given rizatriptan during long-term use. This evaluation can identify patients with unrecognized coronary artery disease.

Maxalt-MLT contains phenylalanine (a component of aspartame). Each 5 mg orally disintegrating tablet contains 1.05 mg phenylalanine and the 10 mg orally disintegrating tablet contains 2.10 mg phenylalanine.

Pregnancy: There are no adequate and well controlled studies in pregnant women. Use only if clearly needed and the potential benefits outweigh the possible hazards to the fetus.

Breastfeeding: It is not known whether rizatriptan appears in breast milk. Because many drugs are excreted in breast milk, caution should be exercised when rizatriptan is given to breastfeeding women.

Children: Not recommended for use in patients younger than 18 years of age.

Drug Interactions:

Tell your doctor or pharmacist if you are taking or if you are planning to take any over-the-counter or prescription medications or dietary supplements while taking this medicine. Doses of one or both drugs may need to be modified or a different drug may need to be prescribed.

- propanolol (eg, *Inderal*)
- ergotamine-containing or ergot-type medications (eg, *Ergomar*, *Sansert*)
- $5\text{–}HT_1$ agonists (eg, sumatriptan, naratriptan, zolmitriptan)
- SSRIs (eg, fluoxetine, fluvoxamine, paroxetine, sertraline)
- MAOIs (eg, phenelzine, moclobemide, tranylcypromine)

Side Effects:

Every drug is capable of producing side effects. Many patients experience no, or minor, side effects. The frequency and severity of side effects depend on many factors including dose, duration of therapy and individual susceptibility. Possible side effects include:

Digestive Tract: Diarrhea; dry mouth; nausea; vomiting.

Nervous System: Decreased mental sharpness; dizziness; exaggerated sense of well being; headache; drowsiness; tremor; anxiety.

Circulatory System: Irregular heartbeat; tightness, heaviness and pain in chest.

Skin: Abnormal skin sensations; flushing; rash, itching, hives.

Other: Cold and warm sensations; pain, pressure, or tightness in neck, throat, or jaw; difficulty breathing; hot flashes; weakness; fatigue; tiredness.

Guidelines for Use:

- This drug is only intended for the acute treatment of migraines (with or without aura) in adults. It does not prevent or reduce the number of attacks. It should not be used for other types of headaches or to prevent a migraine attack.
- *Tablets* — May be taken without regard to food. Take a single dose with fluids as soon as migraine symptoms appear; a second dose may be taken if there is only a partial response or if symptoms return, but no sooner than 2 hours following the first dose. If you do not respond to the first dose, do not take a second tablet without first consulting your doctor. Although the 10 mg dose may provide a greater effect than the 5 mg dose, talk with your doctor about the increased side effects. Do not take more than 30 mg in any 24-hour poriod.
- *Oral disintegrating tablets* — Take without water. Do not remove the tablet from the aluminum foil pouch until ready to take. Peel open with dry hands and place a single dose on the tongue and let dissolve as soon as migraine symptoms appear; a second dose may be taken if there is only a partial reponse or if symptoms return, but no sooner than 2 hours following the first dose. If you do not respond to the first dose, do not take a second tablet without first consulting your doctor. Although the 10 mg dose may provide a greater effect than the 5 mg dose, talk with your doctor about the increased side effects. Do not take more than 30 mg in any 24-hour period.
- *Maxalt-MLT* contains phenylalanine (a component of aspartame). Each 5 mg orally disintegrating tablet contains 1.05 mg phenylalanine and the 10 mg orally disintegrating tablet contains 2.1 mg phenylalanine.
- *Patients taking propranolol* — Do not use more than 3 doses (15 mg) in any 24–hour period.
- *Patients taking SSRI antidepressants* — Although there are no known drug interactions with SSRIs, patients are to keep in close contact with their doctor should any adverse reactions occur during SSRIs/rizatriptan usage.
- Contact your doctor immediately if any of the following occurs: Sudden or severe abdominal pain; shortness of breath; wheezing; swelling of eyelids, face, or lips; skin rash, lumps, or hives; irregular heartbeat; tightness, heaviness, or pain in the chest or throat.
- Some people may experience atypical sensations: Warm, cold, or abnormal skin sensations. Discuss these and any other symptoms with your doctor.
- May cause drowsiness or dizziness. Use caution while driving or performing other tasks that require alertness, coordination, or physical dexterity. Sit or lie down if you feel lightheaded.
- Do not use this medicine if you are pregnant, think you might be pregnant or are not using adequate contraception, unless you have contacted your doctor.
- Do not use any other drug in the same class within 24 hours of use of rizatriptan . These include sumatriptan (*Imitrex*), naratriptan (*Amerge*), or zolmitriptan *(Zomig).*

Guidelines for Use (cont.):

- Do not use within 24 hours of ergotamine/ergot-containing drugs (eg, *Ergomar*, *Sansert*).
- Do not use within 2 weeks of MAOI antidepressants.
- If your medicine has expired, throw it away. If your doctor stops your treatment, throw away any leftover medicine unless otherwise instructed by your doctor.
- Your physician may want to evaluate your cardiovascular system as a precaution before prescribing rizatriptan.
- If you do not receive relief from rizatriptan, or symptoms worsen, contact your doctor.
- The safety of treating more than 4 headaches in a 30-day period is not known.
- Intermittent long-term users who have or develop risk factors for coronary artery disease will need periodic heart tests.
- *First dose:* Your doctor may want you to take the first dose of rizatriptan in the doctor's office if you have any risk factors of coronary artery disease.
- Lab tests or examinations may be required before or during rizatriptan therapy. Be sure to keep appointments.
- Store medicine at a controlled room temperature (59° to 86°F), away from heat, light and moisture. Keep out of the reach of children.

If you have any questions, consult your doctor, pharmacist, or health care provider.

	Generic Name *Brand Name Example*	Supplied As	Generic Available
Rx	**Sumatriptan Succinate**	**Tablets:** 25 mg, 50 mg	No
	Imitrex	**Injection:** 12 mg/mL	No
	Imitrex	**Nasal spray:** 5 mg, 20 mg per acuation	No
	Imitrex		

Type of Drug:

Agent for treating acute migraine headaches in adults.

How the Drug Works:

Sumatriptan constricts blood vessels in the brain, an action that provides relief from migraine headaches.

Uses:

For the acute treatment of migraine attacks in adults with or without aura (pre-attack symptoms).

Unlabeled Use(s): Occasionally doctors may prescribe sumatriptan (injection form only) to treat cluster headaches.

Precautions:

Do not use in the following situations:

- allergy to sumatriptan
- angina
- blood vessel disease, ischemic
- bowel disease, ischemic
- ergotamine-containing preparation, use
- 5-HT_1-containing preparation, use
- heart attack, history
- heart disease, ischemic
- high blood pressure, uncontrolled
- intravenous administration (injection form only)
- MAOI antidepressant use (current or recent)
- migraines, basilar, or hemiplegic
- stroke, history
- transient ischemic attack, history
- vascular ischemia, peripheral

Use with caution in the following situations:

- coronary artery disease, risk or family history
- diabetes
- elderly, older than 65 years of age
- high blood pressure
- high cholesterol
- liver disease
- males older than 40 years of age
- obesity
- renal function, reduced
- smokers
- women, childbearing age
- women, postmenopausal

Medical evaluation: A cardiovascular evaluation may be required in some patients before being given sumatriptan or during long-term use. This evaluation can identify patients with unrecognized coronary artery disease.

First Dose: Your physician may want to have you take your first dose of sumatriptan in his or her office, particularly if there is any concern about unrecognized coronary artery disease.

Pregnancy: Adequate studies have not been done in pregnant women, or animal studies may have shown a risk to the fetus. Use only if clearly needed and potential benefits outweigh the possible hazards to the fetus.

Breastfeeding: Sumatriptan appears in breast milk. Consult your doctor before you begin breastfeeding.

Children: Safety and effectiveness in children have not been established. The use of sumatriptan in patients younger than 18 years of age is not recommended.

Drug Interactions:

Tell your doctor or pharmacist if you are taking or if you are planning to take any over-the-counter or prescription medications or dietary supplements while taking sumatriptan. Doses of one or both drugs may need to be modified or a different drug may need to be prescribed.

- ergot-containing drugs (eg, *Ergomar)*
- 5–HT_1-containing preparations (eg, naratriptan, rizatriptan, zolmitriptan)
- MAOI antidepressants (eg, phenelzine, tranylcypromine, moclobemide)
- SSRI antidepressants (eg, fluoxetine)

Side Effects:

Every drug is capable of producing side effects. Many sumatriptan users experience no, or minor, side effects. The frequency and severity of side effects depend on many factors including dose, duration of therapy, and individual susceptibility. Possible side effects include:

Nasal Spray –

Digestive Tract: Nausea; vomiting.

Nervous System: Dizziness; vertigo (feeling of a whirling motion).

Other: Burning sensation; nasal cavity, sinus or throat discomfort; bad or unusual taste.

Tablets and Injection –

Digestive Tract: Nausea; vomiting; stomach discomfort; diarrhea.

Nervous System: Weakness; dizziness; vertigo (feeling of a whirling motion); drowsiness; fatigue.

Circulatory System: Tightness, pressure, or pain in chest, jaw, neck, or throat; palpitations (pounding in the chest); heart attack; stroke; changes in blood pressure; irregular heartbeat.

Skin: Flushing; sweating.

Other: Nasal cavity, sinus, throat, mouth, or tongue discomfort; light sensitivity; sound sensitivity; pain/redness at injection site; muscle pain; general body discomfort; atypical sensations (eg, tingling, burning, pressure, abnormal skin sensations, hot/cold, tightness); numbness; difficulty breathing; fainting; ringing in ears; hearing loss.

Guidelines for Use:

- This drug is only intended for the acute treatment of migraine attacks in adults. It does not prevent or reduce the number of attacks. It should not be used for other types of headaches without consulting your doctor.
- A patient package insert is available for each of these products.
- *Tablets* — May be taken without regard to food. Take a single dose with fluids as soon as migraine symptoms appear; a second dose may be taken if symptoms return, but no sooner than 2 hours following the first dose. For a given attack, if you have no response to the first tablet, do not take a second tablet without first consulting with your doctor. Do not take more than 200 mg in any 24-hour period.
- *Injection* — Visually inspect injection solution for particles or discoloration before use. Usual dose is a single injection given just below the skin. It should be given as soon as the symptoms of your migraine appear, but it may be given at any time during an attack. A second injection may be given if symptoms come back. Do not have more than 2 injections in any 24-hour period. Allow at least 1 hour between each dose. Pain or redness at injection site usually lasts less than 1 hour. Follow instructions exactly.
- *Nasal Spray* — Usual dose is a single spray administered into one nostril. A second nasal spray may be administered after 2 hours if the headache comes back. For a given attack, if you have no response to the first nasal spray, do not take a second spray without first consulting your doctor. Do not administer more than 40 mg in a 24-hour period.
- Contact your doctor immediately if any of the following occurs: Pain, pressure, or tightness in chest, neck, arms, or throat; sudden or severe abdominal pain; wheezing; shortness of breath; heart throbbing; swelling of eyelids, face, or lips; skin rash; hives; irregular heartbeat.
- Some people may experience atypical sensations: Tingling; flushing; chest pressure; drowsiness; dizziness; tiredness; nausea. Discuss these and any other symptoms with your doctor.
- May cause drowsiness or dizziness. Use caution while driving or performing other tasks that require alertness, coordination, or physical dexterity. Sit or lie down if you feel lightheaded.
- Do not use this medicine if you are pregnant, think you might be pregnant, or are not using adequate contraception, unless you have contacted your doctor.
- Do not use within 24 hours of ergot-containing drugs (eg, *Ergomar)*, or another 5–HT_1 agonist (eg, zolmitriptan, naratriptan).
- Do not use within 2 weeks of taking an MAOI antidepressant.
- The safety of treating more than 4 headaches in a 30-day period is not known.
- Intermittent long-term users who have or develop risk factors for coronary artery disease will need periodic heart tests.
- *First Dose:* Your doctor may want you to take the first dose of sumatriptan in the doctor's office if you have any risk factors of coroary artery disease.

Guidelines for Use (cont.):

- If your medicine has expired, throw it away. If your doctor stops your treatment, throw away any leftover medicine unless otherwise instructed by your doctor.
- Lab tests or examinations may be required before or during sumatriptan therapy. Be sure to keep appointments.
- Store medicine at room temperature (59° to 86°F), away from heat and light. Keep out of the reach of children.

If you have any questions, consult your doctor, pharmacist, or health care provider.

	Generic Name *Brand Name Examples*	Supplied As	Generic Available
Rx	**Zolmitriptan** *Zomig*	**Tablets:** 2.5 mg, 5 mg	No

Type of Drug:

Agent for treating migraine headaches.

How the Drug Works:

Zolmitriptan constricts blood vessels in the brain and inhibits release of inflammatory chemicals, which then provides relief from migraine headaches.

Uses:

For the acute treatment of migraine with or without aura (pre-attack symptoms) in adults. It is not intended to prevent migraine attacks.

Precautions:

Do not use in the following situations:

allergy to zolmitritan or any of its ingredients
coronary artery disease
ergotamine-containing or ergot-type medication, recent use
heart attack, history
heart disease, ischemic
high blood pressure, uncontrolled
5-HT_1 agonist, within 24 hours of use
MAO inhibitor antidepressant use, current or within 2 weeks
migraine, hemiplegic, or basilar
Prinzmetal's angina
Wolff-Parkinson-White syndrome

Use with caution in the following situations:

coronary artery disease, risk of or family history of
diabetes
high cholesterol
irregular heartbeat
liver disease
males, older than 40 years of age with cardiovascular disease
obesity
smokers
women, menopausal

Pregnancy: Adequate studies have not been done in pregnant women. Use only if clearly needed and potential benefits outweigh the possible hazards to the fetus.

Breastfeeding: It is not known if zolmitriptan appears in breast milk. Consult your doctor before you begin breastfeeding.

Children: Safety and effectiveness in children have not been established.

Drug Interactions:

Tell your doctor of pharmacist if you are taking or if you are planning to take any over-the-counter or prescription medications or dietary supplements with zolmitriptan. Doses of one or both drugs may need to be modified or a different drug may need to be prescribed. The following drugs and drug classes interact with zolmitriptan.

cimetidine (eg, *Tagamet*)
ergotamine-containing or ergot-type medications (eg, dihydroergotamine, methysergide)
5–HT_1 agonists (eg, sumatriptan)
MAO inhibitor antidepressants (eg, phenelzine)
SSRIs (eg, fluoxetine, fluvoxamine, paroxetine, sertraline)

Side Effects:

Every drug is capable of producing side effects. Many zolmitriptan users experience no, or minor, side effects. The frequency and severity of side effects depend on many factors including dose, duration of therapy and individual susceptibility. Possible side effects include:

Digestive Tract: Dry mouth; indigestion; difficulty in swallowing; nausea.

Nervous System: Decreased sensitivity to touch; abnormal skin sensations; warm/cold sensations; dizziness; drowsiness; feeling of whirling motion.

Circulatory System: Pounding in the chest; irregular heartbeat; rapid heart rate; high blood pressure.

Other: Chest pain, tightness, pressure, or heaviness; neck, throat, or jaw pain, pressure, or tightness; heaviness, pressure, or tightness other than chest or neck; pain; weakness; muscle pain or weakness; sweating.

Guidelines for Use:

- Usual dose is 2.5 mg. If the headache returns, the dose may be repeated after 2 hours, not to exceed 10 mg in a 24-hour period.
- If the first dose does not relieve the migraine attack, do not take a second dose unless advised to do so by your doctor.
- Safety in treating an average of more than 3 headaches in a 30-day period has not been established.
- Use zolmitriptan only to treat an actual migraine attack. It does not prevent or reduce the number of attacks.
- Talk with your doctor about other medicines which can prevent or reduce the frequency of migraine attacks.
- Inform your doctor if you have high blood pressure, high cholesterol, obesity, diabetes, or a strong family history of heart disease; if you smoke, are postmenopausal, or a male older than 40 years of age.
- Discontinue this medicine and contact your doctor if any of the following occur: Pain or tightness in the chest or throat; shortness of breath; wheeziness; heart throbbing; swelling of eyelids, face or lips; rash; skin lumps or hives.
- Inform your doctor if you are pregnant, become pregnant, are planning to become pregnant, or are breastfeeding.
- Store at controlled room temperature (68° to 77°F). Protect from light and moisture.

If you have any questions, consult your doctor, pharmacist, or health care provider.

	Generic Name *Brand Name Examples*	Supplied As	Generic Available
Rx	**Buclizine HCl**		
	Bucladin-S Softabs[1]	**Tablets:** 50 mg	No
Rx	**Cyclizine**		
	Marezine[2]	**Tablets:** 50 mg	No
	Dimenhydrinate[3]		
otc	*Calm-X, Dramamine, Marmine, Triptone*	**Tablets:** 50 mg	Yes
Rx	*Dimetabs*	**Tablets:** 50 mg	No
otc	*Dramamine*[1]	**Tablets, chewable:** 50 mg	No
otc	*Tega-Vert*	**Capsules:** 50 mg	No
Rx	*Nico-Vert*	**Capsules:** 50 mg	No
otc	*Dramamine*[4]	**Liquid:** 12.5 mg/4 mL	Yes
Rx	*Dramamine*	**Liquid:** 15.62 mg/tsp	No
	Diphenhydramine[3]		
otc	*Banophen, Benadryl 25*	**Capsules:** 25 mg	Yes
Rx	*Banophen, Benadryl, Genahist, Nordryl*	**Capsules:** 25 mg, 50 mg	Yes
otc	*AllerMax, Banophen, Benadryl, Dormarex 2*	**Tablets:** 25 mg, 50 mg	Yes
Rx	*Genahist*	**Tablets:** 50 mg	Yes
otc	*Belix*[3,4]*, Genahist*[4]*, Nidryl*[4]*, Phendry*[4]	**Elixir:** 12.5 mg/tsp	Yes
Rx	*Benadryl*[4]*, Hydramine, Nordryl*[4]	**Elixir:** 12.5 mg/tsp	Yes
otc	*Benylin Cough*[4]*, Diphen Cough, Gen-D-phen*[4]	**Syrup:** 12.5 mg/tsp	Yes
Rx	*Hydramyn*[4]*, Tusstat*[4]	**Syrup:** 12.5 mg/tsp	Yes
	Meclizine		
Rx	*Antivert, Antrizine, Ru-Vert-M*	**Tablets:** 12.5 mg, 25 mg. 50 mg	Yes
otc	*Bonine, Dizmiss*	**Tablets, chewable:** 25 mg	Yes
Rx	*Antivert/25 Chewable*	**Tablets, chewable:** 25 mg	Yes
Rx	*Meni-D*	**Capsules:** 25 mg	No
	Scopolamine		
Rx	*Transderm-Scop*	**Transdermal system:** 1.5 mg	No

	Generic Name *Brand Name Examples*	Supplied As	Generic Available
Rx	**Trimethobenzamide HCl**[1]		
	Tigan, Trimazide	**Capsules:** 100 mg, 250 mg	Yes
	Tebamide, T-Gen, Tigan, Trimazide	**Suppositories, pediatric:** 100 mg	Yes
	Tebamide, T-Gen, Tigan, Trimazide	**Suppositories:** 200 mg	Yes

[1] Contains the dye tartrazine.
[2] This product is also available as an injection.
[3] Some of these products are also available as an injection.
[4] Contains alcohol.

Type of Drug:

Drugs for nausea, vomiting, motion sickness and vertigo (feeling of whirling motion).

How the Drug Works:

Drug-induced vomiting (including drugs, radiation, metabolic disorders) is generally stimulated through the chemoreceptor trigger zone (CTZ), which in turn stimulates the vomiting center (VC) in the brain. Nausea of motion sickness is initiated by stimulation of a mechanism of the ear, which sends impulses to the CTZ. The VC may also be stimulated directly (by stomach irritation, motion sickness, etc). These drugs act on the CTZ, VC, nerve pathways and other centers in the brain to reduce nausea and vomiting.

Uses:

To prevent and treat nausea, vomiting, dizziness and motion sickness.

Meclizine: "Possibly effective" for the management of vertigo associated with diseases affecting the middle ear.

Precautions:

Do not use in the following situations:

- allergy to benzocaine or similar local anesthetics (trimethobenzamide only)
- allergy to the drug
- glaucoma (scopolamine only)
- newborns
- pregnancy (buclizine only)

Use with caution in the following situations:

- abnormal heart rhythm
- asthma
- fever (trimethobenzamide only)
- glaucoma
- kidney disease
- liver disease
- obstruction of the digestive tract
- peptic ulcer
- prostate enlargement
- surgery

Antibiotics: Use dimenhydrinate with caution when giving with antibiotics that may cause ear damage. Dimenhydrinate is capable of masking symptoms of ear damage and irreversible damage may result.

Severe vomiting should not be treated with an antiemetic drug alone. When possible, establish cause of vomiting. Direct primary emphasis toward restoration of body fluids and relief of fever and causative disease process. Avoid excess fluids which may result in water retention and swelling of the brain tissues. Antiemetic effects may impede diagnosis of brain tumors, intestinal obstruction and appendicitis, and may obscure signs of toxicity from overdosage of other drugs.

Scopolamine drug withdrawal: Dizziness, nausea, vomiting, headache and disturbances of equilibrium have been reported in a few patients following discontinuation of the use of the transdermal system. This occurred most often in patients who used the system for more than 3 days.

Pregnancy: Cyclizine, meclizine, dimenhydrinate– Studies in pregnant women have not shown a risk to the fetus. However, no drug should be used during pregnancy unless clearly needed. *Trimethobenzamide, scopolamine–* Adequate studies have not been done in pregnant women. Use only if clearly needed and potential benefits outweigh the possible hazards to the fetus. *Buclizine–* Do not use during pregnancy. The risk of use in a pregnant woman outweighs any possible benefit.

Breastfeeding: Dimenhydrinate and diphenhydramine appear in breast milk. It is now known if cyclizine, meclizine, buclizine, trimethobenzamide and scopolamine appear in breast milk. Consult your doctor before you begin breastfeeding.

Children: Children with acute illnesses (eg, chickenpox, CNS infections, measles) or dehydration seem to be much more susceptible to nervous and muscular system reactions than are adults. In such patients, use antiemetics only under close supervision. Do not dimenhydrinate in children younger than 2 years of age unless directed by a doctor. Do not use cyclizine or meclizine in children younger 12. Scopolamine transdermal system is not recommended for children. Not recommended for uncomplicated vomiting in children. Limit use to prolonged vomiting of known cause for three principal reasons: 1. Although there is no confirmatory evidence, antiemetics may contribute, in combination with viral illnesses (a possible cause of vomiting in children), to the development of Reye's syndrome, a potentially fatal childhood disease. This syndrome follows a nonspecific febrile illness, and is characterized by an abrupt onset of persistent, severe vomiting, lethargy, irrational behavior, progressive degeneration of the brain leading to coma, convulsions and death. 2. Symptoms which can occur secondary to some drugs may be confused with the signs of an undiagnosed disease responsible for the vomiting (eg, Reye's syndrome). 3. Drugs which may be toxic to the liver may unfavorably alter the course of Reye's syndrome. Avoid such drugs in children whose signs and symptoms (vomiting) could represent Reye's syndrome. Aspirin and acetaminophen are toxic to te liver at large doses.

Tartrazine: Some of these products may contain the dye tartrazine (FD&C Yellow No. 5) which can cause allergic reactions in certain individuals. Check package label when available or consult your doctor or pharmacist.

Side Effects:

Every drug is capable of producing side effects. Many anticholinergic antiemetic/antivertigo product users experience no, or minor, side effects.

The frequency and severity of side effects depend on many factors including dose, duration of therapy and individual susceptibility. Possible side effects include:

Dimenhydrinate Only – Sensitivity to light; tingling, heaviness and weakness of the hands; abnormal blood counts; nasal stuffiness; tightness in the chest; wheezing; thickening of respiratory tract secretions.

Digestive Tract: Appetite loss; nausea; vomiting; diarrhea; constipation; stomach upset.

Nervous System: Drowsiness; restlessness; excitation (especially in children); nervousness; sleeplessness; headache; confusion.

Circulatory System: Lowering of blood pressure; pounding in chest (palpitations); increased heart rate.

Urinary Tract: Urinary frequency; difficult urination; urinary retention.

Allergic Reactions: Hives; rash; yellowing of skin and eyes (cyclizine and trimethobenzamide).

Other: Blurred vision; double vision; dry eyes (contact lens wearers); visual and hearing hallucinations; ringing in the ears; dry mouth, nose and throat; muscle cramps and abnormal blood counts (trimethobenzamide only).

Guidelines for Use:

- May cause drowsiness or blurred vision. Use caution while driving or performing other tasks requiring alertness.
- Avoid alcohol and other depressants (eg, sleeping pills, tranquilizers, antianxiety agents, narcotic pain relievers).
- Oral agents may be ineffective if expelled after vomiting has already begun. Consider use of suppositories under such circumstances.
- *Motion sickness*– First dose should be taken 30 minutes before exposure to motion.
- May cause dry mouth.
- *Buclizine*– Tablets can be taken without swallowing water. Place tablet in mouth and allow to dissolve, chew or swallow whole.
- *Transdermal system*– Patient package insert is available with the transdermal products.

  Initiation of therapy– Apply one system on a hairless area behind the ear at least 4 hours before the antiemetic effect is required. Scopolamine will be delivered over 3 days. Wear only one disc at a time. *Handling*– After applying the disc on dry skin behind the ear, wash hands thoroughly with soap and water, then dry them. When removing the disc, discard the removed disc and wash hands and application site thoroughly with soap and water to prevent any traces of scopolamine from coming into direct contact with the eyes. Temporary dilation of the pupils and blurred vision may occur if scopolamine comes in contact with the eyes.

  Continuation of therapy– If the disc is displaced, discard it and place a fresh one behind the other ear. If therapy is required for longer than 3 days, discard the first disc and place a fresh one behind the other ear.

If you have any questions, consult your doctor, pharmacist, or health care provider.

	Generic Name *Brand Name Examples*	Supplied As	Generic Available
C-II	**Dronabinol**		
	Marinol	**Capsules, gelatin:** 2.5 mg, 5 mg, 10 mg	No

Type of Drug:

Marijuana-like agents which reduce nausea and vomiting. Dronabinol also acts to increase appetite in patients with AIDS.

How the Drug Works:

Dronabinol is the principal substance present in *Cannabis sativa L* (marijuana). Non-therapeutic effects of dronabinol are identical to those of marijuana and other cannabinoids. How the cannabinoids decrease nausea and vomiting and stimulate appetite is unknown.

Uses:

To treat nausea and vomiting associated with cancer chemotherapy in patients who have failed to respond adequately to conventional antiemetic treatment. Dronabinol also is used in the treatment of anorexia associated with weight loss in patients with AIDS. Because the cannabinoids may alter the mental state, they are intended for use when the patient can be closely supervised.

Precautions:

Do not use in the following situations:

allergy to marijuana or other cannabinoids
allergy to sesame oil

Use with caution in the following situations:

alcoholism, history of
depression
elderly
heart disease
high blood pressure
mania
schizophrenia

Hazardous tasks: Because of the effects on mental status, do not drive, operate complex machinery or engage in any activity requiring sound judgment and unimpaired coordination while receiving treatment. Effects may persist for an unpredictable period of time. Dronabinol may persist in the body for days.

Supervision is required. Patients receiving cannabinoids should be observed in a doctor's office or hospital. This is especially important during treatment of naive patients. Even in patients experienced with marijuana, however, dronabinol may have serious responses not predicted by prior exposures. Any patient who has a psychotic experience with dronabinol must be monitored until the mental state returns to normal. Additional doses should not be given until the patient has been examined and the circumstances evaluated.

Drug abuse and dependence: Dronabinol is highly abusable. Prescriptions are limited to the amount necessary for a single cycle of chemotherapy or to the amount necessary for the period between clinic visits.

Long-term use of cannabinoids has been associated with disorders of motivation, judgment, and knowledge.

A withdrawal syndrome consisting of irritability, insomnia and restlessness was observed in some subjects within 12 hours following abrupt withdrawal of long-term dronabinol use. The syndrome reached its peak intensity at 24 hours when subjects exhibited hot flashes, sweating, runny nose, loose stools, hiccups, and appetite loss. The syndrome was essentially complete within 48 hours.

Electrocardiogram changes following discontinuation were consistent with a withdrawal syndrome. Several subjects reported disturbed sleep for several weeks after discontinuing high doses.

Pregnancy: Adequate studies have not been done in pregnant women. Use these drugs only if clearly needed.

Breastfeeding: Dronabinol appears in breast milk and is not recommended for use in nursing mothers.

Children: Dronabinol is not recommended for AIDS-related anorexia in children. Caution is recommended in prescribing this drug for children with chemotherapy-induced nausea and vomiting because of its pyschoactive effects.

Elderly: Use with caution in the elderly because of enhanced sensitivity to psychoactive effects.

Drug Interactions:

Tell your doctor or pharmacist if you are taking or planning to take any over-the-counter or prescription medications or dietary supplements with cannabinoids. Doses of one or both drugs may need to be modified or a different drug may need to be prescribed. The following drugs and drug classes interact with cannabinoids.

alcohol
anticholinergic agents (eg, atropine)
barbiturates (eg, phenobarbital)
CNS depressants (benzodiazepines)
disulfiram (eg, *Antabuse)*
fluoxetine *(Prozac)*
sympathomimetic agents (eg, epinephrine)
theophylline (eg, *Theobid)*
tricyclic antidepressants (eg, amitriptyline)

Side Effects:

Every drug is capable of producing side effects. Many cannabinoid users experience no, or minor, side effects. The frequency and severity of side effects depend on many factors including dose, duration of therapy, and individual susceptibility. Possible side effects include:

Digestive Tract: Nausea; vomiting; diarrhea; changes in appetite.

Nervous System: Drowsiness; heightened awareness; dizziness; unsteadiness; depression; weakness; hallucinations; memory loss; confusion; nightmares.

Circulatory System: Increased heart rate; lowered blood pressure.

Other: Dry mouth; vision problems (distortions); flushing.

Guidelines for Use:

- Avoid alcohol and barbiturates. Use other drugs that cause drowsiness (eg, antianxiety agents, narcotic pain relievers) with caution.
- May cause dizziness, drowsiness, and impaired reflexes/judgment. Do not drive or perform hazardous tasks requiring alertness.
- Possible changes in mood and other behavioral effects are possible with these drugs. Do not panic in the event of such manifestations.
- When taking dronabinol to stimulate appetite, take 1 hour before lunch or dinner; do not take before breakfast.
- Remain under supervision of a responsible adult.

If you have any questions, consult your doctor, pharmacist, or health care provider.

	Generic Name *Brand Name Examples*	Supplied As	Generic Available
Rx	**Dolasetron Mesylate**		
	Anzemet	**Tablets**: 50 mg, 100 mg	No
	Anzemet	**Injection**: 12.5 mg/0.625 mL, 20 mg/mL	No
Rx	**Granisetron HCl**		
	Kytril	**Tablets**: 1 mg	No
	Kytril	**Injection**: 1 mg/mL (base)	No
Rx	**Ondansetron HCl**		
	Zofran	**Tablets**: 4 mg, 8 mg, 24 mg (as HCl dihydrate)	No
	Zofran ODT[1]	**Tablets, orally disintegrating**: 4 mg, 8 mg (as base)	No
	Zofran	**Solution, oral**: 4 mg/5 mL (5 mg as HCl dihydrate)	No
	Zofran	**Injection**: 2 mg/mL, 32 mg/50 mL, 40 mg/20 mL (as HCl dihydrate)	No

[1] Contains phenylalanine.

Type of Drug:

Antinauseants; antiemetics; drugs used to prevent nausea and vomiting.

How the Drug Works:

Dolasetron, granisetron, and ondansetron are selective serotonin 5-HT$_3$ receptor antagonists that block serotonin stimulation to prevent nausea and vomiting.

Uses:

Oral doseforms — To prevent nausea and vomiting associated with initial and repeat courses of emetogenic cancer chemotherapy.

Oral dolasetron and ondansetron — To prevent postoperative nausea and vomiting.

Oral granisetron and ondansetron — To prevent nausea and vomiting associated with radiotherapy in patients receiving either total body irradiation, single high-dose fraction, or daily fractions to the abdomen.

Intravenous (IV; into a vein) dolasetron — To prevent and treat postoperative nausea or vomiting.

Unlabeled Use(s): Dolasetron has been used to treat radiotherapy-induced nausea and vomiting. Granisetron has been used for acute nausea and vomiting following surgery. Ondansetron has been used in the treatment of nausea and vomiting associated with acetaminophen poisoning, acute levodopa-induced psychosis, and prostacyclin therapy; to reduce bulimic episodes in patients with bulimia nervosa; to treat patients with social anxiety disorder; and as treatment of spinal or epidural morphine-induced pruritis.

Precautions:

Do not use in the following situations: Allergy to the 5-HT_3 receptor antagonist or any of its ingredients.

Use with caution in the following situations:

- anthracycline therapy, cumulative high dose
- antiarrythmic drug therapy, concurrent
- atrioventricular block II to III (dolasetron only)
- class I or III antiarrythmic agent use, concurrent (dolasetron only)
- congenital QT syndrome
- diuretic use with potential for inducing electrolyte abnormalities
- hypokalemia
- hypomagnesemia
- prolonged QTc, marked (dolasetron only)

Benzyl alcohol: Some of these products contain benzyl alcohol, which has been associated with a fatal "gasping syndrome" in premature infants. Consult your doctor or pharmacist.

Phenylketonuria: Ondansetron orally-disintegrating tablets contain phenylalanine. Consult your doctor or pharmacist.

Pregnancy: There are no adequate and well-controlled studies in pregnant women. Use only if clearly needed and the potential benefits to the mother outweigh the possible hazards to the fetus.

Breastfeeding: Ondansetron appears in breast milk. It is not known if other 5-HT_3 receptor antagonists appear in breast milk. Consult your doctor before you begin breastfeeding.

Children: Safety and effectiveness for use of dolasetron and the injection form of granisetron in children younger than 2 years of age have not been established. Safety and effectiveness for use of the oral form of granisetron in children of any age have not been established. Safety and effectiveness for use of ondansetron in children 3 years of age and younger have not been established.

Drug Interactions:

Tell your doctor or pharmacist if you are taking or if you are planning to take any over-the-counter or prescription medications or dietary supplements while taking a 5-HT_3 receptor antagonist. Doses of one or both drugs may need to be modified or a different drug may need to be prescribed. Rifamycins (eg, rifampin) interact with ondansetron. Antiarrythmic drugs interact with dolasetron.

Side Effects:

Every drug is capable of producing side effects. Many 5–HT_3 receptor antagonist users experience no, or minor, side effects. The frequency and severity of side effects depend on many factors including dose, duration of therapy, and individual susceptibility. Possible side effects include:

Digestive Tract: Diarrhea; nausea; constipation; stomach pain; appetite loss; taste disorder; indigestion; dry mouth.

Nervous System: Headache; drowsiness; weakness; agitation; fatigue; anxiety; stimulation; sleeplessness; dizziness; flushing; shivers; chills; vertigo (feeling of whirling motion); agitation.

Other: Changes in blood pressure; fever; heart rhythm changes; hair loss; abnormal blood counts; muscle, joint, chest, or bone pain; general body discomfort; injection site reaction; cold sensation; rash; tremor; itching; urinary retention; tingling or prickling sensation; deficient oxygenation of the blood.

Guidelines for Use:

- Dosage is individualized. Take exactly as prescribed.
- Do not change the dose or stop taking, unless advised by your doctor.
- *Ondansetron orally-disintegrating tablets* — Remove the tablets from the package just before taking. Peel backing off blister and remove tablet gently. Place tablet on the tongue and swallow with saliva. Tablets disintegrate rapidly on the tongue and do not require water for dissolution or swallowing.
- Contact your doctor immediately if you experience rash, itching, shortness of breath, abnormal heart rhythm, dizziness, fainting, low blood pressure, hives, facial swelling, or difficulty breathing.
- Dolasetron injection can be mixed in apple or apple-grape juice and given orally. The mixed product may be kept up to 2 hours at room temperature (59° to 86°F.
- Store at controlled room temperature (68° to 77°F). Protect from light. Do not freeze injection vials.

If you have any questions, consult your doctor, pharmacist, or health care provider.

	Generic Name *Brand Name Examples*	Supplied As	Generic Available
Rx	**Chlorpromazine**[1]		
	Thorazine	**Tablets:** 10 mg, 25 mg, 50 mg, 100 mg, 200 mg	Yes
	Thorazine Spansules	**Capsules, sustained release:** 30 mg, 75 mg, 150 mg	No
	Thorazine	**Syrup:** 10 mg/tsp	No
	Thorazine	**Concentrate:** 30 mg/mL, 100 mg/mL	Yes
	Thorazine	**Suppositories (as base):** 25 mg, 100 mg	No
Rx	**Perphenazine**[1]		
	Trilafon	**Tablets:** 2 mg, 4 mg, 8 mg, 16 mg	No
	Trilafon[2]	**Concentrate:** 16 mg/tsp	No
Rx	**Prochlorperazine**[1]		
	Compazine	**Tablets:** 5 mg, 10 mg	Yes
	Compazine Spansules	**Capsules, sustained release:** 10 mg, 15 mg	No
	Compazine	**Syrup:** 5 mg/tsp	No
	Compazine	**Suppositories:** 2.5 mg, 5 mg, 25 mg	No
Rx	**Promethazine**[1]		
	Phenergan	**Tablets:** 12.5 mg, 25 mg, 50 mg	Yes
	Phenergan Plain[2], *Phenergan Fortis*[2]	**Syrup:** 6.25 mg/tsp, 25 mg/tsp	Yes
	Phenergan	**Suppositories:** 12.5 mg, 25 mg, 50 mg	Yes
Rx	**Thiethylperazine**[1,3,4]		
	Torecan[3]	**Tablets:** 10 mg	No
Rx	**Triflupromazine HCl**		
	Vesprin[2]	**Injection:** 10 mg/mL 20 mg/mL	No

[1] Some of these products are also available as an injection.
[2] Contains alcohol.
[3] Contains the dye tartrazine.
[4] Contains sulfites.

Type of Drug:

Drugs for nausea and vomiting.

How the Drug Works:

Drug-induced vomiting (including drugs, radiation, metabolic disorders) is generally stimulated through the chemoreceptor trigger zone (CTZ), which in turn stimulates the vomiting center (VC) in the brain. Nausea from motion sickness is initiated by stimulation of a mechanism of the ear, which sends impulses to the CTZ. The VC may also be stimulated directly (by stomach irritation, motion sickness, etc).

These drugs act on the CTZ, VC, nerve pathways and other centers of the brain to reduce nausea and vomiting.

Uses:

To control nausea and vomiting.

Chlorpromazine, Perphenazine – To relieve hiccups.

Promethazine – To treat and prevent motion sickness.

Precautions:

Do not use in the following situations:

- allergy to these drugs
- blood disorders
- bone marrow depression
- brain damage
- coma
- depression of CNS
- liver disease
- pregnancy (thiethylperazine only)
- sedative overdose

Use with caution in the following situations:

- alcohol withdrawal
- asthma
- bladder obstruction
- convulsive disorder, history of
- emphysema
- glaucoma
- heart disease
- hot weather
- kidney disease
- liver disease
- respiratory impairment (due to lung infections, acute)

Sensitivity to light: Rare instances of skin pigmentation have occurred, primarily in females on long-term, high dose therapy. These changes, restricted to exposed areas of the skin, range from almost imperceptible darkening to a slate gray color, sometimes with a violet hue. Pigmentation may fade following drug discontinuation. These effects occur most commonly with chlorpromazine.

May cause photosensitivity. Avoid prolonged exposure to the sun and other ultraviolet light. Use sunscreens and wear protective clothing until tolerance is determined.

Neuroleptic Malignant Syndrome (NMS) is a potentially fatal syndrome associated with phenothiazines. Symptoms include: Increased body heat; muscle rigidity; altered mental abilities, including catatonia; irregular pulse and blood pressure; increased heart rate; sweating; and irregular heart rhythm.

Tardive dyskinesia: Involuntary and uncontrollable movements may develop in patients treated with phenothiazines. Occurrence is highest in the elderly, expecially women. The risk of developing these involuntary movements and the likelihood they will become permanent are increased with long-term use and with high doses. However, it is possible to develop these symptoms after short-term treatment at low doses. The syndrome is characterized by rhythmical involutary movements of tongue, face, mouth, or jaw (eg, protrusion of tongue, puffing of cheeks, puckering of mouth, chewing movements), sometimes accompanied by involuntary movements of the arms and legs. Fine worm-like movement of the tongue may be an early sign of the syndrome. If the medication is stopped at this time, the syndrome may not develop. There is no known treatment for established cases of tardive dyskinesia, although the syndrome may stop, partially or completely, if the drug is withdrawn.

Pregnancy: Safety for use during pregnancy has not been established. Use only when clearly needed and potential benefits outweigh the possible hazards to the fetus.

Thiethylperazine – Do not use during pregnancy. The risk of use in a pregnant woman clearly outweighs any possible benefit.

Breastfeeding: Chlorpromazine appears in breast milk. It is not known if other phenothiazines appear in breast milk. Consult your doctor before you begin breastfeeding.

Children: In general, these products are not recommended for children younger than 12 years of age. Children with acute illnesses (eg, chickenpox, CNS infections, stomach or intestinal irritation, measles) or dehydration appear much more susceptible to neuromuscular reactions than adults. Symptoms can occur and may be confused with the signs of an undiagnosed primary disease responsible for vomiting (eg, Reye syndrome). Avoid these agents in children and adolescents whose signs and symptoms suggest Reye syndrome.

Prochlorperazine, promethazine – Not recommended for children under 20 pounds or younger than 2 years of age. Not for use in pediatric surgery. Children seem more prone to develop reactions, even on moderate doses. Use the lowest effective dose. Occasionally, the patient may react to the drug with signs of restlessness and excitement; if this occurs, do not administer additional doses. Use with caution in children with acute illnesses or dehydration. Not for use in conditions for which children's dosages are not established.

Elderly: Low doses are usually sufficient for elderly patients. These patients are more susceptible to lowered blood pressure and other side effects. Doses should be increased gradually.

Lab tests may be required to monitor treatment. Be sure to keep appointments. Tests may include blood counts and kidney and liver function.

Tartrazine: Some of these products may contain the dye tartrazine (FD&C Yellow No. 5), which can cause allergic reactions in certain individuals. Check package label when available or consult your doctor or pharmacist.

Sulfites: Some of these products may contain sulfite preservatives, which can cause allergic reactions in certain individuals (eg, asthmatics). Check package label when available or consult your doctor or pharmacist.

Drug Interactions:

Tell your doctor or pharmacist if you are taking or if you are planning to take any over-the-counter or prescription medications or dietary supplements with phenothiazines. Doses of one or both drugs may need to be modified or a different drug may need to be prescribed. The following drugs and drug classes interact with phenothiazines.

ACE inhibitors (eg, lisinopril)
alcohol
anorexiants (eg, methamphetamine)
anticholinergics (eg, benztropine)
anticoagulants, oral (eg, warfarin)
atropine
barbiturates (eg, phenobarbital)
beta-blockers (eg, propranolol)
biperiden (*Akineton*)
carbamazepine (eg, *Tegretol*)
charcoal
clidinium (*Quarzan*)
epinephrine (eg, *Adrenalin*)
guanethidine (eg, *Ismelin*)
levodopa (eg, *Larodopa*)
lithium (eg, *Eskalith*)
meperidine (eg, *Demerol*)
methyldopa (*Aldomet*)
metrizamide (*Amipaque*)
metyrosine (*Demser*)
morphine
orphenadrine (*Norflex*)
phenytoin (eg, *Dilantin*)
propranolol (*Inderal*)
trazodone (*Desyrel*)
tricyclic antidepressants (eg, amitriptyline)

Side Effects:

Every drug is capable of producing side effects. Many phenothiazine users experience no, or minor, side effects. The frequency and severity of side effects depend on many factors including dose, duration of therapy and individual susceptibility. Possible side effects include:

Liver: – Yellowing of skin and eyes (jaundice); abnormal liver function tests.

Parkinson Disease-Like Symptoms: – Tremors; drooling; muscle rigidity/restlessness; unusual eye movements; shuffling walk.

Muscular System: Muscle spasms including neck and back muscles; abnormal eye movements; aching and numbness of legs and arms; discoloration; rounding of the tongue; tightness in throat; difficulty swallowing; involuntary movement of tongue, face, mouth or jaw (protrusion of tongue, puffing cheeks, puckering of mouth, chewing movements); weakness; muscular deformation; inability to sit still; fixed eyeballs; exaggerated reflexes; difficulty moving; clumsiness; slurred speech; involuntary movements of arms and legs; agitation; jitteriness.

Circulatory System: Changes in blood pressure; postural hypotension (lightheadedness when rising quickly from a sitting or lying position); ECG changes; cardiac arrest; rapid heartbeat; irregular heart rhythm; change in pulse rate.

Psychiatric: Catatonia; phobia; tiredness; restlessness; hyperactivity; confusion; nightmares; depression; excitement; bizarre dreams; sleeplessness.

Nervous System: Swelling of brain; headache; fatigue; drowsiness; paranoia; lethargy; convulsions; sedation; dizziness; faintness.

Skin: Hives; rash; swelling; redness; itching; sensitivity to light; skin pigmentation; pallor; flushing; sweating; oily skin.

Urinary and Reproductive Tract: Appearance of milk and breast engorgement and aching in women; breast enlargement in men; menstrual irregularities; changes in sex drive; changes in blood sugar levels; infertility and false pregnancy; inhibition of ejaculation.

Eyes or Ocular: Glaucoma; sensitivity to light; blurred vision; changes in pupil size; problems with lens, retina and cornea.

Respiratory System: Tightness of throat in muscular system; nasal congestion; difficulty breathing; asthma.

Digestive Tract: Changes in appetite; nausea; vomiting; constipation; diarrhea, stomach upset; sore throat.

Other: Abnormal blood counts; urinary retention; increased urination; painful erections; impotence (male); swollen glands; thirst; pink or reddish brown urine; dry mouth and nose; ringing in the ears; kidney failure, acute; fever; salivation; sugar in the urine; weight change; swelling of arms, legs and face; urinary retention; inability to control urination; angioneurotic edema; death; swelling of arms, hands and face.

Guidelines for Use:

- *Brand interchange* — Do not change from one brand of this drug to another without consulting your pharmacist or doctor.
- Do not stop taking this medicine without checking with your doctor.
- Oral agents may be ineffective if expelled after vomiting has already begun. Use of suppositories or injection should be considered under such circumstances.
- Take these drugs routinely as directed. They control illness symptoms. They are not addicting.
- May cause drowsiness. Use caution while driving or performing other tasks requiring alertness, coordination, or dexterity.
- Avoid alcohol or other drugs that cause drowsiness.
- *Sensitivity to sunlight* — May cause photosensitivity (sensitivity to sunlight). Avoid prolonged exposure to the sun and other ultraviolet light. Use sunscreens and wear protective clothing until tolerance is determined.
- May discolor the urine pink or reddish-brown. This is not harmful.
- If dizziness or fainting occurs, avoid sudden changes in posture and use caution when climbing stairs, etc. (more common during first week of therapy).
- Use caution in hot weather. These drugs may increase susceptibility to heat stroke.
- Notify your doctor if sore throat, fever, unusual bleeding or bruising, skin rash, weakness, tremors, impaired vision, dark-colored urine, pale stools, jaundice, or involuntary muscle twitching occurs.
- May cause photosensitivity. Avoid prolonged exposure to the sun or other forms of ultraviolet (UV) light (eg, tanning beds). Use sunscreens and wear protective clothing until tolerance is determined.
- Lab tests may be required to monitor treatment. Be sure to keep appointments. Tests may include blood counts and kidney and liver function.

Guidelines for Use (cont.):

- *Liquid concentrates* are light sensitive. They are usually dispensed in amber or opaque bottles and protected from light. These solutions are most conveniently administered by dilution in fruit juices or other liquids. Shake well. Use these solutions immediately after dilution.
- *Liquid concentrates* — Avoid contact with skin (contact dermatitis may occur). Store at room temperature (59° to 86°F). Protect from light.
- *Chlorpromazine* —
  Concentrate: Add desired dosage to 60 mL (2 oz) or more of liquid just prior to use. Suggested liquids are tomato or fruit juice, milk, sugar water, orange syrup, carbonated beverages, coffee, tea, or water. Semisolid foods (soups, puddings, etc) may also be used. The concentrate is intended for institutional use only.
  Sustained release capsules: Do not crush or chew. Swallow whole.
- *Perphenazine —Concentrate:* Dilute only with water, saline, *Seven-Up,*® homogenized milk, carbonated orange drink and pineapple, apricot, prune, orange, *V-8,*® tomato, and grapefruit juices. Do NOT mix with beverages containing caffeine (coffee, cola), tannins (tea), or pectinates (apple juice). Use approximately 60 mL (2 oz) liquid for each 16 mg (5 mL or 1 tsp) concentrate. Store tablets and concentrate at controlled room temperature.
- All dosage forms should be stored between 59° and 77°F. Refrigerate promethazine suppositories between 36° and 46°F.

If you have any questions, consult your doctor, pharmacist, or health care provider.

	Generic Name *Brand Name Examples*	Supplied As	Generic Available
otc	**Phosphorated Carbohydrate** *Emetrol, Nausetrol*	**Solution:** Fructose, dextrose, and phosphoric acid	No

Type of Drug:

Drugs used for nausea and vomiting.

How the Drug Works:

Carbohydrate solutions with phosphoric acid relieve nausea and vomiting by a direct local action on the wall of the digestive tract reducing stomach contractions.

Uses:

For symptomatic relief of nausea and vomiting. Effectiveness has not been proven.

Precautions:

Do not use in the following situations: allergy to the drug

Use with caution in the following situations:
- diabetes
- hereditary fructose intolerance

Pregnancy: Safety for use during pregnancy has not been established. Phosphorated carbohydrate solution has been used for morning sickness.

Breastfeeding: It is not known if these agents appear in breast milk. Consult your doctor before you begin breastfeeding.

Drug Interactions:

Tell your doctor or pharmacist if you are taking or planning to take any over-the-counter or prescription medications or dietary supplements with phosphorated carbohydrate solution. Doses of one or both drugs may need to be modified or a different drug may need to be prescribed.

Side Effects:

Every drug is capable of producing side effects. Many antiemetic/antivertigo agent users experience no, or minor, side effects. The frequency and severity of side effects depend on many factors including dose, duration of therapy and individual susceptibility. Possible side effects include stomach pain and diarrhea.

Guidelines for Use:

- Use exactly as prescribed.
- Do not take for more than 1 hour without consulting your doctor.
- Nausea may signal a serious condition. If symptoms are not relieved or recur often, consult your doctor.
- *Diabetic patients* — Avoid phosphorated carbohydrate solutions because they contain significant amounts of sugar.
- *Phosphorated carbohydrate solutions* — Do not dilute. Do not take oral fluids immediately before the dose, or for at least 15 minutes after the dose.
- Store at room temperature (59° to 86°F).

If you have any questions, consult your doctor, pharmacist, or health care provider.

	Generic Name *Brand Name Example*	Supplied As	Generic Available
Rx	**Midodrine HCl** *ProAmatine*	**Tablets:** 2.5 mg, 5 mg	No

Type of Drug:

Drugs used to elevate blood pressure.

How the Drug Works:

Midodrine causes blood vessels to constrict (become smaller), resulting in an increase in blood pressure.

Uses:

To treat symptoms of orthostatic hypotension (feeling dizzy or lightheaded when rising from a sitting or standing position, or feelings of dizziness while standing). Use only in patients whose lives are considerably impaired despite standard clinical care, such as support stockings, fluid expansion and lifestyle changes.

Unlabeled Use(s): To manage urinary incontinence.

Precautions:

Do not use in the following situations:

heart disease, serious
high blood presure while lying down
hyperthyroidism
kidney disease, acute
pheochromocytoma (tumor of the adrenal gland)
urinary retention

Use with caution in the following situations:

diabetes
fludrocortisone acetate (*Florinef*) use
kidney disease
liver disease
vasoconstrive medications, use
visual problems, history

Supine hypertension is the most potentially serious side effect of midodrine. Supine (lying) and sitting blood pressures should be monitored. Supine hypertension can often be controlled by not lying totally flat (eg, sleeping with the head of the bed elevated).

Pregnancy: Adequate studies have not been done in pregnant women, or animal studies may have shown a risk to the fetus. Use only if clearly needed and potential benefits outweigh the possible hazards to the fetus.

Breastfeeding: It is not known if midodrine appears in breast milk. Consult your doctor before you begin breastfeeding.

Children: Safety and effectiveness are not established.

Lab tests will be required to monitor therapy. Lab tests may include blood pressure tests and kidney and liver function tests.

Drug Interactions:

Tell your doctor or pharmacist if you are taking or planning to take any over-the-counter or prescription medications or dietary supplements while taking this medicine. Doses of one or both drugs may need to be modified or a different drug may need to be prescribed. The following drugs or drug classes may interact with this medicine.

- alpha-adrenergic blockers (eg, doxazoxin)
- cardiac glycosides (eg, digoxin)
- cimetidine (eg, *Tagamet*)
- dihydroergotamine (*D.H.E. 45*)
- ephedrine
- flecainide (*Tambocor*)
- fludrocortisone acetate (*Florinef*)
- metformin (*Glucophage*)
- phenylephrine
- phenylpropanolamine (eg, *Contac*)
- procainamide (eg, *Pronestyl*)
- pseudoephedrine (eg, *Sudafed*)
- quinidine (eg, *Quinora*)
- ranitidine (eg, *Zantac*)
- triamterene (*Dyrenium*)

Side Effects:

Every drug is capable of producing side effects. Many patients experience no, or minor, side effects. The frequency or severity of side effects depend on many factors including dose, duration of therapy and individual susceptibility. Possible side effects include:

Nervous System: Numbness or tingling in scalp, hands or feet; pain; headache; feeling of pressure/fullness in the head; facial flushing; confusion; abnormal thinking; nervousness; anxiety.

Skin: Goosebumps; itching; rash.

Other: Painful or difficult urination; high blood pressure while lying or sitting; chills; dry mouth.

Guidelines for Use:

- Use exactly as prescribed.
- Usual dose is 10 mg, taken three times daily. Take during the daytime hours when you are upright and pursuing daily activities. A suggested dosing schedule of approximately 4 hour intervals is: Shortly before or upon arising in the morning, midday and late afternoon (not later than 6 pm). Doses may be taken in 3 hour intervals if required to control symptoms, but not more frequently. Do not take after the evening meal or less than 4 hours before bedtime.
- If a dose is missed, take it as soon as possible. If several hours have passed or if it is nearing time for the next dose, do not double the dose in order to "catch up" (unless advised to do so by your doctor). If more than one dose is missed or it is necessary to establish a new dosage schedule, contact your doctor or pharmacist.
- Supine (lying down) hypertension can often be controlled by not lying totally flat (eg, sleeping with the head of the bed elevated).
- Tell your doctor or pharmacist about any over-the-counter medications you are taking (eg, cold remedies, diet aids); they can increase the side effects of this medicine.
- Contact your doctor if you experience pounding in the ears, headache, blurred vision, slow pulse, increased dizziness, fainting, cardiac awareness, goosebumps, sensation of coldness or urinary retention.
- Continue taking this medicine, even if your symptoms of low blood pressure are controlled.
- Monitor blood pressure in both the lying and sitting positions.
- Lab tests may be required to monitor therapy. Be sure to keep appointments.
- Store at room temperature (59° to 77°F), out of the reach of children.

If you have any questions, consult your doctor, pharmacist, or health care provider.

	Generic Name *Brand Name Examples*	Supplied As	Generic Available
C-IV	**Alprazolam**		
	Xanax	**Tablets:** 0.25 mg, 0.5 mg, 1 mg, 2 mg	No
C-IV	**Chlordiazepoxide**[1]		
	Librium, Mitran, Reposans,	**Capsules:** 5 mg, 10 mg, 25 mg	Yes
	Libritabs	**Tablets:** 5 mg, 10 mg, 25 mg	No
C-IV	**Clonazepam**		
	Klonopin	**Tablets:** 0.5 mg, 1 mg, 2 mg	No
C-IV	**Clorazepate Dipotassium**	**Capsules:** 3.75 mg, 7.5 mg, 15 mg	Yes
	Gen-Xene, Tranxene	**Tablets:** 3.75 mg, 7.5 mg, 15 mg	Yes
	Tranxene-SD, Tranxene-SD Half Strength	**Tablets, single dose:** 11.25 mg, 22.5 mg	No
C-IV	**Diazepam**[1]		
	Valium	**Tablets:** 2 mg, 5 mg, 10 mg	Yes
	Valrelease	**Capsules, sustained release:** 15 mg	No
	Diazepam, Diazepam Intensol	**Oral solution:** 5 mg/tsp, 5 mg/mL	No
C-IV	**Halazepam**		
	Paxipam	**Tablets:** 20 mg, 40 mg	No
C-IV	**Lorazepam**[1]		
	Ativan	**Tablets:** 0.5 mg, 1 mg, 2 mg	Yes
	Lorazepam Intensol	**Oral solution:** 2 mg/mL	No
C-IV	**Oxazepam**		
	Serax	**Capsules:** 10 mg,15 mg, 30 mg	Yes
	Serax[2]	**Tablets:** 15 mg	Yes
C-IV	**Prazepam**		
	Centrax	**Capsules:** 5 mg, 10 mg, 20 mg	Yes
	Centrax	**Tablets:** 5 mg,10 mg	Yes

[1] Some of these products are also available as an injection.
[2] Contains the dye tartrazine.

Type of Drug:

Agents to relieve nervousness and tension. Sometimes called "minor tranquilizers."

How the Drug Works:

Benzodiazepines affect the brain to calm nervous tension while causing little drowsiness.

Uses:

To treat anxiety disorders and for the short-term relief of the symptoms of anxiety. Anxiety or tension associated with the stress of everyday life does not usually require long-term treatment with an antianxiety agent.

Additional uses:

Alprazolam: To treat panic disorder, with or without agoraphobia and anxiety associated with depression.

Chlordiazepoxide: For symptoms of alcohol withdrawal, preoperative apprehension and anxiety.

Clorazepate: For symptomatic relief of alcohol withdrawal. For management of seizures (with other drugs).

Diazepam: For symptoms of acute agitation, tremor or delirium tremens (DTs). For relief of muscle spasms. For preoperative anxiety (injection only) and with other drugs to help control convulsions.

Lorazepam: To treat anxiety associated with depression. For preoperative anxiety and sedation (injection only).

Oxazepam: To manage anxiety, tension, agitation and irritability in older patients. To treat anxiety associated with alcohol withdrawal or depression.

Unlabeled Use(s): Occasionally doctors may prescribe chlordiazepoxide, diazepam, clorazepate, lorazepam, oxazepam, prazepam or alprazolam for irritable bowel syndrome. Alprazolam and diazepam are occasionally used to treat panic attacks. Alprazolam is occasionally used to treat agoraphobia with social phobia, depression and premenstrual syndrome. Lorazepam is occasionally used to treat chronic insomnia. Lorazepam injection is occasionally used to treat seizures, chemotherapy-induced nausea and vomiting, acute alcohol withdrawal syndrome and psychogenic catatonia.

Precautions:

Do not use in the following situations:

alcoholism, history
allergy to these drugs
children under 6 months, lactation (diazepam only)
drug addiction, history
glaucoma, narrow-angle
intra-arterial administration (lorazepam injection only)
liver disease, significant (clonazepamonly)
psychoses

Use with caution in the following situations:

depression or other psychiatric disorders	kidney disease
	liver disease
elderly and very ill	lung disease (clonazepam only)

Dependence: Prolonged use of benzodiazepines can lead to dependence. A withdrawal syndrome may occur after as little as 4 to 6 weeks of treatment. It is more likely if the drug is short-acting (eg, alprazolam), if it is taken regularly for longer than 3 months, if higher dosages are used and if it is abruptly discontinued.

Onset of withdrawal is within 1 to 10 days; it may last 5 days to a month or more. Symptoms may include: Increased anxiety, sleeplessness, irritability, nausea, headache, muscle tension/cramps, tremor, confusion, abnormal perception of movement, muscle twitching, psychosis and seizures.

Abrupt withdrawal of clonazepam, particularly in patients on long-term, high-dose therapy, may precipitate status epilepticus (a rapid series of convulsions without any periods of consciousness between them). While clonazepam is being gradually withdrawn, the substitution of another anticonvulsant may be indicated. Other symptoms include vomiting, diarrhea and sweating.

When discontinuing therapy, decrease dosage gradually over 4 to 8 weeks to avoid the possibility of withdrawal, especially in patients with a history of seizures, regardless of anticonvulsant drug therapy. Clonidine, propranolol and carbamazepine have been used to treat benzodiazepine withdrawal symptoms.

Unusual reactions: Excitement, stimulation and acute rage have been reported in psychiatric patients and hyperactive aggressive children. These reactions may be secondary to relief of anxiety and usually appear in the first 2 weeks of therapy. Acute hyperexcited states, anxiety, hallucinations, increased muscle spasms and sleep disturbances have been reported. Should these occur, consult your doctor. Anger, hostility and episodes of mania have been reported with alprazolam.

Multiple seizure type: When used in patients in whom several different types of seizure disorders coexist, clonazepam may increase the frequency or precipitate the onset of generalized tonic-clonic (grand mal) seizures. This may require the addition of other anticonvulsants or an increase in dosage.

Diazepam: If an increase in the frequency or severity of grand mal seizures occurs, your doctor may need to increase the dosage of standard anticonvulsant medication.

Pregnancy: Benzodiazepines cross the placenta. Studies have shown a potential effect on the fetus. Use only if clearly needed and potential benefits outweigh the possible hazards to the fetus.

Breastfeeding: Most benzodiazepines appear in breast milk. It is not known if lorazepam appears in breast milk. Do not use these drugs while breastfeeding.

Children: Give the smallest dose possible, as children may be more sensitive to benzodiazepines.

Alprazolam, halazepam, prazepam – Safety and effectiveness have not been established in children younger than 18.

Chlordiazepoxide – Not recommended for use in children younger than 6 (oral) or 12 (injection).

Clorazepate – Not recommended for use in children under 9.

Diazepam – Do not use in children younger than 6 months (oral). Safety and effectiveness have not been established in newborns (injection).

Lorazepam – Safety and effectiveness have not been established in children younger than 12 (oral). Do not use in children younger than 18 (injection).

Elderly: Give the smallest dose possible, as the elderly may be more sensitive to benzodiazepines.

Lab tests : Because of reports of abnormal blood counts and yellowing of the skin or eyes, blood counts, and liver function tests should be performed during long-term therapy.

Tartrazine: Some of these products may contain the dye tartrazine (FD&C Yellow No. 5) which can cause allergic reactions in certain individuals. Check package label when available and consult your doctor or pharmacist.

Drug Interactions:

Tell your doctor or pharmacist if you are taking or planning to take any over-the-counter or prescription medications or dietary supplements with benzodiazepines. Doses of one or both drugs may need to be modified or a different drug may need to be prescribed. The following drugs and drug classes interact with benzodiazepines.

alcohol
antacids
barbiturates (eg, phenobarbital)
cimetidine (*Tagamet*)
contraceptives, oral (eg, *Ortho-Novum*)
digoxin (eg, *Lanoxin*)
disulfiram (eg, *Antabuse*)
fluoxetine *(Prozac)*
isoniazid (eg, *Laniazid*)
ketoconazole *(Nizoral)*
levodopa (eg, *Larodopa*)
metoprolol *(Lopressor)*
narcotic pain relievers (eg, codeine)
neuromuscular blocking agents
phenytoin (eg, *Dilantin*)
probenecid (eg, *Benemid*)
propoxyphene (eg, *Darvon*)
propranolol (eg, *Inderal*)
ranitidine *(Zantac)*
rifampin (eg, *Rifadin*)
scopolamine
theophylline (eg, *Theo-Dur*)
valproic acid (eg, *Depakene*)

Side Effects:

Every drug is capable of producing side effects. Many benzodiazepine users experience no, or minor, side effects. The frequency and severity of side effects depend on many factors including dose, duration of therapy and individual susceptibility. Possible side effects include:

Digestive Tract: Stomach upset; constipation; diarrhea; nausea; change in appetite; vomiting.

Nervous System: Confusion; depression; nervousness; behavior changes; memory loss; drowsiness; fatigue; decreased activity; dizziness; vertigo (feeling of whirling motion); lethargy; apathy; euphoria (exaggerated sense of well being); restlessness; crying; delirium; disorientation; sleep disturbances; incoordination; vivid dreams; headache; seizures; weakness; unsteadiness.

Circulatory System: Changes in heart rate; changes in blood pressure; pounding in the chest (palpitations).

Skin: Hives; itching; rash; hair loss; excessive hair growth; yellowing of skin or eyes.

Senses: Visual disturbances; double vision; decreased hearing; hearing disturbances; nasal congestion; slurred speech; loss of voice.

Urinary and Reproductive Tract: Incontinence; changes in sex drive; urine retention; menstrual problems.

Other: Dry mouth; difficulty swallowing; hiccups; fever; balance problems; tremors and uncontrollable muscle movement; breathing problems; ankle and facial swelling; breast enlargement; production of breast milk; movement difficulties; "glassy-eyed" appearance; increased salivation; sore gums; coated tongue; fluid retention (edema); excessive perspiration; abnormal blood counts; abnormal liver function; joint pain; weight gain or loss; dehydration; swollen lymph nodes; fainting.

Guidelines for Use:

- If a dose is missed, take it as soon as possible. If several hours have passed or if it is nearing time for the next dose, do not double the dose in order to "catch up" (unless advised to do so by your doctor). If more than one dose is missed, or it is necessary to establish a new dosage schedule, contact your doctor or pharmacist. Use exactly as prescribed.
- These drugs can be addictive if used in large doses or for a long time. Do not exceed prescribed dose. Discuss overuse with your doctor.
- Avoid alcohol or other drugs that cause drowsiness while taking these drugs.
- May cause drowsiness. Use caution while driving or performing other tasks requiring alertness.
- May be taken with food or water if stomach upset occurs.
- Patients on long-term or high dosage therapy may experience withdrawal symptoms on abrupt cessation of therapy. Do not discontinue therapy abruptly or change dosage except on advice of your doctor.
- Ingestion of antacids with diazepam and chlordiazepoxide may impair absorption of these drugs.
- *Clonazepam, clorazepate and diazepam–*Carry identification (Medic Alert) if these medications are being used for epilepsy.
- *Intensol solutions–* Mix with liquid or semi-solid food (eg, water, juice, applesauce, pudding).

If you have any questions, consult your doctor, pharmacist, or health care provider.

	Generic Name *Brand Name Example*	Supplied As	Generic Available
Rx	**Buspirone HCl**		
	BuSpar	**Tablets:** 5 mg, 10 mg, 15 mg	No

Type of Drug:

Antianxiety agent; agent to relieve nervousness.

How the Drug Works:

It is not known exactly how buspirone works to relieve anxiety. It is believed that it may react with specific chemical receptors in the brain.

Uses:

For short-term relief of symptoms of anxiety.

To manage anxiety disorders.

Unlabeled Use(s): Occasionally doctors may prescribe buspirone for the symptoms of premenstrual syndrome.

Precautions:

Do not use in the following situations:
allergy to buspirone or any of its ingredients
kidney disease, severe
liver disease, severe
MAOI use, concurrent

Use with caution in the following situations:
kidney disease
liver disease

Improvement in symptoms may occur within 7 to 10 days. Optimum results are generally achieved after 3 to 4 weeks of treatment.

Withdrawal reactions: Patients should be withdrawn from benzodiazepines and other sedative/hypnotic drugs gradually before starting buspirone, especially those who have been using these drugs for a long period of time. Withdrawal symptoms, including irritability, anxiety, agitation, sleeplessness, tremor, stomach cramps, muscle cramps, vomiting, sweating, flu-like symptoms without fever, and occasionally seizures, may occur.

Pregnancy: There are no adequate and well-controlled studies in pregnant women. Use this drug during pregnancy only if clearly needed and the potential benefits to the mother outweigh the possible risks to the fetus.

Breastfeeding: It is not known if buspirone appears in breast milk. Consult your doctor before you begin breastfeeding.

Children: Safety and effectiveness in children younger than 18 years of age have not been established.

Drug Interactions:

Tell your doctor or pharmacist if you are taking or planning to take any over-the-counter or prescription medications or dietary supplements with buspirone. Doses of one or both drugs may need to be modified or a different drug may need to be prescribed. The following drugs and drug classes interact with buspirone:

- alcohol
- azole antifungals (eg, itraconazole)
- cimetidine (eg, *Tagamet*)
- haloperidol (eg, *Haldol)*
- MAOIs (eg, isocarboxazid, phenelzine, tranylcypromine)
- macrolide antibiotics (eg, clarithromycin, erythromycin)
- nefazodone (eg, *Serzone*)
- rifamycins (eg, *Rifabutin*)
- trazodone (eg, *Desyrel)*

Side Effects:

Every drug is capable of producing side effects. Many buspirone users experience no, or minor, side effects. The frequency and severity of side effects depend on many factors including dose, duration of therapy, and individual susceptibility. Possible side effects include:

Digestive Tract: Nausea; stomach upset; diarrhea; constipation; vomiting; dry mouth.

Nervous System: Dizziness; headache; nervousness; lightheadedness; excitement; dream disturbances; drowsiness; fatigue; weakness; sleeplessness; decreased concentration; anger; confusion; depression; numbness; incoordination; tremor; hostility; tingling in hands or feet.

Circulatory System: Chest pain; increased heart rate; pounding in chest.

Senses: Ringing in the ears; sore throat; blurred vision; nasal congestion.

Other: Muscle aches or pains; abnormal skin sensations; sweating or clamminess; rash.

Guidelines for Use:

- Dosage will be individualized according to specific patient needs.
- This medication is designed to be taken every day to prevent anxiety symptoms. It does not work if it is only taken "as needed" or only when anxiety symptoms are present.
- If a dose is missed, take it as soon as possible. If several hours have passed or if it is nearing time for the next dose, do not double the dose in order to catch up, unless advised to do so by your doctor. If more than one dose is missed, or it is necessary to establish a new dosage schedule, contact your doctor or pharmacist. Use exactly as prescribed.
- Inform your doctor if any restlessness or abnormal muscle movements occur (eg, motor restlessness, involuntary repetitive movements of facial or neck muscles).
- May cause drowsiness or dizziness. Use caution while driving or performing other tasks requiring alertness, coordination, and physical dexterity.
- Inform your doctor of any prescription or nonprescription medications, alcohol, or drugs that you are taking, or plan to take, during buspirone treatment.
- Avoid alcohol and other depressant drugs while taking buspirone.
- Inform your doctor if you are pregnant, become pregnant, or are planning to become pregnant while taking buspirone, or if you are breastfeeding.
- Some improvement in symptoms may be seen after 7 to 10 days, but optimum results may take 3 to 4 weeks to develop.
- Store at room temperature (below 86°F). Protect from light.

If you have any questions, consult your doctor, pharmacist, or health care provider.

	Generic Name *Brand Name Examples*	Supplied As	Generic Available
Rx	**Hydroxyzine HCl**		
	Atarax	**Tablets:** 10 mg, 25 mg, 50 mg	Yes
	Atarax 100	**Tablets:** 100 mg	No
	Atarax[1]	**Syrup:** 10 mg/5 mL	Yes
	Hyzine 50	**Injection:** 25 mg/mL, 50 mg/mL	Yes
Rx	**Hydroxyzine Pamoate**		
	Vistaril	**Capsules:** 25 mg, 50 mg, 100 mg	Yes
	Vistaril	**Oral suspension:** 25 mg/5 mL	No
	Vistaril	**Injection:** 25 mg/mL, 50 mg/mL	Yes

[1] Contains alcohol.

Type of Drug:

Antihistamine and agent to relieve nervousness and anxiety.

How the Drug Works:

Hydroxyzine decreases anxiety by suppressing activity in the anxiety centers in the brain. Antihistamine (anti-allergy), bronchodilator, analgesic, and antiemetic properties have also been demonstrated.

Uses:

For short-term (4 months or less) relief of anxiety and tension.

To relieve itching due to allergic conditions (eg, hives, rash, insect bites).

For sedation prior to and following surgery.

Injection – To treat hysteria, alcohol withdrawal symptoms, or delirium tremens. To control vomiting and pain (with other drugs) before and after surgery or delivery. To control nausea and vomiting from causes other than pregnancy.

Precautions:

Do not use in the following situations:

- allergy to hydroxyzine or any of its ingredients
- breastfeeding
- pregnancy

Pregnancy: Do not use during pregnancy. The risk of use in a pregnant woman clearly outweighs any possible benefit.

Breastfeeding: It is not known if hydroxyzine appears in breast milk. Consult your doctor before you begin breastfeeding.

Drug Interactions:

Tell your doctor or pharmacist if you are taking or planning to take any over-the-counter or prescription medications or dietary supplements with hydroxyzine. Doses of one or both drugs may need to be modified or a different drug may need to be prescribed. The following drugs and drug classes interact with hydroxyzine.

alcohol (eg, ethanol)
antihistamines (eg, diphenhydramine)
barbiturates (eg, phenobarbital)
narcotics (eg, morphine)

Side Effects:

Every drug is capable of producing side effects. Many hydroxyzine users experience no, or minor, side effects. The frequency and severity of side effects depend on many factors including dose, duration of therapy, and individual susceptibility. Possible side effects include:

Other: Dry mouth; dizziness; involuntary movements.

Guidelines for Use:

- Dosage will be adjusted according to individual patient response to therapy. Use exactly as prescribed.
- Shake oral suspension vigorously until product is completely resuspended.
- The injection form is only used when tablets, capsules, suspension, or syrup are unable to be taken by the patient.
- The injection form will be prepared and administered by your health care provider.
- Injection solution should be inspected before use. Injection solution should only be administered intramuscularly (IM).
- The effectiveness of hydroxyzine as an antianxiety agent for > 4 months has not been assessed by clinical studies. Your doctor will reassess the usefulness of the drug periodically.
- If a dose is missed, take it as soon as possible. If several hours have passed or if it is nearing time for the next dose, do not double the dose to catch up, unless advised to do so by your doctor. If more than one dose is missed, or it is necessary to establish a new dosage schedule, contact your doctor or pharmacist.
- May cause drowsiness. Use caution while driving or performing other tasks requiring alertness, coordination, or physical dexterity.
- Avoid alcohol or other depressant drugs (eg, narcotics, tranquilizers, antihistamines) while taking hydroxyzine.
- Store tablets and capsules at room temperature (59° to 86°F). Keep tightly closed. Protect from moisture.
- Store oral suspension and syrup below 86°F. Keep tightly closed. Protect from freezing and light.
- Store injection solution at room temperature (59° to 86°F). Protect from light. Discard unused portion of single-dose vial.

If you have any questions, consult your doctor, pharmacist, or health care provider.

Generic Name *Brand Name Examples*	Supplied As	Generic Available
C-IV **Meprobamate**		
Equanil, Miltown	**Tablets:** 200 mg, 400 mg	Yes

Type of Drug:

Agent to relieve nervousness and tension.

How the Drug Works:

Meprobamate works in the brain to relieve anxiety and tension.

Uses:

To provide short-term relief of symptoms of anxiety.

To manage anxiety disorders.

Anxiety or tension associated with stress of everyday life usually does not require treatment with an antianxiety agent.

Precautions:

Do not use in the following situations:

allergy to carisoprodol or related drugs
allergy to meprobamate or any of its ingredients
porphyria, acute or intermittent

Use with caution in the following situations:

addiction, history of
alcoholism
kidney disease
lactation
liver disease
pregnancy
seizure disorder (eg, epilepsy)
suicidal tendencies

Drug dependence: Physical and psychological dependence and abuse may occur. Symptoms of chronic intoxication from prolonged use of greater than recommended doses include incoordination, clumsiness, slurred speech, and veritgo (feeling of whirling motion). Avoid prolonged use. Abrupt discontinuation after prolonged and excessive use may cause a withdrawal syndrome characterized by anxiety, appetite loss, sleeplessness, vomiting, incoordination or clumsiness, tremors, muscle twitching, confusional states, hallucinations, and seizures. Onset of withdrawal symptoms usually begins within 12 to 48 hours after discontinuation of meprobamate and symptoms usually cease within the next 12 to 48 hours.

When excessive dosage has continued for weeks or months the dose should be reduced gradually over a period of 1 or 2 weeks rather than stopping abruptly. Alternatively, a short-acting barbiturate may be substituted, then gradually withdrawn.

Pregnancy: Studies have shown a potential effect to the fetus. Meprobamate passes the placental barrier and an increased risk of birth defects is associated with its use during the first trimester. Use during pregnancy should almost always be avoided. Use with extreme caution. Use only if clearly needed and potential benefits to the mother outweigh the possible hazards to the fetus.

Breastfeeding: Meprobamate appears in breast milk. Consult your doctor before you begin breastfeeding.

Children: Do not use in children younger than 6 years of age.

Elderly: To avoid oversedation, use lowest effective dose.

Drug Interactions:

Tell your doctor or pharmacist if you are taking or planning to take any over-the-counter or prescription medications or dietary supplements with meprobamate. Doses of one or both drugs may need to be modified or a different drug may need to be prescribed. The following drugs and drug classes interact with meprobamate.

- alcohol
- barbiturates (eg, phenobarbital)
- narcotic pain relievers (eg, codeine)

Side Effects:

Every drug is capable of producing side effects. Many meprobamate users experience no, or minor, side effects. The frequency and severity of side effects depend on many factors including dose, duration of therapy, and individual susceptibility. Possible side effects include:

Allergic Reactions: Mild — Rash (over the whole body or only the groin area); abnormal blood counts; purplish or brownish-red discoloration of the skin (either small pin-like or large bruise-like coloring); swelling; swollen glands; fever.

Severe (Rare) — Fever; chills; fluid retention associated with discoloration and rash; difficulty breathing; decreased or lack of urination; skin inflammation; inflammation of the mouth and rectum.

Digestive Tract: Nausea; vomiting; diarrhea.

Nervous System: Drowsiness; dizziness; feeling of whirling motion; incoordination; headache; weakness; overstimulation; exaggerated sense of well being; paradoxical excitement.

Circulatory System: Fast or irregular heartbeat; pounding in chest; low blood pressure; fainting; abnormal heart rhythm.

Skin: Abnormal skin sensations (burning, prickling, tingling); itching.

Other: Slurred speech; fever; impaired vision or vision changes; shortness of breath.

Guidelines for Use:

- Usual adult dosage is 1200 mg to 1600 mg/day in 3 or 4 divided doses. Doses greater than 2400 mg/day are not recommended. Usual dosage for children 6 to 12 years of age is 100 mg to 200 mg 2 to 3 times daily.
- Do not crush or chew tablets due to bitter taste.
- Physical and psychological dependence and abuse may occur.
- Do not suddenly stop taking this drug after long-term use. Consult your doctor.
- Long-term effectiveness (more than 4 months) of meprobamate has not been established. Your doctor will periodically reassess the usefulness of the drug.
- If a dose is missed, take it as soon as possible. If several hours have passed or if it is nearing time for the next dose, do not double the dose in order to catch up, unless advised to do so by your doctor. If more than one dose is missed, or it is necessary to establish a new dosage schedule, contact your doctor or pharmacist. Use exactly as prescribed.
- Inform your doctor if you are pregnant, become pregnant, are planning to become pregnant, or are breastfeeding.
- May cause drowsiness, dizziness, or blurred vision. Use caution while driving or performing other tasks requiring alertness, coordination, or physical dexterity.
- Discontinue use and notify your doctor immediately at first appearance of fever, sore throat, rash, or other signs of allergic reaction. In some instances, rash may be accompanied by more severe allergic reactions (see Side Effects). You may need to begin appropiate symptomatic therapy (eg, epinephrine, antihistamines, corticosteroids), which will be prescribed or administered by your doctor.
- Avoid alcohol and other mental depressants (eg, narcotics, tranquilizers, antihistamines) while taking this medicine.
- Store at controlled room temperature (68° to 77°F). Keep tightly closed. Protect from moisture.

If you have any questions, consult your doctor, pharmacist, or health care provider.

	Generic Name *Brand Name Examples*	Supplied As	Generic Available
Rx	**Bupropion HCl**		
	Wellbutrin	**Tablets:** 75 mg, 100 mg	No
	Wellbutrin SR	**Tablets, sustained release:** 100 mg, 150 mg	No

Type of Drug:

Antidepressant; mood-elevating agent.

How the Drug Works:

The actual antidepressant mechanism of bupropion is not known, but is thought to enhance activity of certain chemicals in the brain (eg, dopamine, norepinephrine, serotonin) which in turn improves depressed mood.

Uses:

To treat depression. Use in treating depression for more than 6 weeks has not been evaluated. Patients who use this drug for extended periods should be periodically re-evaluated by their doctor.

Precautions:

Do not use in the following situations:

- allergy to bupropion or any of its ingredients
- anorexia
- bulimia
- bupropion HCl (eg, *Zyban*), concurrent use for smoking cessation
- monoamine oxidase inhibitor (MAOI) use, concurrent or within 14 days
- seizure disorders

Use with caution in the following situations:

- alcohol
- attempted suicide, history
- brain tumor
- diabetes treated with oral hypoglycemics or insulin
- drug abuse
- head injury, history
- heart attack, recent
- heart disease
- kidney disease
- liver disease
- manic depression, bipolar
- seizure, history or risk of
- therapy that lowers seizure threshold (eg, antipsychotics, antidepressants, theophylline, systemic steroids, benzodiazepine withdrawal)

Pregnancy: Adequate studies have not been done in pregnant women. Use during pregnancy only if clearly needed. Notify your doctor if you are pregnant or intend to become pregnant during therapy.

Breastfeeding: Bupropion HCl is secreted in human in milk. Serious side effects could potentially occur in the nursing infant. Decide whether to discontinue the drug or discontinue breastfeeding, taking into account the importance of the drug to the mother. Consult your doctor before you begin breastfeeding.

Children: Safety and effectiveness have not been established in children younger than 18 years of age.

Elderly: Older patients are known to metabolize drugs more slowly and to be more sensitive to antidepressant drugs. Use the lowest effective dose.

Drug Interactions:

Tell your doctor or pharmacist if you are taking or if you are planning to take any over-the-counter or prescription medications or dietary supplements with bupropion. Doses of one or both drugs may need to be modified or a different drug may need to be prescribed. The following drugs and drug classes interact with bupropion.

antidepressants (eg, fluoxetine, amitriptyline)
antipsychotics (eg, phenothiazines)
carbamazepine (eg, *Tegretol*)
cimetidine (eg, *Tagamet*)
isocarboxazid (*Marplan*)
levodopa (eg, *Sinemet*)
monoamine oxidase inhibitors (eg, phenelzine)
phenobarbital (eg, *Solfoton*)
phenytoin (eg, *Dilantin*)
ritonavir (*Norvir*)
systemic corticosteroids (eg, prednisone)
theophylline (eg, *Slo-Phyllin*)

Side Effects:

Every drug is capable of producing side effects. Many bupropion users experience no, or minor, side effects. The frequency and severity of side effects depend on many factors including dose, duration of therapy, and individual susceptibility. Possible side effects include:

Parkinson's Disease-Like Symptoms: Stumbling gait; movement disorders.

Digestive Tract: Nausea; vomiting; constipation; indigestion; appetite changes; stomach pain; dry mouth; mouth sores.

Nervous System: Seizures; tremor; dizziness; delusions; hallucinations; euphoria (exaggerated sense of well-being); confusion; agitation; hostility; restlessness; anxiety; sedation; sleep disturbances; fatigue; headache; activation of psychosis or mania; sleeplessness; decreased memory.

Circulatory System: Changes in heart rate and rhythm; changes in blood pressure; palpitations (pounding in chest); fast heartbeat; chest pain.

Skin: Rash; itching; excessive sweating; flushing.

Other: Taste changes; blurred vision; hearing problems; impotence; frequent urination; menstrual problems; fever; chills; joint pain; weight changes; decreased sex drive; fainting; urinary urgency; muscle pain; allergic reaction; weakness; abnormal skin sensations; shortness of breath.

Guidelines for Use:

- This medicine should not be used in combination with *Zyban* or any other medication containing bupropion.
- Avoid alcohol to reduce the risk of seizures.
- Do not take in combination with MAO inhibitors or within 14 days of discontinuing treatment with an MAOI.
- The full antidepressant effects of bupropion may take 4 weeks or longer.
- May cause drowsiness. Use caution while driving or performing other tasks requiring alertness, coordination, or physical dexterity.
- Inform your doctor if you are pregnant, become pregnant, are planning to become pregnant, or are breastfeeding.

Bupropion Tablets:

- Usual adult dosage is 300 mg/day given in 3 equally divided doses of 100 mg separated by at least 6 hours. Dosing should begin at 200 mg/day, given as 100 mg twice daily. Based on response, dose may be gradually increased up to 300 mg/day.
- Do not crush or chew tablets. This can cause numbness of the mouth or throat.
- Do not exceed 450 mg bupropion daily. Single doses should not exceed 150 mg due to the risk of seizures.
- If a dose is missed, take it as soon as possible. If several hours have passed or if it is less than 6 hours before your next dose, do not double the dose in order to catch up. Never take more than 150 mg at one time. If more than one dose is missed or it is necessary to establish a new dosage schedule, contact your doctor or pharmacist. Use exactly as prescribed.
- Store at 59° to 77°F. Protect from light and moisture.

Bupropion Sustained Release Tablets:

- Usual adult dosage is 300 mg/day, given in 2 equally divided doses of 150 mg separated by at least 8 hours. Dosing should begin at 150 mg/day given as a single dose in the morning. Based on response, dose may be increased to 150 mg twice daily.
- Do not crush, chew, or divide tablets. Tablets are designed to gradually release medication.
- Do not exceed 400 mg of bupropion sustained release tablets daily. Single doses should not exceed 200 mg due to the risk of seizures.
- If a dose is missed, take it as soon as possible. If several hours have passed or if it is less than 8 hours before your next dose, do not double the dose in order to catch up. Never take more than 200 mg at one time. If more than one dose is missed or it is necessary to establish a new dosage schedule, contact your doctor or pharmacist. Use exactly as prescribed.
- Store at 68° to 77°F. Protect from light and moisture.

If you have any questions, consult your doctor, pharmacist, or health care provider.

Generic Name *Brand Name Example*	Supplied As	Generic Available
Rx **Nefazodone HCl**		
Serzone	**Tablets:** 100 mg, 150 mg, 200 mg, 250 mg	No

Type of Drug:

Antidepressant; mood elevating agent.

How the Drug Works:

The exact mechanism is unknown. Nefazodone appears to block the uptake of serotonin and norepinephrine (chemicals found in the brain). The effect may take a few weeks to be noticed.

Uses:

To treat mental depression in patients older than 18 years of age.

Precautions:

Do not use in the following situations:

- allergy to nefazodone HCl or similar antidepressants (eg, *Desyrel*)
- astemizole use (*Hismanal*)
- monoamine oxidase inhibitor use (eg, *Nardil, Parnate*), current or recent
- terfenadine use (*Seldane*)

Use with caution in the following situations:

- antihypertensive use
- brain blood vessel disease
- drug abuse, history of
- elderly, especially females
- heart attack, recent
- heart disease, unstable
- liver disease
- low blood pressure
- mania (psychological disturbance)
- seizures, history of
- stroke, history of
- suicide attempts, history of

Pregnancy: Adequate studies have not been done in pregnant women. Use only if clearly needed and potential benefits ouweigh the possible hazards to the fetus.

Breastfeeding: It is not known if nefazodone HCl appears in breast milk. Consult your doctor before you begin breastfeeding.

Children: Safety and effectiveness in individuals younger than 18 years of age have not been established.

Elderly: Lower intial doses are recommended for patients over 65.

Drug Interactions:

Tell your doctor or pharmacist if you are taking or if you are planning to take any over-the-counter or prescription medications while taking nefazodone HCl. Doses of one or both drugs may need to be modified or a different drug may need to be prescribed. The following drugs and drug classes interact with nefazodone HCl.

alprazolam (*Xanax*)
astemizole (*Hismanal*)
digoxin (eg, *Lanoxin*)
haloperidol (eg, *Haldol*)
MAOIs (eg, phenelzine)
propranolol (eg, *Inderal*)
terfenadine (*Seldane*)
triazolam (*Halcion*)

Side Effects:

Every drug is capable of producing side effects. Many nefazodone HCl users experience no, or minor, side effects. The frequency and severity of side effects depend on many factors including dose, duration of therapy and individual susceptibility. Possible side effects include:

Digestive Tract: Nausea; constipation; indigestion; diarrhea; appetite changes; vomiting; stomach pain; gas.

Nervous System: Dizziness; sleeplessness; weakness; drowsiness; lightheadedness; confusion; headache; memory loss; incoordination; tremor; anxiety; unstable emotions; depression.

Circulatory System: Low blood pressure; chest pain; pounding in the chest (palpitations); slow heartbeat.

Respiratory System: Cough; runny nose; difficulty breathing; sinus infection; bronchitis; sore throat.

Skin: Itching; rash; abnormal skin sensations; flushing; sweating; decreased sensitivity to touch. *Urinary and Reproductive Tract:* Prolonged or inappropriate erections; decreased sexual drive; changes in urinary frequency; breast pain; painful menstruation; impotence; painful urination.

Other: Dry mouth; vision impairment; eye pain; flu syndrome; chills; fever; stiff neck; swelling in the arms and legs; joint, muscle, back or neck pain; ringing in the ears; abnormal taste sensations; weight gain; swelling; cramping.

Guidelines for Use:

- Take in two divided doses on an empty stomach, or as directed by your doctor.
- Do not discontinue therapy or change the dose unless instructed by your doctor.
- Notify your doctor immediately if you develop a rash, hives, or other type of allergic reaction.
- If a dose is missed, take it as soon as possible. If several hours have passed or if it is nearing time for the next dose, do not double the dose in order to "catch up" (unless advised to do so by your doctor). If more than one dose is missed, contact your doctor or pharmacist.
- Do not use in combination with MAOIs (monoamine oxidase inhibitors) or within 14 days of discontinuing treatment with an MAOI. After stopping this medicine, wait at least 1 week before starting an MAOI.
- Improvement may not be seen for several weeks. Exams may be necessary.
- May impair judgment, thinking or motor skills. Use caution while driving or performing other tasks requiring alertness, coordination or physical dexterity until effects are known.
- Inform your doctor if you are pregnant, become pregnant, are planning to become pregnant or if you are breastfeeding.
- Avoid alcohol while using this medicine.
- Store in a dry place at room temperature.

If you have any questions, consult your doctor, pharmacist, or health care provider.

	Generic Name *Brand Name Examples*	Supplied As	Generic Available
Rx	**Fluoxetine HCl**		
	Prozac	**Tablets**: 10 mg	No
	Prozac	**Pulvules**: 10 mg, 20 mg, 40 mg	No
	Prozac Weekly	**Capsules, delayed-release**: 90 mg	No
	Sarafem	**Pulvules**: 10 mg, 20 mg	No
	Prozac	**Oral solution**: 20 mg/5 mL[1]	Yes

[1] Contains alcohol.

Type of Drug:

Antidepressant; mood elevating agent.

How the Drug Works:

The exact mechanism is not known. It is believed that fluoxetine adjusts or balances how the brain and nervous system produce and respond to their own natural chemicals (called neurotransmitters). Fluoxetine appears to inhibit CNS neuronal uptake of serotonin by the brain. The effect may take a few weeks to be noticed.

Uses:

Prozac: For the treatment of mental depression, bulimia nervosa, and obsessive-compulsive disorder (OCD) in adults.

Sarafem: For the treatment of premenstrual dysphoric disorder (PMDD) in women.

Unlabeled Use(s): Occasionally doctors may prescribe fluoxetine to treat alcoholism, anorexia nervosa, attention-deficit hyperactivity disorder (ADHD), and a wide variety of other mental and physical disorders.

Precautions:

Do not use in the following situations:

allergy to fluoxetine or any of its ingredients
MAOI use, within 14 days
thioridazine use, within 5 weeks

Use with caution in the following situations:

anxiety
diabetes
drug abuse, history of
electroshock therapy
heart attack, recent
heart disease, unstable
insomnia
kidney disease
liver disease
mania/hypomania (psychological disturbances)
seizures, history of
suicide ideation or attempt, history of
weight and appetite, changes in

Diabetes: Decreased blood sugar (glucose) levels (hypoglycemia) have occurred during therapy, and increased blood sugar levels (hyperglycemia) have developed following discontinuation of the drug. The dosage of insulin or the blood glucose-lowering drug may need to be adjusted when fluoxetine is started or discontinued.

Rash and Possible Allergic Events: Approximately 7% of patients have developed a rash or hives. Almost one-third were withdrawn from treatment. Most patients improved promptly with discontinuation of fluoxetine or with treatment with antihistamines or steroids.

Suicidal Tendencies: Data from clinical trial studies have failed to show an increased rate or risk of suicide among patients taking fluoxetine. Because suicide may be a complication of unresponsive depression or OCD, any suicidal thoughts or tendencies should be reported to your doctor.

Pregnancy: Studies in pregnant women have not shown a risk to the fetus. However, the drug should not be used during pregnancy unless clearly needed and the potential benefits to the mother outweigh the possible hazards to the fetus.

Breastfeeding: Fluoxetine appears in breast milk. Use of fluoxetine in nursing mothers is not recommended. Consult your doctor before you begin breastfeeding.

Children: Safety and effectiveness in children have not been established.

Elderly: Fluoxetine has not been sufficiently evaluated in older patients; however, several hundred elderly patients have participated in clinical studies and no unusual adverse age-related problems have been identified.

Drug Interactions:

Tell your doctor or pharmacist if you are taking or if you are planning to take any over-the-counter or prescription medications or dietary supplements while taking fluoxetine. Doses of one or both drugs may need to be modified or a different drug may need to be prescribed. The following drugs and drug classes interact with fluoxetine:

antidepressants (eg, doxepin)
benzodiazepines (eg, diazepam)
carbamazepine (eg, *Tegretol*)
clozapine (eg, *Clozaril*)
cyproheptadine (eg, *Periactin*)
dextromethorphan HBr (eg, *Drixoral*)
haloperidol (eg, *Haldol*)
hydantoins (eg, phenytoin)
lithium (eg, *Eskalith*)
MAOIs (eg, phenelzine)
sumatriptan (eg, *Imitrex*)
thioridazine (eg, *Mellaril*)
tryptophan
warfarin (eg, *Coumadin*)

Side Effects:

Every drug is capable of producing side effects. Many fluoxetine users experience no, or minor, side effects. The frequency and severity of side effects depend on many factors including dose, duration of therapy, and individual susceptibility. Possible side effects include:

Digestive Tract: Stomach upset; indigestion; vomiting; nausea; appetite changes; diarrhea; constipation; gas; dark, bloody stools or vomit; dry mouth.

Nervous System: Tremors; anxiety; nervousness; dizziness; lightheadedness; drowsiness; headache; sleeplessness; fatigue; weakness; decreased concentration; sensation disturbances; abnormal dreams or thinking; memory loss; confusion; psychological disturbances; agitation; twitching.

Circulatory System: Palpitations (pounding in the chest); chest pain; hot flashes; flushing.

Respiratory System: Flu-like syndrome; nasal congestion; sinus headache; sinus infection; cough; yawn; painful or difficult breathing.

Skin: Rash; hives; itching; sweating; acne.

Urinary and Reproductive Tract: Painful menstruation; sexual dysfunction; impotence; changes in sex drive; frequent urination; urinary tract infections.

Rash and Accompanying Events – Fever; edema (fluid retention); carpal tunnel syndrome; respiratory distress; joint pain; protein in urine; abnormal blood counts; swollen lymph nodes; abnormal enzyme levels.

Other: Fever; back, leg, arm, or muscle pain; vision disturbances; taste changes; ringing in the ears; chills; muscle cramps; viral infections; weight changes; accidental injury.

Guidelines for Use:

- Dosage is individualized. Take exactly as prescribed.
- Because this medicine may cause sleeplessness when taken in the evening, take doses as early as possible in the day. Single doses should be taken in the morning. Twice daily doses should be taken in the morning and at noon.
- May be taken with or without food.
- Do not crush, chew, or open delayed-release capsules. Swallow whole.
- If a dose is missed, take it as soon as possible. If several hours have passed or if it is nearing time for the next dose, do not double the dose to catch up unless advised by your doctor. If more than one dose is missed, or it is necessary to establish a new dosage schedule, contact your doctor or pharmacist.
- *Diabetes* — Monitor blood glucose levels daily. Notify your doctor if low blood sugar (fatigue, excessive hunger, profuse sweating, numbness of extremities) occurs, or if excessive thirst, excessive urination, or other symptoms of high blood sugar levels occur (glucose or ketones in the urine or blood).
- Do not use in combination with MAOIs or within 14 days of discontinuing treatment with an MAOI. After stopping fluoxetine, wait at least 5 weeks before starting an MAOI.
- Use with caution in individuals with a history of attempted suicide or suicidal thoughts.
- Avoid using alcohol or other depressants (eg, pain relievers, sedatives, antihistamines) that may cause drowsiness or other side effects.
- May cause drowsiness, dizziness, or impaired judgment. Use caution while driving or performing other tasks requiring alertness, coordination, or physical dexterity.
- Consult your doctor or pharmacist before taking nonprescription or prescription drugs or dietary supplements.
- Notify your doctor if you are pregnant or intend to become pregnant, or if you are breastfeeding.
- Notify your doctor if rash or hives develop, if anxiety or nervousness become troublesome, or if extreme appetite loss develops (especially in underweight patients).
- Improvement may not be seen for several days to a few weeks.
- Store at room temperature (59° to 86°F). Protect from light.

If you have any questions, consult your doctor, pharmacist, or health care provider.

	Generic Name *Brand Name Example*	Supplied As	Generic Available
Rx	**Fluvoxamine Maleate**		
	Luvox	**Tablets**: 25 mg, 50 mg, 100 mg	Yes

Type of Drug:

Antidepressant; mood elevating agent.

How the Drug Works:

It is believed that fluvoxamine maleate adjusts or balances how the brain and nervous system produce and respond to their natural chemicals (called neurotransmitters). Fluvoxamine maleate inhibits the reuptake of serotonin by the brain.

Uses:

For the treatment of obsessions and compulsions in patients with obsessive-compulsive disorder (OCD).

Precautions:

Do not use in the following situations:

- allergy to fluvoxamine or any of its ingredients
- MAOI use (eg, phenelzine), within 14 days
- pimozide use, concurrent
- thioridazine use, concurrent

Use with caution in the following situations:

- attempted suicide, history of
- benzodiazepine (eg, alprazolam) use, concurrent
- elderly
- liver disease
- mania/hypomania, history of
- seizures, history of

Smoking: This medicine may not be as effective if you are a smoker.

Pregnancy: There are no adequate and well-controlled studies in pregnant women. Use only if clearly needed and the potential benefits to the mother outweigh the possible hazards to the fetus.

Breastfeeding: Fluvoxamine appears in breast milk. Consult your doctor before you begin breastfeeding.

Children: Safety and effectiveness are not established in children younger than 8 years of age.

Elderly: Use lower initial doses; then increase gradually if necessary.

Drug Interactions:

Tell your doctor or pharmacist if you are taking or if you are planning to take any over-the-counter or prescription medications or dietary supplements while taking fluvoxamine. Doses of one or both drugs may need to be modified or a different drug may need to be prescribed. The following drugs and drug classes interact with fluvoxamine:

benzodiazepines (eg, alprazolam)
carbamazapine (eg, *Tegretol*)
clozapine (eg, *Clozaril*)
diltiazem (eg, *Cardizem*)
lithium (eg, *Lithobid*)
methadone (eg, *Dolophine*)
MAOIs (eg, phenelzine)
phenytoin (eg, *Dilantin*)
pimozide (*Orap*)
propranolol (eg, *Inderal*)
quinidine (eg, *Quinora*)
sumatriptan (*Imitrex*)
tacrine (*Cognex*)
theophylline (eg, *Theo-Dur*)
thioridazine (eg, *Mellaril*)
tricyclic antidepressants (eg, amitriptyline)
tryptophan
warfarin (eg, *Coumadin*)

Side Effects:

Every drug is capable of producing side effects. Many fluvoxamine users experience no, or minor, side effects. The frequency and severity of side effects depend on many factors including dose, duration of therapy, and individual susceptibility. Possible side effects include:

Digestive Tract: Nausea; vomiting; constipation; indigestion; diarrhea; stomach pain; appetite loss; gas; dry mouth; difficulty swallowing; tooth disorder; sore throat.

Nervous System: Headache; memory loss; apathy; twitching; sleeplessness; nervousness; agitation; anxiety; dizziness; drowsiness; depression; weakness; tremors; mania; unstable emotions; CNS stimulation; abnormal thinking; psychotic reaction.

Circulatory System: Rapid heart beat; changes in blood pressure; fainting; flushing; palpitations (pounding in the chest).

Respiratory System: Nasal congestion; yawn; difficulty breathing; cough; sinus problems; upper respiratory tract infection.

Other: Sweating; taste changes; vision problems; frequent urination; decreased sex drive; inability to achieve orgasm; abnormal ejaculation; painful menstruation; muscular hyperactivity; infection; leg cramps; rash; muscle tension; urinary retention; muscle pain; unusual bruising; nosebleed; abnormal liver enzymes; decreased mobility or movement; general body discomfort; flu-like syndrome; weight changes; chills; swelling of feet, ankles, or hands.

Guidelines for Use:

- Dosage is individualized. Take exactly as prescribed.
- Usual adult starting dose is 50 mg, taken as a single dose at bedtime. The dosage may be increased by 50 mg/day every 4 to 7 days, if necessary, to achieve maximum benefit. The total dosage should not exceed 300 mg/day. Total doses greater than 100 mg should be taken in 2 divided doses. If the doses are not equal, the larger dose should be taken at bedtime.
- Usual pediatric (8 to 17 years of age) starting dose is 25 mg at bedtime. The dosage may be increased by 25 mg/day every 4 to 7 days, if necessary, to achieve maximum benefit. The total dosage should not exceed 200 mg/day. Total doses greater than 50 mg should be taken in 2 divided doses. If the doses are not equal, the larger dose should be given at bedtime.
- Do not discontinue the medication or change the dose unless directed by your doctor.
- May be taken without regard to food.
- If a dose is missed, take it as soon as possible. If several hours have passed or if it is nearing time for the next dose, do not double the dose to catch up, unless advised by your doctor. If more than one dose is missed or it is necessary to establish a new dosage schedule, contact your doctor or pharmacist.
- Contact your doctor if you develop a rash, hives, other allergic reactions, or seizures. Also contact your doctor if nausea, dry mouth, sleeplessness, or drowsiness become troublesome.
- May cause drowsiness, dizziness, or impaired judgement. Use caution while driving or performing other tasks requiring alertness, coordination, or physical dexterity.
- Do not use in combination with MAOIs or within 14 days of discontinuing treatment with an MAOI. After stopping treatment with this medication, wait at least 2 weeks before starting an MAOI.
- Avoid alcohol and smoking while using this medication. Smoking may reduce the effectiveness of the medication.
- Inform your doctor if you are pregnant, become pregnant, are planning to become pregnant, or if you are breastfeeding.
- Store at controlled room temperature (59° to 86°F) in a tightly closed container. Protect from moisture.

If you have any questions, consult your doctor, pharmacist, or health care provider.

	Generic Name *Brand Name Example*	Supplied As	Generic Available
Rx	**Citalopram Hydrobromide**		
	Celexa	**Tablets:** 20 mg, 40 mg	No

Type of Drug:

Antidepressant; mood-elevating agent.

How the Drug Works:

Citalopram blocks the uptake of a chemical found in the brain (serotonin) which increases the activity of this chemical, resulting in improved mood.

Uses:

To treat depression.

Precautions:

Do not use in the following situations:

- allergy to citalopram or any of its ingredients
- monoamine oxidase inhibitor (MAOI) use, concurrent or within 14 days

Use with caution in the following situations:

- alcohol use
- diseases that produce altered metabolic or hemodynamic responses (eg, congestive heart failure)
- kidney disease, severe
- liver disease
- mania, history
- seizure disorder, history
- sodium levels, low
- suicidal tendencies

Pregnancy: Adequate studies have not been done in pregnant women. Use only if clearly needed and potential benefits outweigh the possible hazards to the fetus.

Breastfeeding: Citalopram appears in breast milk. A decision should be made whether to discontinue nursing or discontinue the drug, taking into account the risks to the infant of citalopram exposure (eg, excessive drowsiness, decreased feeding, weight loss) and the importance of the drug to the mother. Consult your doctor before you begin breastfeeding.

Children: Safety and effectiveness in children have not been established.

Elderly: Older individuals may be more sensitive to the effects of citalopram than younger individuals. The recommended dose for most elderly patients is 20 mg/day with titration to 40 mg/day only for nonresponding patients.

Drug Interactions:

Tell your doctor if you are taking or are planning to take any over-the-counter or prescription medications while taking citalopram. Doses of one or both drugs may need to be modified or a different drug may need to be prescribed. The following drugs and drug classes interact with citalopram:

- alcohol
- carbamazepine (eg, *Tegretol*)
- cimetidine (eg, *Tagamet*)
- CNS drugs (eg, antidepressants)
- CYP2C19 inhibitors (eg, omeprazole)
- CYP3A4 inhibitors (eg, ketoconazole, erythromycin)
- imipramine (eg, *Tofranil*)
- lithium (eg, *Lithobid*)
- metoprolol (eg, *Lopressor*)
- monoamine oxidase inhibitors (MAOIs) (eg, phenelzine)
- tricyclic antidepressants (eg, amitriptyline)

Side Effects:

Every drug is capable of producing side effects. Many citalopram users experience no, or minor, side effects. The frequency and severity of side effects depend on many factors including dose, duration of therapy, and individual susceptibility. Possible side effects include:

Digestive Tract: Nausea; dry mouth; vomiting; diarrhea; indigestion; stomach pain; gas; increased salivation; appetite changes.

Nervous System: Dizziness; sleeplessness; drowsiness; agitation; tremor; fatigue; weakness; anxiety; impaired concentration; amnesia; apathy; worsening of depression; suicide attempt; confusion; headache.

Circulatory System: Decreased heart rate; fast heartbeat; postural (standing) low blood pressure; low blood pressure.

Respiratory System: Upper respiratory tract infection; runny nose; sinus infection; coughing.

Urinary and Reproductive Tract: Painful menstruation; absence of menstruation; excessive urination; ejaculation disorder; decreased sex drive; impotence.

Other: Rash; itching; increased sweating; fever; abnormal skin sensations (eg, burning, prickling, tingling); joint or muscle pain; yawning; weight changes; taste pereception changes.

Guidelines for Use:

- Dosage is individualized. Take exactly as prescribed.
- Do not stop taking or change the dose unless directed by your doctor.
- Usual adult starting dose is 20 mg/day as a single dose. If necessary, dose may be increased to 40 mg/day after at least 1 week.
- Take once daily, in the morning or evening, with or without food.
- For most elderly patients and patients with liver disease, 20 mg/day is the recommended dose, with titration to 40 mg/day only for non-responding patients.
- If a dose is missed, inhale it as soon as possible. If several hours have passed or it is nearing time for the next dose, do not double the dose to catch up, unless directed by your doctor. If more than one dose is missed or if it is necessary to establish a new dosage schedule, contact your doctor or pharmacist.
- Contact your doctor if you experience suicidal thoughts, sexual problems, appetite loss, nausea, vomiting, weight gain, restlessness, irritability, confusion, or excessive urination.
- Citalopram should not be used in combination with an MAOI, or within 14 days of discontinuing treatment with an MAOI. At least 14 days should be allowed after stopping citalopram before starting an MAOI.
- May cause drowsiness or dizziness. Use caution while driving or performing other tasks requiring alertness, coordination, or physical dexterity.
- Avoid alcohol while taking citalopram.
- Inform your doctor if you are pregnant, become pregnant, are planning to become pregnant, or are breastfeeding.
- Improvement in depression may be noticed in 1 to 4 weeks. Continue to take citalopram as directed even though your depression has improved.
- Contact your doctor if adverse reactions persist and become bothersome.
- Store at controlled room temperature (59° to 86°F).

If you have any questions, consult your doctor, pharmacist, or health care provider.

	Generic Name *Brand Name Examples*	Supplied As	Generic Available
Rx	**Maprotiline HCl**	**Tablets**: 25 mg, 50 mg, 75 mg	Yes
Rx	**Mirtazapine**		
	Remeron	**Tablets**: 15 mg, 30 mg, 45 mg	No
	Remeron SolTab	**Tablets, orally disintegrating**: 15 mg, 30 mg, 45 mg	No

Type of Drug:

Antidepressant; mood-elevating agent.

How the Drug Works:

The exact mechanism of action is not known. It is believed that tetracyclic antidepressants adjust or balance how the brain and nervous system produce and respond to natural chemicals (neurotransmitters) that elevate mood.

Uses:

Maprotiline: To treat depressive illness in patients with depressive neurosis (dysthymic disorder) and manic-depressive illness (major depressive episode).

Mirtazapine: To treat depression.

Unlabeled Use(s): Maprotiline is also effective for the relief of anxiety associated with depression.

Precautions:

Do not use in the following situations:

allergy to the tetracyclic compound or any of its ingredients
electroshock therapy, concurrent (maprotiline only)
heart attack, acute phase (maprotiline only)
MAOI therapy (eg, phenelzine), within 14 days
seizure disorders, known or suspected (maprotiline only)

Use with caution in the following situations:

abnormal blood counts (mirtazapine only)
alcohol use
anesthetics, general
angina (chest pain), history of
CNS depressant (eg, barbiturates) use
elderly
glaucoma, narrow-angle, history of (maprotiline only)
heart attack, history of
heart disease, significant
high blood pressure therapy
hyperthyroid, history of (maprotiline only)
increased intraocular pressure (maprotiline only)
kidney disease (mirtazapine only)
liver disease (mirtazapine only)
mania or hypomania, history of
seizures, history of
stroke, history of
suicidal tendencies
surgery (maprotiline only)
urinary retention, history of (maprotiline only)

Seizures: Maprotiline use has been associated with seizures. The risk is higher in patients with a history of seizures, in patients taking phenothiazines (eg, promethazine), or when benzodiazepines (eg, alprazolam) are being withdrawn.

Pregnancy: There are no adequate or well-controlled studies in pregnant women. Use only if clearly needed and the potential benefits to the mother outweigh the possible hazards to the fetus.

Breastfeeding: Maprotiline appears in breast milk. It is not known if mirtazapine appears in breast milk. Consult your doctor before you begin breastfeeding.

Children: Safety and effectiveness in children (younger than 18 years of age for maprotiline) have not been established.

Elderly: The elimination of mirtazapine is reduced in elderly patients. In general, lower doses of maprotiline are recommended for patients older than 60 years of age. Use with caution in elderly patients.

Lab tests may be required periodically during treatment. Lab tests may include blood counts and enzyme levels.

Drug Interactions:

Tell your doctor or pharmacist if you are taking or are planning to take any over-the-counter or prescription medications or dietary supplements while taking a tetracyclic compound. Doses of one or both drugs may need to be modified or a different drug may need to be prescribed. The following drugs and drug classes interact with tetracyclic compounds:

alcohol
barbiturates (eg, phenobarbital)
benzodiazepines (eg, alprazolam)
MAOI antidepressants (eg, phenelzine)
phenothiazines (eg, promethazine) (maprotiline only)
thyroid hormones (eg, thyroid desiccated) (maprotiline only)

Side Effects:

Every drug is capable of producing side effects. Many tetracyclic compound users experience no, or minor, side effects. The frequency and severity of side effects depend on many factors including dose, duration of therapy, and individual susceptibility. Possible side effects include:

Digestive Tract: Nausea; vomiting; constipation; dry mouth; thirst; increased appetite; stomach pain; indigestion.

Nervous System: Confusion; anxiety; agitation; abnormal thinking; nervousness; tremor; twitching; drowsiness; clumsiness; dizziness; vertigo (feeling of whirling motion); weakness; fatigue; tiredness; sleeplessness; headache; abnormal dreams; increased sensitivity; apathy; depression; memory loss; numbness or tingling in the hands or feet.

Respiratory System: Difficulty breathing; cough; sinus problems; wheezing.

Circulatory System: Rapid heart rate; irregular heartbeat; increased cholesterol and triglyceride levels; increased blood pressure; low blood pressure on arising.

Skin: Rash; itching; hives; acne; dry skin; flushing; redness; hair loss.

Other: Flu syndrome; general body discomfort; swelling in the hands or feet; blurred vision; muscle, joint, or back pain; frequent urination; urinary tract infection.

Guidelines for Use:

- Dosage is individualized. Take exactly as prescribed.
- Do not stop taking or change the dose unless directed by your doctor.
- *Maprotiline* — May be given as a single daily dose or in divided doses.
- *Mirtazapine* — Take in a single dose, preferably at bedtime. May be taken without regard to food.
- *Remeron SolTabs*— Open tablet blisterpack with dry hands and place the tablet on the tongue. The tablet will disintegrate rapidly and can be swallowed with saliva. No water is needed. Do not chew the tablet, split the tablet, or store the tablet for later use.
- If a dose is missed, take it as soon as possible. If several hours have passed or it is nearing time for the next dose, do not double the dose to catch up, unless advised to do so by your doctor. If more than one dose is missed or it is necessary to establish a new dosage schedule, contact your doctor or pharmacist.
- Avoid the use of alcohol, barbiturates, or other CNS depressants (eg, tranquilizers) while taking this medicine.
- Contact your doctor if you experience sore throat, fever, chills, mouth sores, or other signs of infection. Pay particular attention to any flu-like symptoms or other symptoms that might suggest infection.
- May cause drowsiness or dizziness. Alcohol use may increase this effect. Use caution while driving or performing other tasks requiring alertness, coordination, or physical dexterity.
- Allow at least 14 days between discontinuation of an MAO inhibitor antidepressant (eg, phenelzine) and the start of therapy with this medicine. Also, allow at least 14 days after stopping this medicine before starting an MAO inhibitor.
- Maprotiline has been associated with seizures. This risk is higher in patients with a history of seizures, in patients taking phenothiazines (eg, promethazine) or withdrawing from benzodiazepines (eg, alprazolam).
- Inform your doctor if you are pregnant, become pregnant, are plan to become pregnant, or are breastfeeding.
- *Maprotiline* — Beneficial effects are sometimes seen within 3 to 7 days, although 2 to 3 weeks are usually necessary.
- *Mirtazapine* — Beneficial effects may take 1 to 4 weeks to occur.
- Lab tests may be required to monitor therapy. Be sure to keep appointments.
- Store at room temperature (59° to 86°F) in a tightly closed container, away from light and moisture.

If you have any questions, consult your doctor, pharmacist, or health care provider.

	Generic Name *Brand Name Examples*	Supplied As	Generic Available
Rx	**Isocarboxazid**		
	Marplan	**Tablets:** 10 mg	No
Rx	**Phenelzine**		
	Nardil	**Tablets:** 15 mg	No
Rx	**Tranylcypromine Sulfate**		
	Parnate	**Tablets:** 10 mg	No

Type of Drug:

Antidepressants; mood-elevating agents; MAOIs.

How the Drug Works:

Monoamine oxidase inhibitors (MAOIs) prevent the breakdown of the body's own mood-elevating substances. The effect may take several weeks to be noticed.

Uses:

To treat chronic (long-term) depression in patients who have not responded satisfactorily to other antidepressants. They are rarely used as first-line antidepressant therapy.

Unlabeled Use(s): Occasionally doctors may prescribe MAOIs for bulimia and panic disorder associated with agoraphobia (fear of open or public places) and globus hystericus syndrome (choking sensation associated with hysteria). Phenelzine has been investigated for use as an aid in treating cocaine addiction, night terrors, post-traumatic stress disorder, and migraines resistant to other therapies. Tranylcypromine has been used to treat Binswanger's encephalopathy, seasonal affective disorder, and subjective symptoms of multiple sclerosis.

Precautions:

Do not use in the following situations:

- allergy to MAOIs or any of their ingredients
- cerebrovascular defect, confirmed or suspected (eg, stroke)
- dibenzapine-related agents (eg, tricyclic antidepressants)
- headaches, history of severe or frequent
- heart disease (eg, congestive heart failure)
- high blood pressure
- kidney disease, severe
- liver disease
- liver function tests, abnormal
- other MAOIs, concurrent therapy
- pheochromocytoma (adrenal gland tumor)
- sympathomimetics (eg, amphetamine), concurrent use

Use with caution in the following situations:

- anesthetic agents, concurrent use
- angina, history
- antihypertensives, (eg, thiazide diuretics, rauwolfia alkaloids)
- bupropion, concurrent use

buspirone, concurrent use
caffeine, concurrent use
CNS depressants (eg, alcohol, narcotics, barbiturates)
debilitated patients
dextromethorphan, concurrent use
diabetes
elderly
kidney disease
low blood pressure
meperidine, concurrent use
overactive thyroid
schizophrenia
seizures, history
SSRIs, concurrent use (eg, fluoxetine, sertraline, paroxetine)
suicidal thoughts
tyramine-containing foods (see Precautions)

Drug abuse and dependence: Drug abuse and dependence have been reported in patients using excessive doses of tranylcypromine and isocarboxazid. Some of these patients had a history of substance abuse. The following withdrawal symptoms have been reported: Restlessness; anxiety; depression; confusion; hallucinations; headaches; weakness; diarrhea.

Hypertensive Crisis: Hypertensive crisis (extreme elevations in blood pressure) can result from coadministraton of MAOIs and certain drugs and foods.

Chest pain: MAOIs may suppress chest pain that would otherwise serve as a warning of myocardial ischemia (inadequate circulation of blood to the heart, usually as a result of heart disease).

Liver Dysfunction: Discontinue isocarboxazid use at first sign of liver dysfunction or jaundice (yellowing of skin or eyes).

Depression: Tranylcypromine and isocarboxazid may aggravate coexisting symptoms in depression, such as anxiety and agitation.

Tyramine-containing foods: Do not eat foods with high tyramine, dopamine, or tryptophan content (see the following listing) during or for 2 weeks after the discontinuation of MAOIs. Any high-protein food that is aged or undergoes breakdown by a putrefaction process to improve flavor is suspected of producing a significant increase in blood pressure in patients taking MAOIs. Do not take any new prescription medication without first reviewing it with your doctor or pharmacist. Do not drink alcoholic beverages or self-medicate with dietary supplements, cold, hay fever, or weight-reducing preparations while undergoing therapy. Do not consume excessive amounts of caffeine in any form, and report headache or other unusual symptoms promptly.

***Tyramine-Containing Foods*[1]**

Cheese/Dairy Products: American; blue; boursault; brie; camembert; cheddar; swiss; emmenthaler; gruyere; mozzarella; parmesan; romano; roquefort; stilton; sour cream; yogurt.

Meat/Fish: Beef or chicken liver, other meats, fish (unrefrigerated, fermented, spoiled, smoked, pickled); meats prepared with tenderizer; fermented sausages (bologna, pepperoni, salami, summer sausage); game meat; caviar; dried fish (salted herring); herring (pickled, spoiled); shrimp paste; anchovies; dry sausage; meat extracts.

Alcoholic Beverages (undistilled): Beer (imports, some nonalcoholic); red wine (especially Chianti); cherry; distilled spirits; liqueurs.

Fruit/Vegetables: Avocado (especially overripe); yeast extracts (eg, Marmite); bananas; figs (canned, overripe); dried fruits (eg, raisins, prunes); soy sauce; miso soup; bean curd; sauerkraut; raspberries.

[1] Tyramine contents are not predictable and may vary. The amounts of tyramine are estimated from low to very high.

Other Problem Foods: Broad beans (fava beans, overripe); chocolate; caffeine (eg, coffee, tea, colas); ginseng.

Pregnancy: Safety for use during pregnancy has not been established. Use during pregnancy or in women of childbearing age only when clearly needed and when the potential benefits outweigh the potential hazards to the fetus.

Breastfeeding: Tranylcypromine appears in breast milk. It is not known if the other MAOIs appear in breast milk. Because of the potential for serious adverse effects in the nursing infant, decide whether to discontinue nursing or the drug, taking into account the importance of the drug to the mother. Consult your doctor before you begin breastfeeding.

Children: Use in children younger than 16 years of age is not recommended.

Elderly: The most serious reactions to MAOI use involve changes in blood pressure. Older patients may suffer more problems than younger patients during and following an episode of increased blood pressure or malignant hyperthermia (extremely high fever). Older patients have less compensatory reserve to cope with any serious adverse reactions. Use with caution in the elderly.

Lab tests may be required to monitor therapy. Tests may include periodic liver chemistry (isocarboxazid).

Drug Interactions:

Tell your doctor or pharmacist if you are taking or if you are planning to take any over-the-counter or prescription medications or dietary supplements with MAOIs. Doses of one or both drugs may need to be modified or a different drug may need to be prescribed. The following drugs and drug classes interact with MAOIs:

- anesthetic agents (eg, anesthesia, cocaine)
- anorexiants (eg, amphetamine, phentermine)
- antidiabetic agents (eg, insulin, sulfonylureas, glyburide, tolbutamide)
- antihypertensives (eg, thiazide diuretics, rauwolfia alkaloids)
- beta blockers (eg, metoprolol, nadolol)
- buproprion HCl (eg, *Zyban*)
- buspirone HCl (*BuSpar*)
- caffeine
- CNS depressants (eg, alcohol, narcotics, barbiturates)
- dextromethorphan (eg, *Robitussin DM*)
- dibenzapine-related agents (eg, tricyclic antidepressants, carbamazepine, cyclobenzaprine)
- disulfiram (eg, *Antabuse*)
- guanethidine (eg, *Ismelin*)
- levodopa (eg, *Larodopa*)
- MAOIs, other
- meperidine (eg, *Demerol*)
- methyldopa (eg, *Aldomet*)
- methylphenidate HCl (eg, *Ritalin*)
- metrizamide (*Amipaque*)
- phenylpropanolamine (eg, *Propagest)*
- pseudoephedrine (eg, *Sudafed)*
- selective serotonin reuptake inhibitors (SSRIs) (eg, citalopram, fluoxetine)
- sulfonamides (eg, sulfisoxazole, paroxetine)
- sumatriptan (*Imitrex*)
- sympathomimetics (eg, metaraminol, phenylephrine)
- tyramine-containing foods or beverages (see Precautions)

Side Effects:

Every drug is capable of producing side effects. Many MAOI users experience no, or minor, side effects. The frequency and severity of side effects depend on many factors including dose, duration of therapy, and individual susceptibility. Possible side effects include:

Digestive Tract: Nausea; constipation; diarrhea; stomach pain; appetite loss.

Nervous System: Hyperactivity; tremor; muscle twitching; unusual muscle movements; headache; dizziness; faintness; anxiety; jitteriness; memory impairment; sleep disturbances (eg, sleeplessness, excessively long sleeping periods); weakness; fatigue; drowsiness; restlessness; agitation; exaggerated reflexes; mania (eg, irritability, euphoria, distractability, excitability); abnormal skin sensations; lethargy; sedation.

Circulatory System: Changes in heart rate and rhythm; postural and orthostatic hypotension (dizziness or lightheadedness when rising from a seated or lying position); palpitations (pounding in the chest).

Skin: Rash; itching; sweating; jaundice (yellowing of skin or eyes).

Other: Dilated (widened) pupils; stiff neck; dry mouth; urinary frequency; edema (fluid retention); blurred vision; weight gain; sexual problems; chills; impotence; abnormal blood cell counts; glaucoma; heavy feeling.

Guidelines for Use:

- *Phenelzine* — Recommended initial dosage is 15 mg 3 times daily. Increase dose to at least 60 mg/day at a fairly rapid pace consistent with patient tolerance. It may be necessary to increase dose up to 90 mg/day to obtain sufficient MAO inhibition. Many patients do not show clinical response until treatment at 60 mg has been continued for 4 weeks or more. After maximum benefit is achieved, reduce dose slowly over several weeks. Maintenance dosage may be as low as 15 mg/day or 15 mg every other day; continued for as long as required.
- *Tranylcypromine* — The usual effective dose is 30 mg/day in divided doses. Improvement should be seen within 48 hours to 3 weeks after starting therapy. If there is no improvement after 2 weeks, increase dose in 10 mg/day increments at 1- to 3-week intervals. Dosage range may be extended to a maximum of 60 mg/day from the usual 30 mg/day. Gradually withdraw tranylcypromine when discontinuing therapy.
- *Isocarboxazid* — Recommended initial dosage is 10 mg twice daily. If tolerated, increase by 10 mg every 2 to 4 days to achieve a dose of 40 mg by the end of the first week of treatment. Dose can then be increased by increments of up to 20 mg/week, if needed and tolerated, to a maximum recommended dose of 60 mg/day. Daily dose should be divided into 2 to 4 doses. After a maximum clinical response is achieved, attempt to reduce the dose slowly over a period of several weeks without jeopardizing therapeutic response. Beneficial effect may not be seen in some patients for 3 to 6 weeks. If no response is obtained by then, discontinue therapy. Caution is indicated in patients for whom a dose of 40 mg/day is exceeded.
- Do not discontinue this medication or adjust dosage except on the advice of your doctor. Consult your doctor before taking any other medication, including nonprescription items, while taking an MAOI.
- This medicine may take several weeks to become effective. Continue to take as directed.
- If a dose is missed, take it as soon as possible. If several hours have passed or if it is nearing time for the next dose, do not double the dose in order to catch up, unless advised to do so by your doctor. If more than one dose is missed, or it is necessary to establish a new dosage schedule, contact your doctor.
- Avoid tyramine-containing foods, alcohol, caffeine, and tryptophan (see Precautions).
- May cause drowsiness or blurred vision. Use caution while driving or performing other tasks requiring alertness, coordination, or physical dexterity.
- Dizziness, weakness, or fainting may occur when rising from a lying or sitting position. If this occurs, get up slowly.
- At doses over 30 mg/day, postural hypotension (dizziness or lightheadedness when rising from a seated or lying position) is a major side effect and may result in fainting. Dosage increases will be more gradual in patients showing a tendency toward low blood pressure at the beginning of therapy. Postural hypotension may be relieved by lying down until blood pressure returns to normal.

Guidelines for Use (cont.):

- Hypertensive crises (increase in blood pressure) as a result of concurrent use of MAOI and certain foods or drugs (see Precautions) can occur and are potentially fatal. These crises usually occur within several hours after ingestion of the interacting food or drug. Notify your doctor immediately if you experience a headache that starts in the back of the head and moves forward, pounding in the chest, neck stiffness or soreness, nausea, vomiting, sweating (sometimes with fever or cold, clammy skin), dilated pupils, sensitivity to light, or changes in heart rate with or without chest pain or tightness.
- Notify your doctor if rash or intolerable side effects occur.
- Use may complicate other medical treatment (eg, general anesthesia, surgery). Inform your doctors and dentist about your use of MAOIs. Wear a Medic Alert bracelet or carry a card saying that you are taking an MAOI.
- A waiting period of 10 to 14 days is recommended when switching from one MAOI to another or from a dibenzazepine-related agent. Other medications that interact with MAOIs (eg, fluoxetine) have different waiting periods. Discuss appropriate waiting periods for changes in therapy with your doctor or pharmacist.
- Blood pressure will need to be monitored frequently.
- Lab tests may be required to monitor therapy. Be sure to keep appointments.
- Store at room temperature.

If you have any questions, consult your doctor, pharmacist, or health care provider.

	Generic Name *Brand Name Examples*	Supplied As	Generic Available
Rx	**Paroxetine HCl**		
	Paxil	**Tablets:** 10 mg, 20 mg, 30 mg, 40 mg	No
	Paxil	**Suspension, oral:** 10 mg/5 mL	No
	Paxil CR	**Tablets, controlled-release:** 12.5 mg, 25 mg	No

Type of Drug:

Antidepressant (SSRI); mood-elevating agent.

How the Drug Works:

Paroxetine blocks neuronal reuptake of serotonin in the central nervous system, which potentiates serotogenic activity and combats depression and other behavioral disorders.

Uses:

Tablets/Suspension: To treat mental depression, social anxiety disorder, obsessive-compulsive disorder (OCD), and panic disorder with or without agoraphobia (fear of open places).

Controlled-release tablets: To treat mental depression.

Precautions:

Do not use in the following situations:

- allergy to paroxetine or any of its ingredients
- current or recent (14 days or less) use of a monoamine oxidase inhibitor (MAOI)

Use with caution in the following situations:

- alcohol use
- diuretic therapy, concurrent use
- drug abuse, history of
- illness affecting metabolism or hemodynamic responses (eg, congestive heart failure)
- kidney disease
- liver disease
- mania, history of
- seizures, history of
- suicide, high-risk of

Pregnancy: Adequate studies have not been done in pregnant women. Use only if clearly needed and potential benefits outweigh the possible hazards to the fetus.

Breastfeeding: Paroxetine appears in breast milk. Consult your doctor before breastfeeding.

Children: Safety and effectiveness in children have not been established.

Elderly: Initial dosage in the elderly should be reduced.

Drug Interactions:

Tell your doctor or pharmacist if you are taking or if you are planning to take any over-the-counter or prescription medications or dietary supplements while taking paroxetine. Doses of one or both drugs may need to be modified or a different drug may need to be prescribed. The following drugs and drug classes interact with paroxetine:

- alcohol
- antidepressants (eg, nortriptyline, imipramine, fluoxetine)
- cimetidine (eg, *Tagamet*)
- cyproheptadine (eg, *Periactin*)
- L-tryptophan
- MAOIs (eg, phenelzine)
- phenobarbital (eg, *Solfoton*)
- phenothiazines (eg, thioridazine)
- phenytoin (eg, *Dilantin*)
- procyclidine (*Kemadrin*)
- quinidine (eg, *Quinora*)
- sumatriptan (*Imitrex*)
- theophylline (eg, *Slo-Phyllin*)
- type 1C antiarrhythmics (eg, propafenone)
- warfarin (eg, *Coumadin*)

Side Effects:

Every drug is capable of producing side effects. Many paroxetine users experience no or minor side effects. The frequency and severity of side effects depend on many factors including dose, duration of therapy, and individual susceptibility. Possible side effects include:

Circulatory System: Chest pain; palpitations (pounding in the chest); high blood pressure; rapid heart rate.

Digestive Tract: Nausea; diarrhea; vomiting; constipation; gas; indigestion; appetite changes; dry mouth.

Nervous System: Drowsiness; sleeplessness; agitation; tremor; anxiety; weakness; headache; dizziness; nervousness; confusion; twitching; amnesia; inability to concentrate; abnormal dreams; depression; unstable emotions; vertigo (feeling of whirling motion).

Other: Abnormal ejaculation and other male genital disorders; back pain; joint pain; muscle weakness or pain; tightness in throat; abnormal skin sensations; decreased sex drive; blurred vision; runny nose; taste perversion; urinary frequency; urinary disorder; female genital disorders; chills; general body discomfort; fainting; edema (fluid retention); weight changes.

Respiratory System: Yawning; sore throat; cough; congestion.

Skin: Flushing; sweating; rash; itching.

Guidelines for Use:

- Dosage will be individualized. Small doses are usually used at first and then gradually increased until the desired benefit is obtained. Dosage changes are usually made at intervals more than 1 week.
- Take once daily, preferably in the morning, without regard to meals. Take with food if stomach upset occurs.
- Do not change the dose or stop taking this drug unless advised to do so by your doctor.
- Avoid alcohol when using this drug.
- Do not use in combination with MAOIs (monoamine oxidase inhibitors) or within 14 days of discontinuing treatment with an MAOI. Similarly, at least 2 weeks should be allowed after stopping paroxetine before starting an MAOI.
- May cause drowsiness or dizziness. Use caution while driving or performing other tasks requiring alertness, coordination, or physical dexterity.
- Although improvement may be noticed in 1 to 4 weeks, continue therapy as directed.
- Shake oral suspension well before using.
- Do not chew or crush controlled-release tablets. Swallow whole.
- Consult your doctor or pharmacist before taking any nonprescription or prescription drugs while using paroxetine.
- Inform your doctor if you are pregnant, become pregnant, are planning to become pregnant, or are breastfeeding.
- Significant weight loss may be an undesirable effect of paroxetine therapy.
- Store tablets at controlled room temperature (59° to 86°F).
- Store controlled-release tablets between 68° and 77°F.
- Store suspension at or below 77°F.

If you have any questions, consult your doctor, pharmacist, or health care provider.

Generic Name / *Brand Name Example*	Supplied As	Generic Available
Rx **Sertraline HCl**		
Zoloft	**Tablets:** 25 mg, 50 mg, 100 mg	No

Type of Drug:

Antidepressant; SSRI; mood-elevating agent.

How the Drug Works:

The actual antidepressant mechanism of sertraline is not known. It is presumed that it works by blocking the uptake of serotonin, a chemical found in the brain.

Uses:

To treat mental depression, obsessive-compulsive disorder, panic disorder, and post-traumatic stress disorder.

Precautions:

Do not use in the following situations:

allergy to sertraline
monoamine oxidase inhibitor (MAOI) use, concurrent or within 14 days

Use with caution in the following situations:

attempted suicide, history of
illness, systemic
liver disease
mania
seizures, history of

Pregnancy: There are no adequate and well-controlled studies in pregnant women. Use only if clearly needed and potential benefits to the mother outweigh the possible hazards to the fetus.

Breastfeeding: It is not known if sertraline appears in breast milk. Consult your doctor before you begin breastfeeding.

Children: Safety and effectiveness have not been established.

Drug Interactions:

Tell your doctor or pharmacist if you are taking or if you are planning to take any over-the-counter or prescription medications or dietary supplements with sertraline. Doses of one or both drugs may need to be modified or a different drug may need to be prescribed. The following drugs and drug classes interact with sertraline:

cimetidine (eg, *Tagamet*)
clozapine (eg, *Clozaril*)
diazepam (eg, *Valium*)
digitoxin (*Crystodigin*)
flecainide (*Tambocor*)
hydantoins (eg, phenytoin)
lithium (eg, *Eskalith*)
MAO inhibitors (eg, phenelzine)
propafenone (*Rythmol*)
sumatriptan (*Imitrex*)
tolbutamide (eg, *Orinase*)
tricyclic antidepressants (eg, doxepin)
warfarin (eg, *Coumadin*)

Side Effects:

Every drug is capable of producing side effects. Many sertraline users experience no, or minor, side effects. The frequency and severity of side effects depend on many factors including dose, duration of therapy, and individual susceptibility. Possible side effects include:

Digestive Tract: Nausea; vomiting; diarrhea; indigestion; constipation; gas; appetite changes.

Nervous System: Headache; dizziness; tremor; fatigue; nervousness; anxiety; drowsiness; agitation; sleeplessness; decreased or abnormal skin sensations.

Circulatory System: Pounding in the chest; chest pain.

Other: Dry mouth; runny nose; vision disturbances; ringing in the ears; back pain; muscle pain; sexual problems; excessive sweating; rash; yawning; increased muscle tension; weakness; general body discomfort; flushing.

Guidelines for Use:

- Dosage will be individualized.
- Administer once daily, either in the morning or evening.
- Do not use in combination with MAOIs or within 14 days of treatment with an MAOI.
- If a dose is missed, take it as soon as possible. If several hours have passed or if it is nearing time for the next dose, do not double the dose to catch up unless advised to do so by your doctor. If several doses are missed or it is necessary to establish a new dosage schedule, contact your doctor or pharmacist.
- Avoid alcohol when using this drug.
- May cause drowsiness, dizziness, or blurred vision. Use caution while driving or performing other tasks requiring alertness, coordination, or physical dexterity.
- Significant weight loss may be an undesirable effect of sertraline therapy.
- Store at room temperature (59° to 86°F).

If you have any questions, consult your doctor, pharmacist, or health care provider.

Generic Name *Brand Name Examples*	Supplied As	Generic Available
Rx **Trazodone HCl**		
Desyrel	**Tablets:** 50 mg, 100 mg	Yes
Desyrel Dividose	**Tablets:** 150 mg, 300 mg	Yes

Type of Drug:

Antidepressant; mood-elevating agent.

How the Drug Works:

It is not known how trazodone works to relieve depression. It is believed trazodone modifies the chemical balance in the brain, which changes behavior. It does not stimulate the brain.

Uses:

To relieve mental depression.

Unlabeled Use(s): Occasionally doctors may prescribe trazodone for cocaine withdrawal, to manage aggressive behavior when used with other medications, and to treat patients with panic disorder or agoraphobia (fear of open or public places) with panic attacks.

Precautions:

Do not use in the following situations: Allergy to trazodone or any of its ingredients.

Use with caution in the following situations:

- electroshock therapy, concurrent
- heart attack, recent
- heart disease, preexisting
- heart rhythms, abnormal
- high blood pressure
- suicide attempts, history of

Priapism: If you experience prolonged or painful penile erection, discontinue use immediately and consult your doctor. Permanent damage of normal penis function and impotence have occurred.

Pregnancy: There are no adequate and well-controlled studies in pregnant women. Use only if clearly needed and potential benefits to the mother outweigh the possible hazards to the fetus.

Breastfeeding: It is not known if trazodone appears in breast milk. Consult your doctor before you begin breastfeeding.

Children: Safety and effectiveness in children younger than 18 years of age have not been established.

Lab tests may be required to monitor therapy. Tests include blood counts.

Drug Interactions:

Tell your doctor or pharmacist if you are taking or if you are planning to take any over-the-counter or prescription medications or dietary supplements with trazodone. Doses of one or both drugs may need to be modified or a different drug may need to be prescribed. The following drugs and drug classes interact with trazodone:

- anesthetics
- CNS depressants (eg, alcohol, barbiturates, narcotics)
- digoxin (eg, *Lanoxin*)
- phenytoin (eg, *Dilantin*)
- warfarin (eg, *Coumadin*)

Side Effects:

Every drug is capable of producing side effects. Many trazodone users experience no, or minor, side effects. The frequency and severity of side effects depend on many factors including dose, duration of therapy, and individual susceptibility. Possible side effects include:

Digestive Tract: Upset stomach; nausea; vomiting; diarrhea; constipation; decreased appetite; dry mouth.

Nervous System: Anger; hostility; sleeplessness; nightmares or vivid dreams; confusion; disorientation; decreased concentration; dizziness; drowsiness; excitement; fatigue; headache; tremor; impaired memory; nervousness; incoordination; lightheadedness.

Circulatory System: Changes in blood pressure; pounding in the chest; fast heartbeat.

Senses: Ringing in the ears; blurred vision; red, tired, itching eyes; nasal or sinus congestion.

Other: Shortness of breath; weight changes; swelling; aches and pains; fainting; bad taste in the mouth; abnormal skin sensations; general body discomfort; feeling of heaviness or fullness in the head; prolonged painful erection; decreased sex drive; clamminess; sweating; orthostatic hypotension (dizziness or lightheadedness when rising from a sitting or lying position).

Guidelines for Use:

- Dosage is individualized.
- Dosage will be initiated at a low level and increased gradually by your doctor.
- Take shortly after a meal or snack.
- If a dose is missed, take it as soon as possible. If several hours have passed or if it is nearing time for the next dose, do not double the dose to catch up, unless advised to do so by your doctor. If more than one dose is missed, or it is necessary to establish a new dosage schedule, contact your doctor or pharmacist.
- May cause drowsiness, dizziness, or blurred vision. Use caution while driving or performing other tasks requiring alertness, coordination, or physical dexterity.
- Avoid alcohol or other drowsiness-causing medications (eg, antihistamines, barbiturates, narcotic pain relievers) while taking trazodone.
- Notify your doctor if you experience drowsiness, sore throat, fever, or any signs of infection.
- Male patients with prolonged and painful erections (priapism) should immediately discontinue the drug and consult their doctor.
- Lab tests may be required to monitor therapy. Be sure to keep appointments.
- Store at controlled room temperature (59° to 86°F).

If you have any questions, consult your doctor, pharmacist, or health care provider.

	Generic Name *Brand Name Examples*	Supplied As	Generic Available
Rx	**Venlafaxine HCl**		
	Effexor	**Tablets:** 25 mg, 37.5 mg, 50 mg, 75 mg, 100 mg	No
	Effexor XR	**Capsules, extended-release:** 37.5 mg, 75 mg, 150 mg	No

Type of Drug:

Antidepressant; mood-elevating agent

How the Drug Works:

Venlafaxine inhibits neuronal uptake of serotonin and norepinephrine in the central nervous system, which is believed to combat depression and other behavioral disorders.

Uses:

The treatment of depression. The extended-release form is also used to treat generalized anxiety disorder.

Precautions:

Do not use in the following situations:

allergy to venlafaxine
current or recent (within the past 14 days) use of a monoamine oxidase inhibitor (MAOI)

Use with caution in the following situations:

concomitant systemic illness
liver disease
kidney disease
mania, history of
seizures, history of
suicide, high-risk of

Pregnancy: Adequate studies have not been done in pregnant women. Use only if clearly needed and potential benefits to the mother outweigh the possible hazards to the fetus.

Breastfeeding: Venlafaxine appears in breast milk. A decision should be made to either discontinue nursing or discontinue the drug, taking into account the importance of the drug to the mother.

Children: Safety and effectiveness in children younger than 18 years of age have not been established.

Drug Interactions:

Tell your doctor or pharmacist if you are taking or if you are planning to take any over-the-counter or prescription medications or dietary supplements with venlafaxine HCl. Doses of one or both drugs may need to be modified or a different drug may need to be prescribed. The following drugs and drug classes interact with venlafaxine HCl.

MAOIs (eg, phenelzine)
sibutramine (*Meridia*)

Side Effects:

Every drug is capable of producing side effects. Many venlafaxine HCl users experience no or minor side effects. The frequency and severity of side effects depend on many factors including dose, duration of therapy, and individual susceptibility. Possible side effects include:

Circulatory System: Increased blood pressure; increased heart rate; decreased blood pressure upon rising; flushing.

Digestive Tract: Nausea; constipation; appetite loss; diarrhea; vomiting; indigestion; stomach pain; gas; difficulty swallowing; dry mouth; belching.

Nervous System: Drowsiness; sleeplessness; dizziness; nervousness; headache; vertigo (feeling of whirling motion); migraine; anxiety; tremor; abnormal dreams; abnormal skin sensations; agitation; confusion; impaired memory; depression; abnormal thinking; unstable emotions; lockjaw; twitching; depersonalization; decreased sex drive; muscle stiffness.

Respiratory System: Yawning; bronchitis; difficulty breathing; runny nose; cough.

Senses: Blurred vision; taste changes; ringing in the ears; dilated pupils; ear pain; vision changes.

Skin: Sweating; rash; itching; flushing.

Urinary and Reproductive Tract: Abnormal ejaculation or orgasm; impotence; impaired urination; urinary frequency; menstrual disorders; blood in the urine; painful or difficult urination; irregular bleeding between periods; inflammation of the vagina with itching or abnormal discharge; urinary retention.

Other: Weakness; infection; chills; chest pain; weight gain or loss; accidental injury; general body discomfort; neck pain; muscle pain; joint pain; swelling of hands or feet; unusual bruising.

Guidelines for Use:

- *Tablets* — Usual adult starting dose is 75 mg/day, taken in 2 or 3 divided doses. Dosage may be gradually increased to achieve the desired effect.
- *Extended-release capsules* — Usual adult starting dose is 75 mg/day taken as a single dose.
- Take each dose with food.
- Do not crush, chew, or dissolve extended-release capsules in water. Swallow extended-release capsules whole, with fluid.
- If a dose is missed, take it as soon as possible. If several hours have passed or if it is nearing time for the next dose, do not double the dose to catch up, unless advised to do so by your doctor. If several doses are missed or it is necessary to establish a new dosage schedule, contact your doctor or pharmacist. Use exactly as prescribed.
- Do not change the dose or stop taking venlafaxine unless advised to do so by your doctor.
- If venlafaxine therapy is discontinued, the dose should be gradually reduced over a 2-week period.
- Smaller doses should be used in patients with moderate liver or kidney impairment.
- Venlafaxine should not be used in combination with an MAOI, or within at least 14 days of discontinuing treatment with an MAOI. After stopping venlafaxine, at least 7 days should elapse before starting an MAOI.
- Because any psychoactive drug may impair judgment, thinking, or motor skills, do not operate hazardous machinery, including automobiles, until you are reasonably certain that venlafaxine does not adversely affect your ability to engage in such activities.
- Inform your doctor if you are pregnant, become pregnant, are planning to become pregnant, or if you are breastfeeding during therapy.
- Notify your doctor if rash, hives, or other allergic reactions occur.
- Blood pressure will be monitored during treatment.
- Notify your doctor or pharmacist if you are taking other prescription drugs, over-the-counter drugs, or supplements.
- Avoid alcohol use during venlafaxine therapy.
- Store at room temperature (68° to 77°F). Keep container tightly closed.

If you have any questions, consult your doctor, pharmacist, or health care provider.

	Generic Name *Brand Name Examples*	Supplied As	Generic Available
Rx	**Amitriptyline HCl**		
	Elavil	**Tablets:** 10 mg, 25 mg, 50 mg, 75 mg, 100 mg, 150 mg	Yes
	Elavil	**Injection:** 10 mg/mL	Yes
Rx	**Amoxapine**		
	Asendin	**Tablets:** 25 mg, 50 mg, 100 mg, 150 mg	Yes
Rx	**Clomipramine HCl**		
	Anafranil	**Capsules:** 25 mg, 50 mg, 75 mg	Yes
Rx	**Desipramine HCl**		
	Norpramin	**Tablets:** 10 mg, 25 mg, 50 mg, 75 mg, 100 mg, 150 mg	Yes
Rx	**Doxepin HCl**		
	Sinequan	**Capsules:** 10 mg, 25 mg, 50 mg, 75 mg, 100 mg, 150 mg	Yes
	Sinequan	**Oral concentrate:** 10 mg/mL	Yes
Rx	**Imipramine HCl**		
	Tofranil	**Tablets:** 10 mg, 25 mg, 50 mg	Yes
Rx	**Imipramine Pamoate**		
	Tofranil-PM	**Capsules:** 75 mg, 100 mg, 125 mg, 150 mg	No
Rx	**Nortriptyline HCl**		
	Aventyl Pulvules	**Capsules:** 10 mg, 25 mg	No
	Pamelor	**Capsules:** 10 mg, 25 mg, 50 mg, 75 mg	Yes
	Aventyl, Pamelor[1]	**Oral solution:** 10 mg/5 mL	No
Rx	**Protriptyline HCl**		
	Vivactil	**Tablets:** 5 mg, 10 mg	Yes
Rx	**Trimipramine Maleate**		
	Surmontil	**Capsules:** 25 mg, 50 mg, 100 mg	Yes

[1] Contains alcohol.

Type of Drug:

Antidepressants; mood-elevating agents.

How the Drug Works:

Tricyclic antidepressants (TCAs) appear to adjust or rebalance the brain's own natural chemicals (neurotransmitters), which control mood, feelings, and behaviors. The effect may take a few weeks (1 to 4) to be noticed.

Uses:

For the relief of symptoms of depression (except clomipramine).

Clomipramine: Only for the treatment of obsessive-compulsive disorder.

Doxepin: To treat anxiety.

Imipramine: For the treatment of bedwetting in children 6 years of age and older after possible organic causes have been excluded by appropriate tests.

Unlabeled Use(s): Occasionally doctors may prescribe doxepin, clomipramine, imipramine, or amitriptyline to control chronic pain and to treat bulimia. Imipramine, clomipramine, nortriptyline, and other tricyclic antidepressants have also been used to treat panic disorder. Amitriptyline has been used to prevent the onset of cluster and migraine headaches and to treat pathologic weeping and laughing secondary to forebrain disease. Protriptyline has been used in the treatment of obstructive sleep apnea. Trimipramine and doxepin have been studied in the treatment of peptic ulcer disease and to treat skin disorders. Desipramine has been used to facilitate cocaine withdrawal and to treat bulimia. Clomipramine and nortriptyline have been used to treat panic disorder. Nortriptyline has also been used to treat skin disorders and premenstrual depression.

Precautions:

Do not use in the following situations:

- allergy to TCAs or maprotiline
- glaucoma (doxepin only)
- MAOI antidepressant use, concurrent or within 14 days
- heart attack, recovery phase
- urinary retention (doxepin only)

Use with caution in the following situations:

- electroshock therapy
- glaucoma, angle-closure
- heart disease (eg, heart failure)
- hyperthyroid (overactive thyroid)
- increased intraocular pressure
- irregular heartbeat (imipramine only)
- kidney disease
- liver disease
- mental illness (schizophrenia, mania, paranoia)
- seizure, history
- suicidal tendencies
- surgery
- stroke
- tumor of adrenal medulla
- urinary retention

Tardive Dyskinesia: Involuntary and uncontrollable movements may develop in patients treated with these drugs. Occurrence is highest among the elderly, especially women. The risk of developing these involuntary movements and the likelihood that they will become permanent are increased as the length of treatment and the total amount of drug given increases. However, it is possible to develop these symptoms after short-term treatment at low doses.

Neuroleptic Malignant Syndrome (NMS) is a potentially fatal syndrome associated with use of tricyclic antidepressants. Symptoms include increased body heat, muscle rigidity, altered mental abilities including catatonia, irregular pulse or irregular blood pressure, increased heart rate, sweating, and irregular heart rhythm.

Withdrawal Symptoms: Stopping abruptly after prolonged therapy may produce nausea, headache, dizziness, nightmares, and malaise. Clomipramine may also cause vomiting, sleep disturbances, hyperthermia (abnormally high temperature), and irritability. Gradual dose reduction may produce, within 2 weeks, transient symptoms including irritability, restlessness, dreams, and sleep disturbances.

Sensitivity to sunlight may occur. Avoid prolonged exposure to the sun. Use sunscreens and wear protective clothing until tolerance is determined. These drugs may reduce tolerance to hot weather.

Pregnancy: Adequate studies have not been done in pregnant women. Use only if clearly needed and potential benefits outweigh the possible hazards to the fetus. There have been a few reports of birth defects associated with use of imipramine and amitriptyline. Withdrawal symptoms have been seen in newborns of mothers who have taken clomipramine, desipramine, or imipramine until delivery.

Breastfeeding: Tricyclic antidepressants appear in breast milk. Because of the potential for adverse reactions, a decision should be made whether to discontinue nursing or discontinue the drug, taking into account the importance of the drug to the mother. Consult your doctor before you begin breastfeeding.

Children: Amitriptyline and doxepin are not recommended for patients younger than 12 years of age. Safety and effectiveness have not been established for amoxapine in children younger than 16 years of age. Imipramine HCl use in bedwetting should be limited to children 6 years of age or older. The safety and effectiveness of imipramine HCl in children with conditions other than bedwetting have not been established. Safety and effectiveness have not been established for clomipramine in children < 10 years of age. Trimipramine, nortriptyline, desipramine, imipramine pamoate, and protriptyline are not recommended for use in children.

Elderly: Elderly patients are particularly sensitive to the anticholinergic effects (eg, constipation; difficulty urinating; confusion) of tricyclic antidepressants and may be at increased risk for falls. Lower than normal adult doses are generally used when starting therapy.

Lab tests may be required during treatment with tricyclic antidepressants. Tests may include blood counts, blood sugar levels, ECG, kidney and liver function tests, and drug blood levels.

Drug Interactions:

Tell your doctor or pharmacist if you are taking or if you are planning to take any over-the-counter or prescription medications or duetary supplements with tricyclic antidepressants. Doses of one or both drugs may need to be modified or a different drug may need to be prescribed. The following drugs and drug classes interact with tricyclic antidepressants.

- alcohol
- anorexiants (eg, phentermine)
- anticholinergics (eg, dicyclomine)
- anticoagulants (eg, warfarin)
- azole antifungals (eg, ketoconazole)
- barbiturates (eg, phenobarbital)
- beta blockers (eg, labetalol)
- bupropion (eg, *Zyban*)
- carbamazepine (eg, *Tegretol*)
- catecholamines (*imipramine HCl only*)
- charcoal
- cholestyramine (eg, *Questran*)
- cimetidine (eg, *Tagamet*)
- clonidine (eg, *Catapres*)
- diltiazem (eg, *Cardizem*)
- disulfiram (eg, *Antabuse*)
- ethchlorvynol (*amitriptyline only*)
- food (see below)
- furazolidone (*Furoxone*)
- guanethidine (eg, *Ismelin*)
- guanfacine (*Tenex*)
- hydantoins (eg, phenytoin)
- levodopa (eg, *Larodopa*)
- lithium (eg, *Eskalith*)
- MAOIs (eg, phenelzine)
- methyldopa (eg, *Aldomet*)
- methylphenidate (*Ritalin*)
- phenothiazines (eg, promethazine)
- propafenone (*Rythmol*)
- primidone (eg, *Mysoline*)
- quinidine (eg, *Quinidex Extentabs*)
- quinolones (eg, grepafloxacin, sparfloxacin)
- rifamycins (rifabutin, rifampin)
- sedatives
- SSRI antidepressants (eg, fluoxetine)
- sulfonylureas (eg, chloropropamide, tolazamide)
- sympathomimetics (eg, phenylephrine, ephedrine)
- terbinafine (*Lamisil*)
- thyroid hormones (eg, thyroxine)
- valproic acid and derivatives (eg, divalproex sodium, valproate sodium)
- verapamil (eg, *Calan*)

A high-fiber diet (eg, bran muffins or cereals) may decrease the absorption of TCAs. Patients should avoid consuming excess fiber during drug therapy.

Side Effects:

Every drug is capable of producing side effects. Many tricyclic antidepressant users experience no, or minor, side effects. The frequency and severity of side effects depend on many factors including dose, duration of therapy, and individual susceptibility. Possible side effects include:

Enuretic (Bedwetting) Children: Consider side effects reported with adult use. Most common are nervousness, sleep disorders, tiredness, and mild stomach disturbances. These usually disappear with continued therapy or dosage reduction. Other reported reactions include constipation, convulsions, anxiety, emotional instability, and fainting.

Clomipramine only: Tremors; sleeplessness; nervousness; muscle twitches or spasms; memory impairment; anxiety; impaired concentration; breathing problems; abnormal dreams; irritability; emotional lability; depersonalization; hot flashes; menstrual disorder; vaginal irritation; ejaculation disorder; acne; dry skin; abnormal vision; abnormal tears; muscle aches; back pain; joint pain.

Digestive Tract: Dry mouth; constipation; decreased bowel movement; nausea; vomiting; loss of appetite; diarrhea; stomach discomfort; peculiar taste in mouth; stomach cramps; black tongue; mouth sores.

Nervous System: Confusion with hallucinations (especially in the elderly); disorientation; delusions; anxiety; restlessness; agitation; sleeplessness; tremors; nightmares; hypomania; exacerbation of psychosis; numbness, tingling, and decreased sensations in hands and feet; incoordination; unsteady walking; extrapyramidal symptoms; seizures; ringing in ears; changes in brain wave pattern.

Circulatory System: Increased or decreased blood pressure; increased heart rate; pounding in chest (palpitations); heart attack; abnormal heart rhythms; stroke; dizziness when sitting or standing up.

Skin: Rash; itching; red spots; flushing; hair loss.

Urinary and Reproductive Tract: Urinary retention; decreased urination; dilation of urinary tract.

Other: Blurred vision; problems focusing eyes; dilated pupils; increased pressure in eyes; light sensitivity; face and tongue swelling; decreased blood counts; breast enlargement in men; breast enlargement and milk production in women; increased or decreased sex drive; impotence; testicular swelling; increased or decreased blood sugar; weight gain or loss; perspiration; drowsiness; dizziness; weakness; fatigue; headache; changes in liver function; parotid gland swelling; increased appetite.

Guidelines for Use:

- Use exactly as prescribed.
- Lower dosages are recommended for elderly, adolescent, and outpatients, as compared to hospitalized patients who will be under close supervision. Initiate dosage at a low level and increase gradually, noting carefully the clinical response and any evidence of intolerance. Once depressive symptoms are controlled, maintenance doses will be required for a longer period of time, at the lowest dose that will maintain symptom control.
- For many of these medicines, it is not possible to prescribe a single dosage schedule that is therapeutically effective in all patients. Consequently, the recommended dosage regimens are only a guide, which may be modified by factors such as age, chronic disease, severity of the disease, medical condition of the patient, and degree of psychotherapeutic support.
- If a dose is missed, take it as soon as possible. If several hours have passed or if it is nearing time for the next dose, do not double the dose in order to catch up, unless advised to do so by your doctor. If more than one dose is missed, or it is necessary to establish a new dosage schedule, contact your doctor or pharmacist.
- Once symptoms are controlled, therapy may need to be continued for several months to lessen the chance of relapse.
- Do not change the dose or discontinue therapy unless advised to do so by your doctor.
- These drugs may take 1 to 4 weeks to improve symptoms of depression.
- Do not use in combination with an MAOI or within 14 days of discontinuing treatment with an MAOI. After stopping this medicine, wait at least 2 weeks before starting an MAOI.
- Using these drugs with alcohol or other central nervous system depressants (eg, pain relievers, sedatives, barbiturates) may cause added drowsiness.
- May cause drowsiness or blurred vision. Use caution while driving or performing other tasks requiring alertness, coordination, or physical dexterity.
- Symptoms of nausea, headache, or fatigue may develop after abruptly stopping a tricyclic antidepressant (TCA) after long-term use.
- Notify your doctor if dry mouth, constipation, blurred vision, increased heart rate, impaired coordination, difficult urination, excessive sedation, or seizures occur.
- Notify your doctor if you develop a fever or sore throat.
- Notify your doctor if you experience drowsiness, dizziness, or postural hypotension. Your doctor may need to reduce the dose.
- *Be sure your doctor and pharmacist are aware of the following* —
  Other medical conditions.
  All medications, including nonprescription medicines, that you are taking.
  If you have had an unusual or allergic reaction to any TCA or to maprotiline.
  If you are pregnant or may become pregnant.

Guidelines for Use (cont.):

If you are breastfeeding.

- May cause sensitivity to sunlight. Avoid prolonged exposure to the sun and UV light (eg, tanning beds). Use sunscreens and wear protective clothing until tolerance is determined.
- Taking these drugs at bedtime may help reduce side effects (eg, daytime drowsiness). Discuss this possibility with your doctor or pharmacist.
- Lab tests may be required to monitor therapy. Be sure to keep appointments.
- Store at room temperature in a child-resistant container. Patients should supervise this drug carefully in the home.

Amitriptyline:

- Usual initial adult dosage for outpatients is 75 mg/day in divided doses. If necessary, this may be increased (preferably at bedtime doses) to a total of 150 mg/day. An alternative method is to begin with 50 to 100 mg at bedtime. This may be increased by 25 or 50 mg as necessary in the bedtime dose to a total of 150 mg/day. Smaller initial doses may be needed if side effects appear with higher doses.
- Hospitalized patients may require 100 mg/day initially, which can be increased gradually to 200 mg/day. A small number of patients may need up to 300 mg/day.
- Usual dosage for children and elderly patients is 10 mg 3 times a day with 20 mg at bedtime.
- Usual maintenance dosage is 50 to 100 mg given as a single dose at bedtime.
- *Injection Dosage* — Injection should be used for initial therapy in hospitalized patients who are unable or unwilling to take tablets. Tablets should replace the injection as soon as possible. Usual initial dosage by injection is 20 to 30 mg (2 to 3 ml) 4 times a day. Intramuscular doses may cause the effects to appear more rapidly than with tablets.

Amoxapine:

- Usual starting dosage is 50 mg 2 or 3 times daily. Dosage may be increased to 100 mg 2 or 3 times daily by the end of the first week.
- Increases above 300 mg/day dose should only be made if 300 mg/day had been ineffective during a trial period of at least 2 weeks.
- Usual effective dose is 200 to 300 mg/day. If no response is seen at 300 mg, dosage may be increased to 400 mg/day. Hospitalized patients who have been refractory to antidepressant therapy and who have no history of convulsive seizures may have dosage raised cautiously up to 600 mg/day in divided doses.
- Once the effective dose is established, the daily maintenance dose, if not more than 300 mg, can be given as a single dose at bedtime. If maintenance dose is more than 300 mg per day, then divided doses should be used.

Guidelines for Use (cont.):

Clomipramine:

- During initial titration, clomipramine should be given in divided doses with meals to reduce stomach upset. Maximum benefit may not be achieved until 2 to 3 weeks after dosage change. Therefore, it may be appropriate to wait 2 to 3 weeks between further dosage adjustments.
- Usual adult initial dose is 25 mg daily, gradually increased to 100 mg during the first 2 weeks. Over the next several weeks, the dose may be increased to a daily maximum of 250 mg.
- Usual initial treatment in children is 25 mg daily given with meals. Dose may be increased during the first 2 weeks to a maximum daily dose of 3 mg/kg or 100 mg, whichever is smaller. Over the next several weeks, the dose may be increased to a maximum daily dose of 200 mg.
- After titration, the total daily dose may be given once daily at bedtime to minimize daytime sedation.
- A high incidence of sexual dysfunction in males has been reported. There is also a significant risk of seizures.
- Notify your doctor if you experience drowsiness, dizziness, or postural hypotension (dizziness or lightheadedness when rising from a seated or lying position). Your doctor may need to reduce dose.

Desipramine:

- Usual adult target dose is 100 to 200 mg/day. In some patients, dosage may be increased gradually to 300 mg if necessary. Doses above 300 mg/day are not recommended. Patients needing as much as 300 mg should generally be hospitalized.
- The usual target dose for children and elderly is 25 to 100 mg/day. Usual maximum dosage is 100 mg/day. Doses above 150 mg/day are not recommended.
- Initial therapy may be administered in divided doses or as a single daily dose.
- Maintenance dose may be given on a once-daily schedule.
- Usually start with low doses and gradually increase based on response and tolerance.

Doxepin:

- For most patients with mild-to-moderate illness, starting dose is 75 mg/day. Usual optimum dose is 75 to 150 mg/day.
- In patients with mild symptoms, doses may be as low as 25 to 50 mg/day.
- The total daily dose may be taken on a divided or once-a-day dosage schedule. If the once-a-day schedule is employed, the maximum recommended dose is 150 mg/day, which may be given at bedtime.
- The 150 mg capsule strength is intended for maintenance therapy only and is not recommended for initiation of treatment.

Guidelines for Use (cont.):

- *Oral concentrate* should be diluted just prior to administration with 120 mL (½ cup) of water; whole or skimmed milk; or orange, grapefruit, tomato, prune, or pineapple juice. Doxepin oral concentrate is not compatible with a number of carbonated beverages. For those patients requiring antidepressant therapy who are on methadone maintenance, mix oral concentrate and methadone syrup together with *Gatorade*, lemonade, orange juice, sugar water, *Tang*, or water, but not with grape juice. Preparation and storage of bulk dilution is not recommended.

Imipramine HCl:

- Usual initial adult dose for outpatients is 75 mg/day increased to 150 mg/day. Doses over 200 mg/day are not recommended. Maintenance dose is 50 to 150 mg/day.
- For hospitalized patients, usual initial adult dosage is 100 mg/day in divided doses gradually increased to 200 mg/day as required. If no response occurs after 2 weeks, increase dose to 250 to 300 mg/day.
- For adolescents and elderly patients, usual initial dose is 30 to 40 mg/day, not to exceed 100 mg/day.
- *Childhood bedwetting* — An oral dosage of 25 mg/day given 1 hour before bedtime should be tried in children 6 years of age and older.
- If satisfactory response does not occur within 1 week, increase the dose to 50 mg nightly in children younger than 12 years of age; children older than 12 may receive up to 75 mg nightly.
- Doses larger than 75 mg do not work better and tend to increase the side effects.
- In early night bedwetters, the drug is more effective given earlier and in divided amounts (ie, 25 mg in midafternoon, repeated at bedtime).
- Consider instituting a drug-free period following an adequate therapeutic trial with a favorable response.
- To reduce the tendency to relapse, taper dosage gradually rather than discontinue abruptly.

Imipramine pamoate:

- Initiate adult dose for outpatients at 75 mg/day and increase to 150 mg/day, which is the dose level at which optimum response is usually obtained. If necessary, dose may be increased to 200 mg/day. Doses higher than 75 mg/day may also be administered on a once-a-day basis at bedtime after the optimum dosage and tolerance have been determined.
- Maintenance dosage is usually 75 to 150 mg/day administered on a once-a-day basis, preferably at bedtime.

Nortriptyline:

- Usual adult dosage is 25 mg 3 to 4 times daily. As an alternative regimen, the total daily dose may be given once a day.
- Doses above 150 mg/day per day are not recommended.
- Usual dosage in elderly patients is 30 to 50 mg/day in divided doses.

Guidelines for Use (cont.):

Protriptyline:

- Usual adult dosage is 15 to 40 mg/day divided into 3 or 4 doses. If necessary, dose may be increased to 60 mg/day. Make dose increases with the morning dose.
- Doses above 60 mg/day are not recommended.
- For elderly patients, the usual dosage is 5 mg 3 times a day initially and is increased gradually. The cardiovascular system must be monitored closely if the daily dose exceeds 20 mg.

Trimipramine:

- Usual initial adult dosage for outpatients is 75 mg/day in divided doses. May be increased to 150 mg/day if needed.
- Doses over 200 mg/day are not recommended.
- Hospitalized patients may be given 100 mg/day initially in divided doses, increased gradually in a few days to 200 mg/day. If improvement does not occur in 2 to 3 weeks, the dose may be increased to the maximum recommended dose of 250 to 300 mg/day.
- Usual initial dose for adolescents and elderly patients is 50 mg/day, increasing in gradual increments up to 100 mg/day.

If you have any questions, consult your doctor, pharmacist, or health care provider.

	Generic Name *Brand Name Examples*	Supplied As	Generic Available
Rx	**Chlorpromazine HCl**		
	Thorazine	**Tablets:** 10 mg, 25 mg, 50 mg, 100 mg, 200 mg	Yes
	Thorazine Spansules	**Capsules, sustained release:** 30 mg, 75 mg, 150 mg	No
	Thorazine	**Syrup:** 10 mg/tsp	Yes
	Thorazine	**Concentrate:** 30 mg/mL, 100 mg/mL	Yes
	Thorazine	**Suppositories:** 25 mg, 100 mg	No
	Thorazine[1]	**Injection:** 25 mg/mL	Yes
Rx	**Fluphenazine HCl**		
	Permitil	**Tablets:** 2.5 mg, 5 mg, 10 mg	Yes
	Permitil[2], *Prolixin*[2]	**Concentrate:** 5 mg/mL	No
	Prolixin[2]	**Elixir:** 2.5 mg/tsp	No
	Prolixin	**Injection:** 2.5 mg/ml	No
Rx	**Fluphenazine Enanthate and Decanoate**		
	Prolixin Decanoate	**Injection:** 25 mg/ml	Yes
	Prolixin Enanthate	**Injection:** 25 mg/mL	No
Rx	**Haloperidol**		
	Haldol	**Tablets:** 0.5 mg, 1 mg, 2 mg, 5 mg, 10 mg, 20 mg	Yes
	Haldol	**Concentrate:** 2 mg/mL	Yes
	Haldol	**Injection:** 5 mg/mL	No
	Haldol Decanoate	**Injection:** 50 mg/mL, 100 mg/mL	No
Rx	**Loxapine**		
	Loxitane	**Capsules:** 5 mg, 10 mg, 25 mg, 50 mg	Yes
	Loxitane C	**Concentrate:** 25 mg/mL	No
	Loxitane IM	**Injection:** 50 mg/mL	No
Rx	**Mesoridazine Besylate**		
	Serentil	**Tablets:** 10 mg, 25 mg, 50 mg, 100 mg	No
	Serentil[2]	**Concentrate:** 25 mg/mL	No
	Serentil[3]	**Injection:** 25 mg/mL	No

Rx	**Molindone HCl**		
	Moban	**Tablets:** 5 mg, 10 mg, 25 mg, 50 mg, 100 mg	No
	Moban[1,2]	**Concentrate:** 20 mg/mL	No
Rx	**Perphenazine**		
	Trilafon	**Tablets:** 2 mg, 4 mg, 8 mg, 16 mg	Yes
	Trilafon[2]	**Concentrate:** 16 mg/tsp	No
	Trilafon[1]	**Injection:** 5 mg/mL	No
Rx	**Prochlorperazine**		
	Compazine	**Tablets:** 5 mg, 10 mg	Yes
	Compazine	**Capsules, sustained release:** 10 mg, 15 mg	No
	Compazine	**Suppositories:** 2.5 mg, 5 mg, 25 mg	No
	Compazine	**Syrup:** 5 mg/tsp	No
	Compazine	**Injection:** 5 mg/mL	Yes
Rx	**Promazine HCl**		
	Sparine	**Tablets:** 25 mg, 50 mg, 100 mg	No
	Prozine-50, Sparine	**Injection:** 50 mg/mL	Yes
Rx	**Risperidone**		
	Risperdal	**Tablets:** 1 mg, 2 mg, 3 mg, 4 mg	No
	Risperdal	**Oral Solution:** 1 mg/mL	No
Rx	**Thioridazine HCl**		
	Mellaril	**Tablets:** 10 mg, 15 mg, 25 mg, 50 mg, 100 mg, 150 mg, 200 mg	Yes
	Mellaril[2]	**Concentrate:** 30 mg/tsp, 100 mg/tsp	Yes
	Mellaril-S	**Suspension:** 25 mg/tsp, 100 mg/tsp	No
Rx	**Thiothixene HCl**		
	Navane	**Capsules:** 1 mg, 2 mg, 5 mg, 10 mg, 20 mg	Yes
	Navane[2]	**Concentrate:** 5 mg/mL	Yes
	Navane	**Injection:** 5 mg/mL	No

Rx	**Trifluoperazine HCl**		
	Stelazine	**Tablets:** 1 mg, 2 mg, 5 mg, 10 mg	Yes
	Stelazine[1]	**Concentrate:** 10 mg/mL	Yes
	Stelazine	**Injection:** 5 mg/mL	No
Rx	**Triflupromazine HCl**		
	Vesprin	**Injection:** 10 mg/mL, 20 mg/mL	No

[1] Contains sulfites.
[2] Contains alcohol.
[3] Contains EDTA.

All of the products listed on this table are antipsychotic medications; however, they are not interchangeable. For example, chlorpromazine cannot be used for loxapine. Daily dose may vary depending on individual needs. Do not adjust the dose without consulting your pharmacist or doctor. Clozapine, lithium, olanzapine and pimozide are also used as antipsychotic agents. For more information, see the individual drug monographs in this chapter.

Type of Drug:

Neuroleptic drugs; "major tranquilizers"; antipsychotic agents.

How the Drug Works:

The exact mechanism of action of antipsychotic agents is not fully understood. It is believed antipsychotic agents reduce nerve sensitivity in different areas of the brain. They are not used to treat anxiety but can improve concentration and self control in severely mentally ill (psychotic or schizophrenic) patients.

Uses:

All antipsychotic drugs: To reduce symptoms of psychosis (mental illness). Additional uses for these agents are listed below.

Chlorpromazine: To control the manic phase of manic depression.

To relieve restlessness and apprehension prior to surgery.

To treat tetanus when used with other drugs.

To treat acute intermittent porphyria.

To treat severe behavioral problems in children, including combativeness or explosive hyperactivity, and hyperactivity (short-term).

To control nausea and vomiting.

To relieve intractable hiccups.

Haloperidol: To control tics and vocal utterances in children and adults with Tourette's syndrome.

To treat severe behavioral problems in children, including combativeness or explosive hyperactivity, and hyperactivity (short-term).

Mesoridazine: To treat schizophrenia.

To treat behavioral problems associated with mental deficiency and chronic brain syndrome.

To treat anxiety, tension, depression, nausea and vomiting in alcoholics.

To reduce anxiety and tension associated with neurotic components of many disorders. Also benefits personality disorders in general.

Perphenazine: To control nausea, vomiting and hiccups (injection only).

Prochlorperazine: For short-term treatment of non-psychotic anxiety. Not the drug of choice.

To control severe nausea and vomiting.

Thioridazine: For short-term treatment of depression with variable degrees of anxiety in adults.

To treat multiple symptoms such as agitation, anxiety, depressed mood, tension, sleep disturbances, and fears in the elderly patient.

To treat severe behavioral problems in children, including combativeness or explosive hyperactivity (short-term).

Trifluoperazine: For short-term treatment of non-psychotic anxiety. Not the drug of choice.

Triflupromazine: To control severe nausea and vomiting.

Unlabeled Use(s): Occasionally doctors may prescribe antipsychotic agents to treat Tourette syndrome and to treat some symptoms of dementia (including agitation, hyperactivity, hallucinations, suspiciousness, hostility and uncooperativeness). Other unlabeled uses include:

Chlorpromazine – To treat migraine headaches, symptoms of Huntington's disease, restless leg syndrome, postoperative shivering, opioid withdrawal (in newborns), PCP psychosis.

Fluphenazine – To treat desires of self-mutilation, and symptoms of Huntington's or Lesch-Nyhan disease.

Haloperidol – To treat anxiety disorders, mania, taste disorders, symptoms of Huntington's disease, PCP psychosis, nausea and vomiting, intractable hiccups or sneezing.

Risperidone – To treat AIDS or Parkinsonism-related psychosis.

Precautions:

Do not use in the following situations:

- allergy to these drugs
- blood disorders due to antipsychotics
- blood pressure, extremes (thioridazine only)
- bone marrow depression
- brain damage
- coma
- coronary artery disease
- CNS depressants (alcohol, barbiturates, narcotics), large amounts
- CNS depression, severe
- epilepsy
- glaucoma
- liver disease
- overactive thyroid
- Parkinson's disease (haloperidol only)
- pediatric surgery (prochlorperazine only)
- sedation

Use with caution in the following situations:

- alcohol withdrawal
- angina (trifluoperazine only)
- anticholinergics (eg, atropine) use
- anticonvulsant medications, use (haloperidol only)
- asthma
- brain damage
- breast cancer
- bronchitis, chronic
- circulatory problems
- dehydration (risperidone only)
- depression
- elderly
- electroshock therapy, previous
- emphysema
- exposure to extreme heat or cold
- exposure to organophosphorus insecticides
- glaucoma
- heart disease
- hypovolemia (low blood volume) (risperidone only)
- kidney disease
- lithium (eg, *Lithobid*), use
- liver disease
- lung disease or infection
- myelogram testing (within 24 hrs)
- Neuroleptic Malignant Syndrome, history of
- pheochromocytoma (vascular tumor of adrenal medulla)
- seizures, history
- skin inflammation
- surgery
- urinary retention, tendency
- thyroid, overactive
- thyrotoxicosis (overactivity of thyroid gland) (haloperidol only)

Tardive dyskinesia: Involuntary and uncontrollable movements may develop in patients treated with these drugs. Occurrence is highest among the elderly, especially women. The risk of developing these involuntary movements and the likelihood they will become permanent are increased as the length of treatment and the total amount of drug given is increased. However, it is possible to develop these symptoms after short-term treatment at low doses. The syndrome is characterized by rhythmical involuntary movements of the tongue, face, mouth or jaw (eg, protrusion of tongue, puffing of cheeks, puckering of mouth, chewing movements).

Neuroleptic Malignant Syndrome (NMS) is a potentially fatal syndrome associated with antipsychotic drugs. Symptoms include: Increased body heat, muscle rigidity, altered mental status including irregular pulse and blood pressure, increased heart rate and sweating.

Abrupt withdrawal: These drugs are not known to cause dependence and do not produce tolerance or addiction. However, following abrupt withdrawal of high dose therapy, symptoms such as nausea, vomiting, dizziness, tremors, headache, upset stomach and increased heart rate have been reported. Symptoms occurred in 1 to 4 days and subsided in 1 to 2 weeks. These symptoms can be reduced by a gradual decrease in dosage or by continuing antiparkinson agents for several weeks after the antipsychotic agent is withdrawn.

Skin discoloration: Rare instances of skin pigmentation have occurred, primarily in females on long-term, high dose therapy. These changes, restricted to exposed areas of the skin, range from a very slight darkening to a slate gray color, sometimes with a violet hue. Pigmentation may fade following drug discontinuation. Use caution against exposure to ultraviolet light (eg, tanning booths) or undue exposure to sunlight. These effects occur most commonly with chlorpromazine.

Eye changes: Ocular changes have occasionally occurred in patients receiving long-term, high dose therapy. Eye changes are characterized by deposits of fine particular matter in the lens and cornea. Eye lesions may regress after drug discontinuation. Exposure to light, along with dosage and duration of therapy, seem to be the most significant factor in this reaction.

PKU tests: These drugs may produce false-positive phenylketonuria (PKU) test results.

Lab tests may be required during therapy with antipsychotic drugs. Tests may include: Eye exams, blood counts and kidney and liver function tests.

Sulfites: Some of these products may contain sulfite preservatives which can cause allergic reactions in certain individuals. Check package label when available or consult your doctor or pharmacist.

Pregnancy: Safety for use during pregnancy is not established. Some newborns of women using these medicines have experienced prolonged jaundice and abnormal movements and reflexes. Use only when clearly needed and when the potential benefits outweigh the possible hazards to the fetus.

Breastfeeding: Chlorpromazine, haloperidol and trifluoperazine appear in breast milk. Consult your doctor about these and other antipsychotic agents before you begin breastfeeding.

Children: In general, these products are not recommended for children under 12 years of age. Phenothiazine use in children under 1 year of age may be a factor in sudden infant death syndrome (SIDS). Children with acute illnesses (eg, chickenpox, measles) or dehydration appear much more susceptible to neuromuscular reactions than adults. Symptoms can occur and may be confused with the signs of an undiagnosed primary disease responsible for the vomiting (eg, Reye's syndrome). Avoid antipsychotic agents in children and adolescents whose symptoms (eg, vomiting, hyperactivity, confusion) suggest Reye's syndrome.

Chlorpromazine – Do not use in children under 6 months of age except where potentially life saving. Not for use in conditions for which children's dosages are not established.

Haloperidol – Do not use in children under 3 years of age.

Loxitane – Safety and effectiveness is not established in children under 16 years of age.

Prochlorperazine – Not recommended for children under 20 pounds or under 2 years of age. Not for use in pediatric surgery. Children seem more prone to develop parkinson-like reactions. Use the lowest effective dose. Occasionally, the patient may react to the drug with restlessness and excitement. If this occurs, do not administer additional doses. Use with caution in children with acute illnesses or dehydration. Not for use in conditions for which children's dosages are not established.

Thioridazine – Not recommended for children under 2 years of age.

Trifluoperazine – This drug is for children, aged 6 to 12 years, who are hospitalized or under close supervision. Dosage must be adjusted to the weight of the child and severity of symptoms.

Triflupromazine – Do not use in children under 2½ years of age.

Elderly: Low doses are usually sufficient for elderly patients. These patients are more susceptible to lowered blood pressure and other side effects. Doses should be increased gradually.

Drug Interactions:

Tell your doctor or pharmacist if you are taking or if you are planning to take any over-the-counter or prescription medications or dietary supplements while taking these medicines. Doses of one or both drugs may need to be modified or a different drug may need to be prescribed. The following drugs and drug classes may interact with these medicines.

- ACE inhibitors (eg, captopril)
- alcohol
- aluminum-containing antacids (eg, *Rolaids*)
- anesthetics
- anticholinergics (eg, atropine)
- anticoagulants, oral (eg, warfarin)
- antihistamines (eg, diphenhydramine)
- appetite suppressants (eg, fenfluramine)
- barbiturates (eg, phenobarbital)
- barbiturate anesthetics (eg, methohexital)
- benzodiazepines (eg, lorazepam) (loxapine only)
- beta blockers (eg, propranolol)
- bromocriptine (*Parlodel*)
- carbamazepine (eg, *Tegretol*) (haloperidol only)
- charcoal
- cimetidine (eg, *Tagamet*)
- clonidine (eg, *Catapres*)
- clozapine (*Clozaril*)
- diazoxide (eg, *Proglycem*)
- disulfiram (eg, *Antabuse*)
- dopamine (eg, *Intropin*)
- epinephrine (eg, *Adrenalin*)
- fluoxetine (*Prozac*) (haloperidol only)
- fluvoxamine (*Luvox*) (haloperidol only)
- guanethidine (eg, *Ismelin*)
- hydantoins (eg, phenytoin)
- hydroxyzine (eg, *Atarax*)
- levodopa (eg, *Larodopa*)
- lithium (eg, *Eskalith*)
- meperidine (eg, *Demerol*)
- methyldopa (eg, *Aldomet*)
- metrizamide (*Amipaque*)
- narcotics (eg, codeine)

nefazodone (Serzone) (haloperidol only)
nonsteroidal anti-inflammatory agents (eg, indomethacin) (haloperidol only)
norepinephrine (*Levophed*)
opiates
piperazine (eg, *Antepar*)
polypeptide antibiotics (eg, polymyxin B)
quinidine (eg, *Quinora*)
rifamycins (eg, rifampin) (haloperidol only)
succinylcholine (eg, *Anectine*)
sympathomimetics (eg, phenylpropanolamine)
tetracycline antibiotics (molindone only)
thiazide diuretics (eg, hydrochorothiazides)
trazodone (eg, *Desyrel*)
tricyclic antidepressants (eg, amitriptyline)
valproic acid (eg, *Depakene*)
vitamin C

Side Effects:

Every drug is capable of producing side effects. Many patients experience no, or minor, side effects. The frequency and severity of side effects depend on many factors including dose, duration of therapy and individual susceptibility. Possible side effects include:

Liver – Yellowing of skin and eyes (jaundice); abnormal liver function tests.

Parkinson Disease-Like Symptoms – Tremors; drooling; muscle stiffness; rigidity; shuffling walk; staggering gait; mask-like face; facial grimacing.

Tardive Dyskinesia and Neuroleptic Malignant Syndrome – See Precautions.

Hormones – Appearance of milk and breast engorgement in women; breast enlargement in men; menstrual irregularities; loss of menstruation; changes in sex drive or ability; changes in blood sugar levels; false-positive pregnancy tests; dry vagina.

Muscular System: Muscle spasms or aches; aching and numbness of legs and arms; lockjaw; protrusion, discoloration, aching and rounding of the tongue; tightness in throat; weakness; inability to sit still; exaggeration of reflexes; joint pain or stiffness; difficulty moving.

Digestive Tract: Appetite changes; nausea; vomiting; constipation; diarrhea; stomach pain or upset; fecal impaction; dry mouth; excess salivation; reduced salivation; swallowing difficulty; tongue protrusion; swollen tongue; excessive thirst; reduced thirst; sore mouth or gums; excessive eating.

Circulatory System: Changes in blood pressure; orthostatic hypotension (dizziness or lightheadedness when rising quickly from a sitting or lying position); fainting; changes in heart rate; heart attack.

Psychiatric: Hallucinations; catatonia; restlessness; hyperactivity; confusion; depression; agitation; increased dream activity; bizarre dreams; euphoria (exaggerated sense of well being); excitement; lethargy; paranoid reactions; aggressiveness; sedation.

Nervous System: Headache; drowsiness (about 1 to 2 weeks); increased sleep duration; dizziness; lightheadedness; nervousness; tremors; jitteriness; clumsiness; sleeplessness; anxiety; vertigo (feeling of whirling motion); slurred speech; seizures; fatigue; twitching; tension; numbness.

Respiratory System: Spasms of larynx and bronchial tubes (breathing passages); nasal congestion; increased depth of breathing; painful or difficult breathing; asthma; sore throat; cough; sinus problems; upper respiratory infections.

Skin: Hives; rash; oily skin; red, itching; sensitivity to light; hair loss; pallor; flushing; sweating; discoloration; lesions; swelling; dry skin; yellowing of skin.

Eyes or Ocular: Glaucoma; sensitivity to light; blurred vision; changes in pupil size; cataracts; problems with cornea, lens and retina; abnormal vision; drooping eyelid; brownish coloring of vision, abnormal eye movements; impairment of night vision (thiroridazine only).

Hematologic/Lymphatic: Blood cholesterol level changes; abnormal blood counts; anemia.

Urinary and Reproductive Tract: Urinary retention; increased urination; glucose in urine; lack of bladder control; persistent or painful erections; frequent urination; painful or difficult urination; bedwetting.

Other: Toothache; swelling in hands or feet; weight gain; heatstroke; fever; chills; problems with body temperature regulation; back or chest pain; swollen glands.

Guidelines for Use:

- Use exactly as prescribed.
- *Brand Interchange* — Do not change from one brand of antipsychotics to another without consulting your pharmacist or doctor. Products manufactured by different companies may not be equally effective.
- If a dose is missed, take it as soon as possible. If several hours have passed or if it is nearing time for the next dose, do not double the dose in order to "catch up" (unless advised to do so by your doctor). If more than one dose is missed or it is necessary to establish a new dosage schedule, contact your doctor or pharmacist.
- Oral agents may be ineffective if expelled after vomiting has already begun. Consider use of injection or suppositories under such circumstances.
- Take these drugs routinely as directed. They control illness symptoms. They are not addicting.
- Improvement may not be seen for several weeks.
- May cause drowsiness. Use caution while driving or performing other tasks requiring alertness, coordination or physical dexterity.
- Avoid alcohol or other drugs that cause drowsiness while taking this medicine.
- May cause sensitivity to sunlight. Avoid prolonged exposure to the sun. Use sunscreens and wear protective clothing until tolerance is determined.
- If dizziness or fainting occurs, avoid sudden changes in posture and use caution when climbing stairs, etc (more common after first injection).
- May increase susceptibility to heatstroke. Use caution in hot weather.
- Inform your doctor if you are pregnant, become pregnant, are planning to become pregnant or if you are breastfeeding.
- Contact your doctor if any of the following occurs: Involuntary muscle twitching; involuntary movements of the tongue, stomach cramping; sore throat; fever; lethargy; decreased sensation of thirst; irregular pulse; excessive sweating; soreness of mouth, gums or throat; symptoms of upper respiratory infection; unusual bleeding or bruising; weakness; impaired vision; pale stools; skin rash; tremors; yellowing of skin or eyes.
- *Liquid concentrates* are light sensitive. Keep in amber or opaque bottles and protect from light.
  These solutions are most conveniently used when diluted in fruit juices or other liquids. Use these solutions immediately after dilution.
  Avoid contact with skin (contact dermatitis may occur).
  Shake well before using.
- *Chlorpromazine* —
  Concentrate: Add desired dose to 2 oz or more of liquid just prior to use. Suggested liquids are tomato or fruit juice, milk, simple syrup, orange syrup, carbonated beverages, coffee, tea or water. Semisolid foods (soups, puddings, etc) may also be used.
  Sustained-release capsules: Do not crush or chew. Swallow whole.

Guidelines for Use (cont.):

- *Fluphenazine* —
  Concentrate: Suitable for use only with the following: Water, saline, *Seven-Up*, homogenized milk, carbonated orange beverages, and pineapple, apricot, prune, orange, *V-8*, tomato and grapefruit juices. DO NOT MIX with beverages containing caffeine (coffee, cola), tannics (tea) or pectinates (apple juice).
  Storage: Store oral concentrate between 36° and 86°F.
- *Loxitane* —
  Concentrate: Only use the calibrated dropper which is enclosed in the package for measuring the dose.
  Mix with orange or grapefruit juice shortly before use.
- *Mesoridazine* — Use the calibrated dropper which is enclosed with the package to measure the dose.
  Concentrate may be diluted just prior to use with distilled water, acidified tap water, orange or grape juice. Do not prepare and store in bulk.
- *Molindone* — Tablets contain calcium sulfate. Calcium may interfere with the absorption of medicines such as phenytoin or tetracyclines.
- *Perphenazine* —
  Concentrate: Dilute with only water, saline, *Seven–Up*, homogenized milk, carbonated orange drink and pineapple, apricot, prune, orange, *V-8*, tomato and grapefruit juices. DO NOT MIX with beverages containing caffeine (coffee, cola), tannics (tea) or pectinates (apple juice).
  Use approximately 2 oz liquid for each 1 tsp of concentrate
  Storage: Store concentrate between 36° and 86°F.
- *Risperidone* — Use the calibrated dispensing pipette to measure the dose.
  Mix oral solution with water, coffee, orange juice or lowfat milk. Do not milk with cola or tea.
- *Thioridazine* — Add dose to 2 oz or more just prior to use. Liquids suggested are: Tomato or fruit juices, milk, simple syrup, orange syrup, carbonated beverages, coffee, tea or water. Semisolid foods (soup, puddings, etc) may also be used.
- *Trifluoperazine* — Concentrate is for institutional use only. Use in severe neuropsychiatric conditions when oral medication is preferred and other oral forms are impractical.
  Add concentrate dose to 2 oz or more just prior to use. Liquids suggested are: Tomato or fruit juices, milk, simple syrup, orange syrup, carbonated beverages, coffee, tea or water. Semisolid foods (soup, puddings, etc) may also be used.

Generic Name *Brand Name Example*	Supplied As	Generic Available
Rx **Quetiapine Fumarate**		
Seroquel	**Tablets:** 25 mg, 100 mg, 200 mg	No

Type of Drug:

Antipsychotic.

How the Drug Works:

The exact mechanism is unknown. Drugs of this type usually work by altering nerve transmission in the brain.

Uses:

For the management of the manifestations of psychotic disorders.

Precautions:

Do not use in the following situations: Allergy to the drug or any of its ingredients

Use with caution in the following situations:

- Alzheimer's disease
- cerebrovascular disease
- conduction abnormalities
- decreased plasma levels
- dehydration
- exercise, strenuous
- exposure to extreme heat
- heart attack
- heart disease, ischemic
- heart failure
- long-term use (more than 6 weeks)
- seizures, history of
- suicidal tendency
- underactive thyroid

Neuroleptic malignant syndrome (NMS) is a potentially fatal syndrome associated with quetiapine fumarate. Symptoms include: Increased body heat; muscle rigidity; altered mental abilities, including catatonia; irregular pulse and blood pressure; increased heart rate; sweating; and irregular heart rhythm.

Tardive dyskinesia: Involuntary and uncontrollable movements may develop in patients treated with quetiapine fumarate. Occurrence is highest among the elderly, especially women. The risk of developing these involuntary movements and the likelihood they will become permanent are increased as the length of treatment and the total amount of drug given increases. However, it is possible to develop these symptoms after short-term treatment at low doses.

Pregnancy: Adequate studies have not been done in pregnant women. Use only if clearly needed and potential benefits outweigh the possible risks.

Breastfeeding: It is not known if quetiapine fumarate appears in breast milk. Consult your doctor before you begin breastfeeding.

Children: Safety and effectiveness in children have not been established.

Lab tests or exams may be required to monitor treatment. Be sure to keep appointments.

Drug Interactions:

Tell your doctor or pharmacist if you are taking or if you are planning to take any over-the-counter or prescription medications or dietary supplements with quetiapine fumarate. Doses of one or both drugs may need to be modified or a different drug may need to be prescribed. The following drugs and drug classes interact with quetiapine fumarate.

- antihypertensives (eg, clonidine)
- anticholinergics (eg, benztropine mesylate)
- barbiturates
- carbamazepine (eg, *Tegretol*)
- cimetidine (eg, *Tagamet*)
- erythromycin
- fluconazole (*Diflucan*)
- glucocorticoids
- itraconazole (*Sporanox*)
- ketoconazole (*Nizoral*)
- levodopa (eg, *Larodopa*)
- lorazepam (*Ativan*)
- phenobarbital (*Solfoton*)
- phenytoin (*Dilantin*)
- rifampin (eg, *Rifadin*)
- thioridazine (*Mellaril*)

Side Effects:

Every drug is capable of producing side effects. Many quetiapine fumarate users experience no, or minor, side effects. The frequency and severity of side effects depend on many factors, including dose, duration of therapy and individual susceptibility. Possible side effects include:

Digestive Tract: Difficulty eating; indigestion; stomach pain; constipation; appetite loss.

Nervous System: Altered mental status; orthostatic hypotension (dizziness or lightheadedness when rising quickly from a sitting or lying position); fainting; drowsiness; impaired judgment, thinking or motor skills; headache.

Circulatory System: Irregular heartbeat; changes in blood pressure; palpitations (pounding in the chest); abnormal blood counts.

Respiratory System: Runny nose; sore throat; increased cough; difficulty breathing.

Other: Rash; fever; muscle rigidity; sweating; kidney failure, acute; involuntary and uncontrollable movements; lens problems; dry mouth; weakness; back pain; weight gain; ear pain; tight muscles; joint pain; flu syndrome; swelling of arms and legs.

Guidelines for Use:

- If a dose is missed, take it as soon as possible. If several hours have passed or it is nearing time for the next dose, do not double the dose to catch up. If more than one dose is missed or if it is necessary to establish a new dosage schedule, contact your doctor or pharmacist. Use exactly as prescribed.
- Do not stop taking this medicine without checking with your doctor.
- May cause dizziness, lightheadedness or fainting, especially when rising or standing and during the first 3 to 5 days. If these symptoms should occur, sit or lie down and contact your doctor. Use caution while driving or performing hazardous tasks requiring alertness, coordination or physical dexterity.
- Do not take other medications without your doctor's approval. This includes nonprescription medicines for appetite control, asthma, colds, cough, hay fever or sinus problems.
- Avoid alcohol and other mental depressants (eg, narcotics, tranquilizers, antihistamines) while you are taking this medicine.
- Inform your doctor if you are pregnant, become pregnant, are planning to become pregnant or are breastfeeding.
- Avoid overheating and dehydration.
- *Neuroleptic Malignant Syndrome (NMS)* is a potentially fatal syndrome associated with quetiapine fumarate. Symptoms include: Increased body heat; muscle rigidity; altered mental abilities, including catatonia; irregular pulse and blood pressure; increased heart rate; sweating; and irregular heart rhythm.
- *Tardive dyskinesia* — Involuntary and uncontrollable movements may develop in patients treated with quetiapine fumarate. Occurrence is highest among the elderly, especially women. The risk of developing these involuntary movements and the likelihood they will become permanent are increased as the length of treatment and the total amount of drug given increases. However, it is possible to develop these symptoms after short-term treatment at low doses.

If you have any questions, consult your doctor, pharmacist, or health care provider.

	Generic Name *Brand Name Example*	Supplied As	Generic Available
Rx	**Risperidone**		
	Risperdal	**Tablet**: 0.25 mg, 0.5 mg, 1 mg, 2 mg, 3 mg, 4 mg	No
	Risperdal	**Oral solution**: 1 mg/1 mL	No

Type of Drug:

Benzisoxazole antipsychotic agent; neuroleptic drug; "major tranquilizer."

How the Drug Works:

How risperidone works is not fully understood. It may alter the balance of certain chemicals in the brain that are responsible for thinking and behavior.

Uses:

For the management of manifestations of psychotic disorders (mental illnesses).

Unlabeled Use(s): Bipolar disorder; management of patients with demetia-related psychotic symptoms.

Precautions:

Do not use in the following situations: Allergy to risperidone or any of its ingredients.

Use with caution in the following situations:

Alzheimer's disease	kidney disease
concomitant illness	liver disease
elderly	low blood pressure
heart disease	seizures, history of

Neuroleptic Malignant Syndrome (NMS): NMS is a potentially fatal syndrome associated with risperidone. Symptoms include increased body heat, muscle rigidity, altered mental abilities, irregular pulse and blood pressure, increased heart rate, sweating, and irregular heart rhythm.

Potential for Proarrhythmic Effects: Drugs such as risperidone have been associated with the occurrence of torsades de pointes, a life-threatening abnormal heart rhythm.

Tardive Dyskinesia: Involuntary and uncontrollable muscle movements may develop in patients treated with risperidone. Occurrence is highest among the elderly, especially women. The risk of developing these involuntary movements and the likelihood they will become permanent are increased as the length of treatment and the total amount of drug given increases. However, it is possible to develop these symptoms after short-term treatment at low doses. Tardive dyskinesia is characterized by rhythmical involuntary movements of the tongue, face, mouth, or jaw (eg, protrusion of the tongue, puffing of the cheeks, puckering of the mouth, chewing movements).

Pregnancy: There are no adequate and well-controlled studies in pregnant women. Use only if clearly needed and the potential benefits to the mother outweigh the possible hazards to the fetus.

Breastfeeding: It is not known if risperidone appears in breast milk. Consult your doctor before you begin breastfeeding.

Children: Safety and effectiveness in children have not been established.

Elderly: A lower starting dose is recommend for elderly patients.

Drug Interactions:

Tell your doctor or pharmacist if you are taking or planning to take any over-the-counter or prescription medications or dietary supplements with risperidone. Doses of one or both drugs may need to be modified or a different drug may need to be prescribed. The following drugs and drug classes interact with risperidone:

alcohol
blood pressure-lowering medicines (eg, clonidine)
carbamazepine (eg, *Tegretol*)
clozapine (*Clozaril*)
dopamine (eg, *Intropin*)
fluoxetine (eg, *Prozac*)
levodopa (eg, *Larodopa*)

Side Effects:

Every drug is capable of producing side effects. Many risperidone users experience no, or minor, side effects. The frequency and severity of side effects depend on many factors including dose, duration of therapy, and individual susceptibility. Possible side effects include:

Digestive Tract: Constipation; diarrhea; nausea; indigestion; vomiting; stomach pain; decreased or increased saliva; toothache; appetite loss.

Nervous System: Tremor; restlessness; headache; dizziness; sleeplessness; agitation; anxiety; drowsiness; aggressive reaction; increased sleep duration; increased dream activity; nervousness.

Respiratory System: Upper respiratory infection; sinus irritation; congested or runny nose; coughing; sore throat; difficulty breathing.

Urinary and Reproductive Tract: Frequent urination; heavy menstrual bleeding; difficulty with orgasm; vaginal dryness; difficulty with erection; decreased sexual desire.

Skin: Rash; dry skin; excessively oily skin; dark spots on the skin; sensitivity to sunlight.

Other: Fast heartbeat; back, chest, or joint pain; muscle stiffness or rigidity; difficult or abnormal movement; clumsiness; difficulty walking; involuntary muscle contractions; fatigue; dizziness or lightheadedness upon rising or standing; visual changes; weight gain; fever.

Guidelines for Use:

- Dosage is individualized. Take exactly as prescribed.
- Risperidone can be taken with or without food. Take with food if stomach upset occurs.
- Generally, low starting doses are used and then the dose is increased to achieve the best effects.
- Use the calibrated pipette to measure the dose of the oral solution.
- The oral solution may be taken with water, coffee, orange juice, or low-fat milk; however, it should not be taken with cola or tea.
- Contact your doctor immediately if you experience involuntary muscle movements, muscle rigidity, fever, irregular or fast heartbeat, or profuse sweating.
- May cause dizziness, lightheadedness, or fainting when rising or standing, particularly during initial use. Get up slowly and avoid sudden changes in posture.
- May cause drowsiness. Use caution while driving or performing other tasks requiring alertness, coordination, and physical dexterity.
- Avoid alcohol while you are taking this medicine.
- May cause photosensitivity (sensitivity to sunlight). Avoid prolonged exposure to the sun or other forms of ultraviolet (UV) light (eg, tanning beds). Use sunscreens and wear protective clothing until tolerance is determined.
- Consult your doctor or pharmacist before taking nonprescription or prescription drugs or dietary supplements with risperidone.
- Inform your doctor if you are pregnant, become pregnant, are planning to become pregnant, or are breastfeeding.
- Store tablets at controlled room temperature (59° to 77°F) in a tightly closed container and protect from light. Store the oral solution at controlled room temperature (59° to 77°F) and protect from light. Do not freeze.

If you have any questions, consult your doctor, pharmacist, or health care provider.

Generic Name *Brand Name Examples*	Supplied As	Generic Available
Rx **Olanzapine**		
Zyprexa	**Tablets:** 2.5 mg,[1] 5 mg,[1] 7.5 mg,[1] 10 mg,[1] 15 mg	No
Zyprexa Zydis[2]	**Tablets, disintegrating:** 5 mg, 10 mg	No

[1] Contains crospovidone and lactose.
[2] Contains aspartame.

Type of Drug:

Thienobenzodiazepine antipsychotic agent; neuroleptic drug; "major tranquilizer."

How the Drug Works:

How olanzapine works is not fully understood. It may alter the balance of certain chemicals in the brain that are responsible for thinking and behavior.

Uses:

For the management of symptoms of psychotic disorders (mental illnesses) manifested by delusions or hallucinations.

For short-term treatment of acute manic episodes associated with Bipolar I disorder.

Precautions:

Do not use in the following situations: Allergy to olanzapine or any of its ingredients.

Use with caution in the following situations:

- alcohol ingestion
- Alzheimer dementia
- aspiration pneumonia, at risk
- breast cancer, history of
- cerebrovascular disease
- dehydration, at risk
- elderly (especially women)
- exercise, strenuous
- exposure to extreme heat
- glaucoma, narrow-angle
- heart disease, history of
- high blood pressure medications, concurrent use
- hypovolemia
- intestinal motility, problems with
- liver disease
- neuroleptic malignant syndrome, history of
- prostatic hypertrophy
- seizures, history of
- suicidal tendencies

Orthostatic hypotension: This medicine may cause dizziness, lightheadedness, or fainting, especially when rising or standing. If these symptoms occur, sit or lie down. If these symptoms continue, contact your doctor. Use caution while driving or performing hazardous tasks requiring alertness, coordination, or physical dexterity.

Tardive dyskinesia: Involuntary and uncontrollable movements may develop in patients treated with antipsychotic drugs. Occurrence is highest among the elderly, especially women. The risk of developing these involuntary movements and the likelihood they will become permanent are increased as the length of treatment and the total amount of drug given increases. However, it is possible to develop these symptoms after short-term treatment at low doses. The syndrome is characterized by rhythmical, involuntary movements of the tongue, face, mouth, or jaw (eg, protrusion of tongue, puffing of cheeks, puckering of mouth, chewing movements), sometimes accompanied by involuntary movements of the arms and legs. Fine worm-like movement of the tongue may be an early sign of the syndrome. If the medication is stopped at this time, the syndrome may not develop further. There is no known treatment for established cases of tardive dyskinesia, although the syndrome may stop, partially or completely, if the drug is withdrawn.

Neuroleptic Malignant Syndrome (NMS): NMS is a potentially fatal syndrome associated with antipsychotic drugs. Symptoms include fever, muscle rigidity, altered mental abilities, irregular pulse and blood pressure, fast heartbeat, and profuse sweating.

Pregnancy: Adequate studies have not been done in pregnant women. Use only if clearly needed and the potential benefits to the mother outweigh the possible hazards to the fetus.

Breastfeeding: It is not known if olanzapine appears in breast milk. Consult your doctor before you begin breastfeeding.

Children: Safety and effectiveness in children have not been established.

Elderly: Lower doses may be required, especially if the patient is female and a nonsmoker.

Lab tests may be required to monitor therapy. Tests include liver enzyme levels.

Drug Interactions:

Tell your doctor or pharmacist if you are taking or if you are planning to take any over-the-counter or prescription medications or dietary supplements while taking olanzapine. Doses or one or both drugs may need to be modified or a different drug may need to be prescribed. The following drugs and drug classes may interact with olanzapine:

alcohol
antihypertensive drugs (eg, clonidine)
carbamazepine (eg, *Tegretol*)
charcoal (activated)
diazepam (eg, *Valium*)
dopamine agonists (eg, *Intropin*)
fluvoxamine (*Luvox*)
levodopa (eg, *Larodopa*)
omeprazole (*Prilosec*)
rifampin (eg, *Rifadin*)

Side Effects:

Every drug is capable of producing side effects. Many olanzapine users experience no, or minor, side effects. The frequency and severity of side effects depend on many factors including dose, duration of therapy, and individual susceptibility. Possible side effects include:

Digestive Tract: Constipation; dry mouth; increased appetite; increased salivation; indigestion; vomiting; thirst; dental pain.

Nervous System: Drowsiness; sleeplessness; dizziness; personality disorder; inability to sit still; tremors; difficulty speaking; euphoria (exaggerated sense of well being); twitching; abnormal movements; weakness; suicide attempt; intentional self injury; abnormal dreams; unstable emotions; abnormal skin sensations.

Circulatory System: Lightheadedness or fainting, especially when rising or standing; rapid heart beat; high blood pressure, low blood pressure.

Respiratory System: Cough; sore throat; difficulty breathing; congested or runny nose.

Urinary and Reproductive Tract: Blood in urine; loss of bladder control; urinary tract infection; absence of menstrual bleeding; heavy menstrual bleeding; vaginal itching; abnormal vaginal discharge.

Other: Flu syndrome; fever; back, chest, hand, foot, or joint pain; neck rigidity; swelling in arms or legs; rash; vision problems; unusual bruising; sweating; stiff or rigid muscles; weight changes; decreased libido; eyelid inflammation.

Guidelines for Use:

- Dosage is individualized. Take exactly as prescribed.
- Do not change the dose or stop taking this medicine unless advised by your doctor.
- *Disentegrating tablets* — Do not open until ready to use. Make sure fingers and hands are dry. Open sachet and peel back the foil on the blister; do not push the tablet through the foil. Immediately remove the tablet and place in the mouth. The tablet will dissolve in saliva and can be swallowed with or without liquid.
- A combination of factors, such as people older than 65 years of age, female gender, or nonsmoker, may require dose adjustment.
- May be taken with or without food.
- If a dose is missed, take it as soon as possible. If several hours have passed or if it is nearing time for the next dose, do not double the dose to catch up, unless advised by your doctor. If more than one dose is missed or if it is necessary to establish a new dosage schedule, contact your doctor or pharmacist.
- Avoid alcohol and other mental depressants (eg, narcotics, tranquilizers, antihistamines) while you are taking this medicine.
- Use caution in hot weather; be careful not to become dehydrated. This medicine may increase susceptibility to heat stroke.
- This medicine may cause dizziness, lightheadedness, or fainting, especially when rising or standing. If these symptoms occur, sit or lie down. Contact your doctor if they continue.
- May cause drowsiness. Use caution while driving or performing hazardous tasks requiring alertness, coordination, or physical dexterity.
- Contact your doctor immediately if you experience fever, sweating, muscle rigidity, involuntary movements (of the face, tongue, arms, or legs), abnormal heart rate or rhythm.
- Inform your doctor if you are pregnant, become pregnant, are planning to become pregnant, or if you are breastfeeding.
- Lab tests may be required to monitor therapy. Be sure to keep appointments.
- Store at controlled room temperature (68° to 77°F) away from light and moisture.

If you have any questions, consult your doctor, pharmacist, or health care provider.

	Generic Name *Brand Name Example*	Supplied As	Generic Available
Rx	**Clozapine**		
	Clozaril	**Tablets:** 25 mg, 100 mg	Yes

Type of Drug:

Atypical antipsychotic.

How the Drug Works:

Clozapine reduces nerve sensitivity in many different areas of the brain, helping to modify behavior.

Uses:

For the management of severely ill schizophrenic patients who fail to respond to typical antipsychotic drug treatment. Given only after tho patient has been given at least 2 trials, each with a different antipsychotic drug, at an adequate dose and for an adequate duration.

Precautions:

Do not use in the following situations:

- allergy to clozapine or any of its ingredients
- bone marrow disorders
- coma
- concomitant use with drugs that can cause bone marrow suppression or a decrease in granulocytes
- depression, severe
- epilepsy, uncontrolled
- history of clozapine-induced decrease in granulocytes
- sedation, severe

Use with caution in the following situations:

- alcohol or behavior-modifying drugs, concurrent use of
- decreased white blood cell count (especially granulocytes)
- heart disease
- kidney disease
- liver disease
- narrow angle glaucoma
- prostate enlargement
- seizure, history of

Seizures: Seizures have occurred during therapy with clozapine. The likelihood of seizure becomes greater at higher doses.

Neuroleptic Malignant Syndrome (NMS): NMS is a potentially fatal syndrome associated with antipsychotic drugs. Symptoms include increased body heat, muscle rigidity, altered mental abilities, irregular pulse and blood pressure, increased heart rate, sweating, and irregular heart rhythm.

Tardive dyskinesia: Involuntary and uncontrollable movements may develop in patients treated with some antipsychotic agents. Occurrence is highest in the elderly, especially women. The risk of developing these involuntary movements and the likelihood they will become irreversible are increased with long-term use and with high doses. However, there have been no confirmed cases of tardive dyskinesia associated with clozapine use alone. Nevertheless, without more experience it is not certain that clozapine will not cause this effect. The syndrome is characterized by rhythmical, involuntary movements of tongue, face, mouth, or jaw (eg, sticking out of the tongue, puffing of cheeks, puckering of mouth, chewing movements), sometimes accompanied by involuntary movements of the arms and legs. Fine worm-like movement of the tongue may be an early sign of the syndrome. If the medication is stopped at this time, the syndrome may not develop. There is no known treatment for established cases of tardive dyskinesia, although the syndrome may partially or completely disappear if the drug is withdrawn.

Agranulocytosis: Granulocytes are white blood cells. Clozapine has been shown to decrease the granulocyte count. Symptoms include: Flu-like symptoms (eg, tiredness, weakness, fever, sore throat) and infections.

Pregnancy: Studies in pregnant women or in animals have not shown a risk to the fetus. However, no drug should be used during pregnancy unless clearly needed.

Breastfeeding: Clozapine appears in breast milk and has an effect on the breastfeeding infant. Do not breastfeed while taking clozapine.

Children: Safety and effectiveness in children have not been established.

Lab tests may be required to monitor therapy. Be sure to keep appointments. Weekly blood tests should be performed during clozapine therapy to monitor for the occurrence of decreased granulocytes.

Drug Interactions:

Tell your doctor or pharmacist if you are taking or if you are planning to take any over-the-counter or prescription medications or dietary supplements with clozapine. Doses of one or both drugs may need to be modified or a different drug may need to be prescribed. The following drugs and drug classes interact with clozapine.

- antiarrhythmics (eg, flecainide, quinidine)
- antidepressants (eg, trihexyphenidyl, fluoxetine)
- antihypertensives
- antipsychotics (eg, chlorpromazine)
- carbamazepine (eg, *Tegretol*)
- cimetidine (eg, *Tagamet*)
- epinephrine
- phenothiazines (eg, chlorpromazine)
- warfarin (eg, *Coumadin*)

Side Effects:

Every drug is capable of producing side effects. Many clozapine users experience no, or minor, side effects. The frequency and severity of side effects depend on many factors including dose, duration of therapy and individual susceptibility. Possible side effects include:

Agranulocytosis (decreased white blood count; decreased number of granulocytes): Tiredness, weakness, fever, sore throat.

Digestive Tract: Nausea; vomiting; constipation; stomach pain; diarrhea; loss of appetite.

Nervous System: Seizures; drowsiness; dizziness; headache; tremor; vertigo (feeling of whirling motion); fainting; insomnia; nightmares; restlessness; confusion; impaired movement; agitation; fatigue; inability to sit still; rigidity; weakness; lethargy; clumsiness; slurred speech; depression; anxiety; muscle spasms; decreased mobility or activity.

Circulatory System: Increased heart rate; orthostatic hypotension (dizziness or lightheadedness that occurs when rising quickly from a seated or lying position); heart rhythm changes.

Other: Fever; dry mouth; visual disturbances; increased salivation (especially during sleep); urinary abnormalities; abnormal blood counts; blood disorder; incontinence; throat discomfort; sweating; muscle weakness; difficulty breathing; nasal congestion; rash; abnormal ejaculation; urinary urgency and retention; back, neck, leg, muscle pain; muscle spasm; weight gain; numb tongue; abnormal liver function tests; heartburn.

Guidelines for Use:

- Take only as directed by your doctor. Because of the significant risk of side effects associated with clozapine, patients should be periodically reassessed to determine the need for maintenance treatment.
- May cause drowsiness, dizziness or seizures. Use caution while driving or performing other tasks requiring alertness.
- Orthostatic hypotension (dizziness or drowsiness when rising quickly from a seated or lying position) may occur. Avoid sudden changes in posture.
- Notify your doctor immediately if any of the following symptoms occur: Tiredness, weakness, fever, sore throat, signs of infection, flu-like symptoms or seizures.
- Do not take any prescription or over-the-counter drugs or alcohol with clozapine without first consulting your doctor.
- Notifiy your doctor if you become pregnant or intend to become pregnant during therapy.
- Do not breastfeed during therapy.
- Watch for signs of overdose or toxicity, such as altered states of consciousness, including drowsiness, delirium and coma; increased heart rate; decreased blood pressure; difficulty breathing; and excessive salivation.
- Clozapine is available only through the *Clozaril Patient Management System*, a program that combines white blood cell testing, patient monitoring, pharmacy and drug distribution services, all linked to compliance with required safety monitoring.

If you have any questions, consult your doctor, pharmacist, or health care provider.

	Generic Name *Brand Name Example*	Supplied As	Generic Available
Rx	**Pimozide**		
	Orap	**Tablets:** 2 mg	No

Type of Drug:

Neuroleptic; drugs that modify psychotic behavior.

How the Drug Works:

Pimozide blocks receptors in the nervous system to reduce involuntary motor (movement) and phonic (voice) tics.

Uses:

For the treatment of severely disabling motor and phonic tics in patients with Tourette Disorder who have failed to respond satisfactorily to standard treatment.

Precautions:

Do not use in the following situations:

abnormal heart rhythm, history
allergy to pimozide or other antipsychotic medications
coma
macrolide antibiotic use
tics other than for Tourette's (simple tics)

Use with caution in the following situations:

kidney disease
liver disease
low potassium level
seizures, history of

Tardive dyskinesia: Involuntary and uncontrollable movements may develop in patients treated with pimozide. Occurrence is highest in the elderly, especially women. The risk of developing these involuntary movements and the likelihood they will become irreversible are increased with long-term use and with high doses. However, it is possible to develop these symptoms after short-term treatment at low doses. The syndrome is characterized by rhythmical, involuntary movements of tongue, face, mouth or jaw (eg, protrusion of tongue, puffing of cheeks, puckering of mouth, chewing movements), sometimes accompanied by involuntary movements of the arms and legs. Fine worm-like movement of the tongue may be an early sign of the syndrome. If the medication is stopped at this time, the syndrome may not develop. There is no known treatment for established cases of tardive dyskinexia, although the syndrome may stop, partially or completely, if the drug is withdrawn.

Neuroleptic Malignant Syndrome (NMS) is a potentially fatal syndrome associated with antipsychotic drugs. Symptoms include: Increased body heat, muscle rigidity, altered mental abilities including catatonia, irregular pulse and blood pressure, increased heart rate, sweating and irregular heart rhythm.

Gradual withdrawal: The doctor should periodically attempt to reduce dosage to see if tics persist. Increases of tic intensity and frequency may represent a temporary, withdrawal-related occurrence rather than a return of symptoms. Allow 1 or 2 weeks to elapse before concluding that an increase in tics is due to the underlying disease rather than drug withdrawal.

Pregnancy: Adequate studies have not been done in pregnant women, or animal studies may have shown a risk to the fetus. Use only if clearly needed and potential benefits outweigh the possible hazards to the fetus.

Breastfeeding: It is not known if pimozide appears in breast milk. Consult your doctor before you begin breastfeeding.

Children: Although Tourette Disorder often has its onset between the ages of 2 and 15 years, the use of pimozide in patients under 12 is limited. Pimozide is not recommended for use in any childhood condition other than Tourette Disorder.

Drug Interactions:

Tell your doctor or pharmacist if you are taking or if you are planning to take any over-the-counter or prescription medications or dietary supplements with pimozide. Doses of one or both drugs may need to be modified or a different drug may need to be prescribed. The following drugs and drug classes interact with pimozide:

- alcohol
- antiarrhythmic agents (eg, procainamide)
- phenothiazines (eg, chlorpromazine)
- sedatives (eg, *Dalmane*)
- tricyclic antidepressants (eg, amitriptyline)

Side Effects:

Every drug is capable of producing side effects. Many pimozide users experience no, or minor, side effects. The frequency and severity of side effects depend on many factors including dose, duration of therapy and individual susceptibility. Possible side effects include:

Tardive Dyskinesia and Neuroleptic Malignant Syndrome – See precautions.

Digestive Tract: Diarrhea; constipation; appetite changes; nausea; vomiting; stomach upset; appetite loss; dry mouth; thirst; increased salivation.

Nervous System: Headache; drowsiness; sleeplessness; rigidity; handwriting changes; dizziness; fainting; nervousness; Parkinson disease-like symptoms; muscle restlessness; muscular deformation; inability to sit still; change in posture; impaired movement; abnormal dreams; hyperactivity; depression; sedation; tremor; excitement.

Circulatory System: Changes in blood pressure; increased heart rate; chest pain; pounding in chest; postural hypotension (lightheadedness when rising quickly from sitting or lying position).

Eyes or Ocular: Sensitivity to light; blurred vision; cataracts; swelling around eyes; visual disturbance; unusual eye movements.

Skin: Increased body heat; rash; sweating; skin irritation.

Other: Muscle tightness; speech problems; taste changes; weight changes; impotence; loss of sex drive; decreased accomodation; neck muscle spasms; weakness; difficulty swallowing; muscle pain; excessive urination at night; frequent urination; speech disorder.

Guidelines for Use:

- May cause drowsiness. Use caution while driving or performing other tasks requiring alertness.
- Know the risks of developing tardive dyskinesia with chronic use. Contact the doctor at the earliest sign of tardive dyskinesia or Parkinson-like symptoms. (See Precautions)
- Do not exceed prescribed dose. Sudden, unexpected deaths have occurred in patients taking high doses of pimozide for conditions other than Tourette syndrome.
- The drug should be tapered and withdrawn gradually if therapy has continued for weeks or months.

If you have any questions, consult your doctor, pharmacist, or health care provider.

	Generic Name *Brand Name Examples*	Supplied As	Generic Available
Rx	**Ergoloid Mesylates**	**Tablets, sublingual:** 1 mg	Yes
	Hydergine	**Tablets:** 1 mg	Yes
	Hydergine LC	**Capsules, liquid:** 1 mg	No
	Hydergine[1]	**Liquid:** 1 mg/mL	No

[1] Contains alcohol.

Type of Drug:

Dihydrogenated ergot alkaloids. Drugs used to treat age-related decreases in mental ability.

How the Drug Works:

It is not known how ergoloid mesylates produce beneficial mental effects. It is possible that they may increase brain metabolism, possibly increasing blood flow in the brain.

Uses:

To treat the signs and symptoms of age-related decreases in mental ability, including decreased alertness, short-term memory loss, decreased self-care, and sociability, or age-related changes in mood in patients older than 60 years of age.

Patients who respond may suffer from an aging disorder or have some underlying condition (eg, primary progressive dementia, Alzheimer disease, senile onset, multi-infarct [stroke] dementia).

Precautions:

Do not use in the following situations:

allergy to ergoloid mesylates or any of their ingredients
psychosis

Use with caution in the following situations: Mental decline of unknown origin.

Before prescribing ergoloid mesylates, your doctor may need to rule out other conditions that could cause a decrease in mental ability. Periodic doctor visits may be required after beginning therapy.

Side Effects:

Every drug is capable of producing side effects. Many ergoloid mesylate users experience no, or minor, side effects. The frequency and severity of side effects depend on many factors including dose, duration of therapy, and individual susceptibility. Possible side effects include: Nausea; stomach upset.

Guidelines for Use:

- Use exactly as prescribed.
- Usual starting dosage is 1 mg 3 times daily.
- Allow sublingual tablets to dissolve under your tongue. Do not crush, chew, or swallow sublingual tablets whole.
- Liquid dose form comes with calibrated dropper to measure dose accurately.
- May cause nausea and stomach upset during start of treatment. Take with food if this occurs.
- If a dose is missed, take it as soon as possible. If several hours have passed or if it is nearing time for the next dose, do not double the dose in order to catch up, unless advised to do so by your doctor. If more than one dose is missed, or it is necessary to establish a new dosage schedule, contact your doctor or pharmacist.
- Improvement of symptoms is gradual and may take 3 to 4 weeks to be noticed.
- Treatment for up to 6 months may be necessary to determine effectiveness.
- Do not stop therapy or change the dose unless advised to do so by your doctor.
- Store tablets below 77°F and protect from light. Store liquid capsules between 59° and 77°F, protect from light, and do not freeze. Store liquid below 86°F.

If you have any questions, consult your doctor, pharmacist, or health care provider.

	Generic Name *Brand Name Examples*	Supplied As	Generic Available
Rx	**Lithium Carbonate**	**Tablets:** 300 mg (8.12 mEq lithium)	Yes
		Capsules: 150 mg (4.06 mEq lithium); 300 mg (8.12 mEq lithium); 600 mg (16.24 mEq lithium)	Yes
	Eskalith	**Capsules:** 300 mg (8.12 mEq lithium)	Yes
	Eskalith CR	**Tablets, controlled release:** 450 mg (12.18 mEq lithium)	No
	Lithobid	**Tablets, slow release:** 300 mg (8.12 mEq lithium)	No
Rx	**Lithium Citrate**	**Syrup:** 300 mg (8 mEq lithium carbonate)/5 mL	Yes

Type of Drug:

Antimanic drug.

How the Drug Works:

Lithium reduces the extremes of emotional states, behavior, and feelings during periods of mania by stabilizing nerve and muscle cells.

Uses:

To treat manic episodes of manic-depressive illness (bipolar disorder). Maintenance therapy prevents or decreases the frequency and intensity of subsequent manic episodes.

Unlabeled Use(s): Occasionally doctors may prescribe lithium for cluster headaches, premenstrual tension, postpartum psychosis, eating disorders, alcoholism related to depression, psychosis caused by corticosteroid use, certain movement disorders (eg, tardive dyskinesia), and hyperthyroidism (overactive thyroid); and to increase white blood cell counts in individuals undergoing cancer chemotherapy, AIDS patients taking zidovudine, and in childhood disorders in which white blood cell counts are extremely low.

Precautions:

Do not use in the following situations: Allergy to lithium.

Use with caution in the following situations:

angiotensin-converting enzyme (ACE) inhibitors use
CNS impairment
debilitation, severe
dehydration (fluid loss), severe
diarrhea, chronic
diuretic use
heart disease, moderate-to-severe
infection with fever
kidney disease, severe
low sodium blood level
neuroleptic drug use
organic brain syndrome
pregnancy
psychiatric condition, life-threatening
sweating, chronic and excessive
thyroid function, low
vomiting

Decreased thyroid function (hypothyroidism) may occur with long-term use. Contact your doctor if neck swelling or skin coarsening occurs, or if your activity level decreases. Lithium-induced hypothyroidism may be treated with thyroid hormone therapy.

Chronic lithium therapy may be associated with a reduction in the kidney's concentrating ability, occasionally presenting as nephrogenic diabetes insipidus (thirst and frequent urination). This condition is usually reversible when lithium is discontinued.

Pregnancy: Studies have shown lithium may cause harm to the fetus. Use only if clearly needed and potential benefits to the mother outweigh the possible risks to the fetus. If possible, lithium should be withdrawn for at least the first trimester.

Breastfeeding: Lithium appears in breast milk. Consult your doctor before you begin breastfeeding.

Children: Safety and effectiveness in children younger than 12 years of age have not been established.

Elderly: Because of an increased risk of toxicity, lower doses and more frequent monitoring are necessary.

Lab tests may be required during lithium therapy. Tests may include lithium blood levels, blood counts, urinalysis, electrolytes (eg, sodium, potassium), glucose, electrocardiogram, and thyroid and kidney function tests. Lithium blood levels should be checked twice weekly until dosage is stabilized. When a consistent blood level is reached, testing may be reduced to once weekly. Eventually blood levels will be checked every 2 to 3 months (more frequently in the elderly). See Side Effects.

Drug Interactions:

Tell your doctor or pharmacist if you are taking or if you are planning to take any over-the-counter or prescription medications with lithium. Doses of one or both drugs may need to be modified or a different drug may need to be prescribed. The following drugs and drug classes interact with lithium.

- ACE inhibitors (eg, captopril, lisinopril)
- carbamazepine (eg, *Tegretol)*
- haloperidol *(Haldol)*
- iodide salts (eg, *SSKI*)
- nonsteroidal anti-inflammatory agents (NSAIDS) (eg, ibuprofen)
- succinylcholine (eg, *Anectine)*
- thiazide diuretics (eg, hydrochlorothiazide)
- urinary alkalinizers (eg, sodium bicarbonate)

Side Effects:

Every drug is capable of producing side effects. Many lithium users experience no, or minor, side effects. The frequency and severity of side effects depend on many factors including dose, duration of therapy, and individual susceptibility. Possible side effects include:

Toxicity – The likelihood of toxicity increases with increasing serum lithium levels. Lithium blood levels greater than 1.5 mEq/L carry a greater risk than lower levels. Diarrhea, vomiting, drowsiness, muscle weakness, and lack of coordination may be early signs of lithium toxicity, and can occur at lithium levels below 2 mEq/L. At higher levels, giddiness, blurred vision, ringing in the ears, vertigo (feeling of whirling motion), and a large output of urine may be seen. Serum lithium levels should not be permitted to exceed 2 mEq/L during the acute treatment phase. Fine hand tremor, excessive urination, and mild thirst may occur when starting therapy for the acute manic phase and may persist throughout treatment. Mild nausea and general discomfort may also appear during the first few days of treatment. These side effects are an inconvenience rather than a disabling condition, and usually subside with continued treatment or a temporary dosage reduction.

Digestive Tract: Nausea; appetite loss; vomiting; diarrhea; gastritis; salivary gland swelling; stomach pain; excessive salivation; gas; indigestion; dry mouth; metallic taste; salty taste; taste distortion; swollen lips; thirst.

Nervous System: Tremor; muscle twitches or jerking movement of whole limbs; hypertonicity; incoordination; clumsiness; uncontrolled muscle movement; hyperactive deep tendon reflex; extrapyramidal symptoms (acute dystonia, cogwheel rigidity); blackout spells; seizures; slurred speech; dizziness; feeling of whirling motion; downbeat nystagmus; drowsiness; psychomotor retardation; restlessness; confusion; stupor; coma; uncontrolled tongue movements; tics; ringing in the ears; hallucinations; poor memory; slowed intellectual function; startled response; worsening of organic brain syndromes; pseudotumor cerebri (increased intracranial pressure and papilledema); lethargy; headache; drowsiness; fatigue; giddiness; blurred vision.

Circulatory System: Abnormal heart rhythm; low blood pressure; slow heartbeat; chest tightness.

Skin: Drying and thinning of hair; hair loss; numbness of skin; acne; chronic folliculitis; dry skin; itching; rash; skin ulcers; skin inflammation; hives; worsening of psoriasis.

Urinary and Reproductive Tract: Urinary problems; inability to urinate; increased or decreased urine output; impotence; sexual dysfunction; incontinence of urine or feces.

Laboratory changes: Sugar in urine; decreased kidney function; albumin in urine; increased white blood cell count; increased blood sugar; increased blood calcium.

Other: Transient blind spots; bulging of the eyes; ankle or wrist swelling or painful joints; dental cavities; thyroid abnormalities; fever; weight loss or gain.

Guidelines for Use:

- Use exactly as prescribed.
- Dosage will be individualized according to serum levels and clinical response. Examples of usual doses are as follows:
  Acute mania — 600 mg (capsules, tablets, or syrup) 3 times daily; 900 mg (controlled release, slow release) twice daily.
  Maintenance therapy — 300 mg (capsules, tablets, or syrup) 3 or 4 times daily; 450 mg (controlled release, slow release) twice daily.
- The syrup and immediate release capsules and tablets are usually given 3 to 4 times daily. Controlled and slow release tablets are usually given 2 times daily (every 12 hours), but can be given 3 times daily (every 8 hours).
- Do not crush or chew slow release or controlled release products.
- Take after meals or with food or milk if stomach upset occurs.
- Maintain a normal diet, including salt and adequate fluid intake (8 to 12 glasses of water) daily.
- Watch for signs of overdose or toxicity, such as diarrhea, vomiting, drowsiness, muscle weakness, lack of coordination, giddiness, blurred vision, ringing in the ears, feeling of whirling motion, or increased urination. Stop the medication and contact your doctor immediately.
- May take 2 to 3 weeks to normalize symptoms when used to treat a manic episode.
- If a dose is missed, take it as soon as possible. If several hours have passed or if it is nearing time for the next dose, do not double the dose in order to catch up, unless advised to do so by your doctor. If more than one dose is missed, or it is necessary to establish a new dosage schedule, contact your doctor or pharmacist.
- May cause drowsiness. Use caution while driving or performing other tasks requiring alertness, coordination, or physical dexterity.
- Notify your doctor if you become pregnant or are planning to become pregnant while taking this medicine. Lithium is a potential hazard to the fetus.
- Notify your doctor if sweating and diarrhea occur since this may decrease your tolerance to lithium. Supplemental fluid and salt should be administered under medical supervision until the condition is resolved.
- Lab tests, including lithium blood levels, may be required periodically during treatment. Be sure to keep appointments.
- Lithium blood levels, to be most accurate, should be drawn just before a scheduled dose.
- *Brand interchange* — Do not change from one brand of this drug to another without consulting your pharmacist or doctor. Products manufactured by different companies may not be equally effective.
- Store between 59° to 86°F in a tight, child-resistant container. Protect from moisture.

If you have any questions, consult your doctor, pharmacist, or health care provider.

	Generic Name *Brand Name Examples*	Supplied As	Generic Available
Rx	**Donepezil HCl**		
	Aricept	**Tablets**: 5 mg, 10 mg	No
Rx	**Galantamine HBr**		
	Reminyl	**Tablets**: 4 mg, 8 mg, 12 mg	No
Rx	**Rivastigmine Tartrate**		
	Exelon	**Capsules**: 1.5 mg, 3 mg, 4.5 mg, 6 mg	No
	Exelon	**Solution**: 2 mg/mL	No
Rx	**Tacrine HCl**		
	Cognex	**Capsules**: 10 mg, 20 mg, 30 mg, 40 mg	No

Type of Drug:

Reversible cholinesterase inhibitor used in managing mild to moderate Alzheimer disease-associated dementia.

How the Drug Works:

The exact mechanism is unknown. Cholinesterase inhibitors act by enhancing cholinergic function. Deterioration or loss of cholinergic neurons may be a primary cause of cognitive dysfunction associated with Alzheimer disease. Cholinesterase inhibitors may enhance cholinergic transmission in this setting. If this mechanism of action is correct, the effect of cholinesterase inhibitors may lessen as the disease advances and fewer cholinergic neurons remain functionally intact. There is no evidence that cholinesterase inhibitors alter the course of the underlying dementing process.

Uses:

To treat mild to moderate dementia of the Alzheimer type.

Precautions:

Do not use in the following situations:

- allergy to acridine derivatives (tacrine only)
- allergy to carbamate derivatives (rivastigmine only)
- allergy to a cholinesterase inhibitor or any of its ingredients
- allergy to piperidine derivatives (donepezil only)
- treatment-associated jaundice from previous treatments (tacrine only)

Use with caution in the following situations:

abnormally slow heart rate
anesthesia (succinylcholine type)
asthma, history of
bladder outflow difficulty
cardiac conduction abnormalities
gastrointestinal disease or dysfunction (eg, peptic ulcer, bleeding disorder)
heart disease
kidney disease (galantamine only)
liver disease, active or history of
NSAID use, concurrent
obstructive lung disease, history of
seizures
sick sinus syndrome
ulcers (gastric, duodenal), history of
urinary obstruction

Nicotine: Nicotine use increases the elimination of tacrine from the body.

Gender: Tacrine and galantamine are eliminated from the body more slowly in women.

Pregnancy: There are no adequate and well-controlled studies in pregnant women. Use only if clearly needed and the potential benefits to the mother outweigh possible hazards to the fetus.

Breastfeeding: It is not known if cholinesterase inhibitors are excreted in breast milk. Contact your doctor before you begin breastfeeding.

Children: Safety and effectiveness in children have not been established.

Elderly: Rivastigmine and galantamine are eliminated from the body more slowly in the elderly.

Lab tests will be required to monitor therapy with tacrine. Tests include liver function tests every other week from at least week 4 to week 16, after which monitoring may be decreased to every 3 months, and blood counts.

Drug Interactions:

Tell your doctor or pharmacist if you are taking or if you are planning to take any over-the-counter or prescription medications or dietary supplements with a cholinesterase inhibitor. Doses of one or both drugs may need to be modified or a different drug may need to be prescribed. The following drugs and drug classes interact with cholinesterase inhibitors:

anticholinergics (eg, atropine, scopolamine)
cholinergic agonists (eg, bethanechol)
cholinesterase inhibitors (eg, neostigmine)
cimetidine (eg, *Tagamet*)
erythromycin (eg, *E-mycin*)
fluvoxamine (eg, *Luvox*) (tacrine only)
food (rivastigmine only)
ketoconazole (eg, *Nizoral*)
NSAIDs (eg, ibuprofen)
paroxetine (*Paxil*)
succinylcholine (eg, *Quelicin*)
theophylline (eg, *Theo-Dur*) (tacrine only)

Side Effects:

Every drug is capable of producing side effects. Many cholinesterase inhibitor users experience no, or minor, side effects. The frequency and severity of side effects depend on many factors including dose, duration of therapy, and individual susceptibility. Possible side effects include:

Digestive Tract: Nausea; vomiting; diarrhea; appetite loss; stomach bleeding; black tarry stools; loss of bowel control; bloating; gas; belching; indigestion; stomach pain; weight loss; constipation.

Nervous System: Sleeplessness; fatigue; drowsiness; headache; pain; difficulty moving; dizziness; fainting; depression; abnormal dreams; abnormal thinking; hallucinations; tremors; irritability; numbness or tingling in hands or feet; abnormal skin sensations (eg, burning, prickling, tingling); aggression; feeling of whirling motion; clumsiness; twitching; restlessness; nervousness; anxiety; paranoia; convulsions; weakness; confusion; hostility; difficulty speaking.

Circulatory System: Chest pain; abnormal heartbeat; heart pounding; blood pressure changes; flushing; hot flashes.

Skin: Itching; hives; rash; excessive sweating; unusual bruising or bleeding.

Respiratory System: Difficulty breathing; sore throat; nasal congestion; sinus problems; runny nose; coughing; upper respiratory infection; pulmonary congestion.

Urinary and Reproductive Tract: Loss of bladder control; frequent urination; excessive urination at night; urinary tract infection; blood in the urine.

Other: Flu-like syndrome; chills; fever; general body discomfort; muscle cramps; muscle or joint pain; muscle tension; back pain; swelling in hands or feet; anemia; dehydration; eye irritation; blurred vision; elevated transaminase; accidental trauma; abnormal gait; ringing in the ears; nosebleed.

Guidelines for Use:

- Dosage is individualized. Take exactly as prescribed.
- *Donepezil* — Take in the evening just before bedtime with or without food.
- *Galantamine* — Take during morning and evening meal if possible. Follow recommended dosage and administration. If therapy is interrupted for several days or longer, restart treatment at the lowest dose. Nausea may be reduced by administering with food, antiemetic medication, or ensuring adequate fluid intake.
- *Tacrine* — Take between meals if possible; however, it may be taken with meals to avoid stomach upset. The effect of tacrine is thought to depend upon its administration at regular intervals.
- *Rivastigmine capsules*— Take with food in divided doses in the morning or evening.
- *Rivastigmine solution* — Remove the oral dosing syringe provided in its protective case and, using the provided syringe, withdraw the prescribed amount of rivastigmine. Each dose may be swallowed from the syringe or first mixed with a small glass of water, cold fruit juice, or soda. Stir the mixture before drinking.
- If a dose is missed, take it as soon as possible. If several hours have passed or if it is nearing time for the next dose, do not double the dose to catch up, unless advised by your doctor. If more than one dose is missed or it is necessary to establish a new dosage schedule, contact your doctor or pharmacist.
- *Tacrine* — Do not stop taking this medicine suddenly or change the dosage unless instructed to do so by your doctor. Abrupt discontinuation or large reduction in the total daily dose of tacrine may cause a decline in mental function and behavioral disturbances. Unsupervised increases in the dose of tacrine may also have serious consequences.
- Inform your doctor if you are pregnant, become pregnant, planning to become pregnant, or are breastfeeding before beginning therapy.
- Report any new or worsening side effects to your doctor.
- May cause dizziness or blurred vision. Use caution while driving or performing other tasks requiring alertness, coordination, or physical dexterity.
- *Rivastigmine* — There is a high incidence of nausea and vomiting associated with the use of the drug, along with the possibility of anorexia and weight loss. Monitor for these adverse events and inform your doctor if they occur.
- *Tacrine* — Contact you doctor if you experience side effects that occur soon after taking a dose (eg, nausea, vomiting, loose stools) or develop side effects that are delayed (eg, rash, yellowing of the skin, changes in stool color).
- Lab tests will be required to monitor therapy. Be sure to keep appointments.
- Store capsules and tablets at controlled room temperature (59° to 86°F) away from moisture. Store rivastigmine solution below 77°F in an upright position. Protect from freezing.

If you have any questions, consult your doctor, pharmacist, or health care provider.

	Generic Name *Brand Name Examples*	Supplied As	Generic Available
c-iv	**Chlordiazepoxide and Amitriptyline HCl**	**Tablets:** 5 mg chlordiazepoxide and 12.5 mg amitriptyline	Yes
	Limbitrol[1], *Limbitrol DS*[1]	**Tablets:** 10 mg chlordiazepoxide and 25 mg amitriptyline	Yes
Rx	**Perphenazine and Amitriptyline HCl**	**Tablets:** 4 mg perphenazine and 10 mg amitriptyline; 4 mg perphenazine and 50 mg amitriptyline	Yes
	Etrafon 2-10	**Tablets:** 2 mg perphenazine and 10 mg amitriptyline	Yes
	Etrafon	**Tablets:** 2 mg perphenazine and 25 mg amitriptyline	Yes
	Etrafon Forte	**Tablets:** 4 mg perphenazine and 25 mg amitriptyline	Yes

[1] As hydrochloride salt.

For complete information, see the chlordiazepoxide monograph and the amitriptyline monograph.

Type of Drug:

Amitriptyline is a tricyclic antidepressant, chlordiazepoxide is a benzodiazepine antianxiety agent, and perphenazine is an antipsychotic agent.

How the Drug Works:

Amitriptyline acts on the central nervous system (brain) to exert its antidepressant effects. Chlordiazepoxide acts on the central nervous system to effect emotional responses. Perphenazine acts on the central nervous system to exert its antipsychotic effects.

Uses:

To treat moderate-to-severe depression associated with moderate-to-severe anxiety. Perphenazine and amitriptyline HCl combination is also indicated for anxiety and depression associated with chronic physical disease, depression and anxiety that cannot be clearly differentiated, and schizophrenia with associated symptoms of depression.

Precautions:

Do not use in the following situations:

allergy to these medicines or any of their ingredients
allergy to benzodiazepines or tricyclic antidepressants (chlordiazepoxide and amitriptyline only)
allergy to phenothiazines or tricyclic antidepressants (perphenazine and amitriptyline only)
blood dyscrasias (perphenazine only)
bone marrow depression (perphenazine only)
elective surgery
heart attack, acute recovery phase
liver damage (perphenazine only)
MAOI therapy, concurrent
subcortical brain damage (perphenazine only)

Use with caution in the following situations:

asthma, severe (perphenazine only)
drug addiction, history of
electroshock therapy
emphysema (perphenazine only)
glaucoma, closed angle
heart disease
increased eye pressure (perphenazine only)
kidney impairment
liver impairment
lung disease (perphenazine only)
overactive thyroid
seizure, history of
suicidal tendencies
urinary retention, history of

Neuroleptic Malignant Syndrome (NMS) is a potentially fatal syndrome associated with perphenazine. Symptoms include increased body heat, muscle rigidity, altered mental abilities including catatonia (eg, confusion, withdrawal, unresponsivness), irregular pulse and blood pressure, increased heart rate, and sweating.

Tardive dyskinesia: Involuntary and uncontrollable movements may develop in patients treated with perphenazine. The likelihood that these symptoms will become permanent increases with long-term use and with high doses. However, it is possible to develop these symptoms after short-term treatment at low doses. Occurrence is highest among the elderly. The syndrome is characterized by rhythmical involuntary movements of the tongue, face, mouth, or jaw (eg, protrusion of tongue, puffing of cheeks, puckering of mouth, chewing movements), sometimes accompanied by involuntary movement of the arms and legs. Fine worm-like movements of the tongue may be an early sign of the syndrome. If the medication is stopped at this time, the syndrome may not develop. There is no known treatment for established cases of tardive dyskinesia, although the syndrome may stop, partially or completely, if the drug is withdrawn.

Pregnancy: Safety and effectiveness of psychotherapeutic combinations during pregnancy have not been established. Studies suggest an increased risk of congenital malformations associated with use of minor tranquilizers (chlordiazepoxide, diazepam, meprobamate) during the first trimester of pregnancy. Use of these drugs during pregnancy should almost always be avoided. Use only if clearly needed and potential benefits to the mother outweigh the possible risk to the fetus.

Breastfeeding: It is not known whether these drugs are excreted in human milk. As a general rule, breastfeeding should not be undertaken while on these drugs, because many drugs are excreted in human milk. Consult your doctor before you begin breastfeeding.

Children: Safety and effectiveness of chlordiazepoxide and amitriptyline HCl in children younger than 12 years of age have not been established. Perphenazine and amitriptyline HCl combination is not recommended for use in children.

Elderly: Lowest effective dose is recommended to prevent incoordination, oversedation, confusion, or anticholinergic effects (eg, dry mouth, confusion, blurred vision, constipation, urinary retention).

Lab tests or exams may be required during treatment with psychotherapeutic combinations. Tests may include periodic kidney and liver function tests and blood counts.

Drug Interactions:

Tell your doctor or pharmacist if you are taking or if you are planning to take any over-the-counter or prescription medications or dietary supplements with psychotherapeutic combinations. Doses of one or both drugs may need to be modified or a different drug may need to be prescribed. The following drugs and drug classes interact with psychotherapeutic combinations:

alcohol
anticholinergics (eg, scopolamine) (perphenazine only)
anticoagulants (eg, dicumarol)
antifungal agents (eg, ketoconazole)
beta blockers (eg, propranolol) (chlordiazepoxide only)
carbamazepine (eg, *Tegretol*)
cimetidine (eg, *Tagamet*)
clonidine (eg, *Catapres*)
CNS depressants (eg, barbiturates, narcotics)
contraceptves, oral (eg, *Ortho-Novum*) (chlordiazepoxide only)
disulfiram (eg, *Antabuse*)
drugs metabolized by P450 2D6 (eg, fluoxetine)
ethclorvynol (perphenazine only)
guanethidine (eg, *Ismelin*)
histamine H_2 antagonists (eg, cimetidine, ranitidine)
MAOIs (eg, phenelzine)
quinolones (eg, ciprofloxacin)
rifampin (eg, *Rifadin*)
SSRIs (eg, fluoxetine)
sympathomimetics (eg, epinephrine)
theophyllines (eg, *TheoDur*) (chlordiazepoxide only)
thyroid medications (eg, *Synthroid*)
valproic acid (eg, *Depakote*)

Side Effects:

Every drug is capable of producing side effects. Many patients taking psychotherapeutic combinations experience no, or minor, side effects. The frequency and severity of side effects depend on many factors including dose, duration of therapy, and individual susceptibility. Possible side effects include:

Withdrawal symptoms include convulsions, tremor, stomach and muscle cramps, vomiting, sweating.

Chlordiazepoxide/amitriptyline —

Digestive Tract: Constipation; loss of appetite; bloating; nausea; stomach upset; vomiting; peculiar taste; diarrhea.

Nervous System: Drowsiness; dizziness; vivid dreams; confusion; tremor; fatigue; weakness; restlessness; lethargy; apprehension; poor concentration; delusions; hallucinations; incoordination; clumsiness; numbness; tingling and abnormal skin sensations of the arms and legs; fainting; headache.

Other: Dry mouth; impotence; nasal congestion; fast heartbeat; pounding in the chest; blurred vision; inability to urinate; rash; hives; increased sensitivity to light; itching; excessive or spontaneous flow of breast milk; menstrual irregularities; changes in blood sugar levels; increased sweating; frequent urination; dilated pupils; yellowing of the skin and eyes; hair loss; glandular swelling.

Perphenazine/amitriptyline —

Digestive Tract: Constipation; appetite loss.

Nervous System: Abnormal or involuntary muscle movements; drowsiness; dizziness; vivid dreams; confusion; tremor; fatigue; restlessness; lethargy.

Other: Dry mouth; elevated body temperature; urinary retention; blurred vision; changes in blood pressure; abnormal blood counts; abnormal skin pigmentation.

Guidelines for Use:

- Optimum dosage varies with the severity of the symptoms and the patient response. When satisfactory response is obtained, dosage should be reduced to the smallest amount needed to maintain satisfactory response.
- *Chlordiazepoxide and amitriptyline* — Initial dosage of 3 or 4 tablets daily in divided doses is recommended. The larger portion of the total daily dose may be taken at bedtime. In some patients, a single dose at bedtime may be sufficient.
- *Perphenazine and amitriptyline* — Usual inital dose is 3 to 4 tablets daily in divided doses. Lower inital doses may be used in adolescents and the elderly.
- Take only the amount prescribed by your doctor. Some of these medicines may be habit-forming and may produce dependence. Consult your doctor before increasing the dose or stopping the medicine.
- To avoid withdrawal symptoms after long-term use, a gradual dosage tapering schedule should be followed.
- Do not use in combination with MAOIs or within 14 days of discontinuing treatment with an MAOI. After stopping these medicines, wait at least 14 days before starting an MAOI.
- Avoid alcohol and other mental depressants (eg, narcotics, tranquilizers, antihistamines) while you are taking psychotherapeutic combinations.
- May cause drowsiness. Use caution while driving or performing other tasks requiring alertness, coordination, or physical dexterity.
- Inform your doctor if you are pregnant, become pregnant, are planning to become pregnant, or if you are breastfeeding.
- *Perphenazine and amitriptyline HCl* — Contact your doctor immediately if you notice a rise in body temperature (eg, fever), because this may suggest intolerance to perphenazine. May cause sensitivity to sunlight. Avoid prolonged exposure to the sun or other forms of ultraviolet (UV) light (eg, tanning beds). Use sunscreen and wear protective clothing until tolerance is determined.
- Store at controlled room temperature (36° to 77°F). Keep tightly closed. Protect from light and moisture.

If you have any questions, consult your doctor, pharmacist, or health care provider.

	Generic Name *Brand Name Examples*	Supplied As	Generic Available
C-II	**Amobarbital Sodium**		
	Amytal Sodium	**Powder for Injection:** 500 mg/vial	No
C-III	**Butabarbital Sodium**		
	Butisol	**Tablets:** 15 mg, 30 mg[2], 50 mg[2]	Yes
	Butisol[1,2]	**Elixir**: 30 mg/5 mL	Yes
C-IV	**Mephobarbital**		
	Mebaral	**Tablets:** 32 mg, 50 mg, 100 mg	Yes
	Pentobarbital and Pentobarbital Sodium		
C-II	*Nembutal Sodium*	**Capsules:** 50 mg, 100 mg[2]	No
C-II	*Nembutal*[1]	**Elixir**: 18.2 mg pentobarbital/5 mL[3]	No
C-II	*Nembutal*[1]	**Injection**: 50 mg/mL	Yes
C-III	*Nembutal Sodium*	**Suppositories:** 30 mg, 60 mg, 120 mg, 200 mg	No
C-IV	**Phenobarbital**	**Tablets**: 15 mg, 30 mg, 60 mg, 90 mg, 100 mg	Yes
		Elixir: 20 mg/5 mL[1]	Yes
C-II	**Secobarbital Sodium**		
	Seconal Sodium	**Capsules**: 100 mg	Yes
	Barbiturate Combinations		
C-II	*Tuinal 100 mg Pulvules*	**Capsules:** 50 mg amobarbital sodium, 50 mg secobarbital sodium	No
C-II	*Tuinal 200 mg Pulvules*	**Capsules:** 100 mg amobarbital sodium, 100 mg secobarbital sodium	No

[1] Contains alcohol.
[2] Contains tartrazine dye.
[3] Equivalent to 20 mg pentobarbital sodium/5 mL.

Type of Drug:

Central nervous system (CNS) depressants; sedatives; antianxiety agents; anticonvulsants; "barbs"; "downers."

How the Drug Works:

Barbiturates are capable of producing all levels of CNS mood alternation, from excitation to mild sedation, sleep, and deep coma. They also decrease the severity and or frequency of certain types of seizures. Overdose can produce death. In high therapeutic doses, barbiturates induce anesthesia. Barbiturates depress the sensory cortex, decrease motor activity, alter cerebellar function, and produce drowsiness, sedation, and hypnosis (sleep).

Uses:

To treat sleeplessness by inducing sleep (hypnotic). Do not use for more than 2 weeks. Other drugs have replaced barbiturates as primary sleep aids (all except mephobarbital, phenobarbital).

To calm down (sedate) patients who are agitated (all except pentobarbital injection).

To treat certain seizure disorders. Mephobarbital is indicated for the treatment of grand and petit mal epilepsy. Phenobarbital is indicated for the treatment of generalized and partial seizures. May be used alone or in combination with other medications.

As a preoperative medication (preanesthetic) to lessen anxiety and to assist in induction of anesthesia (amobarbital, secobarbital, and pentobarbital).

Precautions:

Do not use in the following situations:

allergy to barbiturates or any of their ingredients
liver disease, marked
lung disease, severe
porphyria

Use with caution in the following situations:

alcohol use
children
corticosteroid therapy
debilated patients
depression
drug abuse, history of
elderly
heart disease
hypoadrenal function
kidney disease
liver disease
lung disease
pain, acute or chronic
pregnancy
suicidal tendencies

Vitamin D requirements may be increased when taking barbiturates. Long-term barbiturate use may increase the chance for developing rickets or osteoporosis (weakening of bones).

Vitamin K: Bleeding in the early neonatal period due to coagulation defects may follow exposure to anticonvulsant drug *in uterto*; therefore, vitamin K should be given to the mother before delivery or to the child at birth.

Acute or chronic pain: Caution should be exercised when barbiturates are administered to patients with acute or chronic pain because paradoxical excitement could be induced or symptoms could be masked. However, use of barbiturates as sedatives in postoperative surgical period and as adjunct to cancer chemotherapy is well established.

Steroid-dependent patients: Steroids (eg, hydrocortisone, prednisone) may lose some effect when barbiturates are started. Tell your doctor if you take steroid medications regularly.

Barbiturates may be habit forming. Tolerance and dependence may occur with continued use, especially following prolonged use of high doses. To minimize the possibility of overdosage or the development of dependence, the prescribing and dispensing of sedative-hypnotic barbiturates should be limited to the amount required for the interval until the next appointment.

Symptoms of acute intoxication include unsteady walk, slurred speech, and sustained involuntary eye movements. Mental signs of chronic intoxication include confusion, poor judgment, irritability, sleeplessness, and body aches.

Symptoms of dependence are similar to those of chronic alcoholism and include: A strong desire or need to continue taking the drug, tendency to increase the dose, and dependence on the effects of the drug.

Elderly or debilitated patients may be more susceptible to side effects. Lower initial doses may be appropriate.

Pregnancy: Studies have shown a potential effect on the fetus. Withdrawal symptoms may occur in infants born to women who receive barbituates throughout the last trimester of pregnancy. Use only if clearly needed and potential benefits outweigh the possible risks to the fetus.

Breastfeeding: Small amounts of barbiturates appear in breast milk. Drowsiness in the nursing infant has been reported. Consult your doctor before you begin breastfeeding.

Children: Safety and effectiveness have not been established for children younger than 6 years of age. Some children may become irritable, excitable, unexpectedly tearful, or aggressive when taking barbiturates.

Lab tests may be required during long-term therapy. Tests may include blood counts and kidney and liver function tests.

Tartrazine: Some of these products may contain the dye tartrazine (FD&C Yellow No. 5), which can cause allergic reactions in certain individuals. Check package label when available or consult your doctor or pharmacist.

Drug Interactions:

Tell your doctor or pharmacist if you are taking or if you are planning to take any over-the-counter or prescription medications or dietary supplements with barbiturates. Doses of one or both drugs may need to be modified or a different drug may need to be prescribed. The following drugs and drug classes interact with barbiturates.

- alcohol
- anesthetics, general (eg, methoxyflurane)
- anticoagulants (eg, warfarin)
- carbamazepine (eg, *Tegretol)*
- charcoal
- corticosteroids (eg, prednisone)
- contraceptives, oral (eg, *Ortho-Novum)*
- CNS depressant drugs
- divalproex sodium (*Depakote)*
- doxycycline (eg, *Vibramycin)*
- estrogens (eg, estradiol)
- felodipine (*Plendil)*
- griseofulvin (eg, *Grisactin)*
- MAOIs (eg, phenelzine)
- methadone (eg, *Dolophine)*
- metoprolol (eg, *Lopressor)*
- metronidazole (eg, *Flagyl)*
- nifedipine (eg, *Procardia)*
- phenytoin (eg, *Dilantin)*
- propranolol (eg, *Inderal)*
- quinidine (eg, *Quinidex-Extentabs)*
- steroidial hormones (eg, estradiol, estrone, progrestone)
- theophyllines (eg, aminophylline)
- tricyclic antidepressants (eg, amitriptyline)
- valproate
- valproic acid (eg, *Depakene)*

Side Effects:

Every drug is capable of producing side effects. Many barbiturate sedative users experience no, or minor, side effects. The frequency and severity of side effects depend on many factors including dose, duration of therapy, and individual susceptibility. Possible side effects include:

Withdrawal – Symptoms of withdrawal can be severe and may cause death. Minor symptoms may appear 8 to 12 hours after the last dose of a barbiturate and usually appear in the following order: Anxiety, muscle twitching, tremor of hands and fingers, progressive weakness, dizziness, visual perception problems, nausea, vomiting, sleeplessness, and dizziness or lightheadedness when arising from a seated or lying position. Major symptoms, inclusing convulsions and delirium, may occur within 16 hours and last 5 days or less after abrupt stopping of these drugs. Intensity of withdrawal symptoms gradually declines over a period of approxmately 15 days.

Digestive Tract: Nausea; vomiting; constipation.

Nervous System: Drowsiness; agitation; confusion; nightmares; hangover feeling; nervousness; hallucinations; sleeplessness; headache; depression; dizziness; stumbling gait.

Circulatory System: Slowed heart rate; decreased blood pressure.

Respiratory System: Decreased breathing rate; difficulty breathing.

Other: Rash; pain; fever; anemia; injection site reactions; fainting.

Guidelines for Use:

- Doses of barbiturates will be individualized with full knowledge of the patient's particular characteristics, including the patient's age, weight, the condition being treated, and other concurrent medical conditions and medications.
- Take only the amount of drug prescribed by your doctor. Barbiturates may be habit forming both psychologically and physically. Do not change the dose or discontinue therapy unless advised to do so by your doctor.
- *Seizures* — When treating seizures with barbiturates, a barbiturate-induced depression may occur along with a postictal depression once the seizures are controlled; therefore, it is important to use the minimal amount required and to wait for the anticonvulsant effect to develop before administering a second dose.
- Too rapid administration of IV or IM dosing may cause respiratory depression, difficult breathing, larynx spasms, or flushing and redness of the skin with a fall in blood pressure.
- Tell you doctor if you experience pain in the limbs during administration of an injection. This may be a sign of a serious condition. Parenteral solutions of barbiturates are highly alkaline and therefore extreme care should be taken to avoid perivascular extravasation or intra-arterial injection. Results of inappropiate injection may be local tissue damage and pain or gangrene to the limb.
- Tell your doctor if you are pregnant, become pregnant, are planning to become pregnant, or if you are breastfeeding.
- Oral contraceptive effectiveness may be decreased by barbituates. An alternative form of contraceptive (eg, barrier methods) is recommended.
- May decrease alertness or physical ability. Use caution when driving or performing tasks requiring alertness, coordination, or physical dexterity.
- Avoid alcohol and other mental depressants (eg, narcotics, tranquilizers, and antihistamines) while you are taking barbiturates.
- Contact your doctor if you notice fever or excessive sedation.
- Use as an aid to sleep is limited. Do not use for more than 2 weeks.
- *Seizure control* — Do not stop therapy suddenly. Status epilepticus (severe, prolonged seizures) may result from the abrupt discontinuation of mephobarbital or phenobarbital, even when administered in small daily doses for treatment of epilepsy.
- To avoid withdrawal symptoms after long-term use, a gradual dosage tapering schedule should be used.
- Lab tests may be required during prolonged therapy. Be sure to keep appointments.
- Store tablets, capsules, and elixirs at controlled room temperature (68° to 77°F) in a safe place, away from children.

If you have any questions, consult your doctor, pharmacist, or health care provider.

	Generic Name *Brand Name Examples*	Supplied As	Generic Available
c-IV	**Chloral Hydrate**		
	Noctec	**Capsules:** 250 mg, 500 mg	Yes
	Noctec	**Syrup:** 250 mg/tsp, 500 mg/tsp	Yes
	Aquachloral Supprettes, Chloral Hydrate	**Suppositories:** 324 mg[1], 500 mg, 648 mg	No
c-IV	**Estazolam**		
	ProSom	**Tablets:** 1 mg, 2 mg	No
c-IV	**Ethchlorvynol**		
	Placidyl	**Capsules:** 200 mg, 500 mg, 750 mg [1]	No
c-IV	**Flurazepam HCl**		
	Dalmane	**Capsules:** 15 mg, 30 mg	Yes
c-II	**Glutethimide**	**Tablets:** 250 mg, 500 mg	Yes
c-IV	**Paraldehyde**		
	Paral	**Liquid (Oral, Rectal)**	Yes
c-IV	**Quazepam**		
	Doral	**Tablets:** 7.5 mg, 15 mg	No
c-IV	**Temazepam**		
	Restoril	**Capsules:** 15 mg, 30 mg	Yes
c-IV	**Triazolam**		
	Halcion	**Tablets:** 0.125 mg, 0.25 mg	No
c-IV	**Zolpidem Tartrate**		
	Ambien	**Tablets:** 5 mg, 10 mg	No

[1] Contains the dye tartrazine.

Type of Drug:

Central nervous system depressant. Short-term sleep aid.

How the Drug Works:

Nonbarbiturate sedatives and hypnotics cause drowsiness to aid in falling asleep by acting on the central nervous system. They are less likely to cause slower pulse or breathing rate than barbiturate drugs.

Uses:

To treat insomnia for a short period of time (1 to 2 weeks). Long-term use is generally not recommended, and requires periodic medical evaluation.

Should sleeplessness persist, a drug-free interval of 1 or more weeks should elapse before retreatment is considered. An attempt should be made to find alternative nondrug therapy in chronic sleeplessness.

Paraldehyde: To quiet a patient and produce sleep in delirium tremens (DTs) and other psychiatric states characterized by excitement.

Chloral hydrate: To lessen anxiety and produce sleep before surgery. After surgery, chloral hydrate may be used with other medications to control pain.

To prevent or suppress alcohol withdrawal symptoms (rectal).

Unlabeled Use(s): Occasionally doctors may prescribe ethchlorvynol as a sedative at doses of 100 mg to 200 mg 2 or 3 times daily.

Precautions:

Do not use in the following situations:

allergy to the drug
porphyria (ethchlorvynol and glutethimide only)
pregnancy (benzodiazepines only)
sleep apnea (quazepam only)

chloral hydrate only —

gastritis
heart disease, severe,
kidney disease
liver disease

paraldehyde only —

gastroenteritis
liver disease
lung disease
peptic ulcer

Use with caution in the following situations:

depression
disease, preexisting (zolpidem only)
drug addiction
elderly or debilitated patients
esophagitis (chloral hydrate only)
gastritis
impaired respiratory function (benzodiazepines and zolpidem only)
kidney disease
liver disease
porphyria (chloral hydrate only)
suicide attempt, history of
ulcer, duodenal or gastric (chloral hydrate only)

Dependence: Long-term use may result in dependence. Withdrawal symptoms may occur when the drug is stopped.

Triazolam: Short-term episodes of memory loss have been reported with the use of triazolam. Patients, especially the elderly, may become confused, disoriented and may attempt to wander after taking the drug. Upon waking in the morning, the patient may not remember the episode.

Ethchlorvynol: Patients who exhibit unpredictable behavior, restlessness or excitement in response to barbiturates or alcohol may react in this manner to ethchlorvynol. This drug should not be used for the management of sleep loss in the presence of pain, unless sleep loss persists after pain is controlled with pain relievers.

Pregnancy: Adequate studies have not been done in pregnant women. Use only if clearly needed and potential benefits outweigh the possible hazards to the fetus.

Benzodiazepines – Do not use during pregnancy. The risk of use in a pregnant woman clearly outweighs any possible benefit.

Ethchlorvynol – Not recommended for use during the first and second trimesters of pregnancy. Use during the third trimester of pregnancy may produce symptoms in the newborn (eg, jitteriness, hyperactivity, restlessness, irritability, disturbed sleep, hunger).

Breastfeeding: Benzodiazepines, chloral hydrate and zolpidem appear in breast milk. It is not known if the other nonbarbiturate sedatives appear in breast milk. Consult your doctor before you begin breastfeeding.

Children: These drugs are generally not rocommended for children.

Elderly: Use with caution. Elderly patients may be more sensitive to these drugs. There is a risk of oversedation, "morning hangover" (grogginess in the morning), dizziness and confusion. Dose may need to be reduced. See triazolam precaution.

Lab tests may be required during treatment with these drugs. Tests may include: Blood counts and liver and kidney function tests.

Tartrazine: Some of these products may contain the dye tartrazine (FD&C Yellow No. 5) which can cause allergic reactions in certain individuals. Check package label when available or consult your doctor or pharmacist.

Drug Interactions:

Tell your doctor or pharmacist if you are taking or if you are planning to take any over-the-counter or prescription medications with nonbarbiturate sedatives. Doses of one or both drugs may need to be modified or a different drug may need to be prescribed. The following drugs and drug classes interact with nonbarbiturate sedatives:

alcohol
barbiturates (eg, phenobarbital)
narcotic pain relievers

benzodiazepines only—

anticonvulsants (eg, carbamazepine)
antihistamines (eg, diphenhydramine)
cimetidine (*Tagamet)*
contraceptives, oral (eg, *Ortho-Novum)*
digoxin (eg, *Lanoxin)*
disulfiram (eg, *Antabuse)*
erythromycin (eg, *Ery-Tab)*
isocarboxazid (*Marplan)*
isoniazid (eg, *Laniazid)*
neuromuscular blocking agents
nicotine
phenelzine (*Nardil)*
phenothiazines (eg, chlorpromazine)
phenytoin (*Dilantin)*
probenecid (eg, *Benemid)*
rifampin (eg, *Rifadin)*
theophylline (eg, *Theo-Dur)*
tranylcypromine (*Parnate)*
troleandomycin (*Tao)*

chloral hydrate only—

anticoagulants, oral (eg, warfarin)
furosemide (eg, *Lasix)*
hydantoins (eg, phenytoin)

ethchlorvynol only—

anticoagulants, oral (eg, warfarin)

glutethimide only—

anticoagulants, oral (eg, warfarin)
charcoal

paraldehyde only—

disulfiram (eg, *Antabuse)*

Side Effects:

Every drug is capable of producing side effects. Many nonbarbiturate sedative users experience no, or minor, side effects. The frequency and severity of side effects depend on many factors including dose, duration of therapy and individual susceptibility. Possible side effects include.

Digestive Tract: Stomach pain or upset; vomiting; nausea; diarrhea; constipation; indigestion and appetite changes (zolpidem only).

Nervous System: Confusion; excitement; sleep problems (excessive dreaming or nightmares); drowsiness; dizziness; hallucinations (paraldehyde only); headache; anxiety; depression; hysteria (ethchlorvynol only); incoordination; decreased mobility; weakness; facial numbness; disorientation; incoherence; paranoid behavior (chloral hydrate only); zolpidem only amnesia; nervousness; insomnia; euphoria; vertigo (feeling of whirling motion).

Circulatory System: Changes in blood pressure; abnormal blood counts.

Skin: Jaundice (yellowing of skin or eyes); rash; hives; itching; redness; skin and mucous membrane irritation (zolpidem and chloral hydrate only).

Body as a Whole: Allergy; back pain; chest pain; muscle aches; fatigue; flu-like symptoms.

Other: Blurred vision; morning hangover (grogginess); unpleasant taste; unpleasant breath (paraldehyde only); dry mouth; fainting; sleepwalking (chloral hydrate only); prolonged hypnosis (ethchlorvynol only); upper respiratory infections and urinary tract infections (zolpidem only).

Benzodiazepines only –

Digestive Tract: Heartburn; indigestion; appetite loss.

Nervous System: Nervousness; talkativeness; apprehension; irritability; euphoria (exaggerated sense of well being); relaxed feeling; tremor; lack of concentration; memory loss; sleeplessness; restlessness; tiredness; general body discomfort.

Circulatory System: Palpitations (pounding in the chest); chest pain; heart rhythm disturbances.

Other: Ringing in the ears; impairment of the senses; abnormal sensations; sore throat; congestion; joint pain; cramps/pain; stiffness.

Guidelines for Use:

- May cause drowsiness or dizziness. Use caution while driving or performing other tasks requiring mental alertness, coordination or dexterity.
- Avoid alcohol and other drugs which cause drowsiness (eg, pain relievers, sedatives).
- Do not exceed prescribed dosage.
- May be habit forming. Do not discontinue drug abruptly, especially if you have a history of seizures, regardless of other antiseizure medications you may be taking.
- Contact your doctor if visual changes, irregular heartbeats, chest pains, yellowing of skin or eyes, rash or unusual bleeding or bruising occurs.
- *Benzodiazepines* — Nighttime sleep may be disturbed for 1 or 2 nights following stopping of the drug. May cause morning drowsiness, unusual tiredness in the morning or daytime sleepiness after using these medications for sleep. Awakening in the early morning may occur with temazepam and triazolam. Triazolam may cause short-term memory loss (see Precautions). Inform your doctor if you are planning to nurse or to become pregnant or if you become pregnant while taking this medication.
- *Chloral hydrate* — May cause stomach upset. Take capsules with a full glass of water or fruit juice. Swallow capsules whole—do not chew. Dilute syrup in a half glass of water, ginger ale or fruit juice.
- *Ethchlorvynol* — Symptoms of giddiness, incoordination and stomach upset may be reduced if medication is taken with food.
- *Glutethimide* — Contact your doctor if rash occurs.
- *Paraldehyde* — May cause stomach upset. Take with food or mix with milk or iced fruit juice to improve taste. Paraldehyde is irritating to the lining of the digestive tract and must be well diluted. Do not use paraldehyde in any plastic container. Do not dispense with a plastic spoon or syringe. Discard any unused paraldehyde after opening bottle. Do not use if liquid has a brownish color or a strong vinegar odor. Has a strong odor in exhaled air for as long as 24 hours after ingestion. The patient is often unaware of the odor. *Storage* — Upon exposure to light and air, paraldehyde decomposes. Keep away from heat, open flame or sparks. Paraldehyde solidifies at approximately 54°F and must be liquefied before use. Do not store in direct sunlight or expose to temperatures above 77°F. Keep product covered in box until use. Do not use paraldehyde from a container that has been opened for longer than 24 hours.
- *Triazolam* — Do not take when a full night's sleep and elimination of the drug from the body are not possible before the need to be active and functional.

	Brand Name Examples	Supplied As	Generic Available
otc	*Unisom Nighttime Sleep Aid*	**Tablets:** 25 mg doxylamine succinate	No
otc	*Nervine, Nytol QuickCaps, Sominex*	**Tablets:** 25 mg diphenhydramine HCl	Yes
otc	*Sominex Pain Relief*	**Tablets:** 25 mg diphenhydramine HCl and 500 mg acetaminophen	No
otc	*Extra Strength Tylenol PM Geltabs*	**Capsules:** 25 mg diphenhydramine HCl and 500 mg acetaminophen	No
otc	*Maximum Strength Compōz Nighttime Sleep Aid, Maximum Strength Sominex, Twilite*	**Tablets:** 50 mg diphenhydramine HCl	No
otc	*Maximum Strength Compōz Nighttime Sleep Aid, Maximum Strength Nytol QuickGels, Maximum Strength Sleepinal Softgels, Maximum Strength Unisom SleepGels*	**Capsules:** 50 mg diphenhydramine HCl	Yes
otc	*Unisom with Pain Relief*	**Tablets:** 50 mg diphenhydramine HCl and 650 mg acetaminophen	No

Type of Drug:

Nonprescription (over-the-counter) sleep aids.

How the Drug Works:

These drugs contain antihistamines (eg, doxylamine, diphenhydramine) which act on the central nervous system to increase feelings of drowsiness or sleepiness which can help induce and maintain sleep. A few products also contain a pain reliever (eg, acetaminophen) for the relief of minor aches and pains.

Uses:

To treat occasional difficulty in falling asleep.

To relieve sleeplessness with accompanying minor aches, pains, or headache (products containing acetaminophen).

Precautions:

Do not use in the following situations:

- alcohol consumption more than 3 drinks a day
- allergy to these medicines or any of their ingredients
- breastfeeding (doxylamine only)
- pregnancy (doxylamine only)

Use with caution in the following situations:

asthma
breathing problems (eg, emphysema, chronic bronchitis)
difficult urination due to prostate gland enlargement
glaucoma
peptic ulcer, active
prostate gland enlargement
urinary tract obstruction

Pregnancy and breastfeeding: Pregnant or breastfeeding women should not use products containing doxylamine. Consult your doctor before using any of these products during pregnancy or breastfeeding.

Long-term insomnia: Sleep aids should not be used continuously for more than 2 weeks. Contact your doctor if insomnia lasts more than 2 weeks.

Consider all precautions reported for antihistamines when using nonprescription sleep aids. See the Antihistamines monograph in the Respiratory Drugs chapter.

Children: Do not use in children younger than 12 years of age unless directed by a doctor.

Elderly: The elderly may require lower than usual doses. Antihistamines are more likely to cause dizziness, sedation, confusion, and decrease in blood pressure in elderly people.

Drug Interactions:

Tell your doctor or pharmacist if you are taking or if you are planning to take any over-the-counter or prescription medications with nonprescription sleep aids. Doses of one or both drugs may need to be modified or a different drug may need to be prescribed. Alcohol interacts with nonprescription sleep aids. The following drugs or drug classes interact with nonprescription sleep aids containing acetaminophen.

anticoagulants, oral
ethanol (alcohol)
hydantoins (eg, phenytoin)
sulfinpyrazone (eg, *Anturane*)

Side Effects:

Every drug is capable of producing side effects. Many nonprescription sleep aid users experience no, or minor, side effects. The frequency and severity of side effects depend on many factors including dose, duration of therapy, and individual susceptibility. For information on possible side effects of antihistamines. See the Antihistamines monograph in the Respiratory Drugs chapter. Possible side effects include:

Other: Dry mouth; confusion; blurred vision; urinary retention; constipation; drowsiness.

Guidelines for Use:

- Consult individual product information for specific dosage instructions. Do not exceed recommended dosage.
- Take 30 minutes before desired sleep time.
- May cause drowsiness. Use caution while driving or performing tasks which require alertness, coordination, or physical dexterity.
- Do not drink alcoholic beverages while taking any sleep aid. Do not take other sedatives or tranquilizers without first consulting your doctor.
- Do not use nonprescription sleep aids containing acetaminophen if you drink 3 or more alcoholic beverages every day, unless directed to do so by your doctor.
- Do not use nonprescription sleep aids containing acetaminophen for pain for more than 10 days or for fever for more than 3 days, unless directed by your doctor.
- Do not use nonprescription sleep aids containing acetaminophen with other products containing acetaminophen (eg, *Tylenol*) unless advised by your doctor.
- Do not give to children younger than 12 years of age unless directed by your doctor.
- Notify your doctor if your symptoms persist or worsen, if new ones occur, or if sleeplessness continues for more than 2 weeks. Sleeplessness may be a symptom of a serious underlying illness.
- Store at room temperature. Avoid excessive heat or humidity.

If you have any questions, consult your doctor, pharmacist, or health care provider.

Generic Name *Brand Name Examples*	Supplied As	Generic Available
Rx **Acetazolamide**		
Diamox	**Tablets:** 125 mg, 250 mg	Yes
Diamox	**Injection:** 500 mg	Yes
Diamox Sequels	**Capsules, sustained release:** 500 mg	No

Type of Drug:

Anticonvulsant; diuretic or "water pill"; antiglaucoma drug; carbonic anhydrase inhibitor.

How the Drug Works:

Anticonvulsant: Prevents or reduces seizures by slowing abnormal nerve impulses in the brain and central nervous system.

Diuretic: Reduces amount of fluid in the body by increasing urine formation.

Antiglaucoma: Reduces pressure in the eyes by decreasing the formation of fluid inside the eye.

Uses:

To treat petit mal and unlocalized seizures.

To treat edema (excess fluid in tissues) which may accompany congestive heart failure, other circulatory system disorders, or other drug therapy.

Sustained-release capsules: To treat certain types of glaucoma. Usually used in combination with drugs applied directly to the eye.

To prevent or treat the effects of acute mountain sickness.

Precautions:

Do not use in the following situations:

- adrenocortical insufficiency (Addison's disease)
- allergy to acetazolamide
- chronic noncongestive angle-closure glaucoma
- cirrhosis
- electrolyte imbalance (eg, low potassium or sodium levels)
- hyperchloremic acidosis
- kidney disease, severe
- liver disease, severe
- lung obstruction, severe

Use with caution in the following situations:

- allergy to sulfa drugs (eg, *Bactrim*)
- aspirin, high-dose, concurrent
- emphysema
- lung obstruction

Blood disorders can occur while taking this medication. Patients should be routinely monitored to avoid this problem.

Potassium loss: By increasing urine formation, acetazolamide may cause loss of potassium from the body. Low potassium levels may be treated by eating foods and drinking fluids high in potassium, such as citrus (orange) juice, bananas, dates, raisins, melons, and tomatoes. If increasing potassium in the diet does not raise potassium levels to normal, a potassium supplement may be necessary to replace lost potassium.

Pregnancy: Adequate studies have not been done in pregnant women. Use only if clearly needed and potential benefits outweigh the possible hazards to the fetus.

Breastfeeding: Acetazolamide may appear in breast milk. Because of the potential for serious adverse reactions in nursing infants, a decision should be made whether to discontinue nursing or discontinue the drug, taking into account the importance of the drug to the mother. Consult your doctor before you begin breastfeeding.

Children: Safety and effectiveness in children have not been established.

Lab tests are required during treatment with acetazolamide. Tests may include blood counts, electrolytes (eg, potassium, sodium, chloride), and liver and kidney function tests.

Drug Interactions:

Tell your doctor or pharmacist if you are taking or if you are planning to take any over-the-counter or prescription medications or dietary supplements with acetazolamide. Doses of one or both drugs may need to be modified or a different drug may need to be prescribed. The following drugs interact with acetazolamide.

- cyclosporine (eg, *Sandimmune*)
- lithium (eg, *Eskalith*)
- primidone (eg, *Mysoline*)
- quinidine (eg, *Quinidex*)
- salicylates (eg, aspirin, *Arthropan, Doan's, Tusal*)
- salsalate (eg, *Disalcid*)
- steroid therapy (eg, prednisone)

Side Effects:

Every drug is capable of producing side effects. Many acetazolamide users experience no, or minor, side effects. The frequency and severity of side effects depend on many factors including dose, duration of therapy, and individual susceptibility. Possible side effects include:

Digestive Tract: Nausea; vomiting; loss of appetite; diarrhea.

Skin: Unusual bleeding or bruising; rash; red or purple spots under the skin; sensitivity to light.

Other: Fever; tingling or numbness in hands or feet; drowsiness; confusion; allergic reaction; taste alterations; ringing in the ears; hearing dysfunction; excessive urination; electrolyte imbalance; metabolic acidosis; crystals in urine; kidney stones; abnormal blood cell counts; transient nearsightedness; sore throat.

Guidelines for Use:

- *Epilepsy* — Suggested total daily dose is 8 to 30 mg/kg in divided doses. Optimum range appears to be from 375 to 1000 mg daily. When given in combination with other anticonvulsants, the starting dose should be 250 mg once daily in addition to existing medications.
- *Tablets* can be crushed and mixed with sweet foods to mask bitter taste.
- *Capsules* can be opened and contents sprinkled on food, if necessary.
- *Sustained-release capsules* — Do not crush or chew.
- Doses more than 1 g per 24 hours do not produce an increased effect.
- For use of acetazolamide in acute mountain sickness, congestive heart failure, drug-induced edema, and glaucoma, see the Diuretics-Carbonic Anhydrase Inhibitors monograph.
- May cause stomach upset. Take with food.
- May cause drowsiness. Use caution when driving or performing other tasks requiring alertness, coordination, or physical dexterity.
- May cause loss of potassium from the body. Contact your doctor if signs of potassium loss (eg, weakness, muscle cramps, nausea, dizziness) occur.
- Notify your doctor if sore throat, fever, unusual bleeding or bruising, tingling or numbness in the hands or feet, flank or loin pain, or skin rash occurs.
- When using acetazolamide, urination may increase; if possible, take early in the day.
- Temporary nearsightedness (change in vision) has occasionally occurred with this medicine. It subsides when the dose is reduced or the medicine is stopped.
- May cause sensitivity to sunlight. Avoid prolonged exposure to the sun or other forms of ultraviolet (UV) light (eg, tanning beds). Use sunscreens and wear protective clothing until tolerance is determined.
- Store at room temperature (59° to 86°F).

If you have any questions, consult your doctor, pharmacist, or health care provider.

	Generic Name *Brand Name Examples*	Supplied As	Generic Available
Rx	**Carbamazepine**		
	Epitol, Tegretol	**Tablets:** 200 mg	Yes
	Tegretol	**Tablets, chewable:** 100 mg	Yes
	Tegretol	**Suspension:** 100 mg/tsp	No
	Tegretol-XR	**Tablets, extended release:** 100 mg, 200 mg, 400 mg	No

Type of Drug:

Anticonvulsant; drug used to treat a variety of seizure disorders. Analgesic (pain reliever) for certain types of nerve pain (eg, trigeminal neuralgia).

How the Drug Works:

Carbamazepine appears to prevent or reduce the number of seizures by controlling the activity of nerve impulses in the central nervous system. In trigeminal neuralgia, carbamazepine may reduce the activity of nerve impulses in the trigeminal nerve (nerve to the face), decreasing pain transmission.

Uses:

To control partial seizures with complex symptoms (eg, psychomotor, temporal lobe), grand mal and mixed seizures, alone or with other anticonvulsant drugs.

To treat trigeminal neuralgia (tic douloureux), a condition causing severe, stabbing pain in the face. Carbamazepine is not a simple pain reliever and should not be used for the relief of minor aches and pains.

Unlabeled Use(s): Occasionally doctors may prescribe carbamazepine for neurogenic diabetes insipidus; certain psychiatric disorders; restless leg syndrome; nonneuritic pain syndrome (eg, phantom limb pain); and alcohol, cocaine, and benzodiazepine withdrawal management.

Precautions:

Do not use in the following situations:

allergy to carbamazepine
allergy to tricyclic antidepressants (eg, amitriptyline)
bone marrow depression, history
monoamine oxidase inhibitor (eg, phenelzine) use (current or within 14 days)

Use with caution in the following situations:

anemia or other blood disorders, including drug-induced blood disorders
glaucoma
heart disease
kidney disease
liver disease
lupus erythematosus
mixed seizure disorders with atypical absence (petit mal) seizures

Potentially fatal blood cell abnormalities have been reported rarely following treatment with carbamazepine. Early detection of blood changes is important since some abnormalities may be reversible.

Minor pain: Do not use carbamazepine to relieve minor aches and pains.

Pregnancy: Reports suggest an association between use of anticonvulsant drugs by women with epilepsy and an increased number of birth defects in children born to these women. Other factors (eg, genetics or the epileptic condition) may also contribute to the higher incidence of birth defects. Most mothers receiving anticonvulsant medication during pregnancy deliver normal infants. Tests to detect defects should be considered a part of routine prenatal care in childbearing women receiving carbamazepine. Do not abruptly or suddenly discontinue anticonvulsant drugs used to prevent major seizures. This could result in the occurrence of seizures, oxygen deficiency in body tissues, and an increased risk to both the mother and the unborn child. In cases where seizures do not pose a serious threat, your doctor may recommend gradual discontinuation of anticonvulsants prior to and during pregnancy. It is not known whether even minor seizures constitute some risk to the developing embryo or fetus. Use only when clearly needed and when the potential benefits outweigh the potential hazards to the fetus.

Breastfeeding: Carbamazepine appears in breast milk. Consult your doctor before you begin breastfeeding.

Children: Use in children under 6 years of age should be directed by clinicians expert in treating seizure disorders (eg, a neurologist).

Elderly: Carbamazepine may be more likely to cause confusion or agitation in elderly patients than in younger patients. Use with caution.

Lab tests may be required before and during treatment with carbamazepine. Tests may include: Complete blood counts, liver function tests, urinalysis, blood urea nitrogen, eye tests, thyroid tests, and carbamazepine blood levels. Carbamazepine may interfere with thyroid function tests and some pregnancy tests.

Drug Interactions:

Tell your doctor or pharmacist if you are taking or if you are planning to take any over-the-counter or prescription medications or dietary supplements with carbamazepine. Doses of one or both drugs may need to be modified or a different drug may need to be prescribed. The following drugs and drug classes interact with carbamazepine.

acetaminophen (eg, *Tylenol*)
alprazolam (*Xanax*)
anticoagulants, oral (eg, warfarin)
anticonvulsants (eg, valproic acid, phenytoin, phenobarbital, ethosuximide, primidone, felbamate)
azole antifungals (eg, itraconazole)
bupropion HCl (*Wellbutrin*)
charcoal
cimetidine (*Tagamet*)
cisplatin (*Platinol*)
clomipramine HCl (*Anafranil*)
clozapine (*Clozaril*)
contraceptives, oral (eg, *Ortho-Novum*)
cyclosporine (eg, *Neoral*)
danazol (eg, *Danocrine*)
diltiazem (eg, *Cardizem*)
doxycycline (*Vibramycin*)

- doxorubicin (eg, *Rubex*)
- felodipine (*Plendil*)
- fluoxetine (*Prozac*)
- haloperidol (*Haldol*)
- isoniazid (*Nydrazid*)
- lamotrigine (*Lamictal*)
- lithium (eg, *Eskalith*)
- loratadine (*Claritin*)
- macrolide antibiotics (eg, erythromycin)
- muscle relaxants (eg, pancuronium)
- niacinamide
- propoxyphene (eg, *Darvon*)
- rifampin (*Rifadin*)
- theophylline (eg, *Theo-Dur*)
- verapamil (eg, *Calan*)

Side Effects:

Every drug is capable of producing side effects. Many carbamazepine users experience no, or minor, side effects. The frequency and severity of side effects depend on many factors including dose, duration of therapy, and individual susceptibility. Possible side effects include:

Digestive Tract: Nausea; vomiting; stomach upset and pain; diarrhea; constipation; appetite loss; dry mouth or throat; sores on mouth and tongue; sore throat.

Nervous System: Drowsiness; dizziness; incoordination; headache; confusion; mood changes; behavior changes (especially in children); unusual body movements; slurred speech; hallucinations; depression; fatigue.

Circulatory System: Changes in blood pressure; changes in heart rhythm; blood disorder; decreased blood cell counts (eg, platelets, white blood cells); blood clots.

Respiratory System: Difficulty breathing; pneumonia.

Skin: Yellowing of skin or eyes; changes in pigmentation; easy bruising or bleeding; rash; hives; skin lesions; peeling; sensitivity to sunlight; sweating; hair loss.

Eyes or Ocular: Double vision; unusual eye movements; blurred vision; red, itchy eyes.

Urinary and Reproductive Tract: Changes in urinary frequency; urinary retention; kidney failure.

Other: Fainting; fever; chills; sore throat; aches in muscles and joints; leg cramps; swelling of legs or ankles; swollen glands; numbness or tingling in hands or feet; ringing in ears; abnormal sensitivity to sounds; altered liver and kidney function tests; altered thyroid function tests; decreased sexual ability; edema (fluid retention); hemorrhaging or bleeding; aggravation of lupus erythematosus; abnormal skin sensations.

Guidelines for Use:

- Take as directed by your doctor. Daily dose varies depending on individual needs.
- May cause upset stomach. Take with food.
- Shake suspension well before using.
- Suspension should not be administered simultaneously with other liquid medicinal agents or diluents.
- Since the suspension produces higher blood levels than tablets, it is recommended that patients given the suspension be started on lower doses and increased slowly to avoid unwanted side effects.
- Do not use to treat ordinary types of aches or pain. This drug should be used only to treat pain of trigeminal neuralgia.
- *Tegretol-XR* tablets must be swallowed whole and never crushed or chewed. Tablets should be inspected for chips or cracks; damaged tablets should not be consumed. The tablet coating remains in the intestine and is excreted in the stool and may be noticable.
- Carry Medic Alert identification indicating that you are using this drug.
- If you stop taking this drug suddenly, your convulsions may return. Do not stop taking this drug without talking to your doctor.
- If a dose is missed, take it as soon as possible. If several hours have passed or if it is nearing time for the next dose, do not double the dose in order to catch up (unless advised to do so by your doctor). If more than one dose is missed, or it is necessary to establish a new dosage schedule, contact your doctor or pharmacist.
- Stop taking MAO inhibitors at least 14 days before beginning taking carbamazepine.
- Notify your doctor if any of the following occurs: Unusual bleeding or bruising; yellowing of skin or eyes; stomach pain; pale stools; darkened urine; decreased sexual ability; confusion; dizziness; incoordination; hallucinations; excessive sedation; abnormal movements; mood changes; double vision; swelling; fever; chills; sore throat; ulcers in the mouth; rash.
- May cause drowsiness, dizziness, or blurred vision. Use caution when driving or performing other tasks requiring alertness, coordination, or physical dexterity until tolerance is determined.
- Absence (petit mal) seizures do not appear to be controlled by carbamazepine.
- Lab tests will be required before and during treatment, especially during the first 2 months, to make certain the drug is working properly and to screen for possible blood count disorders. Interference with some pregnancy tests had been reported. Be sure to keep appointments.
- Store *Epitol* tablets at room temperature in a tightly sealed, preferably glass container. Protect from moisture. Store *Tegretol* tablets and suspension at room temperature in a tightly sealed, light-resistant container. Protect from moisture.

If you have any questions, consult your doctor, pharmacist, or health care provider.

Generic Name *Brand Name Example*	Supplied As	Generic Available
c-IV **Clonazepam**		
Klonopin	**Tablets:** 0.5 mg, 1 mg, 2 mg	Yes

Type of Drug:

Benzodiazepine. Anticonvulsant; drug used to treat epilepsy (seizures) and panic disorder.

How the Drug Works:

The actual mechanism of clonazepam's action is unknown. However, it is believed that clonazepam prevents or reduces the number of seizures and controls panic attacks by acting on the central nervous system to control the activity of nerve impulses.

Uses:

To control Lennox-Gastaut syndrome (petit mal variant), akinetic, and myoclonic seizures either alone or in combination with other anticonvulsant drugs.

To treat absence (petit mal) seizures when succinimides have failed.

To treat panic disorder with or without agoraphobia (fear of crowds, public places, open areas).

Precautions:

Do not use in the following situations:

allergy to any other benzodiazepine (eg, alprazolam)
allergy to clonazepam or any of its ingredients
glaucoma, acute narrow angle
liver disease

Use with caution in the following situations:

alcoholism
chronic respiratory disease
drug abuse, history of
kidney disease
multiple seizure disorders

Multiple seizure type: When used in patients in whom several different types of seizure disorders coexist, clonazepam may increase the frequency or precipitate the onset of generalized tonic-clonic (grand mal) seizures. This may require the addition of other anticonvulsants or an increase in dosage.

Chronic respiratory disease: Clonazepam may produce respiratory depression and an increase in salivation. In some patients, increased salivation can cause difficulty breathing. Because of these possibilities, use clonazepam with caution in patients with chronic respiratory disease.

Withdrawal syndrome: Withdrawal symptoms (eg, convulsions, psychosis, hallucinations, behavioral disorder, tremor, abdominal and muscle cramps) have occurred following abrupt discontinuation of clonazepam. Severity is related to the degree of dependence and length of time used. The more severe withdrawal symptoms occurred in patients who received excessive doses over an extended period of time. After extended therapy, avoid abrupt discontinuation and follow a gradual dosage tapering schedule.

Drug dependence: Addiction prone individuals (ie, alcoholics, drug addicts) must be closely supervised during clonazepam therapy. Dependence has occurred in such patients.

Pregnancy: Reports suggest an association between use of anticonvulsant drugs by women with epilepsy and an increased number of birth defects in children born to these women. Other factors (eg, genetics or the epileptic condition) may also contribute to the higher incidence of birth defects. Most mothers receiving anticonvulsant medication deliver normal infants. Do not discontinue anticonvulsant drugs used to prevent major seizures. This could result in the occurrence of seizures, oxygen deficiency in body tissues, and an increased risk to both the mother and the unborn child. In cases where seizures do not pose a serious threat, your doctor may recommend discontinuation of anticonvulsants prior to and during pregnancy. It is not known whether even minor seizures constitute some risk to the developing embryo or fetus. In addition, children born to mothers taking benzodiazepines late in pregnancy may exhibit side effects (eg, flaccid muscles, breathing or feeding difficulties) or withdrawal symptoms. Use this medicine during pregnancy only when benefits to the mother outweigh risks to the fetus.

Breastfeeding: Do not breastfeed while receiving clonazepam.

Children: Children being treated for seizure disorder may be more sensitive to the effects of this drug. Consult your doctor. Safety and effectiveness for use in children younger than 18 years of age with panic disorder have not been established.

Lab tests may be required during treatment with clonazepam. Tests may include blood counts and liver function tests.

Drug Interactions:

Tell your doctor or pharmacist if you are taking or if you are planning to take any over-the-counter or prescription medications or dietary supplements with clonazepam. Doses of one or both drugs may need to be modified or a different drug may need to be prescribed. The following drugs and drug classes interact with clonazepam:

- alcohol
- antidepressants (eg, fluvoxamine)
- anticonvulsants, other (eg, carbamazepine)
- azole antifungal agents (eg, ketoconazole)
- cimetidine (eg, *Tagamet*)
- contraceptives, oral (eg, *Ortho-Novum)*
- disulfiram (eg, *Antabuse*)
- indinavir (*Crixivan*)
- MAOIs (eg, phenelzine)
- omeprazole (*Prilosec*)
- rifamycins (eg, rifampin)
- ritonavir (*Norvir*)
- valproic acid (eg, *Depakene*)

Consider all drug interactions reported for benzodiazepines, in the Antianxiety Agents-Benzodiazepines monograph in this chapter when using this drug.

Side Effects:

Every drug is capable of producing side effects. Many clonazepam users experience no, or minor, side effects. The frequency and severity of side effects depend on many factors, including dose, duration of therapy, and individual susceptibility. Possible side effects include:

Digestive Tract: Constipation; diarrhea; nausea; appetite changes.

Nervous System: Drowsiness; incoordination; behavior problems; headache; confusion; depression; memory loss; hysteria; bizarre behavior; mood changes; behavior changes; sleeplessness; tremor; dizziness; vertigo (feeling of whirling motion); partial paralysis; reduced intellectual ability; suicidal thoughts; nightmares; abnormal involuntary body movements; coma; hallucinations.

Respiratory System: Difficult breathing; chest congestion; "runny" nose; coughing; sore throat.

Skin: Rash; excessive growth or loss of hair.

Eyes or Ocular: Blurred vision; double vision; "glassy-eyed" appearance; unusual eye movements.

Other: Fever; fatigue; loss of voice; increased salivation or dry mouth; coated tongue; changes in urination; fluid retention; difficulty speaking; sore gums; swollen lymph nodes; weight changes; increased or decreased sex drive; incontinence of urine or feces; muscle pain or weakness; dehydration; menstruation problems; sexual problems; general deterioration; pounding in the chest; slurred speech.

Guidelines for Use:

- Dosage will be individualized.
- Do not discontinue use or change the dose without first checking with your doctor. If you stop taking this drug suddenly, the frequency of your seizures could increase or you could experience withdrawal symptoms.
- Take with food if stomach upset occurs.
- If a dose is missed, take it as soon as possible. If several hours have passed or if it is nearing time for the next dose, do not double the dose to catch up, unless advised to do so by your doctor. If several doses are missed or it is necessary to establish a new dosage schedule, contact your doctor or pharmacist. Use exactly as prescribed.
- Inform your doctor if you are pregnant, become pregnant, are planning to become pregnant, or if you are breastfeeding.
- May cause drowsiness, dizziness, or blurred vision. Use caution when driving or performing other tasks requiring alertness, coordination, or physical dexterity.
- Using this drug with alcohol or other central nervous system depressants (eg, pain relievers, sedatives) may cause added drowsiness.
- If the drug does not seem to be working as well after taking it for a few weeks, check with your doctor. A dosage adjustment may be needed.
- Carry Medic Alert identification indicating that you are using this drug and have epilepsy.
- Lab tests may be required to monitor therapy. Be sure to keep appointments.
- Store at room temperature (59° to 86°F).

If you have any questions, consult your doctor, pharmacist, or health care provider.

	Generic Name *Brand Name Example*	Supplied As	Generic Available
Rx	**Felbamate**		
	Felbatol[1]	**Tablets:** 400 mg, 600 mg	No
	Felbatol[1]	**Oral suspension:** 600 mg/5 mL	

[1] It has been recommended that use of this drug be discontinued if aplastic anemia or hepatic failure occurs unless, in the judgement of the doctor, continued therapy is warranted. For further information contact Wallace Laboratories at 800-526-3840.

Type of Drug:

Anticonvulsant; antiepileptic.

How the Drug Works:

Felbamate acts on the central nervous system to decrease the frequency of seizures.

Uses:

Felbamate is not indicated as a first-line antiepileptic treatment. Felbamate is recommended for use only in those patients who respond inadequately to alternative treatments and whose epilepsy is so severe that a substantial risk of aplastic anemia or liver failure is deemed acceptable in light of the benefits conferred by its use.

Felbamate is indicated as monotherapy or adjunctive therapy in the treatment of partial seizures with and without generalization in adults with epilepsy.

Also indicated as adjunctive therapy in the treatment of partial or generalized seizures associated with Lennox-Gastaut syndrome in children.

Precautions:

Do not use in the following situations:

- allergy to felbamate or any of its ingredients
- allergy to other carbamates (eg, meprobamate)
- blood disease, history of
- liver dysfunction, history of

Aplastic anemia: This drug should be used only in cases so severe that the risk of aplastic anemia (bone marrow failure) is deemed acceptable.

Liver failure: There have been cases of acute liver failure, some fatal, in association with the use of felbamate.

Discontinuation: Antiepileptic drugs should not be suddenly discontinued because of the risk of increasing seizure frequency.

Sensitivity to light: May cause photosensitivity (sensitivity to sunlight). Avoid prolonged exposure to the sun and other ultraviolet light. Use sunscreens and wear protective clothing until tolerance is determined.

Pregnancy: There are no adequate and well-controlled studies in pregnant women. Use only if clearly needed and potential benefits outweigh the possible hazards to the fetus.

Breastfeeding: Felbamate appears in breast milk. Consult your doctor before you begin breastfeeding.

Children: Safety and effectiveness in children other than those with Lennox-Gastaut syndrome have not been established.

Lab tests may be required to monitor therapy. Tests may include liver function tests (ALT, AST, and bilirubin).

Drug Interactions:

Tell your doctor or pharmacist if you are taking or if you are planning to take any over-the-counter or prescription medications or dietary supplements while taking felbamate. Doses of one or both drugs may need to be modified or a different drug may need to be prescribed. The following drugs and drug classes interact with felbamate:

carbamazepine (eg, *Tegretol)*
hydantoins (eg, phenytoin)
methsuximide (*Celontin*)
phenobarbital (eg, *Solfoton*)
valproic acid (eg, *Depakene)*

Side Effects:

Every drug is capable of producing side effects. Many felbamate users experience no, or minor, side effects. The frequency and severity of side effects depend on many factors including dose, duration of therapy, and individual susceptibility. Possible side effects include:

Digestive Tract: Upset stomach; vomiting; constipation; indigestion; diarrhea; nausea; appetite loss; stomach pain or bloating; hiccough.

Nervous System: Sleeplessness; headache; anxiety; drowsiness; dizziness; nervousness; tremor; depression; abnormal walking; abnormal skin sensations; stupor; confusion; mood changes (especially in children); unstable emotions; abnormal thinking; pinpoint pupils; incoordination; agitation.

Respiratory System: Upper respiratory tract (ie, nose, throat) infection; nasal congestion; sinus inflammation; sore throat; coughing.

Skin: Acne; rash; itching; yellowing of the skin; unusual bruising; sensitivity to light.

Urinary and Reproductive Tract: Urinary incontinence; irregular menstrual bleeding; urinary tract infection.

Other: Aplastic anemia (bone marrow failure); acute liver failure; fatigue; fever; chest pain; palpitations (pounding in the chest); weight fluctuation; face edema (fluid retention or swelling); pain; weakness; impaired vision; changes in taste perception; dry mouth; muscle pain; bleeding or bruising; flu symptoms; general body discomfort; fast heartbeat; middle ear infection; abnormal blood counts; abnormal lab tests.

Guidelines for Use:

- Dosage is individualized. Take exactly as prescribed.
- Do not change the dose or stop taking, unless advised by your doctor.
- May be taken with or without food.
- Shake suspension well before use.
- Do not discontinue use without first checking with your doctor. If you stop taking this drug suddenly, the frequency of your seizures could increase.
- May cause photosensitivity (sensitivity to sunlight). Avoid prolonged exposure to the sun and other ultraviolet (UV) light. Use sunscreens and wear protective clothing until tolerance is determined.
- Notify your doctor immediately if you experience fever, yellowing of the skin or eyes, appetite loss, stomach pain or bloating, weakness, sore throat, unusual bleeding or bruising, rash, or dark urine.
- Lab tests will be required to monitor therapy. Be sure to keep appointments.
- Store at room temperature in a tightly closed container.

If you have any questions, consult your doctor, pharmacist, or health care provider.

	Generic Name *Brand Name Example*	Supplied As	Generic Available
Rx	**Gabapentin**		
	Neurontin	**Capsules**: 100 mg, 300 mg, 400 mg	No
	Neurontin	**Tablets, film coated**: 600 mg, 800 mg	No
	Neurontin	**Solution, oral**: 250 mg/mL	No

Type of Drug:

Anticonvulsant; drug used to treat epilepsy and seizures.

How the Drug Works:

It is not known how gabapentin works to prevent seizures.

Uses:

Used in combination with other anticonvulsant therapy in the treatment of partial seizures with and without secondary generalization in patients older than 12 years of age with epilepsy.

Used in combination with other therapy in the treatment of partial seizures in patients 3 to 12 years of age.

Unlabeled Use(s): Occasionally doctors may prescribe gabapentin for neuropathic pain, tremors associated with multiple sclerosis, bipolar disorder, and migraine prophylaxis.

Precautions:

Do not use in the following situations: Allergy to gabapentin or any of its ingredients.

Use with caution in the following situations:
- kidney disease
- pediatric patients (3 to 12 years of age)

Pregnancy: There are no adequate and well-controlled studies in pregnant women. Use only if clearly needed and the potential benefits to the mother outweigh the possible hazards to the fetus.

Breastfeeding: Gabapentin appears in breast milk. Consult your doctor before you begin breastfeeding.

Children: Safety and effectiveness in children younger than 3 years of age have not been established.

Elderly: Use with caution. Dosage may need to be adjusted.

Drug Interactions:

Tell your doctor or pharmacist if you are taking or if you are planning to take any over-the-counter or prescription medications or dietary supplements while taking gabapentin. Doses of one or both drugs may need to be modified or a different drug may need to be prescribed. Antacids (eg, *Maalox*) interact with gabapentin.

Side Effects:

Every drug is capable of producing side effects. Many gabapentin users experience no, or minor, side effects. The frequency and severity of side effects depend on many factors including dose, duration of therapy, and individual susceptibility. Possible side effects include:

Digestive Tract: Appetite changes; gas; indigestion; constipation; gum inflammation; nausea; vomiting.

Nervous System: Abnormal skin sensations; hyperactivity; change in reflexes; anxiety; nervousness; tremor; hostility; amnesia; vertigo (feeling of whirling motion); depression; abnormal thinking; twitching; drowsiness; dizziness; incoordination; fatigue; emotional lability; concentration problems; difficulty speaking.

Respiratory System: Pneumonia; sore throat; cough; respiratory infection; bronchitis; runny nose.

Skin: Abrasion; itching; bruise-like spots under the skin.

Other: Abnormal vision; joint, back, or muscle pain; weakness; general body discomfort; impotence; high blood pressure; face edema (fluid retention); dry throat or mouth; rapid eye movement; involuntary muscle movements; weight gain; worsening of seizures; abnormal urine tests; viral infection; fever; swelling of the arms or legs; dental abnormalities; abnormal blood counts; bone fracture.

Guidelines for Use:

- Dosage is individualized. Take exactly as prescribed.
- Do not change the dose or stop taking, unless advised by your doctor.
- Take without regard to food.
- Use a dosing spoon or syringe to measure and administer oral solution.
- Convulsions may return or worsen if gabapentin is stopped suddenly.
- Maximum time between doses should not exceed 12 hours.
- If a dose is missed, take it as soon as possible. If several hours have passed or if it is nearing time for the next dose, do not double the dose to catch up, unless advised by your doctor. If more than one dose is missed or it is necessary to establish a new dosage schedule, contact your doctor or pharmacist.
- Small doses are generally used when starting therapy. The dose is then gradually increased as tolerated until an effective dose level is reached.
- Adjust dosage for patients with kidney disease or those undergoing hemodialysis.
- May cause dizziness, drowsiness, or blurred vision. Use with caution while driving or performing other tasks requiring alertness, coordination, and physical dexterity.
- Do not take gabapentin until at least two hours after taking an antacid.
- Carry *MedicAlert* identification indicating that you have epilepsy and the drugs that you are taking.
- Store tablets and capsules at controlled room temperature (59° to 86°F). Store oral solution under refrigeration (36° to 46°F).

If you have any questions, consult your doctor, pharmacist, or health care provider.

	Generic Name *Brand Name Examples*	Supplied As	Generic Available
Rx	**Ethotoin**		
	Peganone	**Tablets:** 250 mg, 500 mg	No
Rx	**Fosphenytoin**		
	Cerebyx	**Injection:** 100 mg, 500 mg	No
Rx	**Mephenytoin**		
	Mesantoin	**Tablets:** 100 mg	No
Rx	**Phenytoin**		
	Dilantin Infatab	**Tablets, chewable:** 50 mg	No
	Dilantin-125[1]	**Oral Suspension:** 125 mg/5 mL	No
Rx	**Phenytoin Sodium, Prompt**[2]		
	Phenytoin Sodium	**Capsules:** 100 mg	Yes
Rx	**Phenytoin Sodium, Extended**		
	Dilantin Kapseals	**Capsules:** 30 mg, 100 mg	Yes
Rx	**Phenytoin Sodium with Phenobarbital**		
	Dilantin with Phenobarbital Kapseals	**Capsules:** 100 mg with 16 mg phenobarbital; 100 mg with 32 mg phenobarbital	No

[1] Contains alcohol.
[2] Also available as an injection.

Type of Drug:

Anticonvulsants; drugs used to treat epilepsy and seizures.

How the Drug Works:

These agents work in the central nervous system to decrease the frequency of seizures.

Uses:

To control grand mal and psychomotor seizures.

Fosphenytoin, Phenytoin: To prevent and treat seizures during or after neurosurgery.

Mephenytoin: To control focal and Jacksonian seizures.

Unlabeled Use(s): Occasionally doctors may use phenytoin to control irregular heartbeats (arrhythmia), trigeminal neuralgia (tic douloureux), recessive dystrophic epidermolysis bullosa and junctional epidermolysis bullosa.

Precautions:

Do not use in the following situations:

- Adams-Strokes syndrome (fosphenytoin, phenytoin)
- allergy to these medicines
- AV block, advanced (phenytoin only)
- blood disorders (ethotoin only)
- liver disease (ethotoin only)
- sino-atrial block (fosphenytoin, phenytoin)
- sinus bradycardia (fosphenytoin, phenytoin)

Use with caution in the following situations:

- AV block, advanced
- cardiac insufficiency (fosphenytoin, phenytoin)
- liver disease
- low blood pressure ((fosphenytoin, phenytoin)
- porphyria, acute, intermittent

Diabetics may experience loss of glucose control. Be prepared to monitor blood sugar more often.

Gum disease occurs frequently with phenytoin. Incidence may be reduced by good oral hygience, including gum massage, frequent brushing and flossing and appropriate dental care.

Pregnancy: Reports suggest an association between use of anticonvulsant drugs by women with epilepsy and an increased number of birth defects in children born to these women. Other factors (eg, genetics or the epileptic condition) may also contribute to the high incidence of birth defects. Most mothers receiving anticonvulsant medication deliver *normal* infants. Do not discontinue anticonvulsant drugs used to prevent major seizures. This could result in the occurrence of severe seizures and an increased risk to both the mother and the unborn child. In cases where seizures do not pose a serious threat, your doctor may recommend discontinuation of anticonvulsants prior to and during pregnancy. It is not known whether even minor seizures constitute some risk to the developing embryo or fetus. Reports suggest that a mother's use of anticonvulsant drugs, particularly barbiturates, is associated with a blood clotting defect in the newborn that may cause a bleeding problem within 24 hours of birth. It has been suggested that vitamin K be given to the mother one month prior to and during delivery, and to the infant immediately after birth. An increase in seizure frequency often occurs during pregnancy because of altered phenytoin absoption or metabolism. Periodic lab tests will be required to measure phenytoin levels during pregnancy and doses may need to be adjusted. After birth, the dosage will probably go back to what it was before pregnancy.

Breastfeeding: Hydantoins appear in breast milk. Because of the potential for serious side effects in breastfed infants, decide whether to discontinue breastfeeding or discontinue the drug. Consult your doctor.

Lab tests may be required to monitor therapy. Tests may include Blood counts, urinalysis, blood sugar levels (especially in diabetics), liver function tests and phenytoin blood levels.

Drug Interactions:

Tell your doctor or pharmacist if you are taking or if you are planning to take any over-the-counter or prescription medications or dietary supplements while taking this medicine. Doses of one or both drugs may need to be modified or a different drug may need to be prescribed. The following drugs and drug classes interact with this medicine.

Increased effects of hydantoins may occur when the following drugs are administered with hydantoins:

- alcohol
- allopurinal (eg, *Zyloprim*)
- amiodarone (*Cordarone*)
- anticoagulants, oral (eg, warfarin)
- barbiturates (eg, phenobarbital)
- benzodiazepines (eg, diazepam)
- chloramphenicol (*Chloromycetin*)
- chlorpheniramine (eg, *Chlor-Trimeton*)
- cimetidine (eg, *Tagamet*)
- clonazepam (*Klonopin*)
- disulfiram (eg, *Antabuse*)
- felbamate (*Felbatol*)
- fluconazole (*Diflucan*)
- fluoxetine (*Prozac*)
- ibuprofen (eg, *Motrin*)
- isoniazid (eg, *Nydrazid*)
- methylphenidate (eg, *Ritalin*)
- metronidazole (eg, *Flagyl*)
- miconazole (eg, *Monistat*)
- omeprazole (*Prilosec*)
- phenacemide (*Phenurone*)
- phenothiazines (eg, chlorpromazine)
- propoxyphene (eg, *Darvon*)
- ranitidine (*Zantac*)
- salicylates (eg, aspirin)
- sodium valproate
- succinimides (eg, ethosuximide)
- sulfonamides (eg, sulfamethoxazole/trimethoprim)
- trazodone (eg, *Desyrel*)
- trimethoprim (eg, *Proloprim*)
- tricyclic antidepressants (eg, imipramine)
- valproic acid (eg, *Depakene*)

Decreased effects of hydantoins may occur when the following drugs are administered with hydantoins:

- alcohol
- antacids containing calcium (eg, *Tums*)
- antineoplastics (eg, methotrexate)
- barbiturates (eg, phenobarbital)
- charcoal
- carbamazepine (eg, *Tegretol*)
- chloral hydrate (eg, *Noctec*)
- clonazepam (*Klonopin*)
- diazoxide (*Proglycem*)
- folic acid (eg, *Folvite*)
- influenza vaccine
- loxapine (eg, *Loxitane*)
- nitrofurantoin (eg, *Furadantin*)
- paroxetin (*Paxil*)
- pyridoxine (eg,vitamin B_6)
- quinolones (eg, ciprofloxacin)
- rifamycins (eg, rifampin)
- sucralfate (*Carafate*)
- theophylline (eg, *Theo-Dur*)

Phenytoin may decrease effects of the following drugs:

acetaminophen (eg, *Tylenol*)
amiodarone (*Cordarone*)
barbiturates (eg, phenobarbital)
carbamazepine (eg, *Tegretol*)
cardiac glycosides (eg, digitoxin)
clonazepam (*Klonopin*)
contraceptives, oral (eg, *Ortho-Novum*)
corticosteroids (eg, prednisone)
cyclosporine (*Sandimmune*)
dicumarol
disopyramide (eg, *Norpace*)
dopamine (eg, *Dopastat*)
doxycycline (eg, *Vibramycin*)
estrogens (eg, estradiol)
furosemide (eg, *Lasix*)
haloperidol (eg, *Haldol*)
itraconazole (*Sporanox*)
levodopa (eg, *Laradopa*)
levonorgestrel (*Norplant System*)
mebendazole (eg, *Vermox*)
meperidine (eg, Dermerol)
methadone (eg, *Dolophine HCl*)
metyrapone
mexiletine (*Mexitil*)
muscle relaxants, nondepolarizing (eg, pancuronium)
phenothiazines (eg, chlorpromazine)
praziquantel (*Biltricide*)
primidone (eg, *Mysoline*)
quinidine (eg, *Quinora*)
sulfonylureas (eg, tolbutamide)
theophylline (eg, *Theo-Dur*)
thyroid hormones (eg, thyroid)
valproic acid (eg, *Depakene*)
verapamil (eg, *Calan*)
vitamin D
warfarin (*Coumadin*)

Other:

enteral nutrition
lithium (eg, *Lithobid*)
warfarin (*Coumadin*)

Side Effects:

Every drug is capable of producing side effects. Many patients experience no, or minor, side effects. The frequency and severity of side effects depend on many factors including dose, duration of therapy and individual susceptibility. Possible side effects include:

Digestive Tract: Nausea; vomiting; diarrhea; constipation.

Nervous System: Clumsiness; slurred speech; confusion; dizziness; sleeplessness; nervousness; twitchings; tiredness; irritability; sleepiness; depression; numbness; tremors; headache

Respiratory System: Sore throat; sinus inflammation; nasal congestion; asthma; coughing; nosebleed; difficulty breathing; chest pain.

Urinary and Reproductive Tract: Difficult, infrequent, painful or excessive urination; loss of bladder control; vaginal infection; genital swelling; kidney failure.

Skin: Rash; hives; yellowing of skin or eyes; irritation at injection site.

Senses: Rapid eye movement; double or impaired vision; light sensitivity; pupil dilation; eye pain or redness; taste changes or loss; distorted sense of smell; tender, bleeding or swollen gums; ear ache; ringing in the ears.

Other: Coarsening of facial features; lip enlargement; hair loss; weight gain; swelling of legs, ankles or hands; joint pain; fever; breast growth in men; swelling of lymph nodes; anemia; high blood sugar levels.

Guidelines for Use:

- Use exactly as prescribed.
- May cause stomach upset. Taking this medicine with or immediately after meals may help prevent stomach discomfort.
- Do not stop taking this medicine suddenly or change the dosage without checking with your doctor.
- *Brand interchange* — Do not change from one brand of this drug to another without consulting your pharmacist or doctor. Products manufactured by different companies may not be equally effective.
- *Phenytoin* — Do not take at the same time with antacids that contain calcium.
- May cause drowsiness, dizziness or blurred vision; alcohol may intensify these effects. Use caution while driving or performing hazardous tasks requiring mental alertness, coordination or physical dexterity.
- Do not stop taking this medicine or change the dose without checking with your doctor. Abrupt stopping of hydantoins in epileptic patients may precipitate seizures.
- It is important to brush and floss your teeth and to see your dentist regularly, in order to reduce the risk of gum swelling.
- *Diabetics* — Monitor blood sugar regularly and report any abnormalities to your doctor.
- Avoid alcohol, antihistamines and other mental depressants (eg, tranquilizers) while taking this medicine.
- Tell your doctor if you are pregnant, become pregnant, are planning to become pregnant or if you are breastfeeding.
- Contact your doctor immediately if rash appears.
- Contact your doctor if any of the following occurs: Drowsiness; slurred speech; clumsiness; rash; severe nausea or vomiting; swollen glands; bleeding, swollen or tender gums; yellowish discoloration of the skin or eyes; joint pain; unexplained fever; sore throat; nosebleed; unusual bleeding or bruising; persistent headache; general body discomfort; bleeding tendencies; pregnancy or any indication of an infection.
- Inform your doctor of any condition in which it is not possible to take this medicine orally (eg, surgery).
- Carry Medic Alert identification indicating that you are have epilepsy and are taking these drugs.
- Lab tests will be required to monitor treatment. Be sure to keep appointments.
- *Capsules* — Do not use if discolored.
- *Dilantin Suspension* — Shake well before use.
- Store at room temperature below 86°F in a tight-fitting container. Protect from freezing, moisture and light.

If you have any questions, consult your doctor, pharmacist, or health care provider.

	Generic Name *Brand Name Example*	Supplied As	Generic Available
Rx	**Trimethadione**		
	Tridione	**Tablets, chewable:** 150 mg	No
	Tridione	**Capsules:** 300 mg	No
	Tridione	**Solution:** 40 mg/mL	No

Because of the potential of these drugs to cause fetal abnormalities and serious side effects, these drugs are used only when less toxic drugs have been found ineffective in controlling petit mal seizures.

Type of Drug:

Anticonvulsants; drug used to treat epilepsy and seizures.

How the Drug Works:

Oxazolidinediones act on the central nervous system to decrease the frequency of seizures.

Uses:

To control absence (petit mal) seizures that do not respond to other antiseizure medications.

Precautions:

Do not use in the following situations: Allergy to these drugs.

Use with caution in the following situations:

- blood disorders
- eye diseases (retina, optic nerve)
- kidney disease
- kidney dysfunction
- liver disease
- porphyria, acute intermittent
- rash (after therapy was started)

Photosensitivity, sensitivity to sunlight, may occur. Therefore, use caution and take protective measures (ie, sunscreens, protective clothing) against exposure to ultraviolet light or sunlight until tolerance is determined.

Pregnancy: Reports suggest an association between use of anticonvulsant drugs by women with epilepsy and an increased number of birth defects in children born to these women. Other factors (eg, genetics or the epileptic condition) may also contribute to the higher incidence of birth defects. Most mothers receiving anticonvulsant medication deliver normal infants. Do not discontinue anticonvulsant drugs used to prevent major seizures. This could result in the occurrence of seizures and oxygen deficiency in body tissues and an increased risk to both the mother and the unborn child. In cases where seizures do not pose a serious threat, your doctor may recommend discontinuation of anticonvulsants prior to and during pregnancy. It is not known whether even minor seizures constitute some risk to the developing embryo or fetus. Reports suggest that mother's use of anticonvulsant drugs, particularly barbiturates, is associated with a blood clotting defect in the newborn that may cause a bleeding problem within 24 hours of birth. It has been suggested that vitamin K be given to the mother one month prior to and during delivery, and to the infant, immediately after birth.

Breastfeeding: It is not known if oxazolidinediones appear in breast milk. Consult your doctor before you begin breastfeeding.

Children: Safety and effectiveness in children under 16 years of age have not been established.

Lab tests may be required during treatment with oxazolidinediones. Be sure to keep appointments. Tests may include blood counts, liver and kidney function tests, eye exams and urinalysis.

Side Effects:

Every drug is capable of producing side effects. Many oxazolidinedione users experience no, or minor, side effects. The frequency and severity of side effects depend on many factors including dose, duration of therapy and individual susceptibility. Possible side effects include:

Digestive Tract: Nausea; vomiting; abdominal pain; appetite loss; gastric distress.

Nervous System: Drowsiness; dizziness; headache; personality changes; irritability; fatigue; sleeplessness; muscle weakness.

Skin: Rash; unusual bleeding or bruising; yellowing of eyes or skin; hair loss; itching; peeling skin.

Other: Vision changes, double vision; sore throat; fever; muscle weakness (especially eyes, eyelids, face, lips, tongue, throat or neck); sensitivity to sunlight; fatigue; abnormal lab tests (see Precautions); weight loss; hiccoughs; blood pressure changes; protein in urine; day blindness; bleeding gums; nosebleeds; vaginal bleeding; blood disorder; decreased blood platelets; anemia; bleeding.

Guidelines for Use:

- If stomach upset occurs, take with food.
- Do not change the dose or stop taking this medication without consulting your doctor.
- Keep scheduled appointments with your doctor, and carry Medic Alert identification listing your medical condition (epilepsy) and medication.
- May cause drowsiness or blurred vision. Use caution while driving or performing other tasks requiring alertness.
- Notify your doctor if any of the following should occur: Visual disturbances, excessive drowsiness or dizziness, sore throat, fever, unusual bleeding or bruising, skin rash, pregnancy, body discomfort or nosebleed.
- Withdraw drug gradually unless serious adverse effects dictate otherwise.
- May cause sensitivity to sunlight. Avoid prolonged exposure to the sun. Use sunscreens and wear protective clothing until tolerance is determined.
- Store capsules below 77°F. Store tablets in refrigerator and keep container tightly closed. Store solution below 86°F.

If you have any questions, consult your doctor, pharmacist, or health care provider.

	Generic Name *Brand Name Example*	Supplied As	Generic Available
Rx	**Oxcarbazepine**		
	Trileptal	**Tablets:** 150 mg, 300 mg, 600 mg	No

Type of Drug:
Anticonvulsant; drug used to treat a variety of seizure disorders.

How the Drug Works:
Oxcarbazepine prevents or reduces some types of seizures by controlling abnormal nerve impulses in the brain.

Uses:
For use alone or in combination therapy for the treatment of partial seizures in adults with epilepsy and as combination therapy for the treatment of partial seizures in children 4 to 16 years of age with epilepsy.

Unlabeled Use(s): Oxcarbazepine has been used for atypical panic disorder.

Precautions:
Do not use in the following situations: Allergy to oxcarbazepine or any of its ingredients.

Use with caution in the following situations:
- allergy to carbamazepine (eg, *Tegretol*)
- blood sodium levels, low
- kidney disease
- liver disease, severe

Pregnancy: There are no adequate and well-controlled clinical studies in pregnant women; however, it is closely related structurally to carbamazepine, which is considered to be teratogenic in humans. Use during pregnancy only if clearly needed and the potential benefits to the mother outweigh the possible hazards to the fetus.

Breastfeeding: Oxcarbazepine and its active metabolite MHD are excreted in human breast milk. Because of the potential for serious adverse reactions, decide whether to discontinue nursing or to discontinue the drug in nursing women, taking into account the importance of the drug to the mother.

Children: Oxcarbazepine has been shown to be effective as adjunctive therapy combined with other drugs for partial seizures in patients 4 to 16 years of age.

Lab tests will be required to monitor therapy. Tests may include blood sodium levels, liver function, kidney function, and blood tests.

Drug Interactions:

Tell your doctor or pharmacist if you are taking or if you are planning to take any over-the-counter or prescription medications or dietary supplements with oxcarbazepine. Doses of one or both drugs may need to be modified or a different drug may need to be prescribed. The following drugs and drug classes interact with oxcarbazepine:

calcium channel blockers (eg, felodipine)
carbamazepine (eg, *Tegretol*)
phenobarbital (eg, *Solfoton*)
phenytoin (eg, *Dilantin*)
oral contraceptives (eg, *Ortho-Novum*)
valproic acid (eg, *Depakene*)

Side Effects:

Every drug is capable of producing side effects. Many oxcarbazepine users experience no, or minor, side effects. The frequency and severity of side effects depend on many factors including dose, duration of therapy, and individual susceptibility. Possible side effects include:

Digestive Tract: Nausea; vomiting; stomach pain; inflammation of the stomach; appetite changes; dry mouth; toothache; diarrhea; indigestion; constipation; rectal bleeding or pain.

Nervous System: Headache; dizziness; drowsiness; anxiety; fatigue; weakness; incoordination; tremors; continual rapid eye movement; abnormal gait; sleeplessness; impaired concentration; amnesia; worsening of seizures; involuntary muscle contractions; unstable emotions; decreased sensation to stimuli; nervousness; agitation; speech disorder; confusion; feeling of whirling motion; abnormal EEG; abnormal thinking.

Respiratory System: Sinus congestion; runny nose; upper respiratory infection; cough; breathing difficulties; sore throat; nosebleed; chest infection.

Skin: Acne; hot flashes; flushing; rash; unusual bruising; increased sweating; itching.

Other: Double vision; abnormal vision; earache; ear infection; fever; allergy; swelling of the legs; chest pain; weight increase; low blood pressure; falling down; swollen lymphnodes; viral infection; urinary tract infection; frequent urination; inflammation or pain of the vagina; low blood sodium levels; thirst.

Guidelines for Use:

- Dosage is individualized. Take exactly as prescribed.
- Do not stop taking or change the dose unless advised to do so by your doctor.
- May be taken without regard to meals.
- Avoid alcohol and other mental depressants (eg, narcotics, tranquilizers, antihistamines) while you are taking this medicine.
- Treatment should be withdrawn gradually to minimize the potential of increased seizure frequency.
- If a dose is missed, take it as soon as possible. If several hours have passed or if it is nearing time for the next dose, do not double the dose to catch up, unless advised by your doctor. If more than one dose is missed, or it is necessary to establish a new dosage schedule, contact your doctor or pharmacist.
- Additional nonhormonal forms of contraception (eg, latex condoms) are recommended because of a reduction in hormonal contraceptive efficacy during therapy.
- Avoid alcohol during therapy; it may cause drowsiness.
- May cause drowsiness, dizziness, or blurred vision. Use caution while driving or performing hazardous tasks requiring alertness, coordination, or physical dexterity until tolerance is determined.
- Store at controlled room temperature (59° to 86°F). Keep tightly closed.

If you have any questions, consult your doctor, pharmacist, or health care provider.

	Generic Name *Brand Name Example*	Supplied As	Generic Available
Rx	**Zonisamide**		
	Zonegran	**Capsules:** 100 mg	No

Type of Drug:

Anticonvulsant; a sulfonamide used to treat a certain type of seizure disorder.

How the Drug Works:

Zonisamide works in the brain to prevent seizures. Its mechanism of action is not fully understood.

Uses:

For adjunctive therapy in the treatment of partial seizures in adults with epilepsy.

Precautions:

Do not use in the following situations:

allergy to zonisamide or any of its ingredients
allergy to sulfonamides

Use with caution in the following situations:

kidney disease
liver disease

Pregnancy: There are no adequate and well-controlled studies in pregnant women. Fetal abnormalities and deaths occured in tested animals. Use only if clearly needed and the potential benefits to the mother outweigh the possible hazards to the fetus.

Breastfeeding: It is not known whether zonisamide is excreted in breast milk. Because of the potential for serious adverse reactions in nursing infants from zonisamide, decide whether to discontinure nursing or the drug, taking into account the importance of the drug to the mother. Consult your doctor before you begin breastfeeding.

Children: Safety and efficacy of zonisamide in patients younger than 16 years of age have not been established. Zonisamide is not approved for pediatric use.

Elderly: Older patients may be more sensitive to the effects of zonisamide. Lower starting doses should be considered.

Lab tests may be required during treatment with zonisamide. Tests may include blood counts and kidney and liver function tests.

Drug Interactions:

Tell your doctor or pharmacist if you are taking or if you are planning to take any over-the-counter or prescription medications or dietary supplements with zonisamide. Doses of one or both drugs may need to be modified or a different drug may need to be prescribed. The following drugs and drug classes interact with zonisamide:

carbamazepine (eg, *Tegretol*)
phenobarbital (eg, *Solfoton*)
phenytoin (eg, *Dilantin*)
valproate (eg, *Depakene*)

Side Effects:

Every drug is capable of producing side effects. Many zonisamide users experience no, or minor, side effects. The frequency and severity of side effects depend on many factors including dose, duration of therapy, and individual susceptiblity. Possible side effects include:

Digestive Tract: Stomach pain; appetite loss; constipation; diarrhea; indigestion; nausea; vomiting.

Nervous System: Agitation or irritability; anxiety; incoordination; confusion; depression; difficulty concentrating; difficulty with memory; dizziness; fatique; headache; sleeplessness; mental slowing; nervousness; continual rapid eye movement; tremor; convulsion; abnormal gait; weakness; unusual thoughts; drowsiness; tiredness; speech problems.

Respiratory System: Sore throat; cough; runny nose.

Skin: Itching; rash; abnormal skin sensations (eg, burning, prickling, tingling).

Other: Dry mouth; unusual bruising; flu symptoms; weight loss; vision problems; ringing in ear; kidney stones; taste changes.

Guidelines for Use:

- Dosage is individualized. Take exactly as prescribed.
- Do not stop taking or change the dose unless advised by your doctor. Abrupt stopping of zonisamide in patients with epilepsy may increase seizure frequency.
- May be taken with or without food.
- Capsules should be swallowed whole.
- Contact your doctor immediately if a child has been taking zonisamide and is not sweating as usual with or without fever.
- Contact your doctor immediately if fever, sore throat, oral ulcers, easy bruising, or rash occur; seizures worsen; or if you experience sudden back pain, stomach pain, or blood in the urine. The latter could be signs of a kidney stone.
- If dose is missed, take as soon as possible. If several hours have passed or if it is nearing time for the next dose, do not double the dose to catch up, unless advised by your doctor. If more than one dose is missed or it is necessary to establish a new dosage schedule, contact your doctor or pharmacist.
- Inform your doctor if you are pregnant, become pregnant, plan on becoming pregnant, or are breastfeeding during zonisamide therapy.
- Women of child-bearing potential who are given zonisamide should use effective contraception.
- May cause drowsiness, dizziness, or blurred vision. Use caution when driving or performing other tasks requiring alertness, coordination, or physical dexterity until tolerance is determined.
- Store at room temperature (59° to 86°F). Protect from moisture and light.

If you have any questions, consult your doctor, pharmacist, or health care provider.

	Generic Name *Brand Name Example*	Supplied As	Generic Available
Rx	**Primidone**		
	Mysoline	**Tablets:** 50 mg, 250 mg	Yes
	Mysoline	**Oral suspension:** 250 mg/tsp	No

Type of Drug:

Anticonvulsant; drug used to treat epilepsy and seizures.

How the Drug Works:

Primidone prevents or reduces the number of seizures by acting on the central nervous system to control the activity of nerve impulses in the brain.

Uses:

To control grand mal, psychomotor or focal epileptic seizures, alone or in combination with other anticonvulsant drugs.

Unlabeled Use(s): Occasionally doctors may prescribe may primidone for benign familial tremor.

Precautions:

Do not use in the following situations:

allergy to phenobarbital
porphyria

Use with caution in the following situations:

kidney disease
liver disease

Pregnancy: Reports suggest an association between use of anticonvulsant drugs by women with epilepsy and an increased number of birth defects in children born to these women. Other factors (eg, genetics or the epileptic condition) may also contribute to the higher incidence of birth defects. Most mothers receiving anticonvulsant medication deliver *normal* infants. Do not discontinue anticonvulsant drugs used to prevent major seizures. This could result in the occurrence of seizures and oxygen deficiency in body tissues and an increased risk to both the mother and the unborn child. In cases where seizures do not pose a serious threat, your doctor may recommend discontinuation of anticonvulsants prior to and during pregnancy. It is not known whether even minor seizures constitute some risk to the developing embryo or fetus. Reports suggest that mother's use of anticonvulsant drugs, particularly barbiturates, is associated with a blood clotting defect in the newborn that may cause a bleeding problem within 24 hours of birth. It has been suggested that vitamin K be given to the mother one month prior to and during delivery, and to the infant, immediately after birth.

Breastfeeding: Primidone appears in breast milk. It may cause the infant to be unusually drowsy or sleepy. Consult your doctor before you begin breastfeeding.

Lab tests may be required during treatment with primidone. Tests may include complete blood counts, liver and kidney function tests and blood levels of primidone.

Drug Interactions:

Tell your doctor or pharmacist if you are taking or if you are planning to take any over-the-counter or prescription medications or dietary supplements with primidone. Doses of one or both drugs may need to be modified or a different drug may need to be prescribed. The following drugs and drug classes interact with primidone.

- acetazolamide (eg, *Diamox)*
- alcohol
- anticoagulants, oral (eg, *Coumadin)*
- carbamazepine (eg, *Tegretol)*
- corticosteroids (eg, prednisone)
- contraceptives, oral (eg, *Ortho Novum)*
- doxycycline (eg, *Vibramycin)*
- griseofulvin (eg, *Grisactin)*
- isoniazid (eg, *Laniazid)*
- methoxyflurane (*Penthrane)*
- metoprolol (*Lopressor)*
- phenytoin (eg, *Dilantin)*
- propranolol (eg, *Inderal)*
- quinidine (eg, *Cin-Quin)*
- theophylline (eg, *Theo-Dur)*
- valproic acid (eg, *Depakene)*

Consider all drug interactions reported for barbiturates in the Sedatives-Barbiturates monograph in this chapter when using this drug.

Side Effects:

Every drug is capable of producing side effects. Many primidone users experience no, or minor, side effects. The frequency and severity of side effects depend on many factors including dose, duration of therapy and individual susceptibility. Possible side effects include:

Digestive Tract: Nausea; vomiting; loss of appetite.

Nervous System: Drowsiness; clumsiness; mood changes; unusual weakness; tiredness; dizziness.

Other: Double vision; blurred vision; unusual movements of the eyes; fever; sore throat; decreased sexual ability; rash.

Guidelines for Use:

- May cause drowsiness or sleepiness. Use caution when driving or performing other tasks requiring alertness.
- May cause stomach upset. May be taken with food.
- Do not stop taking this drug or change the dose without talking with your doctor. If you stop taking this drug suddenly, seizures may suddenly return.
- Carry Medic Alert identification listing your medical condition (epilepsy) and medications.
- Using this drug with alcohol or other central nervous system depressants may cause added drowsiness.
- See your doctor regularly when you begin taking this drug to ensure that you are getting the proper dosage. Lab tests will be needed to monitor therapy. Full effect may not be seen for several weeks.
- Contact your doctor if visual disturbance, rash, fever, sore throat, clumsiness or excessive sleepiness occurs.
- *Oral suspension* — Shake well before using.

If you have any questions, consult your doctor, pharmacist, or health care provider.

	Generic Name *Brand Name Example*	Supplied As	Generic Available
Rx	**Topiramate**		
	Topamax	**Tablets:** 25 mg, 100 mg, 200 mg	No
	Topamax	**Capsules, sprinkle:** 15 mg, 25 mg	No

Type of Drug:

Anticonvulsant; drug used to prevent certain types of seizures.

How the Drug Works:

Topiramate reduces the incidence of seizures by acting on the central nervous system to alter certain neurological transmissions in the brain.

Uses:

To treat adults and children older than 2 years of age with partial onset seizures or primary generalized tonic-clonic seizures and seizures associated with Lennox-Gastaut syndrome in combination with other anticonvulsant drugs.

Precautions:

Do not use in the following situations: Allergy to topiramate or any of its ingredients.

Use with caution in the following situations:

- alcohol ingestion
- glaucoma
- impaired liver function
- kidney failure
- kidney stones

Pregnancy: There are no adequate and well-controlled studies in pregnant women. Use only if clearly needed and the potential benefits to the mother outweigh the possible hazards to the fetus.

Breastfeeding: It is not known if topiramate appears in breast milk. Consult your doctor before you begin breastfeeding.

Children: Safety and effectiveness in children younger than 2 years of age have not been established.

Drug Interactions:

Tell your doctor or pharmacist if you are taking or planning to take any over-the-counter or prescription medications or dietary supplements while taking topiramate. Doses of one or both drugs may need to be modified or a different drug may need to be prescribed. The following drugs and drug classes interact with topiramate:

- carbamazepine (eg, *Tegretol*)
- carbonic anhydrase inhibitors (eg, acetazolamide, dichlorphenamide)
- CNS depressants (eg, narcotics, hypnotics)
- contraceptives, oral (eg, *Ortho-Novum*)
- digoxin (eg, *Lanoxin*)
- phenytoin (eg, *Dilantin*)
- valproic acid (eg, *Depakene*)

Side Effects:

Every drug is capable of producing side effects. Many topiramate users experience no, or minor, side effects. The frequency and severity of side effects depend on many factors including dose, duration of therapy, and individual susceptibility. Possible side effects include:

Digestive Tract: Nausea; indigestion; stomach pain; constipation; diarrhea; vomiting; dry mouth; gingivitis; stomach or intestinal irritation; hemorrhoids; changes in taste sensation.

Nervous System: Dizziness; incoordination; speech disorders; rapid eye movement; abnormal skin sensations; tremor; drowsiness; nervousness; memory difficulty; confusion; depression; appetite loss; agitation; aggressive reaction; hallucination; apathy; slow thinking; difficulty concentrating; anxiety; sleepiness; fatigue; dizziness; mood swings.

Circulatory System: Abnormal blood counts, low blood pressure; AV block; heart rhythm changes.

Respiratory System: Sore throat; upper respiratory infection; sinus infection; difficulty breathing.

Urinary and Reproductive Tract: Breast pain (females); menstrual disorder; blood in urine; urinary tract infection; frequency of urination; urinary incontinence; kidney stones; impotence; difficult or painful urination.

Skin: Rash; itching; increased sweating; acne.

Other: Influenza-like symptoms; hot flushes; body odor; fluid retention; muscle pain or weakness; weight decrease; nosebleed; dehydration; abnormal vision; double vision; joint, bone, back, chest, or leg pain; increased muscle tone; decreased hearing; fever; ringing in the ears.

Guidelines for Use:

- Dosage is individualized. Take exactly as prescribed.
- Do not stop taking or change the dose, unless directed by your doctor.
- May be taken without regard to meals.
- If using the sprinkle capsule, sprinkle contents on a small amount (teaspoonful) of soft food (eg, custard, applesauce, yogurt). Swallow without chewing. Do not store any of the sprinkle capsule/food mixture for later use.
- Because of the bitter taste, tablets should not be broken, crushed, or chewed.
- Maintain adequate fluid intake to decrease the risk of kidney stones.
- Inform your doctor immediately of blurred vision or pain around the eye.
- May cause dizziness, confusion, drowsiness, and difficulty concentrating. Use caution when driving or performing tasks requiring alertness, coordination, or physical dexterity.
- Should be withdrawn gradually to minimize potential of increase in seizures.
- Inform your doctor of prolonged periods of dialysis.
- Consider forms of contraception other than estrogen-containing birth control pills.
- See your doctor regularly to ensure correct dosage is being administered. Lab tests will be needed to monitor therapy.
- Store at 59° to 86°F in a tightly sealed container. Protect from moisture.

If you have any questions, consult your doctor, pharmacist, or health care provider.

	Generic Name *Brand Name Examples*	Supplied As	Generic Available
Rx	**Ethosuximide**		
	Zarontin	**Capsules:** 250 mg	No
	Zarontin	**Syrup:** 250 mg/tsp	Yes
Rx	**Methsuximide**		
	Celontin Kapseals	**Capsules:** 150 mg, 300 mg	No
Rx	**Phensuxide**		
	Milontin Kapseals	**Capsules:** 500 mg	No

Type of Drug:

Anticonvulsants; drugs used to treat epilepsy and seizures

How the Drug Works:

Succinimides acts on the central nervous system to decrease the frequency of seizures.

Uses:

To control absence (petit mal) seizures.

Precautions:

Do not use in the following situations: Allergy to succinimides.

Use with caution in the following situations:

acute intermittent porphyria
blood diseases
kidney diseases
rash (after therapy was started)
liver disease

Lupus: Cases of systemic lupus erythematosus have occurred during treatment with succinimides. Symptoms of this include: Fever, tiredness, skin lesions, pleurisy, headaches and personality changes.

Pregnancy: Reports suggest an association between use of anticonvulsant drugs by women with epilepsy and an increased number of birth defects in children born to these women. Other factors (eg, genetics or the epileptic condition) may also contribute to the higher incidence of birth defects. Most mothers receiving anticonvulsant medication deliver *normal* infants. Do not discontinue anticonvulsant drugs used to prevent major seizures. This could result in the occurrence of seizures and oxygen deficiency in body tissues and an increased risk to both the mother and the unborn child. In cases where seizures do not pose a serious threat, your doctor may recommend discontinuation of anticonvulsants prior to and during pregnancy. It is not known whether even minor seizures constitute some risk to the developing embryo or fetus. Reports suggest that a mother's use of anticonvulsant drugs, particularly barbiturates, is associated with a blood clotting defect in the newborn that may cause a bleeding problem within 24 hours of birth. It has been suggested that vitamin K be given to the mother one month prior to and during delivery, and to the infant, immediately after birth.

Breastfeeding: Consult your doctor concerning use of ethosuximide, methsuximide and phensuximide during breastfeeding.

Lab tests may be required during treatment with succinimides. Tests may include: Blood counts, urinalysis and liver function.

Drug Interactions:

Tell your doctor or pharmacist if you are taking or if you are planning to take any over-the-counter or prescription medications with succinimides. Doses of one or both drugs may need to be modified or a different drug may need to be prescribed. Primidone (eg, *Mysoline*) interacts with succinimides.

Side Effects:

Every drug is capable of producing side effects. Many succinimide users experience no, or minor, side effects. The frequency and severity of side effects depend on many factors including dose, duration of therapy and individual susceptibility. Possible side effects include:

Digestive Tract: Nausea; vomiting; stomach discomfort; loss of appetite; diarrhea; constipation; abdominal pain; weight loss.

Nervous System: Drowsiness; dizziness; mood changes; headache; nervousness; ; euphoria; dream-like feeling; hyperactivity; confusion; sleep disturbances; depression.

Skin: Rash; unusual bleeding or bruising; hives; increased growth and darkening of fine body hairs; hair loss.

Other: Joint pain; fever; sore throat; blurred vision; hiccups; fatigue; impaired coordination; abnormal blood counts; eyes sensitive to light; urinary frequency; blood in urine; muscle weakness; swelling of tongue and gums; swelling around eyes.

Guidelines for Use:

- If stomach upset occurs, take with food or milk.
- Do not change the dose or stop taking this medication without consulting your doctor. Abrupt withdrawal may cause seizures.
- If a dose is missed, take it as soon as possible. If several hours have passed or if it is nearing time for the next dose, do not double the dose in order to "catch up" (unless advised to do so by your doctor). If more than one dose is missed or it is necessary to establish a new dosage schedule, contact your doctor or pharmacist. Use exactly as prescribed.
- Keep scheduled appointments with your doctor and carry Medic-Alert identification listing your medical condition and medicine.
- *Phensuximide* may color the urine pink, red or red-brown. This is not harmful.
- Avoid alcoholic beverages.
- May cause drowsiness, dizziness, or blurred vision. Use caution while driving or performing other tasks requiring alertness.
- Notify your doctor if any of the following occurs: Skin rash, joint pain, unexplained fever, sore throat, unusual bleeding or bruising, drowsiness, dizziness, blurred vision, pregnancy, seizures, depression, aggressiveness or behavioral changes.
- Succinimides, when used alone in mixed types of epilepsy, may increase the frequency of grand mal seizures.

If you have any questions, consult your doctor, pharmacist, or health care provider.

	Generic Name *Brand Name Example*	Supplied As	Generic Available
Rx	**Lamotrigine**		
	Lamictal	**Tablets:** 25 mg, 100 mg, 150 mg, 200 mg	No

Type of Drug:

Anticonvulsant; antiepileptic.

How the Drug Works:

It is not known exactly how lamotrigine works. It is believed that lamotrigine prevents or reduces the number of seizures by acting on stabilizing the brain to control the activity of nerve impulses.

Uses:

As an additional therapy in the treatment of partial seizures in patients older than 16 years of age with epilepsy.

Unlabeled Use(s): Occasionally, doctors may prescribe lamotrigine to adults with generalized clonic-tonic seizures.

Precautions:

Do not use in the following situations:
allergy to lamotrigine or its ingredients
rash in children

Use with caution in the following situations:
anemia
heart disease
kidney disease
liver disease
rash
valproic acid use
visual disorders

Rash may occur during treatment with this medicine and may be a symptom of a serious allergic reaction. If a rash should develop, discontinue lamotrigine if the drug is suspected and contact your doctor immediately. The incidence of severe, potentially life-threatening rash in pediatric patients is very much higher than that reported in adults using lamotrigine. Specifically, reports from clinical trials suggest that as many as 1 in 50 to 1 in 100 pediatric patients develop a potentially life-threatening rash. Thus, lamotrigine is not approved for use in patients below the age of 16.

Pregnancy: Adequate studies have not been done in pregnant women or animal studies may have shown a risk to the fetus. Use only if clearly needed and potential benefits outweigh the possible hazards to the fetus.

Breastfeeding: Lamotrigine appears in breast milk. Breastfeeding while taking lamotrigine is not recommended. Consult your doctor before you begin breastfeeding.

Children: Safety and effectiveness in children younger than 16 years of age have not been established.

Lab tests to monitor the amount of lamotrigine and other seizure drugs in the blood may be needed. Since it is possible that lamotrigine may collect in the tissues of the eyes, testing may be necessary if visual impairment occurs.

Drug Interactions:

Tell your doctor or pharmacist if you are taking or if you are planning to take any over-the-counter or prescription medications or dietary supplements while taking lamotrigine. Doses of one or both drugs may need to be modified or a different drug may need to be prescribed. The following drugs and drug classes interact with lamotrigine:

carbamazepine (eg, *Tegretol)*
folate inhibitors (eg, trimetrexate glucuronate)
phenobarbital (eg, *Solfoton)*
phenytoin (eg, *Dilantin)*
primidone (eg, *Mysoline)*
valproic acid (eg, *Depakene)*

Side Effects:

Every drug is capable of producing side effects. Many lamotrigine users experience no, or minor, side effects. The frequency and severity of side effects depend on many factors including dose, duration of therapy and individual susceptibility. Possible side effects include:

Circulatory System: Hot flashes; pounding in the chest (palpitations); chest pain.

Digestive Tract: Stomachache; nausea; vomiting; diarrhea; indigestion; constipation; dry mouth; loss of appetite; tooth disorder.

Nervous System: Dizziness; incoordination; drowsiness; sleeplessness; tremor; depression; anxiety; nervousness; hostility; convulsions; worsened seizures; irritability; speech disorder; memory loss; confusion; thinking abnormality; unstable emotions; mind racing; rapid eye movement; concentration disturbance; feeling of whirling motion.

Respiratory System: Sore throat; increased cough; difficulty breathing; congestion.

Urinary and Reproductive Tract: Painful menstruation; inflammation of the vagina; absence of menstrual bleeding;

Skin: Rash; itching; hair loss; acne.

Senses: Double vision; blurred vision.

Other: Headache; flu syndrome; fever; neck, joint or back pain; general body discomfort; chills; weakness; abnormal vision; ear pain; ringing in the ears; muscle spasm; accidental injury; infection; weight gain.

Guidelines for Use:

- Use exactly as prescribed.
- May be taken without regard to food.
- For long-term therapy, take in two equally divided doses.
- If a rash should develop, it could be a sign of a serious medical condition. Contact your doctor immediately. Also report any fever or gland swelling.
- Notify your doctor if seizures become worse.
- If a dose is missed, take it as soon as possible. If several hours have passed or if it is nearly time for the next dose, do not double the dose to "catch up" (unless advised to do so by your doctor). If more than one dose is missed or it is necessary to establish a new dosage schedule, contact your doctor or pharmacist.
- May cause dizziness and drowsiness. Avoid driving or performing other tasks requiring alertness or coordination until effects are known, then use caution.
- Do not discontinue medication or change the dose without first consulting with your doctor. Seizures could increase. Unless safety concerns require a faster withdrawal, the dose of lamotrigine should be tapered over 2 weeks.
- Inform your doctor if you are pregnant, become pregnant, are planning to become pregnant during therapy, or if you are breastfeeding or intend to breastfeed an infant.
- Lab tests may be required to monitor therapy. Be sure to keep appointments.
- Store in a dry place at room temperature; protect from light.

If you have any questions, consult your doctor, pharmacist, or health care provider.

Generic Name *Brand Name Examples*	Supplied As	Generic Available
Rx **Tiagabine HCl**		
Gabitril Filmtab	**Tablets:** 4 mg, 12 mg, 16 mg, 20 mg	No

Type of Drug:

Anticonvulsant; drug used to treat seizures.

How the Drug Works:

It is not known exactly how tiagabine works. It is believed that tiagabine prevents or reduces the number of seizures by altering chemicals in the brain to inhibit nerve impulses which cause certain types of seizures.

Uses:

As an additional therapy in the treatment of partial seizures in patients older than 12 years of age.

Precautions:

Do not use in the following situations: Allergy to tiagabine or any of its ingredients.

Use with caution in the following situations:

EEG abnormalities
change of epilepsy drugs
liver disease
non-induced patients
preexisting cognitive/neuropsychiatric disorders
withdrawal, abrupt

Pregnancy: Adequate studies have not been done in pregnant women. Use only if clearly needed and potential benefits outweigh the possible hazards to the fetus.

Breastfeeding: It is not known if tiagabine appears in breast milk. Consult your doctor before you begin breastfeeding.

Children: Safety and effectiveness in children younger than 12 years of age have not been established.

Lab tests may be required with tiagabine.

Drug Interactions:

Tell your doctor or pharmacist if you are taking or if you are planning to take any over-the-counter or prescription medications or dietary supplements with tiagabine. Doses of one or both drugs may need to be modified or a different drug may need to be prescribed. The following drugs and drug classes interact with tiagabine.

carbamazepine (eg, *Tegretol*)
CNS depressants (eg, diazepam, alcohol, tranquilizers, hypnotics)
ethanol
phenobarbitol (eg, *Solfoton*)
phenytoin (eg, *Dilantin*)
primidone (eg, *Mysoline*)
triazolam
valproate (eg, *Depakote*)

Side Effects:

Every drug is capable of producing side effects. Many tiagabine users experience no, or minor, side effects. The frequency and severity of side effects depend on many factors including dose, duration of therapy and individual susceptibility. Possible side effects include:

Digestive Tract: Nausea; stomach pain; diarrhea; vomiting; increased appetite; mouth sores; constipation; appetite loss; dry mouth; gas; indigestion; inflammation of the gums.

Nervous System: Dizziness; lightheadedness; drowsiness; nervousness; irritability; tremor; abnormal thinking; difficulty concentrating; depression; confusion; incoordination; sleeplessness; speech disorder; difficulty with memory; abnormal skin sensations; unstable emotions; abnormal walk; hostility; continual rapid eye movement; language problems; agitation; accidental injury; anxiety; depersonalization; slurred speech; headache; fainting; exaggerated sense of well-being; hallucinations; excessive or decreased movement; decreased sensitivity to touch; muscle twitching; migraine; paranoid reaction; personality disorder; decreased reflexes; stupor; feeling of whirling motion.

Circulatory System: High blood pressure; pounding in the chest (palpitations); rapid heartbeat.

Respiratory System: Bronchitis; difficulty breathing; nosebleed; pneumonia; increased cough.

Skin: Flushing; rash; itching; unusual bruising; acne; hair loss; dry skin; sweating.

Other: Weakness/lack of energy; pain; muscle weakness; sore throat; chest pain; flu-like syndrome; sinus infection; back pain; fever; vision problems; eye irritation; urinary tract infection; urinary frequency; infection; allergic reaction; chills; cyst; neck pain; general body discomfort; swelling; swelling of arms and legs; weight gain or loss; joint pain; weak or tight muscles; ear pain; ringing in the ears; ear infection; painful menstruation; painful or difficult urination; irregular menstruation; inability to control urination; inflammation of the vagina with itching and vaginal discharge; lymph node disorder.

Guidelines for Use:

- Usual starting dose is 4 mg once daily.
- Take with food.
- Take as directed by your doctor. The daily dose varies depending on individual needs. Do not adjust the dose or discontinue therapy without consulting your doctor. This could have serious adverse effects.
- If a dose is missed, take it as soon as possible. If several hours have passed or if it is nearing time for the next dose, do not double the dose in order to "catch up" (unless advised by your doctor). If more than one dose is missed or it is necessary to establish a new dosage schedule, contact your doctor or pharmacist. Use exactly as prescribed.
- This medicine may cause drowsiness or dizziness. Use caution while driving or performing other tasks requiring mental alertness, coordination or physical dexterity.
- Avoid alcohol and other mental depressants (eg, narcotics, tranquilizers, antihistamines) while you are taking this medicine.
- Inform your doctor if you are pregnant, become pregnant, are planning to become pregnant or if you are breastfeeding.
- Withdraw tiagabine gradually to minimize the potential of increased seizure frequency, unless safety concerns require a more rapid withdrawal.
- Keep scheduled appointments with your doctor and carry Medic Alert identification listing your medical condition and medicine.
- Lab tests may be required to monitor treatment. Be sure to keep appointments.
- Store at controlled room temperature (68° to 77°F). Protect from light and moisture.

If you have any questions, consult your doctor, pharmacist, or health care provider.

	Generic Name *Brand Name Example*	Supplied As	Generic Available
Rx	**Levetiracetam**		
	Keppra	**Tablets**: 250 mg, 500 mg, 750 mg	No

Type of Drug:

Anticonvulsant; antiseizure agent.

How the Drug Works:

Although the precise mechanism of action is not known, it appears that levetiracetam inhibits bursts of neural impulses and propagation of seizure activity.

Uses:

For adjunctive therapy in the treatment of partial onset seizures in adults with epilepsy.

Precautions:

Do not use in the following situations: Allergy to levetiracetam or any of its ingredients.

Use with caution in the following situations: Moderate to severe kidney disease.

Pregnancy: There are no adequate and well-controlled studies in pregnant women. Use only if clearly needed and the potential benefits to the mother outweigh the possible risks to the fetus.

Breastfeeding: It is not known if levetiracetam appears in breast milk. Consult your doctor before you begin breastfeeding.

Children: Safety and effectiveness in patients younger than 16 years of age have not been established.

Drug Interactions:

Tell your doctor or pharmacist if you are taking or planning to take any over-the-counter or prescription medications or dietary supplements while taking levetiracetam. Doses of one or both drugs may need to be modified or a different drug may need to be prescribed.

Side Effects:

Every drug is capable of producing side effects. Many patients experience no, or minor, side effects. The frequency and severity of side effects depend upon many factors including dose, duration of therapy, and individual susceptibility. Possible side effects include:

Nervous System: Drowsiness; incoordination; dizziness; depression; nervousness; vertigo (feeling of whirling motion); amnesia; anxiety; hostility; emotional lability; hostility; fatigue.

Respiratory System: Sore throat; runny nose; increased cough; sinus irritation.

Other: Abnormal skin sensations; weakness; headache; infection; pain; appetite loss; double vision

Guidelines for Use:

- Dosage is individualized.
- Do not change the dose or stop taking unless advised to do so by your doctor.
- May be taken without regard to meals or snacks.
- If a dose is missed, take it as soon as possible. If several hours have passed or if it is nearing time for the next dose, do not double the dose in order to catch up, unless advised to do so by your doctor. If several doses are missed, or it is necessary to establish a new dosage schedule, contact your doctor or pharmacist.
- May cause dizziness or drowsiness. Use caution while driving or performing other tasks requiring alertness, coordination, or physical dexterity.
- Notify your doctor if you experience drowsiness, fatigue, coordination difficulties, or behavior abnormalities.
- Notify your doctor if you are pregnant, become pregnant, or are planning to become pregnant while undergoing therapy with levetiracetam.
- Store at controlled room temperature (59° to 86°F).

If you have any questions, consult your doctor, pharmacist, or health care provider.

	Generic Name *Brand Name Examples*	Supplied As	Generic Available
Rx	**Valproic Acid**		
	Depakene	**Capsules**: 250 mg	Yes
	Depakene	**Syrup**: 250 mg/5 mL	Yes
	Depakote	**Capsules, sprinkle**: 125 mg (as divalproex sodium)	No
	Depakote	**Tablets, delayed-release**: 125 mg, 250 mg, 500 mg (as divalproex sodium)	No
	Depakote ER	**Tablets, extended-release**: 500 mg (as divalproex sodium)	No
	Depacon	**Injection**: 100 mg/mL	No

Type of Drug:

Anticonvulsant; drug used to treat epilepsy, seizures, and other conditions.

How the Drug Works:

Valproic acid prevents or reduces the number of seizures by controlling the abnormal activity of nerve impulses in the brain and central nervous system. Sodium valproate and divalproex sodium are converted to valproic acid in the body.

Uses:

Used alone or in combination with other anticonvulsants to control simple (petit mal) and complex absence seizures alone or in combination with other anticonvulsant drugs.

To treat manic episodes associated with bipolar disorder (divalproex sodium delayed-release tablets).

For the prevention of migraine headaches (divalproex sodium delayed-release and extended-release tablets).

Unlabeled Use(s): Occasionally doctors may prescribe valproic acid for other types of seizures including grand mal seizures, myoclonic seizures; infantile spasm seizures and recurrent febrile (fever) seizures in children; minor incontinence after intestinal tract surgery; anxiety disorders/panic attacks; and patients with intractable status epilepticus who have not responded to other therapies.

Precautions:

Do not use in the following situations:

allergy to valproic acid, sodium valproate, or divalproex
liver disease/dysfunction

Use with caution in the following situations:

acute head trauma
blood/bleeding disorders
children younger than 2 years of age

congenital metabolic disorders
kidney disease
liver disease, history
multiple anticonvulsant use
organic brain disorder
pregnancy
severe seizure disorders with mental retardation
suicidal thoughts

Liver disease: Liver failure resulting in death has occurred in patients receiving valproic acid and its derivatives. Children younger than 2 years of age are at an increased risk of developing fatal liver toxicity, especially those on multiple anticonvulsants, those with congenital metabolic disorders, those with severe seizure disorders accompanied by mental retardation, and those with organic brain disease. Use with extreme caution and as a sole agent. The incidence of liver toxicity decreases considerably in progressively older patient groups. These incidents usually have occurred during the first 6 months of treatment. Serious liver problems may be preceded by nonspecific symptoms such as loss of seizure control, general feeling of ill health, weakness, drowsiness, facial swelling, appetite loss, yellowing of skin and eyes, or vomiting.

Pancreatitis: Cases of life-threatening pancreatitis have been reported in children and adults receiving valproate. Some of the cases have been described as hemorrhagic with a rapid progression from initial symptoms to death. Abdominal pain, nausea, vomiting, or anorexia can be symptoms of pancreatitis that require prompt medical evaluation.

Pregnancy: Studies have shown a potential risk to the fetus. Using these drugs during pregnancy may result in birth defects. If you are pregnant, or are planning to become pregnant, discuss with your doctor the possible risks to the unborn infant. Use only if clearly needed and the potential benefits outweigh the possible risks.

Breastfeeding: Valproic acid appears in breast milk. Consult your doctor before you begin breastfeeding.

Children: Children younger than 2 years of age may be particularly sensitive to the possible liver damage caused by valproic acid, especially if taking other anticonvulsant drugs at the same time. Safety and effectiveness have not been established in children under 18 years of age for treatment of acute mania. Safety and efficacy of divalproex sodium for the prevention of migraines has not been established in children under 16 years of age. Divalproex sodium extended-release tablets are not recommended in children. Consult your doctor. See *Liver disease.*

Elderly: Elderly patients may be at an increased risk of drowsiness and tremor.

Lab tests will be required during treatment with valproic acid. Tests may include liver function, blood counts, prothrombin, and other tests for blood-clotting mechanisms and blood levels of valproic acid.

Drug Interactions:

Tell your doctor or pharmacist if you are taking or if you are planning to take any over-the-counter or prescription medications or dietary supplements with valproic acid. Doses of one or both drugs may need to be modified or a different drug may need to be prescribed. The following drugs and drug classes interact with valproic acid:

- anticoagulants, oral (eg, warfarin)
- barbiturates (eg, phenobarbital)
- carbamazepine (eg, *Tegretol*)
- charcoal
- chlorpromazine (eg, *Thorazine*)
- cimetidine (eg, *Tagamet*)
- clonazepam (eg, *Klonopin*)
- diazepam (eg, *Valium*)
- ethanol
- ethosuximide (eg, *Zarontin*)
- felbamate (*Felbatol*)
- hydantoins (eg, phenytoin)
- lamotrigine (*Lamictal*)
- phenobarbital (eg, *Solfoton*)
- primidone (eg, *Mysoline*)
- rifampin (eg, *Rifadin*)
- salicylates (eg, aspirin)
- tricyclic antidepressants (eg, amitriptyline)
- warfarin (eg, *Coumadin*)
- zidovudine (AZT; *Retrovir*)

Side Effects:

Every drug is capable of producing side effects. Many valproic acid users experience no, or minor, side effects. The frequency and severity of side effects depend on many factors including dose, duration of therapy, and individual susceptibility. Possible side effects include:

Senses: Abnormal vision; eye redness/pain; blurred vision; double vision; spots before the eyes; unusual eye movements; dry eyes; hearing loss; ear pain/disorder; ringing in the ears; taste perversion.

Digestive Tract: Changes in appetite; nausea; vomiting; stomach cramps; indigestion; diarrhea; fecal incontinence; constipation; gas; tongue inflammation.

Nervous System: Weakness; tiredness; nervousness; forgetfulness; clumsiness; drowsiness; behavior changes; depression; headache; tremors; hallucinations; dizziness; slurred speech; abnormal dreams; abnormal thinking; agitation; abnormal gait; twitching; abnormal skin sensations (eg, burning, prickling, tingling); feeling of whirling motion; exagerated sense of well-being; decreased sense of stimulation; difficulty moving; increased reflexes; confusion; sleeplessness.

Circulatory System: Changes in blood pressure; palpitations (pounding in the chest); postural hypotension (dizziness or lightheadedness when rising from a sitting or lying position); fast heartbeat; flushing; chest pain.

Skin: Yellowing of skin or eyes; unusual bleeding or bruising; sensitivity to light; rash; itching; dry or oily skin; skin redness; hair follicle infection.

Other: Swelling of the face, hands, or feet; weight changes; flushing; abscessed teeth; joint or chest pain; leg cramps; tight muscles; back pain; difficulty breathing; cough; runny nose; painful or difficult urination; loss of bladder control; sensitivity to sunlight; Stevens-Johnson syndrome; pancreatitis; chills; fever; neck pain or stiffness; changes in menstrual periods; painful menstruation; hair loss; injection site reactions; inflammation of the tongue; sore throat; flu-like syndrome; sweating.

Guidelines for Use:

- Dosage is individualized. Take exacly as prescribed.
- May cause stomach upset. Take with food.
- *Tablets and capsules* — Swallow whole; do not chew or crush. Chewing or crushing tablets or capsules may cause irritation in the mouth or throat.
- *Sprinkle capsules* — May be swallowed whole or may be taken by opening the capsule and sprinkling the contents on a small amount (teaspoonful) of soft foods such as applesauce or pudding. Swallow quickly without chewing. Do not store drug/food mixture for future use.
- *Injection* — For IV use only. Administer a 60-minute infusion with same frequency as the oral products. Rapid infusion of valproate has been associated with an increase in adverse events.
- May cause dizziness, drowsiness, or sleepiness. Use caution when driving or performing other tasks requiring alertness, coordination, or physical dexterity. Taking at bedtime may help decrease drowsiness. Consult your doctor.
- Consult your doctor immediately if you experience loss of seizure control, weakness, swelling of the face, unusual bleeding or bruising, skin reactions, lethargy, general body discomfort, loss of appetite, yellowing of skin or eyes, vomiting, nausea, abdominal pain, or anorexia.
- Do not stop taking this medicine without checking with your doctor. If you stop taking this medicine suddenly, your seizures may suddenly begin again.
- If dose is missed, take as soon as possible. If several hours have passed or if it is nearing time for the next dose, do not double the dose to catch up, unless advised by your doctor. If more than one dose if missed or it is necessary to establish a new dosage schedule, contact your doctor or pharmacist.
- When you first begin taking this medicine, see your doctor regularly. The doctor may want to adjust the dose you are taking to make sure it is the best dose to control your condition and minimize side effects. Checkups are particularly important if you are taking other anticonvulsant drugs with valproic acid.
- Inform your doctor if you are pregnant, become pregnant, plan on becoming pregnant, or are breatfeeding during valproic acid therapy.
- *Diabetes* — These drugs may interfere with urine tests for ketones and may give inaccurate test results.
- Using these drugs with alcohol or other central nervous system depressants (eg, narcotic pain relievers, sedatives) may cause additional drowsiness.
- Carry Medic Alert identification indicating that you are taking these drugs and have epilepsy.
- May cause photosensitivity (sensitivity to sunlight). Avoid prolonged exposure to the sun and other ultraviolet light. Use sunscreens and wear protective clothing until tolerance is determined.
- Store capsules below 77°F. Store tablets and syrup below 86°F. Store vials at controlled room temperature (59° to 86°F).

If you have any questions, consult your doctor, pharmacist, or health care provider.

	Generic Name *Brand Name Examples*	Supplied As	Generic Available
Rx	**Baclofen**		
	Lioresal	**Tablet**: 10 mg, 20 mg	Yes
	Lioresal Intrathecal	**Injection**: 10 mg/20 mL (500 mcg/mL), 10 mg/5 mL (2000 mcg/mL)	No

Type of Drug:

Skeletal muscle relaxant.

How the Drug Works:

Baclofen reduces the frequency and severity of muscle spasms that occur as a result of neurological disorders such as multiple sclerosis.

Uses:

Tablets: To relieve the spasticity, pain, and rigidity from muscle spasms due to multiple sclerosis. May help with spinal cord injuries and other spinal cord diseases.

Injection: To manage severe spasticity of spinal cord origin in patients who do not respond to or have side effects from the tablets.

Unlabeled Use(s): Occasionally doctors may prescribe oral baclofen for trigeminal neuralgia (tic douloureux), tardive dyskinesia in combination with neuroleptics, and intractable hiccoughs; the injection form may reduce spasticity in cerebral palsy in children.

Precautions:

Do not use in the following situations:

- allergy to baclofen or any of its ingredients
- cerebral palsy (tablet only)
- muscle spasms due to rheumatic disorders (tablet only)
- Parkinson's disease (tablet only)

Use with caution in the following situations:

- autonomic dysreflexia (lesions on the spinal cord)
- epilepsy
- kidney disease
- infection (injection only)
- psychotic disorders
- stroke (tablet only)

Epilepsy: Increased frequency of seizures has occurred in epileptic patients taking baclofen. Frequent physical exams and neurological tests may be required.

Abrupt withdrawal: Hallucinations and seizures have occurred when treatment with baclofen has been stopped suddenly. Except in cases of serious side effects, the dose must be reduced slowly when the drug is discontinued.

Ovarian cysts: Ovarian cysts are sometimes found in women who have taken baclofen for up to one year. The cysts often disappear despite continued treatment.

Pregnancy: There are no adequate and well-controlled studies in pregnant women. Use only if clearly needed and potential benefits to the mother outweigh the possible hazards to the fetus.

Breastfeeding: Oral baclofen appears in breast milk. It is not known if injectable baclofen appears in breast milk. Consult your doctor before you begin breastfeeding.

Children: Safety and effectiveness in children younger than 12 years of age (oral) and in children younger than 4 years of age (injection) have not been established.

Drug Interactions:

Tell your doctor or pharmacist if you are taking or if you are planning to take any over- the-counter or prescription medications or dietary supplements while taking this medicine. Doses of one or both drugs may need to be modified or a different drug may need to be prescribed. The following drugs and drug classes interact with this medicine.

alcohol
morphine
narcotic pain relievers (eg, *Percodan)*
sleep aids (eg, flurazepam)
tricyclic antidepressants (eg, amitriptyline)

Side Effects:

Every drug is capable of producing side effects. Many patients experience no, or minor, side effects. The frequency and severity of side effects depend on many factors including dose, duration of therapy and individual susceptibility. Possible side effects include:

Digestive Tract: Nausea; constipation; vomiting.

Nervous System: Drowsiness; dizziness; lightheadedness; weakness; tiredness; headache; seizures; sleeplessness; numbness; tingling; slurred speech.

Skin: Rash; itching; excessive sweating.

Other: Visual disturbances; ankle swelling (edema); weak muscles; weight gain; nasal congestion; difficulty breathing; frequent urination; low blood pressure.

Guidelines for Use:

- Use exactly as prescribed.
- If a dose is missed, take it as soon as possible. If several hours have passed or if it is nearing time for the next dose, do not double the dose in order to "catch up" (unless advised to do so by your doctor). If more than one dose is missed or it is necessary to establish a new dosage schedule, contact your doctor or pharmacist.
- May cause drowsiness, dizziness and tiredness. Use caution when driving or performing other tasks requiring alertness. Avoid alcohol and other drugs that cause drowsiness during use of baclofen.
- Sudden discontinuation of baclofen can result in hallucinations. Discontinue only under doctor's supervision.
- Notify your doctor if frequent urges to urinate, painful urination, constipation, nausea, headache, insomnia, confusion, palpitations or chest pain occurs and persists.
- *Injections* — Not for IV, IM, subcutaneous, or epidermal use. Visually inspect solutions for particles or discoloration.
- Store at room temperature. Do not freeze. Do not heat or sterilize solution.

If you have any questions, consult your doctor, pharmacist, or health care provider.

Generic Name *Brand Name Example*	Supplied As	Generic Available
Rx **Dantrolene Sodium**		
Dantrium	**Capsules**: 25 mg, 50 mg, 100 mg	No
Dantrium Intravenous	**Powder for injection**: 20 mg/vial	No

Type of Drug:

Skeletal muscle relaxant.

How the Drug Works:

Dantrolene relaxes skeletal muscle by acting directly on the muscle.

In rare cases, the use of anesthetics in certain individuals can lead to a life-threatening rapid rise in body temperature known as "malignant hyperthermia". It may be due to anesthetics triggering a complex series of events in the muscles that ultimately lead to very high body temperatures. Dantrolene is used to treat or prevent malignant hyperthermia because it is thought that it interferes with the necessary sequence of events which lead to malignant hyperthermia.

Uses:

To treat muscle spasms (spasticity) due to certain nerve disorders (eg, cerebral palsy, multiple sclerosis, spinal cord injury or stroke). It is best used for individuals with reversible spasms and in whom the spasms interfere with rehabilitation. It may also be used on a long-term basis for some individuals in whom the spasms are painful or disabling. It should not be used in individuals for whom spastic movements are important for gaining or sustaining upright posture or balance or for moving about, or for treatment of spasm resulting from rheumatism.

To treat or prevent malignant hyperthermia (life-threatening rapid rises in body temperature resulting from the use of an anesthetic). These reactions usually occur in the operating room during the course of an operation. Dantrolene is given intravenously in these situations. However, certain individuals considered at risk for malignant hyperthermia from an anesthetic will often be given dantrolene orally prior to an operation. In addition, dantrolene may be given intravenously after malignant hyperthermia has occurred during an operation to prevent a recurrence.

Unlabeled Use(s): Occasionally doctors may prescribe dantrolene for exercise-induced muscle pain, neuroleptic malignant syndrome and heat stroke.

Precautions:

Do not use in the following situations:

allergy to dantrolene
liver disease (eg, cirrhosis, hepatitis)
rheumatic disorder

Use with caution in the following situations:

females	lung disease
heart disease	patients older than 35 years of age
long-term use	

Liver: Serious liver disorders, including some that were fatal, have occurred as a result of using dantrolene. Risk of hepatitis appears to be greatest in women, in patients older than 35 and in patients taking other drugs in addition to dantrolene. It is important that liver function be checked routinely by physical exam and blood tests.

Photosensitivity: May cause photosensitivity (sensitivity to sunlight). Avoid prolonged exposure to the sun or other forms of ultraviolet (UV) light (eg, tanning beds). Use sunscreens and wear protective clothing until tolerance is determined.

Pregnancy: Adequate studies have not been done in pregnant women, or animal studies may have shown a risk to the fetus. Use only if clearly needed and potential benefits outweigh the possible hazards to the fetus.

Breastfeeding: Do not use dantrolene during breastfeeding.

Children: Safety and effectiveness in children under 5 have not been established. Use is not recommended.

Drug Interactions:

Tell you doctor or pharmacist if you are taking or planning to take any over-the-counter or prescription medications or dietary supplements while taking this medicine. Doses of one or both drugs may need to be modified or a different drug may need to be prescribed. The following drugs and drug classes interact with this medicine.

anticoagulants, oral (eg, warfarin)
clofibrate (eg, *Atromid-S)*
estrogens (eg, *Premarin)*

Side Effects:

Every drug is capable of producing side effects. Many patients experience no, or minor, side effects. The frequency and severity of side effects depend on many factors including dose, duration of therapy and individual susceptibility. Possible side effects include:

Urinary and Reproductive Tract: Change in frequency of urination; blood in urine; loss of urine control (incontinence); difficulty obtaining erection; painful urination; difficulty with urination; frequent urination at night.

Digestive Tract: Diarrhea; constipation; black, tarry stools; loss of appetite; difficulty swallowing; upset stomach; abdominal cramps.

Nervous System: Drowsiness; dizziness; difficulty with speech; seizures; headache; lightheadedness; sleeplessness; depression; confusion; anxiety (nervousness); weakness; tiredness.

Circulatory System: Rapid heart rate; changes in blood pressure; swelling, redness, pain and tenderness over a vein (phlebitis).

Skin: Unusual hair growth; rash; itching; hives; redness; sweating; yellowing of skin and eyes.

Other: Hepatitis; general feeling of ill health; vision problems; double vision; taste changes; sore muscles; backache; chills and fever; feeling of suffocation; excessive tearing; difficulty breathing; chest pain.

Guidelines for Use:

- Use exactly as prescribed.
- If a dose is missed, take it as soon as possible. If several hours have passed or if it is nearing time for the next dose, do not double the dose in order to "catch up" (unless advised to do so by your doctor). If more than one dose is missed or it is necessary to establish a now dosage schedule, contact your doctor or pharmacist.
- If no apparent benefit is observed after 45 days of treatment, the drug should be stopped.
- May cause drowsiness, dizziness or lightheadedness. Use caution when driving or performing other tasks requiring alertness, coordination or physical dexterity.
- Avoid alcohol and other drugs that can cause drowsiness, dizziness or lightheadedness.
- May cause weakness, tiredness, nausea, diarrhea and a general feeling of ill health. A decrease in grip strength and weakness of leg muscles (particularly when walking down stairs) may occur after receiving dantrolene intravenously. Notify your doctor if any of these symptoms persist.
- Use caution while eating because choking and difficulty swallowing can occur on the day dantrolene is administered.
- May cause photosensitivity (sensitivity to sunlight). Avoid prolonged exposure to sunlight or other forms of ultraviolet (UV) light (eg, tanning beds). Use sunscreens and wear protective clothing until tolerance is determined.
- Notify your doctor if skin rash, itching, bloody or black tarry stools, or yellowish discoloration of the skin or eyes occurs.
- Store at room temperature. Protect from light.

If you have any questions, consult your doctor, pharmacist, or health care provider.

	Generic Name *Brand Name Example*	Supplied As	Generic Available
Rx	**Tizanidine HCl** *Zanaflex*	**Tablets:** 4 mg	No

Type of Drug:

Centrally acting muscle relaxant.

How the Drug Works:

Tizanidine activates chemical receptors in the brain which inhibit nerve stimulation of muscles.

Uses:

For acute and intermittent treatment of increased muscle tone associated with spasticity.

Precautions:

Do not use in the following situations: Allergy to tizandine or any of its ingredients.

Use with caution in the following situations:

antihypertensive drug therapy
cardiac rhythm disturbance
elderly
females taking oral contraceptives
kidney disease
liver disease
long-term use
low blood pressure

Liver injury: Tizanidine occasionally causes liver injury which is usually reversible when the medicine is stopped. Liver enzyme testing is used to identify this problem. Report any symptoms of nausea, vomiting, appetitie loss or jaundice (yellowing of skin or eyes) to your doctor.

Pregnancy: Adequate studies have not been done in pregnant women. Use only if clearly needed and potential benefits outweigh the possible hazards to the fetus.

Breastfeeding: It is not known if tizanidine appears in breast milk.

Children: Safety and effectiveness in children have not been established.

Elderly: Use with caution in elderly patients.

Lab tests may be required to monitor treatment. Be sure to keep appointments. Tests may include: Liver function and kidney function.

Drug Interactions:

Tell your doctor or pharmacist if you are taking or if you are planning to take any over-the-counter or prescription medications or dietary supplements with tizanidine. Doses of one or both drugs may need to be modified or a different drug may need to be prescribed. The following drugs and drug classes interact with tizanidine.

alcohol
acetaminophen (eg, *Tylenol*)
alpha-adrenergic agonists (eg, clonidine)
antihypertensives (eg, prazosin)
baclofen (*Lioresal*)
CNS depressants (eg, benzodiazepines)
oral contraceptives (eg, *Ortho-Novum 1/35)*

Side Effects:

Every drug is capable of producing side effects. Many tizanidine users experience no, or minor, side effects. The frequency and severity of side effects depend on many factors including dose, duration of therapy and individual susceptibility. Possible side effects include:

Digestive Tract: Dry mouth; constipation; vomiting; stomach pain; diarrhea; indigestion.

Nervous System: Sedation; drowsiness; hallucinations; increased spasms; dizziness; nervousness; depression; anxiety; abnormal skin sensations.

Circulatory System: Low blood pressure; slow or irregular heartbeat.

Endocrine: Rash; sweating; skin ulcer.

Other: Abnormal liver function tests; general body weakness; urinary tract infection; infection; speech disorder; blurred vision; urinary frequency; flu-like syndrome; difficulty moving; sore throat; fever; muscle weakness; back pain; nasal congestion; runny nose.

Guidelines for Use:

- Usual starting dose is 4 mg daily to reduce side effects. Gradual increases in dose will be made to maximize muscle relaxant effect.
- Each dose can be taken as needed every 6 to 8 hours up to three times a day.
- May be taken with or without food.
- If a dose is missed, take it as soon as possible. If several hours have passed or it is nearing time for the next dose, do not double the dose to "catch up" (unless advised by your doctor). If more than one dose is missed or it is necessary to establish a new dosage schedule, contact your doctor or pharmacist.
- If dry mouth, drowsiness or weakness occurs, contact your doctor immediately.
- May cause dizziness, lightheadedness or fainting, especially when rising or standing. If these symptoms should occur, sit or lie down and contact your doctor. Use caution while driving or performing hazardous tasks requiring alertness, coordination or physical dexterity.
- This medicine may cause some other medicines (eg, benzodiazepines, baclofen) and alcohol to have increased sedative or drowsiness effects.
- Inform you doctor if you are pregnant, become pregnant, are planning to become pregnant or if you are breastfeeding.
- Inform your doctor if you are taking oral contraceptives so that necessary dosage adjustments may be made.
- Limited information exists regarding long-term use of this medicine.
- Lab tests or exams may be required to monitor treatment. Be sure to keep appointments. Tests may include: Liver function and kidney function.
- Store at 59° to 86°F.

If you have any questions, consult your doctor, pharmacist, or health care provider.

	Generic Name *Brand Name Examples*	Supplied As	Generic Available
Rx	**Carisoprodol**		
	Soma	**Tablets**: 350 mg	Yes
Rx	**Chlorphenesin Carbamate**		
	Maolate[1]	**Tablets**: 400 mg	No
Rx	**Chlorzoxazone**		
	Paraflex Caplets, Remular-S	**Tablets**: 250 mg	Yes
	Parafon Forte DSC Caplets	**Tablets**: 500 mg	Yes
Rx	**Cyclobenzaprine**		
	Flexeril	**Tablets**: 10 mg	Yes
c-iv	**Diazepam**[2]		
	Valium	**Tablets**: 2 mg, 5 mg, 10 mg	Yes
	Diazepam	**Oral solution**: 5 mg/tsp	Yes
	Diazepam Intensol	**Oral solution, concentrated**: 5 mg/mL	Yes
Rx	**Metaxalone**		
	Skelaxin	**Tablets**: 400 mg	No
Rx	**Methocarbamol**[2]		
	Robaxin, Robaxin-750	**Tablets**: 500 mg, 750 mg	Yes
Rx	**Orphenadrine Citrate**[2]	**Tablets**: 100 mg	Yes
	Norflex	**Tablets, sustained release**: 100 mg	No

[1] Contains the dye tartrazine.
[2] Some of these products are available as an injection.

Type of Drug:

Skeletal muscle relaxants.

How the Drug Works:

These drugs indirectly affect nerves that cause muscle tension or spasm. They also have sedative effects on the central nervous system.

Uses:

To relieve muscle discomfort due to strain, sprain or injury. These agents are not a substitute for rest or physical therapy needed for proper healing. Sometimes given in combination with other pain relieving drugs (such as aspirin or acetaminophen).

Diazepam is also used for spasticity caused by upper motor neuron disorders (eg, cerebral palsy, paraplegia); athetosis; stiff-man syndrome.

Methocarbamol and injectable diazepam may have a beneficial effect for tetanus.

Unlabeled Use(s): Occasionally doctors may prescribe these medicines for other conditions. Cyclobenzaprine may be useful as an adjunct in managing fibrositis syndrome; orphenadrine citrate taken at bedtime may be beneficial in treating leg cramps.

Precautions:

Do not use in the following situations:

- abnormal heartbeats
- allergy to the drug
- allergy to meprobamate (carisoprodol only)
- anemia (metaxolone only)
- bladder neck obstruction (orphenadrine only)
- congestive heart failure (CHF)
- gastrointestinal obstruction (orphenadrine only)
- hyperthyroidism (overactive thyroid)
- MAOI use
- myasthenia gravis (orphenadrine only)
- peptic ulcer (orphenadrine only)
- porphyria
- prostate enlargement (orphenadrine only)

Use with caution in the following situations:

- addiction-prone individuals
- epilepsy
- glaucoma (increased intraocular pressure)
- kidney disease
- liver disease
- long-term use
- urine retention

Pregnancy: Adequate studies have not been done in pregnant women, or animal studies may have shown a risk to the fetus. Use only if clearly needed and potential benefits outweigh the possible hazards to the fetus.

Diazepam – Studies have shown a potential adverse effect on the fetus. Use only if clearly needed and potential benefits outweigh the possible risks.

Breastfeeding: Carisoprodol appears in breast milk. It is not known if the other skeletal muscle relaxants appear in breast milk. Consult your doctor before you begin breastfeeding.

Children: Use in children is generally not recommended. Usage may vary. Consult your doctor.

Elderly: In elderly and debilitated patients, it is recommended that dosage of diazepam be limited to the smallest effective amount to guard against development of incoordination and sedation.

Lab tests may be required to monitor therapy. Be sure to keep appointments. Tests may include: Urinalysis, blood counts, liver and kidney function tests.

Tartrazine: Some of these products may contain the dye tartrazine (FD&C Yellow No. 5) which can cause allergic reactions in certain individuals. Check package label when available or consult your doctor or pharmacist.

Sulfites: Some of these products contain sulfite preservatives which can cause allergic reactions in certain individuals (eg, asthmatics). Check package label when available or consult your doctor or pharmacist.

Drug Interactions:

Tell your doctor or pharmacist if you are taking or if you are planning to take any over-the-counter or prescription medications or dietary supplements while taking this medicine. Doses of one or both drugs may need to be modified or a different drug may need to be prescribed. The following drugs and drug classes interact with this medicine.

alcohol
anticholinergic drugs (eg, atropine)
barbiturates (eg, phenobarbital)
narcotic analgesics (eg, codeine)
monoamine oxidase inhibitors (eg, phenylzine)
phenothiazines (eg, promethazine)
propoxyphene (eg, *Darvon)*

orphenadrine citrate only:

amantadine (eg, *Symadine)*
haloperidol (eg, *Haldol)*

Consider all drug interactions reported for benzodiazepines (see the Antianxiety Agents-Benzodiazepines monograph in this chapter) when using diazepam as a muscle relaxant.

Side Effects:

Every drug is capable of producing side effects. Many patients experience no, or minor, side effects. The frequency and severity of side effects depend on many factors including dose, duration of therapy and individual susceptibility. Possible side effects include:

Because of cyclobenzaprine's similarity to tricyclic antidepressants (TCAs), consider all side effects for TCAs listed in the monograph in this chapter.

Allergic Reactions: Rash; itching; redness; hives; asthma attack; eye discomfort; breathing problems; fever.

Digestive Tract: Stomach upset; constipation; indigestion; nausea; vomiting.

Nervous System: Tremor; dizziness; drowsiness; headache; nervousness; depression; fatigue; sleeplessness; confusion; weakness; slurred speech; irritability; incoordination; paralysis.

Circulatory System: Changes in heartbeat; lightheadedness after standing quickly from a sitting or lying position; fainting; abnormal heartbeat; pounding in the chest; heart attack; low blood pressure.

Skin: Yellowing of skin or eyes; unusual bleeding or bruising; flushing; hives; rash.

Other: Stuffy nose; sore throat; fever; balance problems; discolored urine; blurred vision; dry mouth; anemia; hiccups; general body discomfort; overstimulation; double vision; rapid eye movement; hallucinations; decreased urination; loss of bladder control; discoloration of urine; temporary vision loss; pupil dilation; increased tension in eyes; sloughing, pain or inflammation at injection site; taste changes.

Guidelines for Use:

- Use exactly as prescribed.
- May cause stomach upset. Take with food.
- If a dose is missed, take it as soon as possible. If several hours have passed or if it is nearing time for the next dose, do not double the dose in order to "catch up" (unless advised to do so by your doctor). If more than one dose is missed or it is necessary to establish a new dosage schedule, contact your doctor or pharmacist.
- May cause dry mouth, difficult urination, constipation, headache or stomach upset. Notify your doctor if these effects persist, or if skin rash or itching, yellowing of skin or eyes, fever, nasal congestion, rapid heart rate, palpitations or confusion occurs.
- *Orthostatic hypotension* — Dizziness or lightheadedness may occur if you stand up too fast from a lying or sitting position. If this occurs, get up slowly and avoid sudden changes in posture.
- *Chlorzoxazone* may discolor urine orange or purple-red.
- *Methocarbamol* may darken urine to brown, black or green.
- These drugs make an injury temporarily feel better. Do not push your recovery. Lifting or exercising too soon may further damage muscles.
- Muscle relaxants are related to tranquilizers. With the exception of diazepam, they are not considered to be addictive. They should not be used to treat other general body pain.
- May cause drowsiness, dizziness or lightheadedness. Use caution when driving or performing other tasks requiring alertness, coordination or physical dexterity.
- Avoid alcohol or other drugs that cause drowsiness during treatment with skeletal muscle relaxants.
- Do not use a larger dose or use more often than prescribed.
- Store at room temperature.

If you have any questions, consult your doctor, pharmacist, or health care provider.

SKELETAL MUSCLE RELAXANT COMBINATIONS

	Generic Name *Brand Name Examples*	Supplied As	Generic Available
Rx	**Methocarbamol w/ASA**		
	Robaxisal	**Tablets**: 400 mg methocarbamol and 325 mg aspirin	Yes
	Carisoprodol Compound		
Rx	*Sodol Compound, Soma Compound*	**Tablets**: 200 mg carisoprodol and 325 mg aspirin	Yes
c-III	*Soma Compound w/Codeine*	**Tablets**: 200 mg carisoprodol, 325 mg aspirin and 16 mg codeine phosphate	No
Rx	**Chlorzoxazone w/APAP**		
	Flexaphen	**Capsules**: 250 mg chlorzoxazone and 300 mg acetaminophen	No
Rx	**Orphenadrine Citrate w/ASA**		
	Norgesic	**Tablets**: 25 mg orphenadrine citrate, 385 mg aspirin and 30 mg caffeine	No
	Norgesic Forte	**Tablets**: 50 mg orphenadrine citrate, 770 mg aspirin and 60 mg caffeine	No

Type of Drug:

Skeletal muscle relaxant combinations.

Uses:

As adjuncts to rest, physical therapy and other measures for relief of discomfort associated with acute, painful musculoskeletal conditions. The other combinations are classified as "probably effective" for this indication. Components of these combinations include:

Muscle relaxants: Methocarbamol; chlorzoxazone; carisoprodol; orphenadrine citrate.

Analgesics: Acetaminophen; aspirin; codeine.

Caffeine used as a CNS stimulant, also has minor analgesic activity. It increases the pain relieving effects and helps the medication begin working faster.

See the corresponding monographs for more information on these components.

Guidelines for Use:

- Use exactly as prescribed.
- If stomach upset occurs, take with food.
- If a dose is missed, take it as soon as possible. If several hours have passed or if it is nearing time for the next dose, do not double the dose in order to "catch up" (unless advised to do so by your doctor). If more than one dose is missed or it is necessary to establish a new dosage schedule, contact your doctor or pharmacist.
- May cause dry mouth, difficult urination, constipation, headache or stomach upset. Notify your doctor if these effects persist, or if skin rash or itching, yellowing of skin or eyes, fever, nasal congestion, rapid heart rate, pounding in the chest or confusion occurs.
- *Orthostatic hypotension* — Dizziness or lightheadedness may occur if you stand up too fast from a sitting or lying position. If this occurs, get up slowly and avoid sudden changes in posture.
- *Chlorzoxazone* may discolor urine orange or purple-red.
- *Methocarbamol* may darken urine to brown, black or green.
- These drugs make an injury temporarily feel better. Do not push your recovery. Lifting or exercising too soon may further damage muscles.
- Muscle relaxants are related to tranquilizers. They are not considered to be addictive. They should not be used to treat other general body pain.
- May cause drowsiness, dizziness or lightheadedness. Use caution when driving or performing other tasks requiring alertness, coordination or physical dexterity.
- Avoid alcohol or other drugs that cause drowsiness during treatment with these drugs.
- Do not use a larger dose or use more often than prescribed.
- Store at room temperature.

If you have any questions, consult your doctor, pharmacist, or health care provider.

	Generic Name *Brand Name Examples*	Supplied As	Generic Available
Rx	**Benztropine Mesylate**[1]		
	Cogentin	**Tablets:** 0.5 mg, 1 mg, 2 mg	No
Rx	**Biperiden**[1]		
	Akineton	**Tablets:** 2 mg	No
	Diphenhydramine[1]		
otc	*Banophen, Benadryl, Benadryl Allergy Kapseals, Benadryl Dye Free Allergy Liqui Gels*	**Capsules:** 25 mg, 50 mg	Yes
Rx	*Banophen, Benadryl, Benadryl Kapseals, Genahist*	**Capsules:** 25 mg, 50 mg	Yes
otc	*AllerMax, Banophen, Benadryl Allergy, Benadryl 25, Diphenhist Captabs, Dormarex 2*	**Tablets:** 25 mg, 50 mg	Yes
Rx	*Genahist*	**Tablets:** 25 mg	Yes
Rx	*Diphenhydramine HCl*	**Tablets:** 50 mg	Yes
otc	*Benadryl Allergy*	**Tablets, chewable:** 12.5 mg	No
otc	*Banophen*[2], *Belix*[2,3], *Diphenhist, Genahist*[2], *Nidryl*[2], *Phendry*[2], *Siladryl*[2]	**Elixir:** 12.5 mg/tsp	Yes
Rx	*Benadryl*[2]	**Elixir:** 12.5 mg/tsp	Yes
otc	*Benadryl Allergy, Benadryl Dye Free, Scot-Tussin Allergy*	**Liquid:** 6.25 mg/tsp, 12.5 mg/tsp	No
otc	*Benylin Cough*[2], *Diphen Cough*	**Syrup:** 12.5 mg/tsp	Yes
Rx	*Hydramyn*[2], *Tusstat*[2]	**Syrup:** 12.5 mg/tsp	Yes
Rx	**Ethopropazine**		
	Parsidol	**Tablets:** 10 mg, 50 mg	No
Rx	**Procyclidine**		
	Kemadrin	**Tablets:** 5 mg	No

	Generic Name *Brand Name Examples*	Supplied As	Generic Available
Rx	**Trihexyphenidyl HCl**		
	Artane, Trihexy-2, Trihexy-4	**Tablets:** 2 mg, 5 mg	Yes
	Artane Sequels	**Capsules, sustained release:** 5 mg	No
	Artane[2]	**Elixir:** 2 mg/tsp	No

[1] Some of these products are also available as an injection.
[2] Contains alcohol.
[3] Sugar free.

Type of Drug:

Antiparkinson agents.

How the Drug Works:

Parkinsonism is a neurological disease with a variety of origins characterized by tremor, rigidity, and disorders of posture and equilibrium. The onset is slow and progressive with symptoms advancing over months to years.

The group of drugs known as "anticholinergic agents" can reduce the frequency and severity of the symptoms of parkinsonism by restoring the chemical imbalance that causes Parkinson disease. The effectiveness of anticholinergics for parkinsonism is not dependent on the origin of the symptoms. These agents are typically used for milder cases of parkinsonism.

Uses:

To reduce the frequency and severity of the symptoms of parkinsonism and to control drug-induced parkinsonism-like disorders. Used alone or with other antiparkinson agents. Anticholineric agents do *not* cure the causes of these symptoms.

Precautions:

Do not use in the following situations:

allergy to anticholinergic agents
children younger than 3 years of age
glaucoma
myasthenia gravis
prostate enlargement
stomach or intestinal disorders (eg, obstruction, ulcers)
urinary bladder obstruction

Use with caution in the following situations:

constipation
digestive tract obstruction
elderly (older than 60 years of age)
heat intolerance
heart rate, irregular or rapid
high blood pressure
kidney disease
liver disease
low blood pressure
pounding sensation in chest
psychiatric disorder
urinary difficulties

Pregnancy: Adequate studies have not been done in pregnant women. Use only if clearly needed and potential benefits outweigh the possible hazards to the fetus.

Breastfeeding: Anticholinergic agents appear in breast milk and may reduce milk production. Consult your doctor before you begin breastfeeding.

Children: Do not use benztropine in children younger than 3 years old. Safety and effectiveness in older children have not been established.

Elderly: Geriatric patients, particularly over 60, frequently develop increased sensitivity to anticholinergic drugs and require strict dosage monitoring. Use with caution. Mental confusion and disorientation, agitation, hallucinations and psychotic-like symptoms may develop. Administer carefully to elderly patients with hardening of the arteries because side effects may be more severe.

Drug Interactions:

Tell your doctor or pharmacist if you are taking or if you are planning to take any over-the-counter or prescription medications or dietary supplements with anticholinergic agents. Doses of one or both drugs may need to be modified or a different drug may need to be prescribed. The following drugs and drug classes interact with anticholinergic agents.

antihistamines (eg, diphenhydramine)
chlorpromazine (eg, *Thorazine)*
digoxin (eg, *Lanoxin)*
haloperidol (eg, *Haldol)*
levodopa (eg, *Larodopa)*
narcotic pain relievers (eg, *Percodan)*
phenothiazines (eg, promethazine)
quinidine (eg, *Cin-Quin)*
tricyclic antidepressants (eg, amitriptyline)

Side Effects:

Every drug is capable of producing side effects. Many anticholinergic users experience no, or minor, side effects. The frequency and severity of side effects depend on many factors including dose, duration of therapy and individual susceptibility. Possible side effects include:

Possible Side Effects Specific to Ethopropazine – Seizures; brain wave changes, blood disorders; hormone disorders; yellow discoloration of skin and eyes (jaundice); and hallucinations.

Digestive Tract: Nausea; vomiting; stomach pain; constipation.

Nervous System: Disorientation; confusion; memory loss; hallucinations; lightheadedness; dizziness; weakness; agitation; nervousness; paranoia; delusions; delirium; excessive elation; excitement; depression.

Circulatory System: Rapid heart rate; pounding of chest (palpitations); low blood pressure; lightheadedness and dizziness upon rising quickly from a lying position.

Skin: Rash; flushing; decreased sweating; hives.

Eyes or Ocular: Blurred vision; double vision; widened pupils; visual disturbances; glaucoma.

Other: Difficulty urinating; painful urination; muscle weakness; cramping; dry mouth; fever; numbness of fingers; difficulty achieving or maintaining erection; blood disorders (orphenadrine citrate); swollen glands.

Guidelines for Use:

- May cause drowsiness, dizziness, or blurred vision. Use caution when driving or performing other tasks requiring alertness.
- Avoid alcohol and other drugs that cause drowsiness when using anticholinergic agents.
- Stomach upset may occur. Take with food.
- Sucking on hard candy, drinking fluids, or maintaining good dental hygiene can relieve the dry mouth that can result from taking any of the anticholinergic agents.
- Difficult urination and constipation can occur. Use "stool softeners" if necessary. Notify your doctor if either difficult urination or constipation persist.
- Notify your doctor if a rapid heartbeat, pounding sensation in chest, confusion, eye pain, or rash occurs.
- Anticholinergic agents can reduce the ability to sweat, an important function by which overheating is prevented. Avoid excess sun or exercise which may cause excessive sweating.
- Elderly patients may be highly sensitive to anticholinergic drugs. Use with caution. See Precautions.

If you have any questions, consult your doctor, pharmacist, or health care provider.

	Generic Name *Brand Name Examples*	Supplied As	Generic Available
Rx	**Amantadine HCl**	**Capsules:** 100 mg	Yes
	Symmetrel	**Tablets:** 100 mg	No
	Symmetrel	**Syrup:** 50 mg/5 mL	Yes
Rx	**Bromocriptine Mesylate**		
	Parlodel SnapTabs	**Tablets:** 2.5 mg	No
	Parlodel	**Capsules:** 5 mg	No
Rx	**Carbidopa**		
	Lodosyn	**Tablets:** 25 mg	No
Rx	**Levodopa**		
	Larodopa	**Tablets:** 100 mg, 250 mg, 500 mg	No
Rx	**Carbidopa/Levodopa**		
	Sinemet 10-100, Sinemet 25-100, Sinemet 25-250	**Tablets:** 10 mg carbidopa, 100 mg levodopa; 25 mg carbidopa, 100 mg levodopa; 25 mg carbidopa, 250 mg levodopa	Yes
	Sinemet CR	**Tablets, sustained-release:** 25 mg carbidopa, 100 mg levodopa; 50 mg carbidopa, 200 mg levodopa	No

For more information, see the amantadine monograph in the Anti-infectives chapter and the bromocriptine monograph in the Miscellaneous chapter.

Type of Drug:

Antiparkinson agents.

How the Drug Works:

Parkinsonism is a neurological disease with a variety of causes characterized by tremor, rigidity, and disorders of posture and balance. The onset is slow and progressive, with symptoms advancing over months to years. Currently, there is no cure for the disease. The goal of therapy is to provide symptomatic relief and attempt to maintain the independence and mobility of the patient.

It is thought that the involuntary muscle movements (shaking) of Parkinson's disease are due to reduced amounts of the chemical transmitter dopamine in the nervous system. Levodopa is transformed by the body and the nervous system into dopamine. Carbidopa prevents levodopa from being broken down outside the nervous system. Bromocriptine stimulates dopamine receptors. The action of amantadine is not fully understood. It may increase dopamine concentrations in the nervous system or make the nervous system more sensitive to dopamine.

Uses:

To treat Parkinson's disease, which may develop spontaneously or follow injury to the nervous system. Amantadine is also used for drug-induced extrapyramidal reactions (symptoms of Parkinson's disease caused by medication).

Unlabeled Use(s): Occasionally doctors may prescribe levodopa for herpes zoster (shingles) and restless legs syndrome.

Precautions:

Do not use in the following situations:

- allergy to ergot alkaloids (bromocriptine only)
- allergy to these drugs or any of their ingredients
- angle-closure (narrow angle) glaucoma, untreated (amantadine, levodopa only)
- high blood pressure, uncontrolled (bromocriptine only)
- melanoma, history of (levodopa only)
- monoamine oxidase inhibitor (MAOI) therapy, concurrent or within the previous 14 days (carbidopa/levodopa only)
- skin cancer, possibility of (levodopa only)

Use with caution in the following situations:

- bronchial asthma (levodopa only)
- depression
- endocrine gland disease (levodopa only)
- glaucoma, chronic wide-angle (levodopa only)
- heart attack, history of (bromocriptine, levodopa only)
- heart disease, history of
- irregular heartbeat (bromocriptine, levodopa only)
- kidney disease
- liver disease
- lung disease, severe (levodopa only)
- orthostatic hypotension (drop in blood pressure when standing up)
- peptic ulcer, history of (levodopa only)
- peripheral edema, history of
- postpartum period (bromocriptine only)
- psychiatric disorders, history of
- psychoses
- recurrent eczema, history of (amantadine only)
- seizures, history of
- substance abuse, history of

Carbidopa: Carbidopa had no antiparkinsonian effect when given alone. It is always used in combination with levodopa or carbidopa/levodopa products.

Neuroleptic malignant-like syndrome (NMS): NMS, including muscular rigidity, involuntary movements, altered consciousness, elevated body temperature, fast heartbeat, changes in blood pressure, mental changes, and increased serum enzymes, has been reported when antiparkinson agents were stopped suddenly. Do not abruptly reduce the dosage or discontinue use of amantadine or levodopa without consulting your doctor.

"On-off" phenomenon: Some patients who initially respond to levodopa therapy may develop the "on-off" phenomenon, a condition in which patients suddenly swing between an improved condition to a worsened condition. This effect may occur within minutes or hours and is asso-

ciated with long-term levodopa therapy. Other patients may experience a deteriorating response. These conditions can be managed. Contact your doctor.

Pregnancy: There are no adequate and well-controlled studies in pregnant women. Use only if clearly needed and potential benefits to the mother outweigh the possible hazards to the fetus.

Breastfeeding: Use of amantadine, bromocriptine, and levodopa while breastfeeding is not recommended. It is not known if carbidopa appears in breast milk. Consult your doctor before you begin breastfeeding.

Children: Safety and effectiveness of amantadine in children younger than 1 year of age have not been established. Safety and effectiveness of bromocriptine in children younger than 15 years of age have not been established. Safety and effectiveness of carbidopa/levodopa in children younger than 18 years of age have not been established.

Elderly: Elderly patients may require less amantadine or carbidopa/levodopa than younger patients.

Lab tests will be required to monitor therapy. Tests may include blood counts, eye tests, pituitary tests, blood pressure monitoring, and liver, kidney, and heart function tests.

Drug Interactions:

Tell your doctor or pharmacist if you are taking or planning to take any over-the-counter or prescription medications or dietary supplements with dopaminergic agents. Doses of one or both drugs may need to be modified or a different drug may need to be prescribed. The following drugs and drug classes interact with dopaminergic agents:

Amantadine —

anticholinergics (eg, belladonna)
triamterene/hydrochlorothiazide (eg, *Dyazide*)

Bromocriptine —

antihypertensives (eg, diltiazem)
ergot alkaloids (eg, ergotamine)
erythromycin (eg, *Ilosone*)

Carbidopa/levodopa —

antihypertensives (eg, diltiazem)
hydantoins (eg, phenytoin)
iron salts (eg, ferrous fumarate)
phenelzine (*Nardil*)
pyridoxine (vitamin B_6)
tranylcypromine (*Parnate*)

Side Effects:

Every drug is capable of producing side effects. Many dopaminergic users experience no, or minor, side effects. The frequency and severity of side effects depend on many factors including dose, duration of therapy, and individual susceptibility. Possible side effects include:

Digestive Tract: Nausea; vomiting; diarrhea; constipation; gas; appetite loss; stomach pain or cramps; gastrointestinal bleeding; indigestion; heartburn.

Nervous System: Uncontrolled movement (twitching) of face, eyelids, mouth, hands, or legs; abnormally slow movement; mood swings; mental changes; anxiety; fatigue; euphoria (exaggerated sense of well-being); delusions; hallucinations; abnormal dreams; confusion; weakness; agitation; nervousness; dizziness; fainting; orthostatic hypotension (dizziness or lightheadedness when rising quickly from a sitting or lying position); headache; depression; increased tremor; incoordination; sleeplessness; faintness; "on-off" phenomenon; falling; dementia; lightheadedness; irritability; drowsiness; vertigo (feeling of whirling motion).

Circulatory System: Palpitations (pounding in the chest); irregular heartbeat; chest pain; changes in blood pressure.

Skin: Flushing; rash; increased sweating; hives; itching; hair loss; abnormal skin sensations.

Other: Difficult urination; urinary incontinence; difficulty swallowing; numbness; increased salivation; dry mouth or nose; grinding of the teeth; difficulty opening mouth; taste changes; bitter taste; burning tongue; general body discomfort; hot flashes; double vision; blurred vision; dilated pupils; weight changes; dark sweat, saliva, or urine; abnormal blood counts; abnormal liver, kidney, and heart function tests; back, leg, or shoulder pain; abnormal or difficult breathing; suicidal ideation; vein inflammation; visual disturbances; shortness of breath; fluid retention; frequent urination; persistent erection of the penis, accompanied by pain and tenderness; urinary retention; nasal congestion; throat pain; intestinal ulcer; cough; hoarseness; sense of stimulation; hiccups.

Guidelines for Use:

- Dosage is individualized.
- Be patient. Take this drug routinely as directed. It may take several weeks to a few months to notice benefit from use because the dose is carefully adjusted over time.
- May upset stomach. Take with food at regular intervals.
- Do not change the dose or stop taking unless advised by your doctor. Suddenly stopping treatment may induce neuroleptic malignant-like syndrome (ie, muscle stiffness, involuntary movement, altered consciousness, elevated body temperature, fast heartbeat, changes in blood pressure, mental changes).
- Do not crush or chew sustained-release products.
- *Sustained-release carbidopa/levodopa* — The onset of effect of the first morning dose may be delayed for up to 1 hour. Notify your doctor if this delayed response poses a problem.
- Avoid alcohol during therapy. It may increase the potential for nervous system effects such as dizziness, confusion, lightheadedness, or dizziness when standing up.
- Discontinue MAOIs ≤ 14 days before starting levodopa or carbidopa/levodopa therapy.
- *Diabetic patients* — Levodopa may interfere with urine tests for sugar or ketones. Report any abnormal results to your doctor before adjusting dosage of antidiabetic medications.
- Gradually increase physical activity as symptoms of Parkinson's disease improve.
- Notify your doctor if you experience uncontrollable movements of the face, eyelids, mouth, tongue, neck, arms, hands, or legs; mood or mental changes; difficult urination; severe or persistent nausea and vomiting; swelling of the arms or legs; or shortness of breath.
- Do not get up quickly after sitting or lying down. Notify your doctor if you experience dizziness or lightheadedness when you rise from a sitting or lying position.
- May cause dizziness, drowsiness, or blurred vision. Use with caution while driving or performing other tasks requiring alertness, coordination, and physical dexterity.
- Levodopa may darken urine, saliva, or sweat. This is not harmful.
- Do not take levodopa along with vitamins containing vitamin B_6 (pyridoxine). This vitamin can reduce drug benefits. Carbidopa-containing products may be taken with vitamin B_6.
- Using carbidopa together with levodopa may allow a smaller dose of levodopa to be used and reduce its side effects (eg, nausea, vomiting).
- Lab tests will be required to monitor therapy. Be sure to keep appointments.
- Store at controlled room temperature (59° to 86°F). Store bromocriptine below 77°F.

If you have any questions, consult your doctor, pharmacist, or health care provider.

Generic Name *Brand Name Example*	Supplied As	Generic Available
Rx **Pramipexole Dihydrochloride**		
Mirapex	**Tablets:** 0.125 mg, 0.25 mg, 1 mg, 1.5 mg	No

Type of Drug:

Antiparkinson agent.

How the Drug Works:

Parkinsonism is a neurological disease with a variety of origins characterized by tremor, rigidity and disorders of posture and balance. The onset is slow and progressive with symptoms advancing over months to years. There is no cure for the disease. The goal of therapy is to provide relief from the symptoms, and to attempt to maintain the independence and mobility of the patient.

It is thought that the involuntary muscle movements (shaking) of Parkinson disease are caused by reduced amounts of dopamine in the nervous system. Pramipexole may exert its effects by stimulating the dopamine receptors in the nervous system.

Uses:

To manage or treat signs and symptoms of Parkinson disease. May be used with levodopa in the later stages of the disease.

Precautions:

Do not use in the following situations: Allergy to pramipexole

Use with caution in the following situations:

hallucinations
low blood pressure
kidney disease
movement difficulty
retinal disease (of the eye)

Pregnancy: Adequate studies have not been done in pregnant women. Use only if clearly needed and potential benefits outweigh the possible hazards to the fetus.

Breastfeeding: It is not known if pramipexole appears in breast milk. Consult your doctor before you begin breastfeeding.

Children: Safety and effectiveness have not been established.

Elderly: Elderly patients have a greater tendency to develop hallucinations.

Drug Interactions:

Tell your doctor or pharmacist if you are taking or if you are planning to take any over-the-counter or prescription medications or dietary supplements with pramipexole dihydrochloride. Doses of one or both drugs may need to be modified or a different drug may need to be prescribed. The following drugs and drug classes interact with pramipexole.

butyrophenones (eg, haloperidol)
cimetidine (eg, *Tagamet)*
diltiazem(eg, *Cardizem)*
metoclopramide (eg, *Reglan)*
phenothiazines (eg, chlorpromazine)
quinidine (eg, *Quinora)*
quinine (eg, quinine sulfate)
ranitidine (eg, *Zantac)*
thioxanthenes (eg, chlorprothixene)
triamterene (*Dyrenium)*
verapamil (eg, *Calan)*

Side Effects:

Every drug is capable of producing side effects. Many pramipexole users experience no, or minor, side effects. The frequency and severity of side effects depend on many factors including dose, duration of therapy and individual susceptibility. Possible side effects include:

Digestive Tract – Nausea; constipation; appetite loss; difficulty swallowing; dry mouth; gas; diarrhea; vomiting; indigestion; stomach pain.

Nervous System – Dizziness; drowsiness; sleeplessness; hallucinations; confusion; amnesia; reduced skin sensations; muscle tone abnormalities; inability to sit still; thinking abnormalities; decreased sex drive; muscle twitches; movement disorders; dream abnormalities; walking abnormalities; stiffness; paranoid reaction; delusions; sleep disorders; headache; nervousness; leg cramps; tremor.

Circulatory System – Low blood pressure.

Respiratory System – Difficulty breathing; sinus infection; runny nose/ congestion; pneumonia.

Urinary and Reproductive Tract – Impotence; increased urination; urinary tract infection; inability to control urination.

Skin – Skin disorders; rash.

Senses – Vision abnormalities; double vision; abnormal taste.

Other – Weakness; swelling; general body discomfort; fever; decreased weight; accidental injury; chest pain; joint pain; muscle weakness; pain; back pain; fainting; depression; sore throat; sweating; flushing; flu syndrome; increased saliva; tooth disease; increased cough; allergic reaction; voice alteration.

Guidelines for Use:

- Take pramipexole only as directed by your doctor.
- Taking pramipexole with food may reduce nausea.
- Dosage will be started low and gradually increased to achieve maximum effect. Do not change dose sooner than recommended.
- Do not change the dose or discontinue unless advised to do so by your doctor.
- It is recommended that pramipexole be discontinued gradually over a period of a week.
- Hallucinations may occur, especially in the elderly.
- Dizziness or lightheadedness may occur if you stand up too fast from a lying or sitting position. If this occurs, get up slowly and avoid sudden changes in posture.
- Kidney disease patients may need dosage adjustments.
- This medication may cause drowsiness or dizziness. Use caution while driving or performing other tasks requiring mental alertness, coordination or physical dexterity.
- Caution should be used when taking other CNS depressants (eg, alcohol, sedatives) in combination with pramipexole.
- Inform your doctor if you are pregnant, become pregnant, are planning to become pregnant or if you are breastfeeding.
- Store at controlled room temperature (59° to 86° F) and protect from light.

If you have any questions, consult your doctor, pharmacist, or health care provider.

	Generic Name *Brand Name Examples*	Supplied As	Generic Available
Rx	**Ropinirole HCl**		
	Requip	**Tablets:** 0.25 mg, 0.5 mg, 1 mg, 2 mg, 5 mg	No

Type of Drug:

Antiparkinson agent.

How the Drug Works:

Parkinsonism is a neurological disease with a variety of origins characterized by tremor, rigidity and disorders of posture and balance. The onset is slow and progressive with symptoms advancing over months to years. There is no cure for the disease. The goal of therapy is to provide relief from the symptoms, and to attempt to maintain the independence and mobility of the patient.

It is thought that the involuntary muscle movements (shaking) of Parkinson disease are caused by reduced amounts of dopamine in the nervous system. Ropinirole may exert its effects by stimulating the dopamine receptors in the nervous system.

Uses:

To treat signs and symptoms of Parkinson disease. May be used with levodopa in the later stages of the disease.

Precautions:

Do not use in the following situations: Allergy to ropinirole.

Use with caution in the following situations:

- fainting
- hallucinations
- kidney impairment, severe
- liver impairment, severe
- low blood pressure
- pulmonary (lung) disease
- movement difficulty
- neuroleptic malignant syndrome
- retinal disease (of the eye)

Pregnancy: Adequate studies have not been done in pregnant women. Use only if clearly needed and potential benefits outweigh the possible hazards to the fetus.

Breastfeeding: It is not known if ropinirole appears in breast milk. Consult your doctor before you begin breastfeeding.

Children: Safety and effectiveness have not been established.

Elderly: Elderly patients have a greater tendency to develop hallucinations.

Drug Interactions:

Tell your doctor or pharmacist if you are taking or if you are planning to take any over-the-counter or prescription medications or dietary supplements with ropinirole. Doses of one or both drugs may need to be modified or a different drug may need to be prescribed. The following drugs and drug classes interact with ropinirole:

- butyrophenones (haloperidol)
- cipofloxacin (eg, *Cipro*)
- estrogens (eg, *Premarin*)
- L-dopa (*Sinemet*)
- metoclopramide (eg, *Reglan*)
- phenothiazines (eg, chlorpromazine)
- thioxanthenes (chlorprothixene)

Side Effects:

Every drug is capable of producing side effects. Many ropinirole users experience no, or minor, side effects. The frequency and severity of side effects depend on many factors including dose, duration of therapy and individual susceptibility. Possible side effects include:

Digestive Tract: Constipation; stomach pain; appetite loss; indigestion; gas; nausea; vomiting.

Nervous System: Flushing; dry mouth; increased sweating; dizziness; hyperactivity; decreased sensitivity to touch; whirling feeling; inability to sleep; anxiety; nervousness.

Circulatory System: High blood pressure; low blood pressure; orthostatic symptoms (dizziness when rising quickly); fainting; premature heart beat; pounding in the chest; fast heart beat; slow heart beat; high blood sugar.

Respiratory System: Bronchitis; difficulty breathing; sore throat; sinus infection; cough.

Skin: Abnormal sensations; rash.

Other: Weakness; chest pain; fluid accumulation in the lower extremities; fatigue; feeling poorly; pain; headache; increased alkaline phosphatase; amnesia; impaired concentration; confusion; hallucination; drowsiness; yawning; impotence; viral infection; urinary tract infection; cold feet and hands; abnormal vision; double vision; night blindness; joint pain; tremor; back pain; difficulty moving; aggravated Parkinsonism; depression; falls; muscle pain; leg cramps; arthritis; weight loss; muscle spasm; joint degeneration; abnormal dreams; muscular deformation; increased salivation; gout; gum inflammation; blood in the urine; rigidity; inability to control urine; pus in the urine; ringing in the ears.

Guidelines for Use:

- Take ropinirole only as directed by your doctor (three times daily).
- May be taken with or without food. Taking with food may reduce nausea.
- Dosage will be increased to achieve maximum effect.
- Do not discontinue or change the dose unless advised to do so by your doctor.
- Hallucinations may occur, especially in the elderly.
- Dizziness or lightheadedness may occur if you stand up too fast from a lying or sitting position. If this occurs, get up slowly and avoid sudden changes in posture.
- Caution should be used when taking other CNS depressants (eg, antidepressants) or alcohol.
- This medication may cause drowsiness or dizziness. Use caution while driving or performing other tasks requiring mental alertness, coordination or physical dexterity.
- Inform your doctor if you are pregnant, become pregnant, are planning to become pregnant or if you are breastfeeding.
- Store at controlled room temperature (59° to 77°F) and protect from light.

If you have any questions, consult your doctor, pharmacist, or health care provider.

	Generic Name *Brand Name Example*	Supplied As	Generic Available
Rx	**Pergolide Mesylate**		
	Permax	**Tablets:** 0.05 mg, 0.25 mg, 1 mg	No

Type of Drug:

Antiparkinson agent.

How the Drug Works:

Parkinsonism is a neurological disease characterized by tremor, rigidity, and disorders of posture and equilibrium. It has multiple causes. The onset is slow and progressive with symptoms advancing over months to years.

It is thought that the involuntary muscle movements (shaking) of Parkinson disease are due to reduced amounts of the chemical dopamine in the central nervous system (brain). Pergolide may exert its effects by directly stimulating the dopamine receptors in the brain.

Uses:

To manage the signs and symptoms of Parkinson's disease. Used along with levodopa and carbidopa.

For complete information on levodopa and carbidopa as antiparkinson agents, see the Antiparkinson-Dopaminergic Agents monograph in this chapter.

Precautions:

Do not use in the following situations: Allergy to pergolide or other ergot derivatives.

Use with caution in the following situations:

abnormal heart rhythms
confusion, recent
hallucinations, recent
hypotension (low blood pressure)
movement disorders

Neuroleptic Malignant-like Syndrome (NMS): NMS, including muscular rigidity, elevated body temperature, mental changes, and increased serum enzymes, has been reported when antiparkinson agents were stopped suddenly. Therefore, do not reduce the dosage of pergolide abruptly or discontinue it without consulting your doctor.

Pregnancy: There are no adequate and well-controlled studies in pregnant women. Use during pregnancy only if clearly needed.

Breastfeeding: It is not known if pergolide appears in breast milk. Consult your doctor before you begin breastfeeding.

Children: Safety and effectiveness have not been established.

Drug Interactions:

Tell your doctor or pharmacist if you are taking or planning to take any over-the-counter or prescription medications or dietary supplements with pergolide mesylate. Doses of one or both drugs may need to be modified or a different drug may need to be prescribed. The following drugs and drug classes interact with pergolide mesylate:

butyrophenones (eg, haloperidol)
metoclopramide (eg, *Reglan)*
phenothiazines (eg, chlorpromazine)
thioxanthines (eg, thiothixene)

Side Effects:

Every drug is capable of producing side effects. Many pergolide users experience no, or minor, side effects. The frequency and severity of side effects depend on many factors including dose, duration of therapy, and individual susceptibility. Possible side effects include:

Digestive Tract: Nausea; vomiting; constipation; diarrhea; indigestion; stomach pain; appetite loss; difficulty swallowing.

Nervous System: Hallucinations; difficult or abnormal movement; restlessness; twitching; confusion; dizziness; drowsiness; fainting; sleeplessness; anxiety; tremor; depression; abnormal dreams; personality changes; headache; weakness; incoordination; difficulty walking.

Circulatory System: High or low blood pressure; orthostatic hypotension (dizziness or lightheadedness when arising from a seated or lying position); palpitations (pounding in the chest); irregular heartbeat; heart attack.

Respiratory System: Runny nose; difficulty breathing.

Skin: Rash; sweating; abnormal skin sensations.

Other: Dry mouth; taste changes; general body pain; joint, muscle, or nerve pain; abnormal vision; double vision; frequent urination; urinary tract infections; blood in urine; edema (fluid retention); back, neck, and chest pain; flu-like symptoms; nosebleed; hiccups; weight gain; chills; difficulty speaking; anemia.

Guidelines for Use:

- Dosage will be individualized.
- Do not change the dose or stop taking this medicine unless advised to do so by your doctor.
- If a dose is missed, take it as soon as possible. If several hours have passed or it is nearing time for the next dose, do not double the dose to catch up, unless advised by your doctor. If more than one dose is missed or it is necessary to establish a new dosage schedule, contact your doctor or pharmacist.
- Notify your doctor if you experience confusion, hallucinations, pounding in the chest, irregular heart rate, or difficulty in movement.
- *Orthostatic hypotension* — Dizziness or lightheadedness may occur when arising quickly from a seated or lying position. Avoid sudden changes in posture while taking pergolide.
- May cause drowsiness. Use caution while driving or performing other tasks requiring alertness, coordination, or physical dexterity.
- Inform your doctor if you are pregnant, become pregnant, are planning to become pregnant, or if you are breastfeeding.
- Store at controlled room temperature (59° to 86°F).

If you have any questions, consult your doctor, pharmacist, or health care provider.

	Generic Name *Brand Name Examples*	Supplied As	Generic Available
Rx	**Selegiline HCl**		
	Eldepryl	**Capsules:** 5 mg	No
	Carbex	**Tablets:** 5 mg	Yes

Type of Drug:

Monoamine oxidase type B inhibitor, (MAOI); drug used to treat Parkinson's disease.

How the Drug Works:

Selegiline prolongs the anti-Parkinson activity of levodopa and interferes with normal enzyme activities.

Uses:

To treat Parkinson disease in conjunction with levodopa/carbidopa in patients whose response to levodopa/carbidopa is deteriorating. There is no evidence that it has any benefit without the concurrent use of levodopa.

Tyramine-containing foods: Avoid foods which can interact with monoamine oxidase inhibitors (isocarboxazid, phenelzine, tranylcypromine).

Tyramine-Containing Foods[1]
Cheese/Dairy Products: American, processed; blue; Boursault; brick, natural; Brie; Camembert; cheddar; Emmenthaler; Gruyere; mozzarella; Parmesan; Romano; Roquefort; Stilton; sour cream; yogurt.
Meat/Fish: Beef or chicken liver, other meats, fish (unrefrigerated, fermented); meats prepared with tenderizer; fermented sausages (bologna, pepperoni, salami, summer sausage); game meat; caviar; dried fish (especially salted herring); herring (pickled or spoiled).
Alcoholic Beverages (undistilled): Beer and ale (imports); red wine (especially Chianti); sherry.
Fruit/Vegetables: Avocado (especially overripe); yeast extracts (eg, marmite); bananas; figs, canned (overripe); raisins; soy sauce.
Other Foods: Fava beans (overripe); chocolate; caffeine (eg, coffee, tea, colas).

[1] Tyramine contents are not predictable and may vary. The amounts of tyramine are estimated from low to very high.

Precautions:

Do not use in the following situations:

allergy to selegiline
meperidine (eg, *Demerol*) use, concurrent
tyramine-containing foods

Use with caution:

antidepressant (eg, amitriptyline) use, concurrent or recent
SSRI (eg, fluxetine) use, concurrent or recent

Pregnancy: There are no adequate or well-controlled studies in pregnant women. It is not known if this drug can harm the fetus or interfere with reproduction. Use only if clearly needed and if potential benefit to the mother justifies the potential risk to the fetus.

Breastfeeding: It is not known if selegiline appears in breast milk. Consult your doctor before you begin breastfeeding.

Children: Safety and effectiveness have not been established.

Drug Interactions:

Tell your doctor or pharmacist: if you are pregnant, are planning to become pregnant, or are breastfeeding; and if you are taking, will be taking, or stop taking any prescrition or nonprescription medications or dietary supplements. Dosage of levodopa may need to be decreased after you begin taking selegiline.

contraceptives, oral (eg, *Ortho-Novum*)
meperidine (eg, *Demerol*)
SSRIs (eg, fluoxetine)
sympathomimetics (eg, ephedrine)
tricyclic antidepressants (eg, amitriptyline)

Side Effects:

Every drug is capable of producing side effects. Many selegiline users experience no, or minor, side effects. The frequency and severity of side effects depend on many factors including dose, duration of therapy, and individual susceptibility. Possible side effects include:

Other: Increased or decreased urination (especially at night); difficult urination.

Digestive Tract: Nausea; vomiting; diarrhea; constipation; loss of appetite; stomach pain; heartburn; difficulty swallowing; dry mouth.

Nervous System: Weakness; confusion; anxiety; dreams and nightmares; headache; depression; affected speech; tremor; restlessness; sleeplessness; involuntary or abnormal movements; agitation; loss of balance; spasms of eyelid; hallucinations.

Circulatory System: Dizziness when arising quickly from a seated or lying position (orthostatic hypotension); changes in blood pressure; pounding of the chest (palpitations); irregular pulse; angina (chest pain); irregular heartbeats; fainting.

Respiratory System: Shortness of breath; asthma.

Skin: Increased sweating; hair loss; sensitivity to sunlight; facial hair growth; rash; bruising.

Guidelines for Use:

- Dosage is individualized.
- To avoid interference with sleep, take as a single dose with breakfast or in 2 divided doses with breakfast and lunch.
- Do not exceed the recommended daily dose of 10 mg.
- Dosage of levodopa may need to be decreased after the patient begins to take selegiline. Discuss this possibility with your doctor. Do not change the dosage unless advised to do so by your doctor.
- Immediately report any severe headaches or unusual symptoms to your doctor.
- Do not change the dose or stop taking unless advised to do so by your doctor.
- Store at controlled room temperature (59° to 86°F)

If you have any questions, consult your doctor, pharmacist, or health care provider.

	Generic Name *Brand Name Example*	Supplied As	Generic Available
Rx	**Entacapone**		
	Comtan	**Tablets, film-coated:** 200 mg	No

Type of Drug:

Antiparkinson agent; catechol-O-methyltransferase (COMT) inhibitor.

How the Drug Works:

Entacapone interferes with one of the enzymes (COMT) in the body responsible for eliminating levodopa. It is used in combination with levodopa/carbidopa (eg, *Sinemet*) to prolong the beneficial effects of levodopa in treating symptoms of Parkinson's disease. Entacapone has no antiparkinsonian effects of its own and must always be administered in combination with levodopa/carbidopa.

Uses:

Entacapone is used in combination with levodopa/carbidopa to treat patients with idiopathic Parkinson's disease who experience the signs and symptoms of end-of-dose "wearing-off" (worsening of Parkinson's symptoms between doses of levodopa/carbidopa). The effectiveness of entacapone has not been evaluated in patients with idiopathic Parkinson's disease who do not experience end-of-dose "wearing-off."

Precautions:

Do not use in the following situations: Allergy to entacapone or any of its ingredients.

Use with caution in the following situations:

dyskinesia, pre-existing
liver disease
low blood pressure

Pregnancy: There are no adequate and well-controlled studies in pregnant women. Use only if clearly needed and potential benefits outweigh the possible hazards to the fetus.

Breastfeeding: It is not known if entacapone appears in breast milk. Consult your doctor before you begin breastfeeding.

Children: Safety and effectiveness for use in children have not been established.

Drug Interactions:

Tell your doctor or pharmacist if you are taking or planning to take any over-the-counter or prescription medications or dietary supplements while taking entacapone. Doses of one or both drugs may need to be modified or a different drug may need to be prescribed. The following drugs and drug classes interact with entacapone:

ampicillin (eg, *Omnipen*)
apomorphine
bitolterol (*Tornalate*)
chloramphenicol (eg, *Chloromycetin*)
cholestyramine (eg, *Questran*)

dobutamine (*Dobutrex*)
dopamine (eg, *Intropin*)
epinephrine (eg, *Epipen*)
erythyromycin (eg, *E-mycin*)
isoetherine
isoproterenol (eg, *Isuprel*)
MAO inhibitors (eg, phenelzine)
methyldopa (eg, *Aldomet*)
norepinephrine (*Levophed*)
probenecid
rifampin (eg, *Rifadin*)

Side Effects:

Every drug is capable of producing side effects. Many entacapone users experience no, or minor side effects. The frequency and severity of side effects depend on many factors including dose, duration of therapy, and individual susceptibility. Possible side effects include:

Digestive Tract: Nausea; diarrhea; stomach pain; constipation; vomiting; dry mouth; indigestion; gas; gastritis.

Nervous System: Difficulty moving; abnormal movements; muscular hyperactivity; muscle pain; slow mobility; dizziness; hallucinations; anxiety; agitation; drowsiness.

Other: Difficulty breathing; elevated body temperature; increased sweating; unusual bleeding or bruising; little red spots under the skin; brown-orange discoloration of urine; back pain; altered taste; fatigue; weakness; bacterial infection.

Guidelines for Use:

- Dosage is individualized. Use exactly as prescribed.
- Do not change the dose or stop taking this medicine unless advised to do so by your doctor.
- May be taken without regard to meals or snacks.
- Your doctor may reduce your levodopa/carbidopa dose while taking this medicine.
- Each dose is taken at the same time as a dose of levodopa/carbidopa.
- If you experience hallucinations, severe or persistent nausea, or difficult or abnormal movement, contact your doctor immediately.
- May cause dizziness, lightheadedness, or fainting when rising or standing, particularly during initial use. Get up slowly and avoid sudden changes in posture.
- Do not drive a car or operate complex machinery until the effects of entacapone on your mental or motor performance can be gauged.
- Urine color may change to a brownish-orange discoloration. This is normal and of no concern.
- Inform your doctor if you are pregnant, become pregnant, are planning to become pregnant, or are breastfeeding.
- This medicine should not be stopped suddenly. If a decision is made to discontinue this medicine, the dose should be reduced slowly if possible.
- Store at controlled room temperature (59° to 86°F).

If you have any questions, consult your doctor, pharmacist, or health care provider.

Antacids, 917

Antacid Combinations, 921

Anticholinergics/Antispasmodics, 931

Anticholinergic Combinations, 936

Mouth and Throat Products
- Doxycycline, 939

H. Pylori Agents
- Ranitidine Bismuth Citrate, 942
- Bismuth Subsalicylate/Metronidazole/Tetracycline HCl, 944
- Lansoprazole/Amoxicillin/Clarithromycin, 947

Histamine H_2 Antagonists, 950

Anti-Ulcer
- Misoprostol, 955
- Sulcrafate, 957

Antiflatulents, 959

Digestive Aids
- Digestive Enzymes, 961
- Metoclopramide, 965
- Proton Pump Inhibitors, 968
- Miscellaneous Digestive Products, 971

Gallstone Dissolving Agents
- Oral, 973
- Infusion, 975

Laxatives
- Bulk Reducing, 977
- Glycerin, 981
- Lactulose, 983
- Mineral Oil, 985
- Saline, 988
- Stimulant, 991
- Stool Softeners, 995
- Laxative Combinations, 998

Bowel Evacuants
- Polyethylene Glycol, 1003
- Bowel Evacuant Kits, 1005

Antidiarrheals
- Bismuth Subsalicylate, 1007
- Difenoxin and Diphenoxylate, 1010
- Lactobacillus, 1013
- Loperamide, 1014
- Antidiarrheal Combination Products, 1016

5-Aminosalicylate (5-ASA) Agents, 1019

Infliximab, 1022

Anti-obesity Agents
- Orlistat, 1025

	Generic Name *Brand Name Examples*	Supplied As	Generic Available
otc	**Aluminum Carbonate Gel, Basic**		
	Basaljel	**Capsules:** Equivalent to 608 mg dried aluminum hydroxide gel or 500 mg aluminum hydroxide	No
	Basaljel	**Tablets:** Equivalent to 608 mg dried aluminum hydroxide gel or 500 mg aluminum hydroxide	No
otc	**Aluminum Hydroxide Gel**		
	Alu-Cap	**Capsules:** 400 mg	No
	Amphojel	**Tablets:** 300 mg, 600 mg	No
	Alu-Tab	**Tablets:** 500 mg	No
	ALternaGEL, Amphojel	**Suspension:** 320 mg/5 mL, 600 mg/5 mL	Yes
otc	**Calcium Carbonate**	**Tablets:** 500 mg, 600 mg, 648 mg, 1250 mg	Yes
		Suspension: 1250 mg/5 mL	Yes
	Gastro-Relief	**Tablets, chewable:** 250 mg	No
	Amitone	**Tablets, chewable:** 350 mg	No
	Mallamint	**Tablets, chewable:** 420 mg	No
	Alkets, Antacid Tablets, Chooz[1]*, Tums*	**Tablets, chewable:** 500 mg	Yes
	Extra Strength Alkets, Extra Strength Antacid Tablets, Tums E-X[2]	**Tablets, chewable:** 750 mg	Yes
	Alka-Mints	**Tablets, chewable:** 850 mg	No
	Tums Ultra[2]	**Tablets, chewable:** 1000 mg	No
	Calci-Chew	**Tablets, chewable:** 1250 mg	Yes
otc	**Magaldrate (Aluminum Magnesium Hydroxide Sulfate)**		
	Iosopan, Lowsium	**Suspension:** 540 mg/5 mL	Yes
otc	**Magnesia (Magnesium Hydroxide)**		
	Phillips' Milk of Magnesia	**Tablets, chewable:** 311 mg	No
	Milk of Magnesia, Phillips' Milk of Magnesia	**Suspension:** 400 mg/5 mL	Yes

	Generic Name *Brand Name Examples*	Supplied As	Generic Available
	Concentrated Phillips' Milk of Magnesia	**Suspension:** 800 mg/5 mL	No
otc	**Magnesium Oxide**	**Tablets:** 500 mg	Yes
	Uro-Mag	**Capsules:** 140 mg	No
	Mag-Ox 400	**Tablets:** 400 mg	Yes
otc	**Sodium Bicarbonate**	**Tablets:** 325 mg, 650 mg	Yes
	Bell/ans	**Tablets:** 520 mg	No
otc	**Sodium Citrate**		
	Citra pH	**Solution:** 450 mg/5 mL	No

[1] Contains phenylalanine.
[2] Contains tartrazine.

Type of Drug:

Antacids.

How the Drug Works:

Antacids neutralize stomach acid and increase the pH of the stomach. This action also inhibits activity of pepsin, a digestive enzyme that can be irritating to the stomach lining. They also increase the tone of the muscular valve between the stomach and the esophagus, which helps prevent stomach acids from getting into the esophagus and causing heartburn.

Uses:

To treat upset stomach due to excessive acid production (including heartburn, acid indigestion, and sour stomach).

To treat excess acid secretion associated with peptic ulcer (ulcers in the stomach or intestine).

Aluminum carbonate: To treat or control hyperphosphatemia.

Calcium carbonate, magnesium oxide: To treat calcium or magnesium deficiencies, respectively.

Magnesium hydroxide: To relieve occasional constipation (irregularity).

Unlabeled Use(s): Occasionally doctors may prescribe aluminum hydroxide, aluminum carbonate, and calcium carbonate to reduce phosphorus levels in certain kidney conditions. Aluminum hydroxide or aluminum hydroxide with magnesium hydroxide may be used to prevent stress ulcer bleeding (stress ulcers occur with serious illnesses such as life-threatening infections or blood loss).

Precautions:

Use with caution in the following situations:

kidney disease (magnesium-containing products only)
stomach-emptying disorders (aluminum-containing products only)
upper digestive tract hemorrhage (aluminum hydroxide only)

Sodium content: Some antacids have a high sodium content. Select a low-sodium antacid product if you have high blood pressure, heart conditions, kidney disease, fluid retention, or are on a low-sodium diet. Check package label when available or consult your doctor or pharmacist.

Sodium bicarbonate: Sodium bicarbonate products can alter normal blood chemistry if used for long periods of time or in excessive doses.

Phenylketonuria: Some of these products contain phenylalanine. Check package label when available or consult your doctor or pharmacist.

Pregnancy: There are no adequate and well-controlled studies in pregnant women. Use only if clearly needed and the potential benefits to the mother outweigh the possible risks to the fetus.

Breastfeeding: It is not known if antacids appear in breast milk. Consult your doctor before you begin breastfeeding.

Tartrazine: Some of these products may contain the dye tartrazine (FD&C Yellow No. 5), which can cause allergic reactions in certain individuals. Check package label when available or consult your doctor or pharmacist.

Drug Interactions:

Tell your doctor or pharmacist if you are taking or if you are planning to take any over-the-counter or prescription medications or dietary supplements with antacids. Doses of one or both drugs may need to be modified or a different drug may need to be prescribed. The following drugs and drug classes interact with antacids:

allopurinol (eg, *Zyloprim*) (aluminum products only)
chloroquine (eg, *Aralen*) (aluminum products only)
digoxin (eg, *Lanoxin*) (aluminum products only)
ethambutol (*Myambutol*) (aluminum products only)
hydantoins (eg, phenytoin)
iron salts (eg, ferrous fumarate)
isoniazid (eg, *Nydrazid*) (aluminum products only)
ketoconazole *(Nizoral)*
levothyroxine (eg, *Synthroid*)
penicillamine (eg, *Cuprimine*) (aluminum products only)
quinidine (eg, *Cin-Quin*)
quinolone antibiotics (eg, ciprofloxacin)
salicylates (eg, aspirin)
sodium polystyrene sulfonate (eg, *Kayexalate)*
tetracyclines (eg, doxycycline) (aluminum products only)
valproic acid (eg, *Depakote*)

Side Effects:

Every drug is capable of producing side effects. Many antacid users experience no, or minor, side effects. The frequency and severity of side effects depend on many factors including dose, duration of therapy, and individual susceptibility. Possible side effects include:

Aluminum-containing antacids: Constipation; high aluminum blood levels; low phosphorus levels.

Calcium-containing antacids: Appetite loss; nausea; vomiting; dry mouth; increased urination; constipation; stomach pain; thirst; confusion; high blood calcium levels.

Magnesium-containing antacids: Diarrhea; high magnesium blood levels; muscle weakness; slow reflexes.

Guidelines for Use:

- Consult individual product labeling for dosage. Antacids contain a variety of different ingredients. Do not exceed the maximum recommended dosage.
- *Chewable tablets* — Chew thoroughly before swallowing. May be followed with a glass of water.
- *Suspensions* — Shake well before using.
- *Product choice* — Liquid products work faster and have greater activity than other forms. Tablets and capsules may be more acceptable and convenient, particularly when you are away from home or when the liquid would be inconvenient to carry.
- Antacids reduce acidity for about 30 to 60 minutes when taken on an empty stomach. Acidity is reduced for about 2 to 3 hours when antacids are taken 1 hour after meals.
- Antacids can interfere with the absorption of some drugs. Do not take medication within 2 hours of taking the antacid.
- Notify your doctor if "coffee-ground" vomiting or black, tarry stools occur.
- Taking too much of these products can cause the stomach to secrete excess stomach acid. Consult your doctor or pharmacist about the appropriate dose.
- *Long-term use* — Do not take for longer than 2 weeks for the relief of indigestion, unless advised to do so by your doctor. If discomfort continues, consult your doctor.
- Store at room temperature (59° to 86°F) in a dry place. Refrigeration of liquid antacids may improve the flavor. Avoid freezing. If the taste of one antacid product is not satisfactory, talk to your doctor or pharmacist about switching to another product.

If you have any questions, consult your doctor, pharmacist, or health care provider.

<table>
<tr><th>Brand Name Examples</th><th>Aluminum Hydroxide</th><th>Magnesium Hydroxide</th><th>Calcium Carbonate</th><th>Other Content</th><th>Sodium (mg)[2]</th></tr>
<tr><td>otc Tempo</td><td>133</td><td>81</td><td>414</td><td rowspan="4">20 mg simethicone</td><td>3</td></tr>
<tr><td>otc Maalox</td><td rowspan="10">200</td><td rowspan="10">200</td><td rowspan="10"></td><td></td></tr>
<tr><td>otc Mintox</td><td></td></tr>
<tr><td>otc Rulox #1</td><td></td></tr>
<tr><td>otc Almacone</td><td>20 mg simethicone</td><td></td></tr>
<tr><td>otc Mylanta</td><td></td><td>0.77</td></tr>
<tr><td>otc Gelusil</td><td rowspan="5">25 mg simethicone</td><td>< 5</td></tr>
<tr><td>otc Maalox Plus</td><td></td></tr>
<tr><td>Magalox Plus</td><td></td></tr>
<tr><td>otc Mintox Plus</td><td></td></tr>
<tr><td>otc RuLox</td><td></td></tr>
<tr><td>otc Entra Strength Maalox</td><td rowspan="2">350</td><td rowspan="2">350</td><td rowspan="2"></td><td rowspan="2">30 mg simethicone</td><td></td></tr>
<tr><td>otc Extra Strength Maalox Plus</td><td></td></tr>
<tr><td>otc Rulox #2</td><td rowspan="2">400</td><td rowspan="2">400</td><td rowspan="2"></td><td></td><td rowspan="2"></td></tr>
<tr><td>otc Mylanta Double Strength</td><td>40 mg simethicone</td></tr>
<tr><td>otc Calcium Rich Rolaids</td><td></td><td>80</td><td>412</td><td></td><td>0.4</td></tr>
<tr><td>otc Advanced Formula Di-Gel</td><td></td><td>128</td><td>280</td><td>20 mg simethicone</td><td></td></tr>
</table>

ANTACID COMBINATIONS — CAPSULES AND TABLETS

Brand Name Examples	Aluminum Hydroxide	Magnesium Hydroxide	Calcium Carbonate	Other Content	Sodium (mg)[2]
otc *Foamicon*	80			20 mg magnesium trisilicate, sodium bicarbonate	18.4
otc *Genaton*					
otc *Gaviscon*					
otc *Double Strength Gaviscon-2*	160			Alginic acid, sodium bicarbonate, 40 mg magnesium trisilicate	36.8
otc *Extra Strength Genaton*	160			105 mg magnesium carbonate, alginic acid, sodium bicarbonate	29.9
otc *Gaviscon Extra Strength Relief Formula*					
otc *Gas-Ban*			300	40 mg simethicone	
otc *Mylanta Gelcaps*			311	232 mg magnesium carbonate	
otc *Mylagen Gelcaps*					
otc *Calglycine*[2]			420	150 mg glycine	
otc *Titralac*[2]					0.3
otc *Titralac Plus*				21 mg simethicone	1.1
otc *Alkets*			500		≤ 2
otc *Marblen*			520	400 mg magnesium carbonate	
otc *Titralac Extra Strength*[2]			750		0.6

	Brand Name Examples	Aluminum Hydroxide	Magnesium Hydroxide	Calcium Carbonate	Other Content	Sodium (mg)[2]
otc	*Riopan Plus*	†			480 mg magaldrate, 20 mg simethicone	
otc	*Riopan Plus Double Strength*				1080 mg magaldrate, 20 mg simethi-cone	

† See Other Content column.
[1] Content given in mg per capsule, tablet or wafer.
[2] Sugar free.

Type of Drug:

Antacid combinations.

Uses:

To treat upset stomach due to too much acid secretion (including heartburn, gastroesophageal reflux, acid indigestion and sour stomach).

To treat excess acid secretion associated with peptic ulcer, irritation of the stomach, irritation of the esophagus or hiatal hernia.

Unlabeled Use(s): To prevent significant stress ulcer bleeding. To treat duodenal and gastric ulcers.

Guidelines for Use:

- *Chewable tablets* — Chew before swallowing. Follow with a glass of water.
- If you are currently taking a prescription drug or other medications, do not take an antacid without checking with your doctor or pharmacist.
- Magnesium-containing products may cause diarrhea; aluminum and calcium-containing products may cause constipation.
- Antacids reduce acidity for about 30 minutes when taken on an empty stomach and for about 3 hours when taken 1 hour after meals.
- Notify your doctor if "coffee-ground" vomiting or black, tar-like stools occur.
- Taking too much of these products can cause the stomach to secrete excess stomach acid. Consult your doctor or pharmacist about the appropriate dose.
- *Long-term use* — Do not take for longer than 2 weeks for the relief of indigestion. If discomfort continues, consult your doctor.

If you have any questions, consult your doctor, pharmacist, or health care provider.

	Brand Name Examples	Aluminum Hydroxide	Magnesium Hydroxide	Calcium Carbonate	Other Content	Sodium (mg)[2]
otc	Almacone	200	200		20 mg simethicone	
otc	Di-Gel					
otc	Gelusil				25 mg simethicone	
otc	Mi-Acid				20 mg simethicone	
otc	Mygel Suspension					
otc	Mylagen					<1.25
otc	Mylanta					0.68
otc	Alumina, Magnesia, and Simethicone Suspension	213	200		20 mg simethicone	
otc	Alamag Suspension	225	220			<1.25
otc	Alamag Plus Suspension				25 mg simethicone	
otc	Antacid Suspension					
otc	Maalox Suspension					
otc	Magnalox					
otc	Magnox Suspension					
otc	Rulox Suspension					

	Brand Name Examples	Aluminum Hydroxide	Magnesium Hydroxide	Calcium Carbonate	Other Content	Sodium (mg)[2]
otc	*Aludrox Suspension*	307	103		Simethicone	
otc	*Almacone II Double Strength Suspension*	400	400		40 mg simethicone	
otc	*Gas-Ban DS*					
otc	*Mygel II Suspension*					
otc	*Mylagen II*					< 1.25
otc	*Mylanta Double Strength*	400	400		40 mg simethicone	
otc	*Extra Strength Maalox Suspension*	500	450			
otc	*Extra Strength Maalox Plus Suspension*					
otc	*Extra Strength Mintox Plus*					
otc	*Kudrox Double Strength Suspension*					
otc	*Rulox Plus Suspension*					
otc	*Maalox Therapeutic Concentrate Suspension*	600	300			

	Brand Name Examples	Aluminum Hydroxide	Magnesium Hydroxide	Calcium Carbonate	Other Content	Sodium (mg)[2]
otc	*Genaton*	31.7			137.3 mg magnesium carbonate, sodium alginate, EDTA	13
otc	*Gaviscon*				119.3 mg magnesium carbonate, sodium alginate, EDTA	13
otc	*Gaviscon Extra Strength Relief Formula*	254			237.5 mg magnesium carbonate, simethicone	
otc	*Nephrox*	320			10% mineral oil	
otc	*Titralac Plus*[2]			500	20 mg simethicone	0.15
otc	*Marblen*			520	400 mg magnesium carbonate	
otc	*Lowsium Plus Suspension*	††			540 mg magaldrate, mg simethicone	
otc	*Magaldrate Plus Suspension*					
otc	*Riopan Plus Suspension*					

	Brand Name Examples	Aluminum Hydroxide	Magnesium Hydroxide	Calcium Carbonate	Other Content	Sodium (mg)[2]
otc	*Riopan Plus Double Strength Suspension*				1080 mg magaldrate and 40 mg simethicone	
otc	*Maalox Heart-burn Relief*				140 mg aluminum hydroxide-magnesium carbonate, 175 mg magnesium carbonate	

† See Other Content column.
[1] Content given in mg per 5 mL.
[2] Sugar free.

Type of Drug:

Antacid combinations.

Uses:

To treat upset stomach due to too much acid secretion (including heartburn, gastroesophageal reflux, acid indigestion and sour stomach).

To treat excess acid secretion associated with peptic ulcer, irritation of the stomach, irritation of the esophagus or hiatal hernia.

Unlabeled Use(s): To prevent significant stress ulcer bleeding. To treat duodenal and gastric ulcers.

Guidelines for Use:

- *Suspension* — Shake well before using.
- If you are currently taking a prescription drug or other medications, do not take an antacid without checking with your doctor or pharmacist.
- Magnesium-containing products may cause diarrhea; aluminum and calcium-containing products may cause constipation.
- *Refrigeration* of liquid antacids may improve the flavor (avoid freezing). Talk to your doctor or pharmacist about switching to another product if the taste is not satisfactory.
- Antacids reduce acidity for about 30 minutes when taken on an empty stomach and for about 3 hours when taken 1 hour after meals.
- Notify your doctor if "coffee-ground" vomiting or black, tar-like stools occur.
- Taking too much of these products can cause the stomach to secrete excess stomach acid. Consult your doctor or pharmacist about the appropriate dose.
- *Long-term use* — Do not take for longer than 2 weeks for the relief of indigestion. If discomfort continues, consult your doctor.

If you have any questions, consult your doctor, pharmacist, or health care provider.

	Brand Name Examples	Supplied As
otc	*Citrocarbonate*[1]	**Effervescent granules:** 780 mg sodium bicarbonate, 1820 mg sodium citrate and 700.6 mg sodium per dose
otc	*Bromo Seltzer*	**Effervescent granules:** 2781 mg sodium bicarbonate, 325 mg acetaminophen, 2224 mg citric acid and 761 mg sodium per dose
otc	*Gold Alka-Seltzer*	**Effervescent tablets:** 958 mg sodium bicarbonate, 832 mg citric acid, 312 mg potassium bicarbonate and 311 mg sodium
otc	*Alka-Seltzer*	**Effervescent tablets:** 1700 mg sodium bicarbonate, 1000 mg citric acid, 9 mg phenylalanine, 325 mg aspirin and 506 mg sodium
otc	*Original Alka-Seltzer*	**Effervescent tablets:** 1916 mg sodium bicarbonate (heat treated), 1000 mg citric acid, 325 mg aspirin and 567 mg sodium
otc	*Extra Strength Alka-Seltzer*	**Effervescent tablets:** 1985 mg sodium bicarbonate (heat treated), 1000 mg citric acid, 500 mg aspirin and 588 mg sodium

[1] Sugar free.

Type of Drug:

Antacid combinations.

Uses:

To treat upset stomach due to too much acid secretion (including heartburn, gastroesophageal reflux, acid indigestion and sour stomach).

To treat excess acid secretion associated with peptic ulcer, irritation of the stomach, irritation of the esophagus or hiatal hernia.

Unlabeled Use(s): To prevent significant stress ulcer bleeding. To treat duodenal and gastric ulcers.

Guidelines for Use:

- *Effervescent tablets* — Allow to completely dissolve in water. Allow most of the bubbling to stop before drinking.
- If you are currently taking a prescription drug or other medications, do not take an antacid without checking with your doctor or pharmacist.
- Magnesium-containing products may cause diarrhea; aluminum and calcium-containing products may cause constipation.
- Antacids reduce acidity for about 30 minutes when taken on an empty stomach and for about 3 hours when taken 1 hour after meals.
- Notify your doctor if "coffee-ground" vomiting or black, tar-like stools occur.
- Taking too much of these products can cause the stomach to secrete excess stomach acid. Consult your doctor or pharmacist about the appropriate dose.
- *Long-term use* — Do not take for longer than 2 weeks for the relief of indigestion. If discomfort continues, consult your doctor.

If you have any questions, consult your doctor, pharmacist, or health care provider.

	Generic Name *Brand Name Examples*	Supplied As	Generic Available
Rx	**Dicyclomine**[1]		
	Bentyl[1,2]	**Capsules:** 10 mg	Yes
	Bentyl[1,2]	**Tablets:** 20 mg	Yes
	Bentyl[1,3]	**Syrup:** 10 mg/5 mL	Yes
Rx	**Hyoscyamine Sulfate**		
	Anaspaz[4], *Cystospaz*[2], *Levsin*[1,5], *Donnamar*	**Tablets:** 0.125 mg, 0.15 mg	No
	Cystospaz-M, Levsinex Timecaps	**Capsules, timed release:** 0.375 mg	No
	Levsin Drops[6]	**Solution:** 0.125 mg/ml	No
	Levsin[6]	**Elixir:** 0.125 mg/5 mL	No
Rx	**Glycopyrrolate**		
	Robinul	**Tablets:** 1 mg	Yes
	Robinul Forte	**Tablets:** 2 mg	Yes
Rx	**Mepenzolate Bromide**		
	Cantil[2,7]	**Tablets:** 25 mg	No
Rx	**Methscopolamine Bromide**		
	Pamine[2]	**Tablets:** 2.5 mg	No
Rx	**Propantheline Bromide**		
	Pro-Banthine[2]	**Tablets:** 7.5 mg, 15 mg	Yes

[1] This product also available as an injection.
[2] Contains lactose.
[3] Contains parabens.
[4] Contains lactose, mannitol.
[5] Contains sugar, lactose.
[6] Contains alcohol.
[7] Contains the dye tartrazine.

Type of Drug:

Drugs used to treat stomach and intestinal disorders; anticholinergic; antispasmodic.

How the Drug Works:

These drugs inhibit actions of nerves in smooth muscle, secretory glands and the central nervous system. They slow certain activity of the stomach and intestines and reduce cramping, reduce secretions (acids, enzymes, etc) of the stomach and intestines, relax the urinary bladder (reduce spasm) and promote closure of the sphincter valve (these actions tend to cause urinary retention). They also slow or increase the heart rate, block sweating (causing the body temperature to rise), reduce salivary gland secretions (causing dry mouth), widen the pupils of the eyes and reduce the ability of the eyes to focus.

Uses:

To treat peptic ulcers.

To treat diarrhea.

To treat irritable bowel syndrome (spastic colon).

To treat irritation or inflammation of the stomach and intestines (eg, colitis).

To treat infant colic.

To treat spasms of the bile and urinary tracts.

To treat frequent urination problems and bedwetting.

To reduce symptoms of runny or congested nose.

Precautions:

Do not use in the following situations:

- allergy to these drugs or any of their ingredients
- diarrhea
- enlarged colon
- enlarged prostate
- glaucoma (narrow-angle)
- heart problems (eg, ischemia, rapid or irregular heart rate)
- infants less than 6 months of age (dicyclomine only)
- intestinal obstructions
- lack of intestinal muscle tone in elderly or debilitated patients
- myasthenia gravis
- nursing mothers (dicyclomine)
- ulcerative colitis, severe
- urinary obstruction

Use with caution in the following situations:

- abnormal heart rhythm
- asthma
- bile duct disorders
- congestive heart failure
- colon problems (eg, ulcerative colitis)
- coronary artery disease
- dementia, elderly
- drowsiness, blurred vision
- elderly
- esophagitis, reflux
- gastric or duodenal ulcers
- heart disease
- hiatal hernia with gastric reflux
- high blood pressure
- hot weather
- hyperthyroidism (overactive thyroid)
- kidney disease
- liver disease
- nerve disorder
- prostate gland problems
- psychosis

Exposure to heat: These drugs can reduce sweating if you are exposed to hot weather. This can cause heat prostration, fever and heatstroke.

Diarrhea can be an early symptom of incomplete intestinal obstruction. Check with your doctor or pharmacist before self-medicating diarrhea with these drugs.

Contact lens use: These products can cause drying of the eyes. Contact lens wearers should use an appropriate lubricating solution while taking these products.

Anticholinergic psychosis has been reported in sensitive individuals given anticholinergic drugs. CNS signs and symptoms include confusion, disorientation, short-term memory loss, hallucinations, slurred speech, incoordination, coma, exaggerated sense of well-being, decreased anxiety, fatigue, sleeplessness, agitation and inappropriate affect. These CNS signs and symptoms usually resolve within 12 to 24 hours after discontinuation of the drug.

Pregnancy: Studies in pregnant women or in animals have been judged not to show a risk to the fetus in patients taking dicyclomine and mepenzolate bromide. Adequate studies have not been done in pregnant women in association with the other listed drugs. Use only if clearly needed and potential benefits outweigh the possible hazards to the fetus.

Breastfeeding: These drugs appear in breast milk. They may reduce milk production and cause side effects in the infant. Breastfeeding is contraindicated in patients taking dicyclomine. Consult your doctor before you begin breastfeeding.

Children: Safety and effectiveness in children have not been established. Hyoscyamine has been used in infant colic. Some infant deaths have been associated with the use of dicyclomine. Dicyclomine is not recommended for use in children under 6 months of age.

Elderly: These drugs can cause agitation and mental confusion in older patients.

Lab tests may be required during therapy including upper gastrointestinal contrast radiology or endoscopy, as well as tests for blood in the stool. Be sure to keep appointments.

Tartrazine: Some of these products may contain the dye tartrazine (FD&C Yellow No. 5) which can cause allergic reactions in certain individuals. Check package label when available or consult your doctor or pharmacist.

Drug Interactions:

Tell your doctor or pharmacist if you are taking or if you are planning to take any over-the-counter or prescription medications or dietary supplements with gastrointestinal anticholinergics or antispasmodics. Doses of one or both drugs may need to be modified or a different drug may need to be prescribed. The following drugs and drug classes interact with gastrointestinal anticholinergics or antispasmodics.

amantadine (eg, *Symmetrel*)
antacids (eg, *Maalox)*
anticholinergics, other (eg, belladonna alkaloids)
benzodiazepines (eg, diazepam)
beta blockers (eg, atenolol)
cholinergics (eg, pilocarpine)
cholinesterase inhibitors (eg, physostigmine)
corticosteroids (eg, prednisone)
digoxin (eg, *Lanoxin)*
haloperidol (eg, *Haldol)*
isocarboxazid *(Marplan)*
levodopa (eg, *Dopar*)
MAO inhibitors (eg, phenelzine)
meperidine (eg, *Demerol)*
metoclopramide (eg, *Reglan)*
nitrates (eg, nitroglycerin)
phenothiazines (eg, promethazine)
selegiline *(Eldepryl)*

sympathomimetics (eg, epinephrine)
thioxanthenes (eg, thiothixene)
tranylcypromine *(Parnate)*
tricyclic antidepressants (eg, amitriptyline)

Side Effects:

Every drug is capable of producing side effects. Many anticholinergic or antispasmodic users experience no, or minor, side effects. The frequency and severity of side effects depend on many factors including dose, duration of therapy and individual susceptibility. Possible side effects include:

Digestive Tract: Nausea; vomiting; bloating; constipation; abdominal pain; appetite loss; difficulty swallowing.

Nervous System: Confusion; excitement; restlessness; hallucinations; headache; nervousness; drowsiness; dizziness; lightheadedness; tingling; numbness; difficulty moving; fainting; disorientation; short-term memory loss; slurred speech; incoordination; coma; exaggerated sense of well-being; decreased anxiety; tiredness; speech disturbance; weakness; sleeplessness; fever; tremor.

Circulatory System: Pounding in the chest (palpitations); fast or irregular heartbeat.

Respiratory System: Difficulty breathing; nasal stuffiness; nasal congestion.

Skin: Rash; itching; flushing; decreased sweating; hives; skin disorder.

Other: Difficult urination; muscle weakness; visual problems; blurred vision; dry mouth; taste changes; urinary retention; impotence; reduced breast milk production and flow; enlarged pupils; eye sensitivity to light; increased eye pressure.

Guidelines for Use:

- Take exactly as prescribed.
- Take 30 minutes before meals. Take mepenzolate with meals and at bedtime.
- If a dose is missed, take it as soon as possible. If several hours have passed or if it is nearing time for the next dose, do not double the dose to "catch up" (unless advised by your doctor). If more than one dose is missed or it is necessary to establish a new dosage schedule, contact your doctor or pharmacist.
- May cause drowsiness, dizziness or blurred vision. Use caution when driving or performing other tasks requiring mental alertness, coordination or physical dexterity.
- Notify your doctor if skin rash, flushing, rapid heartbeat, urinary retention, blurred vision or eye problems occur.
- May cause dry mouth, difficulty in urination or constipation, or increased sensitivity to light. Notify your doctor if these effects persist or become severe.
- If symptoms of fever, heatstroke and decreased sweating occur, discontinue the drug and contact a doctor immediately.
- Signs of overdosage with these drugs include: Headache, nausea, vomiting, dizziness, dry mouth, blurred vision, rapid heartbeat or loss of heart rhythm, dry skin, fever, difficulty in swallowing, excitation, tiredness, stupor, coma, respiratory depression and paralysis. Contact your doctor if these instances occur.
- Avoid alcohol and medicines (eg, tranquilizers, sedating antihistamines) that cause drowsiness.
- Sucking on hard sugarless candy, drinking fluids and maintaining good oral hygiene can relieve dry mouth.
- Inform your doctor if you are pregnant, become pregnant, are planning to become pregnant or are breastfeeding.
- Store at room temperature.

If you have any questions, consult your doctor, pharmacist, or health care provider.

	Generic Name *Brand Name Examples*	Anticholinergic	Sedative
Rx	**Atropine-containing Combinations**		
	Barbidonna No. 2[1]	**Tablets:** 0.025 mg atropine sulfate, 0.0074 mg scopolamine HBr, 0.1286 mg hyoscyamine HBr or SO_4	32 mg phenobarbital
	Barbidonna[1]		16 mg phenobarbital
	Donnatal	**Tablets:** 0.0194 mg atropine sulfate, 0.0065 mg scopolamine HBr, 0.1037 mg hyoscyamine HBr or SO_4	16.2 mg phenobarbital
	Donnatal Extentabs	**Tablets, sustained release:** 0.0582 mg atropine sulfate, 0.0195 mg scopolamine HBr, 0.3111 mg hyoscyamine sulfate	48.6 mg phenobarbital
	Donnatal	**Capsules:** 0.0194 mg atropine sulfate, 0.0065 mg scopolamine HBr, 0.1037 mg hyoscyamine HBr or SO_4	16.2 mg phenobarbital
	Donnatal[2], *Hyosophen*[2], *Belladonna Alkaloids with Phenobarbital*[2]	**Elixir:** 0.0194 mg atropine sulfate, 0.0065 mg scopolamine HBr, 0.1037 mg hyoscyamine HBr or SO_4/5 mL	16.2 mg phenobarbital/5 mL
Rx	**Belladonna-containing Combinations**		
	Butibel	**Tablets:** 15 mg belladonna extract	15 mg butabarbital sodium
	Chardonna-2	**Tablets:** 15 mg belladonna extract	15 mg phenobarbital
	Bellergal-S[3]	**Tablets, sustained release:** 0.2 mg l-alkaloids of belladonna	40 mg phenobarbital

	Generic Name *Brand Name Examples*	Anticholinergic	Sedative
	Butibel[2]	**Elixir:** 15 mg belladonna extract/5 mL	15 mg butabarbital sodium/5 mL
Rx	**L-hyoscyamine-containing Combinations**		
	Levsin w/Phenobarbital	**Tablets:** 0.125 mg hyoscyamine sulfate	15 mg phenobarbital
	Levsin-PB Drops[2]	**Elixir:** 0.125 mg hyoscyamine sulfate/mL	15 mg phenobarbital/mL
Rx	**Clidinium Bromide-containing Combinations**		
	Librax, Chlordiazepoxide and Clidinium Bromide	**Capsules:** 2.5 mg clidinium bromide	5 mg chlordiazepoxide HCl

[1] Contains lactose.
[2] Contains alcohol.
[3] Contains 0.6 mg ergotamine tartrate.

Type of Drug:

Gastrointestinal anticholinergic combinations.

Uses:

Combination anticholinergic preparations may include the following components:

Antihistamines: May be included for antihistaminic effects, sedative or anticholinergic side effects. For more information, see the Antihistamines monograph in the Respiratory Drugs chapter.

Ergotamine tartrate: Provides inhibition of the nervous system. For more information, see the Agents for Migraine-Migraine Combinations monograph in the CNS Drugs chapter.

Kaolin: Used for its adsorbent properties.

Sedatives and antianxiety agents: For more information, see the individual monographs in the CNS Drugs chapter.

Guidelines for Use:

- Dosage is individualized. Take exactly as prescribed.
- Do not stop taking or change the dose unless directed by your doctor.
- Some agents must be taken 30 minutes before meals. Consult your doctor or pharmacist.
- May cause drowsiness. Use caution when driving or performing other tasks requiring alertness, coordination, or physical dexterity.
- Notify your doctor if you experience skin rash, flushing, or eye pain.
- May cause dry mouth, difficult urination, constipation, blurring of vision, headache, nausea, vomiting, dilated pupils, dry skin, dizziness, difficulty swallowing, or increased sensitivity to light. Notify your doctor if these effects persist or become severe.
- Barbiturates may be habit-forming; tolerance, psychological dependence, and physical dependence may occur following prolonged use of high doses.

If you have any questions, consult your doctor, pharmacist, or health care provider.

	Generic Name *Brand Name Example*	Supplied As	Generic Available
Rx	**Doxycycline**		
	Periostat	**Tablets**: 20 mg (as hyclate)	No

Type of Drug:

Antibiotic; tetracycline.

How the Drug Works:

Doxycycline reduced elevated collagenase activity in the gingival crevicular fluid of adult patients with periodontitis.

Uses:

As an adjunct to tooth scaling and root planing to promote attachment level gain and to reduce pocket depth in patients with adult periodontitis.

Precautions:

Do not use in the following situations:

acutely abscessed periodontal pocket
allergy to doxycycline or any of its ingredients
breastfeeding
infancy and childhood (up to 8 years of age)
pregnancy

Use with caution in the following situations:

esophageal or peptic ulcer disease, preexisting
oral candidiasis, history of or predisposition to

Tooth discoloration: Use of a tetracycline during tooth development (last half of pregnancy, infancy, and childhood up to 8 years of age) may cause permanent discoloration of the teeth (yellow-gray-brown). This is more common during long-term use but has been observed following repeated short-term courses. Enamel hypoplasia has also been reported. Do not use a tetracycline in this age group or in pregnant or nursing mothers unless the potential benefits outweigh the possible risks.

Superinfection: Use of broad spectrum antibiotics (especially prolonged or repeated therapy) may result in bacterial or fungal overgrowth. Such overgrowth may lead to a second infection. The tetracycline may need to be stopped and another antibiotic may need to be prescribed for the second infection.

Pseudotumor cerebri: Tetracyclines have been associated with pseudotumor cerebri (benign intracranial hypertension). Early signs and symptoms include headache, nausea, vomiting, and blurred vision. If these symptoms develop, stop the drug immediately and contact your doctor.

Cross resistance: Antimicrobial activity of the tetracyclines is similar. Resistance to one tetracycline may mean resistance to most or all of the others.

Pregnancy: May cause harm when administered to a pregnant woman. Do not use during pregnancy. The risk of use in a pregnant woman clearly outweighs any possible benefit.

Breastfeeding: Tetracyclines are excreted in breast milk. Do not use while breastfeeding because of the potential for serious adverse effects in nursing infants.

Children: Tetracyclines should not be used in children under 8 years of age, unless other drugs are not likely to be effective or are not advised.

Lab tests may be required during long-term treatment with tetracyclines. Tests may include blood counts and liver and kidney function tests.

Drug Interactions:

Tell your doctor or pharmacist if you are taking or if you are planning to take any over-the-counter or prescription medications or dietary supplements with doxycycline. Doses of one or both drugs may need to be modified or a different drug may need to be prescribed. The following drugs and drug classes interact with tetracyclines:

- aluminum salts (eg, aluminum hydroxide)
- anticoagulants (eg, warfarin)
- barbiturates (eg, phenobarbital)
- bismuth salts (eg, bismuth subsalicylate)
- calcium salts (eg, calcium citrate)
- carbamazepine (eg, *Tegretol*)
- charcoal
- contraceptives, oral (eg, *Ortho-Novum*)
- digoxin (eg, *Lanoxin*)
- iron salts (eg, ferrous fumarate)
- magnesium salts (eg, magnesium hydroxide)
- methoxyflurane (*Penthrane*)
- penicillins (eg, amoxicillin)
- phenytoin (eg, *Dilantin*)
- rifampin (eg, *Rifadin*)
- sodium bicarbonate
- tricalcium phosphate (eg, *Posture*)
- urinary alkalinizers (eg, sodium bicarbonate)
- zinc salts (eg, zinc gluconate)

Side Effects:

Every drug is capable of producing side effects. Many doxycycline users experience no, or minor, side effects. The frequency and severity of side effects depend on many factors including dose, duration of therapy, and individual susceptibility. Possible side effects include:

Digestive Tract: Acid indigestion; appetite loss; vomiting; diarrhea; nausea; mouth sores; sore throat; toothache; tooth disorder; swollen gums.

Respiratory System: Bronchitis; cough; sinus congestion; sinus headache; runny nose.

Other: Backache; common cold; flu-like symptoms; headache; infection; injury; joint or muscle pain; menstrual cramps; vaginal candidiasis; pain; rash; hives; sensitivity to light; anemia.

Guidelines for Use:

- Dosage will be individualized. Take exactly as prescribed.
- Do not stop taking or change the dose unless directed by your doctor.
- Take 1 tablet 2 times daily at 12 hour intervals, preferably 1 hour before or 2 hours after a meal. Therapy lasts for up to 9 months.
- If a dose is missed, take it as soon as possible. If several hours have passed or it is nearing time for the next dose, do not double the dose to catch up, unless advised to do so by your doctor. If more than one dose is missed, or it is necessary to establish a new dosage schedule, contact your doctor or pharmacist.
- To prevent irritation or ulceration of the esophagus (food pipe), take with a full glass of water or other nondairy liquid. Do not lie down for at least 30 minutes after a dose.
- Do not use during pregnancy or breastfeeding.
- Do not use in children under 8 years of age unless other drugs are not likely to be effective or are inadvisable. Use during tooth development may cause permanent discoloration and inadequate hardening of baby and permanent teeth.
- Avoid use of tetracyclines with antacids, laxatives, alcohol, dairy products (eg, milk, cheese), or iron-containing products. If any of these products must be taken, take at least 2 hours before or after tetracyclines.
- May cause photosensitivity (sensitivity to sunlight). Avoid prolonged exposure to the sun and other sources of ultraviolet (UV) light (eg, tanning beds). Use sunscreens and wear protective clothing until tolerance is determined.
- Concurrent use of tetracyclines with oral contraceptives (eg, *Ortho-Novum*) may cause the oral contraceptives to be less effective. Discuss alternative contraceptive methods with your doctor.
- Notify your doctor if you experience skin redness, flushing, itching, or hives.
- *Do not use outdated tetracyclines.* Outdated tetracyclines may be highly toxic to the kidneys.
- Lab tests may be required to monitor therapy. Be sure to keep appointments.
- Store at controlled room temperature (59° to 86°F).

If you have any questions, consult your doctor, pharmacist, or health care provider.

	Generic Name *Brand Name Examples*	Supplied As	Generic Available
Rx	**Ranitidine Bismuth Citrate**		
	Tritec	**Tablets:** 400 mg	No

Type of Drug:

H. pylori agent; anti-ulcer drug.

How the Drug Works:

This drug, when combined with other drugs, acts as an anti-infective to help eliminate the bacteria that is responsible for many cases of peptic ulcer disease.

Uses:

Used in combination with clarithromycin to treat active duodenal ulcers caused by *H. pylori* infection. Do not use ranitidine bismuth citrate alone.

Precautions:

Do not use in the following situations:
- allergy to this medicine or its ingredients
- hangover

Use with caution in the following situations:
- kidney disease
- porphyria
- urine tests (may give false results)

Clarithromycin therapy: If *H. pylori* infection is not eradicated after ranitidine bismuth citrate and clarithromycin treatment, the infection may be resistant to clarithromycin. Any patients who do not respond to this therapy should not be retreated with a regimen containing clarithromycin.

Darkening of the tongue: The bismuth may cause a temporary and harmless darkening of the tongue or stool. Stool darkening should not be confused with blood in the stool.

Pregnancy: Adequate studies have not been done in pregnant women, or animal studies may have shown a risk to the fetus. Use only if clearly needed and potential benefits outweigh possible risks to the fetus.

Breastfeeding: It is not known if ranitidine bismuth citrate appears in breast milk. Consult your doctor before you begin breastfeeding.

Children: Safety and effectiveness in children have not been established.

Drug Interactions:

Tell your doctor or pharmacist if you are taking or planning to take any over-the-counter or prescription medications or dietary supplements while taking this medicine. Doses of one or both drugs may need to be modified or a different drug may need to be prescribed. The following drugs and drug classes interact with this medicine:

antacids
aspirin

Side Effects:

Every drug is capable of producing side effects. Many patients experience no, or minor, side effects. The frequency and severity of side effects depend on many factors including dose, duration of therapy and individual susceptibility. Possible side effects include:

Digestive Tract: Diarrhea; nausea; vomiting; constipation.

Nervous System: Headache; dizziness.

Other: Itching; gynecological problems; taste changes; sleep problems; chest pain.

Guidelines for Use:

- The usual dose of ranitidine bismuth citrate is 400 mg twice a day for 4 weeks in conjunction with clarithromycin 500 mg three times a day for the first 2 weeks.
- Both ranitidine bismuth citrate and clarithromycin may be taken without regard to food.
- If a dose is missed, take it as soon as possible. If several hours have passed or if it is nearing time for the next dose, do not double the dose in order to "catch up" (unless advised to do so by your doctor). If more than one dose is missed or it is necessary to establish a new dosage schedule, contact your doctor or pharmacist. Use exactly as prescribed.
- The bismuth may cause a temporary and harmLess darkening of the tongue or stool. Stool darkening should not be confused with blood in the stool.
- May cause dizziness. Use caution while driving or performing other tasks which require alertness, coordination or physical dexterity.
- Avoid alcohol, aspirin and NSAIDS (eg, ibuprofen) while taking this medicine.
- Store at room temperature or in the refrigerator (36° to 86°F). Protect from moisture and light.

If you have any questions, consult your doctor, pharmacist, or health care provider.

Generic Name *Brand Name Examples*	Supplied As	Generic Available
Rx **Bismuth Subsalicylate, Metronidazole, Tetracycline HCl**		
Helidac	**Tablets:** 262.4 mg bismuth subsalicylate **Tablets:** 250 mg metronidazole **Capsules:** 500 mg tetracycline HCl	No

Type of Drug:

H. pylori agents; anti-ulcer drug.

How the Drug Works:

The three drugs used in this combination treatment are used to eliminate the H. pylori bacteria known to cause certain kinds of ulcers.

Uses:

Used in combination with an H_2 antagonist to treat active duodenal ulcers cause by *H. pylori* infection.

Precautions:

Do not use in the following situations:

- allergy to bismuth subsalicylate, metronidizole or other nitroimidazole derivatives, any of the tetracyclines, aspirin or salicylates
- breastfeeding
- children
- kidney disease
- liver disease
- pregnancy

Use with caution in the following situations:

- blood disorders
- blurred vision
- candidiasis infection
- headache
- nervous system diseases

Dark tongue/stools: The bismuth may cause a temporary and harmLess darkening of the tongue and stool. Stool darkening should not be confused with blood in the stool.

Children (over 8) and teenagers who have or who are recovering from chicken pox or flu should not use this medicine to treat nausea and vomiting. If nausea and vomiting are present, contact your doctor because this could be an early sign of Reye syndrome.

Superinfection: Use of antibiotics (especially prolonged or repeated therapy) may result in bacterial or fungal overgrowth. Such overgrowth may lead to a second infection. This medicine may need to be stopped and another antibiotic may need to be prescribed for the second infection.

Photosensitivity: May cause photosensitivity (risk of sunburn). Avoid prolonged exposure to the sun or other forms of ultraviolet (UV) light (eg, tanning beds). Use sunscreens and wear protective clothing until tolerance is determined.

Pregnancy: Do not use this combination during pregnancy.

Breastfeeding: Metronidazole and tetracycline appear in breast milk. Do not breastfeed while taking this medicine. Consult your doctor.

Children: Do not use this medicine in children under 8 years of age. Tetracycline may cause discoloration and damage to developing teeth. Safety and effectiveness in children with *H. Pylori* have not been established.

Elderly: Use with caution in elderly patients because of potential kidney and liver dysfunction.

Drug Interactions:

Tell your doctor or pharmacist if you are taking or planning to take any over-the-counter or prescription medications or dietary supplements while taking this medicine. Doses of one or both may need to be modified or another drug may need to be prescribed. See the individual Bismuth Subsalicylate, Metronidazole and Tetracyclines monographs for further information.

Side Effects:

Every drug is capable of producing side effects. Many patients experience no, or minor, side effects. The frequency and severity of side effects depend on many factors including dose, duration of therapy and individual susceptibility. Possible side effects include:

Digestive Tract: Diarrhea; nausea; vomiting; stomach pain; dark bloody stools; anal discomfort; appetite loss; constipation.

Nervous System: Dizziness; abnormal skin sensations; weakness; sleeplessness; pain.

Guidelines for Use:

- Use exactly as prescribed.
- Each dose contains four pills: two pink round chewable tablets (bismuth subsalicylate), one white tablet (metronidazole) and one pale orange and white capsule (tetracycline). Take each dose four times a day with meals and at bedtime. Chew and swallow the bismuth subsalicylate (pink) tablets, and swallow the metronidazole (white) tablets and tetracycline (pale orange and white) capsules whole with a full glass of water (8 ounces). Do not take with milk or other dairy products.
- Drink adequate amounts of fluid, especially with the bedtime tetracycline dose to reduce the risk of irritation and ulceration of the esophagus.
- If a dose is missed, continue the normal dosing schedule until the medication is gone. Do not double the dose in order to "catch up." If more than four doses are missed, contact your doctor or pharmacist.
- This treatment includes salicylates. If ringing in the ears occurs while taking with aspirin, consult your doctor about stopping the aspirin therapy until treatment is completed.
- Using tetracyclines may render oral contraceptives less effective. Use a different or additional form of contraception. Breakthrough bleeding has been reported.
- Inform your doctor if you are pregnant, become pregnant, are planning to become pregnant or if you are breastfeeding.
- Avoid alcohol while taking metronidazole and for one day afterward.
- This medication may cause dizziness. Use caution while driving or performing other tasks requiring alertness, coordination or physical dexterity.
- May cause photosensitivity (sensitivity to sunlight). Avoid prolonged exposure to the sun or other forms of ultraviolet light (eg, tanning beds). Use sunscreens and wear protective clothing until tolerance is determined.
- Bismuth subsalicylate may cause temporary and harmLess darkening of the tongue and stool. Stool darkening should not be confused with blood in the stool.
- Store at room temperature.

If you have any questions, consult your doctor, pharmacist, or health care provider.

	Generic Name *Brand Name Examples*	Supplied As	Generic Available
Rx	**Lansoprazole/Amoxicillin/Clarithromycin**		
	Prevpac	**Capsules and Tablets**: 30 mg[1]/500 mg[2]/500 mg[3]	No

[1] Lansoprazole (contains sucrose).
[2] Amoxicillin.
[3] Clarithromycin (contains povidone).

Type of Drug:

A combination of drugs used to reduce the risk of duodenal (stomach/intestinal) ulcer recurrence caused by infection with *H. pylori.*

How the Drug Works:

Lansoprazole reduces gastric (stomach) acid secretion by blocking the final step of gastric acid production. Amoxicillin kills bacteria by preventing the production of the bacterial cell wall. Clarithromycin suppresses the formation of vital proteins by bacteria, slowing bacterial growth.

Uses:

For the treatment of *H. pylori* infection and duodenal (stomach/intestinal) ulcers (active or 1-year history of a duodenal ulcer) to eradicate *H. pylori* and prevent ulcer recurrence.

Precautions:

Do not use in the following situations:

allergy to any ingredients
astemizole (*Hismanal* therapy)
cisapride (*Propulsid* therapy)
macrolide antibiotic allergy (eg, erythromycin)
penicillin allergy (eg, ampicillin)
pimozide (*Orap* therapy)

Use with caution in the following situations:

kidney impairment, severe
pregnancy (clarithromycin)

Diarrhea: If diarrhea develops during lansoprazole/amoxicillin/clarithromycin use, pseudomembranous colitis must be considered. This inflammatory condition of the colon is due to overgrowth of bacteria that are not killed by lansoprazole/amoxicillin/clarithromycin. The primary cause is a toxin produced by a bacteria known as *Clostridia difficile*. Colitis symptoms may range in severity from mild to life-threatening. Mild cases usually respond by stopping the antibiotic. In more severe cases, other antibiotics may need to be used.

Pregnancy: Adequate studies have not been done in pregnant women. Use only if clearly needed and potential benefits outweigh the possible hazards to the fetus.

Breastfeeding: Amoxicillin appears in breast milk. Because of the potential for serious adverse effects, decide whether to discontinue nursing or discontinue the drug. Consult your doctor.

Children: Safety and effectiveness in children have not been established.

Drug Interactions:

Tell your doctor or pharmacist if you are taking or if you are planning to take any over-the-counter or prescription medications or dietary supplements while taking this medicine. Doses of one or both drugs may need to be modified or a different drug may need to be prescribed. The following drugs and drug classes interact with this medicine.

Amoxicillin only

allopurinol (eg, *Zyloprim*)
contraceptives, oral (eg, *Ortho-Novum*, *Ovral*)
probenecid (*Benemid*)
tetracyclines (eg, tetracycline HCl)

Clarithromycin only

anticoagulants, oral (eg, warfarin)
astemizole (*Hismanal*)
benzodiazepines (eg, alprazolam, diazepam, midazolam, triazolam)
buspirone (*Buspar*)
cisapride (*Propulsid*)
cyclosporine (eg, *Neoral*, *Sandimmune*)
dihydroergotamine or ergotamine (eg, *Ergomar*)
disopyramide (*Norpace*)
fluconazole (*Diflucan*)
HMG-CoA reductase inhibitors (eg, atorvastatin, fluvastatin, simvastatin)
pimozide (*Orap*)
rifabutin (*Mycobutin*)
rifampin (*Rifadin*, *Rimactane*)
tacrolimus (*Prograf*)

Lansoprazole only

ampicillin (eg, *Omnipen*)
cyanocobalamin (eg, *Crystamine*)
drugs metabolized by the cytochrome P 450 system (eg, diazepam, ibuprofen, indomethacin, phenytoin, prednisone, propanolol)
iron salts
ketoconazole (*Nizoral*)
sucralfate (*Carafate*)

Lansoprazole and Clarithromycin only

carbamazepine (eg, *Tegretol*)
digoxin (eg, *Lanoxin*)
theophylline (eg, *Theo-Dur*)

Side Effects:

Every drug is capable of producing side effects. Many patients experience no, or minor, side effects. The frequency and severity of side effects depend on many factors including dose, duration of therapy, and individual susceptibility. Possible side effects include:

Digestive Tract: Diarrhea; taste changes; nausea; dark stools; sore tongue; mouth sores; tongue discoloration; dry mouth; thirst; indigestion; stomach pain or irritation; vomiting; rectal itching.

Urinary and Reproductive Tract: Vaginal inflammation; vaginal infection.

Nervous System: Headache; confusion; dizziness.

Other: Muscle pain; itching; rash; hives.

Guidelines for Use:

- Take exactly as prescribed.
- Each medication packet contains enough medication for 2 doses.
- Usual adult dose is 30 mg lansoprazole (1 pink and black capsule), 1 g amoxicillin (2 maroon and light pink capsules), and 500 mg clarithromycin (1 yellow tablet) taken together twice daily before eating (morning and evening) for 14 days. Swallow each pill whole.
- Failure to complete full course of therapy may allow the infection to return.
- If a dose is missed, take it as soon as possible. If several hours have passed or if it is nearing time for the next dose, do not double the dose in order to catch up unless advised to do so by your doctor. If more than 1 dose is missed, or if it is necessary to establish a new dosage schedule, contact your doctor or pharmacist.
- Discontinue therapy immediately and contact your doctor if any of the following occurs: Rash; hives; difficulty breathing; swelling of the eyelids, face, tongue, or lips.
- Notify your doctor if diarrhea develops while taking this medicine or shortly after completing therapy.
- This product contains a penicillin. Tell your doctor if you have a penicillin allergy.
- Decreased dosage or dosing intervals of clarithromycin may be necessary for patients with severe kidney impairment and will be determined by your doctor.
- Store at controlled room temperature (59° to 86°F). Protect from light and moisture.

If you have any questions, consult your doctor, pharmacist, or health care provider.

	Generic Name *Brand Name Examples*	Supplied As	Generic Available
	Cimetidine[1]		
otc	*Tagamet HB 200*	**Tablets**: 200 mg	Yes
Rx	*Tagamet*	**Tablets**: 200 mg, 300 mg, 400 mg, 800 mg	Yes
otc	*Tagamet HB 200*	**Suspension**: 200 mg/20 mL	No
Rx	*Tagamet*	**Liquid**: 300 mg/5 mL	Yes
	Famotidine[1]		
otc	*Pepcid AC*	**Tablets**: 10 mg	Yes
Rx	*Pepcid*	**Tablets**: 20 mg, 40 mg	Yes
otc	*Pepcid AC*[2]	**Tablets, chewable**: 10 mg	No
Rx	*Pepcid RPD*[2]	**Tablets, orally disintegrating**: 20 mg, 40 mg	No
otc	*Pepcid AC*	**Gelcaps**: 10 mg	Yes
Rx	*Pepcid*	**Powder for oral suspension**: 40 mg/5 mL	No
	Nizatidine		
Rx	*Axid Pulvules*	**Capsules**: 150 mg, 300 mg	No
otc	*Axid AR*	**Tablets**: 75 mg	No
	Ranitidine[1]	**Capsules**: 150 mg, 300 mg	Yes
otc	*Zantac 75*	**Tablets**: 75 mg	Yes
Rx	*Zantac 150*	**Tablets:** 150 mg	Yes
Rx	*Zantac 300*	**Tablets**: 300 mg	Yes
Rx	*Zantac 150 EFFERdose*[2]	**Tablets, effervescent:** 150 mg	No
Rx	*Zantac 150 EFFERdose*[2]	**Granules, effervescent**: 150 mg	No
Rx	*Zantac*	**Syrup:** 15 mg/mL	Yes
otc	**Famotidine/Calcium Carbonate/Magnesium Hydroxide**		
	Pepcid Complete	**Tablets, chewable**: 10 mg famotidine/800 mg calcium carbonate/165 mg magnesium hydroxide	No

[1] This product is also available as an injection.
[2] Contains phenylalanine.

Type of Drug:

Anti-ulcer drugs.

How the Drug Works:

Histamine H_2 antagonists reduce acid in the stomach by blocking one of the chemical transmitters (histamine) that is responsible for stimulating the production of stomach acid.

Uses:

To treat and prevent recurrence of duodenal (first part of small intestine) ulcers.

To treat gastric (stomach) ulcers.

To prevent recurrence of gastric (stomach) ulcers (ranitidine only).

To treat hypersecretory (increased acid secretion) conditions (eg, Zollinger-Ellison syndrome).

To treat erosive gastroesophageal reflux disease (GERD) (reflux of stomach acid into the food pipe, which causes heartburn).

To treat (over-the-counter cimetidine, famotidine, and nizatidine only) or prevent (over-the-counter cimetidine, famotidine, and nizatidine only) heartburn, acid indigestion, or sour stomach.

Unlabeled Use(s): Occasionally doctors may prescribe:

Cimetidine – To prevent stress-induced or peptic ulcers and certain types of respiratory complications (aspiration pneumonia) during anesthesia. It may be used to treat hyperparathyroidism (overactive parathyroid gland), indigestion, ringworm, herpes virus infections, chronic warts, chronic hives, allergic skin reactions, acetaminophen overdose, colorectal cancer, and abnormal hair growth in women.

Famotidine – To prevent stress-induced or peptic ulcers and certain types of respiratory conditions (aspiration pneumonia) during anesthesia. It may also be used to treat bleeding of the stomach or intestines.

Nizatidine – To treat peptic ulcers.

Ranitidine – To prevent stomach and intestinal damage associated with long-term nonsteroidal anti-inflammatory drug therapy (eg, ibuprofen), stress-induced or peptic ulcers, certain types of respiratory complications (aspiration pneumonia) during anesthesia, and to treat bleeding of the stomach or intestines.

Precautions:

Do not use in the following situations: Allergy to the histamine H_2 antagonist or any of its ingredients.

Use with caution in the following situations:

immunocompromised patients	liver disease
kidney disease	porphyria, acute (ranitidine only)

Phenylketonuric patients: Some of these products contain phenylalanine. Consult your doctor or pharmacist.

Pregnancy: There are no adequate and well-controlled studies in pregnant women. Use only if clearly needed and the potential benefits to the mother outweigh the possible hazards to the fetus.

Breastfeeding: Cimetidine, famotidine, nizatidine, and ranitidine appear in breast milk. Consult your doctor before you begin breastfeeding.

Children: Safety and effectiveness of nizatidine in children have not been established. Safety and effectiveness of famotidine in children under 1 year of age and of ranitidine in children under 1 month of age have not been established. Cimetidine use is not usually recommended in children less than 16 years of age. Over-the-counter cimetidine, famotidine, nizatidine, or ranitidine use is not recommended in children under 12 years of age.

Elderly: Safety and effectiveness are similar to younger patients. Elderly patients may have reduced kidney function. Smaller cimetidine doses may be prescribed.

Lab tests may be required to monitor therapy. Tests may include liver function tests.

Drug Interactions:

Tell your doctor or pharmacist if you are taking or if you are planning to take any over-the-counter or prescription medications or dietary supplements while taking histamine H_2 antagonists. Doses of one or both drugs may need to be modified or a different drug may need to be prescribed. The following drugs and drug classes interact with histamine H_2 antagonists:

cimetidine-

aminoquinolones (eg, chloroquine)
anticoagulants, oral (eg, warfarin)
beta-blockers (eg, propranolol)
benzodiazepines (except lorazepam, oxazepam, temazepam)
carbamazepine (eg, *Tegretol*)
carmustine (*BiCNU*)
dofetilide (*Tikosyn*)
hydantoins (eg, phenytoin)
ketoconazole (eg, *Nizoral*)
lidocaine (eg, *Xylocaine*)
metformin (eg, *Glucophage*)
moricizine (*Ethmozine*)
nifedipine (eg, *Procardia*)
pentoxifylline (*Trental*)
praziquantel (*Biltricide*)
procainamide (eg, *Pronestyl*)
quinidine (eg, *Quinora*)
theophylllines (eg, aminophylline)
tricyclic antidepressants (eg, amitriptyline)

famotidine and ranitidine-

ketoconazole (eg, *Nizoral*)

nizatidine-

charcoal
ketoconazole (eg, *Nizoral*)
ketoprofen (eg, *Orudis*)

Side Effects:

Every drug is capable of producing side effects. Many histamine H_2 antagonist users experience no, or minor, side effects. The frequency and severity of side effects depend on many factors including dose, duration of therapy, and individual susceptibility. Possible side effects include:

Digestive Tract: Diarrhea; constipation; stomach pain.

Nervous System: Confusion; hallucinations; fatigue; dizziness; sleepiness; headache.

Other: Impotence; breast enlargement (males).

Guidelines for Use:

- Dosage is individualized. Take exactly as prescribed or as directed by the package label.
- Do not stop taking or change the dose, unless directed by your doctor.
- May be taken without regard to meals.
- If a dose is missed, take it as soon as possible. If several hours have passed or it is nearing time for the next dose, do not double the dose to catch up, unless advised to do so by your doctor. If more than one dose is missed or it is necessary to establish a new dosage schedule, contact your doctor or pharmacist.
- It may be necessary to make lifestyle changes to assist in the treatment and prevention of ulcers and other digestive problems. These changes may include stress-reduction programs, exercise, and dietary changes.
- Notify your doctor if you experience diarrhea, dizziness, confusion, anxiety, depression, disorientation, agitation, or hallucinations.
- Notify your doctor if you experience any symptoms that suggest a bleeding ulcer, such as black, tarry stools or "coffee-ground" vomit.
- Antacids can be used at the same time to help control acid symptoms. Stagger doses of antacids and cimetidine or ranitidine.
- May cause dizziness or drowsiness. Use caution while driving or performing other tasks requiring alertness, coordination, or physical dexterity.
- *Over-the-counter products* — Contact your doctor if you have trouble swallowing or persistent stomach pain. Do not take maximum daily dosage for > 2 weeks continuously except under the advice and supervision of your doctor.
- *Famotidine suspension* — Shake well before using. Do not freeze. Discard unused suspension after 30 days.
- *Famotidine orally disintegrating tablets* — Keep tablets in unopened package until time of use. Open tablet blister pack with dry hands and place tablet on tongue to dissolve and be swallowed with saliva. No water is needed for taking the tablet.
- *Pepcid Complete* — Do not swallow tablets whole; chew completely before swallowing.
- *Ranitidine effervescent tablets or granules* — Dissolve in 6 to 8 oz of water before drinking.
- Inform your doctor if you are pregnant, become pregnant, are planning to become pregnant, or are breastfeeding.
- Lab tests or exams may be required to monitor therapy. Be sure to keep appointments.
- Store at room temperature in a tight container away from light.

If you have any questions, consult your doctor, pharmacist, or health care provider.

	Generic Name *Brand Name Example*	Supplied As	Generic Available
Rx	**Misoprostol**		
	Cytotec	**Tablets**: 100 mcg, 200 mcg	No

Type of Drug:

Anti-ulcer drug; prostaglandin.

How the Drug Works:

Misoprostol reduces the amount of acid secreted by the stomach. It also helps to protect the stomach lining.

Uses:

To prevent formation of stomach ulcers in patients who are taking nonsteroidal anti-inflammatory drugs (NSAIDs), including aspirin. For high-risk individuals taking NSAIDs who are at greater risk for developing ulcers or who are at greater risk for complications from ulcers (eg, elderly, patients with a history of ulcers, patients with other debilitating diseases).

Unlabeled Use(s): Occasionally doctors may prescribe misoprostol to treat duodenal ulcers or to reduce the risk of organ rejection in kidney transplants.

Precautions:

Do not use in the following situations:

allergy to misoprostol or any of its ingredients
allergy to prostaglandins
pregnancy

Use with caution in the following situations:

kidney disease
women of childbearing age

Diarrhea: Usually develops early in the course of therapy and resolves after approximately 8 days. Discontinuation may be required.

Pregnancy: Do not use during pregnancy. The risk of use in a pregnant woman clearly outweighs any possible benefit. Women of childbearing potential should not receive the drug unless the patient requires NSAIDs and is at high risk of complications from stomach ulcers associated with the use of NSAIDs, or is at high risk of developing stomach ulceration. Such patients may use misoprostol if the following criterla are met:

- The patient is capable of complying with effective contraceptive measures.
- The patient has received both oral and written warnings of the hazards of misoprostol, the risk of possible contraception failure, and the danger to other women of childbearing potential should the drug be taken by mistake.
- The patient has a negative serum pregnancy test within 2 weeks prior to beginning therapy.
- The patient will begin therapy only on the second or third day of the next normal menstrual period.

Breastfeeding: It is unlikely that misoprostol is excreted in breast milk. It is not known if active metabolites are excreted in breast milk. Do not use while breastfeeding; the drug may cause significant diarrhea in nursing infants.

Children: Safety and effectiveness in children under 18 years of age have not been established.

Drug Interactions:

Tell your doctor or pharmacist if you are taking or if you are planning to take any over-the-counter or prescription medications or dietary supplements with misoprostol. Doses of one or both drugs may need to be modified or a different drug may need to be prescribed. Antacids interact with misoprostol.

Side Effects:

Every drug is capable of producing side effects. Many misoprostol users experience no, or minor, side effects. The frequency and severity of side effects depend on many factors including dose, duration of therapy and individual susceptibility. Possible side effects include:

Digestive Tract: Diarrhea; nausea; vomiting; constipation; abdominal pain; gas; indigestion.

Other: Menstrual irregularities; painful menstruation; vaginal bleeding or spotting; headache.

Guidelines for Use:

- Take misoprostol for the duration of NSAID therapy.
- Contraceptive measures (birth control) are recommended during therapy.
- If a dose is missed, take it as soon as possible. If several hours have passed or if it is nearing time for the next dose, do not double the dose in order to "catch up" (unless advised to do so by your doctor). If more than one dose is missed, or it is necessary to establish a new dosage schedule, contact your doctor or pharmacist. Use exactly as prescribed.
- Diarrhea may occur early in the course of therapy. It may be minimized by taking after meals and at bedtime.
- Discontinue the drug and notify your doctor immediately if pregnancy is suspected. Misoprostol produces contractions of the uterus that may cause a miscarriage (see Precautions).
- Avoid magnesium-containing antacids.
- Never give your misoprostol tablets to anyone else.

If you have any questions, consult your doctor, pharmacist, or health care provider.

	Generic Name Brand Name Example	Supplied As	Generic Available
Rx	**Sucralfate**		
	Carafate	**Tablets:** 1 g	No
		Suspension: 10 mL/2 tsp.	No

Type of Drug:

Anti-ulcer drug.

How the Drug Works:

Sucralfate helps ulcers heal by forming a protective layer on the ulcer to serve as a barrier against acid, bile salts and enzymes present in the stomach and duodenum.

Uses:

For short-term treatment (up to 8 weeks) of duodenal ulcers.

For maintenance therapy for duodenal ulcer patients at reduced dosage after healing of acute ulcers.

Unlabeled Use(s): Occasionally doctors may prescribe sucralfate for oral and esophageal ulcers caused by chemotherapy or radiation, drug-induced digestive tract irritation, prevention of stress ulcers, long-term treatment of gastric (stomach) ulcers or inflammation of the esophagus. Sucralfate has also been shown to speed the healing of gastric ulcers.

Precautions:

Use with caution in the following situations:

dialysis
kidney disease

Pregnancy: Adequate studies have not been done in pregnant women. Use only if clearly needed and potential benefits outweigh the possible hazards to the fetus.

Breastfeeding: It is not known if sucralfate appears in breast milk. Consult your doctor before you begin breastfeeding.

Children: Safety and effectiveness in children have not been established.

Drug Interactions:

Tell your doctor or pharmacist if you are taking or if you are planning to take any over-the-counter or prescription medications or dietary supplements with sucralfate. Doses of one or both drugs may need to be modified or a different drug may need to be prescribed. The following drugs and drug classes interact with sucralfate.

antacids (aluminum-containing)
cimetidine (eg, *Tagamet)*
ciprofloxacin (eg, *Cipro)*
digoxin (eg, *Lanoxin)*
ketoconazole (eg, *Nizoral)*
norfloxacin (eg, *Noroxin)*
penicillamine (eg, *Cuprimine)*
phenytoin (eg, *Dilantin)*
rantidine (eg, *Zantac)*
tetracycline (eg, *Sumycin)*
theophylline (eg, *Theolair)*
warfarin (eg, *Coumadin)*

Side Effects:

Every drug is capable of producing side effects. Many sucralfate users experience no, or minor, side effects. The frequency and severity of side effects depend on many factors including dose, duration of therapy and individual susceptibility. Possible side effects include:

Other: Red or black stools; coughing up or vomiting bright red or "coffee ground-like" material.

Digestive Tract: Constipation; diarrhea; nausea; stomach discomfort; indigestion.

Skin: Rash; itching; hives.

Other: Dry mouth; back pain; dizziness; sleepiness; facial swelling; difficulty breathing.

Guidelines for Use:

- Take on an empty stomach at least 1 hour before meals and at bedtime.
- Do not take antacids 30 minutes before or after taking sucralfate.
- If a dose is missed, take it as soon as possible. If several hours have passed or if it is nearing time for the next dose, do not double the dose in order to "catch up" (unless advised to do so by your doctor). If more than one dose is missed, or it is necessary to establish a new dosage schedule, contact your doctor or pharmacist. Use exactly as prescribed.
- If red or black stools, coughing up or vomiting bright red or "coffee ground-like" material occur, contact your doctor.
- Duodenal ulcer is a chronic recurrent disease. While a single course of therapy of 4 to 8 weeks may completely heal the ulcer, ulcers may occur again and may be more severe.
- *Suspension* — Shake well before using.

If you have any questions, consult your doctor, pharmacist, or health care provider.

	Generic Name *Brand Name Examples*	Supplied As	Generic Available
otc	**Charcoal**		
	Charcoal	**Tablets:** 325 mg	No
	Charcoal	**Capsules:** 260 mg	No
	Charcocaps	**Capsules:** 260 mg activated charcoal	No
otc	**Simethicone**		
	Phazyme, Phazyme 95	**Tablets:** 60 mg, 95 mg	No
	Extra Strength Gas-X, Gas-X, Mylicon, Mylicon-125	**Tablets, chewable:** 40 mg, 80mg, 125 mg	No
	Phazyme 125	**Capsules:** 125 mg	No
	Flatulex, Mylicon, Phazyme	**Drops:** 40 mg/0.6 mL	Yes

Type of Drug:

Anti-gas agents.

How the Drug Works:

"Flatulence" refers to excessive amounts of air or gases in the stomach or intestines that result in abdominal discomfort (eg, pain, fullness, bloating). The air or gases are trapped in small bubbles. Simethicone relieves discomfort due to flatulence by helping the formation of larger gas bubbles which are easier to eliminate by belching or passing rectally.

Excessive air and gases that can accumulate in the stomach or intestines will bind to charcoal. As the charcoal is eliminated from the body, the air and gases are also eliminated, resulting in relief.

Other substances that bind to charcoal include certain poisons, drugs and naturally occurring substances. By binding to charcoal, absorption of these substances into the bloodstream is reduced. This can be an advantage in the treatment of poisonings but a disadvantage when it interferes with the effects of a drug.

Uses:

Charcoal: For relief of intestinal gas, diarrhea and intestinal distress associated with indigestion.

For prevention of itching associated with kidney dialysis treatment and intestinal motility testing.

To treat certain poisonings and drug overdoses by decreasing absorption into the bloodstream and speeding up removal of the poisons and drugs from the body.

Simethicone: To relieve abdominal discomfort due to excess air or gases in the stomach, intestines or both. Conditions where antiflatulents may be helpful include: Surgery, peptic ulcer, air swallowing, spastic or irritable bowel, acid indigestion and diverticulitis.

Precautions:

Children: Do not use charcoal in children under 3.

Drug Interactions:

Tell your doctor or pharmacist if you are taking or if you are planning to take any over-the-counter or prescription medications or dietary supplements with charcoal. Doses of one or both drugs may need to be modified or a different drug may need to be prescribed. The following drugs and drug classes interact with charcoal.

acetaminophen (eg, *Tylenol)*
barbiturates (eg, phenobarbital)
carbamazepine (eg, *Tegretol)*
digitoxin (eg, *Crystodigin)*
digoxin (eg, *Lanoxin)*
furosemide (eg, *Lasix)*
glutethimide
hydantoins (eg, phenytoin)
methotrexate (eg, *Rheumatrex)*
nizatidine (*Axid)*
phenothiazines (eg, chlorpromazine)
propoxyphene (eg, *Darvon)*
salicylates (eg, aspirin)
sulfonamides (eg, sulfisoxazole)
sulfones
sulfonylureas (eg, glipizide)
tetracyclines (eg, doxycycline)
theophyllines (eg, aminophylline)
tricyclic antidepressants (eg, amitriptyline)
valproic acid (eg, *Depakene)*

Guidelines for Use:

Charcoal:

- Take either 2 hours before or 1 hour after taking other oral drugs, because many drugs bind to charcoal in the stomach or intestines and never reach the bloodstream.
- Swallow 2 tablets whole after eating, as needed. Do not chew. Do not exceed 20 tablets per day.
- Stool will turn black. This is normal.

Simethicone:

- Take 1 to 2 tablets as needed after each meal and at bedtime. Do not exceed 4 tablets in 24 hours unless directed by your doctor.
- *Gas-X* — Do not exceed 6 tablets in 24 hours.
- *Phazyme* — Do not exceed 3 softgels per day.
- Swallow softgels whole with water.
- Drops — Shake well before using.
- Chewable tablets — Chew thoroughly before swallowing.
- Store at room temperature. Protect from moisture. Keep out of reach of children.

If you have any questions, consult your doctor, pharmacist, or health care provider.

	Generic Name *Brand Name Examples*	Pancreatin (mg)	Lipase (units)	Protease (units)	Amylase (units)
otc	**Pancreatin**				
	Donnazyme Tablets[1]	500	1000	12,500	12,500
	Hi-Vegi-Lip Tablets[2]	600	4800	60,000	60,000
	Pancreatin 4X Tablets[1], *Pancrezyme 4X Tablets*[2]	2400	12,000	60,000	60,000
	Pancreatin 8X Tablets[1]	7200	22,500	180,000	180,000
Rx	**Pancrelipase**				
	Cotazym Capsules[1]		8000	30,000	30,000
	Cotazym-S Capsules[1]		5000	20,000	20,000
	Creon 5 Capsules[1]		5000	18,750	16,600
	Creon 10 Capsules[1]		10,000	37,500	33,200
	Creon 20 Capsules[1]		20,000	75,000	66,400
	Lipram 4500 Capsules[1], *Ultrase Capsules*[1]		4500	25,000	20,000
	Lipram-CR10 Capsules[1]		10,000	37,500	33,200
	Lipram-CR20 Capsules[1]		20,000	75,000	66,400
	Lipram-PN10 Capsules[1]		10,000	30,000	30,000
	Lipram-PN16 Capsules[1]		16,000	48,000	48,000
	Lipram-UL12 Capsules[1], *Ultrase MT 12 Capsules*[1]		12,000	39,000	39,000
	Lipram-UL18 Capsules[1], *Ultrase MT 18 Capsules*[1]		18,000	58,500	58,500
	Lipram-UL20 Capsules[1], *Ultrase MT 20 Capsules*[1]		20,000	65,000	65,000
	Pancrease Capsules[1]		4500	25,000	20,000
	Pancrease MT 4 Capsules[1]		4000	12,000	12,000
	Pancrease MT 10 Capsules[1]		10,000	30,000	30,000

Generic Name *Brand Name Examples*	Pancreatin (mg)	Lipase (units)	Protease (units)	Amylase (units)
Pancrease MT 16 Capsules[1]		16,000	48,000	48,000
Pancrease MT 20 Capsules[1]		20,000	44,000	56,000
Zymase Capsules[1]		12,000	24,000	24,000

[1] Derived from pork.
[2] Derived from vegetables.

Type of Drug:

Digestive enzymes.

How the Drug Works:

Pancreatic enzymes (lipase, protease, and amylase) help digest and absorb the fats, proteins, and carbohydrates (starches and sugars) from food. Lipase accelerates the breakdown of fat, protease accelerates the breakdown of protein, and amylase accelerates the breakdown of starch. Pancreatin and pancrelipase, derived from pork or vegetable sources, contain all three of these enzymes.

Uses:

To replace pancreatic enzymes in patients who do not produce normal amounts (eg, patients with cystic fibrosis, chronic pancreatitis, removal of the pancreas, obstruction of the pancreatic duct, and pancreatic insufficiency).

To treat excess fat in a bowel movement due to malabsorption syndrome or stomach bypass surgery.

To test pancreatic function.

Precautions:

Do not use in the following situations:

allergy to pork (pork source products)
allergy to these medicines or any of their ingredients
pancreatic disease, chronic acute exacerbation
pancreatitis, acute

Powder: Do not inhale or spill powder on skin because it may irritate skin or mucous membranes. Inhalation can precipitate an allergic reaction, coughing spell, bronchospasm, nasal irritation, watery eyes, or asthma attack. If it is necessary to open the capsules, wear a mask and gloves.

Pregnancy: Adequate studies have not been done in pregnant women. Use only if clearly needed and potential benefits to the mother outweigh the possible hazards to the fetus.

Breastfeeding: It is not known if pancreatin or pancrilipase are excreted in human milk. Consult your doctor before you begin breastfeeding.

Lab tests may be required during treatment. Tests may include stool fat content.

Drug Interactions:

Tell your doctor or pharmacist if you are taking or if you are planning to take any over-the-counter or prescription medications or dietary supplements with digestive enzymes. Doses of one or both drugs may need to be modified or a different drug may need to be prescribed. The following drugs and drug classes interact with digestive enzymes:

calcium carbonate (eg, *Tums*)
iron supplements (eg, *Feosol*)
magnesium hydroxide (eg, *Milk of Magnesia*)

Side Effects:

Every drug is capable of producing side effects. Many digestive enzyme users experience no, or minor, side effects. The frequency and severity of side effects depend on many factors including dose, duration of therapy, and individual susceptibility. Possible side effects include:

Digestive Tract: Nausea; stomach cramps; diarrhea; constipation; vomiting; stomach pain or burning; belching; gas; intestinal obstruction; anal irritation; stool abnormalities (eg, green stool); bloating.

Other: Abnormal smell and taste; rash; mouth sores; abnormal blood counts; fainting; sore throat; mouth irritation.

Guidelines for Use:

- Consult your doctor and product labeling for individual dosing instructions. Do not exceed the recommended dosage.
- Take with meals and snacks. Do not take on an empty stomach.
- Do not inhale or spill powder on skin. Inhaling may cause an allergic reaction, coughing spell, bronchospasm, nasal irritation, or asthma attack.
- Do not crush or chew coated tablets or capsules. If an intact capsule cannot be swallowed whole, it may be opened and the contents taken with a small amount of food that does not require chewing and has a pH less than 5.5 (eg, applesauce). Do not mix with dairy products. Consume immediately after mixing. Wear a mask and gloves while handling open capsules.
- Drink a full glass of water or juice with medicine to insure swallowing.
- Avoid using antacids or supplements containing calcium carbonate or magnesium hydroxide while taking digestive enzymes. Antacids may negate the beneficial effect of the enzymes.
- Maintain an adequate fluid intake (at least 64 ounces per day) while taking this medicine.
- Pancrelipase may interfere with the absorption of folic acid. Women who are pregnant or planning to become pregnant during treatment with this medicine should take folic acid supplements.
- Do not change the dose or stop taking unless advised to do so by your doctor.
- Do not change brands without consulting with your pharmacist or doctor.
- Discontinue use and notify your doctor if allergy symptoms (eg, rash, wheezing, shortness of breath) develop.
- Vegetarians or patients with allergies to pork can use the *Hi-Vegi-Lip* tablets or *Pancrezyme 4X* tablets, which are of vegetable origin.
- Lab tests may be required to monitor therapy. Be sure to keep appointments.
- Store at room temperature (59° to 86°F) in a cool, dry place.

If you have any questions, consult your doctor, pharmacist, or health care provider.

	Generic Name Brand Name Examples	Supplied As	Generic Available
Rx	**Metoclopramide**[1]		
	Clopra, Maxolon, Octamide, Reclomide, Reglan	**Tablets:** 10 mg	Yes
	Reglan[2]	**Syrup:** 5 mg/tsp	No
	Metoclopramide Intensol	**Concentrated solution:** 10 mg/mL	No

[1] Some of these products may be available as an injection.
[2] Sugar free.

Type of Drug:

Digestive tract (gastrointestinal) stimulant.

How the Drug Works:

These drugs stimulate the contractions/movements of the stomach and small intestine.

Uses:

To treat symptoms of diabetic gastroparesis (eg, nausea, vomiting, heartburn, persistent fullness after meals and appetite loss).

To treat the nausea and vomiting associated with cancer chemotherapy.

To treat gastroesophageal reflux (reflux of stomach contents into the throat).

Unlabeled Use(s): Occasionally doctors may prescribe metoclopramide to improve breast milk secretion, to improve response to migraine medications, for nausea and vomiting, to treat anorexia nervosa, to treat gastric ulcers, for intestinal blockage after operations, diabetic cystoparesis (weak bladder), and bleeding from the esophagus.

Precautions:

Do not use in the following situations:
- allergy to metoclopramide
- epilepsy or seizure conditions
- intestinal obstruction or perforation
- pheochromocytoma (adrenal tumor)
- stomach or intestinal bleeding

Use with caution in the following situations:
- breast cancer, history
- diabetes

Diabetics: Metoclopramide affects the movement of food from the stomach to the intestines and also the absorption of food. Insulin dose may need to be adjusted.

Pregnancy: Metoclopramide crosses the placenta. Studies in pregnant women have not shown a risk to the fetus. However, no drug should be used during pregnancy unless clearly needed.

Breastfeeding: Metoclopramide appears in breast milk. Consult your doctor before you begin breastfeeding.

Children: Metoclopramide has been used in children. However, muscle spasms of the neck, face and jaw, and involuntary movement of the eyes have been reported more commonly in children.

Drug Interactions:

Tell your doctor or pharmacist if you are taking or if you are planning to take any over-the-counter or prescription medications or dietary supplements with metoclopramide. Doses of one or both drugs may need to be modified or a different drug may need to be prescribed The following drugs and drug classes interact with metoclopramide.

acetaminophen (eg, *Tylenol)*
alcohol
anticholinergics (eg, atropine)
butyrophenone (eg, *Haldol)*
cimetidine (*Tagamet)*
cyclosporine (eg, *Sandimmune)*
digoxin (eg, *Lanoxin)*
hypnotics (eg, phenobarbital)
insulin
levodopa (eg, *Larodopa)*
narcotic pain relievers (eg, codeine)
phenothiazines (eg, promethazine)
sedatives (eg, flurazepam)
succinylcholine (eg, *Anectine)*
tetracycline (eg, *Sumycin)*
thioxanthene(eg, *Navane)*
tranquilizers (eg, *Valium)*

Side Effects:

Every drug is capable of producing side effects. Many metoclopramide users experience no, or minor, side effects. The frequency and severity of side effects depend on many factors including dose, duration of therapy and individual susceptibility. Possible side effects include:

Digestive Tract: Nausea; diarrhea.

Nervous System: Restlessness; drowsiness; fatigue; weakness; involuntary trembling, jerky movements; shaking muscle spasms; dizziness; anxiety; sleeplessness; headache; depression; hallucinations; facial grimacing; slurred speech; teeth grinding.

Other: Increased blood pressure; excessive or spontaneous flow of breast milk; stopping of menstrual period; nipple tenderness; breast enlargement in males; impotence in males; rash; asthma-like symptoms; impaired vision; uncontrolled urination or bowel movements; difficult breathing; decreased blood pressure; neuroleptic malignant syndrome (NMS).

Guidelines for Use:

- May cause drowsiness. Use caution when driving or performing other tasks requiring alertness.
- Take 30 minutes before each meal.
- Notify your doctor if involuntary movement of the eyes, face or limbs occurs.

If you have any questions, consult your doctor, pharmacist, or health care provider.

	Generic Name *Brand Name Examples*	Supplied As	Generic Available
Rx	**Esomeprazole Magnesium**		
	Nexium	**Capsules, delayed-release**: 20 mg, 40 mg	No
Rx	**Lansoprazole**		
	Prevacid	**Capsules, delayed-release**: 15 mg, 30 mg	No
Rx	**Omeprazole**		
	Prilosec	**Capsules, delayed-release**: 10 mg, 20 mg, 40 mg	No
Rx	**Pantoprazole Sodium**		
	Protonix[1]	**Tablets, delayed-release**: 20 mg, 40 mg	No
Rx	**Rabeprazole Sodium**		
	Aciphex	**Tablets, delayed-release**: 20 mg	No

[1] Also available as an injection.

Type of Drug:

Proton pump inhibitors (PPIs); gastric (stomach) acid secretion inhibitors.

How the Drug Works:

PPIs reduce gastric acid secretion by blocking the final step of acid production by the stomach lining.

Uses:

For short-term treatment (less than or equal to 8 weeks) of gastroesophageal reflux disease (GERD, the reflux of stomach contents into the food pipe, which can cause heartburn); and to maintain healing and reduce relapse rates of heartburn symptoms in patients with erosive or ulcerative GERD.

For short-term treatment (4 to 8 weeks for omeprazole; less than or equal to 4 weeks for lansoprazole and rabeprazole) of active duodenal ulcers; to maintain healing of duodenal ulcers (lansoprazole only).

For short-term treatment (4 to 8 weeks for omeprazole; less than or equal to 8 weeks for lansoprazole) of active benign gastric ulcers; to treat and reduce the risk of gastric ulcers associated with the use of nonsteroidal anti-inflammatory drugs (NSAIDs) (lansoprazole only).

For short-term treatment (4 to 8 weeks for esomeprazole and omeprazole; less than or equal to 8 weeks for lansoprazole) or to maintain healing of inflammation and erosion of the food pipe (erosive esophagitis).

In combination therapy with antibiotics for treatment and elimination of *Helicobacter pylori* infection and associated active duodenal ulcer and to reduce the risk of ulcer recurrence (esomeprazole, omeprazole, and lansoprazole only).

For long-term treatment of hypersecretory (increased acid secretion) conditions (eg, Zollinger-Ellison syndrome) (omeprazole, lansoprazole, and rabeprazole only).

Unlabeled Use(s): These agents may increase the effectiveness of pancreatic enzyme replacements used to treat the "fatty stools" of patients with cystic fibrosis. Omeprazole has been prescribed to treat laryngitis.

Precautions:

Do not use in the following situations: Allergy to the PPI or any of its ingredients.

Use with caution in the following situations:
Asian patients (omeprazole only)
liver disease, severe

Pregnancy: There are no adequate and well-controlled studies in pregnant women. Use only if clearly needed and the potential benefits to the mother outweigh the possible hazards to the fetus.

Breastfeeding: It is not known if proton pump inhibitors appear in breast milk. Consult your doctor before you begin breastfeeding.

Children: Safety and effectivenss in children have not been established.

Drug Interactions:

Tell your doctor or pharmacist if you are taking or planning to take any over-the-counter or prescription medications or dietary supplements with PPIs. Doses of one or both drugs may need to be modified or a different drug may need to be prescribed. The following drugs and drug classes interact with PPIs:

benzimidazoles (eg, albendazole) (rabeprazole only)
benzodiazepines (eg, diazepam) (omeprazole only)
cyclosporine (eg, *Neoral*)
digoxin (eg, *Lanoxin*)
iron salts (eg, ferrous sulfate)
ketoconazole (eg, *Nizoral*)
phenytoin (eg, *Dilantin*) (omeprazole only)
sucralfate (eg, *Carafate*)
theophylline (eg, *Theo-Dur*) (omeprazole only)

Side Effects:

Every drug is capable of producing side effects. Many PPI users experience no, or minor, side effects. The frequency and severity of side effects depend on many factors including dose, duration of therapy, and individual susceptibility. Possible side effects include:

Digestive Tract: Diarrhea; nausea; vomiting; stomach pain; constipation; gas; belching; dry mouth.

Nervous System: Dizziness; headache; weakness; sleeplessness.

Other: Rash; back pain; upper respiratory tract infection; cough; high blood sugar.

Guidelines for Use:

- Dosage is individualized. Take exactly as prescribed.
- Do not change the dose or stop taking this medicine unless advised to do so by your doctor.
- Usually taken once daily, at least 1 hour before a meal. Dosages and dosing regimens may vary depending on condition being treated.
- Take rabeprazole after the morning meal when treating duodenal ulcers.
- Take pantoprazole with or without regard to food.
- These medicines must be taken daily to be effective in treating and preventing acid-related gastrointestinal diseases. Do not take on an "as needed" basis.
- Antacids may be used as needed with these medicines.
- Do not chew, crush, or split capsules or tablets. Swallow whole. If you have difficulty swallowing esomeprazole or lansoprazole capsules, they may be opened, sprinkled on 1 tablespoon of applesauce, *Ensure* pudding, cottage cheese, yogurt, or strained pears, and swallowed immediately without chewing the granules. Lansoprazole capsules can also be emptied into a small glass of either orange or tomato juice (60 mL; approximately 2 oz), mixed briefly, and swallowed immediately. To ensure complete ingestion, rinse the glass with 4 or more ounces of juice and swallow the contents immediately.
- If a dose is missed, take it as soon as possible. If several hours have passed or it is nearing time for the next dose, do not double the dose to catch up, unless advised to do so by your doctor. If more than one dose is missed, or it is necessary to establish a new dosage schedule, contact your doctor or pharmacist.
- Inform your doctor if you are pregnant, become pregnant, plan on becoming pregnant, or are breastfeeding.
- PPIs should be taken at least 30 minutes prior to taking sucralfate.
- Store at controlled room temperature (59° to 86°F) in a tightly closed container. Protect from light and moisture.

If you have any questions, consult your doctor, pharmacist, or health care provider.

	Brand Name Examples	Supplied As
Rx	*Ku-Zyme*	**Capsules**: 30 mg amylase, 6 mg protease, 1200 USP units lipase, 2 mg cellulase
Rx	*Kutrase*	**Capsules**: 30 mg amylase, 6 mg protease, 1200 USP units lipase, 2 mg cellulase, 0.0625 mg hyoscyamine sulfate, 15 mg phenyltoloxamine citrate
otc	*Papaya Enzyme*	**Tablets, chewable**: 15 mg papain (from papaya leaves or fruit), 2 mg protease, 2 mg amylase

Type of Drug:

Miscellaneous digestive products; digestive enzymes.

How the Drug Works:

Components of these combinations include:

Digestive enzymes: Papain aids in protein digestion. Pancreatic enzymes (eg, amylase, protease, lipase) aid in the intestinal digestion of starch, protein, and fats, respectively (see the Digestive Enzymes monograph in this chapter). Cellulase aids in fiber digestion.

Anticholinergics: (eg, hyoscyamine) relieve spasm and reduce diarrhea and cramping (see the Anticholinergics/Antispasmodics monograph in this chapter).

Antihistamines: Phenyltoloxamine citrate is used for its sedative effects.

Uses:

For the symptomatic treatment of various digestive problems, to supplement deficiencies of natural digestive enzymes, and for a variety of vague digestive disorders (eg, nervous indigestion).

Precautions:

Do not use in the following situations:

- allergy to the digestive enzyme or any of its ingredients (eg, pork protein)
- chronic pancreatic disease, acute exacerbation of
- glaucoma (*Kutrase* only)
- intestinal atony, elderly and debilitated patients (*Kutrase* only)
- myasthenia gravis (*Kutrase* only)
- obstructive disease of the gastrointestinal tract (*Kutrase* only)
- pancreatitis, acute
- paralytic ileus (*Kutrase* only)
- toxic megacolon complicating ulcerative colitis (*Kutrase* only)
- ulcerative colitis, severe
- unstable cardiovascular states in acute hemorrhage (*Kutrase* only)
- urinary obstruction (*Kutrase* only)

Use Kutrase with caution in the following situations:

autonomic neuropathy
cardiac arrythmia (abnormal heart rhythm)
congestive heart failure
coronary artery disease
hiatal hernia associated with reflux esophagitis
hypertension (high blood pressure)
hyperthyroidism (overactive thyroid)
kidney disease
tachycardia (fast heartbeat)

Pregnancy: There are no adequate and well-controlled studies in pregnant women. Use only if clearly needed and the potential benefits to the mother outweigh the possible hazards to the fetus.

Breastfeeding: Hyoscyamine sulfate appears in breast milk. It is not known if the digestive enzymes or phenytoloxamine appear in breast milk. Consult your doctor.

Drug Interactions:

Tell your doctor or pharmacist if you are taking or if you are planning to take any over-the-counter or prescription medications or dietary supplements while taking a digestive product. Doses of one or both drugs may need to be modified or a different drug may need to be prescribed.

Side Effects:

Every drug is capable of producing side effects. Many digestive product users experience no, or minor, side effects. The frequency and severity of side effects depend on many factors including dose, duration of therapy, and individual susceptibility. Possible side effects include: Dizziness; drowsiness; blurred vision; urinary retention; dry mouth; loose stools; allergic reaction.

Guidelines for Use:

- Dosage is individualized. Check package labeling or consult your doctor or pharmacist.
- Take with or after meals or snacks.
- If capsules are opened, avoid inhalation of the powder. Sensitive patients could experience an allergic reaction.
- If a dose is missed, wait until the next meal to take. Do not double the dose to catch up, unless advised to do so by your doctor.
- Reduce dose if loose stools occur.
- *Kutrase* may cause drowsiness, dizziness, or blurred vision. Use caution while driving or performing other tasks requiring alertness, coordination, or physical dexterity.
- Inform your doctor if you are pregnant, become pregnant, plan on becoming pregnant, or are breastfeeding.
- Store at room temperature (59° to 86°F) in a tight-fitting container.

If you have any questions, consult your doctor, pharmacist, or health care provider.

GALLSTONE DISSOLVING AGENTS, ORAL

Generic Name *Brand Name Example*	Supplied As	Generic Available
Rx **Ursodiol (Ursodeoxycholic Acid)**		
Actigall	**Capsules**: 300 mg	Yes

Type of Drug:

Gallstone dissolving agent.

How the Drug Works:

Ursodiol helps dissolve cholesterol gallstones. It is most effective if the gallstones are small or "floatable." Patients must have a working gallbladder.

Uses:

To dissolve cholesterol gallstones smaller than 20 mm in diamoter in patients who are not good candidates for surgery because of systemic disease, advanced age, or reaction to general anesthesia.

For the prevention of gallstones in obese patients experiencing rapid weight loss.

Precautions:

Do not use in the following situations:

- allergy to bile acids
- allergy to ursodiol or any of its ingredients
- biliary-gastrointestinal fistula
- biliary obstruction
- calcified cholesterol gallstones
- cholangitis
- cholecystitis, acute and unremitting
- gallstone pancreatitis
- liver disease, chronic
- radiolucent bile pigment stones
- radiopaque stones

Use with caution in the following situations: Liver disease.

Gallstone recurrence: Treatment requires months of therapy. Complete dissolution does not always occur and recurrence within 5 years has been observed in less than or equal to 50% of patients. Consider alternative therapy if possible.

Pregnancy: There are no adequate and well-controlled studies in pregnant women. Use only if clearly needed and the potential benefits to the mother outweigh the possible hazards to the fetus.

Breastfeeding: It is not known if ursodiol appears in breast milk. Consult your doctor before you begin breastfeeding.

Children: Safety and effectiveness have not been established.

Lab tests will be required during treatment. Tests include liver function.

Drug Interactions:

Tell your doctor or pharmacist if you are taking or planning to take any over-the-counter or prescription medications or dietary supplements with ursodiol. Doses of one or both drugs may need to be modified or a different drug may need to be prescribed. The following drugs and drug classes interact with ursodiol:

antacids, aluminum-based (eg, aluminum hydroxide)
bile acid sequestrants (eg, cholestyramine)
clofibrate (eg, *Atromid-S*)
contraceptives, oral (eg, *Ortho-Novum*)
estrogens (eg, estradiol)

Side Effects:

Every drug is capable of producing side effects. Many patients experience no, or minor, side effects. The frequency and severity of side effects depend on many factors including dose, duration of therapy and individual susceptibility. Possible side effects include.

Digestive Tract: Nausea; vomiting; diarrhea; severe abdominal pain (especially in upper right side); indigestion; constipation; gas; gallbladder inflammation; inflammation of the mouth.

Nervous System: Headache; fatigue; anxiety; depression; sleep problems.

Skin: Rash; itching; hives; dry skin; sweating; hair thinning.

Other: Metallic taste; joint and muscle pain; cough; runny nose; back pain; mouth sores.

Guidelines for Use:

- Use exactly as prescribed. Otherwise, the gallstones may dissolve very slowly or not at all.
- If a dose is missed, take it as soon as possible. If several hours have passed or if it is nearing time for the next dose, do not double the dose in order to "catch up" (unless advised to do so by your doctor). If more than one dose is missed or it is necessary to establish a new dosage schedule, contact your doctor or pharmacist.
- Carefully follow the diet your doctor has prescribed.
- Contact your doctor if diarrhea, stomach pain, severe sudden pain in upper right side, nausea or vomiting occurs.
- Therapy usually takes months. Complete dissolving of gallstones does not occur in all patients, and recurrence within 5 years occurs in up to 50% of patients.
- The long-term effects (more than 24 months) of this medicine are not known.
- Lab tests will be required to monitor therapy. Be sure to keep appointments.
- Store below 86°F.

If you have any questions, consult your doctor, pharmacist, or health care provider.

Generic Name *Brand Name Examples*	Supplied As	Generic Available
Monoctanoin		
Rx *Moctanin*	**Infusion**	No

Type of Drug:

Gallstone dissolving agent.

How the Drug Works:

Monoctanoin is a liquid given through a catheter into the bile duct. Gallstones (found in the gallbladder or bile duct) may remain in the bile duct after surgical removal of the gallbladder. If these stones are made of cholesterol and are too large to pass out of the body on their own, monoctanoin may help dissolve them. Complete dissolution is more likely when there is a single stone than when there are multiple stones.

Uses:

To dissolve cholesterol gallstones that remain in the bile duct after the gallbladder has been removed. Used when other means of removing the stones have failed, or in patients who are not good candidates for surgery.

Precautions:

Do not use in the following situations:

- biliary tract infection, significant
- duodenal ulcer, recent
- jejunitis, history
- liver disease
- pancreatitis, acute
- porto-systemic shunting

Use with caution in the following situations: Obstructive jaundice.

Pregnancy: Adequate studies have not been done in pregnant women, or animal studies may have shown a risk to the fetus. Use only if clearly needed and potential benefits outweigh the possible hazards to the fetus.

Breastfeeding: It is not known if monoctanoin appears in breastmilk. Consult your doctor before you begin breastfeeding.

Children: Safety and effectiveness have not been established.

Lab tests may be required to monitor therapy. Lab tests include liver function tests.

Side Effects:

Every drug is capable of producing side effects. Many patients experience no, or minor, side effects. The frequency and severity of side effects depend on many factors including dose, duration of therapy and individual susceptibility. Possible side effects include: Stomach pain; nausea; vomiting; diarrhea; appetite loss; loose stools; indigestion; fever.

GALLSTONE DISSOLVING AGENT, INFUSION

Guidelines for Use:

- This agent must be given by your doctor through a catheter or tube into the bile duct. It is given continuously for 2 to 10 days.
- Tell your doctor immediately if stomach pain, nausea, diarrhea, vomiting, fever, appetite loss, chills, severe pain in the upper right side, or yellowing or skin or eyes occurs.

If you have any questions, consult your doctor, pharmacist, or health care provider.

	Generic Name *Brand Name Examples*	Supplied As	Generic Available
otc	**Methylcellulose**		
	Citrucel	**Powder:** 2 g/heaping tbsp	No
	Citrucel Sugar Free[1]	**Powder:** 2 g, 52 mg phenylalanine/heaping tbsp	No
	Unifiber	**Powder**	No
otc	**Barley Malt Extract**		
	Maltsuprex	**Tablets:** 750 mg	No
	Maltsuprex	**Powder:** 8 g/tbsp	No
	Maltsuprex	**Liquid:** 16 g/tbsp	No
otc	**Polycarbophil**		
	Equalactin, Fiberall, Mitrolan	**Tablets, chewable:** 500 mg, 1250 mg	No
	FiberCon[2]*, Fiber-Lax, FiberNorm, Konsyl Fiber*	**Tablets:** 500 mg, 625 mg	No
otc	**Psyllium**		
	Fiberall Natural Flavor[1]*, Fiberall Orange Flavor*[1]	**Powder:** 3.4 g with wheat bran, < 10 mg sodium, < 60 mg potassium, < 6 calories/dose	No
	Hydrocil Instant[1]	**Powder:** 3.5 g	No
	Konsyl[1]	**Powder:** 100% psyllium	No
	Konsyl-Orange	**Powder:** 3.4 g/tbsp	No
	Maalox Daily Fiber Therapy	**Powder:** ≈ 3.4 g, sucrose, 35 calories/12 g	No
	Metamucil	**Powder:** ≈ 3.4 g, 3.5 g carbohy-drates, < 10 mg sodium, 31 mg potassium, 14 calories/dose	No
	Metamucil Orange Flavor	**Powder:** ≈ 3.4 g, 7.1 g carbohydrates, < 10 mg sodium, 31 mg potassium, 30 calories/dose	No
	Metamucil Sugar Free[1]	**Powder:** ≈ 3.4 g, 0.3 g carbohydrates, < 10 mg sodium, 31 mg potassium, 1 calorie/dose	No
	Mylanta Natural Fiber Supplement	**Powder:** 3.4 g	No
	Restore[4]	**Powder:** 3.4 g/dose, orange flavor, saccharine, sucrose	

Generic Name *Brand Name Examples*	**Supplied As**	**Generic Available**
Metamucil	**Wafers:** ≈ 1.7 g, 18 g carbohydrate, 18 mg sodium, 4.5 g fat, 96 calories/dose	No
Fiberall	**Wafers:** 3.4 g, 0.03 g sodium, 78 calories/wafer	No
Alramucil [3]	**Effervescent powder:** 3.6 g, citric acid, sucrose, saccharin, potassium bicarbonate, sodium bicarbonate, 4 calories, < 0.01 g sodium/packet	No
Effer-syllium	**Effervescent powder:** 3 g/rounded tsp	No
Metamucil Lemon-Lime Flavor	**Effervescent powder:** ≈ 3.4 g, sodium and potassium bicarbonate, < 10 mg sodium, calcium carbonate, 290 mg potassium, 1 calorie/dose	No
Metamucil Orange Flavor	**Effervescent powder:** ≈ 3.4 g, sodium and potassium bicarbonate, < 10 mg sodium, 310 mg potassium, 1 calorie/dose	No
Perdiem Fiber [5]	**Granules:** 4.03 g 1.8 mg sodium, 36.1 mg potassium, 4 calories/rounded tsp	No
Serutan	**Granules:** 2.5 g, < 0.03 g sodium/heaping tsp	No
Siblin	**Granules:** 2.5 g/rounded tsp	No

[1] Sugar free.
[2] Sodium free.
[3] Also available in orange flavor.
[4] Also available sugar free.
[5] Dye free.

Laxatives promote bowel emptying. Nonprescription laxatives are frequently misued due to lack of understanding of normal bowel function. Restrict self-medication to short-term therapy of constipation. Chronic use of laxatives (particularly stimulants) may lead to dependence. Prior to laxative use, consider living habits affecting bowel function including disease state and drug history. Rational therapy and prevention of constipation include: Adequate fluid intake (4 to 6 glasses of water daily), proper dietary habits including sufficient bulk or roughage, responding to the urge to defecate and daily exercise.

Type of Drug:

Bulk laxative.

How the Drug Works:

Bulk laxatives hold water in the stool and dissolve and swell in the intestinal fluids to stimulate intestinal activity. They are considered to be the safest laxative products for the treatment of constipation and to help maintain normal bowel function in some digestive disorders.

Uses:

For short-term treatment of constipation.

Psyllium: To treat irritable bowel syndrome, diverticular disease, spastic colon and hemorrhoids.

Polycarbophil: To treat acute nonspecific diarrhea or diarrhea associated with conditions such as diverticulitis or irritable bowel syndrome.

Unlabeled Use(s): Occasionally doctors may prescribe psyllium in combination with a dietary program for the reduction of cholesterol levels.

Precautions:

Do not use in the following situations:

allergy to any ingredients of these products
abdominal pain, undiagnosed
abdominal surgery
appendicitis symptoms (nausea, vomiting, stomach pain)
intestinal obstruction
intestinal ulcers, stenosis or adhesions
stool impaction

Use with caution in the following situations:

kidney stones

Rectal bleeding or failure of the laxative to produce a bowel movement can indicate a more serious condition which requires medical attention.

Laxatives that contain sodium should be used with caution by patients with heart
disease, high blood pressure, conditions in which swelling occurs, or patients who are on low-sodium diets.

Long-term use: These products should not be used over one week except by the advice of your doctor.

Failure to drink adequate fluids with these products can result in intestinal obstruction or fecal impaction.

Pregnancy: Bulk laxatives may be used during pregnancy, but only under the direction of a doctor.

Drug Interactions:

Tell your doctor or pharmacist if you are taking or if you are planning to take any over-the-counter or prescription medications or dietary supplements with this medicine. Doses of one or both drugs may need to be modified or a different drug may need to be prescribed. Tetracycline (eg, *Achromycin V*) interacts with polycarbophil.

Side Effects:

Every drug is capable of producing side effects. Many patients experience no, or minor, side effects. The frequency and severity of side effects depends on many factors including dose, duration of therapy and individual susceptibility. Possible side effects include:

Digestive Tract: Diarrhea; nausea; vomiting; rectal irritation; bloating; gas; stomach pain; intestinal or rectal obstruction.

Other: Dizziness; weakness; fainting; sweating; pounding in the chest.

Guidelines for Use:

- Use exactly as prescribed.
- Take with a full glass of water or juice.
- Do not use if abdominal pain, nausea or vomiting occurs.
- Contact your doctor if unrelieved constipation, rectal bleeding, muscle cramps or pain, weakness, or dizziness occurs.
- Bulk laxatives are the safest laxatives. However, laxative use is only a temporary measure. When normal bowel habits return, stop use of these products unless instructed otherwise by your doctor. Prolonged, frequent or excessive use may result in dependence or electrolyte imbalance.

If you have any questions, consult your doctor, pharmacist, or health care provider.

	Generic Name *Brand Name Examples*	Supplied As	Generic Available
	Glycerin, USP		
otc	*Sani-Supp*	**Suppositories:** Glycerin and sodium stearate	Yes
	Glycerin Rectal Liquid		
otc	*Fleet Babylax*	**Liquid:** 4 mL glycerin applicators	No

Laxatives promote bowel emptying. Nonprescription laxatives are frequently misued due to lack of understanding of normal bowel function. Restrict self-medication to short-term therapy of constipation. Chronic use of laxatives (particularly stimulants) may lead to dependence. Prior to laxative use, consider living habits affecting bowel function including disease state and drug history. Rational therapy and prevention of constipation include: Adequate fluid intake (4 to 6 glasses of water daily), proper dietary habits including sufficient bulk or roughage, responding to the urge to defecate and daily exercise.

Type of Drug:

Hyperosmolar laxatives.

How the Drug Works:

Glycerin irritates the colon and draws water into the colon, stimulating bowel movements.

Uses:

For short-term treatment of constipation.

To treat constipation in infants and children.

Precautions:

Do not use in the following situations:

- abdominal surgery
- allergy to any ingredient of these products
- appendicitis symptoms (nausea, vomiting, abdominal pain)
- intestinal obstruction
- stool impaction

Frequent use of laxatives and inadequate fluid can cause an imbalance in fluid and electrolyte levels. Symptoms may include muscle cramps, muscle weakness or dizziness.

Rectal bleeding or failure of the laxative to produce a bowel movement can indicate a more serious condition which requires medical attention.

Children: Physical manipulation of a glycerin suppository in infants will usually promote bowel movements. Because of this, side effects are usually minimal.

Side Effects:

Every drug is capable of producing side effects. Many patients experience no, or minor, side effects. The frequency and severity of side effects depends on many factors including dose, duration of therapy and individual susceptibility. Possible side effects include:

Circulatory System: Pounding of the chest (palpitations).

Other: Bowel cramping; stomach cramps; irritation of the rectal area; diarrhea; nausea; vomiting; weakness; dizziness; fainting; sweating; bloating; gas; excessive bowel activity.

Guidelines for Use:

- Laxative use is only a temporary measure. Do not use longer than one week. Stop use of these products when normal bowel habits return. Prolonged, frequent or excessive use may result in dependence or electrolyte imbalance.
- *Suppositories* — Insert one suppository high in the rectum and retain 15 minutes. It does not need to melt to produce laxative action.
- *Rectal liquid* — With gentle, steady pressure, insert stem with tip pointing towards naval. Squeeze unit until nearly all the liquid is expelled. Remove. A small amount of liquid will remain in unit.
- Do not use if abdominal pain, nausea or vomiting occurs.
- Contact your doctor if unrelieved constipation, rectal bleeding, muscle cramps or pain, weakness or dizziness occurs.
- Effects usually occur within 30 minutes.

If you have any questions, consult your doctor, pharmacist, or health care provider.

Generic Name *Brand Name Examples*	**Supplied As**	**Generic Available**
Lactulose *Cephulac, Cholac, Chronulac, Constilac, Constulose, Duphalac, Enulose*	**Syrup:** 10 g/tbsp	Yes

Laxatives promote bowel emptying. Nonprescription laxatives are frequently misused due to lack of understanding of normal bowel function. Restrict self-medication to short-term therapy of constipation. Chronic use of laxatives (particularly stimulants) may lead to dependence. Prior to laxative use, consider living habits affecting bowel function including disease state and drug history. Rational therapy and prevention of constipation include: Adequate fluid intake (4 to 6 glasses of water daily), proper dietary habits including sufficient bulk or roughage, responding to the urge to defecate and daily exercise.

Type of Drug:

Laxative.

How the Drug Works:

Lactulose draws water into the colon to create bulk and stimulate a bowel movements.

Uses:

Chronulac, Constilac, Duphalac — For the treatment of constipation.

Cephulac, Cholac, Enulose — To prevent and treat portal-systemic encephalopathy (liver disease), including the stages of hepatic precoma and coma.

Precautions:

Do not use in the following situations:
- allergy to any ingredient in these products
- low galactose-sugar diet

Use with caution in the following situations:
- diabetes
- electrocautery procedures
- other laxatives, use

Lab tests: Elderly or debilitated patients who receive lactulose for more than 6 months should have electrolyte levels (eg, potassium chloride, carbon dioxide) done periodically.

Diabetes: This product contains sugar. Use with caution.

Pregnancy: Studies in pregnant women or in animals have been judged not to show a risk to the fetus. However, no drug should be used during pregnancy unless clearly needed.

Breastfeeding: It is not known if lactulose appears in breastmilk. Consult your doctor before you begin breastfeeding.

Children: Safety and effectiveness have not been established.

Drug Interactions:

Tell your doctor or pharmacist if you are taking or if you are planning to take any over-the-counter or prescription medications or dietary supplements while taking this medicine. Doses of one or both drugs may need to be modified or a different drug may need to be prescribed. The following drugs and drug classes interact with this medicine.

antacids
neomycin (eg, *Mycifradin*)

Side Effects:

Every drug is capable of producing side effects. Many patients experience no, or minor, side effects. The frequency and severity of side effects depends on many factors including dose, duration of therapy and individual susceptibility. Possible side effects include: Gas and belching; stomach pain; bowel cramping; diarrhea; nausea; vomiting.

Guidelines for Use:

- *Chronulac, Constilac, Duphalac* — Usual adult dose is 1 to 2 tablespoonfuls (15 to 30 mL) daily. Do not take more than 4 tablespoonfuls (60 mL) daily.
- *Cephulac, Cholac, Enulose* — Usual adult dose is 2 to 3 tablespoonfuls (30 to 45 mL) three to four times daily. Adjust dosage every day or two to produce 2 or 3 soft stools daily.
- May be mixed with fruit juice, water or milk to improve taste.
- May cause belching, gas or cramps. Notify your doctor if these effects become bothersome or if unusual diarrhea occurs.
- Do not take other laxatives while on lactulose therapy.
- Prevention of constipation includes: Adequate fluid intake (4 to 6 glasses of water daily), proper dietary habits including sufficient bulk or roughage, responding to the urge to defecate and daily exercise.
- Effects may not be seen for 24 to 48 hours.
- *Duphalac* — Darkening of syrup may occur. This is not significant.
- Store below 86°F. Do not freeze.

If you have any questions, consult your doctor, pharmacist, or health care provider.

Generic Name / *Brand Name Examples*	Supplied As	Generic Available
otc **Mineral Oil**		
Mineral Oil	**Liquid, heavy**	Yes
Neo-Cultol	**Jelly:** Refined mineral oil	No
Milkinol	**Emulsion:** Mineral oil in an emulsifying base	No
Kondremul Plain[1]	**Emulsion:** Mineral oil with Irish moss, acacia and glycerin	No

[1] Sugar free.

Laxatives promote bowel emptying. Nonprescription laxatives are frequently misused due to lack of understanding of normal bowel function. Restrict self-medication to short-term therapy of constipation. Chronic use of laxatives (particularly stimulants) may lead to dependence. Prior to laxative use, consider living habits affecting bowel function including disease state and drug history. Rational therapy and prevention of constipation include: Adequate fluid intake (4 to 6 glasses of water daily), proper dietary habits including sufficient bulk or roughage, responding to the urge to defecate and daily exercise.

Type of Drug:

Lubricant or emollient laxative, liquid petrolatum.

How the Drug Works:

Mineral oil lubricates the colon and softens feces by coating it and holding water in the fecal mass.

Uses:

For short-term treatment of constipation, or relief of fecal impaction.

To prevent straining at the stool in patients who have heart conditions or who have had recent rectal surgery.

Precautions:

Do not use in the following situations:

abdominal surgery
allergy to any ingredient in these products
appendicitis symptoms (nausea, vomiting, abdominal pain)
docusate use
intestinal obstruction

Frequent use of laxatives and inadequate fluid can cause an imbalance in fluid and electrolyte levels. Symptoms may include muscle cramps, muscle weakness or dizziness.

Rectal bleeding or failure of the laxative to produce a bowel movement can indicate a more serious condition which requires medical attention.

Lipid pneumonia can occur if mineral oil is accidentally inhaled into the lunges, especially when the patient is lying down. Patients who are young, elderly or have difficulty swallowing are at greater risk for this problem.

Anal or rectal surgery: Mineral oil can leak from the rectum and cause itching, hemorrhoids irritation and discomfort.

Pregnancy: Mineral oil can decrease absorption of fat-soluable vitamins (A, D, E, K) from the diet or from vitamin tablets. Consult your doctor before using these products.

Drug Interactions:

Tell your doctor or pharmacist if you are taking or if you are planning to take any over-the-counter or prescription medications while taking this medicine. Doses of one or both drugs may need to be modified or a different drug may need to be prescribed. The following drugs and drug classes interact with this medicine.

surfactant laxatives (eg, docusate)
vitamin A
vitamin D
vitamin E
vitamin K

Side Effects:

Every drug is capable of producing side effects. Many patients experience no, or minor, side effects. The frequency and severity of side effects depends on many factors including dose, duration of therapy and individual susceptibility. Possible side effects include:

Digestive Tract: Nausea; vomiting; diarrhea; stomach pain; bloating; gas; bowel cramping.

Nervous System: Weakness; dizziness; fainting.

Other: Irritation, itching or bleeding of rectal area; hemorrhoids; anal seepage; sweating; pounding of the chest (palpitations); muscle cramps or pain.

Guidelines for Use:

- The usual adult dose is 5 to 45 mL.
- Take with a full glass or water or juice.
- These products are most effective when taken on an empty stomach.
- Although the usual directions are to give the dose at bedtime, caution is advised because of lipid pneumonia (see Precautions).
- Laxative use is only a temporary measure. Do not use longer than one week. Stop use of these products when normal bowel habits return. Prolonged, frequent or excessive use may result in dependence or electrolyte imbalance.
- Do not use if abdominal pain, nausea or vomiting occurs.
- Contact your doctor if unrelieved constipation, rectal bleeding, muscle cramps or pain, weakness or dizziness occurs.
- Mineral oil may seep from the rectum, soiling clothing and causing itching, irritation, hemorrhoids and rectal discomfort. This is less likely to happen with the emulsion.
- Prevention of constipation includes: Adequate fluid intake (4 to 6 glasses of water daily), proper dietary habits including sufficient bulk or roughage, responding to the urge to defecate and daily exercise.
- Effects usually occur in 6 to 8 hours. Plan accordingly.

If you have any questions, consult your doctor, pharmacist or healthcare provider.

	Generic Name *Brand Name Examples*	Supplied As
	Brand Name Examples	Supplied As
otc	*Citrate of Magnesia*	**Solution:** Magnesium citrate
otc	*Epsom Salt*	**Granules:** Magnesium sulfate
otc	*Fleet Phospho-soda*[1], *Sodium Phosphates*[1]	**Solution:** 18 g sodium phosphate and 48 g sodium biphosphate/100 mL
otc	*Milk of Magnesia - Concentrated, Phillips' Milk of Magnesia, Concentrated*	**Liquid:** Magnesium hydroxide
otc	*Milk of Magnesia, Phillips' Milk of Magnesia*	**Liquid:** Magnesium hydroxide, 7% to 8.5% aqueous suspension

[1] Sugar free.

Laxatives promote bowel emptying. Nonprescription laxatives are frequently misued due to lack of understanding of normal bowel function. Restrict self-medication to short-term therapy of constipation. Chronic use of laxatives (particularly stimulants) may lead to dependence. Prior to laxative use, consider living habits affecting bowel function including disease state and drug history. Rational therapy and prevention of constipation include: Adequate fluid intake (4 to 6 glasses of water daily), proper dietary habits including sufficient bulk or roughage, responding to the urge to defecate and daily exercise.

Type of Drug:

Saline laxatives.

How the Drug Works:

Saline laxatives cause water to accumulate in the intestine, thereby increasing pressure in the intestine and causing bowel movements.

Uses:

For short-term treatment of constipation.

To clean out the bowel before bowel examinations or bowel surgery.

Precautions:

Do not use in the following situations:

abdominal surgery
allergy to any ingredient in these products
appendicitis symptoms (nausea, vomiting, abdominal pain)
intestinal obstruction
stool impaction

Use with caution in the following situations:

congestive heart failure
high blood pressure
kidney disease
sodium-restricted diet
swelling/water retention

Frequent use of laxatives and inadequate fluid can cause an imbalance in fluid and electrolyte levels. Symptoms may include muscle cramps, muscle weakness or dizziness.

Rectal bleeding or failure of the laxative to produce a bowel movement can indicate a more serious condition which requires medical attention.

Pregnancy: Saline laxatives can cause an electrolyte imbalance (eg, potassium). Use of a bulk or stool-softening laxative is preferred. Consult your doctor.

Drug Interactions:

Tell your doctor or pharmacist if you are taking or if you are planning to take any over-the-counter or prescription medications while taking this medicine. Doses of one or both drugs may need to be modified or a different drug may need to be prescribed. Tetracyclines interact with magnesium-containing products.

Side Effects:

Every drug is capable of producing side effects. Many patients experience no, or minor, side effects. The frequency and severity of side effects depends on many factors including dose, duration of therapy and individual susceptibility. Possible side effects include:

Digestive Tract: Nausea; vomiting; diarrhea; stomach pain; bloating; gas; bowel cramping; griping.

Nervous System: Weakness; dizziness; fainting.

Other: Irritation of rectal area; sweating; pounding of the chest (palpitations); sweating; rectal bleeding; muscle cramps or pain; electrolyte imbalance (eg, potassium).

Guidelines for Use:

- Take with a full glass of water or juice.
- Laxative use is only a temporary measure. Do not use longer than one week. Stop use of these products when normal bowel habits return. Prolonged, frequent or excessive use may result in dependence or electrolyte imbalance.
- Do not use if abdominal pain, nausea or vomiting occurs.
- Contact your doctor if unrelieved constipation, rectal bleeding, muscle cramps or pain, weakness or dizziness occurs.
- Prevention of constipation includes: Adequate fluid intake (4 to 6 glasses of water daily), proper dietary habits including sufficient bulk or roughage, responding to the urge to defecate and daily exercise.
- Effects usually occur in 30 minutes to 3 hours.
- Store magnesium citrate solutions in the refrigerator to retain potency and to improve taste.

If you have any questions, consult your doctor, pharmacist or healthcare provider.

	Generic Name *Brand Name Examples*	How Supplied	Generic Available
otc	**Bisacodyl**		
	Feen-a-mint	**Tablets:** 5 mg	No
	Dulcagen, Dulcolax, Fleet	**Tablets, enteric coated:** 5 mg	Yes
	Bisacodyl Uniserts, Bisco-Lax, Dulcagen, Dulcolax, Fleet	**Suppositories:** 10 mg	Yes
otc	**Calcium Salts of Sennosides A & B**		
	Ex-Lax Gentle Nature, Senexon	**Tablets:** 5.6 mg, 20 mg	No
otc	**Cascara Sagrada**	**Tablets:** 325 mg	Yes
	Cascara Sagrada Aromatic Fluid Extract[1]	**Liquid**	Yes
otc	**Castor Oil**	**Liquid**	Yes
	Purge	**Liquid:** 95%	Yes
	Emulsoil[2]	**Emulsion:** 95%	No
	Fleet Flavored Castor Oil	**Emulsion:** 67%	No
	Neoloid[2]	**Oil:** 36.4%	No
otc	**Phenolphthalein**		
	Alophen Pills, Espotabs, Ex-Lax Maximum Relief, Ex-Lax Unflavored, Feen-a-mint, Lax Pills, Laxative Pills, Modane, Prulet	**Tablets:** 60 mg, 90 mg, 97.2 mg, 130 mg, 135 mg	No
	Evac-U-Gen, Ex-Lax Chocolated, Feen-a-mint, Feen-a-mint Chocolated, Medilax	**Tablets, chewable:** 65 mg, 90 mg, 97.2 mg, 120 mg	No
	Evac-U-Lax Tablets	**Wafers, chewable:** 80 mg	No
	Feen-a-mint	**Gum:** 97.2 mg	No
otc	**Senna**		
	Black-Draught, Senexon, Senna-Gen, Senolax, Senokot, Senokotxtra	**Tablets:** 8.6 mg, 217 mg, 374 mg, 600 mg	No
	Black-Draught[3]*, Gentlax, Senokot*	**Granules:** 15 mg/tsp, 1.65 g/½ tsp	No
	Senokot	**Suppositories:** 652 mg	No
	Dosalax[1]*, Senokot*[1]	**Syrup:** 8.8 mg/tsp	No

Generic Name *Brand Name Examples*	How Supplied	Generic Available
Dr. Caldwell Senna[1], *Fletcher's Castoria*[1]	**Liquid:** 33.3 mg/mL	No

[1] Contains alcohol.
[2] Sugar free.
[3] Contains the dye tartrazine.

Laxatives promote bowel emptying. Nonprescription laxatives are frequently misued due to lack of understanding of normal bowel function. Restrict self-medication to short-term therapy of constipation. Chronic use of laxatives (particularly stimulants) may lead to dependence. Prior to laxative use, consider living habits affecting bowel function including disease state and drug history. Rational therapy and prevention of constipation include: Adequate fluid intake (4 to 6 glasses of water daily), proper dietary habits including sufficient bulk or roughage, responding to the urge to defecate and daily exercise.

Type of Drug:

Irritant or stimulant laxatives.

How the Drug Works:

Stimulant laxatives act directly on the intestines, irritating the digestive tract lining and stimulating intestinal activity.

Uses:

For short-term treatment of constipation.

To clean out the bowel before bowel examinations or bowel surgery.

Precautions:

Do not use in the following situations:

- abdominal pain, undiagnosed
- abdominal surgery
- allergy to any ingredient of these products
- appendicitis symptoms (nausea, vomiting, abdominal pain)
- children under 10 years of age (bisacodyl only)
- intestinal obstruction
- stool impaction
- ulcerative lesions of colon (bisacodyl only)

Use with caution in the following situations:

- multiple enemas (bisacodyl only)

Frequent use of laxatives and inadequate fluid can cause an imbalance in fluid and electrolyte levels. Symptoms may include muscle cramps, muscle weakness or dizziness.

Rectal bleeding or failure of the laxative to produce a bowel movement can indicate a more serious condition which requires medical attention.

Discoloration of the urine (yellow-brown, pink-red, red-violet or red-brown) may occur with phenolphthalein, cascara sagrada or senna.

Tartrazine: Some of these products may contain the dye tartrazine (FD&C Yellow No. 5) which can cause allergic reactions in certain individuals. Check package label when available or consult your doctor or pharmacist.

Pregnancy: Adequate studies have not been done in pregnant women, or animal studies may have shown a risk to the fetus. Use only if clearly needed and potential benefits outweigh the possible hazards to the fetus. Improper use of these products can cause a dangerous electrolyte imbalance. Use of a bulk or stool-softening laxative is preferred. *Castor oil* — Do not use during pregnancy. It can produce premature labor.

Breastfeeding: Cascara sagrada appears in breast milk. Use can result in diarrhea in the infant. Consult your doctor before you begin breastfeeding.

Children: Do not use bisacodyl tannex in children under 10 years of age.

Drug Interactions:

Tell your doctor or pharmacist if you are taking or if you are planning to take any over-the-counter or prescription medications or dietary supplements while taking these products. Doses of one or both drugs may need to be modified or a different drug may need to be prescribed. Antacids and milk interact with bisacodyl.

Side Effects:

Every drug is capable of producing side effects. Many patients experience no, or minor, side effects. The frequency and severity of side effects depends on many factors including dose, duration of therapy and individual susceptibility. Possible side effects include:

Digestive Tract: Nausea; vomiting; stomach pain; bowel cramping; diarrhea; bloating; gas.

Nervous System: Weakness; dizziness; fainting.

Other: Irritation of the rectal area; sweating; pounding of the chest (palpitations).

Guidelines for Use:

- Use exactly as prescribed.
- Laxative use is only a temporary measure. Do not use longer than one week. Stop use of these products when normal bowel habits return. Prolonged, frequent or excessive use may result in dependence or electrolyte imbalance.
- Take with a full glass of water or juice.
- *Bisacodyl* — Swallow tablets whole (do not crush). Do not take within 1 hours of antacids or milk.
- *Suspensions and emulsions* — Shake well before use.
- Do not use if abdominal pain, nausea or vomiting occurs.
- Contact your doctor if unrelieved constipation, rectal bleeding, muscle cramps or pain, weakness or dizziness occurs.
- *Phenolphthalein* may cause a skin reaction. Stop using if this occurs.
- *Biscodyl suppositories* may cause proctitis and inflammation. Do not take these for long-term use.
- Pink-red, red-violet, yellow-brown or red-brown discoloration of the urine may occur, particularly with phenophthalein, senna or cascara sagrada.
- Some of these products may contain the dye tartrazine (FD&C Yellow No. 5) which can cause allergic reactions in certain individuals. Check package label when available or consult your doctor or pharmacist.
- Prevention of constipation includes: Adequate fluid intake (4 to 6 glasses of water daily), proper dietary habits including sufficient bulk or roughage, responding to the urge to defecate and daily exercise.
- Effects usually occur in 6 to 10 hours with most of these products, except castor oil (2 to 4 hours) and bisacodyl suppositories (15 to 60 minutes). Plan accordingly.
- Store at room temperature.

If you have any questions, consult your doctor, pharmacist, or health care provider.

	Generic Name *Brand Name Examples*	How Supplied	Generic Available
otc	**Docusate Calcium**		
	Correctol, Correctol Extra Gentle	**Tablets:** 5 mg	No
	Correctol, DC Softgels, Pro-Cal-Sof, Surfak Liquigels[1]*, Sulfalax Calcium*	**Capsules:** 5 mg, 50 mg, 240 mg	Yes
	Correctol	**Capsules, soft gel:** 100 mg	No
otc	**Docusate Potassium**		
	Diocto-K, Kasof	**Capsules:** 100 mg, 240 mg	No
otc	**Docusate Sodium**		
	Dialose	**Tablets:** 100 mg	No
	Colace, Colace-T, Disonate, Dioeze, DOK, DOS Softgel, D-S-S, Modane Soft, Pro-Sof Capsules, Regulax SS	**Capsules:** 50 mg, 100 mg, 240 mg, 250 mg	Yes
	Colace[1]*, Diocto, Disonate, DOK, Silace*	**Syrup:** 50 mg/Tsb, 60 mg/Tsb	Yes
	Colace, Diocto, Disonate, DOK	**Liquid:** 150 mg/Tsb	Yes
	Doxinate[1]	**Solution:** 50 mg/mL	No

[1] Contains alcohol.

Laxatives promote bowel emptying. Nonprescription laxatives are frequently misued due to lack of understanding of normal bowel function. Restrict self-medication to short-term therapy of constipation. Chronic use of laxatives (particularly stimulants) may lead to dependence. Prior to laxative use, consider living habits affecting bowel function including disease state and drug history. Rational therapy and prevention of constipation include: Adequate fluid intake (4 to 6 glasses of water daily), proper dietary habits including sufficient bulk or roughage, responding to the urge to defecate and daily exercise.

Type of Drug:

Surfactant laxatives; fecal softeners.

How the Drug Works:

Fecal softeners soften the stool by mixing fat and water into fecal matter. They are helpful when feces are hard or dry, or in conditions where passage of a firm stool is painful.

Uses:

For short-term treatment of constipation.

To soften the stool in patients who should not strain at the stool (eg, patients who have had a heart attack or recent rectal surgery).

Precautions:

Do not use in the following situations:

- abdominal pain, undiagnosed
- abdominal surgery
- allergy to any ingredient of these products
- appendicitis symptoms (nausea, vomiting, abdominal pain)
- intestinal obstruction
- mineral oil use (docusate sodium only)
- stool impaction

Frequent use of laxatives and inadequate fluid can cause an imbalance in fluid and electrolyte levels. Symptoms may include muscle cramps, muscle weakness or dizziness.

Rectal bleeding or failure of the laxative to produce a bowel movement can indicate a more serious condition which requires medical attention.

Pregnancy: Adequate studies have not been done in pregnant women, or animal studies may have shown a risk to the fetus. Use only if clearly needed and potential benefits outweigh the possible hazards to the fetus.

Breastfeeding: It is not known if docusate sodium appears in breast milk. Consult your doctor before you begin breastfeeding.

Drug Interactions:

Tell your doctor or pharmacist if you are taking or if you are planning to take any over-the-counter or prescription medications or dietary supplements while taking these products. Doses of one or both drugs may need to be modified or a different drug may need to be prescribed. Mineral oil interacts with docusate.

Side Effects:

Every drug is capable of producing side effects. Many patients experience no, or minor, side effects. The frequency and severity of side effects depends on many factors including dose, duration of therapy and individual susceptibility. Possible side effects include:

Digestive Tract: Nausea; vomiting; stomach pain; bowel cramping; diarrhea; bloating; gas.

Other: Weakness; dizziness; fainting; irritation of the rectal area; sweating; pounding of the chest (palpitations).

Guidelines for Use:

- Use exactly as prescribed.
- Laxative use is only a temporary measure. Do not use longer than one week. Stop use of these products when normal bowel habits return. Prolonged, frequent or excessive use may result in dependence or electrolyte imbalance.
- Take with a full glass of water or juice.
- Do not use if abdominal pain, nausea or vomiting occurs.
- Contact your doctor if unrelieved constipation, rectal bleeding, muscle cramps or pain, weakness or dizziness occurs.
- *Liquid* — Give in milk, fruit juice or infant formula to mask taste.
- *Enemas* — Add 1 or 2 tsp liquid to a retention or flushing enema.
- Prevention of constipation includes: Adequate fluid intake (4 to 6 glasses of water daily), proper dietary habits including sufficient bulk or roughage, responding to the urge to defecate and daily exercise.
- Effects usually occur in 24 to 72 hours with most of these products. Plan accordingly.
- Store at room temperature.

If you have any questions, consult your doctor, pharmacist, or health care provider.

LAXATIVE COMBINATIONS – CAPSULES AND TABLETS

	Brand Name Examples	Docusate (mg)	Senna Combinations (mg)	Phenophthalein (mg)	Casanthranol (mg)	Cascara Sagrada (mg)	Sodium Carboxy-methylcellulose (mg)	Generic Available
otc	*Gentlax S Tablets*	50[1]	8.6[2]					No
otc	*Senokot-S Tablets*	50[1]	187					No
otc	*Doxidan Capsules, Docucal-P Softgels*	60[3]		65				No
otc	*Ex-Lax Extra Gentle Pills*	75[1]		65				No
otc	*Phillip's LaxCaps, Phillip's Laxative Gelcaps*	83[1]		90				No
otc	*Colax Tablets, Correctol Tablets, Dialoce Plus Capsules and Tablets, Disolan Capsules, Feen-a-mint Pills, Femilax Tablets, Modane Plus Tablets*	100[1]		65				No
otc	*Unilax Capsules*	230[1]		130				No
otc	*Disanthrol Capsules, Doxidan LiquiGels, Genasoft Plus Softgels ,Peri-Colace Capsules, Peri-Dos Softgels, Pro-Sof Plus Capsules, Regulace Capsules*	100[1]			30			Yes
otc	*Dialose Plus Capsules, Diocto-K Plus Capsules, Dioctolose Plus Capsules, DSMC Plus Capsules*	100[4]			30			Yes
otc	*Disoplex Capsules*	100[1]					400	No
otc	*Disolan Forte Capsules*	100[1]			30		400	No
otc	*Herbal Laxative Tablets*[8]		125[5]			20[6]		No

	Brand Name Examples	Docusate (mg)	Senna Combinations (mg)	Phenophthalein (mg)	Casanthranol (mg)	Cascara Sagrada (mg)	Sodium Carboxy-methylcellulose (mg)	Generic Available
otc	*Veracolate Tablets*			32.4		75[7]		No
otc	*Nature's Remedy Tablets*					150		No

[1] As sodium.
[2] As sennosides.
[3] As calcium.
[4] As potassium.
[5] As senna leaves.
[6] As cascara sagada bark.
[7] As extract.
[8] Sugar free.

Laxatives promote bowel emptying. Nonprescription laxatives are frequently misued due to lack of understanding of normal bowel function. Restrict self-medication to short-term therapy of constipation. Chronic use of laxatives (particularly stimulants) may lead to dependence. Prior to laxative use, consider living habits affecting bowel function including disease state and drug history. Rational therapy and prevention of constipation include: Adequate fluid intake (4 to 6 glasses of water daily), proper dietary habits including sufficient bulk or roughage, responding to the urge to defecate and daily exercise.

Type of Drug:

Laxative combinations.

Uses:

To treat constipation.

For more information on laxative ingredients, see docusate, and senna and phenolphthalein. Casanthranol is a stimulant laxative used in laxative combinations.

Guidelines for Use:

- Use exactly as prescribed.
- Take 1 or 2 at bedtime with a full glass of water.
- Do not use in the presense of abdominal pain, nausea or vomiting.
- Laxative use if only a tempeorary measure; do not use longer than 1 week. When regularity returns, discontiue use. Prolonged, frequent or excessive use may result in dependence or electrolyte imbalance.
- Contact your doctor if unrelieved constipation rectal bleeding or symptoms of electrolyte imbalance (eg, muscle cramps or pain, weakness, dizziness) occurs.
- Pink-red, red-violet or red-brown discoloration of alkaline urine may occur with cascara sagrada, phenolphthalein or senna.
- Prevention of constipation includes: Adequate fluid intake (4 to 6 glasses of water daily), proper dietary habits including sufficient bulk or roughage, responding to the urge to defecate and daily exercise.

If you have any questions, consult your doctor, pharmacist, or health care provider.

	Brand Name Examples	Supplied As	Generic Available
otc	*Agoral*[1]	**Emulsion:** 4.2 m mineral oil and 0.2 g phenolphthalein per Tbsp in an emlulsion with agar, tragacanth, egg albumin, acacia and glycerin	No
otc	*Haley's M-O*[1]	**Emulsion:** 900 magnesium hydroxide and 3.75 mL mineral oil/Tbsp	No
otc	*Kondremul w/Phenolphthalein*	**Emulsion:** 55% mineral oil and 150 mg phenolphthalein per Tbsp with Irish moss as an emulsifier	No
otc	*Liqui-Doss*[1,2]	**Emulsion:** Mineral oil in an emulsifying base	No
otc	*Black-Draught*[3,4]	**Syrup:** 90 mg per Tbsp casanthranol with senna extract, fluid rhubarb aromatic, methyl salicylate and menthol	No
otc	*Diocto C*[3], *Peri-Colace*[3]	**Syrup:** 60 mg docusate sodium and 30 mL casanthranol/Tbsp	Yes
otc	*Silace-C*[3]	**Syrup:** 30 mg casanthranol and 60 mL docusate sodium per Tsb	No

[1] Sugar free.
[2] Alcohol free.
[3] Contains alcohol.
[4] Contains the dye tartrazine.

Laxatives promote bowel emptying. Nonprescription laxatives are frequently misued due to lack of understanding of normal bowel function. Restrict self-medication to short-term therapy of constipation. Chronic use of laxatives (particularly stimulants) may lead to dependence. Prior to laxative use, consider living habits affecting bowel function including disease state and drug history. Rational therapy and prevention of constipation include: Adequate fluid intake (4 to 6 glasses of water daily), proper dietary habits including sufficient bulk or roughage, responding to the urge to defecate and daily exercise.

Type of Drug:

Laxative combinations.

Uses:

To treat constipation.

For more information on laxative ingredients, see docusate, and senna and phenolphthalein. Casanthranol is a stimulant laxative used in laxative combinations.

Guidelines for Use:

- Use exactly as prescribed.
- Take 5 to 45 mL (1tsp to 3 Tbs) at bedtime with a full glass of water.
- Do not use in the presence of abdominal pain, nausea or vomiting.
- Laxative use if only a temporary measure; do not use longer than 1 week. When regularity returns, discontinue use. Prolonged, frequent or excessive use may result in dependence or electrolyte imbalance.
- Contact your doctor if unrelieved constipation rectal bleeding or symptoms of electrolyte imbalance (eg, muscle cramps or pain, weakness, dizziness) occurs.
- Pink-red, red-violet or red-brown discoloration of alkaline urine may occur with cascara sagrada, phenolphthalein or senna.
- Some of these products may contain the dye tartrazine (FD&C Yellow No. 5) which can cause allergic reactions in certain individuals. Check package label when available or consult your doctor or pharmacist.
- Prevention of constipation includes: Adequate fluid intake (4 to 6 glasses of water daily), proper dietary habits including sufficient bulk or roughage, responding to the urge to defecate and daily exercise.
- Store at room temperature.

If you have any questions, consult your doctor, pharmacist, or health care provider.

	Generic Name *Brand Name Examples*	**Supplied As**	**Generic Available**
Rx	**Polyethylene Glycol**		
	Colyte, Colyte Flavored	**Powder for oral solution:** **1 gal:** 227.1 g polyethylene glycol 3350 **4 L:** 240 g polyethylene glycol 3350	No
	GoLYTELY	**Powder for oral solution:** 236 g polyethylene glycol 3350/4 L jug	No
	OCL	**Oral solution:** 6 g polyethylene glycol 3350/100 mL	No

Type of Drug:

Bowel-cleansing agent administered prior to a diagnostic procedure on the lower portion of the colon.

How the Drug Works:

Oral polyethylene glycol induces a diarrhea (onset, 30 to 60 minutes) that rapidly cleanses the bowel, usually within 4 hours. The electrolytes contained in the solution allow for the use of large volumes of this solution without significant changes in water or electrolyte balance.

Uses:

For bowel cleansing prior to diagnostic examination of the lower portion of the colon.

Precautions:

Do not use in the following situations:

- allergy to polyethylene glycol or any of its ingredients
- bowel perforation
- ileus
- obstruction of digestive tract
- retention of stomach contents
- toxic colitis
- toxic megacolon

Use with caution in the following situations:

- impaired gag reflex
- regurgitation- or aspiration-prone
- ulcerative colitis, severe
- unconscious or semiconscious patients

Pregnancy: Safety for use during pregnancy has not been established. Use only if clearly needed and the potential benefits outweigh the possible hazards to the fetus.

Children: Safety and effectiveness in children have not been established.

Drug Interactions:

Tell your doctor or pharmacist if you are taking or if you are planning to take any over-the-counter or prescription medications or dietary supplements while using polyethylene glycol. Doses of one or both drugs may need to be modified or a different drug may need to be prescribed. Do not take oral medications within 1 hour of starting polyethylene glycol solution.

Side Effects:

Every drug is capable of producing side effects. Many polyethylene glycol users experience no, or minor, side effects. Possible side effects include: Nausea; stomach fullness; bloating; stomach cramps; vomiting; anal irritation.

Guidelines for Use:

- Recommended adult dosage is 4 liters of solution prior to the exam. Drink 8 oz every 10 minutes until the watery stool is clear and free of solid matter or until the 4 liters are consumed. Rapid drinking of each portion is preferred to drinking small amounts continuously. The first bowel movement should occur in about 1 hour.
- *Preparation of solution from powder* — Lukewarm tap water may be used. Shake container vigorously several times to ensure that the powder is completely dissolved. Prepare solution ahead of time and store in refrigerator since solution is more palatable if chilled.
- Do not add additional ingredients (eg, flavorings) to the solution before use.
- Polyethylene glycol is usually administered orally but may be given via nasogastric tube to patients who are unwilling or unable to drink the solution. Nasogastric tube administration is at the rate of 20 to 30 mL/minute. The first bowel movement should occur approximately 1 hour after the start of administration.
- Fasting 3 to 4 hours before drinking the solution produces the best results. However, do not eat solid foods < 2 hours before solution is administered.
- For midmorning examination, allow 3 hours for drinking and 1 hour to complete bowel evacuation, or drink the solution the evening before the examination, particularly if you are to have a barium enema.
- No foods except clear liquids are permitted after administration of the solution.
- You may experience some stomach bloating and discomfort before the bowels start to move. If severe discomfort or distention occur, stop drinking temporarily or drink each portion at longer intervals until these symptoms disappear.
- Oral medication administered within 1 hour of the start of administration of the solution may be flushed from the gastrointestinal tract and not absorbed.
- Store powder at controlled room temperature (59° to 86°F). Refrigerate the reconstituted solution. Use within 48 hours. Discard unused portion. Store *OCL* solution at room temperature (59° to 86°F). Protect from excessive heat and freezing.

If you have any questions, consult your doctor, pharmacist, or health care provider.

	Brand Name Examples	Supplied As
otc	*Evac-Q-Kwik*	300 mL magnesium citrate 3 bisacodyl tablets (5 mg/tablet)[1,2] 1 bisacodyl suppository (10 mg)
otc	*Fleet Prep Kit # 1*	45 mL phospho-soda (21.6 g monobasic sodium phosphate, 8.1 g dibasic sodium phosphate) 4 bisacodyl tablets (5 mg/tablet) 1 bisacodyl suppository (10 mg)
otc	*Fleet Prep Kit # 2*	45 mL phospho-soda (21.6 g monobasic sodium phosphate, 8.1 g dibasic sodium phosphato) 4 bisacodyl tablets (5 mg/tablet) 1 bagenema
otc	*Fleet Prep Kit # 3*	45 mL phospho-soda (21.6 g monobasic sodium phosphate, 8.1 g dibasic sodium phosphate) 4 bisacodyl tablets (5 mg/tablet) 30 mL bisacodyl enema (10 mg)
otc	*Tridrate Dry Bowel Cleansing System*	19 g magnesium citrate powder 3 bisacodyl tablets (5 mg/tablet) 1 bisacodyl suppository (10 mg)
otc	*X-Prep Bowel Evacuant Kit-1*	74 mL extract of senna concentrate (130 mg sennosides)[3,4] 2 tablets (8.6 mg sennosides, 50 mg docusate sodium per tablet)[1] 1 bisacodyl suppository (10 mg)
otc	*X-Prep Bowel Evacuant Kit-2*	74 mL extract of senna concentrate (130 mg sennosides)[3,4,5] 30 g granules (8 g magnesium citrate, 5.3 g magnesium sulfate)[4,6] 1 bisacodyl suppository (10 mg)
otc	*X-Prep Senna Liquid Bowel Evacuant*	74 mL extract of senna concentrate (130 mg sennosides, 50 g sugar)[3,4]

[1] Contains lactose.
[2] Contains sugar.
[3] Contains parabens.
[4] Contains sucrose.
[5] Contains alcohol.
[6] Contains saccharin.

Type of Drug:

Bowel-cleansing drugs.

Uses:

For bowel cleansing prior to examination or surgery of the digestive tract.

Precautions:

Do not use in the following situations:

kidney disease (*Fleet Prep Kits # 1, 2, and 3; Evac-Q-Kwik; Tridrate; X-Prep Bowel Evacuant Kit-2*)

magnesium-restricted diet (*Evac-Q-Kwik, X-Prep Bowel Evacuant Kit-2; Tridrate*)

megacolon

sodium-restricted diet (*Fleet Prep Kits # 1, 2, and 3*)

Children: Safety and effectiveness in children under 5 years of age have not been established.

Side Effects:

Every drug is capable of producing side effects. Many bowel evacuant kit users experience no, or minor, side effects. The frequency and severity of side effects depend on many factors including dose, duration of therapy, and individual susceptibility, Possible side effects include:

Other: Stomach discomfort; faintness; rectal burning; stomach cramps.

Guidelines for Use:

- Review kit insert for complete instructions. Instructions include eating guidelines, minimum fluid requirements, and timing of use of bowel evacuant kit components. Follow directions exactly to ensure best results and to avoid the need for repeat examination.
- Take with a glass of water.
- Do not use for longer than 1 week unless directed by your doctor.
- Consult a doctor before use if you notice a sudden change in bowel habits that persists > 2 weeks.
- Consult your doctor if you are pregnant, planning to become pregnant, or are breastfeeding.
- Do not use when abdominal pain, nausea, or vomiting are present unless directed to do so by your doctor.
- Notify your doctor immediately if you experience rectal bleeding or a failure to respond to the bowel evacuant.
- Continue to take prescription medications as scheduled, unless advised differently by your doctor.

If you have any questions, consult your doctor, pharmacist, or health care provider.

	Generic Name *Brand Name Examples*	Supplied As	Generic Available
otc	**Bismuth Subsalicylate**		
	Pepto-Bismol[1,2]	**Tablets:** 262 mg	No
	Pepto-Bismol[1,2]	**Tablets, chewable:** 262 mg	Yes
	Pepto-Bismol[1,2]	**Suspension:** 262 mg/15 mL	Yes
	Pepto-Bismol, Maximum Strength[1,2]	**Suspension:** 525 mg/15 mL	No

[1] Low sodium.
[2] Sugar free.

Type of Drug:

Antidiarrheal; drug for indigestion.

How the Drug Works:

The exact mechanism of action of bismuth subsalicylate is not known; however, it appears to reduce stomach secretions, reduce inflammation, and inhibit some bacterial and viral organisms capable of producing intestinal tract diseases.

Uses:

To control diarrhea, including traveler's diarrhea (generally within 24 hours).

To treat indigestion (eg, upset stomach, heartburn) without causing constipation.

To treat nausea.

To relieve stomach cramps.

Unlabeled Use(s): Occasionally doctors and pharmacist may recommend bismuth subsalicylate to prevent traveler's diarrhea and to treat infantile diarrhea.

Precautions:

Do not use in the following situations:
allergy to bismuth subsalicylate
allergy to salicylates (aspirin)

Use with caution in the following situations:
chickenpox (children)
flu (children)
radiologic (x-ray) examinations of GI tract

Pregnancy: This product contains salicylates. Do not take bismuth subsalicylate during pregnancy, especially during the third trimester.

Breastfeeding: Salicylates appear in breast milk. If bismuth subsalicylate is needed, the patient should stop breastfeeding.

Children: Impaction (severe constipation) may occur in infants. Consult your doctor before using in children < 3 years of age.

Drug Interactions:

Tell your doctor or pharmacist if you are taking or if you are planning to take any over-the-counter or prescription medications or dietary supplements with bismuth subsalicylate. Doses of one or both drugs may need to be modified or a different drug may need to be prescribed. The following drugs and drug classes interact with bismuth subsalicylate.

- anticoagulants, oral (eg, warfarin)
- corticosteroids (eg, hydrocortisone)
- insulin (*Humulin*, *Iletin*)
- methotrexate (eg, *Rheumatrex*)
- salicylates (eg, aspirin)
- spironolactone (eg, *Aldactone)*
- sulfinpyrazone (eg, *Anturane)*
- tetracyclines (eg, doxycycline)
- valproic acid (eg, *Depakene)*

Side Effects:

Every drug is capable of producing side effects. Many bismuth subsalicylate users experience no, or minor, side effects. Possible side effects include severe constipation, darkening of tongue, and darkening of stools.

Consider all side effects and drug interactions reported for salicylates when using bismuth subsalicylate. See Analgesics – Aspirin and Salicylates monograph in the CNS drugs chapter.

Guidelines for Use:

- Dosage for tablets and chewable tablets for adults is 2 tablets. For children ages 9 to 12 years old, 1 tablet; children 6 to 9 years old, 2/3 of a tablet; and children 3 to 6 years old 1/3 of a tablet.
- Dosing for suspension for adults is 2 tbsp (30 mL). For children ages 9 to 12, 1 tbsp (15 mL); children 6 to 9 years old, 2 tsp (10 mL); and children 3 to 6, 1 tsp (5 mL).
- Dose may be repeated every 30 to 60 minutes if needed. Do not take more than 8 doses in 24 hours (regular strength) or 4 doses in 24 hours (maximum strength).
- Shake suspension well before using.
- Chewable tablets may be chewed or allowed to dissolve in mouth. Do not swallow whole.
- Swallow regular tablets whole with a glass of water. Do not chew regular tablets.
- Drink plenty of fluids to prevent dehydration which may accompany diarrhea.
- May cause temporary and harmLess darkening of the tongue or stool.
- If taken with other salicylate-containing products (eg, aspirin), and ringing in the ears occurs, discontinue use.
- Contact your doctor if diarrhea is accompanied by high fever or if diarrhea continues for more than 2 days.
- Do not use to treat nausea or vomiting in children or teenagers with the flu or chickenpox without consulting a doctor. If nausea or vomiting is present, consult a doctor because this could be an early sign of Reye syndrome, a rare but serious illness.
- *Suspension:* Store at room temperature. Refrigeration may improve taste. Avoid excessive heat and protect from freezing.
- *Tablets:* Avoid excessive heat.

If you have any questions, consult your doctor, pharmacist, or health care provider.

	Generic Name *Brand Name Examples*	Supplied As	Generic Available
C-IV	**Difenoxin with Atropine Sulfate**		
	Motofen	**Tablets:** 1 mg difenoxin, 0.025 mg atropine sulfate	No
C-V	**Diphenoxylate with Atropine Sulfate**		
	Lomotil, Lonox	**Tablets:** 2.5 mg diphenoxylate, 0.025 mg atropine sulfate	Yes
	Lomotil	**Liquid:** 2.5 mg diphenoxylate, 0.025 mg atropine sulfate/5 mL	Yes

Type of Drug:

Antidiarrheal.

How the Drug Works:

Difenoxin and diphenoxylate, related to the narcotic pain reliever meperidine, act on intestinal tract muscles and slow intestinal motility. Atropine is present to discourage deliberate misuse of these drugs.

Uses:

To relieve diarrhea.

Precautions:

Do not use in the following situations:

- allergy to the drug or any of its ingredients
- children under 2 years of age
- diarrhea associated with antibiotic therapy (eg, pseudomembranous colitis)
- diarrhea associated with enterotoxin-producing bacteria (eg, toxigenic *E. coli*, *Salmonella*, *Shigella*)
- jaundice (yellowing of skin or eyes)

Use with caution in the following situations:

- children (diphenoxylate only)
- dehydration
- Down's syndrome (diphenoxylate only)
- drug addiction, history
- kidney disease
- liver disease
- MAOI use, concurrent
- patients receiving addictive drugs
- ulcerative colitis, acute

Diphenoxylate can be habit forming. If you have been taking large doses and suddenly stop taking the medication, symptoms of withdrawal may occur. These symptoms include muscle cramps, stomach cramps, "goose bumps," unusual sweating, nausea, vomiting, and shaking or trembling. Recommended doses used to treat diarrhea do not cause addiction.

Pregnancy: Adequate studies have not been done in pregnant women. Use only if clearly needed and potential benefits outweigh the possible hazards to the fetus.

Breastfeeding: Difenoxin and diphenoxylate may appear in breast milk. Atropine appears in breast milk. Because of the potential for serious side effects in nursing infants, a decision should be made whether to discontinue nursing or to discontinue the drug, taking into account the importance of the drug to the mother.

Children: Do not use difenoxin tablets or diphenoxylate liquid in children < 2 years of age. Do not use diphenoxylate tablets in children < 13 years of age. Safety and effectiveness of difenoxin tablets have not been established in children < 12 years of age. Use with caution in children with Down's syndrome due to presence of atropine.

Drug Interactions:

Tell your doctor or pharmacist if you are taking or if you are planning to take any over-the-counter or prescription medications or dietary supplements with antidiarrheals containing difenoxin, diphenoxylate, or atropine sulfate. Doses of one or both drugs may need to be modified or a different drug may need to be prescribed. The following drugs and drug classes interact with antidiarrheals containing difenoxin, diphenoxylate, or atropine sulfate.

alcohol
barbiturates (eg, phenobarbital)
MAOIs (eg, isocarboxazid, phenelzine, tranylcypromine, selegiline)
narcotic pain relievers (eg, meperidine)
tranquilizers (eg, benzodiazepines)

Side Effects:

Every drug is capable of producing side effects. Many antidiarrheal users experience no, or minor, side effects. The frequency and severity of side effects depend on many factors including dose, duration of therapy, and individual susceptibility. Possible side effects include:

Both: Nausea; vomiting; dizziness; drowsiness; headache.

Difenoxin only: Constipation; lightheadedness; dry mouth; stomach pain.

Diphenoxylate only: Stomach ache; appetite loss; toxic megacolon; paralytic ileus; pancreatitis; restlessness; confusion; depression; exaggerated sense of well-being; itching; hives; swelling of gums; numbness of arms or legs; general body discomfort; allergic reaction.

Atropine only: Dry skin; flushing; fever; fast heartbeat; urinary retention.

Guidelines for Use:

- *Difenoxin* — Starting dose in adults is 2 mg by mouth, then 1 mg after each loose stool or 1 mg every 3 to 4 hours as needed. Total dose in any 24-hour period should not exceed 8 mg.
- *Diphenoxylate* — Initial dosage in adults is 2 tablets by mouth 4 times daily or 10 mL (2 tsp) of liquid 4 times daily (20 mg/day). Once control of diarrhea is achieved, reduce the dose to the lowest possible level (eg, 2 tablets daily) to maintain control. Do not use tablets for children < 13 years of age. Only use the plastic dropper included with the liquid to measure doses for children. Doses for children must be carefully determined. Talk to your doctor or pharmacist about the correct dose for your child.
- If clinical improvement of acute diarrhea is not observed within 48 hours, do not continue the medication. If improvement of chronic diarrhea is not seen within 10 days of using diphenoxylate (with a maximum daily dose of 20 mg), symptoms are unlikely to be controlled by further administration.
- Do not take more than the prescribed dose.
- Appropriate fluid and electrolyte therapy should be used in conjunction with diphenoxylate therapy in the treatment of diarrhea in children.
- Avoid alcohol and other sedatives that may cause drowsiness.
- May cause drowsiness or dizziness. Use caution when performing tasks requiring alertness, coordination, or physical dexterity.
- May cause dry mouth. Chew sugarless gum or suck sugarless hard candies if desired.
- Keep out of reach of children because accidental overdose may result in severe, even fatal, breathing problems.
- Notify your doctor if diarrhea persists or if fever, rapid heart rate, or stomach swelling occur.
- Store at room temperature (59° to 86°F) in a child resistant container. Protect diphenoxylate from light.

If you have any questions, consult your doctor, pharmacist, or health care provider.

	Generic Name *Brand Name Examples*	Supplied As	Generic Available
otc	**Lactobacillus**		
	Bacid	**Capsules:** Cultured strain of not less than 500 million viable L-acidophilus with 100 mg sodium carboxymethylcellulose	No
	Lactinex	**Granules**	No
	Lactinex	**Chewable tablets**	No
	More-Dophilus[1]	**Powder:** 4 billion units of acidophilus-carrot derivative/g	No

[1] Sugar free.

Type of Drug:

Antidiarrheal.

How the Drug Works:

Lactobacillus creates a more normal bacterial environment in the digestive tract and prevents the growth of unfavorable bacteria that may contribute to diarrhea.

Uses:

To treat uncomplicated diarrhea, including diarrhea due to long-term antibiotic therapy.

To treat fever blisters (cold sores).

Precautions:

Do not use in the following situations:

allergy to milk or lactose

Use with caution in the following situations:

children under 3 years of age
presence of high fever

Guidelines for Use:

- Some of the availabie products need to be refrigerated. Check package label.
- Do not use for more than 2 days unless directed by your doctor.
- If high fever is present, do not use unless directed by your doctor.

If you have any questions, consult your doctor, pharmacist, or health care provider.

	Generic Name *Brand Name Examples*	Supplied As	Generic Available
	Loperamide HCl		
Rx	*Imodium*	**Capsules:** 2 mg	No
otc	*Imodium A-D Caplets, Kaopectate II Caplets, Maalox Anti-Diarrheal Caplets*	**Tablets:** 2 mg	No
otc	*Imodium A-D*[1], *Pepto Diarrhea Control*	**Liquid:** 1 mg/tsp	Yes

[1] Contains alcohol.

Type of Drug:

Antidiarrheal.

How the Drug Works:

Loperamide decreases movement of the digestive tract. This allows more time for reabsorption of water and electrolytes from the stool.

Uses:

For relief of nonspecific acute diarrhea, chronic diarrhea associated with inflammatory bowel disease and for Traveler's diarrhea.

To deacrease the volume of discharge from ileostomies.

Precautions:

Do not use in the following situations:

allergy to loperamide
blood in the stools
high fever

Use with caution in the following situations:

diarrhea associated with antibiotic therapy
liver disease
ulcerative colitis

Pregnancy: There are no adequate and well-controlled studies in pregnant women. Safety for use during pregnancy has not been established. Use only when clearly needed and when the potential benefits outweigh the potential hazards to the fetus.

Breastfeeding: It is not known if loperamide appears in breast milk. Consult your doctor before you begin breastfeeding.

Children: Not recommended in children under 6. Use with caution and consult your doctor.

Drug Interactions:

Tell your doctor or pharmacist if you are taking of if you are planning to take any over-the-counter or prescription medications or dietary supplements with loperamide. Doses of one or both drugs may need to be modified or a different drug may need to be prescribed. Cholestyramine (*Questran*) interacts with loperamide.

Side Effects:

Every drug is capable of producing side effects. Many loperamide users experience no, or minor, side effects. The frequency and severity of side effects depend on many factors including dose, duration of therapy and individual susceptibility. Possible side effects include:

Digestive Tract: Constipation; nausea; vomiting; appetite loss; stomach ache; abdominal distention or bloating.

Other: Dry mouth; fever; rash; drowsiness, dizziness.

Guidelines for Use:

- Do not take more than the prescribed dose.
- May cause drowsiness or dizziness. Use caution when driving or performing other tasks requiring alertness, coordination or physical dexterity.
- Drink plenty of clear fluids to help prevent dehydration, which may accompany diarrhea.
- May cause dry mouth. Chew sugarless gum or suck sugarless hard candies if desired.
- Notify your doctor if diarrhea does not stop after a few days or if abdominal pain, distention or fever occurs.

If you have any questions, consult your doctor, pharmacist, or health care provider.

ANTIDIARRHEAL COMBINATION PRODUCTS

Generic Name *Brand Name Examples*	Supplied As	Generic Available
Opiate-containing combinations		
c-III Diabismul	**Tablets:** 1.23 mg powdered opium, 125 mg bismuth subcarbonate and 125 mg calcium carbonate	No
c-III B.P.P.-Lemmon	**Tablets:** 1.2 mg powdered opium, 120 mg kaolin, 15 mg pectin, 120 mg bismuth subgallate and 15 mg zinc phenolsulfonate	No
c-III KBP/O	**Capsules:** 3 mg powdered opium, 350 mg kaolin, 60 mg bismuth subcarbonate in a pectin base	No
c-V Dia-Quel[1]	**Liquid:** 18 mg opium, 0.9 mg homatropine MBr and 144 mg pectin/2 tbsp	No
c-V Banatol[1] *Infantol Pink*[1]	**Liquid:** 15 mg opium, bismuth subsalicylate, pectin, zinc phenolsulfonate and extract Irish moss/2 tbsp	No
c-V Kaodene with Codeine	**Suspension:** 32.4 mg codeine phosphate, 3.9 g kaolin, 194.4 mg pectin, sodium carboxymethylcellulose and bismuth subsalicylate/2 tbsp	No
c-V Amogel PG[1], *Donnagel-PG*[1], *Donnapectolin-PG*[1], *Kaodonna-PG*[1], *Kapectolin PG*[1], *Quiagel PG*[1]	**Suspension:** 24 mg powdered opium, 6 g kaolin, 142.8 pectin, 0.1037 mg hyoscyamine sulfate, 0.0194 mg atropine sulfate and 0.0065 mg scopolamine HBr/2 tbsp	Yes
c-V Parepectolin[1], *Kapectolin w/Paregoric*[1]	**Suspension:** 15 mg opium, 5.5 g kaolin and 162 mg pectin/2 tbsp	No
c-V Diabismul	**Suspension:** 14 mg opium and 5 g kaolin/2 tbsp	No
c-V Corrective Mixture w/Paregoric[1,2]	**Suspension:** 3.6 mL paregoric, 270 mg pepsin, 60 mg zinc sulfocarbolate, 132 mg phenyl salicylate and 510 mg bismuth subsalicylate, 0.78 mEq sodium/2 tbsp	No

	Generic Name *Brand Name Examples*	Supplied As	Generic Available
c-v	*Kaodene with Paregoric*	**Suspension:** 1.5 mg anhydrous morphine, 3.9 g kaolin, 194.4 mg pectin, bismuth subsalicylate and sodium carboxymethylcellulose/2 tbsp	No
otc	**Opiate-free combinations**		
	Rheaban	**Tablets:** 750 mg colloidal activated attapulgite	No
	Diar-Aid	**Tablets:** 750 mg activated attapulgite and 150 mg pectin	No
	Diasorb[1]	**Tablets:** 750 mg activated attapulgite	No
	Kaopectate	**Tablets:** 600 mg attapulgite	No
	Devrom	**Tablets, chewable:** 200 mg bismuth subgallate	No
	Kaopectate Concentrate	**Liquid:** 8.7 g kaolin and 195 mg pectin/2 tbsp	No
	Diasorb[1]	**Liquid:** 750 mg activated attapulgite/tsp	No
	Dia-Eze	**Suspension:** 11 g kaolin and 300 mg bismuth subgallate/2 tbsp	No
	Kapectolin Gell with Belladonna[1], *Donnagel*[2], *Quiagel*	**Suspension:** 6 g kaolin, 142.8 mg pectin, 0.1037 mg hyoscyamine sulfate, 0.0194 mg atropine sulfate and 0.0065 mg scopolamine HBr/2 tbsp	Yes
	Kaolin w/Pectin, Kao-tin, Kapectolin, Kaopectate, K-Pek	**Suspension:** 5.85 g kaolin and 130 mg pectin/2 tbsp	Yes
	K-P	**Suspension:** 5.2 g kaolin and 260 mg pectin /2 tbsp	No
	K-C	**Suspension:** 5.2 g kaolin, 260 mg pectin, and 260 mg bismuth subcarbonate/2 tbsp	
	Kaodene Non-Narcotic	**Suspension:** 3.9 g kaolin, 194.4 mg pectin, sodium carboxymethylcellulose and bismuth subsalicylate/2 tbsp	No

[1] Sugar free.
[2] Contains alcohol.

ANTIDIARRHEAL COMBINATION PRODUCTS

Type of Drug:

Antidiarrheal combination products.

How the Drug Works:

These drugs reduce intestinal movement, absorb fluid, reduce the severity of intestinal inflammation and modify intestinal bacteria.

Uses:

To treat the symptoms of diarrhea. Adequate controlled studies demonstrating the effectiveness of these antidiarrheal combinations are lacking. In these preparations:

Opium (tincture, powder, or paregoric) and codeine phosphate are used to reduce the intestinal activity, to relieve the urge to have a bowel movement without success and to relieve the pain associated with diarrhea.

Belladonna alkaloids and homatropine methylbromide are used to control hyperactivity and increased secretion in the digestive tract.

Activated attapulgite, kaolin and *pectin* are used for their absorbent actions to bind up and remove digestive tract irritants.

Aluminum hydroxide and bismuth salts have antacid and absorbent properties.

Zinc phenosulfonates and *zinc sulfocarbolate* have been used as intestinal antiseptics and astringents.

Bacterial cultures are used to favorably modify intestinal bacteria.

Guidelines for Use:

- Do not use agents which slow digestive tract motility for diarrhea associated with antibiotic-caused colitis or in diarrhea caused by bacteria.
- Do not use these preparations for more than 2 days, in the presence of high fever, or in infants and children under 3, except under a doctor's direction.
- Salicylate absorption may occur from bismuth subsalicylate. Observe caution in patients with bleeding disorders or aspirin sensitivity and in children.
- *Liquids* — Shake well before using.

	Generic Name *Brand Name Examples*	Supplied As	Generic Available
Rx	**Balsalazide Disodium**		
	Colazal	**Capsules**: 750 mg	No
Rx	**Mesalamine (5-ASA)**		
	Asacol	**Tablets, delayed-release**: 400 mg	No
	Rowasa	**Suppositories**: 500 mg	Yes
	Rowasa[1]	**Suspension, rectal**: 4 g/60 mL	No
Rx	**Olsalazine Sodium**		
	Dipentum	**Capsules**: 250 mg	No

[1] Contains sulfites.

Type of Drug:

Intestinal anti-inflammatory agents.

How the Drug Works:

The exact mechanism of action of the 5-aminosalicyclic acid (5-ASA) agents is unknown. They appear to work topically, reducing inflammation of the colon by preventing the production of substances involved in the inflammatory process.

Uses:

Balsalazide Disodium: To treat mild to moderate active ulcerative colitis (inflammation of the colon or rectum).

Mesalamine: To treat mild to moderate inflammation of the colon or rectum (eg, ulcerative colitis) and to reduce chances of reoccurance (delayed-release tablets).

To treat active mild to moderate distal ulcerative colitis, proctosigmoiditis, or proctitis (rectal suppositories and suspension).

Olsalazine Sodium: To reduce the chances that ulcerative colitis will reoccur in patients who cannot take sulfasalazine.

Precautions:

Do not use in the following situations:
allergy to the 5-ASA agent or any of its ingredients
allergy to salicylates (eg, aspirin)

Use with caution in the following situations:
allergy to sulfasalazine, history of
kidney disease
pyloric stenosis (tablets and capsules only)
sulfite sensitivity (rectal suspension only)

Intolerance: Mesalamine can cause an intolerance syndrome characterized by cramping, acute stomach pain, bloody diarrhea, fever, headache, and rash. Prompt withdrawal is required. Consult your doctor.

Worsening of symptoms: Worsening of symptoms of colitis (thought to have been caused by mesalamine or sulfasalazine) has occurred.

Pregnancy: There are no adequate and well-controlled studies in pregnant women. Use during pregnancy only if clearly needed and the potential benefits to the mother outweigh the possible hazards to the fetus.

Breastfeeding: Oral mesalamine appears in breast milk. It is not known if rectal mesalamine, balsalazide, or olsalazine appear in breast milk. Consult your doctor before you begin breastfeeding.

Children: Safety and effectiveness in children have not been established.

Sulfites: Some of these products contain sulfite preservatives that can cause allergic reactions in certain individuals. Check package label when available or consult your doctor or pharmacist.

Drug Interactions:

Tell your doctor or pharmacist if you are taking or if you are planning to take any over-the-counter or prescription medications or dietary supplements with 5-ASA. Doses of one or both drugs may need to be modified or a different drug may need to be prescribed. Thiopurines (eg, mercaptopurine) and anticoagulants (eg, warfarin) interact with olsalazine.

Side Effects:

Every drug is capable of producing side effects. Many 5-ASA users experience no, or minor, side effects. The frequency and severity of side effects depend on many factors including dose, duration of therapy, and individual susceptibility. Possible side effects include:

Digestive Tract: Diarrhea; constipation; frequent stools; indigestion; heartburn; bloating; gas; stomach pain or cramps; nausea; vomiting; belching; worsening of colitis; appetitie loss; rectal bleeding; mouth inflammation.

Nervous System: Dizziness; headache; tiredness; weakness; disorientation; sleeplessness; fatigue; drowsiness; depression; vertigo (feeling of whirling motion); lightheadedness.

Other: Sweating; chills; hair loss; fever; flu-like symptoms; cough; muscle pain, cramps, or tension; general pain; painful urination; fever; leg, back, chest, joint, or rectal pain; hemorrhoids; sore throat; edema (fluid retention); general body discomfort; dry mouth; sore throat; congestion; runny nose; sinus inflammation; upper respiratory infection; painful menstruation; eye inflammation; hives; rash; itching; acne; increased bowel swelling; urinary tract infection.

Guidelines for Use:

- Dosage is individualized. Take exactly as prescribed.
- If a dose is missed, take it as soon as possible. If several hours have passed or if it is nearing time for the next dose, do not double the dose to catch up, unless advised by your doctor. If more than one dose is missed, or it is necessary to establish a new dosage schedule, contact your doctor or pharmacist.
- Inform your doctor if you are pregnant, become pregnant, planning to become pregnant, or are breastfeeding.

Mesalamine:

- Tablets — Swallow whole. Do not break outer coating. Intact or partially intact tablets may appear in stool. Contact your doctor if this occurs repeatedly.
- Rectal suspension — For rectal use only. Review the patient instructions included. Shake bottle well. Remove protective sheath from the applicator tip. Holding the bottle at the neck will not allow medication to be discharged. The position most often used is to lie on the left side (to help flow into the sigmoid colon), with the lower leg extended and the upper right leg bent forward for balance. An alternative is the knee-chest position. Gently insert the applicator tip in the rectum pointing toward the navel. A steady squeezing of the bottle will discharge most of the preparation. After administering, withdraw and discard the bottle. Remain in position for at least 30 minutes.
- Suspension should be given once daily, preferably at bedtime. The drug should be retained in the rectum all night if possible.
- Suppositories — Usual dosage is twice daily. The drug should be retained in the rectum for 1 to 3 hours or longer. Review the patient instructions included for the proper insertion technique.
- Improvement may not be seen for up to 3 weeks. Usual treatment is one enema or 2 suppositories daily for 3 to 6 weeks.
- Contents of suspension and suppositories can cause staining of clothes, sheets, or flooring. Choose a location where this will not be a problem.
- Store tablets at controlled room temperature (68° to 77°F); store suspension at room temperature (59° to 86°F); store suppositories at a temperature of 66° to 79°F.

Olsalazine sodium:

- Take with food. Take in evenly divided doses.
- May cause diarrhea in some patients. Contact your doctor if diarrhea occurs.
- Contact your doctor before stopping treatment. Abrupt withdrawal may cause adverse effects.
- Store at room temperature (59° to 86°F).

Balsalazide disodium:

- Store at room temperature (59° to 86°F).

If you have any questions, consult your doctor, pharmacist, or health care provider.

Generic Name *Brand Name Example*	Supplied As	Generic Available
Rx **Infliximab** *Remicade*	**Powder for Injection:** 100 mg/20 mL vial	No

Type of Drug:

Immunomodulator; monoclonal antibody.

How the Drug Works:

Inhibits the TNF alpha (tissue necrosis factor) receptor binding responsible for inflammatory and immune responses.

Uses:

For the reduction of signs and symptoms of moderately to severely active Crohn disease in patients who have had an inadequate response to conventional therapy. For reduction in the number of draining abdominal fistula in fistulizing Crohn disease.

For use in combination with methotrexate to reduce signs and symptoms of rheumatoid arthritis in patients who have had an inadequate response to methotrexate alone.

Precautions:

Do not use in the following situations:
allergy to infliximab or any of its ingredients
live vaccinations, concurrent

Use with caution in the following situations:
CNS demyelinating disease, current or history of
human antichimeric antibody (HACA) development
immunosuppression
infection
malignancy

Autoimmune antibodies: Auto antibodies may develop and, rarely, a lupus-like syndrome (eg, difficulty breathing, chest pain, joint pain) may occur.

Pregnancy: It is not known whether infliximab can cause fetal harm when administered to a pregnant woman. Use only if clearly needed and the potential benefits to the mother outweigh the possible hazards.

Breastfeeding: It is not known if infliximab appears in breast milk. Consult your doctor before you begin breastfeeding.

Children: Safety and effectiveness in children have not been established.

Elderly: There is a higher incidence of infections in the elderly population in general. Use caution when administering infliximab to elderly patients.

Drug Interactions:

Tell your doctor or pharmacist if you are taking or if you are planning to take any over-the-counter or prescription medications or dietary supplements with infliximab. Doses of one or both drugs may need to be modified or a different drug may need to be prescribed. Specific studies on interactions with infliximab have not been conducted; however, immunosuppressants and live vaccines may interact with infliximab.

Side Effects:

Every drug is capable of producing side effects. Many infliximab users experience no, or minor, side effects. The frequency and severity of side effects depend on many factors including dose, duration of therapy, and individual susceptibility. Possible side effects include:

Digestive Tract: Diarrhea; nausea; abdominal pain or swelling; vomiting; indigestion; intestinal obstruction; intestinal perforation; intestinal constriction; pancreatitis; gastric ulcers; gallstones; appendicitis; intestinal bleeding; rectal pain.

Nervous System: Headache; fatigue; drowsiness; dizziness; anxiety; depression; confusion; delerium; spinal narrowing; brain lesions.

Circulatory System: Chest pain; anemia; fainting; fast heartbeat; abnormal heart rhythm; palpitations (pounding in the chest); slow heartbeat; unusual bruising; decreased platelets; heart failure; stroke; spleen disease; leukopenia; kidney disease or failure; gallbladder disease.

Respiratory System: Difficulty breathing; upper or lower respiratory tract infection; congested or runny nose; sinus infection; cough; sore throat; throat inflammation; difficulty swallowing; adult respiratory distress syndrome.

Skin: Itching; hives; rash; abnormal skin sensations; acne; hair loss; fungal skin infection; redness; dry skin; hot flushes; skin tumors.

Other: Sweating; infections; muscle pain; swelling; general body discomfort; conjunctivitis; joint pain; back pain; abscess; painful or difficult urination; increased frequency of urination; dehydration; weight decrease; edema (fluid retention); lymphoma; tendon injury; bone fracture; joint degredation; urinary tract infection; breast tumors; endometriosis; adenocarcinoma.

Infusion Reactions – Fever; chills; itching; rash; hives; chest pain; low blood pressure; high blood pressure; difficulty breathing.

Guidelines for Use:

- This medicine will be prepared and administered by your health care provider in a medical setting.
- Dosage is individualized.
- *Crohn disease* — Recommended dose is 5 mg/kg given as a single intravenous infusion. Safety and efficacy of therapy beyond a single dose have not been established.
- *Fistulizing Crohn disease* — An initial 5 mg/kg dose should be followed with additional 5 mg/kg doses at 2 and 6 weeks after the first infusion. Safety and efficacy of therapy beyond 3 doses have not been studied.
- *Rheumatoid arthritis* — Recommended dose is 3 mg/kg given as an IV infusion followed with additional 3 mg/kg doses at 2 to 6 weeks after the first infusion, then every 8 weeks thereafter. Give infliximab in combination with methotrexate.
- Inform your doctor if you are pregnant, become pregnant, planning to become prenant, or are breatfeeding before beginning therapy.
- Severe rash, hives, difficulty breathing, low blood pressure, or other signs of an allergic reaction can occur.

If you have any questions, consult your doctor, pharmacist, or health care provider.

	Generic Name *Brand Name Examples*	Supplied As	Generic Available
Rx	**Orlistat**		
	Xenical	**Capsules**: 120 mg	No

Type of Drug:

Lipase inhibitor.

How the Drug Works:

Inhibits enzyme in intestine (lipase) which breaks down dietary fats into small absorbable particles. By preventing breakdown and absorption of fat in the intestine and increasing its subsequent loss in the stool, fewer calories are absorbed, which may result in weight loss.

Uses:

For obesity management including weight loss and weight maintenance when used in conjunction with a reduced-calorie diet. Orlistat is indicated for obese patients with an initial body mass index (BMI) ≥ 30 kg/m^2 or ≥ 27 kg/m^2 in the presence of other risk factors (eg, high blood pressure, diabetes, dyslipidemia).

To reduce the risk of weight regain after prior loss.

Precautions:

Do not use in the following situations:

- allergy to orlistat or any of its ingredients
- cholestasis
- chronic malabsorption syndrome

Use with caution in the following situations:

- anorexia nervosa
- bulimia
- cyclosporine therapy, concomitant
- high fat diet
- hyperoxaluria, history
- hypothyroidism
- kidney stones
- warfarin therapy, concomitant

Diabetes: Weight loss induction by orlistat may be accompanied by improved metabolic control in diabetic patients, which might require a reduction in dose of oral hypoglycemic medication (eg, sulfonylureas, metformin) or insulin.

Organic causes of obesity (eg, hypothyroidism) should be excluded before orlistat is prescribed.

Pregnancy: There are no adequate and well-controlled studies in pregnant women. Orlistat is not recommended for use during pregnancy.

Breastfeeding: It is not known if orlistat appears in breast milk. Therefore, orlistat should not be taken by nursing women. Consult your doctor before you begin breastfeeding.

Children: Safety and effectiveness of orlistat in children have not been established.

Drug Interactions:

Tell your doctor or pharmacist if you are taking or plan to take any over-the-counter or prescription medications or dietary supplements while taking orlistat. Doses of one or both drugs may need to be modified or a different drug may need to be prescribed. The following drugs and drug classes interact with orlistat:

- beta-carotene
- cyclosporine (eg, *Sandimmune*)
- pravastatin (*Pravachol*)
- vitamin E acetate
- warfarin (eg, *Coumadin*)

Side Effects:

Every drug is capable of producing side effects. Many orlistat users experience no, or minor, side effects. The frequency and severity of side effects depend on many factors including dose, duration of therapy, and individual susceptibility. Possible side effects include:

Digestive Tract: Oily spotting; gas with discharge; fecal urgency; fatty or oily stool; oily evacuation; stomach pain or discomfort; nausea; infectious diarrhea; rectal pain or discomfort; tooth disorder; gum disorder; nausea; vomiting; inability to control bowel movements; increased frequency of bowel movements.

Nervous System: Headache; dizziness; fatigue; sleep disorder; anxiety; depression.

Respiratory System: Flu; upper or lower respiratory tract infection; ear, nose, and throat symptoms.

Skin: Rash; dry skin.

Other: Back pain; pain in legs or feet; swollen feet; joint pain; muscle pain; joint disorder; tendonitis; menstrual irregularity; inflammation of the vagina with itching or abnormal discharge; urinary tract infection; ear infection.

Guidelines for Use:

- The recommended dose of orlistat is 120 mg (1 capsule) 3 times daily with each main meal containing fat (during or up to 1 hour after the meal). Doses > 120 mg 3 times daily have not been shown to provide additional benefit.
- If a meal is occasionally missed or contains no fat, the dose of orlistat can be omitted.
- Eat a nutritionally balanced, reduced-calorie diet that contains ≈ 30% of calories from fat. Gastrointestinal events may increase when orlistat is taken with a diet high in fat (> 30% total daily calories from fat). The daily intake of fat, carbohydrate, and protein should be distributed over 3 main meals. If orlistat is taken with any one meal very high in fat, the possibility of gastrointestinal adverse effects increases.
- Take a multivitamin supplement that contains fat-soluble vitamins (A, D, E, and K) to ensure adequate nutrition, because orlistat has been shown to reduce the absorption of some fat-soluble vitamins. Take the multivitamin supplement (with food to reduce gastrointestinal discomfort) once a day at least 2 hours before or after the administration of orlistat, such as at bedtime.
- Based on fecal fat measurements, the effect of orlistat is seen as soon as 24 to 48 hours after dosing. Upon discontinuation of therapy, fecal fat content usually returns to pretreatment levels within 48 to 72 hours.
- Safety and effectiveness of orlistat beyond 2 years have not been established.
- Store between 59° to 86°F in a tightly closed container. Do not use after expiration date.

If you have any questions, consult your doctor, pharmacist, or health care provider.

Antibiotics
- Aminoglycosides, Oral, 1031
- Aztreonam, 1034
- Cephalosporins, 1037
- Chloramphenicol, 1045
- Lincosamides, 1048
- Macrolides, 1052
- Spectinomycin HCl, 1059
- Erythromycin, Topical, 1061
- Vancomycin, 1063
- Oxalodinones, 1066
- Fluoroquinolones, 1069
- Carbapenem Antibiotics – Meropenem, 1074
- Imipenem-Cilastatin, 1076
- Metronidazole, 1079
- Mupirocin, 1082
- Penicillins, Oral, 1084
- Tetracyclines, 1089
- Tetracyclines, Topical, 1094
- Trimethoprim (TMP), 1096
- Topical, Miscellaneous, 1098

Sulfonamides
- Sulfonamides,1101
- Erythromycin Ethylsuccinate/ Sulfisoxazole, 1104
- Trimethoprim/Sulfamethoxazole (TMP-SMZ), 1108
- Vaginal Anti-infectives, 1111

Antifungals
- Clotrimazole, 1114
- Fluconazole, 1116
- Griseofulvin, 1118
- Itraconazole, 1121
- Ketoconazole, 1124
- Nystatin, 1128
- Topical Preparations, 1130
- Topical Combinations, 1135
- Vaginal Preparations, 1138

Antimalarials
- Aminoquinolines, 1141
- Mefloquine, 1144
- Pyrimethamine, 1147
- Sulfadoxine/Pyrimethamine, 1149
- Halofantrine HCl, 1152
- Atovaquone/Proguanil HCl, 1154
- Quinine Sulfate, 1156

Antiviral Agents
- Foscarnet, 1158
- Ganciclovir, 1161
- Antiherpes Virus Agents, 1164
- Amantadine, 1167
- Cidofovir, 1170
- Ribavirin, 1173
- Rimantadine, 1176
- Zanamivr, 1178
- Oseltamivir Phosphate, 1180

Antiretroviral Agents
- Protease Inhibitors, 1182
- Nucleotide Analog Reverse Transcriptase Inhibitors, 1187
- Nucleoside Reverse Transcriptase Inhibitors, 1190
- Non-Nucleoside Reverse Transcriptase Inhibitors, 1195

Antiparasitics
- Albendazole, 1199
- Mebendazole, 1201
- Pyrantel, 1203
- Thiabendazole, 1205
- Ivermectin, 1207

Urinary Anti-infectives
- Methenamine/Methenamine Salts, 1209
- Fosfomycin Tromethamine, 1212
- Nalidixic Acid, 1214
- Nitrofurantoin, 1216
- Combinations, 1219

Miscellaneous Anti-infectives
- Antituberculosis Drugs, 1222
- Atovaquone, 1232
- Pentamidine Isethionate, 1234
- Interferon Alfa-n3, 1237
- Interferon Alfacon-1, 1239
- Interferon Gamma-1b, 1242
- Scabicides/Pediculicides, 1244

	Generic Name *Brand Name Examples*	Supplied As	Generic Available
Rx	**Kanamycin Sulfate**		
	Kantrex	**Capsules:** 500 mg	No
Rx	**Neomycin Sulfate**	**Tablets:** 500 mg	Yes
	Neo–fradin	**Solution, oral:** 125 mg/5 mL	No
Rx	**Paromomycin Sulfate**		
	Humatin	**Capsules:** 250 mg	No

The aminoglycosides are antibiotics with a broad spectrum of activity and effectiveness. The oral aminoglycosides are not significantly absorbed and are used primarily to suppress bacteria within the digestive tract. The injectable aminoglycosides (eg, neomycin, streptomycin, kanamycin, gentamicin, tobramycin, amikacin, netilmicin) are used in the treatment of serious infections. The following monograph discusses only the oral aminoglycosides.

For detailed information regarding injectable aminoglycosides and their uses, contact your pharmacist or doctor.

Type of Drug:

Anti-infective; antibiotic used to suppress the growth of bacteria normally found in the digestive tract.

How the Drug Works:

Aminoglycosides inhibit production of essential proteins in bacteria, causing bacterial cell death.

Uses:

Capsules and tablets: To suppress growth of intestinal bacteria.

In combination with other therapies to manage hepatic coma.

Neomycin oral solution: Used in hepatic coma to reduce ammonia-formulating bacteria in the intestinal tract. This reduction in blood ammonia has resulted in neurological improvement.

Paromomycin: To treat intestinal amebiasis (parasites).

Precautions:

Do not use in the following situations:

allergy to these drugs or any of their ingredients
inflammation or ulceration of digestive tract
obstruction of digestive tract

Use with caution in the following situations:

hearing loss
kidney disease
liver disease
myasthenia gravis
parkinsonism
ulcerative lesions, bowel (paromomycin only)

Hearing and kidney toxicity: Aminoglycosides (particularly the injectable products) can cause significant hearing and kidney damage. Toxicity may develop with routine doses, particularly in people with preexisting kidney disease and preexisting hearing loss. Evidence of toxicity requires discontinuation of the drug.

Superinfection: Use of antibiotics (especially prolonged or repeated therapy) may result in bacterial or fungal overgrowth of nonsusceptible organisms (secondary infection). The aminoglycoside may need to be stopped and another antibiotic may need to be prescribed.

Pregnancy: Safety for use during pregnancy has not been established. Some aminoglycosides (eg, neomycin) can cause fetal harm. Use only when clearly needed and when potential benefits outweigh the possible hazards to the fetus.

Breastfeeding: Most aminoglycosides appear in breast milk. It is not known if neomycin appears in human breast milk. Because of the potential for serious adverse reactions from the aminoglycosides in nursing infants, a decision should be made whether to discontinue nursing or to discontinue the drug, taking into account the importance of the drug to the mother.

Children: Safety and efficacy in patients under 18 years of age have not been established. If treatment is necessary, use with caution. Do not exceed a treatment period of 3 weeks because of absorption from the gastrointestinal tract.

Elderly: Patients may have reduced kidney function that is not evident in the results of routine screening tests. Monitoring of kidney function and hearing during treatment is very important if oral therapy is prolonged.

Lab tests may be required during treatment with aminoglycosides. Tests may include blood counts, hearing tests, kidney function tests, and urine tests.

Drug Interactions:

Tell your doctor or pharmacist if you are taking or if you are planning to take any over-the-counter or prescription medications with aminoglycosides. Doses of one or both drugs may need to be modified or a different drug may need to be prescribed. The following drugs and drug classes interact with aminoglycosides.

- 5-fluorouracil (eg, *Adrucil*)
- aminoglycosides, other
- anticoagulants, oral (eg, warfarin)
- antimicrobial drugs, ototoxic or nephrotoxic (eg, gentamicin)
- digitalis (eg, digoxin)
- diuretics (eg, furosemide)
- mannitol (eg, *Osmitrol*)
- methotrexate (eg, *Rheumatrex*)
- neuromuscular blocking agents (eg, tubocurarine)
- penicillin V potassium (eg, *Veetids*)
- polypeptide antibiotics (eg, polymyxin B)
- vitamin A
- vitamin B_{12}, oral

Side Effects:

Every drug is capable of producing side effects. Many aminoglycoside users experience no, or minor, side effects. The frequency and severity of side effects depend on many factors including dose, route of administration, duration of therapy, and individual susceptibility. Possible side effects include:

Kidney problems – Blood and protein in urine; increased urination; problems urinating; abnormal kidney function tests; destruction of kidney cells.

Hearing loss (May be no warning) – Ringing in the ears; hearing impairment; ear problems; dizziness.

Other: Rash; itching; nausea; vomiting; diarrhea; fatty stools; abdominal cramps; malaborption syndrome (increased fecal fat, decreased serum carotene, fall in xylose absorption).

Guidelines for Use:

- Complete full course of therapy.
- *Kanamycin sulfate* – As an adjunct to mechanical cleansing of the large bowel in short-term therapy, usual dosage is 1 g (2 capsules) every hour for 4 hours followed by 1 g (2 capsules) every 6 hours for 36 to 72 hours.
  As an adjunct in extended therapy of hepatic coma, usual dosage is 8 g to 12 g (16 to 24 capsules) per day in divided doses.
- *Neomycin sulfate* – As an adjunct to mechanical cleansing of the bowel before bowel surgery, usual dosage is 1 g (2 tablets) with 1 g erythromycin at 19 hours, 18 hours, and again at 11 hours before surgery.
  As an adjunct in extended therapy of hepatic coma, usual dosage is 4 g (8 tablets) per day in divided doses.
  For oral solution management of hepatic coma, withdraw protein from diet, avoid the use of diuretic agents, and give supportive therapy (eg, blood products). Recommended dosage is 4 g to 12 g/day in divided doses over 5 to 6 days, during which protein should be returned incrementally to the diet.
- *Paromomycin sulfate* – For intestinal amebiasis in adults and children, usual dosage is 25 mg to 35 mg/kg body weight daily, administered in 3 doses with meals, for 5 to 10 days.
  For management of hepatic coma in adults, usual dosage is 4 g daily in divided doses, given at regular intervals for 5 to 6 days.
- If a dose is missed, take it as soon as possible. If several hours have passed or if it is nearing time for the next dose, do not double the dose in order to catch up (unless advised to do so by your doctor). If more than one dose is missed or it is necessary to establish a new dosage schedule, contact your doctor or pharmacist.
- May cause nausea, vomiting, or diarrhea.
- Notify your doctor if ringing in the ears, hearing impairment, rash, problems urinating, or dizziness occurs.
- Drink plenty of fluids.
- Lab tests may be required. Be sure to keep appointments.
- Store at room temperature (59° to 86°F) and protect from moisture.

If you have any questions, consult your doctor, pharmacist, or health care provider.

Generic Name *Brand Name Examples*	Supplied As	Generic Available
Rx **Aztreonam**		
Azactam	**Powder for Injection:** 500 mg, 1 g, 2 g	No

Type of Drug:

Synthetic anti-infective, antibiotic.

How the Drug Works:

Aztreonam kills susceptible bacteria by interfering with formation of the bacterial cell wall. This increases the likelihood that the cell wall will rupture and result in cell death. Aztreonam is a particularly effective antibiotic against susceptible gram-negative bacteria.

Uses:

To treat serious infections caused by susceptible bacteria. Aztreonam may be particularly useful in treating urinary tract infections (eg, bladder infections), lower respiratory tract infections (eg, pneumonia), septicemia (blood poisoning), skin infections, abdominal infections, and gynecologic infections caused by gram-negative bacteria.

Unlabeled Use(s): Occasionally doctors may prescribe aztreonam to treat gonorrhea.

Precautions:

Do not use in the following situations:

allergy to aztreonam or any of its ingredients

Use with caution in the following situations:

allergy to beta-lactam antibiotics (eg, cephalosporins, penicillins)
aminoglycoside use, concurrent (eg, gentamicin)
kidney disease
liver disease

Elderly patients and patients with decreased kidney function: Drug may not be eliminated as rapidly in these patients. Dosage of the drug may be decreased or dosage interval altered in some instances.

Superinfection: Use of antibiotics (especially prolonged or repeated therapy) may result in bacterial or fungal overgrowth of organisms (secondary infection). Aztreonam may need to be stopped and another antibiotic prescribed for the second infection.

Diarrhea: If diarrhea develops during aztreonam use, pseudomembranous colitis must be considered. This inflammatory condition of the colon is due to overgrowth of bacteria that are not killed by aztreonam. The primary cause is a toxin produced by a bacteria known as *Clostridia difficile.* Colitis symptoms may range in severity from mild to life-threatening. Mild cases usually respond by stopping the antibiotic. In more severe cases, other antibiotics may need to be used.

Pregnancy: Adequate studies have not been done in pregnant women. Use only if clearly needed and potential benefits outweigh the possible hazards to the fetus.

Breastfeeding: Aztreonam appears in breast milk. Consult your doctor before you begin breastfeeding.

Children: The safety and effectiveness of aztreonam have been established in children 9 months to 16 years of age. It is not known whether aztreonam is safe and effective in children less than 9 months of age or in any child with septicemia (blood poisoning) or skin infections due to some types of organisms.

Lab tests may be required. Be sure to keep appointments.

Drug Interactions:

Tell your doctor or pharmacist if you are taking or if you are planning to take any over-the-counter or prescription medications with aztreonam. Doses of one or both drugs may need to be modified or a different drug may need to be prescribed. Beta-lactamase-inducing antibiotics (eg, cefoxitin) interact with aztreonam.

Side Effects:

Every drug is capable of producing side effects. Many aztreonam users experience no, or minor, side effects. The frequency and severity of side effects depend on many factors including dose, duration of therapy, and individual susceptibility. Possible side effects include:

Local: Inflammation of the vein (IV); discomfort, pain, redness, or swelling at injection site (IM).

Digestive Tract: Nausea; vomiting; diarrhea.

Other: Rash; fever; hives; itching; difficulty breathing; wheezing; dizziness; vaginal itching; headache.

Guidelines for Use:

- Aztreonam is usually administered by health care professionals in a health care setting.
- Aztreonam may occasionally be prescribed for home therapy. If so, carefully follow the storage, preparation, administration, and disposal directions given to you by your doctor.
- Given intramuscularly (IM) or intravenously (IV) only.
- The IV route of administration is preferred in patients requiring single doses greater than 1 g or in bacterial septicemia (blood poisoning), localized abscess, peritonitis (inflammation of the lining of the abdomen), and other severe or life-threatening infections.
- Duration of therapy depends on severity of infection. Usually continued for 48 hours after symptoms disappear or evidence of bacterial absence is confirmed. Persistent infections may require therapy for several days to several weeks.
- If diarrhea occurs, notify your doctor immediately. This could be a symptom of a severe side effect (pseudomembranous colitis) requiring immediate medical attention. Mild cases of colitis usually respond by stopping the drug. In more severe cases, other antibiotics may need to be used.
- Aztreonam may cause abnormal liver, kidney, and blood tests.
- Lab tests may be required. Be sure to keep appointments.
- Store at room temperature. Avoid excessive heat.

If you have any questions, consult your doctor, pharmacist, or health care provider.

	Generic Name *Brand Name Examples*	Supplied As	Generic Available
Rx	**Cefaclor**		
	Ceclor	**Capsules:** 250 mg, 500 mg	Yes
	Ceclor	**Oral suspension:** 125 mg/5 mL, 187 mg/5 mL, 250 mg/5 mL, 375 mg/5 mL	Yes
	Ceclor CD	**Tablets, extended release:** 375 mg, 500 mg	No
Rx	**Cefadroxil**		
	Duricef	**Capsules:** 500 mg	Yes
	Duricef	**Tablets:** 1 g	Yes
	Duricef	**Oral suspension:** 125 mg/5 mL, 250 mg/5 mL, 500 mg/5 mL	No
Rx	**Cefazolin Sodium**		
	Ancef, Kefzol	**Injection:** 500 mg, 1 g, 5 g, 10 g	Yes
	Ancef[1]	**Injection, (frozen):** 500 mg, 1 g	No
Rx	**Cefdinir**		
	Omnicef	**Capsules:** 300 mg	No
	Omnicef[2]	**Oral suspension:** 125 mg/5 mL	No
Rx	**Cefepime Hydrochloride**		
	Maxipime	**Injection:** 500 mg, 1 g, 2 g	No
Rx	**Cefixime**		
	Suprax	**Tablets:** 200 mg, 400 mg	No
	Suprax	**Oral suspension:** 100 mg/5 mL	No
Rx	**Cefmetazole Sodium**		
	Zefazone	**Injection:** 1 g, 2 g	No
	Zefazone	**Injection (frozen):** 1g/50 mL, 2 g/50 mL	No
Rx	**Cefonicid Sodium**		
	Monocid	**Powder for Injection, lyophilized:** 500 mg, 1 g, 10 g	No
Rx	**Cefoperazone Sodium**		
	Cefobid	**Injection:** 1 g, 2 g, 10 g	No
	Cefobid	**Injection (frozen):** 1 g/50 mL, 2 g/50 mL	No

	Generic Name *Brand Name Examples*	**Supplied As**	**Generic Available**
Rx	**Cefotaxime Sodium**		
	Claforan	**Injection:** 500 mg, 1 g, 2 g, 10 g	No
	Claforan	**Injection (frozen):** 1 g/50 mL, 2 g/50 mL	No
Rx	**Cefotetan Disodium**		
	Cefotan	**Injection:** 1 g, 2 g, 10 g	No
	Cefotan	**Injection (frozen):** 1 g/50 mL, 2 g/50 mL	No
Rx	**Cefoxitin Sodium**		
	Mefoxin	**Injection:** 1 g, 2 g, 10 g	No
	Mefoxin	**Injection (frozen):** 1 g, 2 g	No
Rx			
	Vantin	**Tablets:** 100 mg, 200 mg	No
	Vantin	**Oral suspension:** 50 mg/5 mL, 100 mg/5 mL	No
Rx	**Cefprozil**		
	Cefzil	**Tablets:** 250 mg, 500 mg	No
	Cefzil[β]	**Oral suspension:** 125 mg/ 5 mL, 250 mg/5 mL	No
Rx	**Ceftazidime**		
	Ceptaz, Fortaz, Tazicef, Tazidime	**Injection:** 500 mg, 1 g, 2 g, 6 g, 10 g	No
	Fortaz, Tazicef	**Injection (frozen):** 1 g, 2 g	No
Rx	**Ceftibuten**		
	Cedax	**Capsules:** 400 mg	No
	Cedax	**Oral suspension:** 90 mg/5 mL, 180 mg/5 mL	No
Rx	**Ceftizoxime Sodium**		
	Cefizox	**Injection:** 500 mg, 1 g, 2 g, 10 g	No
	Cefizox	**Injection (frozen):** 1 g	No
Rx	**Ceftriaxone Sodium**		
	Rocephin	**Injection:** 250 mg, 500 mg, 1 g, 2 g, 10 g	No
	Rocephin	**Injection (frozen):** 1 g, 2 g	No

	Generic Name *Brand Name Examples*	Supplied As	Generic Available
Rx	**Cefuroxime**		
	Ceftin	**Tablets:** 125 mg, 250 mg, 500 mg	No
	Ceftin	**Oral suspension:** 125 mg/ 5 mL, 250 mg/5 mL	No
	Kefurox, Zinacef	**Injection:** 750 mg, 1.5 g, 7.5 g	Yes
	Zinacef	**Injection (frozen):** 750 mg, 1.5 g	No
Rx	**Cephalexin HCl Monohydrate**		
	Keftab	**Tablets:** 500 mg	No
Rx	**Cephalexin Monohydrate**		
	Keflex	**Capsules:** 250 mg, 500 mg	Yes
		Tablets: 250 mg, 500 mg, 1 g	Yes
		Oral suspension: 125 mg/ 5 mL, 250 mg/5 mL	Yes
Rx	**Cephapirin Sodium**		
	Cefadyl	**Injection:** 500 mg, 1 g, 2 g, 4 g, 20 g	No
Rx	**Cephradine**		
	Velosef	**Capsules:** 250 mg, 500 mg	Yes
	Velosef	**Oral suspension:** 125 mg/ 5 mL, 250 mg/5 mL	Yes
	Velosef	**Injection:** 250 mg, 500 mg, 1 g, 2 g	No
Rx	**Loracarbef**		
	Lorabid	**Capsules:** 200 mg, 400 mg	No
	Lorabid	**Oral suspension:** 100 mg/5 mL, 200 mg/5 mL	No

[1] Contains dextrose.
[2] Contains sucrose (2.86 g/5 mL).
[3] Contains sucrose, aspartame, and phenylalanine (28 mg/5 mL).

Type of Drug:

Anti-infective; antibiotic.

How the Drug Works:

Cephalosporins kill susceptible bacteria by preventing the formation and maintenance of the normal bacterial cell wall. This increases the likelihood that the cell wall will rupture. Effectiveness of the cephalosporins depends on factors such as dose, concentration of drug in blood, other body fluids and tissue, and the susceptibility of the organism. They are most effective when organisms are growing rapidly.

Uses:

To treat infections caused by various susceptible bacteria. Cephalosporins are particularly useful in treating respiratory tract infections (eg, bronchitis, pneumonia, otitis media), middle ear infections, skin and skin structure infections, urinary tract infections, bone and joint infections, blood poisoning, inflammation of the heart, sore throat (pharyngitis and tonsillitis), central nervous system infections (eg, meningitis), gynecologic infections, genital infections, abdominal infections, early Lyme disease, and sexually transmitted diseases.

Some cephalosporins are used before, during, and after surgery to reduce the risk of developing an infection. Certain injectable cephalosporins may be used in combination with other antibiotics to treat serious infections, but careful monitoring of kidney function is required.

Unlabeled Use(s): Ceftriaxone may be used to treat nervous system complications, joint pain, or inflammation of the heart associated with Lyme disease in patients who cannot use penicillin G.

Precautions:

Do not use in the following situations:

- allergy to cephalosporins or any of their ingredients
- hemolytic anemia, cephalosporin-associated

Use with caution in the following situations:

- allergy to penicillins
- bleeding disorders
- breastfeeding
- elderly
- gallbladder disease, symptoms
- kidney disease (especially in conjunction with dialysis)
- liver disease
- malnourished
- prolonged or repeated cephalosporin therapy
- stomach or intestinal disease, history (eg, colitis)

Superinfection: Use of antibiotics (especially prolonged or repeated therapy) may result in bacterial or fungal overgrowth (secondary infection). The cephalosporin may need to be stopped and another antibiotic prescribed for the second infection.

Bleeding complications: Bleeding complications seen with use of certain injectable cephalosporins (eg, cefmetazole, cefoperazone, cefotetan, ceftriaxone) are not generally a problem with oral therapy. Factors which may increase risk of bleeding complications are liver and kidney disease, low blood platelet count, poor nutrition, concurrent cancer, use of anticoagulants or aspirin, and use in elderly or debilitated patients.

Penicillin allergy: Penicillin-allergic patients should use cephalosporins cautiously. If a patient is allergic to penicillins, he or she may also be allergic to cephalosporins and vice versa. Cephalosporins are not an absolutely safe alternative to penicillins in the penicillin-allergic patient. Consult your doctor or pharmacist.

Serum sickness-like reactions: Serum sickness-like reactions (skin rashes with inflammation, joint pain, and fever) have been reported, usually following a second course of therapy and usually occur more frequently in children than adults. Symptoms usually occur a few days after beginning therapy and resolve after the drug is discontinued. Antihistamines and corticosteroids may be helpful in managing symptoms.

Coomb's test: Positive direct Coomb's tests may be caused by cephalosporins.

Immune mediated hemolytic anemia: Immune mediated hemolytic anemia has been observed in patients receiving cephalosporins. Rare cases of severe hemolytic anemia, including fatalities, have been reported. If a patient develops anemia any time within 2 to 3 weeks after the administration of a cephalosporin, consider the diagnosis of a cephalosporin-associated anemia and stop the drug until the cause is determined. Periodically monitor patients receiving prolonged courses of a cephalosporin for treatment of infections for signs and symptoms of hemolytic anemia.

Disulfiram-like reactions: Disulfiram-like reactions such as flushing, sweating, headache, and fast heartbeat may occur when alcoholic beverages are ingested within 72 hours after the use of certain cephalosporins (cefazolin, cefmetazole, cefoperazone, cefotetan).

Diarrhea: If diarrhea develops during cephalosporin use, pseudomembranous colitis must be considered. This inflammatory condition of the colon is due to overgrowth of bacteria that are not killed by cephalosporins. The primary cause is a toxin produced by a bacteria known as *Clostridia difficile.* Colitis symptoms may range in severity from mild to life-threatening. Mild cases usually respond to stopping the antibiotic. In more severe cases, other antibiotics may need to be used.

Seizures: Certain cephalosporins (usually injectables) may cause convulsions (seizures) in patients with decreased kidney function if the dose is not reduced. If seizures occur, the drug should be discontinued.

Pregnancy: There are no adequate and well controlled studies in pregnant women. Use only if clearly needed and the possible benefits outweigh the possible risks to the fetus.

Breastfeeding: Cephalosporins appear in breast milk. The nursing infant is at risk for certain cephalosporin-induced side effects. Caution should be exercised when administered to a nursing woman. Consult your doctor before you begin breastfeeding.

Children: Cephalosporins have been used in children. However, safety and effectiveness of the various cephalosporins are dependent on the age of the child and the organism being treated. Refer to individual package labeling and consult your doctor.

Lab tests may be needed to monitor therapy. Tests may include kidney and liver function tests, blood cell counts, and prothrombin time or International Normalized Ratio (INR) (blood-clotting tests).

Drug Interactions:

Tell your doctor or pharmacist if you are taking or if you are planning to take any over-the-counter or prescription medications while taking cephalosporins. Doses of one or both drugs may need to be modified or a different drug may need to be prescribed. The following drugs and drug classes interact with cephalosporins.

- alcohol
- aminoglycosides (eg, neomycin)
- antacids, aluminum- or magnesium-containing
- anticoagulants, oral (eg, warfarin)
- carbamazepine (eg, *Tegretol*)
- chloramphenicol (eg, *Chloromycetin)*
- diuretics (eg, furosemide)
- H_2-receptor antagonists (eg, cimetidine) (cefpodoxime and ceftibuten only)
- iron supplements (eg, ferrous sulfate)
- nephrotoxic drugs (eg, gentamicin)
- probenecid

Side Effects:

Every drug is capable of producing side effects. Many cephalosporin users experience no, or minor, side effects. The frequency and severity of side effects depend on many factors including dose, duration of therapy, and individual susceptibility. Possible side effects include:

Allergic Reactions: Rash; hives; itching; fever; joint pain; edema (fluid retention); difficulty breathing; Stevens-Johnson syndrome; toxic epidermal necrolysis; low blood pressure; skin inflammation; weakness; abnormal skin sensations; fainting; flushing; skin redness.

Serum sickness-like reactions: Rash; joint pain; fever.

Local: Pain, hardness, burning, tenderness, swelling, bleeding, or bruising at injection site; phlebitis (vein inflammation).

Digestive Tract: Nausea; vomiting; diarrhea; stomach pain; appetite loss; gas; indigestion; loose, reddish, or frequent stools; oral thrush; swollen tongue; excessive salivation; stomach inflammation.

Nervous System: Headache; dizziness; hot flashes; hallucinations; confusion; drowsiness; fatigue; agitation; nervousness; sleeplessness; seizures; irritability; chills; hyperactivity.

Other: Fever; nosebleed; low blood pressure; secondary fungal infection, particularly in the mouth, rectal, vaginal, and intestinal areas; taste changes; changes in color perception; abnormal lab tests including liver and kidney function tests, blood counts, urine and blood glucose, urine protein, bilirubin, and creatinine levels; itching in genital, vaginal, and anal areas; anemia; aggravation of myasthenia gravis; chest tightness or pain; yellowing of skin and eyes; difficulty breathing; joint pain and swelling; decreased platelets; transient hepatitis; back pain; kidney dysfunction; bleeding; runny nose; liver dysfunction; thirst; cough; swelling around the eyes; positive Coomb's tests; decreased phosphorus levels; painful or difficult urination; symptoms of gallbladder disease; lockjaw; neck muscle spasm; kidney pain; vaginal discharge; viral illness; arthritis; painful menstruation; flu syndrome.

Guidelines for Use:

- Use exactly as prescribed by your doctor.
- May be taken with food or milk if stomach upset occurs.
- *Ceftin* oral suspension, *Ceclor CD* tablets, and *Vantin* tablets should be administered with meals. Tablets should not be cut, crushed, or chewed.
- *Cefpodoxime* — Take with food to enhance absorption
- *Ceftibuten and loracarbef* — Take ceftibuten at least 2 hours before or 1 hour after a meal. Take loracarbef on an empty stomach, at least 1 hour before or 2 hours after a meal.
- *Cefuroxime tablets* — Swallow whole; do not crush or chew. Children who cannot swallow the tablet whole should receive the oral suspension.
- Take at prescribed intervals. Do not skip doses.
- Continue use until all of the prescribed drug has been taken. Failure to take a full course of therapy may prevent complete elimination of bacteria, allowing the infection to return. Continue the antibiotic even after a fever or other symptoms disappear.
- Iron supplements, including multivitamins that contain iron, interfere with the absorption of cefdinir. If iron supplements are required during cefdinir therapy, cefdinir should be taken at least 2 hours before or after the iron supplement.
- If a dose is missed, take or inject it as soon as possible. If several hours have passed or if it is nearing time for the next dose, do not double the dose in order to catch up (unless advised to do so by your doctor). If more than one dose is missed, or it is necessary to establish a new dosage schedule, contact your doctor or pharmacist.
- If diarrhea occurs, contact your doctor immediately. This could be a symptom of a severe side effect (pseudomembranous colitis) requiring immediate medical attention. Mild cases of colitis usually respond to stopping the drug. In more severe cases, other antibiotics may need to be used.
- Cephalosporins may cause allergic reactions. These may vary from mild itching and rash to a life-threatening reaction. Report prior allergic reactions to cephalosporins, penicillins, and any other drugs to your doctor. If you experience rash, hives, nausea, severe diarrhea, itching, fever, joint or muscle pain, chest tightness, fluid retention, urinary problems, chills, unusual bleeding or bruising, or difficulty breathing, contact your doctor immediately.
- May trigger seizures, especially in patients with kidney disease. Discontinue use and notify your doctor if seizures occur.
- Notify your doctor if you are breastfeeding. Cephalosporins appear in breast milk.
- May interact with other drugs. Consult your pharmacist or doctor before taking another drug while taking a cephalosporin.
- *Diabetes* — May interfere with urine tests for glucose and may give false test results. Notify your doctor before changing diet or dosage of diabetes medication.
- Some cephalosporins interact adversely with recent alcohol use (before or up to 72 hours after administration).

Guidelines for Use (cont.):

- A minimum of 10 days of treatment is recommended for any infection caused by group A beta-hemolytic streptococci. This is the bacteria that causes strep throat. This treatment period is necessary to prevent rheumatic fever (and possible heart damage) or kidney inflammation and damage.
- Ceftriaxone is indicated in the treatment of chancroid; uncomplicated gonococcal infections of the cervix, urethra, throat, rectum, and conjunctiva; bacteremia; gonococcal meningitis and endocarditis; ophthalmic neonatorum caused by *N. gonorrheae*; prophylactic treatment of infants whose mothers have a gonococcal infection; arthritis; epididymitis; pelvic inflammatory disease; proctitis; proctocolitis; and enteritis.
- Cefoxitin and cefotan are indicated in the treatment of pelvic inflammatory disease (PID).
- Cefixime, cefotetan, cefoxitin, and cefotaxime are indicated in the treatment of gonococcal infections.
- Ceftriaxone is indicated in the treatment of gonococcal meningitis and endocarditis.
- Cefotetan and cefoxitin are indicated for the treatment of pelvic inflammatory disease.
- Refer to product labeling for specific storage information.
- *Injections* — Carefully follow preparation, administration, and storage instructions provided by your health care provider regarding injections. Do not use injectable solutions if they are discolored or contain particles.
- *Oral suspensions* — Store in refrigerator (except cefixime and loracarbef). Do not freeze. Shake well before using. Check expiration date. May be kept for 14 days without significant loss of potency. Cefixime and loracarbef may be kept at room temperature. Cefuroxime may be kept for 10 days, either in the refrigerator or at room temperature.

If you have any questions, consult your doctor, pharmacist, or health care provider.

	Generic Name *Brand Name Examples*	Supplied As	Generic Available
Rx	**Chloramphenicol**	**Capsules:** 250 mg	Yes
	Chloromycetin Sodium Succinate	**Powder for Injection:** 100 mg/mL	Yes

Type of Drug:

Anti-infective; antibiotic.

How the Drug Works:

Chloramphenicol interferes with or prevents protein production in susceptible bacteria, slowing their growth.

Uses:

To treat serious infections in children and adults for which potentially less-harmful drugs are ineffective or not recommended.

To treat acute infections of typhoid fever. Not recommended for the routine treatment of the typhoid "carrier state."

To treat certain infections in patients with cystic fibrosis.

Precautions:

Do not use in the following situations:

- allergy to chloramphenicol or any of its ingredients
- bacterial infections, prophlaxis
- minor infections (eg, colds, influenza, throat infections)
- premature or newborn infants

Use with caution in the following situations:

- bone marrow depression, drugs causing
- glucose-6-phosphate dehydrogenase (G-6-PD, an enzyme) deficiency
- kidney disease
- liver disease
- porphyria (high concentrations of iron-free pigment)

Blood disorders: Serious and even fatal blood disorders have occurred after chloramphenicol use. There have been reports of aplastic anemia (severe form of anemia), granulocytopenia (decreased white blood count, causing increased risk of infections), and thrombocytopenia (decreased platelet count, causing bleeding or bruising). Blood disorders have occurred after short-term as well as long-term use. Monitoring of blood counts will be required frequently during treatment.

Superinfection: Use of antibiotics (especially prolonged or repeated therapy) may result in bacterial or fungal overgrowth. Such overgrowth of nonsusceptible organisms may lead to a secondary infection. Chloramphenicol may need to be stopped and another antibiotic prescribed for the second infection.

Pregnancy: There are no studies to establish the safety of this drug in pregnancy. Because chloramphenicol readily crosses the placental barrier, cautious use is particularly important during pregnancy at term or during labor because of potential toxic effects on the fetus (gray syndrome). Use only if clearly needed and potential benefits outweigh the possible hazards to the fetus.

Breastfeeding: Chloramphenicol appears in breast milk. Use with caution, if at all, while breastfeeding, because of the possibility of toxic effects on the nursing infant. Consult your doctor before you begin breastfeeding.

Children: Use with caution and in smaller doses in premature and full-term infants to avoid gray syndrome toxicity.

Lab tests are required to monitor treatment. Tests include bacterial cultures, blood counts, and chloramphenicol blood levels.

Drug Interactions:

Tell your doctor or pharmacist if you are taking or if you are planning to take any over-the-counter or prescription medications while taking chloramphenicol. Doses of one or both drugs may need to be modified or a different drug may need to be prescribed. The following drugs and drug classes interact with chloramphenicol.

- anticoagulants, oral (eg, warfarin)
- barbiturates (eg, phenobarbital)
- cyclophosphamide (eg, *Cytoxan*)
- hydantoins (eg, phenytoin)
- iron salts (eg, ferrous sulfate)
- penicillins (eg, amoxacillin)
- rifampin (eg, *Rifadin*)
- sulfonylureas (eg, glipizide)
- vitamin B_{12}

Side Effects:

Every drug is capable of producing side effects. Many chloramphenicol users experience no, or minor, side effects. The frequency and severity of side effects depend on many factors including dose, duration of therapy, and individual susceptibility. Possible side effects include:

Gray syndrome is a potentially life-threatening condition that can occur in premature infants and newborns given high doses of chloramphenicol during the first 48 hours of life. Symptoms include: Swelling of abdomen; ashen (pale) color; vomiting; shock; difficulty breathing; refusal to suck; loose green stools; limp muscles; decreased temperature.

Hematologic: Blood disorders (eg, bone marrow suppression, anemia) are the most serious side effects associated with chloramphenicol. Potentially fatal blood disorders may occur. Symptoms include: Fever, difficulty breathing; rash; numb or tingling hands or feet.

Digestive Tract: Nausea; vomiting; diarrhea; inflammation of the mouth or tongue.

Skin: Rash; hives; itching; unusual bleeding or bruising.

Other: Bone marrow depression; fever; confusion; depression; delirium; headache; fatigue; changes in vision; difficulty breathing.

Guidelines for Use:

- Dosage is individualized. Use exactly as prescribed.
- Usually taken every 6 hours around the clock.
- The injectable intravenous (IV; into a vein) form will usually be prepared and administered by a health care provider in a medical setting. It may occasionally be prescribed for home therapy.
- An oral dosage form of chloramphenicol will be substituted for the IV form as soon as possible by your health care provider.
- Take the oral dose on an empty stomach (at least 1 hour before or 2 hours after a meal). It may be taken with food if stomach upset occurs.
- Continue use until all of the prescribed medicine has been taken. Failure to take all of the medicine may prevent complete elimination of bacteria, allowing the infection to return.
- If a dose is missed, take it as soon as possible. If several hours have passed or it is nearing time for the next dose, do not double the dose to catch up unless advised to do so by your doctor. If more than one dose is missed or it is necessary to establish a new dosage schedule, contact your doctor or pharmacist.
- The use of this antibiotic, as with other antibiotics, may result in an overgrowth of nonsusceptible organisms, including fungi (secondary infection). If infections caused by nonsusceptible organisms appear during therapy, the chloramphenicol may need to be stopped and another antibiotic prescribed for the second infection.
- Doses are variable and depend on factors such as type of infection, age, liver function, and kidney function.
- Contact your doctor immediately if you experience fever, sore throat, mouth sores, tiredness, unusual bleeding or bruising, visual disturbances, diarrhea, or unusual sensations in hands or feet.
- Gray Syndrome may occur in premature infants and newborns, particularly if chloramphenicol is given during the first 48 hours of life. Symptoms appear after 3 to 4 days of continual higher-dose treatment and may include swelling of the abdomen, ashen (pale) color, vomiting, shock, difficulty breathing, refusal to suck, loose green stools, limp muscles, and decreased temperature. Death may occur within hours of onset of the symptoms. Death occurs in approximately 40% of patients. Stopping therapy when symptoms first appear increases the chance for complete recovery.
- Do not continue treatment with chloramphenicol longer than necessary. Avoid repeating a course of therapy with chloramphenicol, if possible.
- Do not use to treat minor infections such as colds, flu, or throat infections.
- Do not use to prevent an infection.
- Lab tests are required to monitor treatment. Be sure to keep appointments.
- Store capsules below 86°F. Protect from moisture and excessive heat. Store injection below 104°F, preferably at room temperature (59° to 86°F).

If you have any questions, consult your doctor, pharmacist, or health care provider.

	Generic Name *Brand Name Examples*	Supplied As	Generic Available
Rx	**Clindamycin HCl**		
	Cleocin HCl	**Capsules:** 75 mg[1], 150 mg[1], 300 mg	Yes
	Cleocin Pediatric	**Granules, flavored:** 75 mg/ 5 mL	No
	Cleocin Phosphate	**Injection:** 150 mg/mL	Yes
Rx	**Clindamycin, Topical**		
	Cleocin T	**Gel:** 10 mg/g (1%)	Yes
	Cleocin T	**Lotion:** 10 mg/mL	Yes
	Cleocin T, Clinda-Derm	**Solution, topical:** 10 mg/mL (1%)	Yes
Rx	**Lincomycin**		
	Lincocin	**Capsules:** 500 mg	No
	Lincocin[2], *Lincorex*[2]	**Injection:** 300 mg/mL	Yes

[1] Contains tartrazine dye.
[2] Contains benzyl alcohol.

Type of Drug:

Anti-infective; antibiotic.

How the Drug Works:

Systemic clindamycin and lincomycin cause bacterial cell death by suppressing protein production in susceptible bacteria.

Topical clindamycin treats acne by reducing the skin bacterial count and reducing the presence of free fatty acids that irritate the skin surface.

Uses:

Oral or injectable: To treat serious infections caused by susceptible bacteria. Use should be reserved for those allergic to penicillin or for use when penicillin or erythromycin is not appropriate. Less toxic agents should be used first whenever possible.

Topical: To treat acne.

Unlabeled Use(s): Occasionally doctors may prescribe topical clindamycin for rosacea. Clindamycin has been used to treat bacterial vaginosis due to *Gardenella vaginalis* and pelvic inflammatory disease.

Precautions:

Do not use in the following situations:

- allergy to lincosamides or any of their ingredients
- infections, minor bacterial or viral
- meningitis (clindamycin only)

Use with caution in the following situations:

- asthma or significant allergies, history of
- colitis or other digestive tract diseases, history of
- diarrhea
- kidney disease
- liver disease, moderate to severe

Benzyl alcohol: Some of these injectable products contain benzyl alcohol, which has been associated with fatal "gasping syndrome" in premature infants.

Superinfection: Use of antibiotics (especially prolonged or repeated therapy) may result in bacterial or fungal overgrowth (secondary infection) of nonsusceptible organisms. Clindamycin or lincomycin may need to be stopped and another antibiotic may need to be prescribed for the second infection.

Diarrhea: If diarrhea develops during lincosamide use, consider pseudomembranous colitis. This inflammatory condition of the colon is due to overgrowth of bacteria that are not killed by lincosamides. The primary cause is a toxin produced by a bacteria known as *Clostridia difficile.* Colitis symptoms may range from mild to life-threatening. Mild cases usually respond by stopping the antibiotic. In more serious cases, another antibiotic may need to be used.

Pregnancy: Clindamycin and lincomycin cross the placenta. There are no adequate and well-controlled studies in pregnant women. Use only if clearly needed and the potential benefits outweigh the possible hazards to the fetus.

Breastfeeding: Oral and injectable clindamycin and lincomycin appear in breast milk. It is not known if topical clindamycin appears in breast milk. Consult your doctor before you begin breastfeeding.

Children:

Oral and injectable lincosamides – Use of lincomycin in newborns is not recommended. Use caution when administering clindamycin to newborns and infants and carefully monitor when administering to children under 16 years of age.

Topical clindamycin – Safety and effectiveness in children under 12 years of age have not been determined.

Elderly: Use with caution. Older patients with severe illness may not tolerate drug-associated diarrhea well. Watch for changes in frequency of bowel movements.

Lab tests may be required during long-term treatment with lincosamides. Tests may include liver and kidney function tests, blood counts, and bacterial cultures.

Tartrazine: Some of these products may contain tartrazine dye (FD&C Yellow No. 5), which can cause allergic reactions in certain individuals. Check package label when available or consult your doctor or pharmacist.

Drug Interactions:

Tell your doctor or pharmacist if you are taking or planning to take any over-the-counter or prescription medications or dietary supplements while taking lincosamides. Doses of one or both drugs may need to be modified or a different drug may need to be prescribed. The following drugs and drug classes interact with lincosamides:

erythromycin (eg, *E-Mycin*)
kaolin-pectin (eg, *Kaopectate*)
neuromuscular blocking agents (eg, pancuronium bromide)

Side Effects:

Every drug is capable of producing side effects. Many lincosamide users experience no, or minor, side effects. The frequency and severity of side effects depend on many factors including dose, duration of therapy, and individual susceptibility. Possible side effects include:

Digestive Tract: Nausea; vomiting; diarrhea; bloody stools; anal itching; stomach pain or cramps; mouth or tongue sores; sore throat; unpleasant taste; heartburn.

Skin: Rash; hives; itching; red, dry, flaking, peeling, burning, or oily skin (topical clindamycin only).

Other: Ringing in the ears; feeling of whirling motion; vaginal infection; yellowing of skin or eyes; pain or irritation at injection site; abnormal liver function tests; abnormal blood cell counts; difficulty breathing; joint pain; kidney dysfunction including infrequent urination; low blood pressure.

Guidelines for Use:

- Dosage is individualized. Use exactly as prescribed.
- *Oral —*
  Lincomycin — Take on an empty stomach (except for water) at least 1 to 2 hours before or after meals. Take each dose with a full glass of water (6 to 8 oz).
  Clindamycin — Take without regard to food. Take each dose with a full glass of water (6 to 8 oz).
  Store at room temperature (59° to 86°F). Do not refrigerate the pediatric solution. Discard after 2 weeks.
- *Topical clindamycin* — For external use only. Shake lotion well immediately before use.
  If using solution with pledget applicator, remove pledget from foil just before use. Discard after single use.
  Apply a thin layer of the gel, lotion, or solution to the affected area twice daily.
  Make sure the area is clean and dry before application.
  Avoid contact with the eyes, nose, mouth, or other mucous membranes and damaged skin. Burning or irritation may occur.
  In case of contact with the eye, damaged skin, or mucous membranes, bathe the area with large amounts of cool tap water for several minutes.
  Store at room temperature (59° to 86°F). Protect from freezing. Keep container tightly closed.
- *Injections —*
  This medication will usually be prepared and administered by your health care provider in a medical setting. This medicine may occasionally be prescribed for home therapy. If so, carefully follow the storage, preparation, administration, and disposal techniques taught to you by your health care provider. Do not use if solution is discolored or contains particles.
- If a dose is missed, apply, take, or inject it as soon as possible. If several hours have passed or it is nearing time for the next dose, do not double the dose to catch up, unless directed by your doctor. If more than one dose is missed or it is necessary to establish a new dosage schedule, contact your doctor or pharmacist.
- Discontinue use and contact your doctor immediately if you experience severe diarrhea, stomach pain or cramps, bloody stools, unusual bleeding, bruising, joint pain, itching, hives, rash, or difficulty breathing. These could be symptoms of severe side effects requiring immediate medical attention. Do not treat diarrhea without consulting your doctor.
- Continue use until all of the prescribed medicine has been taken. Failure to take all of the medicine may prevent complete elimination of bacteria, allowing the infection to return.
- Lab tests may be required during long-term treatment. Be sure to keep appointments.

If you have any questions, consult your doctor, pharmacist, or health care provider.

	Generic Name *Brand Name Examples*	Supplied As	Generic Available
Rx	**Azithromycin**		
	Zithromax	**Tablets:** 250 mg, 600 mg	No
		Suspension, when reconstituted: 100 mg/5 mL (as dihydrate), 200 mg/5 mL (as dihydrate)	No
		Powder for Injection, lyophilized:100 mg/mL	No
Rx	**Clarithromycin**		
	Biaxin	**Tablets:** 250 mg, 500 mg	No
		Granules for oral suspension: 125 mg/5 mL, 250 mg/5 mL	No
Rx	**Dirithromycin**		
	Dynabac	**Tablets, enteric coated:** 250 mg	No
Rx	**Erythromycin Base**[1]	**Capsules, delayed release:** 250 mg, 500 mg	Yes
		Tablets, film coated: 250 mg, 500 mg	Yes
	E–base	**Tablets, delayed release:** 333 mg, 500 mg	Yes
	E-Mycin	**Tablets, delayed release:** 250 mg, 333 mg	Yes
	Ery-Tab	**Tablets, enteric coated:** 250 mg, 333 mg, 500 mg,	Yes
	PCE Dispertab	**Tablets with polymer coated particles:** 333 mg, 500 mg	No
	Eryc	**Capsules, delayed release:** 250 mg	Yes
Rx	**Erythromycin Estolate**	**Oral suspension:** 200 mg/5 mL, 250 mg/5 mL, 400 mg/5 mL	Yes
	Ilosone Pulvules	**Capsules:** 250 mg	Yes
Rx	**Erythromycin Ethylsuccinate**		
	Ery-Ped	**Tablets, chewable:** 200 mg	No
	E.E.S. 400	**Tablets, film coated:** 400 mg	Yes
	E.E.S. Granules	**Powder for oral suspension:** 200 mg/5 mL	No
	Ery-Ped Drops	**Suspension:**100 mg/2.5 mL	No
	E.E.S. 200, Ery-Ped 200	**Suspension:** 200 mg/5 mL	Yes
	E.E.S. 400, Ery-Ped 400	**Suspension:** 400 mg/5 mL	Yes

	Generic Name *Brand Name Examples*	Supplied As	Generic Available
Rx	**Erythromycin Gluceptate**		
	Ilotycin Gluceptate	**Injection:** 1 g	Yes
Rx	**Erythromycin Lactobionate**		
	Erythrocin Lactobionate	**Injection, lyophilized:** 500 mg, 1 g, 500 mg piggyback	Yes
Rx	**Erythromycin Stearate**		
	Erythrocin Stearate	**Tablets, film coated:** 250 mg, 500 mg	Yes
Rx	**Troleandomycin**		
	TAO	**Capsules:** 250 mg	No

[1] Some of these products are also available as an injection.

Type of Drug:

Antibiotic; anti-infective.

How the Drug Works:

Macrolide antibiotics suppress the formation of protein by bacteria, slowing bacterial growth or causing bacterial cell death.

Uses:

All (except Troleandomycin): To treat mild to moderate infections (eg, pharyngitis, tonsillitis, chronic bronchitis, pneumonia, skin infections) caused by susceptible bacteria.

Azithromycin: To treat lower and upper respiratory tract infections, pharyngitis or tonsillitis, skin infections, middle ear infections (children only), and certain sexually transmitted diseases caused by susceptible organisms.

Clarithromycin: To treat lower and upper respiratory tract infections, pharyngitis or tonsillitis, skin infections, sinusitis, middle ear infections (children only); to prevent spread of *Mycobacterium avium* complex (MAC) in patients with advanced HIV infection; and to treat stomach and intestinal ulcers caused by *Helicobacter pylori.*

Dirithromycin: To treat chronic bronchitis, secondary acute bronchitis, community-aquired pneuomnia, pharyngitis or tonsillitis, and skin infections.

Erythromycin: To treat *Mycoplasma pneumoniae* (respiratory tract infection), Legionnaire's disease, intestinal dysenteric amebiasis, pelvic inflammatory disease, whooping cough, diphtheria, erythrasma, and certain sexually transmitted diseases (eg, syphilis, gonorrhea, urethritis). Also used to prevent recurrent attacks of rheumatic fever and to prevent bacterial endocarditis. As an *alternative drug* in penicillin or tetracycline allergy or when penicillin or tetracycline is not recommended or not tolerated to treat susceptible organisms.

Troleandomycin: To treat lower and upper respiratory tract infections.

Unlabeled Use(s): Occasionally doctors may prescribe erythromycin prior to surgery.

Precautions:

Do not use in the following situations:

All – allergy to azithromycin, erythromycin, or any of the macrolide antibiotics

Azithromycin – moderate to severe pneumonia with other risk factors such as cystic fibrosis, immunodeficiency, functional asplenia, elderly or debilitated patients, hospital-acquired infections, patients requiring hospitalization, unknown or suspected bacteremia (blood poisoning)

Clarithromycin – patients receiving astemizole (*Hismanal*), cisapride, or pimozide

Erythromycin – astemizole, cisapride, liver disease

Use with caution in the following situations:

Azithromycin – kidney disease, liver disease

Clarithromycin – kidney disease, severe

Dirithromycin – bacteremias (blood poisoning), diarrhea, liver disease

Erythromycin – liver disease, myasthenia gravis

Diarrhea – If diarrhea develops during use, pseudomembranous colitis must be considered. This inflammatory condition of the colon is due to overgrowth of bacteria that are not killed by macrolide antibiotics. The primary cause is a toxin produced by a bacteria known as *Clostridia difficile.* Mild cases usually respond to stopping the antibiotic. Severe cases may require treatment with a different antibiotic.

Superinfection – Use of antibiotics (especially prolonged and repeated therapy) may result in bacterial or fungal overgrowth (secondary infection). Macrolide antibiotics may need to be stopped and another antibiotic may need to be prescribed for the second infection.

Pregnancy: Safety for use during pregnancy has not been established for many of these medications. Adequate studies have not been done with azithromycin, dirithromycin, erythromycin, and troleandomycin. Use these medications only if clearly needed and potential benefits to the mother outweigh the possible hazards to the fetus. Clarithromycin should not be used in pregnant women. There is a risk to the fetus.

Breastfeeding: Erythromycin appears in breast milk. It is not known if other macrolide antibiotics appear in breast milk. Consult your doctor before you begin breastfeeding.

Children: Safety and efficacy of erythromycin have not been established. Azithromycin is not recommended for middle ear infections in children under 6 months of age and is not recommended for pharyngitis or tonsillitis in children under 2 years of age. Injectable form of azithromycin is not recommended in children under 16 years of age. Clarithromycin is not recommended in children under 6 months of age for treatment of mycobacterial infections, or in children under 20 months of age. Dirithromycin is not recommended in children under 12 years of age. Troleandomycin is safe for children.

Elderly: Clarithromycin dosage should be reduced in elderly patients with severe kidney disease.

Lab tests may be required to monitor therapy. Tests may include cultures, blood cell counts, and kidney or liver tests.

Drug Interactions:

Tell your doctor or pharmacist if you are taking or if you are planning to take any over-the-counter or prescription medications with a macrolide antibiotic. Doses of one or both drugs may need to be modified or a different drug may need to be prescribed. The following drugs and drug classes interact with macrolide antibiotics.

carbamazepine (eg, *Tegretol*)
cyclosporine (eg, *Sandimmune*)
ergot-containing drugs (eg, *Ergomar*)
pimozide (*Orap*)

Azithromycin –

antacids, aluminum- or magnesium-containing (eg, *Rolaids*)
HMG-CoA reductase inhibitors (eg, lovastatin)
phenytoin (eg, *Dilantin*)
theophylline (eg, *Theo-Dur*)
triazolam (*Halcion*)

Clarithromycin–

anticoagulants, oral (eg, warfarin)
astemizole (*Hismanal*)
buspirone (*Buspar*)
cisapride (*Propulsid*)
digoxin (eg, *Lanoxin*)
disopyramide (eg, *Norpace*)
HMG-CoA reductase inhibitors (eg, lovastatin)
omeprazole (*Prilosec*)
rifabutin (*Mycobutin*)
rifampin (eg, *Rifadin*)
tacrolimus (*Prograf*)
theophylline (eg, *Theo-Dur*)
zidovudine (*Retrovir*)

Dirithromycin–

antacids, aluminum- or magnesium-containing (eg, *Rolaids*)
contraceptives, oral
digoxin (eg, *Lanoxin*)
theophylline (eg, *Theo-Dur*)

Erythromycin –

antacids, aluminum- or magnesium-containing (eg, *Rolaids*)
anticoagulants, oral (eg, warfarin)
alfentanil (*Alfenta*)
astemizole (*Hismanal*)
benzodiazepines (eg, diazepam)
bromocriptine (eg, *Parlodel*)
buspirone (*Buspar*)
carbamazepine (eg, *Tegretol*)
cisapride (*Propulsid*)
corticosteroids (eg, methylprednisolone)
cyclosporine (eg, *Sandimmune*)
digoxin (eg, *Lanoxin*)
disopyramide (eg, *Norpace*)
ethanol
felodipine (*Plendil*)
grepafloxacin (*Raxar*)
HMG-CoA reduce inhibitors (eg, lovastatin)
iron salts (eg, ferrous sulfate)
rifabutin (*Mycobutin*)
rifampin (eg, *Rifabutin*)
sparfloxacin (*Zagam*)
sucralfate (*Carafate*)
sulfonamides (eg, sulfisoxazole)
tacrolimus (*Prograf*)
theophylline (eg, *Theo-Dur*)
valproate (eg, *Depakote*)
vinblastine (eg, *Velban*)

Troleandomycin –

astemizole (*Hismanal*)
benzodiazepines (eg, diazepam)
buspirone (*Buspar*)
cisapride (*Propulsid*)
methylprednisolone (eg, *Medrol*)
oral contraceptives containing estrogen
rifabutin (*Mycobutin*)
rifampin (eg, *Rifabutin*)
tacrolimus (*Prograf*)
theophylline (eg, *Theo-Dur*)

Side Effects:

Every drug is capable of producing side effects. Many macrolide antibiotic users experience no, or minor, side effects. The frequency and severity of side effects depend on many factors including dose, duration of therapy, and individual susceptibility. Possible side effects include:

Digestive Tract: Nausea, diarrhea, vomiting, stomach pain; upset stomach.

Other: Hives, rash.

Azithromycin – Vaginal infection; headache; itching; dizziness; appetite loss; injection site pain and inflammation.

Clarithromycin – Stomach discomfort; headache; taste changes.

Dirithromycin – Stomach problems; indigestion; gas; headache; weakness; dizziness; feeling of a whirling motion; sleeplessness; cough; itching; vaginal inflammation.

Erythromycin – Stomach cramps or discomfort; severe stomach pain; yellowing of eyes or skin; liver dysfunction; abnormal liver function tests.

Guidelines for Use:

- Use exactly as prescribed.
- Take tablets or capsules with a full glass of water (6 to 8 oz).
- Contact your doctor if nausea, vomiting, diarrhea, stomach cramps, unusual tiredness, severe abdominal pain, yellow discoloration of skin or eyes, rash, dark urine, or pale stools occurs.
- If diarrhea occurs, contact your doctor immediately. This could be a symptom of a severe side effect requiring immediate medical attention. Do not treat diarrhea without consulting your doctor.
- If a dose is missed, take or inject it as soon as possible. If several hours have passed or if it is nearing time for the next dose, do not double the dose in order to catch up (unless advised to do so by your doctor). If more than one dose is missed or it is necessary to establish a new dosage schedule, contact your doctor or pharmacist.
- Continue use until all of the prescribed medicine has been taken, even if fever or other symptoms have disappeared. Failure to take all of the medicine may prevent complete elimination of bacteria, allowing the infection to return.
- If chest pain, difficulty breathing, mouth sores, rash, hives, itching, or sensitivity to light occur, contact your doctor immediately. These may be signs of a serious allergic reaction. The medicine should be discontinued and appropriate therapy instituted.
- *Azithromycin* – Take capsules and suspension at least 1 hour before or 2 hours after a meal. Tablets can be taken without regard to meals. If stomach upset occurs, tablets can be taken with food.

  The recommended IV dosage for adult patients is 500 mg as a single dose for at least 2 days. IV therapy should be followed by oral azithromycin as a single daily dose to complete a 7-day course of therapy. Your health care professional will determine the change in doseform.

  At the recommended dose, azithromycin should not be relied upon to treat syphilis. The Center for Disease Control (CDC) recommends azithromycin for the treatment of recurrent or persistent urethritis and chlamydial infection in adults and children weighing more than 45 kg. Azithromycin is also recommended for treatment of nongonococcal urethritis and uncomplicated gonococcal infections of cervix, pharynx, urethra, and rectum.

  Do not take aluminum- or magnesium-containing antacids 1 hour before or 2 hours after taking this medicine.

  May cause sensitivity to sunlight. Avoid prolonged exposure to the sun and other sources of ultraviolet light (eg, tanning beds). Use sunscreens and wear protective clothing until tolerance is determined.

  Store capsules and tablets between 59° to 86°F.

  IV form – Inspect solution prior to administration. Do not use if solution contains particles or is discolored. IV should be infused over a period of at least 60 minutes. Injection should not be given rapidly or intramuscularly.

  Store suspension in a tightly sealed container between 41° to 86°F. Use suspension within 10 days. Shake well before each use. Discard remaining suspension after treatment course is completed.Do not freeze. When diluted, azithromycin injection is stable for 24 hours at or below room temperature (86°F), or for 7 days if refrigerated (41°F).

Guidelines for Use (cont.):

- *Clarithromycin* – May be taken without regard to food. Take with food if stomach upset occurs.
  Follow each dose of the suspension with 6 to 8 oz of fluid.
  Take at evenly spaced intervals throughout the day, preferably every 12 hours.
  Adequate birth control is necessary with this product. If pregnancy occurs while taking this medication, the patient should be told of the potential hazard to the fetus.
  Store tablets at room temperature (59° to 86°F); protect from light in a tightly closed container. Shake suspension well before each use. Do not refrigerate. After mixing suspension, store at room temperature (59° to 86°F) away from light. Use within 14 days. Discard any unused medication.
- *Dirithromycin* – Take with food or within 1 hour of eating. Do not cut, chew, or crush the tablets. Store at room temperature (59° to 86°F).
- *Erythromycin* – Take on an empty stomach, 1 hour before or 2 hours after meals. If stomach upset occurs, take with food. The estolate, ethylsuccinate, and enteric coated forms of erythromycin are not significantly affected by food.
  Take at evenly spaced intervals throughout the day, preferably around the clock.
  Patients receiving intravenous injection should be transferred to the oral doseform as soon as possible.
  Erythromycin may not reach the fetus in adequate concentration to prevent congenital syphilis. Infants born to women treated for syphilis during pregnancy with oral erythromycin should be treated with an appropriate penicillin regimen.
  The CDC recommends erythomycin base products for the treatment of urethritis, infant pneumonia caused by *C. trachomatis*, and for the treatment chlamydial infection in pregnant women and children weighing less than 45 kg. Erythromycin base products are recommended as an alternative regimen for chlamydial infection in adults and nongonococcal urethritis.
  The CDC recommends erythromycin ethylsuccinate for treatment of urethritis and as alternative regimen for nongonococcal urethritis and chlamydial infection in adults and pregnant women.
  Some of these products may contain benzyl alcohol which has been reported to be associated with fatal "gasping syndrome" in premature infants and an increased incidence of neurological and other complications.
  After reconstitution of drops, liquid, and suspension, store at or below 77°F. Shake suspension well before using. Use within 14 days. Refrigerate to maintain the best taste.
- *Troleandomycin* – Dosage depends on condition being treated and its severity. Dosage should be within 250 mg to 500 mg 4 times a day for adults and 125 mg to 250 mg every 6 hours for children.

If you have any questions, consult your doctor, pharmacist, or health care provider.

	Generic Name *Brand Name Examples*	Supplied As	Generic Available
Rx	**Spectinomycin Hydrochloride**		
	Trobicin	**Powder for Injection:** 2 g vial	No

Type of Drug:

Anti-infective; antibiotic.

How the Drug Works:

Spectinomycin inhibits protein synthesis in bacterial cells resulting in the death of the bacteria.

Uses:

To treat acute gonorrheal urethritis and proctitis in men and acute gonorrheal cervicitis and proctitis in women due to susceptible strains of *Neisseria gonorrhoeae*, the bacteria that causes gonorrhea. Also used to treat men and women recently exposed to gonorrhea.

Precautions:

Do not use in the following situations: allergy to spectinomycin or any of its ingredients.

Use with caution in the following situations: patients with a history of atopy.

Syphilis: Spectinomycin is not effective in the treatment of syphilis. Antibiotics used in high doses for short periods of time to treat gonorrhea may mask or delay the symptoms of incubating syphilis. All patients with gonorrhea should have a serologic test for syphilis at the time of diagnosis and a follow up test after 3 months.

Benzyl alcohol: Spectinomycin contains benzyl alcohol which has been reported to be associated with fatal "gasping syndrome" in premature infants and an increased incidence of neurologic and other complications.

Pregnancy: Adequate studies have not been done in pregnant women. Use only if clearly needed and potential benefits to the mother outweigh the possible risk to the fetus.

Breastfeeding: It is not known if spectinomycin appears in breast milk. Consult your doctor before you begin breastfeeding.

Children: Safety and effectiveness in children have not been established.

Drug Interactions:

Tell your doctor or pharmacist if you are taking or planning to take any over-the-counter or prescription medications while taking spectinomycin. Doses of one or both drugs may need to be modified or a different drug may need to be prescribed.

Side Effects:

Every drug is capable of producing side effects. Many spectinomycin users experience no, or minor, side effects. The frequency and severity of side effects depend on many factors including dose, duration of therapy, and individual susceptibility. Possible side effects include: Soreness at injection site; nausea; dizziness; decreased urination; itching; hives; rash; chills; fever; sleeplessness; acute allergic reactions (eg, difficulty breathing, decreased blood pressure).

Guidelines for Use:

- This medication will be prepared and administered by a health care professional.
- To alleviate pain or soreness at injection site, apply warm compresses and take over-the-counter analgesics (eg, acetaminophen, ibuprofen).
- Not effective for syphilis. Antibiotics used in high doses for a short period of time to treat gonorrhea may mask or delay the symptoms of incubating syphilis.
- Contains benzyl alcohol which has been reported to be associated with fatal “gasping syndrome” in premature infants and an increased incidence of neurologic and other complications.
- Patients treated with spectinomycin should have a follow-up blood test for syphilis after 3 months.

If you have any questions, consult your doctor, pharmacist, or health care provider.

Generic Name *Brand Name Examples*	Supplied As	Generic Available
Rx **Erythromycin, Topical** [1]		
Staticin	**Solution:** 1.5%	No
A/T/S, Del-Mycin, Erycette, Eryderm 2%, Erymax, Erythra-Derm, Theramycin Z, T-Stat	**Solution:** 2%	Yes
A/T/S, Emgel, Erygel	**Gel:** 2%	Yes
Rx **Erythromycin Topical Combination** [1]		
Benzamycin	**Gel:** 30 mg erythromycin and 50 mg benzoyl peroxide/g	No

[1] Contains ethyl alcohol.

Type of Drug:

Topical antibiotic; acne medicine applied to the skin.

How the Drug Works:

The mechanism by which topical erythromycin treats acne is not known. Reduction of inflammatory lesions is presumably related to its antibiotic action.

Uses:

For the topical treatment of acne vulgaris.

Precautions:

Do not use in the following situations:

allergy to erythromycin or any of its ingredients
ophthalmic (eye) use

Superinfection: Use of antibiotics (especially long-term or repeated therapy) may result in bacterial or fungal overgrowth of nonsusceptible organisms (secondary infection). Contact your doctor if you suspect an infection unrelated to acne vulgaris.

Diarrhea: If diarrhea develops during topical erythromycin use, pseudomembranous colitis must be considered. This inflammatory condition of the colon is due to overgrowth of bacteria that are not killed by topical erythromycin. The primary cause is a toxin produced by a bacteria known as *Clostridia difficile*. Mild cases usually respond to stopping the antibiotic.

Pregnancy: There are no adeqate and well controlled studies in pregnant women. Use only when clearly needed and when the potential benefits outweigh the possible hazards to the fetus.

Breastfeeding: It is not known if erythromycin appears in breast milk after topical administration. Consult your doctor before you begin breastfeeding.

Children: Safety and efficacy in children have not been established.

Drug Interactions:

Tell your doctor or pharmacist if you are taking or if you are planning to take any over-the-counter or prescription medications while using topical erythromycin. Doses of one or both drugs may need to be modified or a different drug may need to be prescribed.The following drugs and drug classes interact with topical erythromycin.

acne therapy, topical (eg, abrasive, desquamating, or peeling agents)
clindamycin (eg, *Cleocin T*)

Side Effects:

Every drug is capable of causing side effects. Many patients experience no, or minor, side effects. The frequency and severity of side effects depend on many factors including dose, duration of therapy, and individual susceptibility. Possible side effects include:

Skin: Flushing, redness, peeling, burning, or tenderness in treated area; dryness; itching; oily skin; eye irritation; skin discoloration; inflammation of the face, eyes, or nose; hives.

Guidelines for Use:

- For topical use only. Do not use in the eyes.
- Keep away from eyes, nose, mouth, and other mucous membranes. If contact occurs, flush with water.
- Apply topical erythromycin to the affected areas in the morning and evening. Wash affected areas with soap and water, rinse well, and pat dry before applying the drug.
- Reduce frequency of application to once a day if excessive drying and peeling occur.
- Apply gels with fingertips. Spread medication lightly. Do not rub into skin.
- Apply solutions with applicator pad or fingertips. Wash hands after application.
- If excessive skin irritation or diarrhea occurs, discontinue use and consult your doctor.
- If there has been no improvement after 6 to 8 weeks, or if condition worsens, discontinue treatment and contact your doctor.
- Use additional topical acne therapy with caution because a cumulative irritant effect may occur.
- *Combination gel* — May bleach hair or colored fabric. Store combination gel in refrigerator (36° to 46°F). Do not freeze. Discard unused drug after 3 months.
- Store all erythromycin products (except combination gel) at room temperature (59° to 77°F). Keep tightly closed.

If you have any questions, consult your doctor, pharmacist, or health care provider.

	Generic Name *Brand Name Examples*	Supplied As	Generic Available
Rx	**Vancomycin HCl**		
	Vancocin	**Pulvules:** 125 mg, 250 mg	Yes
	Vancocin	**Solution, oral:** 1 g, 10 g	Yes
	Vancocin, Vancoled	**Powder for injection:** 500 mg, 1 g, 5 g, 10 g	Yes

Type of Drug:

Anti-infective; antibiotic.

How the Drug Works:

Vancomycin inhibits RNA production and interferes with the formation of the bacterial cell wall in susceptible bacteria.

Uses:

To treat staphylococcal enterocolitis and antibiotic-associated pseudomembranous colitis caused by *Clostridia difficile* (oral use only). The injection solution may also be given orally for this use. Oral use of vancomycin is not effective for other types of infection.

To treat serious, resistant, or severe infections (particularly staphylococcal infections) not treatable with other antimicrobials, including penicillins and cephalosporins (injection only).

To prevent bacterial inflammation of the heart (endocarditis) in penicillin-allergic patients who have congenital heart disease or rheumatic or other acquired or valvular heart disease when these patients undergo dental procedures or surgery of the upper respiratory tract (injection only).

Precautions:

Do not use in the following situations: Allergy to vancomycin or any of its ingredients.

Use with caution in the following situations:

excessive dose requirements
hearing loss
intestinal lining inflammation
kidney disease
low blood pressure
nephrotoxic agent therapy, concurrent (eg, aminoglycosides)
ototoxic agent therapy, concurrent (eg, aminoglycosides)

Superinfection: Use of antibiotics (especially prolonged or repeated therapy) may result in bacterial or fungal overgrowth (secondary infection). Vancomycin may need to be stopped and another antibiotic may need to be prescribed for the second infection.

Pseudomembranous colitis/diarrhea: If diarrhea develops during IV use of vancomycin injection, pseudomembranous colitis must be considered. This inflammatory condition of the colon is due to overgrowth of bacteria that are not killed by vancomycin. Mild cases usually respond to stopping the antibiotic.

Pregnancy: There are no adequate and well-controlled studies in pregnant women. Use only if clearly needed and the potential benefits to the mother outweigh the possible hazards to the fetus.

Breastfeeding: Vancomycin appears in breast milk. A decision should be made whether to discontinue nursing or discontinue the drug, taking into account the importance of the drug to the mother.

Children: Dosage may need to be adjusted, especially in premature neonates and young infants.

Elderly: Dosage may need to be adjusted, especially when kidney disease is also present.

Lab tests may be required to monitor therapy. Tests include hearing tests, kidney function, vancomycin blood levels, and blood count tests.

Drug Interactions:

Tell your doctor or pharmacist if you are taking or planning to take any over-the-counter or prescription medications or dietary supplements while taking vancomycin. Doses of one or both drugs may need to be modified or a different drug may need to be prescribed. The following drugs and drug classes interact with vancomycin:

- anesthetics (especially in children)
- nephrotoxic agents (eg, aminoglycosides, amphotericin B, cisplatin, bacitracin, polymyxin B)
- nondepolarizing muscle relaxants (eg, tubocurarine)
- ototoxic agents (eg, aminoglycosides)

Side Effects:

Every drug is capable of producing side effects. Many vancomycin users experience no, or minor, side effects. The frequency and severity of side effects depend upon many factors including dose, duration of therapy, and individual susceptibility. Possible side effects include:

Injection and oral: Kidney dysfunction or failure; hearing loss; abnormal blood cell counts; hives; itching; diarrhea; nausea; chills; rash; fever; ringing in the ears; dizziness; feeling of a whirling sensation.

Injection only: Pain, tenderness, or inflammation at the injection site; low blood pressure; difficulty breathing; wheezing; pain and muscle spasm of chest and back; flushing of upper body; blood vessel inflammation.

Guidelines for Use:

- Dosage is individualized. Take exactly as prescribed.
- Do not change the dose or stop taking, unless directed by your doctor.
- *Oral Solution* — Mix thoroughly to dissolve the dose. May be further diluted with 1 oz of water. Common flavoring syrups may be added to the solution to improve the taste. The diluted solution may be administered via nasogastric tube.
- *Injection* — For intravenous (IV; into a vein) use only. Visually inspect solutions for particles or discoloration before use. Follow the injection procedure taught to you by your health care provider. Administer dose over no less than 60 minutes to avoid rapid-infusion-related reactions.
- If a dose is missed, take or inject it as soon as possible. If several hours have passed or it is nearing time for the next dose, do not double the dose to catch up, unless advised by your doctor. If more than one dose is missed or it is necessary to establish a new dosage schedule, contact your doctor or pharmacist.
- Continue use until all of the prescribed medicine has been taken, even if fever or other symptoms have disappeared. Failure to use all of the medicine may prevent complete elimination of bacteria, allowing the infection to return.
- Dosage reduction may be necessary in patients with kidney function impairment and in premature neonates and young infants.
- If diarrhea develops during intravenous vancomycin use, pseudomembranous colitis must be considered. Contact your doctor immediately.
- Contact your doctor immediately if you experience sudden dizziness or lightheadedness with or without rash over the face and body, or hearing loss.
- Lab tests may be required to monitor therapy. Be sure to keep appointments.
- *Pulvules* — Store at controlled room temperature (59° to 86°F).
- *Oral Solution* — Store in the refrigerator. May be refrigerated for up to 2 weeks.
- *Injection* — Prior to reconstitution, store at room temperature (59° to 86°F). After reconstitution, store in the refrigerator. When reconstituted with 5% Dextrose Injection or 0.9% Sodium Chloride Injection, the injection may be kept for 14 days. When reconstituted with any other solution, the injection may stored for 96 hours (4 days).

If you have any questions, consult your doctor, pharmacist, or health care provider.

	Generic Name *Brand Name Example*	Supplied As	Generic Available
Rx	**Linezolid**[1]		
	Zyvox[2]	**Tablets**: 400 mg, 600 mg	No
	Zyvox[2,3]	**Suspension, oral**: 100 mg/5 mL	No

[1] Also available as an intravenous injection
[2] Contains sodium.
[3] Contains phenylalanine.

Type of Drug:

Anti-infective; antibiotic.

How the Drug Works:

This drug inhibits bacterial protein synthesis, preventing bacterial reproduction.

Uses:

For the treatment of vancomycin-resistant *Enterococcus faecium* infections, nosocomial pneumonia, complicated and uncomplicated skin and skin structure infections, and community-acquired pneumonia caused by susceptible bacteria.

Precautions:

Do not use in the following situations: Allergy to linezolid or any of its ingredients.

Use with caution in the following situations: History of high blood pressure.

Phenylketonuria: Each 5 mL of linezolid oral suspension contains 20 mg phenylalanine. Consult your doctor or pharmacist.

Myelosuppression: Myelosuppression has been reported in patients receiving linezolid. Monitor blood counts weekly, particularly in those who receive linezolid for longer than 2 weeks, those with preexisting myelosuppression, those receiving drugs that produce bone marrow suppression, or those with a chronic infection who have received previous or concomitant antibiotic therapy. Consider stopping linezolid therapy in patients who develop or have worsening myelosuppression.

Pseudomembranous colitis/diarrhea: If diarrhea develops during linezolid use, pseudomembranous colitis must be considered. This inflammatory condition of the colon is due to overgrowth of bacteria that are not killed by linezolid. Mild cases usually respond when drug use is discontinued.

Tyramine-containing foods: Avoid large quantities of food or beverages with high tyramine content while taking linezolid. Quantities of tyramine consumed should be less than 100 mg/meal. Foods high in tyramine content include those that may have undergone protein changes by aging, fermentation, pickling, or smoking to improve flavor, such as aged cheeses (0 to 15 mg tyramine/oz), fermented or air-dried meats (0.1 to 8 mg tyramine/oz), sauerkraut (8 mg tyramine/8 oz), soy sauce (5 mg tyramine/1 tsp), tap beers (4 mg tyramine/12 oz), and red wines (0 to

6 mg tyramine/8 oz). The tyramine content of any protein-rich food may be increased if stored for long periods or improperly refrigerated.

Pregnancy: There are no adequate and well-controlled studies in pregnant women. Use only if clearly needed and the potential benefits to the mother outweigh the possible hazards to the fetus.

Breastfeeding: It is not known if linezolid appears in breast milk. Consult your doctor before you begin breastfeeding.

Children: Safety and effectiveness have not been established.

Lab tests may be required to monitor therapy. Tests include weekly blood counts.

Drug Interactions:

Tell your doctor or pharmacist if you are taking or planning to take any over-the-counter or prescription medications or dietary supplements while taking linezolid. Doses of one or both drugs may need to be modified or a different drug may need to be prescribed. The following drugs or drug classes interact with linezolid:

- adrenergic agents (eg, epinephrine, pseudoephedrine)
- selective serotnin reuptake inhibitors (eg, fluoxetine)
- MAOIs (eg, phenelzine)

Side Effects:

Every drug is capable of producing side effects. Many linezolid users experience no, or minor, side effects. The frequency and severity of side effects depend on many factors including dose, duration of therapy, and individual susceptibility. Possible side effects include:

Digestive Tract: Diarrhea; nausea; vomiting; taste sensation altered; tongue discoloration; constipation.

Other: Abnormal blood counts; headache; dizziness; rash; fever; changes in blood pressure; vaginal infection; fungal infection; abnormal lab tests; sleeplessness; itching.

Guidelines for Use:

- Dosage is individualized. Take exactly as prescribed.
- Do not change or stop taking the dose, unless directed by your doctor.
- May be taken without regard to meals.
- Notify your doctor if you experience frequent and persistent diarrhea.
- Do not vigorously shake the oral suspension before use. Gently invert the bottle a few times to mix.
- Inform your doctor if you are taking medications containing pseudoephedrine, such as cold remedies and decongestants.
- Inform your doctor if you are taking selective serotonin reuptake inhibitors or other antidepressants.
- Avoid eating large quantities of food or beverages with a high tyramine content.
- Lab tests may be required to monitor therapy. Be sure to keep appointments.
- Store at room temperature (59° to 86°F) in a tightly-closed container. Protect from light. Use oral suspension within 21 days.

If you have any questions, consult your doctor, pharmacist, or health care provider.

	Generic Name *Brand Name Examples*	Supplied As	Generic Available
Rx	**Ciprofloxacin**[1]		
	Cipro	**Suspension, oral:** 5 g/100 mL, 10 g/100 mL	No
	Cipro	**Tablets:** 100 mg, 250 mg, 500 mg, 750 mg	No
Rx	**Gatifloxacin**[1]		
	Tequin	**Tablets**: 200 mg, 400 mg	No
Rx	**Levofloxacin**[1]		
	Levaquin	**Tablets:** 250 mg, 500 mg, 750 mg	No
Rx	**Lomefloxacin HCl**		
	Maxaquin	**Tablets, film-coated:** 400 mg	No
Rx	**Moxifloxacin HCl**[1]		
	Avelox	**Tablets**: 400 mg	No
Rx	**Norfloxacin**		
	Noroxin	**Tablets:** 400 mg	No
Rx	**Ofloxacin**[1]		
	Floxin	**Tablets:** 200 mg, 300 mg, 400 mg	No
Rx	**Sparfloxacin**		
	Zagam	**Tablets:** 200 mg	No
Rx	**Trovafloxacin Mesylate**[2]		
	Trovan	**Tablets:** 100 mg, 200 mg	No

[1] Also available as an injection.
[2] Alatrofloxacin mesylate is available as an injection.

Type of Drug:

Anti-infectives; antibiotics.

How the Drug Works:

Fluoroquinolones cause an inhibition of DNA production of susceptible bacteria, resulting in inability to reproduce and bacterial cell death.

Uses:

Ciprofloxacin: To treat acute sinusitis, lower respiratory tract infections (eg, bronchitis), nosocomial pneumonia, skin and skin structure infections, bone and joint infections, urinary tract infections, infectious diarrhea, typhoid fever, acute uncomplicated cystitis in women, chronic prostate infection, complicated intra-abdominal infections (in combination therapy), inhalation anthrax (postexposure), and uncomplicated cervical, rectal, and urethral gonorrhea caused by susceptible bacteria. Also used as empirical therapy for febrile neutropenic patients.

Gatifloxacin: To treat chronic bronchitis, acute sinusitis, community-acquired pneumonia, complicated and uncomplicated urinary tract infections, pyelonephritis, uncomplicated urethral and cervical gonorrhea, and acute, uncomplicated rectal infections in women.

Levofloxacin: To treat sinus infections, lower respiratory system infections (eg, chronic bronchitis, community-acquired pneumonia), complicated and uncomplicated skin and skin structure infections, complicated and uncomplicated urinary tract infections, and acute pyelonephritis.

Lomefloxacin: To treat lower respiratory infections (except chronic bronchitis caused by *Streptococcus pneumoniae*) and urinary tract infections. Also used for preoperative prevention of infection in certain types of surgery.

Moxifloxacin: To treat acute bacterial sinusitis, acute bacterial exacerbation of chronic bronchitis, community-acquired pneumonia, and uncomplicated skin structure infections.

Norfloxacin: To treat sexually transmitted diseases (eg, uncomplicated gonorrhea), urinary tract infections, and prostate infections.

Ofloxacin: To treat lower respiratory infections (eg, chronic bronchitis, community-acquired pneumonia), sexually transmitted diseases (eg, uncomplicated gonorrhea, nongonococcal urethritis and cervicitis, acute pelvic inflammatory disease), skin and skin structure infections, uncomplicated cystitis, complicated urinary tract infections, and prostate infections.

Sparfloxacin: To treat community-acquired pneumonia and acute bacterial exacerbations of chronic bronchitis.

Trovafloxacin/alatrofloxacin: For use as initiating therapy in in-patient health care facilities to treat serious life- or limb-threatening infections such as community-acquired pneumonia, nosocomial pneumonia, complicated intra-abdominal infections, gynecologic and pelvic infections, and skin and skin structure infections.

Unlabeled Use(s): Occasionally doctors may prescribe fluoroquinolones for traveler's diarrhea, gonorrheal complications, ear infections, joint infections, bacterial meningitis, blood infections, bronchitis, pneumonia, prostate infections, osteomyelitis, prevention in urological surgery, pelvic inflammatory disease (PID), sinus infections, and endocarditis (inflammation of the lining of the heart).

Precautions:

Do not use in the following situations:

- allergy to any fluoroquinolone antibiotic or any of its ingredients
- allergy to quinolones
- low blood potassium
- tendon rupture associated with quinolone use, history of tendonitis
- QT_C prolongation (abnormal heartbeat, electrocardiogram abnormality) (gatifloxacin, moxifloxacin only)
- QT_C prolonging antiarrythmic drug (eg, disopyramide, amiodarone) therapy, concurrent

Use with caution in the following situations:

- kidney disease
- liver disease
- myasthenia gravis
- nervous system disorders, known or suspected (eg, epilepsy)

CNS stimulant toxicity: May produce seizures, psychosis, tremors, restlessness, light-headedness, confusion, hallucinations, paranoia, depression, nightmares, and sleeplessness.

Pseudomembranous colitis/diarrhea: If diarrhea develops during fluoroquinolone use, pseudomembranous colitis must be considered. This inflammatory condition of the colon is due to overgrowth of bacteria that are not killed by fluoroquinolones. Mild cases usually respond to stopping the antibiotic.

Sensitivity to light: May cause photosensitivity (sensitivity to sunlight), especially in patients using ciprofloxacin, lomefloxacin, ofloxacin, sparfloxacin, or trovafloxacin. Avoid prolonged exposure to the sun and other ultraviolet (UV) light sources (eg, tanning beds). Use sunscreens and wear protective clothing until tolerance is determined.

Superinfection: Use of antibiotics (especially prolonged or repeated therapy) may result in bacterial or fungal overgrowth. Such overgrowth may lead to a second infection. Fluoroquinolones may need to be stopped and another antibiotic may need to be prescribed for the second infection.

Syphilis testing: These medicines may mask or delay symptoms of syphilis during treatment for gonorrhea. At the time of gonorrhea diagnosis, patients should also be tested for syphilis. Patients should also have a follow-up test for syphilis after 3 months.

Tendonitis: Discontinue taking medicine, notify your doctor, rest, and refrain from exercise if you experience joint or muscle pain, inflammation, or rupture of a tendon.

Pregnancy: There are no adequate and well-controlled studies in pregnant women. Use only if clearly needed and the potential benefits to the mother outweigh the possible hazards to the fetus.

Breastfeeding: Ciprofloxacin, ofloxacin, sparfloxacin, and trovafloxacin appear in breast milk. It is not known if other fluoroquinolones appear in breast milk. Because of the potential for serious adverse reactions, decide whether to discontinue nursing or discontinue the drug, taking into account the importance of the drug to the mother. Consult your doctor before you begin breastfeeding.

Children: Safety and effectiveness in children have not been established. Use in patients under 18 years of age is not recommended.

Elderly: Elderly patients may require adjusted dosages, particularly if moderate to severe kidney impairment exists.

Lab tests may be required to monitor therapy. Tests include blood counts, liver, pancreas, and kidney function tests, blood glucose monitoring, and blood pressure monitoring.

Drug Interactions:

Tell your doctor or pharmacist if you are taking or if you are planning to take any over-the-counter or prescription medications or dietary supplements while taking a fluoroquinolone. Doses of one or both drugs may need to be modified or a different drug may need to be prescribed. The following drugs and drug classes interact with fluoroquinolones although not every fluoroquinolone may interact similarly:

- antacids with aluminum, calcium, or magnesium (eg, *Amphojel*, *Tums*, *Milk of Magnesia*)
- antiarrythmic agents (eg, amiodarone, quinidine)
- anticoagulants (eg, warfarin)
- caffeine
- cyclosporine (eg, *Neoral*)
- didanosine (*Videx*)
- disopyramide (eg, *Norpace*)
- glyburide (eg, *Micronase*)
- iron salts (eg, ferrous fumarate)
- macrolide antibiotics (eg, erythromycin)
- nitrofurantoin (*Furadantin*)
- NSAIDs (eg, ibuprofen)
- phenothiazines (eg, promethazine)
- phenytoin (eg, *Dilantin*)
- procainamide (eg, *Pronestyl*)
- sotalol (eg, *Betapace*)
- sucralfate (eg, *Carafate*)
- theophyllines (eg, aminophylline)
- tricyclic antidepressants (eg, amitriptyline)
- warfarin (eg, *Coumadin*)
- zinc salts

Side Effects:

Every drug is capable of producing side effects. Many fluoroquinolone users experience no, or minor, side effects. The frequency and severity of side effects depend on many factors including dose, duration of therapy, and individual susceptibility. Possible side effects include:

Digestive Tract: Nausea; vomiting; diarrhea; stomach pain; appetite loss; constipation; heartburn; gas; dry or painful mouth; indigestion; taste sensation changes; pseudomembranous colitis; oral fungal infection; mouth sores.

Nervous System: Dizziness; drowsiness; headache; sleeplessness; sleep disturbances; vertigo (feeling of whirling motion); nervousness; weakness; fatigue; psychotic reactions; hallucinations; seizures; confusion; depression; anxiety; light-headedness; paranoia; agitation; abnormal dreams; tremor.

Circulatory System: Abnormal heart rhythm; fast heartbeat; heart murmur; blood sugar changes; changes in blood pressure; palpitations (pounding in the chest).

Skin: Rash; hives; itching; photosensitivity; external vaginal itching; dry skin; sweating; pain and redness at injection site.

Other: Restlessness; vaginal irritation or discharge; lack of energy; general body discomfort; fever; vision disturbances; hearing loss; fainting; chills; swelling; abnormal lab tests; ringing in the ears; painful or difficult urination; blood in the urine; sore throat; exacerbated signs of myasthenia gravis; joint pain or stiffness; jaw, arm, back, neck, or chest pain; gout flare up; tingling of the fingers; difficulty breathing; tremor; sweating; runny nose; facial swelling; thirst; leg cramps; fainting; liver damage (trovafloxacin, alatrofloxacin only).

Guidelines for Use:

- Dosage is individualized. Take exactly as prescribed.
- Do not change the dose or stop taking, unless directed by your doctor.
- Take norfloxacin on an empty stomach, 1 hour before or 2 hours after meals. All other fluoroquinolones may be taken without regard to meals.
- Drink plenty of liquids while taking this medicine.
- Do not consume caffeine-containing products (eg, certain drugs, coffee, tea, certain carbonated beverages) during therapy with fluorquinolones (other than sparfloxacin).
- Do not take antacids containing magnesium, calcium, or aluminum or products containing citric acid buffered with sodium citrate, iron, magnesium, zinc, or didanosine chewable/buffered tablets or buffered solution, or the pediatric powder for oral solution simultaneously or within 6 hours before or 2 hours (8 hours for moxifloxacin) after taking a fluoroquinolone.
- If a dose is missed, take it as soon as possible. If several hours have passed or it is nearing time for the next dose, do not double dose to catch up, unless advised to do so by your doctor. If more than one dose is missed, or it is necessary to establish a new dosage schedule, contact your doctor or pharmacist.
- May cause dizziness or light-headedness. Use caution when driving or performing other tasks requiring alertness, coordination, or physical dexterity until tolerance is determined.
- Stop taking at first appearance of rash, facial swelling, rapid heartbeat, difficulty breathing, or other allergic signs. Report nausea, vomiting, or diarrhea to your doctor.
- Continue use until all of the prescribed drug has been taken, even if fever or other symptoms of infection have disappeared. Failure to take a full course of therapy may prevent complete elimination of bacteria, causing a relapse of infection.
- Discontinue medication and notify your doctor if you experience tremors; light-headedness; appetite loss; yellowing of the skin or eyes; dark urine; pale stools; confusion; hallucinations; palpitations (pounding in the chest); fainting spells; paranoia; depression; nightmares; insomnia; or pain, inflammation, or rupture of a tendon.
- Patients with a history of seizures or other nervous system disorders should consult their doctor before use.
- Diabetic patients should monitor blood sugar regularly while taking a fluoroquinolone. Notify your doctor immediately if you experience a hypoglycemic or hyperglycemic reaction.
- May cause sensitivity to sunlight. Avoid prolonged exposure to sun or other ultraviolet (UV) light (eg, tanning beds). Use sunscreens and wear protective clothing. Discontinue use if you experience burning sensation, redness, swelling, blisters, rash, or itching.
- Lab tests may be required to monitor therapy. Be sure to keep appointments.
- Store as directed by the package labeling.

If you have any questions, consult your doctor, pharmacist, or health care provider.

	Generic Name *Brand Name Example*	Supplied As	Generic Available
Rx	**Meropenem**		
	Merrem I.V.	**Powder for injection:** 500 mg, 1 g	No

Type of Drug:

Carbapenem antibiotic.

How the Drug Works:

Meropenem kills certain bacteria by interfering with formation of the bacterial cell wall.

Uses:

To treat serious infections caused by susceptible bacteria that produce complicated intra-abdominal infections and bacterial meningitis (in children 3 months of age and older).

Precautions:

Do not use in the following situations:

allergy to meropenem or any of its ingredients
allergy to other carbapenem antibiotics
anaphylactic reaction to β-lactams (eg, penicillin)

Use with caution in the following situations:

allergy to cephalosporins
bacterial meningitis
brain lesions
colitis, active
compromised kidney function
diarrhea, active
multiple allergies, history of
seizures, history of

Kidney function impairment: A dosage adjustment is required in patients with kidney function impairment.

Pseudomembranous colitis/diarrhea: If diarrhea develops during meropenem use, pseudomembranous colitis must be considered. This inflammatory condition of the colon is due to overgrowth of bacteria not killed by meropenem. Mild cases usually respond to stopping the antibiotic.

Superinfection: Use of antibiotics (especially prolonged or repeated therapy) may result in bacterial or fungal overgrowth. Such overgrowth may lead to a secondary infection. Meropenem may need to be stopped and another antibiotic prescribed for the secondary infection.

Pregnancy: There are no adequate and well-controlled studies in pregnant women. Use only if clearly needed and the potential benefits to the mother outweigh the possible hazards to the fetus.

Breastfeeding: It is not known if meropenem appears in breast milk. Consult your doctor before you begin breastfeeding.

Children: The safety and effectiveness of meropenem have been established in patients 3 months of age and older. Use of meropenem in pediatric patients with bacterial meningitis or intra-abdominal infections is supported by evidence from adequate and well-controlled studies.

Elderly: A dosage adjustment is recommended in elderly patients with diminished kidney function.

Lab tests may be required to monitor therapy. Be sure to keep appointments. Tests may include: Periodic assessment of organ function, including kidney, liver and blood function.

Drug Interactions:

Tell your doctor or pharmacist if you are taking or if you are planning to take any over-the-counter or prescription medications with meropenem. Doses of one or both drugs may need to be modified or a different drug may need to be prescribed. Probenecid interacts with meropenem; avoid concurrent use.

Side Effects:

Every drug is capable of producing side effects. Many meropenem users experience side effects. The frequency and severity of side effects depend on many factors including dose, duration of therapy and individual susceptibility. Possible side effects include:

Digestive Tract: Diarrhea; nausea; vomiting; constipation; blood in stools; mouth infection; inflammation of the tongue.

Skin: Hives; rash; itching.

Other: Headache; nosebleeds; difficulty breathing; inflammation at injection site; vein inflammation; abnormal lab tests.

Guidelines for Use:

- Any rash, itching, shortness of breath, dizziness, or disorientation should be reported to a physician.
- Diarrhea should be reported to a physician.
- Use with caution in patients with a seizure disorder.
- The dose and duration of therapy is based on location and severity of infection, age and kidney function.
- This drug is given by injection. Solutions for injection must be prepared using appropriate aseptic techniques.
- This drug should not be added to solutions containing other drugs.
- If a dose is missed, inject it as soon as possible. If several hours have passed or if it is nearing time for the next dose, do not double the dose in order to "catch up" (unless advised to do so by your doctor). If more than one dose is missed or it is necessary to establish a new dosage schedule, contact your doctor or pharmacist. Use exactly as prescribed.
- It is best to administer freshly prepared solution; however, solutions remain stable for 1 to 4 hours at room temperature or for 2 to 24 hours if refrigerated depending on the solution in which it is mixed. Check product literature for specific storage guidelines.

If you have any questions, consult your doctor, pharmacist, or health care provider.

	Generic Name *Brand Name Example*	Supplied As	Generic Available
	Imipenem-Cilastatin		
Rx	*Primaxin I.V.*[1] *Primaxin I.M.*[2]	**Injection:** 250 mg imipenem equivalent and 250 mg cilastatin equivalent; 500 mg imipenem equivalent and 500 mg cilastatin equivalent; 750 mg cilastatin equivalent and 750 mg imipenem equivalent	No

[1] Contains 3.2 mEq/g.
[2] Contains 2.8 mEq/g.

Type of Drug:

Anti-infection drug; antibiotic.

How the Drug Works:

Imipenem-cilastatin kills certain bacteria by interfering with formation of the bacterial cell wall.

Uses:

To treat serious infections caused by susceptible bacteria that produce the following types of infections: Lower respiratory tract infections, intra-abdominal infections, gynecological infections and skin infections.

Primaxin I.V. only: To treat urinary tract infections, bacterial septicemia (blood poisoning), bone and joint infections, endocarditis (inflammation of the lining of the heart), polymicrobic infections (infections due to several species of organisms) and to treat infections resistant to other antibiotics (eg, cephalosporins, penicillins, aminoglycosides).

Precautions:

Do not use in the following situations:

allergy to any component of this drug
allergy to local anesthetics of the amide type (I.M. form only)
severe shock or heart block due to use of lidocaine HCl diluent (I.M. form only)

Use with caution in the following situations:

allergy to penicillins, cephalosporins or other beta-lactams
brain injury or disease
hemodialysis patients
kidney disease
nervous system disorder (eg, seizures)

Superinfection: Use of antibiotics (especially prolonged or repeated therapy) may result in bacterial or fungal overgrowth. Such overgrowth may lead to a secondary infection. Imipenem-cilastatin may need to be stopped and another antibiotic prescribed for the secondary infection.

Diarrhea: If diarrhea develops during imipenem-cilastatin use, pseudomembranous colitis must be considered. This inflammatory condition of the colon is due to overgrowth of bacteria that are not killed by imipenem-cilastatin. The primary cause is a toxin produced by a bacteria known as Clostridia difficile. Mild cases usually respond to stopping the antibiotic.

Lab tests may be required to monitor treatment. Be sure to keep appointments. Tests may include: Blood counts, liver and kidney function tests.

Pregnancy: Adequate studies have not been done in pregnant women, or animal studies may have shown a risk to the fetus. Use only if clearly needed and potential benefits outweigh the possible hazards to the fetus.

Breastfeeding: It is not known if imipenem-cilastatin or lidocaine HCl (diluent) appear in breast milk. Consult your doctor before you begin breastfeeding.

Children: Safety and effectiveness in children under 12 years of age have not been established.

Drug Interactions:

Tell your doctor or pharmacist if you are taking or if you are planning to take any over-the-counter or prescription medications while taking this medicine. Doses of one or both drugs may need to be modified or a different drug may need to be prescribed. The following drugs and drug classes interact with this medicine:

ganciclovir *(Cytovene)* (I.V. form only)
probenecid (eg, *Benemid*)

Side Effects:

Every drug is capable of producing side effects. Many patients experience no, or minor, side effects. The frequency and severity of side effects depend on many factors including dose, duration of therapy and individual susceptibility. Possible side effects include:

Local: Vein and injection site inflammation; pain, redness at injection site.

Other: Weakness; fever; difficulty breathing; itching; rash; seizures; drowsiness; low blood pressure; nausea; vomiting; diarrhea.

Guidelines for Use:

- Any rash, itching, shortness of breath, dizziness or disorientation should be reported to a physician.
- The initial dose is based on location and severity of infection, susceptibility of bacteria to the drug and patient characteristics (eg, age, weight, kidney function). Duration of therapy depends on the condition being treated and its severity. Therapy should not be stopped without consulting your doctor.
- If a dose is missed, inject it as soon as possible. If several hours have passed or if it is nearing time for the next dose, do not double the dose to "catch up" (unless advised to do so by your doctor). If more than one dose is missed, contact your doctor or pharmacist.
- See product literature for storage and mixing guidelines.
- *Primaxin I.M.* — Intramuscular injection should be administered in the thigh or buttocks only. Use within 1 hour after preparation. Keep refrigerated; do not freeze.
- *Primaxin I.V.* — Maintains potency for 4 hours at room temperature and for 24 hours when refrigerated. Do not freeze.

If you have any questions, consult your doctor, pharmacist, or health care provider.

	Generic Name *Brand Name Examples*	Supplied As	Generic Available
	Metronidazole[1]		
Rx	*Flagyl, Protostat*	**Tablets:** 250 mg, 500 mg	Yes
Rx	*Flagyl 375*	**Capsules:** 375 mg	No
Rx	*MetroGel*	**Gel:** 0.75%	No

[1] Some of these products are also available as an injection.

Type of Drug:

Anti-infection drug active against various bacteria and protozoa; antibiotic.

How the Drug Works:

Metronidazole enters the bacterial or protozoal cell, impairing production of essential chemicals, leading to cell death.

Uses:

Oral: To treat serious infections caused by susceptible bacteria. These infections may include: Abdominal infections (peritonitis, abscess); skin infections; gynecologic infections (eg, endometritis); infections of the blood; bone and joint infections; meningitis and brain abscess; lower respiratory infections (eg, pneumonia); and endocarditis.

To treat amebiasis and trichomoniasis (protozoal infections).

Topical: To treat inflammatory papules and pustules of rosacea (acne).

Unlabeled Use(s): Occasionally doctors may prescribe metronidazole to reduce infection rates in gynecologic and abdominal surgery and to treat hepatic encephalopathy, Crohn's disease, antibiotic-associated colitis, bacterial vaginosis, bed sores, giardia infections and stomach ulcers caused by certain bacteria.

Precautions:

Do not use in the following situations:

allergy to metronidazole, parabens, other ingredients or similar drugs
pregnancy, first trimester in patients with trichomoniasis

Use with caution in the following situations:

blood disorders
central nervous system disorders (eg, seizures)
fungal infections (eg, candidiasis)
liver disease

Nervous system effects: Seizures and numbness or tingling of the hands and feet have been reported. Stop taking this medicine if such symptoms occur. In some cases, the symptoms are not reversible.

Pregnancy: Adequate studies have not been done in pregnant women. Use only during the second and third trimesters if alternative treatment has been inadequate and only if clearly needed and potential benefits outweigh the possible hazards to the fetus.

Breastfeeding: Metronidazole appears in breast milk. A nursing mother should express and discard any breast milk produced while on the drug and resume breastfeeding 24 to 48 hours after the drug is stopped.

Children: Except for amebiasis, safety and effectiveness have not been established.

Lab tests may be required to monitor treatment. Be sure to keep appointments. Tests may include: White blood cell counts, protime tests for patients taking oral anticoagulants and lithium level tests for patients taking lithium.

Drug Interactions:

Tell your doctor or pharmacist if you are taking or if you are planning to take any over-the-counter or prescription medications with metronidazole. Doses of one or both drugs may need to be modified or a different drug may need to be prescribed. The following drugs and drug classes interact with metronidazole.

alcohol
anticoagulants, oral
(eg, *Coumadin*)
cimetidine (eg, *Tagamet*)
disulfiram (eg, *Antabuse*)
phenobarbital
phenytoin (eg, *Dilantin*)

Side Effects:

Every drug is capable of producing side effects. Many metronidazole users experience no, or minor, side effects. The frequency and severity of side effects depend on many factors including dose, duration of therapy and individual susceptibility. Possible side effects include:

Oral –

Digestive Tract: Nausea; vomiting; diarrhea; appetite loss, stomach ache; constipation.

Nervous System: Seizures; vertigo (feeling of whirling motion); depression; lack of coordination; confusion; irritability; weakness; inability to sleep; headache; dizziness.

Skin: Rash; hives; flushing.

Other: Dry mouth; joint pain; metallic taste; nasal congestion; abnormal blood cell count; painful and frequent urination; darkened urine; overgrowth of Candida (yeast); tingling in hands and feet; numbness; abnormal skin sensations; furry tongue; inflammation of the mouth or tongue; fever; bladder problems and inflammation; urinary problems; sense of pelvic pressure; pain during sex; decreased sex drive; dryness of vagina or vulva; inflammation of prostate.

Topical – Tearing of eyes (if drug is applied too close to the eye); redness; mild dryness, burning and irritation of the skin.

Guidelines for Use:

Oral:

- Avoid alcoholic beverages. Concurrent use of alcohol and metronidazole may produce abdominal pain, nausea, vomiting, headache and flushing. Do not consume alcohol for at least 1 full day after therapy with tablets is stopped and for at least 3 days after therapy with capsules is stopped.
- Take the full course of therapy to produce the best response.
- May cause a darkening of the urine.
- Some patients report a metallic taste while taking metronidazole.
- Sexual partners of patients with trichomoniasis should be treated simultaneously, whether they have symptoms or not.
- Stop taking this medication and notify your doctor if seizures, numbness or tingling in arms or legs occur.

Topical:

- Wash area before application. Rub on a thin film twice daily.
- For external use only. Avoid contact with the eyes.

If you have any questions, consult your doctor, pharmacist, or health care provider.

	Generic Name *Brand Name Example*	Supplied As	Generic Available
	Mupirocin		
Rx	*Bactroban, Bactroban Nasal*	**Ointment:** 2%	No

Type of Drug:

Topical anti-infective; externally used antibiotic.

How the Drug Works:

Mupirocin inhibits bacterial protein production by interfering with formation of RNA, causing bacterial cell death in susceptible organisms.

Uses:

Topical: To treat impetigo.

Nasal: To eradicate nasal colonization with methicillin-resistant *Staphylococcus aureus* in adult patients and healthcare workers as part of a comprehensive infection control program to reduce the risk of infection among high-risk patients during institutional outbreaks of infections with this pathogen.

Precautions:

Do not use in the following situations:
- allergy to any component of the ointment
- in the eyes

Superinfection: Use of antibiotics (especially prolonged or repeated therapy) may result in bacterial or fungal overgrowth. Such overgrowth may lead to a secondary infection. Mupirocin may need to be stopped and another antibiotic prescribed for the secondary infection.

Pregnancy: Studies in pregnant women have not shown a risk to the fetus. However, no drug should be used during pregnancy unless clearly needed.

Breastfeeding: It is not known if mupirocin appears in breast milk. Consult your doctor before you begin breastfeeding.

Children:

Nasal – Safety in children under 12 years of age has not been established.

Drug Interactions:

Tell your doctor or pharmacist if you are taking or planning to take any over-the-counter or prescription medication while taking mupirocin. Doses of one or both drugs may need to be modified or a different drug may need to be prescribed.

Side Effects:

Every drug is capable of producing side effects. Many mupirocin users experience no, or minor, side effects. The frequency and severity of side effects depend on many factors including dose, duration of therapy and individual susceptibility. Possible side effects include:

Skin: Burning; stinging; pain; itching.

Other: Sinus infection, congestion; headache; respiratory disorder; sore throat; throat inflammation; taste perversion; cough.

Guidelines for Use:

Topical:

- Apply a small amount of ointment to the affected area 3 times daily. A loose gauze dressing may be used to cover the area, if desired.
- If improvement of impetigo is not seen in 3 to 5 days, contact the doctor.
- Do not use in or near the eyes.
- If an inflammatory reaction persists, it may be due to a chemical irritation or an allergic reaction to the drug. Stop using mupirocin and consult your doctor.

Nasal:

- Application should be made in the morning and evening for 5 days.
- Apply half of the ointment into one nostril and the other half into the other nostril.
- Discard the tube. Do not re-use.
- Press the sides of the nose together and gently massage for about 1 minute to spread the ointment throughout the insides of the nostrils.
- Do not use in or near the eyes.
- Do not use any other nasal products at the same time.
- If an inflammatory reaction persists, it may be due to a chemical irritation or an allergic reaction to the drug. Stop using mupirocin and consult your doctor.

If you have any questions, consult your doctor, pharmacist, or health care provider.

	Generic Name *Brand Name Examples*	Supplied As	Generic Available
Rx	**Amoxicillin**		
	Amoxil	**Tablets:** 500 mg, 875 mg	No
	Amoxil, Trimox	**Tablets, chewable:** 125 mg, 200 mg, 250 mg, 400 mg	Yes
	Amoxil, Trimox	**Capsules:** 125 mg, 250 mg, 500 mg	Yes
	Amoxil, Trimox	**Oral suspension:** 125 mg/5 mL, 200 mg/5 mL, 250 mg/5 mL, 400 mg/5 mL	Yes
	Amoxil Pediatric Drops, Trimox Pediatric Drops	**Oral suspension:** 50 mg/mL	No
Rx	**Amoxicillin and Potassium Clavulanate**		
	Augmentin	**Tablets:** 250 mg amoxicillin, 125 mg clavulanic acid; 500 mg amoxicillin, 125 mg clavulanic acid; 875 mg amoxicillin, 125 mg clavulanic acid	No
	Augmentin	**Tablets, chewable:** 125 mg amoxicillin, 31.25 mg clavulanic acid; 200 mg amoxicillin, 28.5 mg clavulanic acid; 250 mg amoxicillin, 62.5 mg clavulanic acid; 400 mg amoxicillin, 57 mg clavulanic acid	No
	Augmentin	**Oral suspension:** 125 mg amoxicillin, 31.25 mg clavulanic acid/5 mL; 200 mg amoxicillin, 28.5 mg clavulanic acid/5 mL; 250 mg amoxicillin, 62.5 mg clavulanic acid/5 mL; 400 mg amoxicillin, 57 mg clavulanic acid/5 mL	No
Rx	**Ampicillin**		
	Principen, Totacillin	**Capsules:** 250 mg; 500 mg	Yes
	Principen, Totacillin	**Oral suspension:** 125 mg/5 mL; 250 mg/5 mL	Yes
Rx	**Bacampicillin HCl**		
	Spectrobid	**Tablets:** 400 mg	No
Rx	**Carbenicillin Indanyl Sodium**		
	Geocillin	**Tablets, film coated:** 382 mg	No

Rx	**Cloxacillin Sodium**	**Capsules:** 250 mg, 500 mg	Yes
		Oral solution: 125 mg/5 mL	Yes
Rx	**Dicloxacillin Sodium**		
	Dycill, Dynapen	**Capsules:**125 mg, 250 mg, 500 mg	Yes
	Dynapen	**Oral suspension:** 62.5 mg/ 5 mL	No
Rx	**Oxacillin Sodium**	**Capsules:** 250 mg, 500 mg	Yes
		Oral solution: 250 mg/5 mL	Yes
Rx	**Penicillin V Potassium**		
	Beepen-VK, Veetids	**Tablets:** 250 mg, 500 mg	Yes
	Beepen-VK, Veetids	**Oral solution:** 125 mg/5 mL, 250 mg/5 mL	Yes

Penicillins are antibiotics with a broad spectrum of activity and effectiveness. The injectable penicillins (eg, penicillin G, penicillin G procaine, penicillin G benzathine, methicillin sodium, nafcillin sodium, oxacillin sodium, ampicillin sodium, carbenicillin disodium, ticarcillin disodium) are used in the treatment of serious infections. The following monograph discusses only oral penicillins.

For detailed information regarding injectable penicillins and their use, contact your pharmacist or doctor.

Type of Drug:

Antibiotics; anti-infection drugs; penicillins.

How the Drug Works:

Penicillins kill susceptible bacteria by preventing the production of the bacterial cell wall. They are most effective in killing bacteria when bacteria are rapidly multiplying.

Uses:

To treat mild-to-moderate infections caused by penicillin-sensitive bacteria.

Precautions:

Do not use in the following situations:

- allergy to any penicillin or any of its ingredients
- cholestatic jaundice, drug-induced, history of (amoxicillin and clavulanate potassium only)
- infection caused by penicillinase-producing organisms (amoxicillin, ampicillin, bacampicillin, penicillin V only)
- liver dysfunction, drug-induced, history of (amoxicillin and clavulanate potassium only)
- mononucleosis (amoxicillin, ampicillin, bacampicillin only)

Use with caution in the following situations:

- allergies, history of
- allergy to cephalosporins
- asthma, history of
- cardiospasm
- gastric dilation
- hay fever, history of
- intestinal hypermotility
- kidney impairment
- liver disease (amoxicillin and clavulanate potassium only)
- nausea
- rash, history of
- severe illness
- vomiting

Superinfection: Use of antibiotics (especially for prolonged or repeated therapy) may result in bacterial or fungal overgrowth. Such overgrowth may lead to a second infection. The penicillin may need to be stopped and another antibiotic prescribed to treat the second infection.

Diarrhea: If diarrhea develops during penicillin use, pseudomembranous colitis must be considered. This inflammatory condition of the colon is due to overgrowth of bacteria that are not killed by penicillins. The primary cause is a toxin produced by a bacteria known as *Clostridia difficile*. Mild cases usually respond to stopping the antibiotic.

Penicillin V: Penicillin V is preferred over penicillin G for oral therapy. Penicillin V achieves blood levels 2 to 5 times higher than the same dose of penicillin G. Penicillin V is also stable in stomach acid, while penicillin G is not.

Clavulanic acid: Oral penicillins may be combined with clavulanic acid, a drug that inactivates enzymes produced by bacteria that destroy the penicillin. Clavulanic acid extends the effectiveness of penicillins.

Allergy: A person allergic to one penicillin may be allergic to other penicillins. Reactions to penicillin vary from mild itching and rashes to life-threatening reactions. All allergic reactions to any drug or food should be reported to your doctor.

Cephalosporins are a distinct group of antibiotics closely related to the penicillins. Due to the similarity, people allergic to penicillins may also be allergic to cephalosporins, and people allergic to cephalosporins may also be allergic to penicillins.

Cross resistance: Bacteria may become resistant to penicillin. If resistance develops to one of these drugs, it may result in resistance to most, if not all, penicillins.

Pregnancy: There are no adequate and well-controlled studies in pregnant women. Use only if clearly needed and the potential benefits to the mother outweigh the possible risks to the fetus.

Breastfeeding: Penicillins appear in breast milk. Consult your doctor before you begin breastfeeding.

Children: Use with caution in patients under 3 months of age. Safety and effectiveness of carbenicillin in children have not been established.

Lab tests may be required to monitor therapy. Tests may include blood counts, kidney and liver function tests, and bacteriologic studies.

Drug Interactions:

Tell your doctor or pharmacist if you are taking or if you are planning to take any over-the-counter or prescription medications with penicillins. Doses of one or both drugs may need to be modified or a different drug may need to be prescribed. The following drugs and drug classes interact with penicillins:

allopurinol (eg, *Zyloprim*)
amiloride (*Midamor*) (amoxicillin only)
aminoglycosides (eg, amikacin)
anticoagulants (eg, warfarin)
beta blockers (eg, atenolol)
chloramphenicol (eg, *Chloromycetin*)
contraceptives, oral (eg, *Ortho-Novum*)
disulfiram (eg, *Antabuse*)
food
macrolides (eg, erythromycin)
methotrexate (eg, *Rheumatrex*)
probenecid (eg, *Benemid*)
sulfonamides (eg, sulfisoxazole)
tetracyclines (eg, doxycycline)

Side Effects:

Every drug is capable of producing side effects. Many penicillin users experience no, or minor, side effects. The frequency and severity of side effects depend on many factors including dose, duration of therapy, and individual susceptibility. Possible side effects include:

Allergy — Side effects are more likely to occur in individuals with a history of previous allergic reactions. In penicillin-sensitive individuals with a history of allergy, asthma, hay fever, or hives, the reactions may be immediate and severe.

Allergic symptoms include nausea, vomiting, low blood pressure, shortness of breath, swollen joints, flushing, redness, wheezing, hives, itching, spasms in throat and breathing tubes, joint and muscle pain, difficulty breathing, chills, fever, fluid retention, skin rashes, and exhaustion.

Digestive Tract: Nausea; vomiting; diarrhea; stomach upset; gas; stomach pain or cramps; inflammation of the tongue or mouth; black, hairy tongue; loose stools.

Skin: Hives; itching; rash.

Other: Taste changes; abnormal liver function tests and blood counts; vaginal infection.

Guidelines for Use:

- Use exactly as prescribed. Dosage and duration of therapy will take into account severity of infection, susceptibility of bacteria to the drug, and general health of the patient.
- Take at even intervals, preferably around the clock.
- Absorption of most oral penicillins is decreased by food. These drugs are best taken on an empty stomach (1 hour before or 2 hours after a meal) with a full glass of water. Penicillin V, amoxicillin, and bacampicillin are exceptions and may be taken with food.
- Continue until all the prescribed drug has been taken even if symptoms of infection have disappeared. Failure to take a full course of therapy may prevent complete elimination of bacteria, causing a relapse of the infection.
- A minimum of 10 days of treatment is recommended for any infection caused by group A beta-hemolytic streptococci. This treatment period is necessary to prevent rheumatic fever or kidney inflammation and damage.
- If a dose is missed, take it as soon as possible. If several hours have passed or if it is nearing time for the next dose, do not double the dose to catch up, unless advised to do so by your doctor. If more than one dose is missed or it is necessary to establish a new dosage schedule, contact your doctor or pharmacist.
- Notify your doctor immediately if shortness of breath, wheezing, skin rash, mouth irritation, black tongue, sore throat, itching, nausea, vomiting, severe diarrhea, fever, swollen joints, unusual bleeding or bruising, flushing, redness, hives, or skin inflammation occurs.
- Contact your doctor immediately if severe diarrhea, stomach pain or cramps, or bloody stools occur. These could be symptoms of a serious side effect requiring immediate medical attention. Do not treat diarrhea without consulting your doctor.
- Use of antibiotics (especially prolonged or repeated therapy) may result in bacterial or fungal overgrowth. Such overgrowth may lead to a second infection. The penicillin may need to be stopped and another antibiotic prescribed for the second infection.
- Do not take any additional medications while taking a penicillin without your doctor's approval, including nonprescription drugs such as antacids, laxatives, and vitamins.
- If you have previously experienced an allergic reaction to penicillin, consider wearing a medical identification tag or bracelet documenting this reaction.
- Lab tests may be required to monitor therapy. Be sure to keep appointments.
- *Oral suspensions and solutions* — Do not freeze. Shake well before using. Check expiration date. Discard any liquid forms of penicillin after 7 days if stored at room temperature, or after 14 days if refrigerated.
- *Tablets and capsules* — Store at controlled room temperature (59° to 86°F) in a tightly closed container.

If you have any questions, consult your doctor, pharmacist, or health care provider.

	Generic Name *Brand Name Examples*	Supplied As	Generic Available
Rx	**Demeclocycline HCl**		
	Declomycin	**Tablets:** 150 mg, 300 mg	No
Rx	**Doxycycline**		
	Ed-DOXY Caps, Periostat, Vibramycin	**Capsules (as hyclate):** 20 mg, 50 mg, 100 mg	Yes
	Monodox	**Capsules (as monohydrate):** 50 mg, 100 mg	No
	Vibra-Tabs	**Tablets (as hyclate):** 100 mg	Yes
	Doryx	**Capsules, coated pellets (as hyclate):** 100 mg	No
	Vibramycin[1]	**Oral suspension (as monohydrate):** 25 mg/5 mL	No
	Vibramycin	**Syrup (as calcium):** 50 mg/5 mL	No
	Vibramycin	**Injection (as hyclate):** 100 mg/vial	Yes
Rx	**Minocycline HCl**		
	Dynacin, Minocin, Vectrin	**Capsules:** 50 mg, 75 mg, 100 mg	Yes
	Minocin[1]	**Oral suspension:** 50 mg/5 mL	No
	Minocin	**Injection:** 100 mg/vial	No
Rx	**Oxytetracycline HCl**		
	Terramycin	**Capsules:** 250 mg	Yes
	Terramycin	**Injection:** 50 mg/mL, 100 mg/2 mL, 250 mg/2 mL	No
Rx	**Tetracycline HCl**		
	Sumycin 250, Sumycin 500	**Capsules:** 250 mg, 500 mg	Yes
	Sumycin 250, Sumycin 500	**Tablets:** 250 mg, 500 mg	Yes
	Sumycin Syrup[1]	**Oral suspension:** 125 mg/5 mL	Yes

[1] Contains sulfites (metabisulfites).

Type of Drug:

Antibiotics; anti-infection drugs; antibacterial drugs.

How the Drug Works:

Tetracyclines inhibit susceptible bacteria's production of proteins necessary for their growth. This slows and prevents the bacteria's growth and reproduction while body defense mechanisms (eg, white blood cells) destroy them.

Uses:

To treat a wide variety of infections caused by susceptible bacteria.

As alternative drugs for certain types of infection when penicillin cannot be used (eg, penicillin allergy).

For treatment of uncomplicated urethral, endocervical, or rectal infections caused by *Chlamydia trachomatis.*

To treat severe acne and inclusion conjunctivitis.

Used with amebicides (antiparasitic drugs) to treat acute intestinal amebiasis (parasites).

Doxycycline: For use as a preventative against certain types of malaria in short-term (less than 4 months) travelers.

Also used as an adjunct to scaling and root planing to promote attachment level gain and to reduce pocket depth in patients with adult periodontitis (*Periostat* only).

Minocycline: To treat uncomplicated infections of the rectal and genitourinary tract caused by *Ureaplasma urealyticum.*

Unlabeled Use(s): Occasionally doctors may prescribe tetracyclines for other uses.

Demeclocycline – Used in patients with decreased blood sodium associated with the syndrome of inappropriate antidiuretic hormone (SIADH) secretion.

Doxycycline – To prevent “traveler's diarrhea.”

Minocycline – Used as an alternative to sulfonamides in nocardiosis.

Tetracycline – Used in specialized procedures for certain types of lung cancer. Tetracycline used with gentamicin has been recommended for wound infections or infections caused by eating contaminated seafood. Tetracycline suspension has been used as a mouthwash in the treatment of mouth ulcers and canker sores.

Tetracycline and doxycycline – Recommended for early Lyme disease.

Precautions:

Do not use in the following situations: Allergy to any tetracycline or any of its ingredients

Use with caution in the following situations:

children under 8 years of age
kidney disease
liver disease (injectable forms only)
oral candidiasis, predisposition or history of (*Periostat* only)
pregnancy

Bone: Tetracycline binds to calcium in bone. A decrease in growth rate has been observed in premature infants given oral tetracycline. This effect was reversible when the drug was discontinued.

Teeth: Use during tooth development (last half of pregnancy, infancy, and childhood to 8 years of age) may cause permanent discoloration (yellow-gray-brown) and inadequate calcification (hardening) of baby and permanent teeth. This reaction is more common if use is long term or repeated. Doxycycline and oxytetracycline may be less likely to affect teeth than other tetracyclines.

Pseudotumor cerebri: Tetracyclines have been associated with pseudotumor cerebri (benign intracranial hypertension). Early signs and symptoms include headache, nausea, vomiting, and blurred vision. Bulging fontanels ("soft spots") have been associated with tetracycline use in infants. If these symptoms develop, stop the drug immediately and contact your doctor.

Demeclocycline: Demeclocycline has resulted in the appearance of diabetes insipidus syndrome (eg, increased urination, increased thirst, and craving for ice water) in some patients on long-term therapy. The syndrome is reversible when therapy is discontinued.

Superinfection: Use of broad spectrum antibiotics (especially prolonged or repeated therapy) may result in bacterial or fungal overgrowth. Such overgrowth may lead to a second infection. The tetracycline may need to be stopped and another antibiotic may need to be prescribed for the second infection.

Cross resistance: Antimicrobial activity of the tetracyclines is similar. Resistance to one tetracycline may mean resistance to most or all of the others.

Pregnancy: Do not use during pregnancy. The risk of use in a pregnant woman clearly outweighs any possible benefit (see Children).

Breastfeeding: Tetracyclines appear in breast milk. Consult your doctor before you begin breastfeeding.

Children: Tetracyclines should not be used in children under 8 years of age, unless other drugs are not likely to be effective or are not advised.

Lab tests may be required during long-term treatment with tetracyclines. Tests may include blood counts and liver and kidney function tests.

Sulfites: Some of these products may contain sulfite preservatives that can cause allergic reactions in certain individuals. (eg, asthmatics). Check package label when available or consult your doctor or pharmacist.

Drug Interactions:

Tell your doctor or pharmacist if you are taking or if you are planning to take any over-the-counter or prescription medications with tetracyclines. Doses of one or both drugs may need to be modified or a different drug may need to be prescribed. The following drugs and drug classes interact with tetracyclines:

- aluminum salts (eg, aluminum carbonate)
- anticoagulants (eg, warfarin)
- bismuth salts (eg, bismuth subsalicylate)
- calcium salts (eg, calcium citrate)
- charcoal
- colestipol (*Colestid*)
- contraceptives, oral (eg, *Ortho-Novum*)
- digoxin (eg, *Lanoxin)*
- food
- insulin
- iron salts (eg, ferrous sulfate)
- lithium (eg, *Eskalith*)
- magnesium salts (eg, magnesium sulfate)
- penicillins (eg, penicillin V)
- urinary alkalinizers (eg, sodium bicarbonate)
- zinc salts (eg, zinc gluconate)

Side Effects:

Every drug is capable of producing side effects. Many tetracycline users experience no, or minor, side effects. The frequency and severity of side effects depend on many factors including dose, duration of therapy, and individual susceptibility. Possible side effects include:

Diabetes Insipidus Syndrome (demeclocycline): Weakness; excessive urination; excessive thirst.

Digestive Tract: Nausea; vomiting; appetite loss; diarrhea; indigestion; tongue inflammation; difficulty swallowing; indigestion; black, hairy tongue.

Skin: Rash; hives; sensitivity to sunlight; red or purple spots under the skin.

Other: Joint pain; anemia; decreased platelets; abnormal liver or kidney function tests and blood counts; mouth sores; teeth staining (in children); headache; lightheadedness (minocycline); pancreatic inflammation; exacerbation of lupus; pseudotumor cerebri; dizziness; common cold; sinus congestion; sinus headache; menstrual cramps; pain; decreased hearing; skin inflammation in the anal and genital region; feeling of whirling motion (minocycline); blurred vision.

Guidelines for Use:

- Dosage will be individualized. Use exactly as prescribed. Do not change the dose or stop taking unless advised to do so by your doctor.
- Injectable tetracyclines are used when oral dosage forms are not suitable.
- If a dose is missed, take it as soon as possible. If several hours have passed or if it is nearing time for the next dose, do not double the dose in order to catch up, unless advised to do so by your doctor. If more than one dose is missed, or it is necessary to establish a new dosage schedule, contact your doctor or pharmacist.
- Continue use until all the prescribed drug has been taken, even if symptoms of infection are gone. Failure to take a full course of therapy may prevent complete elimination of bacteria, causing a relapse of the infection.
- Do not use during pregnancy.
- Do not use in children younger than 8 years of age unless other drugs are not likely to be effective or are inadvisable. Use during tooth development may cause permanent discoloration and inadequate hardening of baby and permanent teeth.
- Take oral doseforms on an empty stomach at least 1 hour before or 2 hours after a meal. Exceptions are doxycycline and minocycline, which are not affected by food or milk.
- *Periostat* — Take at least 1 hour before the morning and evening meals.
- To prevent irritation of the esophagus (food pipe), take capsules or tablets with a full glass of water or other non-dairy liquid. Do not lie down for at least 30 minutes after a dose.
- Shake oral suspensions and syrups well before using.
- Avoid use of tetracyclines with antacids, laxatives, alcohol, dairy products (eg, milk, cheese) or iron-containing products. If any of these products must be taken, take at least 2 hours before or after tetracyclines.
- May cause photosensitivity (sensitivity to sunlight). Avoid prolonged exposure to the sun and other ultraviolet light. Use sunscreens and wear protective clothing until tolerance is determined.
- Concurrent use of tetracyclines with oral contraceptives (eg, *Ortho-Novum*) may cause the oral contraceptives to be less effective. Discuss alternative contraceptive methods with your doctor.
- Notify your doctor if you experience skin redness or flushing.
- *Do not use outdated tetracyclines.* Outdated tetracyclines may be highly toxic to the kidneys.
- *Minocycline* — Minocycline may cause lightheadedness, dizziness and vertigo (feeling of whirling motion). Use caution while driving or performing other tasks requiring alertness.
- Lab tests may be required to monitor therapy. Be sure to keep appointments.
- Store at controlled room temperature (59° to 86°F). Do not freeze oral suspensions or syrups. Check expiration date.

If you have any questions, consult your doctor, pharmacist, or health care provider.

ANTIBIOTICS — TETRACYCLINES, TOPICAL

	Generic Name *Brand Name Examples*	Supplied As	Generic Available
Rx	**Meclocycline Sulfosalicylate**		
	Meclan	**Cream:** 1%	No
	Tetracycline		
Rx	*Topicycline*	**Topical solution:** 2.2 mg/mL	No
otc	*Achromycin*	**Ointment:** 3%	No

Type of Drug:

Externally applied antibiotic.

How the Drug Works:

The mechanism by which topical tetracycline treats acne is not well defined. It is probably related, in large part, to its antibacterial activity.

Uses:

To treat acne vulgaris.

To prevent infection in minor skin abrasions and to treat superficial infections of the skin.

Precautions:

Do not use in the following situations: Allergy to tetracyclines or other ingredients in the formulation

Use with caution in the following situations:
- kidney disease
- liver disease

Pregnancy: Safety for use during pregnancy has not been established. Use only when clearly needed and when the potential benefits outweight the potential hazards to the fetus.

Breastfeeding: Safety for use while breastfeeding has not been established. Consult your doctor.

Children: Safety and effectiveness in children under 11 have not been established.

Sulfites: Some of these products may contain sulfite preservatives, which can cause allergic reactions in certain individuals. Check package label when available or consult your doctor or pharmacist.

Side Effects:

Every drug is capable of producing side effects. Many topical tetracycline users experience no, or minor, side effects. The frequency and severity of side effects depend on many factors including dose, duration of therapy and individual susceptibility. Possible side effects include: Irritation of skin; burning after application; rash; itching; slight yellow staining of skin or hair follicles.

Guidelines for Use:

- For external use only.
- Avoid contact with the eyes and lining of the nose and mouth.
- Apply to the affected area 2 times daily (morning and evening) for best results. Less frequent applications may be used if the response is good.
- Apply generously until the affected skin is thoroughly wet or covered.
- Stinging or burning may occur but should only last for a few minutes. If stinging or burning persists, contact your doctor.
- Excessive use of the cream may stain some fabrics.
- A slight yellowing of the skin may occur. This is not harmful and may be removed by washing.
- Normal use of cosmetics is permissible.

If you have any questions, consult your doctor, pharmacist, or health care provider.

	Generic Name *Brand Name Examples*	Supplied As	Generic Available
Rx	**Trimethoprim**		
	Proloprim	**Tablets:** 100 mg, 200 mg	Yes

Type of Drug:

Anti-infective agent.

How the Drug Works:

Trimethoprim (TMP) blocks production of folic acid which is needed by bacteria. Decreased folic acid interferes with the production of protein by the bacterial cell resulting in slowed bacterial growth or cell death.

Uses:

To treat urinary tract infections caused by susceptible bacteria.

Precautions:

Do not use in the following situations:

allergy to trimethoprim
anemia due to folic acid deficiency

Use with caution in the following situations:

folic acid deficiency
infants under 2 months
kidney disease
liver disease

Pregnancy: Adequate studies have not been done in pregnant women. Use only if clearly needed and potential benefits outweigh the possible hazards to the fetus.

Breastfeeding: Trimethoprim appears in breast milk. Consult your doctor before you begin breastfeeding.

Children: Safety in infants under 2 months has not been established. Effectiveness when taken alone in children under 12 has not been established.

Drug Interactions:

Tell your doctor or pharmacist if you are taking or if you are planning to take any over-the-counter or prescription medications with trimethoprim. Doses of one or both drugs may need to be modified or a different drug may need to be prescribed. Phenytoin (eg, *Dilantin)* interacts with trimethoprim.

Side Effects:

Every drug is capable of producing side effects. Many trimethoprim users experience no, or minor, side effects. The frequency and severity of side effects depend on many factors including dose, duration of therapy and individual susceptibility. Possible side effects include:

Digestive Tract: Stomach upset; nausea; vomiting.

Skin: Rash; inflammation; itching; swelling; redness; peeling skin.

Other: Inflammation of the tongue; fever; yellowing of skin or eyes; anemia; abnormal liver or kidney function tests.

Guidelines for Use:

- Take medication until it is gone. Do not stop without consulting your doctor.
- Do not use if you have anemia due to folic acid deficiency.
- Notify your doctor immediately if you develop any unusual bleeding or bruising, sore throat, fever, fatigue or skin reactions.
- May cause photosensitivity (sensitivity to sunlight). Avoid prolonged exposure to the sun or other forms of ultraviolet (UV) light (eg, tanning beds). Use sunscreens and wear protective clothing until tolerance is determined.

If you have any questions, consult your doctor, pharmacist, or health care provider.

ANTIBIOTICS — TOPICAL, MISCELLANEOUS

	Generic Name *Brand Name Examples*	Supplied As	Generic Available
otc	**Bacitracin**		
	Baciguent	**Ointment:** 500 units/g	Yes
Rx	**Chloramphenicol**		
	Chloromycetin	**Cream:** 1% in a water miscible ointment base	No
Rx	**Erythromycin**		
	Akne-mycin	**Ointment:** 2%	No
Rx	**Gentamicin**		
	Garamycin	**Ointment:** 0.1% (as 1.7 mg sulfate/g)	Yes
	Garamycin	**Cream:** 0.1% (as 1.7 mg sulfate/g)	Yes
otc	**Neomycin Sulfate**		
	Myciguent	**Ointment:** 0.5% (5 mg neomycin sulfate/g, equal to 3.5 mg neomycin/g)	Yes
	Myciguent	**Cream:** 0.5% (5 mg neomycin sulfate/g, equal to 3.5 mg neomycin/g)	No
otc	**Multiple Antibiotics**		
	Neosporin	**Cream:** 10,000 units polymyxin B sulfate and 3.5 mg neomycin base/g	No
	Polysporin	**Ointment:** 10,000 units polymyxin B sulfate and 500 units zinc bacitracin/g	No
	Polysporin	**Aerosol:** 200,000 units polymyxin B sulfate and 10,000 units zinc bacitracin/90 g	No
	Spectrocin	**Ointment:** 2.5 mg neomycin base (as sulfate) and 0.25 mg gramicidin/g	No
	Terramycin w/Polymyxin B Sulfate	**Powder:** 30 mg oxytetracycline and 10,000 units polymyxin B sulfate/g	No
	Terramycin w/Polymyxin B Sulfate	**Ointment:** 30 mg oxytetracycline and 10,000 units polymyxin B sulfate/g	No

	Generic Name *Brand Name Examples*	Supplied As	Generic Available
otc	**Triple Antibiotic**		
	N.B.P., Neomac, Septa	**Ointment:** 5000 units polymyxin B sulfate, 3.5 mg neomycin base and 400 units bacitracin/g	Yes
otc	*Lanabiotic*	**Ointment:** 5000 units polymyxin B, 3.5 mg neomycin base, 500 units bacitracin and 40 mg lidocaine/g	No
otc	*Mycitracin Triple Antibiotic*	**Ointment:** 5000 units polymyxin B, 3.5 mg neomycin base and 400 units zinc bacitracin/g	No
otc	*Neomixin, Neosporin*	**Ointment:** 5000 units polymyxin B sulfate, 3.5 mg neomycin base and 400 units zinc acitracin/g	No
otc	*Polysporin*	**Powder:** 10,000 units polymyxin B sulfate and 500 units zinc bacitracin/g	No

Type of Drug:

Externally applied antibiotics.

How the Drug Works:

Topical antibiotics exert their antibacterial action by different mechanisms with the same effect. The choice of antibiotic(s) depends on the nature of the wound and the suspected bacterial infection.

Uses:

To prevent infections after minor skin lacerations (cuts) or abrasions (scrapes).

To treat superficial infections of the skin caused by susceptible bacteria.

Precautions:

Do not use in the following situations:

allergy to any component of the formulation
in the eyes
in the outer ear canal (if eardrum is perforated)

Use with caution in the following situations:

deep skin infections
if redness, swelling, inflammation or pain worsens while using the drug

Neomycin sensitivity – Frequent application of neomycin sulfate to inflamed skin increases the chance of sensitivity developing. Reddening, swelling, dry scaling and itching may occur. Consult your doctor.

Superinfection – Use of antibiotics (especially prolonged or repeated therapy) may result in bacterial or fungal overgrowth. Such overgrowth may lead to a second infection. The topical antibiotic may need to be stopped and another antibiotic prescribed for the second infection.

Side Effects:

Every drug is capable of producing side effects. Many miscellaneous topical antibiotic users experience no, or minor, side effects. The frequency and severity of side effects depend on many factors including dose, duration of therapy and individual susceptibility. Possible side effects include:

Skin: Rash; itching; burning; redness; swelling; sensitivity to sunlight (gentamicin).

Other: Hearing loss (neomycin); kidney damage (neomycin); sensitivity to neomycin (see Precautions).

Guidelines for Use:

- Apply a small amount of drug in a thin layer on the affected area 1 to 5 times daily. Cover the area with a loose gauze dressing, if desired.
- Clean the affected area prior to applying the drug.
- Deeper skin infections may require oral or injectable antibiotic therapy in addition to topical treatment.
- Do not use in or near the eyes.
- If rash or irritation develops or worsens where the antibiotic is applied, contact your doctor.

If you have any questions, consult your doctor, pharmacist, or health care provider.

	Generic Name *Brand Name Examples*	Supplied As	Generic Available
Rx	**Sulfadiazine**	**Tablets:** 500 mg	Yes
Rx	**Sulfamethizole**		
	Thiosulfil Forte	**Tablets:** 500 mg	No
Rx	**Sulfamethoxazole**		
	Gantanol, Gantanol DS, Urobak	**Tablets:** 500 mg, 1 g	Yes
	Gantanol	**Oral suspension:** 500 mg/tsp	No
Rx	**Sulfasalazine**		
	Azulfidine	**Tablets:** 500 mg	Yes
	Azulfidine EN-tabs	**Tablets, enteric coated:** 500 mg	Yes
	Azulfidine	**Oral suspension:** 250 mg/tsp	No
Rx	**Sulfisoxazole**		
	Gantrisin	**Tablets:** 500 mg	Yes
	Gantrisin	**Syrup:** 500 mg acetyl sulfisoxazole/tsp	No
	Gantrisin	**Pediatric suspension:** 500 mg acetyl sulfisoxazole/tsp	No
Rx	**Multiple Sulfonamides**		
	Triple Sulfa	**Tablets:** 167 mg sulfadiazine, 167 mg sulfamerazine and 167 mg sulfamethazine	Yes
	Triple Sulfa No. 2	**Tablets:** 162 mg sulfadiazine, 162 mg sulfamerazine and 162 mg sulfamethazine	Yes
	Triple Sulfa	**Suspension:** 167 mg sulfadiazine, 167 mg sulfamerazine and 167 mg sulfamethazine/tsp	Yes

Type of Drug:

Anti-infection drugs; sulfa drugs.

How the Drug Works:

Sulfonamides inhibit the use of Para-aminobenzoic acid (PABA) by the bacterial cell. PABA is an essential component in folic acid production and bacterial cell function.

Uses:

To treat infections caused by susceptible bacteria. Infections may include: Urinary tract infections (pyelonephritis, pyelitis, cystitis), chancroid, inclusion conjunctivitis, trachoma, nocardiosis, toxoplasmosis, malaria, middle ear infections, meningitis, rheumatic fever and dermatitis herpetiformis.

Sulfasalazine is prescribed for treatment of ulcerative colitis.

Unlabeled Use(s): Occasionally doctors may prescribe sulfasalazine for rheumatoid arthritis, collagenous colitis, and Crohn's disease. Sulfisoxazole has been used to prevent recurrences of middle ear infections.

Precautions:

Do not use in the following situations:

- allergy to salicylates or aspirin (sulfasalazine only)
- allergy to sulfonamides or related drugs (oral antidiabetic drugs or thiazide diuretics)
- breastfeeding
- infants under age 2 (sulfasalazine only)
- infants under 2 months (except pyrimethamine to treat toxoplasmosis)
- intestinal or urinary obstruction (sulfasalazine only)
- porphyria
- pregnancy at term

Use with caution in the following situations:

- acid urine
- blood disorders
- bronchial asthma
- glucose-6-phosphate dehydrogenase (G-6-PD) deficiency
- kidney disease
- liver disease
- pregnancy prior to term
- streptococcus infections (eg, strep throat)

Sensitivity to light: Sulfonamides may cause sensitivity to light. Avoid prolonged exposure to the sun. Use sunscreens and wear protective clothing until tolerance is determined.

Avoid drugs which may acidify the urine in large doses (such as vitamin C, ammonium chloride). Sulfonamides crystallize in an acid urine. This may cause serious complications in the kidneys. Adequate fluid (eg, water) intake is recommended to increase urine flow.

Pregnancy: Safety for use during pregnancy has not been established. Sulfonamides cross the placenta and studies have shown a potential effect to the fetus. Consult your doctor if pregnancy is suspected.

Breastfeeding: Sulfonamides appear in breast milk. Although the actual amount of drug that a breastfed infant would receive appears to be low, sulfonamides are not recommended while breastfeeding. Consult your doctor.

Children: Do not use sulfasalazine in children under 2.

Tartrazine: Some of these products may contain the dye tartrazine (FD&C Yellow No. 5) which can cause allergic reactions in certain individuals. Check package label when available or consult your doctor or pharmacist.

Drug Interactions:

Tell your doctor or pharmacist if you are taking or if you are planning to take any over-the-counter or prescription medications with sulfonamides. Doses of one or both drugs may need to be modified or a different drug may need to be prescribed. The following drugs and drug classes interact with sulfonamides.

chlorpropamide (eg, *Diabinese)*
contraceptives, oral (eg, *Ortho-Novum)*
digoxin (eg, *Lanoxin)*
folic acid
iron
local anesthetics (eg, benzocaine)
methotrexate (eg, *Moxate)*
nonsteroidal anti-inflammatory agents (eg, ibuprofen)
PABA (eg, *Potaba)*
phenylbutazone (eg, *Butazolidin)*
phenytoin (eg, *Dilantin)*
probenecid (eg, *Benemid)*
salicylates (eg, aspirin)
thiazide diuretics (eg, hydrochlorothiazide)
tolbutamide (eg, *Orinase)*
warfarin (eg, *Coumadin)*

Side Effects:

Every drug is capable of producing side effects. Many sulfonamide users experience no, or minor, side effects. The frequency and severity of side effects depend on many factors including dose, duration of therapy and individual susceptibility. Possible side effects include:

Digestive Tract: Nausea; vomiting; diarrhea; appetite loss; stomach ache.

Nervous System: Headache; vertigo (feeling of whirling motion); depression; seizures; sleeplessness; drowsiness.

Skin: Rash; itching; hives; chills; unusual bleeding or bruising; yellowing of skin or eyes.

Other: Blood disorders, abnormal blood counts; abnormal urine tests; numbness or tingling in hands or feet; ringing in the ears; liver damage; hepatitis; sensitivity to light; kidney damage; fever; joint pain; difficult breathing.

Guidelines for Use:

- Complete full course of therapy for the best response.
- Take on an empty stomach. Take with a full glass of water.
- *Sulfasalazine*— Take at evenly spaced intervals after meals.
- *Sulfasalazine* may cause an orange-yellow discoloration of the urine.
- Sensitivity to light — Avoid prolonged exposure to the sun. Use sunscreens and wear protective clothing until tolerance is determined.
- *Oral suspensions*— Shake well before using. Keep bottle tightly closed. Refrigerate after opening. Discard unused portion after 14 days.
- Notify your doctor if any of the following occurs: Blood in urine, yellowing of skin or eyes, easy bruising, rash, ringing in ears, difficulty in breathing, fever, sore throat or chills.

If you have any questions, consult your doctor, pharmacist, or health care provider.

Generic Name *Brand Name Example*	Supplied As	Generic Available
Rx **Erythromycin Ethylsuccinate and Sulfisoxazole**		
Eryzole	**Oral suspension:** Erythromycin ethylsuccinate (equivalent to 200 mg erythromycin) and sulfisoxazole acetyl (equivalent to 600 mg sulfisoxazole)/5 mL	Yes

Type of Drug:

Antibiotic combination; combination sulfonamide - erythromycin anti-infective.

Uses:

To treat acute middle ear infections (acute otitis media) in children older than 2 months of age caused by susceptible strains of *Haemophilus influenzae.*

Precautions:

Do not use in the following situations:

- allergy to erythromycin
- allergy to sulfonamides or related drugs (oral anti-diabetic drugs or thiazide diuretics)
- breastfeeding of infants under 2 months of age
- infants under 2 months of age
- pregnancy at term (after 36 weeks)
- concomitant use of terfenadine (not available in the US)

Use with caution in the following situations:

- glucose-6-phosphate dehydrogenase (G6PD) deficiency
- kidney disease
- liver disease
- myasthenia gravis
- severe allergies or bronchial asthma

Avoid the following: Drugs or vitamins that may acidify the urine in large doses (eg, vitamin C, ammonium chloride). Sulfonamides crystallize in an acid urine. This may cause serious complications in the kidneys. Adequate fluid (eg, water) intake is strongly recommended to increase urine flow.

Diarrhea: If diarrhea develops during erythromycin ethylsuccinate/sulfixoxazole use, pseudomembranous colitis must be considered. This inflammatory condition of the colon is due to overgrowth of bacteria that are not killed by erythromycin ethylsuccinate/sulfisoxazole. The primary cause is a toxin produced by a bacteria known as *Clostridium difficile.* Mild cases usually respond to stopping the antibiotic. More severe cases may need to be treated with another antibiotic.

Superinfection: Use of antibiotics (especially for prolonged or repeated therapy) may result in bacterial or fungal overgrowth. Such overgrowth may lead to a second infection. Erythromycin ethylsuccinate/sulfisoxazole may need to be stopped and another antibiotic may need to be prescribed for the second infection.

Pregnancy: Adequate studies have not been done in pregnant women. Use only if clearly needed and potential benefits to the mother outweigh the possible hazards to the fetus.

Breastfeeding: These drugs appear in breast milk. Consult your doctor before you begin breastfeeding. A decision should be made whether to discontinue nursing or discontinue the drug, taking into account the importance of the drug to the mother.

Children: Do not give to infants under 2 months of age. Sulfonamides are not recommended for this age group.

Lab tests may be required during treatment. Tests may include complete blood counts, urinalysis, and kidney function tests.

Drug Interactions:

Tell your doctor or pharmacist if you are taking or if you are planning to take any over-the-counter or prescription medications with erythromycin ethylsuccinate/sulfisoxazole. Doses of one or both drugs may need to be modified or a different drug may need to be prescribed. The following drugs and drug classes interact with erythromycin ethylsuccinate/sulfisoxazole:

- alfentanil (*Alfenta*)
- anticoagulants, oral (eg, warfarin)
- benzodiazepines (eg, midazolam, triazolam)
- bromocriptine (*Parlodel*)
- carbamazepine (eg, *Tegretol*)
- cyclosporine (eg, *Neoral*)
- digoxin (eg, *Lanoxin*)
- dihydroergotamine (*D.H.E. 45*)
- disopyramide (eg, *Norpace*)
- ergotamine (eg, *Ergomar*)
- hexobarbital (not available in the US)
- lovastatin (*Mevacor*)
- methotrexate (eg, *Rheumatrex*)
- phenytoin (eg, *Dilantin*)
- sulfonylureas (eg, chlorpropamide)
- terfenadine (not available in the US)
- theophylline (eg, *Theo-Dur*)
- thiopental (eg, *Pentothal*)

Side Effects:

Every drug is capable of producing side effects. Many erythromycin ethylsuccinate/sulfisoxazole users experience no, or minor, side effects. The frequency and severity of side effects depend on many factors including dose, duration of therapy, and individual susceptibility. Possible side effects include:

Digestive Tract: Nausea; vomiting; stomach pain; diarrhea; appetite loss; inflammation of the liver; intestinal bleeding; dark, bloody stools; gas; inflammation and redness of the mouth and tongue.

Nervous System: Headache; dizziness; abnormal skin sensations; convulsions; ringing in the ears; vertigo (feeling of whirling motion); incoordination.

Circulatory System: Fast heartbeat; pounding in the chest; fainting; bluish discoloration of skin; irregular heart rhythm; inflammation of blood vessels or heart tissue.

Urinary and Reproductive Tract: Blood in the urine; infrequent or frequent urination; inability to urinate.

Skin: Serious immediate allergic reaction; delayed allergic reaction (days or weeks); giant hives or skin inflammation; rash; itching; mild skin eruption; sensitivity to light.

Other: Reversible hearing loss; low blood sugar levels; abnormal blood counts; red or purple spots/patches under the skin; low iron or blood counts sometimes resulting in fatigue; clotting disorders; mental disorder; hallucinations; disorientation; anxiety; depression; inflammation of the eye; cough; shortness of breath; fluid retention; fever; drowsiness; weakness; fatigue; yellowing of the skin or eyes; inflammation of lung tissue; rigidity; chills; flushing; sleeplessness.

Guidelines for Use:

- Dosage will be individualized.
- Doses should be equally divided into 3 or 4 daily doses and administered for 10 days. Continue therapy for entire 10 days even if symptoms of infection have disappeared.
- Shake well before using.
- May be administered without regard to meals.
- Maintain an adequate fluid intake to prevent formation of crystals in the urine and kidney stones.
- Do not stop taking the drug or change the dose unless advised to do so by your doctor.
- *Superinfection* — Use of antibiotics (especially for prolonged or repeated therapy) may result in bacterial or fungal overgrowth. Such overgrowth may lead to a second infection. Erythromycin ethylsuccinate/sulfisoxazole may need to be stopped and another antibiotic may need to be prescribed for the second infection.
- Discontinue use and contact your doctor immediately at first appearance of a rash.
- Contact your doctor immediately if severe diarrhea, stomach pain/cramps, or bloody stools occur. This could be a symptom of a serious side effect requiring medical attention. Do not treat diarrhea without first consulting your doctor.
- May cause sensitivity to ultraviolet (UV) light. Avoid prolonged exposure to the sun. Use sunscreens and wear protective clothing until tolerance is determined.
- May cause nausea, vomiting, diarrhea, unusual tiredness, or stomach pain. Contact your doctor if effects persist and are bothersome.
- Contact your doctor immediately if sore throat, fever, pallor, rash, darkened urine, unusual bleeding or bruising, yellowing of eyes or skin, or difficulty breathing occurs.
- Lab tests or exams may be required to monitor treatment. Be sure to keep appointments.

If you have any questions, consult your doctor, pharmacist, or health care provider.

SULFONAMIDES — TRIMETHOPRIM AND SULFAMETHOXAZOLE (TMP-SMZ)

	Generic Name *Brand Name Examples*	Supplied As	Generic Available
Rx	**Trimethoprim and Sulfamethoxazole**, **TMP-SMZ**[1]		
	Bactrim, Bethaprim SS, Cotrim, Septra, Sulfatrim, Uroplus SS	**Tablets:** 80 mg trimethoprim and 400 mg sulfamethoxazole	Yes
	Bactrim DS, Bethaprim DS, Cotrim DS, Septra DS, Sulfatrim DS, Uroplus DS	**Tablets, double strength:** 160 mg trimethoprim and 800 mg sulfamethoxazole	Yes
	Bactrim[2] *Bethaprim*[2], *Cotrim Pediatric, Septra* [2], *Sulfatrim, Sulmeprim*	**Oral suspension:** 40 mg trimethoprim and 200 mg sulfamethoxazole/tsp	Yes

[1] Also available as an injection.
[2] Contains alcohol.

For more information, see the trimethoprim and sulfonamides monographs.

Type of Drug:

Combination sulfonamide-trimethoprim anti-infective; TMP-SMZ, Co-trimoxazole.

How the Drug Works:

Trimethoprim (TMP) and sulfamethoxazole (SMZ) block the production of folic acid. Decreased folic acid interferes with the production of critical nucleic acids and proteins of bacteria.

Uses:

To treat certain urinary tract infections; intestinal infections caused by *Shigella; Pneumocystis carinii* pneumonia; middle ear infections; chronic bronchitis.

Unlabeled Use(s): Occasionally doctors may prescribe TMP-SMZ for cholera, salmonella-type infections, to prevent urinary tract infections (women), nocardiosis and "traveler's diarrhea," and to prevent infections in patients with a compromised immune system with *Pneumocystis carinii* infections or leukemia.

Precautions:

Do not use in the following situations:

allergy to sulfonamides or related drugs (oral antidiabetic drugs or thiazide diuretics)
allergy to trimethoprim
anemia due to folic acid deficiency
breastfeeding
infants less than 2 months of age
pregnancy at term

Use with caution in the following situations:

AIDS patients with *carinii* pneumonitis
alcoholism
allergy, severe
anticonvulsant therapy
asthma
folic acid deficiency
glucose-6-phosphate dehydrogenase (G-6-PD) deficiency
kidney disease
liver disease
malnutrition
strep throat

Avoid drugs that may acidify the urine in large doses (such as vitamin C, ammonium chloride) when taking sulfonamides. Sulfonamides crystallize in an acid urine. This may cause serious complications in the kidneys. Adequate fluid intake (eg, water) is recommended to increase urine flow.

AIDS patients may not tolerate or respond to TMP-SMZ because of their abnormally functioning immune systems.

Superinfection: Use of antibiotics (especially prolonged or repeated therapy) may result in bacterial or fungal overgrowth. Such overgrowth may lead to a second infection. TMP-SMZ may need to be stopped and another antibiotic prescribed for the second infection.

Pregnancy: Do not use at term (after 36 weeks). Adequate studies have not been done in pregnant women. Use only if clearly needed and potential benefits outweigh the possible hazards to the fetus.

Breastfeeding: TMP-SMZ appears in breast milk. Do not use TMP-SMZ during breastfeeding. Consult your doctor.

Children: Use in children less than 2 months is not recommended.

Elderly: Patients may be at an increased risk for side effects, particularly when complicating conditions exist (such as kidney or liver disease). Dosage must be adjusted accordingly.

Sulfites: Some of these products may contain sulfite preservatives which can cause allergic reactions in certain individuals. Check package label when available or consult your doctor or pharmacist.

Drug Interactions:

Tell your doctor or pharmacist if you are taking or if you are planning to take any over-the-counter or prescription medications with TMP-SMZ. Doses of one or both drugs may need to be modified or a different drug may need to be prescribed. The following drugs and drug classes interact with TMP-SMZ.

acetohexamide (eg, *Dymelor)*
anticoagulants, oral (eg, *Coumadin)*
chlorpropamide (eg, *Diabinese)*
cyclosporine *(Sandimmune)*
methotrexate (eg, *Mexate)*
phenytoin (eg, *Dilantin)*
thiazide diuretics (eg, hydrochlorothiazide)
tolazamide (eg, *Tolinase)*
tolbutamide (eg, *Orinase)*

Consider all drug interactions reported for sulfamethoxazole when using this drug.

Side Effects:

Every drug is capable of producing side effects. Many TMP-SMZ users experience no, or minor, side effects. The frequency and severity of side effects depend on many factors including dose, duration of therapy and individual susceptibility. Possible side effects include:

Digestive Tract: Nausea; vomiting; appetite loss; stomach pain; diarrhea.

Nervous System: Headache; depression; seizures; hallucinations; weakness; nervousness; meningitis; insomnia; vertigo (feeling of whirling motion); sleeplessness.

Skin: Rash; peeling of skin; yellowing of the skin or eyes; sensitivity to light; hives; itching.

Other: Inflammation of the tongue and mouth; fever; chills; inflammation of the eyes; ringing in the ears; abnormal liver and kidney function tests; joint or muscle pain.

Guidelines for Use:

- Take on an empty stomach. If upset stomach occurs, take with food.
- Take with a full glass of water.
- Treat initial, uncomplicated urinary tract infections with a single antibacterial. Use this combination for more complicated infections resistant to more traditional therapy.
- Complete the full course of therapy for best results and to decrease the risk of a relapse.
- Consult your doctor immediately if sore throat, fever, chills, pale skin, yellowing of skin or eyes, rash or unusual bleeding or bruising occurs.

If you have any questions, consult your doctor, pharmacist, or health care provider.

Generic Name / *Brand Name Examples*	Supplied As	Generic Available
Rx **Sulfanilamide**		
AVC	**Vaginal cream:** 15%	Yes
AVC	**Vaginal suppositories:** 1.05 g	No
Rx **Tripe Sulfa**		
Sultrin Triple Sulfa	**Vaginal tablets:** 172.5 mg sulfathiazole, 143.75 mg sulfacetamide, 184 mg sulfabenzamide and urea	No
Dayto Sulf, Gyne-Sulf, Sulfa-Trip, Sultrin Triple Sulfa, Trysul, V.V.S.	**Vaginal cream:** 3.42% sulfathiazole, 2.86% sulfacetamide, 3.7% sulfabenzamide and 0.64% urea	Yes
Rx **Vaginal Anti-infective Combinations**		
Terramycin w/Polymyxin B Sulfate	**Vaginal tablets:** 100 mg oxytetracycline and 100,000 units polymyxin B sulfate	Yes
Vagisec Plus	**Vaginal suppositories:** 6 mg aminacrine HCl, 5.25 mg polyoxyethylene nonyl phenol, 0.66 mg EDTA and 0.07 mg docusate sodium	No
Cantri	**Vaginal cream:** 10% sulfisoxazole, 0.2% aminacrine HCl and 2% allantoin	No
Nil	**Vaginal cream:** 15% sulfanilamide, 0.2% aminacrine HCl and 1.5% allantoin	No
Alasulf, Benegyn, Deltavac, D.I.T.1-2	**Vaginal cream:** 15% sulfanilamide, 0.2% aminacrine HCl and 2% allantoin	No
Cleocin[1]	**Vaginal cream:** 2% clindamycin phosphate	No
MetroGel	**Vaginal gel:** 0.75% metronidazole	No

[1] Contains mineral oil.

Type of Drug:

Vaginal anti-infection products.

Uses:

In these combinations:

Antibiotics: For infections due to susceptible organisms. Consult monographs on individual agents.

Triple Sulfa: For treatment of bacterial vaginosis.

Sulfanilamide: For the treatment of *Candida albicans* vulvovaginitis (monilia, yeast) only.

Sulfonamides: For infections due to susceptible organisms.

Estrogens: To aid in the return of the vaginal mucosa to normal.

Metronidazole: For the treatment of bacterial vaginosis.

Oxyquinoline benzoate and aminacrine: For use as antiseptics.

Allantoin: Aids in the surgical removal of dead tissue and in tissue regeneration.

Polyoxyethylene nonyl phenol, alkyl aryl sulfonate, sodium lauryl sulfate, and docusate sodium: Used as wetting agents.

Precautions:

Do not use in the following situations:

- alcohol use (metronidazole only)
- allergy to lincomycin (clindamycin only)
- allergy to the vaginal anti-infective or any of its ingredients
- colitis, antibiotic-associated (clindamycin only)
- disulfiram therapy, within 2 weeks (metronidazole only)
- inflammation of the intestine, history of (clindamycin only)
- kidney disease (sulfonamides only)
- ulcerative colitis (clindamycin only)

Use with caution in the following situations:

- CNS diseases (metronidazole only)
- impaired liver function (metronidazole only)
- pregnancy

Drug Interactions:

Tell your doctor or pharmacist if you are taking or if you are planning to take any over-the-counter or prescription medications or dietary supplements with vaginal anti-infectives. Doses of one or both drugs may need to be modified or a different drug may need to be prescribed. Anticoagulants (eg, warfarin) and disulfiram (eg, *Antabuse)* interact with metronidazole.

Side Effects:

Every drug is capable of producing side effects. Many vaginal anti-infective users experience no, or minor, side effects. The frequency and severity of side effects depend on many factors including dose, duration of therapy, and individual susceptibility. If local irritation, rash, or itching develops, discontinue treatment and contact your doctor. Cramps, stomach pain, and a change in white blood cell count may occur with metronidazole use.

Guidelines for Use:

- Patient instructions are included with product.
- Dosage is individualized. Use exactly as prescribed.
- Do not stop taking or change the dose unless directed by your doctor. Complete full course of therapy.
- Use the applicator provided to insert high into the vagina. An applicator may not be recommended during pregnancy. Use only on the advice of your doctor.
- Notify your doctor if burning, itching, irritation, or an allergic reaction occurs.
- Mineral oil may weaken latex or rubber products such as condoms or diaphragms. Do not use such products within 72 hours following treatment with mineral oil-containing products.
- Do not engage in vaginal sexual intercourse during treatment.
- Avoid contact with the eyes.

If you have any questions, consult your doctor, pharmacist, or health care provider.

	Generic Name *Brand Name Examples*	Supplied As	Generic Available
	Clotrimazole		
Rx	*Lotrimin*	**Cream**: 1%	Yes
otc	*Cruex, Lotrimin AF*	**Cream**: 1%	Yes
Rx	*Lotrimin*	**Lotion**: 1%	No
otc	*Lotrimin AF*	**Lotion**: 1%	No
Rx	*Fungoid, Lotrimin*	**Solution**: 1%	Yes
otc	*Lotrimin AF*	**Solution**: 1%	No
Rx	*Mycelex*	**Troches**: 10 mg	No

Type of Drug:

Topical antifungal.

How the Drug Works:

Fungi apparently bind to the drug. The cell membrane of fungi is altered, allowing fungal cell contents to leak out, resulting in cell death. The troche binds to the oral mucosa (lining of the mouth) and provides a long-term concentration in saliva.

Uses:

Solutions, creams, and lotions: To treat tinea pedis (athlete's foot), tinea cruris (jock itch), and tinea corporis (ringworm).

Troche (hard lozenge): To treat thrush (oral candidiasis) or reduce the incidence of thrush in immuncompromised patients.

Rx products: To treat tinea versicolor (pityriasis) and candidiasis (yeast).

Precautions:

Do not use in the following situations: Allergy to clotrimazole or any of its ingredients.

Use with caution in the following situations: Liver disease.

Pregnancy: There are no adequate and well-controlled studies in pregnant women. Use only if clearly needed and the potential benefits to the mother outweigh the possible hazards to the fetus.

Breastfeeding: It is not known if clotrimazole appears in breast milk. Consult your doctor before you begin breastfeeding.

Children: Do not use in children under 2 years of age, unless directed by your doctor. Supervise use in children under 12 years of age.

Side Effects:

Every drug is capable of producing side effects. Many clotrimazole users experience no, or minor, side effects. The frequency and severity of side effects depend on many factors including dose, duration of therapy, and individual susceptibility. Possible side effects include:

Troche: Nausea; vomiting; abnormal liver function tests; unpleasant mouth sensations; itching.

Topical: Redness; stinging; burning; blistering; peeling; swelling; itching; hives; general skin irritation.

Guidelines for Use:

- Dosage is individualized. Use exactly as prescribed.
- Do not stop taking or change the dose, unless directed by your doctor.
- Avoid contact with eyes. Do not use on scalp or nails.
- Avoid use of occlusive wrappings or dressings.
- If condition persists or worsens, or if irritation, redness, burning, blistering, swelling, oozing, or itching occurs, discontinue use and notify your doctor.
- If a dose is missed, take it as soon as possible. If several hours have passed or it is nearing time for the next dose, do not double the dose in order to catch up, unless advised to do so by your doctor. If more than one dose is missed or it is necessary to establish a new dosage schedule, contact your doctor or pharmacist.
- Continue use until a full course of therapy is completed. Failure to use all of the medicine may prevent complete elimination of the fungi, causing the infection to return.
- Contact your doctor or pharmacist if symptoms persist after a course of treatment is completed.
- Do not use for treating fungal infection other than in the mouth (troches only) or on the skin (creams, lotions, solutions).
- *Troches* — Slowly dissolve in the mouth for maximum effect.
- *Lotions, creams, and solutions* — Apply after cleansing the affected area, unless directed otherwise by your doctor. Apply twice daily, morning and evening. Improvement should be seen within 1 week.
- Avoid sources of infection or reinfection.
- Avoid contact with eyes.

If you have any questions, consult your doctor, pharmacist, or health care provider.

	Generic Name *Brand Name Example*	Supplied As	Generic Available
Rx	**Fluconazole**[1]		
	Diflucan	**Tablets:** 50 mg, 100 mg, 150 mg, 200 mg	No
	Diflucan	**Oral Suspension:** 50 mg/5 mL, 200 mg/5 mL	No

[1] Also available as an injection.

Type of Drug:

Antifungal agent.

How the Drug Works:

Fluconazole interferes with the formation of the cell membrane of fungi. This causes leakage of cellular contents, resulting in fungal cell death.

Uses:

To treat candidiasis (yeast) infections of the mouth, throat, and vagina.

To treat other serious candidal infections such as urinary tract infection, peritonitis (inflammation of the lining of the abdomen and pelvis), and pneumonia.

To treat cryptococcal meningitis (caused by yeast-like organisms affecting the brain).

To decrease the incidence of candidiasis (yeast) infections in patients undergoing bone marrow transplants who receive chemotherapy or radiation therapy.

Precautions:

Do not use in the following situations: Allergy to fluconazole or any of its ingredients.

Use with caution in the following situations:

allergy to other azole antifungals (eg, ketoconazole)
kidney disease
liver disease
weakened immune system or other serious underlying conditions (eg, AIDS, cancer)

Pregnancy: There are no adequate and well-controlled studies in pregnant women. Use only if clearly needed and the potential benefits to the mother outweigh the possible hazards to the fetus.

Breastfeeding: Fluconazole appears in breast milk. Consult your doctor before you begin breastfeeding.

Children: Safety and effectiveness have not been established in infants under 6 months of age.

Drug Interactions:

Tell your doctor or pharmacist if you are taking or if you are planning to take any over-the-counter or prescription medications while taking this medicine. Doses of one or both drugs may need to be modified or a different drug may need to be prescribed.The following drugs and drug classes interact with this medicine.

anticoagulants, oral (eg, warfarin)
antihistamines, nonsedating (eg, *Seldane*)
cimetidine (eg, *Tagamet*)
cyclosporine (eg, *Sandimmune*)
hydrochlorothiazide (eg, *Esidrix*)
oral contraceptives (eg, *Ortho-Novum*)
phenytoin (eg, *Dilantin*)
rifampin (eg, *Rifadin*)
sulfonylureas (eg, glipizide)
tacrolimus *(Prograf)*
theophylline (eg, *Theo-Dur*)
zidovudine *(Retrovir)*

Side Effects:

Every drug is capable of producing side effects. Many patients experience no, or minor, side effects. The frequency and severity of side effects depend on many factors including dose, duration of therapy, and individual susceptibility. Possible side effects include:

Digestive Tract: Nausea; vomiting; diarrhea; indigestion; stomach ache; changes in taste.

Other: Headache; dizziness; rash.

Guidelines for Use:

- Use exactly as prescribed.
- Continue use until all of the prescribed medicine has been taken. Failure to take or use all of the medicine may prevent complete elimination of the fungi, causing the infection to return.
- If a dose is missed, take or inject it as soon as possible. If several hours have passed or if it is nearing time for the next dose, do not double the dose in order to "catch up" (unless advised to do so by your doctor). If more than one dose is missed or it is necessary to establish a new dosage schedule, contact your doctor or pharmacist.
- Contact your doctor if rash, yellowing of skin or eyes, nausea, weakness, difficulty breathing or facial swelling develops.
- *Intravenous solution* — Do not use if solution is cloudy or contains particles. Follow the administration procedure taught to you by your healthcare provider. Do not remove unit from overwrap until ready for use. Store at room temperature (bottles, 41° to 86°F; bags, 41° to 77°F).
- *Oral suspension* — Shake well before use. Store at room temperature (41°to 86°F) and discard unused portion after 2 weeks. Protect from freezing.
- *Tablets* — Store at room temperature (below 86°F).

If you have any questions, consult your doctor, pharmacist, or health care provider.

	Generic Name *Brand Name Examples*	Supplied As	Generic Available
Rx	**Griseofulvin Microsize**		
	Grisactin	**Capsules:** 250 mg	No
	Fulvicin-U/F, Grifulvin V, Grisactin	**Tablets:** 250 mg, 500 mg	No
	Grifulvin V	**Oral suspension:** 125 mg/tsp	No
Rx	**Griseofulvin Ultramicrosize**		
	Fulvicin P/G, Grisactin Ultra, Gris-PEG	**Tablets:** 125 mg, 165 mg, 250 mg, 330 mg	Yes

Type of Drug:

Antifungal agent.

How the Drug Works:

Griseofulvin is deposited into the skin. Diseased skin tissue gradually flakes off and is replaced by noninfected tissue that contains griseofulvin. The new skin cells become highly resistant to further fungal infections.

Uses:

To treat ringworm (fungal) infections of the hair, skin and nails.

To treat athlete's foot.

Precautions:

Do not use in the following situations:

- allergy to griseofulvin
- liver failure
- porphyria (high concentrations of iron-free pigments)
- pregnancy
- to treat minor infections which will respond to skin-applied agents alone

Use with caution in the following situations:

- allergy to penicillin
- long-term therapy
- lupus erythematosus

Sensitivity to light: May cause photosensitivity (sensitivity to sunlight). Avoid prolonged exposure to the sun and other ultraviolet light. Use sunscreens and wear protective clothing until tolerance is determined.

Males: Males should wait at least 6 months after therapy before trying to father a child.

Lab Tests: Patients on long-term griseofulvin therapy may be required to have complete blood counts and liver and kidney function tests done periodically. Be sure to keep appointments.

Pregnancy: Do not use during pregnancy. The risk of use in pregnant women clearly outweighs any possible benefit.

Children: Safety and effectiveness have not been established in children under 2 years of age.

Drug Interactions:

Tell your doctor or pharmacist if you are taking or if you are planning to take any over-the-counter or prescription medications while taking this medicine. Doses of one or both drugs may need to be modified or a different drug may need to be prescribed.The following drugs and drug classes interact with this medicine.

alcohol
anticoagulants, oral (eg, warfarin)
barbiturates (eg, phenobarbital)
contraceptives, oral (eg, *Ortho-Novum)*
cyclosporine (eg, *Sandimmune)*
estrogens (eg, *Premarin)*
salicylates (eg, aspirin)

Side Effects:

Every drug is capable of producing side effects. Many patients experience no, or minor, side effects. The frequency and severity of side effects depend on many factors including dose, duration of therapy and individual susceptibility. Possible side effects include:

Digestive Tract: Nausea; vomiting; diarrhea; stomach ache; whiteness in mouth.

Other: Headache; fatigue; dizziness; confusion; sleeplessness; impaired coordination; rash; hives; itching.

Guidelines for Use:

- Use exactly as prescribed.
- Take with food high in fat content (eg, peanut butter).
- Shake suspension well before using.
- If a dose is missed, take it as soon as possible. If several hours have passed or if it is nearing time for the next dose, do not double the dose in order to "catch up" (unless advised to do so by your doctor). If more than one dose is missed or it is necessary to establish a new dosage schedule, contact your doctor or pharmacist.
- Beneficial effects may not be apparent for several weeks. Continue use until all of the prescribed medicine has been taken, even if symptoms have disappeared. Failure to take all of the medicine may prevent complete elimination of fungi, causing the infection to return.
- Observe good hygiene during treatment to help control infection and prevent reinfection.
- Contact your doctor if any of the following occurs: Sore throat, skin rash, facial swelling, yellowing of skin/eyes, difficulty breathing, fatigue, fever or weight loss.
- Inform your doctor if you are pregnant, become pregnant or are planning to become pregnant. Males should wait at least 6 months after therapy before trying to father a child.
- Topical antifungal therapy may accompany oral therapy. Topical therapy is especially useful in athlete's foot (tinea pedis) and jock itch (tinea cruris).
- May cause photosensitivity (sensitivity to sunlight). Avoid prolonged exposure to the sun and other ultraviolet light. Use sunscreens and wear protective clothing until tolerance is determined.
- Lab tests may be necessary to monitor therapy. Be sure to keep appointments.
- *Tablets*— Store at room temperature (59° to 86°F) in a tightly closed container.
- *Oral suspension* — Store at room temperature (59° to 86°F) in a light-resistant container.

If you have any questions, consult your doctor, pharmacist, or health care provider.

	Generic Name *Brand Name Examples*	Supplied As	Generic Available
Rx	**Itraconazole**		
	Sporanox	**Capsules:** 100 mg	No

Type of Drug:

Antifungal agent.

How the Drug Works:

Itraconazole inhibits the formation of the cell membrane of fungi. This causes leakage of cellular contents, resulting in fungal cell death.

Uses:

For treatment of fungal infections due to blastomycosis, histoplasmosis, aspergillosis (in patients intolerant of or who do not respond to amphotericin B) and onychomycosis (when due to dermatophytes of the toenail). Occasionally doctors may prescribe this medicine for other fungal infections.

Precautions:

Do not use in the following situations:

- allergy to itraconazole
- astemizole (*Hismanal)* use
- cisapride (*Propulsid)* use
- midazolam (oral) use
- pregnant woman with onychomycosis (fungal nail disease), treatment of
- terfenadine (*Seldane)* use
- triazolam (*Halcion)* use

Use with caution in the following situations:

- allergy to similar antifungals
- liver disease

Lab Tests: Liver enzyme test values should be monitored in patients with pre-existing liver function abnormalities and in patients receiving itraconazole treatment for over 1 month. Be sure to keep appointments.

Pregnancy: Adequate studies have not been done in pregnant women, or animal studies may have shown a risk to the fetus. Use only if clearly needed and the potential benefits outweigh the possible hazards to the fetus. Effective contraception (birth control) must be used throughout itraconazole therapy and for 2 months following treatment.

Onychomycosis (fungal nail disease) treatment – Do not use itraconazole during pregnancy. The risk of use in a pregnant woman clearly outweighs any possible benefit.

Breastfeeding: Itraconazole appears in breast milk. Do not use while breastfeeding.

Children: Safety and effectiveness in children have not been established.

Drug Interactions:

Tell your doctor or pharmacist if you are taking or if you are planning to take any over-the-counter or prescription medications while taking this medicine. Doses of one or both drugs may need to be modified or a different drug may need to be prescribed. The following drugs and drug classes interact with this medicine.

anticoagulants (eg, warfarin)
antidiabetic drugs, oral (eg, glipizide)
astemizole (*Hismanal*)
calcium channel blockers (dihydropyridine class eg, nifedipine)
carbamazepine (eg, *Tegretol*)
cisapride (*Propulsid*)
cyclosporine (eg, *Sandimmune*)
didanosine (*Videx*)
digoxin (eg, *Lanoxin*)
HMG-CoA reductase inhibitors (eg, lovastatin)
H_2 antagonists (eg, cimetidine)
isoniazid (eg, *Laniazid*)
midazolam, oral
phenytoin (eg, *Dilantin*)
quinidine (eg, *Quinora*)
rifampin (eg, *Rifadin*)
tacrolimus (*Prograf*)
terfenadine (*Seldane*)
triazolam (*Halcion*)
vincristine (eg, *Oncovin*)

Side Effects:

Every drug is capable of producing side effects. Many patients experience no, or minor, side effects. The frequency and severity of side effects depend on many factors including dose, duration of therapy, and individual susceptibility. Possible side effects include:

Digestive Tract: Nausea; vomiting; stomach pain; diarrhea; appetite loss.

Nervous System: Headache; dizziness; fatigue; sleepiness; drowsiness; feeling of whirling motion.

Skin: Rash; hives; itching.

Other: Fever; general body discomfort; muscle pain; decreased sexual drive; impotence; edema (fluid retention); difficulty breathing; high blood pressure; dizziness or lightheadedness when rising quickly from a sitting or lying position; abnormal lab values; dark urine; pale stools; yellowing of the skin or eyes.

Guidelines for Use:

- Use exactly as prescribed.
- Usual dose is 200 mg once daily, taken after a full meal.
- Continue use until all of the prescribed drug has been taken, even if symptoms have disappeared. Failure to take a full course of therapy may prevent complete elimination of fungi, causing the infection to return.
- If a dose is missed, take it as soon as possible. If several hours have passed or if it is nearing time for the next dose, do not double the dose in order to "catch up" (unless advised to do so by your doctor). If more than one dose is missed, contact your doctor or pharmacist.
- Contraceptive measures (birth control) are recommended during treatment and for 2 months following treatment. Inform your doctor if you are pregnant, become pregnant, are planning to become pregnant, or if you are breastfeeding.
- Lab tests may be required to monitor therapy. Be sure to keep appointments.
- Contact your doctor if any of the following occurs: Unusual fatigue, appetite loss, nausea, vomiting, yellowing of skin or eyes, dark urine, pale stools, rash, itching, hives or difficulty breathing.
- Store at room temperature (59° to 86°F) away from moisture and light.

If you have any questions, consult your doctor, pharmacist, or health care provider.

	Generic Name *Brand Name Examples*	Supplied As	Generic Available
Rx	**Ketoconazole**		
	Nizoral[1]	**Cream:** 2%	No
	Nizoral	**Shampoo:** 2%	No
	Nizoral	**Tablets:** 200 mg	No

[1] Contains sulfites.

Type of Drug:

Antifungal agent.

How the Drug Works:

Ketoconazole interferes with the formation of the cell membrane of fungi. This causes leakage of cellular contents, resulting in fungal cell death.

Uses:

Cream: For topical treatment of ringworm, jock itch, athlete's foot, tinea versicolor (pityriasis), candidiasis (yeast) infections of the skin and seborrheic dermatitis (inflamed scaling skin).

Shampoo: To reduce scaling due to dandruff.

Tablets: To treat systemic (internal) fungal infections. Also used to treat severe fungal infections of the skin or mouth that have not responded to topical therapy or oral griseofulvin, or in patients who are unable to take griseofulvin.

Precautions:

Do not use in the following situations:

All doseforms—

allergy to ketoconazole

Tablets only—

astemizole *(Hismanal)* use
cisapride *(Propulsid)* use
fungal meningitis
terfenadine *(Seldane)* use
triazolam *(Halcion)* use

Use with caution in the following situations:

lack of adequate stomach acid (tablets only)
liver disease (tablets only)
prostatic cancer (tablets only)

Liver disease – This medication has caused liver disease in some patients. The injury is usually reversible if treatment is discontinued as soon as symptoms occur. Stop taking this medicine and contact your doctor immediately if any of the following occurs: Fatigue, appetite loss, nausea, vomiting, yellowing of skin or eyes, dark urine or pale stools.

Pregnancy: Adequate studies have not been done in pregnant women, or animal studies may have shown a risk to the fetus. Use only if clearly needed and potential benefits outweigh the possible hazards to the fetus.

Breastfeeding: Oral ketoconazole probably appears in breast milk. Do not breastfeed during oral ketoconazole treatment. It is not known if ketoconazole cream appears in breast milk. The shampoo does not appear in breast milk. Exercise caution when applying topical ketoconazole to a nursing woman.

Children: Safety and effectiveness of topical and oral ketoconazole have not been established in children under 2 years of age. Do not use in children unless the potential benefits outweigh the risks.

Lab tests may be required to monitor therapy with oral ketoconazole. Be sure to keep appointments. Lab tests may include liver function tests.

Sulfites: Some of these products may contain sulfite preservatives which can cause allergic reactions in certain individuals (eg, asthmatics). Check package label when available or consult your doctor or pharmacist.

Drug Interactions:

Tell your doctor or pharmacist if you are taking or if you are planning to take any over-the-counter or prescription medications while taking this medicine. Doses of one or both drugs may need to be modified or a different drug may need to be prescribed.The following drugs and drug classes interact with this medicine.

All doseforms:

alcohol
antacids
anticholinergics (eg, atropine)
didanosine *(Videx)*
digoxin (eg, *Lanoxin*)
H_2 antagonists (eg, cimetidine)
isoniazid (eg, *Laniazid*)
theophylline (eg, *Theo-Dur*)

Tablets only:

anticoagulants, oral (eg, warfarin)
antidiabetic agents, oral (eg, sulfonylureas)
astemizole *(Hismanal)*
cisapride *(Propulsid)*
corticosteroids (eg, methyl-prednisolone)
cyclosporine (eg, *Sandimmune*)
midazolam *(Versed)*
phenytoin (eg, *Dilantin*)
rifampin (eg, *Rifadin*)
tacrolimus *(Prograf)*
terfenadine *(Seldane)*
triazolam *(Halcion)*

Side Effects:

Every drug is capable of producing side effects. Many patients experience no, or minor, side effects. The frequency and severity of side effects depend on many factors including dose, duration of therapy and individual susceptibility. Possible side effects include:

Topical cream – Skin irritation; itching; stinging.

Tablets – Nausea; vomiting; stomach ache; itching; skin reactions.

Shampoo – Hair loss; loss of curl in hair; skin irritation or dryness.

Guidelines for Use:

- Use exactly as prescribed.
- If a dose is missed, take or apply it as soon as possible. If several hours have passed or if it is nearing time for the next dose, do not double the dose in order to "catch up" (unless advised to do so by your doctor). If more than one dose is missed or it is necessary to establish a new dosage schedule, contact your doctor or pharmacist.
- Continue use until all of the prescribed medicine has been taken or used. Failure to use all of the medicine may prevent complete elimination of the fungi, causing the infection to return.
- *Cream*—
  For external use only.
  Apply once daily, covering the affected and surrounding area. (For seborrheic dermatitis, apply twice daily for 4 weeks or until clearing has occurred.)
  Avoid contact with the eyes.
  Discontinue use and contact your doctor if irritation occurs.
  Improvement may be seen soon after treatment is begun. Jock itch, yeast infections and ringworm should be treated for 2 weeks to reduce the possibility of recurrence. Patients with tinea versicolor usually require 2 weeks of treatment; patients with athlete's foot usually require 6 weeks.
  If no clinical improvement is seen after the treatment period, consult your doctor.
  Store at room temperature. Do not freeze.
- *Shampoo*—
  For external use only.
  Moisten hair and scalp thoroughly with water. Apply enough shampoo to produce enough lather to wash the scalp and hair, and gently massage it over entire scalp area for 1 minute. Rinse hair thoroughly with warm water. Repeat, leaving shampoo on scalp for an additional 3 minutes. After the second thorough rinse, dry hair with towel or hair dryer.
  Shampoo twice a week for 4 weeks with at least 3 days between each shampooing and then intermittently as needed to maintain control.
  Avoid contact with the eyes.
  Discontinue use and contact your doctor if irritation occurs.
  Occasionally the use of the shampoo has resulted in removal of curl from permanently waved hair.
  Store below 77°F away from light.
- *Tablets*—
  Usual dose is 200 mg once daily.
  If stomach upset occurs, take with food.
  In cases of achlorhydria (low stomach acidity), dissolve tablets in a 4 mL (approximately 1 teaspoon) solution of 0.2 N HCl. Use a glass or plastic straw to avoid contact with the teeth. Follow with a glass of water.
  Do not take with antacids, anticholinergics or H_2-blockers (eg, *Tagamet*). Wait at least 2 hours after having taken the ketoconazole before taking these products.

Guidelines for Use (cont.):

- *Tablets*— (cont.)
  Contact your doctor if any of the following occurs: Fatigue, appetite loss, nausea, vomiting, yellowing of skin or eyes, dark urine, pale stools, rash or difficulty breathing.
  May cause dizziness, drowsiness or headache. Use caution while driving or performing other tasks requiring alertness, coordination or physical dexterity.
  Lab tests may be required to monitor treatment. Be sure to keep appointments.
  Store at room temperature (59° to 86°F) away from moisture.

If you have any questions, consult your doctor, pharmacist, or health care provider.

Generic Name *Brand Name Examples*	Supplied As	Generic Available
Rx **Nystatin**		
Mycostatin,, Nilstat	**Tablets:** 500,000 Units	Yes
Mycostatin[1], *Nilstat, Nystex*[1]	**Oral suspension:** 100,000 units/mL	Yes
Mycostatin Pastilles	**Troches (Lozenges):** 200,000 units	No
Mycostatin, Nilstat, Nystex	**Cream:** 100,000 units/g	Yes
Mycostatin, Nilstat, Nystex	**Ointment:** 100,000 units/g	Yes
Mycostatin,, Pedi-Dri	**Powder:** 100,000 units/g	Yes
Nilstat	**Powder:** 50 million units, 150 million units, 500 million units, 1 billion units, 2 billion units, 5 billion units	Yes

[1] Contains alcohol.

Type of Drug:

Antifungal agent.

How the Drug Works:

Nystatin interferes with the formation of the cell membrane of fungi. This causes leakage of cellular contents, resulting in fungal cell death.

Uses:

To treat oral (thrush), intestinal, skin or mucous membrane fungal infections due to *Candida* species (yeast).

Precautions:

Do not use in the following situations: Allergy to this medicine

Pregnancy: Adequate studies have not been done in pregnant women, or animal studies may have shown a risk to the fetus. Use only if clearly needed and potential benefits outweigh the possible hazards to the fetus.

Breastfeeding: Since it is not known whether nystatin appears in breast milk, it should be used with caution. Contact your doctor before you begin breastfeeding.

Children: Safety and effectiveness have not been established.

Side Effects:

Every drug is capable of producing side effects. Many patients experience no, or minor, side effects. The frequency and severity of side effects depend on many factors including dose, duration of therapy and individual susceptibility. Possible side effects include: Nausea; vomiting; diarrhea; stomach ache.

Guidelines for Use:

- Use exactly as prescribed.
- Avoid contact with the eyes.
- If a dose is missed, take or apply it as soon as possible. If several hours have passed or if it is nearing time for the next dose, do not double the dose in order to "catch up" (unless advised to do so by your doctor). If more than one dose is missed or it is necessary to establish a new dosage schedule, contact your doctor or pharmacist.
- Continue use until all of the prescribed medicine has been taken. Failure to use all of the medicine may prevent complete elimination of the fungi, causing the infection to return.
- Discontinue use and contact your doctor if mouth or skin irritation occurs.
- *Tablets*— Usually taken 3 times a day. Store at room temperature protected from light and moisture.
- *Oral Suspension*— Shake well before using. Swish thoroughly (as long as possible) in mouth before swallowing. Store at room temperature protected from light. Avoid freezing. Doses vary depending upon age. Keep out of the reach of children.
- *Troches (Lozenges/Pastilles)*— Dissolve slowly in the mouth. Do not chew or swallow whole. Good oral hygiene, including proper care of dentures, is of the utmost importance. Store refrigerated (36° to 46°F).
- *Cream and Ointment*— Apply liberally after cleansing the affected area (unless otherwise directed) until healing is complete. These medications do not stain skin or mucous membranes. Store at room temperature. Do not freeze.
- *Children*— Nystatin has been specially compounded by pharmacists and administered in the form of flavored frozen popsicles to improve oral retention. Consult your doctor or pharmacist.

If you have any questions, consult your doctor, pharmacist, or health care provider.

ANTIFUNGALS, TOPICAL PREPARATIONS

	Generic Name *Brand Name Examples*	Supplied As	Generic Available
Rx	**Amphotericin B**		
	Fungizone	**Cream**: 3%	No
	Fungizone	**Lotion**: 3%	No
Rx	**Ciclopirox Olamine**		
	Loprox	**Cream**: 0.77%	No
	Loprox	**Lotion**: 0.77%	No
	Loprox	**Gel**: 0.77%	No
	Penlac Nail Lacquer	**Solution**: 8%	No
	Clotrimazole		
otc	*Cruex, Desenex, Lotrimin AF*	**Cream**: 1%	Yes
otc	*Lotrimin AF*	**Lotion**: 1%	No
Rx	*Fungoid*	**Solution**: 1%	Yes
otc	*Lotrimin AF*	**Solution**: 1%	No
Rx	**Econazole Nitrate**		
	Spectazole	**Cream:** 1%	No
otc	**Gentian Violet**	**Solution:** 1%	Yes
	Miconazole Nitrate		
otc	*Micatin*	**Cream:** 2%	Yes
Rx	*Monistat-Derm*	**Cream:** 2%	No
otc	*Lotrimin AF, Micatin, Zeasorb-AF*	**Powder:** 2%	No
otc	*Fungoid Tincture*	**Solution:** 2%	No
otc	*Lotrimin AF, Micatin*	**Spray:** 2%	No
otc	*Cruex, Desenex, Lotrimin AF, Micatin, Ting*	**Spray powder:** 2%	No
Rx	**Naftifine Hydrochloride**		
	Naftin	**Cream:** 1%	No
	Naftin	**Gel:** 1%	No
Rx	**Nystatin**		
	Pedi-Dri	**Powder**: 100,000 U/g	No
Rx	**Oxiconazole Nitrate**		
	Oxistat	**Cream:** 1%	No
	Oxistat	**Lotion:** 1%	No

	Generic Name *Brand Name Examples*	Supplied As	Generic Available
Rx	**Sulconazole Nitrate**		
	Exelderm	**Cream:** 1%	No
	Exelderm	**Solution:** 1%	No
otc	**Terbinafine Hydrochloride**		
	Lamisil AT	**Cream:** 1%	No
otc	**Tolnaftate**		
	NP•27, Tinactin	**Cream:** 1%	Yes
	Odor-Eaters, Quinsana Plus, Tinactin	**Powder**: 1%	Yes
	Aftate for Athlete's Foot, Aftate for Jock Itch, Tinactin, Tinactin for Jock Itch	**Spray powder**: 1%	Yes
	Absorbine Jr., Aftate for Athlete's Foot, Odor-Eaters, Tinactin, Ting	**Spray liquid**: 1%	No
	Absorbine Jr., Dr. Scholl's Fungi Solution, Tinactin	**Solution**: 1%	Yes
	Absorbine Jr.	**Gel**: 1%	No
	Tinactin	**Wipes**: 1%	
otc	**Undecylenic Acid and Derivatives**		
	Breezee Mist	**Powder**: Undecylenic acid	No
	FungiCure	**Liquid**: 10% undecylenic acid	No

Type of Drug:

Topical antifungals; drugs used to treat fungal infections of the skin or nails.

How the Drug Works:

Topical antifungals exert their action by different mechanisms and treat a wide variety of fungi. The choice of topical antifungal depends on the nature of the infection.

ANTIFUNGALS, TOPICAL PREPARATIONS

Uses:

Products and their uses are listed in the following table:

Generic Name	Uses: Athlete's Foot	Jock Itch	Ring-worm	Tinea versicolor (pityriasis)	Other
Amphotericin B					Candidiasis[1]
Ciclopirox	✔	✔	✔	✔	Candidiasis[1] infections on skin
Clotrimazole	✔	✔	✔	✔	Candidiasis,[1] seborrheic dermatitis of scalp; see clotrimazole monograph in this chapter
Econazole	✔	✔	✔	✔	Candidiasis[1] infections on skin
Gentian Violet					Anti-infective and antifungal dye
Miconazole	✔	✔	✔	✔	Candidiasis[1] infections on skin
Naftifine	✔	✔	✔		
Nystatin					Candidiasis[1]; see nystatin monograph in this chapter
Oxiconazole	✔	✔	✔	✔	
Sulconazole	✔	✔	✔	✔	
Terbinafine	✔	✔	✔	✔[2]	Candidiasis[1] infections on skin[2]
Tolnaftate	✔	✔	✔	✔	Adjunctive therapy in other fungal infections
Undecylenic Acid	✔	✔			Prickly heat, diaper rash, itching, burning and chafing, excessive perspiration and irritation in the groin area, foul-smelling perspiration

[1] Also called canida, moniliasis, albicans, or yeast.
[2] Unlabeled use.

Precautions:

Do not use in the following situations: Allergy to the topical antifungal or any of its ingredients.

Use with caution in the following situations:
blistered, raw, or oozing areas of skin
worsening skin irritation during drug therapy

Pregnancy: There are no adequate and well-controlled studies in pregnant women. Use only if clearly needed and the potential benefits to the mother outweigh the possible hazards to the fetus.

Breastfeeding: Some topical antifungals may appear in breast milk. Consult your doctor before you begin breastfeeding. Avoid direct application of terbinafine to the breast.

Children: Do not use undecylenic acid, clotrimazole, miconazole, or tolnaftate on children under 2 years of age. Amphotericin B and nystatin can be used in infants. Safety and effectiveness for use of the other topical antifungals in children under 10 years of age have not been established.

Side Effects:

Every drug is capable of producing side effects. Many topical antifungal users experience no, or minor, side effects. The frequency and severity of side effects depend on many factors including dose, duration of therapy, and individual susceptibility. Possible side effects include: Allergic contact dermatitis; burning; hives; blistering; peeling; itching; stinging; redness; swelling; dryness.

Guidelines for Use:

- Use exactly as directed.
- For external use only. Avoid contact with the eyes, nose, or mouth or other mucous membranes.
- Cleanse and dry the area to be treated before application.
- Avoid inhalation of spray products.
- Apply with caution to blistered or raw skin, oozing skin, or skin over a deep puncture wound.
- Wash hands before and after applying.
- Avoid the use of occlusive wraps or dressings unless directed by your health care provider.
- Patients with decreased circulation, including diabetic patients, should consult their doctor or pharmacist before using undecylenic acid.
- Allergic reactions may occur. If the condition being treated worsens or irritation, burning, redness, swelling, or stinging persists, discontinue use and inform your health care provider.
- Frequency of application and duration of therapy is dependent on the condition being treated, its location, the drug, the strength of the drug, and the doseform used. For assistance in drug selection and dosage guidelines, consult your pharmacist or doctor.
- Amphotericin B and gentian violet may stain fabric, skin, or hair.
- For athlete's foot, wear well-fitting and ventilated shoes. Change socks at least once a day.
- Use these medications for the full treatment time, even after the symptoms improve.
- Notify your physician if there is no improvement after 4 weeks.
- Shake ciclopirox lotion well before each use.
- Spray powders and liquids and tolnaftate solution and gel are flammable. Do not use near heat or open flame.
- *Penlac Nail Lacquer* — Do not shower or bathe for at least 8 hours after applying the solution. Do not use polish or other nail cosmetic products on treated nails. Product is flammable. Do not use near heat or open flame. Must be used as part of a comprehensive management program including the removal of the unattached, infected nails. Store in the original carton after each use to protect from light.
- Store at room temperature (68° to 77°F). Avoid freezing.

If you have any questions, consult your doctor, pharmacist, or health care provider.

	Brand Name Examples	Supplied As
otc	*Blis-To-Sol*	**Liquid:** Undecylenic acid and salicylic acid **Powder:** Benzoic acid and salicylic acid
otc	*Castaderm*	**Liquid:** Resorcinol, boric acid, acetone, basic fuchsin, phenol and 9% alcohol
Rx	*Castellani Paint*	**Solution:** Basic fuchsin, phenol, resorcinol, acetone and alcohol. Also available as a colorless solution without basic fuchsin
otc	*Castel Minus*	**Liquid:** 10% resorcinol, acetone, basic fuchsin, hydroxyethylcelluose and 11.5% alcohol
otc	*Castel Plus*	**Liquid:** 10% resorcinol, acetone, basic fuchsin, hydroxyethylcellulose and 11.5% alcohol
otc	*Dermasept Antifungal*	**Liquid:** 6.098% tannic acid, 5.081% zinc chloride, 2.032% benzocaine, 3.049% methylbenzethonium HCl, 1.017% tolnaftate, 5.081% undecylenic acid, 58.539% ethanol 38B, phenyl, benzyl alcohol, benzoic acid, coal tar, camphor, menthol
otc	*Fungi•Nail*	**Liquid:** 10% undecylenic acid, 5% salicylic acid, 70% isopropyl alcohol
Rx	*Gordochom*	**Liquid:** 25% undecylenic acid and 3% chloroxylenol in an oil base
Rx	*Mycolog-II*	**Cream:** 100,000 units nystatin and 1 mg triamcinolone acetonide per gram **Ointment:** 100,000 units nystatin and 1 mg triamcinolone acetonide per gram
otc	*Neo-Castaderm*	**Liquid:** Resorcinol, boric acid, acetone, sodium bisulfite, phenol and 9% alcohol

	Brand Name Examples	Supplied As
otc	*Prophyllin*	**Ointment:** 5% sodium propionate and 0.0125% chlorophyll derivatives
		Powder: Makes a solution containing 1% sodium propionate and 0.0025% water soluble chlorophyllin
otc	*SteriNail*	**Solution:** Undecylenic acid, tolnaftate, propylene glycol, acetone, acetic acid, propionic acid, benzyl alcohol, eucalyptol and benzyl acetate, *Steri-Scrub*and *Steri-Brush*included
otc	*Ting*	**Powder:** Benzoic acid, boric acid, zinc oxide, zinc stearate and propylene glycol
		Cream: Benzoic acid, boric acid, zinc oxide, zinc stearate, sodium stearate, titanium dioxide and 19% alcohol
Rx	*Tinver*	**Lotion:** 25% sodium thiosulfate, 1% salicylic acid, 10% isopropyl alcohol, menthol, propylene glycol, EDTA and colloidal alumina
otc	*Whitfield's*	**Ointment:** 6% benzoic acid and 3% salicylic acid

Type of Drug:

Antifungal agents. Drugs used to treat fungal infections.

How the Drug Works:

Topical antifungals exert their action by different mechanisms and treat a wide variety of fungi. The choice of topical antifungal depends on the nature of the infection.

Uses:

The principal active components of these formulations include:

Antifungal agents—

Undecylenic acid
Nystatin
Iodochlorhydroxyquin
Parachlorometaxylenol
Sodium propionate, sodium caprylate, zinc caprylate, zinc propionate, zinc stearate, benzoic acid, sodium thiosulfate, phenol and resorcinol
Tolnaftate
Triamcinolone acetonide

Other components include:

Salicylic acid for its topical keratolytic (softening or peeling).
Tannic acid as an astringent (agent that causes shrinking or puckering of tissue, eg, styptic pencil).
Boric acid as an astringent and antiseptic.
Zinc oxide for its astringent, antiseptic and protective properties.
Chloroxylenol as an antiseptic.
Benzocaine as an anesthetic.
Menthol for its anti-itch, anesthetic and antiseptic effects.
Chlorophyll derivatives to promote healing, relieve pain and inflammation and reduce smell in wounds, burns, surface ulcers, cuts, scrapes and skin irritations.
Basic fuchsin for its antifungal and antibacterial activity.

In general, powders are used with other products. Ointments, creams and liquids are used as primary therapy in very mild conditions or as preventative agents, especially in moist areas. In addition, powders with a cornstarch base may be preferred over those with a talc base.

Guidelines for Use:

- For external use only. Avoid contact with the eyes, nose, mouth or other mucous membranes.
- Cleanse and dry the area to be treated before application.
- Avoid the use of occlusive dressings, unless directed by the doctor.
- Allergic reactions may occur. If the condition being treated worsens or irritation, burning, redness, swelling or stinging persists, do not reapply the drug and contact your doctor.
- *Undecylenic acid* - Patients with decreased circulation, including diabetics, should consult their doctor before use.
- Frequency of application and duration of therapy is dependent on the condition being treated, its location, the drug, the strength of the drug and the dosage form used. For assistance in drug selection and dosage guidelines, consult your pharmacist or doctor.

If you have any questions, consult your doctor, pharmacist, or health care provider.

ANTIFUNGALS — VAGINAL PREPARATIONS

	Generic Name *Brand Name Examples*	Supplied As	Generic Available
Rx	**Butoconazole Nitrate**		
	Femstat	**Vaginal cream:** 2%	No
	Clotrimazole		
otc	*Femcare, Gyne-Lotrimin, Mycelex-7, Sweent'n fresh clotrimazole-7*	**Vaginal tablets:** 100 mg	Yes
Rx	*Mycelex-G*	**Vaginal tablets:** 500 mg	No
otc	*Gyne-Lotrimin Combination Pack*	**Cream:** 1% **Tablets:** 500 mg	No
Rx	*Mycelex Twin Pack*	**Cream:** 1% **Tablets:**500 mg	No
otc	*Femcare, Gyne-Lotrimin, Mycelex-7, Sweent'n fresh clotrimazole-7*	**Vaginal cream:** 1%	Yes
Rx	**Gentian Violet**		
	Genapax	**Tampons:** 5 mg	No
	Miconazole Nitrate		
otc	*Monistat 7*	**Vaginal suppositories:** 100 mg	No
Rx	*Monistat 3*	**Vaginal suppositories:** 200 mg	No
otc	*Monistat 7*	**Vaginal cream:** 2%	Yes
otc	*Monistat 7 Combination Pack*	**Cream:** 2% **Vaginal suppositories:** 100 mg	No
Rx	*Monistat-Derm*	**Topical Cream;** 2%	No
Rx	*Monistat Dual-Pak*	**Cream:** 2% **Vaginal suppositories:** 200 mg	No
Rx	**Nystatin**		
	Mycostatin	**Vaginal tablets:** 100,000 units	Yes
Rx	**Terconazole**		
	Terazol 3	**Vaginal suppositories:** 80 mg	No
	Terazol 3, Terazol 7	**Vaginal cream:** 0.4%, 0.8%	No
Rx	**Tioconazole**		
	Vagistat-1	**Vaginal ointment:** 6.5%	No

Type of Drug:

Vaginal antifungal agents.

How the Drug Works:

These drugs apparently weaken the cell membrane and allow leakage of cellular contents, producing cell death.

Uses:

To treat vaginal candidiasis (monilia or "yeast" infections.

Precautions:

Do not use in the following situations: Allergy to the drug or any of its ingredients.

Pregnancy: Adverse effects or complications have not been reported in infants born to women treated with these agents. Avoid use of a vaginal applicator during pregnancy. Insertion of tablets by hand is preferred. Use only on advice of your doctor. Because small amounts of these drugs may be absorbed from the vagina, use during the first trimester only when essential. Use butoconazole during the second and third trimesters only. Possible exposure of the fetus through direct transfer of terconazole from an irritated vagina may occur.

Breastfeeding: It is not known if vaginal antifungals appear in breast milk. Consult your doctor before you begin breastfeeding.

Children: Safety and effectiveness of terconazole and tioconazole have not been established.

Side Effects:

Every drug is capable of producing side effects. Many vaginal antifungal users experience no, or minor, side effects. The frequency and severity of side effects depend on many factors including dose, duration of therapy, and individual susceptibility. Possible side effects include:

General: Vaginal irritation; burning; itching.

Clotrimazole: Stomach cramps; bloating; vaginal rash; painful intercourse.

Miconazole: Pelvic cramps; headache; hives; skin rash.

Butoconazole: Vaginal swelling, discharge, or soreness.

Terconazole: Headache; body aches; local irritation; sensitivity to light; painful menstruation; stomach pain; fever; genital pain.

Tioconazole: Vaginal discharge, pain, dryness, or scaling; vulvar edema and swelling; excessive urination at night; difficult urination; painful intercourse.

Guidelines for Use:

- Patient instructions for proper use are enclosed in each package and should be strictly followed.
- *Vaginal tablets, creams, and suppositories* — Insert high into the vagina, except during pregnancy.
- Complete a full course of therapy. Use continuously, even during the menstrual period.
- If the vaginal medication causes burning or irritation, or if symptoms worsen, contact your doctor.
- Refrain from sexual intercourse during treatment or use condoms to avoid the risk of reinfection.
- A sanitary napkin or minipad may be used to prevent staining of clothing due to seepage or leakage. Do not use a tampon.
- Concurrent use (up to 72 hours) with certain latex products (eg, condoms, diaphragms) is not recommended.
- If candidiasis is chronic and recurrent, other factors may be involved. Factors that increase the risk of candidiasis include diabetes, chronic antibiotic therapy, pregnancy, steroid use, and oral contraceptive use.

If you have any questions, consult your doctor, pharmacist, or health care provider.

	Generic Name *Brand Name Examples*	Supplied As	Generic Available
Rx	**Chloroquine Hydrochloride**		
	Aralen HCl	**Injection**: 50 mg/mL	No
Rx	**Chloroquine Phosphate**		
	Aralen	**Tablets**: 250 mg, 500 mg	Yes
Rx	**Hydroxychloroquine Sulfate**		
	Plaquenil	**Tablets**: 200 mg	Yes
Rx	**Primaquine Phosphate**	**Tablets**: 26.3 mg	Yes

Type of Drug:

Antimalarial anti-infectives.

How the Drug Works:

The actual mechanism of action of aminoquinoline antimalarial drugs is unknown. They may destroy malaria parasites by inhibiting normal metabolism inside the parasite.

These drugs can treat and cure malarial infections caused by susceptible strains of *Plasmodium falciparum* but do not cure infections caused by *P. vivax* or *P. malariae*. Their use may lengthen the time period between treatment and relapse in cases that are not cured.

Uses:

To prevent and treat acute attacks of malaria caused by *Plasmodium vivax, P. malariae, P. ovale*, and susceptible strains of *P. falciparum.*

Chloroquine is also used as an amebicide.

Chloroquine HCl injection is used to treat acute attacks caused by *P. vivax*, *P. malariae*, *P. ovale*, and susceptible strains of *P. falciparum*.

Hydroxychloroquine is also used to treat acute or chronic rheumatoid arthritis and chronic discoid and systemic lupus erythematosus.

Primaquine is used only for the prevention of relapse of *P. vivax*, or following termination of chloroquine suppressive therapy in an area where *P. vivax* is endemic.

Unlabeled Use(s): Occasionally doctors may prescribe chloroquine to suppress rheumatoid arthritis, or to treat discoid and systemic lupus erythematosus, scleroderma, pemphigus, lichen planus, polymyositis, sarcoidosis, and porphyria cutanea tarda.

Precautions:

Do not use in the following situations:

allergy to aminoquinolines or any of their ingredients
retinal or visual field changes (eg, dark holes in vision)

Primaquine only —
- bone marrow depressants, concurrent use
- granulocytopenia tendency
- hemolytic drugs, concurrent use
- quinacrine, recent or concurrent use

Use with caution in the following situations:
- alcohol abuse
- children
- favism, history of or family history of (primaquine only)
- glucose-6 phosphate dehydrogenase (G-6-PD) deficiency
- liver disease
- nicotinamide adenine dinucleotide (NADH) methemoglobin reductase deficiency (primaquine only)
- porphyria
- psoriasis
- hepatoxic (toxic to the liver) drugs, concurrent use

Pregnancy: Use only if clearly needed and the potential benefits to the mother outweigh the possible hazards to the fetus.

Breastfeeding: Aminoquinolines appear in breast milk. Safety for use during breastfeeding has not been established. Consult your doctor before you begin breastfeeding.

Children: Children are especially sensitive to aminoquinoline compounds. Deaths following accidental ingestion of relatively small doses and sudden deaths from injections of chloroquine have been reported. Hydroxychloroquine is not for long-term therapy in children.

Lab tests will be required to monitor therapy. Tests including reflex and vision assessments and blood counts may be required.

Drug Interactions:

Tell your doctor or pharmacist if you are taking or planning to take any over-the-counter or prescription medications with aminoquinolines. Doses of one or both drugs may need to be modified or a different drug may need to be prescribed. The following drugs and drug classes interact with aminoquinolines:
- cimetidine (eg, *Tagamet*)
- magnesium salts (eg, magnesium carbonate)

Side Effects:

Every drug is capable of producing side effects. Many aminoquinoline users experience no, or minor, side effects. The frequency and severity of side effects depend on many factors including dose, duration of therapy, and individual susceptibility. Possible side effects include:

Eyes or Ocular: Visual disturbances; blurred vision; difficulty focusing; "foggy" vision; night blindness; abnormal retina found during eye examinations.

Digestive Tract: Nausea; vomiting; diarrhea; stomach upset or cramps; appetite loss.

Skin: Rash; itching; pigment changes; hair loss.

Other: Ringing in the ears; hearing loss; dizziness; seizures; headache; abnormal blood counts; low blood pressure; darkening of the urine.

Guidelines for Use:

- Dosage is individualized. Take exactly as prescribed for the full course of therapy.
- Do not change the dose or stop taking unless advised by your doctor.
- May cause stomach upset. Take with food.
- Notify your doctor if you experience any change in vision, ringing in the ears, rash, muscle weakness, or hearing impairment.
- *Primaquine* — Notify your doctor immediately if you experience darkening of the urine.
- Overdosage can be especially severe and is extremely dangerous in children. Keep this medication in a childproof container and out of the reach of children.
- May cause nausea, vomiting, stomach pain, diarrhea, appetite loss, irregular heartbeat, or low blood pressure. Notify your doctor if these persist or become bothersome.
- Irreversible damage to the retina of the eye, usually with long-term, high-dose use, has been reported. When long-term use is expected, periodic eye exams should be performed. Retinal changes and visual disturbances may continue even after stopping therapy.
- Chloroquine HCl injection is used when oral therapy is not possible. It will be prepared and administered by your health care provider.
- Lab tests will be required to monitor therapy. Be sure to keep appointments.
- Store at controlled room temperature (59° to 86°F). Protect from light.

If you have any questions, consult your doctor, pharmacist, or health care provider.

	Generic Name *Brand Name Example*	Supplied As	Generic Available
Rx	**Mefloquine Hydrochloride**		
	Lariam	**Tablets:** 250 mg	No

Type of Drug:

Antimalarial anti-infective.

How the Drug Works:

It is not known exactly how mefloquine acts to inhibit malaria-causing organisms (*Plasmodium falciparum, P. vivax*) in the blood. This drug does not eliminate the liver phase of *P. vivax* parasite growth. To prevent relapses in this situation, aminoquinoline drugs (eg, primaquine) must be used.

Uses:

To prevent (prophylax) and malaria caused by susceptible strains of *Plasmodium falciparum* or by *P. vivax.* Also used to treat mild to moderate malarial infections caused by susceptible strains of *P. falciparum* or *P. ovale.*

Precautions:

Do not use in the following situations:

allergy to mefloquine or related drugs (eg, quinine, quinidine)
depression
epilepsy, history of
halofantrine, concurrent with or after mefloquine
psychosis, history of

Use with caution in the following situations:

heart disease
liver disease

Discontinue use: Discontinue use if unexplained anxiety, depression, restlessness, or confusion appears during use. These symptoms may signal a more serious problem. Contact your doctor immediately.

Pregnancy: Adequate studies have not been done in pregnant women. Use only if clearly needed and potential benefits to the mother outweigh the possible hazards to the fetus. Women of childbearing age who travel to areas of the world where malaria exists should avoid becoming pregnant and use reliable contraception for 2 months after the last dose.

Breastfeeding: Mefloquine appears in breast milk. Consult your doctor before you begin breastfeeding.

Children: Safety and effectiveness in children under 6 months of age have not been established.

Lab tests and periodic doctor visits will be required during long-term treatment with mefloquine. Liver function tests, blood counts (platelets and white blood cells), and eye examinations may be required.

Drug Interactions:

Tell your doctor or pharmacist if you are taking or planning to take any over-the-counter or prescription medications with mefloquine. Doses of one or both drugs may need to be modified or a different drug may need to be prescribed. The following drugs and drug classes interact with mefloquine:

- anticonvulsants (eg, valproic acid)
- beta-blockers (eg, propranolol)
- chloroquine (eg, *Aralen*)
- halofantrine (*Halfan*)
- quinidine (eg, *Quinora*)
- quinine
- typhoid vaccine, live attenuated oral

Side Effects:

Every drug is capable of producing side effects. Many mefloquine users experience no, or minor, side effects. The frequency and severity of side effects depend on many factors including dose, duration of therapy, and individual susceptibility. Possible side effects include:

Digestive Tract: Nausea; vomiting; diarrhea; stomach pain; appetite loss.

Nervous System: Dizziness; headache; fatigue; seizures; vertigo (feeling of whirling motion); confusion; anxiety; depression; fainting; loss of balance; drowsiness; sleeplessness; abnormal dreams.

Other: Ringing in the ears; chills; rash; fever; muscle aches; visual disturbances; abnormal blood tests; changes in blood pressure.

Guidelines for Use:

- Dose and duration of therapy depend on the drug, patient's age, and situation being treated. Take specifically as prescribed for the full course of therapy. Contact your doctor if you are not able to take as prescribed or cannot complete the full course of therapy.
- Take with food to prevent stomach upset.
- Take with at least 8 oz. of water.
- May cause dizziness. Use caution when driving or performing other tasks requiring alertness, coordination, or physical dexterity.
- Side effects of mefloquine may decrease with prolonged therapy. However, if side effects do occur and do not decrease, they may persist up to several weeks after the last dose.
- If a dose is missed, take it as soon as possible. If several hours have passed or if it is nearing time for the next dose, do not double the dose to catch up. If more than one dose is missed or it is necessary to establish a new dosage schedule, contact your doctor or pharmacist.
- Discontinue use and contact your doctor if you experience unexplained anxiety, depression, restlessness, or confusion.
- If you are a woman of childbearing age who travels to areas where malaria exists, avoid becoming pregnant.
- Lab tests may be required to monitor therapy. Be sure to keep appointments.
- Store at controlled room temperature (59° to 86°F).

If you have any questions, consult your doctor, pharmacist, or health care provider.

	Generic Name *Brand Name Example*	Supplied As	Generic Available
Rx	**Pyrimethamine**		
	Daraprim	**Tablets:** 25 mg	No

Type of Drug:

Antimalarial anti-infective.

How the Drug Works:

This drug works primarily by inhibiting key enzymes critical to the life of susceptible strains of the organisms causing malaria.

Uses:

In susceptiblo strains of plasmodia only. It is not suitable as a preventative agent for travelers to most areas because of prevalent resistance worldwide.

Used with a sulfonamide (eg, sulfadoxine) to treat toxoplasmosis.

In conjunction with a sulfonamide to initiate transmission control and suppression for susceptible strains of plasmodia. Fast-acting antimalarial drugs (eg, chloroquine, quinine) are preferable for the treatment of acute malaria attacks.

Precautions:

Do not use in the following situations:

allergy to pyrimethamine or any of its ingredients
megaloblastic anemia due to folate deficiency

Use with caution in the following situations:

alcohol abuse
convulsive disorders
folate deficiency
folate-reducing therapies (eg, methotrexate, phenytoin)
G-6-PD deficiency
kidney disease
liver disease
malabsorption syndrome

Pregnancy: There are no adequate and well-controlled studies in pregnant women. Use only if clearly needed and potential benefits to the mother outweigh the possible hazards to the fetus.

Breastfeeding: Pyrimethamine is excreted in breast milk. Consult your doctor before you begin breastfeeding.

Lab tests may be required during treatment. Tests may include blood and platelet counts.

Drug Interactions:

Tell your doctor or pharmacist if you are taking or if you are planning to take any over-the-counter or prescription medications or dietary supplements while taking pyrimethamine. Doses of one or both drugs may need to be modified or a different drug may need to be prescribed. The following drugs and drug classes interact with pyrimethamine:

antifolic drugs (eg, methotrexate, sulfonamides, trimethoprim-sulfamethoxazole)
lorazepam (eg, *Ativan*)

Side Effects:

Every drug is capable of producing side effects. Many pyrimethamine users experience no, or minor, side effects. The frequency and severity of side effects depend on many factors including dose, duration of therapy, and individual susceptibility. Possible side effects include:

Digestive Tract: Appetite loss; vomiting; inflammation and redness of the tongue.

Circulatory System: Irregular heart rhythm; abnormal blood counts; blood in the urine.

Other: Rash; redness.

Guidelines for Use:

- Dosage is individualized. Take exactly as prescribed.
- Do not exceed the recommended dose.
- Taking with meals may minimize appetite loss and vomiting.
- Discontinue use and notify your doctor immediately at the first appearance of a rash.
- Sore throat, lethargy, pale skin, unusual bruising, or inflamed or reddened tongue may be early signs of a serious disorder. Contact your doctor immediately to determine whether you should discontinue taking the drug and seek medical treatment.
- Contraceptive measures (birth control) are recommended during treatment.
- Inform your doctor if you are pregnant, become pregnant, are planning to become pregnant, or are breastfeeding.
- Lab tests may be required to monitor treatment. Be sure to keep appointments.
- Store in a dry place at room temperature (59° to 77°F). Protect from light.

If you have any questions, consult your doctor, pharmacist, or health care provider.

	Generic Name *Brand Name Example*	Supplied As	Generic Available
Rx	**Sulfadoxine and Pyrimethamine**		
	Fansidar	**Tablets:** 500 mg sulfadoxine and 25 mg pyrimethamine	No

Type of Drug:
Antimalarial anti-infective.

How the Drug Works:
The combination of these drugs inhibits the normal enzymatic metabolism within a parasite causing malaria.

Uses:
For the treatment of *Plasmodium falciparum* malaria for patients in whom chloroquine resistance is suspected.

For prevention of *P. falciparum* malaria for travelers to areas where chloroquine-resistant malaria is endemic.

Precautions:
Do not use in the following situations:

- allergy to pyrimethanmine or sulfonamides
- blood dyscrasias
- infants under 2 months of age
- kidney disease, severe
- liver disease, severe (for prevention only)
- megalobastic anemia due to folate deficiency
- nursing mothers
- pregnancy (at term)

Use with caution in the following situations:

- allergy, severe
- bronchial asthma
- folate deficiency
- kidney disease
- liver disease

Stevens-Johnson Syndrome and Toxic Epidermal Necrolysis: Fatalities, though rare, have been associated with the administration of this medicine. Discontinue this medicine and consult your doctor immediately at the first appearance of skin rash, reduction in the count of any formed blood elements, or occurrence of bacterial or fungal infections.

Pregnancy: There are no adequate and well-controlled studies in pregnant women, but women should be cautioned against becoming pregnant during use. Use only if clearly needed and potential benefits to the mother outweigh the possible hazards to the fetus.

Breastfeeding: Sulfonamides appear in breast milk. Women should not breastfeed during therapy.

Children: This medicine should not be given to infants under 2 months of age.

Lab tests may be required during treatment. Tests may include periodic blood counts, analysis of urine, and organ function (eg, liver, kidney) tests.

Drug Interactions:

Tell your doctor or pharmacist if you are taking or planning to take an over-the-counter or prescription medications or dietary supplements with sulfadoxine and pyrimethamine. Doses of one or both drugs may need to be modified or a different drug may need to be prescribed. The following drugs and drug classes interact with sulfadoxine and pyrimethamine:

antifolic drugs (eg, sulfonamides, trimethoprim-sulfamethoxazole)
chloroquine (eg, *Aralen*)

Side Effects:

Every drug is capable of producing side effects. Many sulfadoxine and pyrimethamine users experience no, or minor, side effects. The frequency and severity of side effects depend on many factors including dose, duration of therapy, and individual susceptibility. Possible side effects include:

Digestive Tract: Inflammation and redness of the tongue or mouth; nausea; vomiting; stomach pain; hepatitis; liver damage; diarrhea; pancreatitis.

Nervous System: Headache; inflammation of peripheral nerves; tingling sensation; depression; convulsions; incoordination or clumsiness; hallucinations; ringing in the ears; dizziness; insomnia; apathy; fatigue; muscle weakness; nervousness.

Hematologic: Abnormal blood counts; anemia; decreased blood platelets; red or purple spots or patches under the skin; easy bruising or bleeding.

Respiratory System: Cough; shortness of breath; difficulty breathing.

Allergic Reactions: Flushing or redness of skin; skin eruptions; hives; rash; redness; itching; flaking and sloughing of skin; pale or yellowing of skin; swelling; sensitivity to light.

Other: Joint pain; fever; chills; abnormal kidney function.

Guidelines for Use:

- Dosage is individualized.
- Keep out of reach of children.
- Discontinue this medicine and seek medical attention immediately at the first appearance of a skin rash.
- Notify your doctor immediately if you experience sore throat, fever, joint pain, cough, shortness of breath, pale or yellow skin, unusual bruising, or inflammation or redness of the tongue or mouth. These symptoms may be early indications of a serious disorder that requires immediate treatment.
- Adequate fluid intake must be maintained in order to prevent crystal formation in the urine and stone formation in the kidneys.
- Contraceptive measures (birth control) are recommended during treatment to avoid birth defects should pregnancy occur. Contact your doctor if you suspect you are pregnant.
- Nursing mothers should not breastfeed their infants during treatment with this medicine.
- Lab tests may be required to monitor treatment. Be sure to keep appointments.

If you have any questions, consult your doctor, pharmacist, or health care provider.

	Generic Name *Brand Name Example*	Supplied As	Generic Available
Rx	**Halofantrine HCl**		
	Halfan	**Tablets:** 250 mg	No

Type of Drug:

Antimalarial anti-infective.

How the Drug Works:

The mechanism of antimalarial activity of halofantrine is not known. This drug does not eliminate the liver phase of *Plasmodium vivax* parasite growth. To prevent relapses after initial treatment, aminoquinoline drugs (eg, primaquine) must be used to eradicate hepatic phase parasites.

Uses:

For the treatment of adults who can tolerate oral medication and who have mild to moderate malaria caused by *P. falciparum* or *P. vivax*.

Precautions:

Do not use in the following situations:

allergy to halofantrine or any of its ingredients
AV conduction disorders
fainting, unexplained
family history of congenital QT_c prolongation
heart disease, known or suspected
mefloquine, used concurrently or after halofantrine

Pregnancy: There are no adequate and well-controlled studies in pregnant women. Use only if clearly needed and potential benefits to the mother outweigh the possible hazards to the fetus.

Breastfeeding: It is not known if halofantrine appears in breast milk. Consult your doctor before you begin breastfeeding.

Children: Safety and effectiveness in children have not been established.

Drug Interactions:

Tell your doctor or pharmacist if you are taking or if you are planning to take any over-the-counter or prescription medications or dietary supplements while taking halofantrine. Doses of one or both drugs may need to be modified or a different drug may need to be prescribed. The following drugs, drug classes, and foods interact with halofantrine:

high-fat foods
mefloquine (*Lariam*)

Side Effects:

Every drug is capable of producing side effects. Many halofantrine users experience no, or minor, side effects. The frequency and severity of side effects depend on many factors including dose, duration of therapy, and individual susceptibility. Possible side effects include:

Digestive Tract: Stomach pain; appetite loss; diarrhea; nausea; vomiting.

Other: Dizziness; headache; coughing; itching; shakiness; chills; muscle pain.

Guidelines for Use:

- Dosage is individualized. Take exactly as prescribed.
- Take on an empty stomach at least 1 hour before or 2 hours after food.
- May cause dizziness. Use caution while driving or performing other tasks requiring alertness, coordination, or physical dexterity.
- Inform your doctor if you are pregnant, become pregnant, are planning to become pregnant, or are breastfeeding
- If you are a woman of childbearing age who travels to areas where malaria exists, avoid becoming pregnant.
- May cause photosensitivity (sensitivity to sunlight). Avoid prolonged exposure to the sun or other forms of ultraviolet (UV) light (eg, tanning beds). Use sunscreens and wear protective clothing until tolerance is determined.
- Store at room temperature (68° to 77°F). Protect from light.

If you have any questions, consult your doctor, pharmacist, or health care provider.

	Generic Name *Brand Name Examples*	Supplied As	Generic Available
Rx	**Atovaquone and Proguanil HCl**		
	Malarone	**Tablets:** 250 mg atovaquone and 100 mg proguanil HCl	No
	Malarone Pediatric	**Tablets:** 62.5 mg atovaquone and 25 mg proguanil HCl	No

Type of Drug:

Antimalarial anti-infective.

How the Drug Works:

Atovaquone and proguanil alter the biochemistry of *Plasmodium falciparum*, causing death of the malaria-producing organism.

Uses:

For the prevention and treatment of *P. falciparum* malaria, including areas where chloroquine, halofantrine, mefloquine, and amodioquine resistance has been reported.

Precautions:

Do not use in the following situations: Allergy to atovaquone, proguanil HCl, or any of the ingredients in this medicine.

Use with caution in the following situations: Kidney failure.

Pregnancy: There are no adequate and well-controlled studies in pregnant women. Use only if clearly needed and potential benefits to the mother outweigh the possible hazards to the fetus.

Breastfeeding: Proguanil appears in breast milk. It is not known if atovaquone appears in breast milk. Consult your doctor before you begin breastfeeding.

Children: Safety and effectiveness for use in children who weigh less than 24 pounds (11 kilograms) have not been established.

Elderly: Cautious dose selection for elderly patients is recommended.

Lab tests may be required during treatment.

Drug Interactions:

Tell your doctor or pharmacist if you are taking or if you are planning to take any over-the-counter or prescription medications or dietary supplements while taking atovaquone or proguanil. Doses of one or both drugs may need to be modified or a different drug may need to be prescribed. The following drugs, foods, and drug classes interact with atovaquone or proguanil:

high-fat foods
metoclopramide (eg, *Reglan*)
rifampin (eg, *Rifadin*)
tetracycline (eg, *Sumycin*)

Side Effects:

Every drug is capable of producing side effects. Many atovaquone or proguanil users experience no, or minor, side effects. The frequency and severity of side effects depend on many factors including dose, duration of therapy, and individual susceptibility. Possible side effects include:

Digestive Tract: Stomach pain; inflamed stomach; nausea; vomiting; appetite loss; indigestion; diarrhea.

Nervous System: Headache; dizziness; weakness.

Other: Itching; fever; muscle pain; cough; abnormal liver tests.

Guidelines for Use:

- Dosage is individualized. Take exactly as prescribed.
- Do not change the dose or stop taking this medicine unless advised by your doctor.
- Take this medicine at the same time each day with food or a milk drink.
- Take a repeat dose if vomiting occurs within 1 hour of taking the medicine.
- Talk to your doctor about other forms of malaria prevention if this medicine is prematurely discontinued.
- Use of protective clothing, insect repellents, and bednets are important in preventing malaria.
- Preventative treatment should be started 1 or 2 days before entering a malaria-endemic area and continued daily during the stay and for 7 days after returning.
- Because medicines are not always 100% effective, seek medical attention for illnesses that occur during or after return from a malaria-endemic area.
- Inform your doctor if you are pregnant, become pregnant, are planning to become pregnant, or are breastfeeding.
- Pregnant women should talk with their doctors prior to traveling to malaria-endemic areas.
- Store at controlled room temperature (59° to 86°F).

If you have any questions, consult your doctor, pharmacist, or health care provider.

	Generic Name	Supplied As	Generic Available
Rx	**Quinine Sulfate**	**Capsules:** 200 mg, 325 mg	Yes
		Tablets: 260 mg	Yes

Type of Drug:

Antimalarial anti-infective.

How the Drug Works:

The antimalarial activity of quinine is unclear. It appears to kill the malaria-causing parasite by disrupting its metabolism.

Uses:

To treat chloroquine-resistant *Plasmodium falciparum* malaria. Used either alone, with pyrimethamine and a sulfonamide, or with a tetracycline. It is also considered alternative therapy for chloroquine-sensitive strains of *P. falciparum, P. malariae, P. ovale*, and *P. vivax*. Mefloquine and clindamycin may also be used with quinine, depending on where the malaria was acquired (eg, Southeast Asia, Bangladesh, East Africa).

Unlabeled Use(s): Doctors may occasionally prescribe quinine sulfate for the prevention and treatment of nocturnal recumbency (nighttime) leg cramps.

Precautions:

Do not use in the following situations:

- allergy to quinine sulfate or any of its ingredients
- blackwater fever, history of
- glucose-6-phosphate dehydrogenase (G-6-PD) deficiency
- inflammation of optic nerve
- pregnancy
- ringing in the ears
- thrombocytopenic purpura with previous quinine use

Use with caution in the following situations: Irregular heartbeat.

Allergy: Discontinue quinine if there is any evidence of allergy. Flushing, itching, rash, fever, stomach pain, difficulty breathing, ringing in the ears, and vision problems may occur, even with only small doses of quinine. Extreme flushing of the skin with intense itching over most of the body is most common.

Pregnancy: Do not use during pregnancy. The risk of use in a pregnant woman clearly outweighs any possible benefit. Birth defects have been reported with large doses.

Breastfeeding: Quinine appears in breast milk. Consult your doctor before you begin breastfeeding.

Drug Interactions:

Tell your doctor or pharmacist if you are taking or planning to take any over-the-counter or prescription medications with quinine sulfate. Doses of one or both drugs may need to be modified or a different drug may need to be prescribed. The following drugs and drug classes interact with quinine sulfate:

anticoagulants, oral (eg, warfarin)
antihistamines, nonsedating (eg, loratadine)
digoxin (eg, *Lanoxin)*
nondepolarizing muscle relaxants (eg, pancuronium)
rifamycins (eg, rifampin)
succinylcholine (eg, *Anectine)*

Side Effects:

Every drug is capable of producing side effects. Many quinine sulfate users experience no, or minor, side effects. The frequency and severity of side effects depend on many factors including dose, duration of therapy, and individual susceptibility. Possible side effects include:

Cinchonism: Ringing in the ears; headache; diarrhea; nausea; disturbed vision.

Eyes or Ocular: Disturbed color vision and perception; sensitivity to light; blurred vision; night blindness; double vision; dilated pupil; optic nerve damage.

Digestive Tract: Nausea; vomiting; stomach ache.

Nervous System: Headache; vertigo (feeling of whirling motion); restlessness; confusion; excitement; apprehension; delirium; dizziness; convulsions.

Other: Ringing in the ears; fever; hepatitis; blood cell disorders; lowered body temperature; chest pain; thrombocytopenia purpura; deafness; fainting; rash; itching; flushing.

Guidelines for Use:

- Dosage is individualized.
- Do not change the dose or stop taking unless advised by your doctor.
- May cause stomach upset. Take with food or after meals.
- May cause nausea, vomiting, diarrhea, stomach cramps or pain, or ringing in the ears. Contact your doctor if these symptoms persist.
- May cause blurred vision or dizziness. Use caution when driving or performing other tasks requiring alertness, coordination, and physical dexterity.
- Notify your doctor immediately if you experience any evidence of allergy such as flushing, itching, rash, fever, stomach pain, difficulty breathing, ringing in the ears, or vision problems.
- Store at controlled room temperature (59° to 86°F). Protect from light and moisture.

If you have any questions, consult your doctor, pharmacist, or health care provider.

	Generic Name *Brand Name Example*	Supplied As	Generic Available
Rx	**Foscarnet Sodium (Phosphonoformic acid; PFA)**		
	Foscavir	**Injection:** 24 mg/mL	No

Type of Drug:

Antiviral drug.

How the Drug Works:

Foscarnet exerts its antiviral activity by selective inhibition of virus-specific DNA. Foscarnet is not necessarily a cure for cytomegalovirus (CMV) retinitis or herpes simplex virus (HSV) infections.

Uses:

To treat CMV retinitis (infection in lining of eyeball) in patients with acquired immunodeficiency syndrome (AIDS) and acyclovir-resistant mucocutaneous HSV infections in immunocompromised patients only. Safety and effectiveness have not been established for treatment of other CMV infections (eg, pneumonitis, gastroenteritis), other HSV infections (eg, retinitis, encephalitis), congenital or neonatal CMV or HSV disease, or nonimmunocompromised individuals. Also used as combination therapy with ganciclovir for patients who have relapsed after monotherapy with either drug.

Precautions:

Do not use in the following situations: Allergy to foscarnet sodium or any of its ingredients.

Use with caution in the following situations:

- anemia
- drugs affecting serum calcium levels, concurrent use of
- heart disease
- kidney disease
- mineral and electrolyte levels, abnormal (eg, low blood calcium)
- seizures

Pregnancy: There are no adequate and well-controlled studies in pregnant women. Use only if clearly needed and the potential benefits to the mother outweigh the possible hazards to the fetus.

Breastfeeding: The Centers for Disease Control and Prevention (CDC) recommends that HIV-infected mothers not breastfeed their infants to avoid risking postnatal transmission of HIV. It is not known if foscarnet is excreted in breast milk. Consult your doctor before you begin breastfeeding.

Children: Safety and effectiveness have not been established. Foscarnet may affect the development of teeth and bones. Use only after careful evaluation and if the potential benefits outweigh the possible risks.

Elderly: Monitor kidney function carefully before and during treatment with foscarnet and adjust dosage as necessary.

Lab tests will be required to monitor treatment. Tests include kidney function, plasma minerals and electrolytes, serum creatinine, and eye examinations.

Drug Interactions:

Tell your doctor or pharmacist if you are taking or planning to take any over-the-counter or prescription medications or dietary supplements while taking foscarnet. Doses of one or both drugs may need to be modified, or a different drug may need to be prescribed. The following drugs and drug classes interact with foscarnet:

aminoglycosides (eg, gentamycin)
amphotericin B (eg, *Fungizone*)
didanosine (*Videx*)
pentamidine isethionate (*Pentam 300*)
ritonavir (*Norvir*)
saquinavir (*Invirase*)
zidovudine (*Retrovir*)

Foscarnet decreases serum levels of ionized calcium. Use caution when other drugs known to influence serum calcium levels are used.

Side Effects:

Every drug is capable of producing side effects. Many foscarnet users experience side effects. The frequency and severity of side effects depend on many factors including dose, duration of therapy, and individual susceptibility. Possible side effects include:

Digestive Tract: Nausea; vomiting; diarrhea; stomach pain; appetite loss; taste sensation changes; constipation; indigestion; gas; dark or bloody stool; inflammation of pancreas; mouth infection; dry mouth; rectal bleeding.

Nervous System: Headache; dizziness; abnormal skin sensations; tremor; muscle spasms; seizures; decreased sensitivity to touch; dementia; clumsiness; stupor; sense disturbances; confusion; drowsiness; depression; anxiety; sleeplessness; fatigue; weakness; nervousness; agitation; memory loss; aggressive behavior; hallucinations; abnormal speech; incoordination.

Circulatory System: Blood pressure changes; chest pain; palpitations (pounding in the chest); rapid heartbeat; cerebrovascular disorder; blood clots; abnormal heart rhythm.

Respiratory System: Cough; difficult breathing; pneumonia; sinus inflammation; sore throat; nasal congestion; wheezing; bronchospasm; spitting up blood.

Skin: Rash; sweating; itching; flushing; ulcers; discoloration; redness; seborrhea.

Urinary and Reproductive Tract: Protein in urine; decreased urination; painful or difficult urination; urinary tract infections.

Other: Fever; general body discomfort; back pain; bacterial or fungal infections; chills; pain or inflammation at injection site; general ill health; flu-like symptoms; abscess; edema (fluid retention); facial swelling; abnormal vision; eye pain; inflammation of eye; abnormal levels of minerals and electrolytes; weight loss; thirst; joint and muscle pain; leg cramps; difficulty swallowing; bone marrow suppression; anemia; abnormal blood counts; abnormal kidney function; death.

Guidelines for Use:

- Dosage is individualized according to kidney function. Take exactly as prescribed.
- Usual dose is injected intravenously (IV; into a vein) 2 to 3 times daily for 2 to 3 weeks. Take in evenly spaced intervals throughout the day.
- Do not exceed recommended dosage, frequency, or rate of infusion.
- Follow the injection procedure taught to you by your health care provider.
- If a dose is missed, inject it as soon as possible. If several hours have passed or if it is nearing time for the next dose, do not double the dose to catch up, unless advised to do so by your doctor. If more than one dose is missed or it is necessary to establish a new dosage schedule, contact your doctor or pharmacist.
- Drink plenty of fluids.
- Foscarnet is not a cure for CMV retinitis or HSV. You may continue to experience effects of retinitis during or following treatment. While complete healing of HSV may occur, relapse occurs in most patients. Patients should remain under the care of a doctor.
- Foscarnet does not reduce the risk of transmitting HIV to others through sexual contact or blood contamination.
- HIV-infected mothers should not breastfeed because of the risk of transmitting the HIV infection to the infant.
- Kidney function may be impaired during foscarnet therapy. Patients with abnormal kidney function should use with caution. Dose modifications and possible discontinuation may be required.
- Discontinue immediately and contact your doctor if tingling around the mouth, urination problems, numbness in the extremities, or abnormal sensations such as burning or prickling occurs during or after infusion.
- Lab tests and eye exams are required to monitor therapy. Be sure to keep appointments.
- Store at room temperature (59° to 86°F). Do not freeze.

If you have any questions, consult your doctor, pharmacist, or health care provider.

	Generic Name / *Brand Name Example*	Supplied As	Generic Available
Rx	**Ganciclovir Sodium**[1]		
	Cytovene	**Capsules:** 250 mg, 500 mg	No

[1] Also available as an intravenous injection.

Type of Drug:

Antiviral drug to treat and prevent cytomegalovirus (CMV) infections.

How the Drug Works:

It is believed that ganciclovir interferes with the ability of cytomegalovirus (CMV) to reproduce by stopping the production of important proteins needed by the virus to grow.

Uses:

Ganciclovir capsules are used as an alternative to intravenous ganciclovi-rfor maintenance treatment of CMV retinitis in immunocompriomised patients, including patients with AIDS, in whom retinitis is stable following treatment with intravenous ganciclovir and for whom the risk of more rapid progression is balanced by the benefit associated with avoiding daily IV infusions. Ganciclovir capsules are also used to prevent CMV disease in transplant recipients.

Intravenous ganciclovir is used for the treatment of CMV retinitis (inflammation of the retina) in patients with immunocompromised (weakened) immune systems, including patients with acquired immunodeficiency syndrome (AIDS). It is also used to prevent CMV disease in transplant patients at risk for CMV disease.

Unlabeled Use(s): Occasionally doctors may prescribe ganciclovir for CMV pneumonia in transplant patients, CMV gastroenteritis in patients with irritable bowel disease, and for CMV pneumonitis.

Precautions:

Do not use in the following situations:

- allergy to acyclovir or ganciclovir, or any of its ingredients
- nonimmunocomromised patients
- treatment of congenital or newborn CMV disease
- treatment of other CMV infections

Use with caution in the following situations:

- cytopenias (low blood cell counts), preexisting
- cytopenic reactions to other drugs, chemicals, or radiation therapy, history of
- kidney disease
- transplant recipients

Pregnancy: There are no adequate and well-controlled studies in pregnant women. Use only if clearly needed and the potential benefits to the mother outweigh the possible hazards to the fetus. Women of childbearing potential should avoid becoming pregnant during ganciclovir therapy.

Breastfeeding: The Centers for Disease Control and Prevention (CDC) recommends that HIV-infected mothers not breastfeed their infants to avoid risking postnatal transmission of HIV. It is not known if ganciclovir is excreted in breast milk. Do not breastfeed while taking ganciclovir. Consult your doctor before you begin breastfeeding.

Children: Safety and effectiveness have not been established. Use only after careful evaluation and if the potential benefits outweigh the possible risks.

Elderly: Monitor kidney function carefully before and during treatment with ganciclovir and adjust dosage as necessary.

Lab tests will be required to monitor treatment. Tests may include blood cell counts, eye exams, and kidney function tests.

Drug Interactions:

Tell your doctor or pharmacist if you are taking or if you are planning to take any over-the-counter or prescription medications or dietary supplements while taking ganciclovir. Doses of one or both drugs may need to be modified or a different drug may need to be prescribed. The following drugs and drug classes interact with ganciclovir:

- cell growth inhibitors (eg, dapsone, pentamidine, flucytosine, vincristine, vinblastine, adriamycin, amphotericin B, trimethoprim/sulfamethoxazole)
- didanosine (*Videx*)
- imipenem-cilastatin (*Primaxin*)
- nephrotoxic drugs (eg, aminoglycosides)
- probenecid
- zidovudine (*Retrovir*)

Side Effects:

Every drug is capable of producing side effects. Many ganciclovir users experience no, or minor, side effects. The frequency and severity of side effects depend on many factors including dose, duration of therapy, and individual susceptibility. Possible side effects include:

Hematologic: Granulocytopenia (neutropenia), usually within first or second week of therapy; thrombocytopenia.

Digestive Tract: Nausea; vomiting; diarrhea; appetite loss.

Nervous System: Headache; abnormal sensations in arms or legs.

Skin: Itching; sweating.

Other: Infections; fever; chills; general body pain; inflammation at injection site; fertility problems; impaired kidney function; abnormal liver function tests; retinal detachment; vision changes; phlebitis; abnormal blood cell counts.

Guidelines for Use:

- Dosage is individualized. Take exactly as prescribed.
- Do not change the dose or stop taking, unless directed by your doctor.
- The injectable form of ganciclovir is prepared and administered intravenously (IV; into vein) by your health care provider in a medical setting.
- Take capsules with food to maximize effectiveness. Do not open, crush, or chew capsules.
- *Capsules* — If a dose is missed, take it as soon as possible. If several hours have passed or it is nearing time for the next dose, do not double the dose to catch up, unless advised to do so by your doctor. If more than one dose is missed or it is necessary to establish a new dosage schedule, contact your doctor or pharmacist.
- Avoid contact of broken or crushed capsules with skin, mouth or nasal tissues, or eyes. If contact occurs, wash skin thoroughly with soap and water and rinse eyes thoroughly with plain water.
- Notify your doctor immediately if you experience fever or other signs of infection, sore throat, or unusual bleeding or bruising.
- Ganciclovir is not a cure for CMV retinitis. You may continue to experience effects of retinitis during or following treatment. Patients should remain under the care of a doctor.
- Contraceptive (birth control) measures are recommended for men and women during therapy. Men should use barrier contraception during and for at least 90 days following ganciclovir treatment.
- HIV-infected mothers should not breastfeed because of the risk of transmitting the infection to the infant.
- Lab tests and eye exams will be required to monitor therapy. Be sure to keep appointments.
- Store capsules between 41°F and 77°F.

If you have any questions, consult your doctor, pharmacist, or health care provider.

	Generic Name *Brand Name Examples*	Supplied As	Generic Available
Rx	**Acyclovir**[1]		
	Zovirax	**Tablets:** 400 mg, 800 mg	Yes
	Zovirax	**Capsules:** 200 mg	Yes
	Zovirax	**Oral suspension:** 200 mg/ 5 mL	Yes
	Zovirax	**Ointment:** 5%	No
Rx	**Famciclovir**		
	Famvir	**Tablets**: 125 mg, 250 mg, 500 mg	No
Rx	**Valacyclovir**		
	Valtrex	**Tablets**: 500 mg, 1 g	No

[1] Also available as an intravenous injection.

Type of Drug:

Antiviral drug used to treat herpes zoster infections (shingles), genital herpes, and chickenpox.

How the Drug Works:

Acyclovir prevents the herpes virus from reproducing, reducing the time needed to recover from the infection and the time for the lesion to heal. Acyclovir does not eliminate the virus and is not a cure. It does not prevent transmission of the virus to others.

Uses:

Oral: To treat initial episodes and manage recurrent episodes of genital herpes infections. Also for acute treatment of herpes zoster (shingles) and treatment of chickenpox.

Topical: To treat initial episodes of genital herpes infections and limited non-life-threatening HSV skin infections in immunocompromised patients.

Unlabeled Use(s): Occasionally doctors may prescribe acyclovir for cytomegalovirus and herpes simplex infections following bone marrow or kidney transplants, disseminated primary eczema herpeticum, herpes infections other than those affecting the genitals (eg, infection of the brain, eye, rectum, finger), infectious mononucleosis and chickenpox-related pneumonia. Valacyclovir has also been used as prophylactic treatment for prevention of cytomegalovirus (CMV) disease in patients with advanced HIV and in patients postrenal transplant.

Precautions:

Do not use in the following situations: Allergy to the antiherpes virus agent or any of its ingredients.

Use with caution in the following situations:

drugs potentially toxic to the kidneys
kidney disease

Pregnancy: There are no adequate and well-controlled studies in pregnant women. Use only if clearly needed and the potential benefits to the mother outweigh the possible hazards to the fetus.

Breastfeeding: Acyclovir appears in breast milk. Consult your doctor before you begin breastfeeding.

Children: Safety and effectiveness of acyclovir in children younger than 2 years of age have not been established. Saftey and effectiveness of famciclovir have not been established in children younger than 18 years of age. Safety and effectiveness of valcyclovir in children have not been established.

Drug Interactions:

Tell your doctor or pharmacist if you are taking or if you are planning to take any over-the-counter or prescription medications or dietary supplements with an antiherpes virus agent. Doses of one or both drugs may need to be modified or a different drug may need to be prescribed. The following drugs and drug classes interact with antiherpes virus agents:

cimetidine (eg, *Tagamet*)
digoxin (eg, *Lanoxin*)
interferon (*Roferon)*
methotrexate (eg, *Mexate)*
probenecid
theophylline (eg, *Theo-Dur*)
zidovudine (*Retrovir)*

Side Effects:

Every drug is capable of producing side effects. Many antiherpes virus agent users experience no, or minor, side effects. The frequency and severity of side effects depend on many factors including dose, duration of therapy, and individual susceptibility. Possible side effects include:

Digestive Tract: Nausea; vomiting; diarrhea.

Skin: Burning; stinging; itching (ointment only); rash.

Other: Headache; abnormal skin sensations; weakness; numbness or tingling; general body discomfort.

Guidelines for Use:

- Dosage is individualized. Take exactly as prescribed. Do not exceed recommended dosage, frequency or length of treatment.
- Antiherpes virus agents are not cures for herpes simplex infections.
- Avoid sexual intercourse when lesions (sores) are present to prevent infecting your partner.
- Notify your doctor if lesions appear more frequently or become worse.
- *Oral* — Patient information from the manufacturer is included with product.
  If a dose is missed, take it as soon as possible. If several hours have passed or it is nearing time for the next dose, do not double the dose to catch up, unless advised to do so by your doctor. If more than one dose is missed or it is necessary to establish a new dosage schedule, contact your doctor or pharmacist.
- *Topical* —Begin therapy as early as possible following the onset of symptoms.
  Apply to all lesions every 3 hours, 6 times per day for 7 days.
  A one-half inch ribbon of ointment will generally cover about 4 square inches.
  If an application is missed, apply as soon as possible, but not if it is almost time for the next application.
  Ointment must thoroughly cover all lesions.
  To reduce the risk of spreading the infection, use a finger cot or rubber glove to apply the ointment.
  Some burning, stinging or itching may occur. If these symptoms are persistent, consult your doctor.
  Acyclovir ointment is of little benefit in treating recurrent attacks.
  Do not use chronically to prevent recurrences.
  Do not use in or near eyes.

If you have any questions, consult your doctor, pharmacist, or health care provider.

Generic Name *Brand Name Example*	Supplied As	Generic Available
Rx **Amantadine HCl**	**Capsules:** 100 mg	Yes
Symmetrel	**Tablets**: 100 mg	No
Symmetrel	**Syrup:** 50 mg/5 mL	Yes

Type of Drug:

Antiviral drug for influenza A virus; antiparkinson agent.

How the Drug Works:

It is not known exactly how amantadine acts to treat and prevent influenza A infection or symptoms of Parkinson disease.

Uses:

To prevent and treat respiratory tract infections caused by influenza A virus (flu) in high-risk patients with heart, lung, muscle-nerve, or immunodeficiency diseases, and for people in close contact with patients with influenza type A illness.

A flu shot (immunization) is the best way to prevent influenza type A infection. Amantadine may be used when flu shots are not possible or unavailable.

Recommendations for use for prevention of influenza type A virus:
- During an influenza A outbreak, when the flu shot may not be effective.
- To aid late immunization of high-risk individuals.
- To reduce the spread of the virus to high-risk persons during influenza type A outbreaks.
- To treat high-risk patients during the flu season when a flu shot is not possible because of allergy to the vaccine.
- To supplement vaccination protection in those with impaired immune responses.

To treat Parkinson disease and drug-induced extrapyramidal reactions (movement disorders). See the Antiparkinson-Dopaminergic Agents monograph in the CNS Drugs chapter.

Precautions:

Do not use in the following situations: Allergy to amantadine or any of its ingredients.

Use with caution in the following situations:

congestive heart failure
eczema, recurrent, history of
edema (fluid retention)
elderly
glaucoma, narrow angle
kidney disease
liver disease
mental illness (eg, psychosis)
seizure conditions (eg, epilepsy)
substance abuse, current or history of

Abrupt discontinuation: Do not abruptly stop taking amantadine. A few patients with Parkinson disease have experienced a parkinsonian crisis (tremors, rigidity, etc.) when this drug was stopped suddenly.

Mental problems: Amantadine can exacerbate mental problems in patients with a history of psychiatric disorders or substance abuse. Suicide attempts have been reported in patients treated with amantadine. Discontinue use and immediately notify your doctor if mood or personality changes are noted.

Other respiratory tract illnesses: Amantidine is not effective for preventing or treating viral respiratory tract illnesses other than influenza A.

Pregnancy: There are no adequate and well-controlled studies in pregnant women. Use only if clearly needed and the potential benefits to the mother outweigh the possible hazards to the fetus.

Breastfeeding: Amantadine appears in breast milk. Consult your doctor before you begin breastfeeding.

Children: Safety and effectiveness in children younger than 1 year of age have not been established.

Elderly: Patients 65 years of age and older may need lower doses than other individuals.

Drug Interactions:

Tell your doctor or pharmacist if you are taking or planning to take any over-the-counter or prescription medications or dietary supplements with amantadine. Doses of one or both drugs may need to be modified or a different drug may need to be prescribed. The following drugs and drug classes interact with amantadine:

anticholinergics (eg, trihexyphenidyl)
CNS stimulants (eg, phentermine)
quinidine (eg, *Quinora*)
quinine
thiazide diuretics (eg, hydrochlorothiazide)
triamterene (eg, *Dyrenium*)
trimethoprim/sulfamethoxazole (eg, *Bactrim*)

Side Effects:

Every drug is capable of producing side effects. Many amantadine users experience no, or minor, side effects. The frequency and severity of side effects depend on many factors including dose, duration of therapy, and individual susceptibility. Possible side effects include:

Digestive Tract: Nausea; constipation; appetite loss; diarrhea.

Nervous System: Dizziness; lightheadedness; depression; hallucinations; confusion; abnormal dreams; anxiety; irritability; headache; incoordination; sleeplessness; drowsiness.

Other: Skin mottling; edema (fluid retention); dry mouth; fatigue; orthostatic hypotension (dizziness or lightheadedness when rising quickly from a sitting or lying position).

Guidelines for Use:

- Dosage is individualized. Take exactly as prescribed.
- Do not stop taking or change the dose, unless directed by your doctor.
- May be taken without regard to food. Take with food if stomach upset occurs.
- *For treatment of symptoms of influenza A virus* — Start as soon as possible after onset of symptoms and continue for 24 to 48 hours after symptoms disappear.
- *For prevention of influenza A virus* — Start in anticipation of contact or as soon as possible after exposure. Continue daily for at least 10 days. The infectious period extends from shortly before to one week after the onset of symptoms.
- If used in combination with the influenza vaccine (flu shot), take amantadine for 2 to 4 weeks after the vaccine has been given (until protective antibody responses to the vaccine have developed).
- If the flu vaccine is unavailable or cannot be taken, amantadine should be taken for up to 90 days.
- Therapy may not result in protection for all individuals.
- If a dose is missed, take it as soon as possible. If several hours have passed or it is nearing time for the next dose, do not double the dose to catch up, unless advised to do so by your doctor. If more than one dose is missed or it is necessary to establish a new dosage schedule, contact your doctor or pharmacist.
- This medicine may cause drowsiness, dizziness, or blurred vision. Use caution while driving or performing other tasks requiring alertness, coordination, or physical dexterity.
- If dizziness or lightheadedness occurs, avoid sudden changes in posture. Notify your doctor of this effect if this continues.
- Contact your doctor if you experience mood changes, swelling of hands or feet, difficult urination, or shortness of breath.
- Avoid excessive alcohol intake while taking amantadine. It may increase potential for dizziness, confusion, and lightheadedness.
- Store at controlled room temperature (59° to 86°F) in a tightly closed container. Protect tablets and capsules from moisture.

If you have any questions, consult your doctor, pharmacist, or health care provider.

	Generic Name *Brand Name Example*	Supplied As	Generic Available
Rx	**Cidofovir**		
	Vistide	**Injection:** 75 mg/mL	No

Type of Drug:

Antiviral drug to treat cytomegalovirus (CHV) infections.

How the Drug Works:

Cidofovir interferes with the ability of cytomegalovirus (CMV) to reproduce by stopping the production of important proteins needed by the virus to grow.

Uses:

To treat CMV retinitis (infection in lining of eyeball) in patients with acquired immunodeficency syndrome (AIDS). It must be used in combination with oral probenecid.

The safety and efficacy of cidofovir have not been established for the treatment of other CMV infections (such as pneumonitis or gastroenteritis), congenital or neonatal CMV disease, or CMV disease in non-HIV-infected individuals.

Precautions:

Do not use in the following situations:
- allergy to cidofovir or any of its ingredients
- allergy to probenecid or other sulfa-containing medications
- direct intraocular injection (injection into eye)
- kidney disease, moderate to severe
- nephrotoxic agents (eg, gentamicin), concurrent use

Use with caution in the following situations:
- elderly
- kidney disease

Kidney impairment: Kidney toxicity has occurred with cidofovir. Intravenous prehydration with normal saline and oral administration of probenecid will be used with each cidofovir infusion. Blood and urine tests will be performed no more than 48 hours before each dose of cidofovir.

Pregnancy: There are no adequate and well-controlled studies in pregnant women. Use only if clearly needed and potential benefits outweigh the possible hazards to the fetus. Advise against pregnancy during and for at least 1 month following the use of this medicine.

Breastfeeding: The Centers for Disease Control and Prevention (CDC) recommends that HIV-infected mothers not breastfeed their infants to avoid risking postnatal transmission of HIV. It is not known if cidofovir appears in breast milk. Do not breastfeed while taking this medicine.

Children: Safety and effectiveness in children have not been established.

Elderly: Use with caution in elderly patients. Dosage adjustments may be necessary.

Lab tests will be required to monitor therapy. Lab tests will include blood counts, kidney function tests, urine protein tests, and eye exams.

Drug Interactions:

Tell your doctor or pharmacist if you are taking or if you are planning to take any over-the-counter or prescription medications or dietary supplements while taking cidofovir. Doses of one or both drugs may need to be modified or a different drug may need to be prescribed. The following drugs and drug classes may interact with cidofovir:

amphotericin B (eg, *Fungizone*)
aminoglycosides (eg, gentamicin)
foscarnet (*Foscavir*)
NSAIDs (eg, ibuprofen)
pentamidine (eg, *Pentam 300*)
vancomycin (eg, *Vancocin*)

Side Effects:

Every drug is capable of producing side effects. Many cidofovir users experience no, or minor, side effects. The frequency and severity of side effects depend on many factors including dose, duration of therapy, and individual susceptibility. Possible side effects include:

Digestive Tract: Nausea; vomiting; diarrhea; appetite loss; mouth sores.

Urinary and Reproductive Tract: Protein in urine; elevated serum creatinine.

Other: Rash; hair loss; headache; weakness; fever; infections; chills; difficulty breathing; pneumonia; anemia; decreased white blood cell counts; low intraocular pressure (pressure of fluid inside eye); increased cough.

Guidelines for Use:

- This medication will be prepared and administered by your health care provider in a medical setting.
- Usual dose is administered once weekly for 2 consecutive weeks, and then once every 2 weeks. The dose may be changed by your doctor as a result of lab test results.
- Probenecid may cause headache, nausea, vomiting, or allergic reactions (eg, rash, fever, chills, difficulty breathing). Taking probenecid after a meal or using antiemetics may decrease the nausea. Antihistamines or acetaminophen (eg, *Tylenol*) may be used to lessen the allergic reactions.
- *Zidovudine (AZT; Retrovir)* — Patients taking AZT should temporarily discontinue its administration or decrease its dose by half (50%) on the days of the cidofovir administration. Talk with your doctor about which would be best for you.
- Cidofovir is not a cure for CMV retinitis. You may continue to experience effects of retinitis during or following treatment. Patients should remain under the care of a doctor.
- HIV-infected mothers should not breastfeed because of the risk of transmitting the HIV infection or this drug to the infant.
- Contraceptive (birth control) measures are recommended for men and women during therapy. Men should use barrier contraception during and for at least 90 days following treatment. Women should use effective contraception during and for 30 days following treatment. Inform your doctor if you are pregnant, suspect pregnancy, or are planning to become pregnant.
- Kidney impairment is the major toxicity of cidofovir. Have blood tests and kidney function tests performed at least 48 hours before each dose of cidofovir.
- Lab tests and eye exams will be required to monitor therapy. Be sure to keep appointments.

If you have any questions, consult your doctor, pharmacist, or health care provider.

	Generic Name *Brand Name Examples*	Supplied As	Generic Available
Rx	**Ribavirin**		
	Rebetol	**Capsules**: 200 mg	No
	Virazole	**Powder for reconstitution, aerosol:** 6 g/100 mL (20 mg/ mL when reconstituted)	No

Type of Drug:

Antiviral drug for inhalation treatment of respiratory syncytial virus (RSV) infections, anti-hepatitis C virus (HCV) drug.

How the Drug Works:

Ribavirin inhibits the growth of the respiratory syncytial virus. The exact mechanism of action is not known.

Uses:

Rebetol — To treat chronic hepatitis C in patients with compensated liver disease. Only use in combination with interferon alfa-2b (*Intron A*).

Virazole — To treat certain hospitalized infants and young children with severe lung infections due to RSV. Adults are rarely treated with ribavirin by inhalation. Treatment early in the course of RSV infection is desirable for optimal effect.

Precautions:

Do not use in the following situations:

- adults (*Virazole* only)
- allergy to ribavirin or any of its ingredients
- heart disease, unstable (*Rebetol* only)
- hemoglobin abnormalities (eg, sickle cell anemia) (*Rebetol* only)
- hepatitis, autoimmune
- kidney disease, severe (*Rebetol* only)
- male partners of pregnant women
- pregnancy or during periods when one may become pregnant

Use with caution in the following situations:

- heart disease (*Rebetol* only)
- kidney disease (*Rebetol* only)
- mechanical ventilation (*Virazole* only)

Other viral infections: Ribavirin capsules are not effective for treating viral infections (eg, HIV, hepatitis B, influenza) other than hepatitis C.

Secondary exposure hazard: Avoid direct care of patient if you are a mother or health care provider who is pregnant or planning to become pregnant. Aerosolized ribavirin is given in rooms with special ventilation. Wear appropriate respirator masks. The aerosol machine should be turned off 5 to 10 minutes before prolonged patient contact.

Pregnancy: Do not use during pregnancy. The risk of use in pregnant women clearly outweighs any possible benefit. Women of child-bearing potential, including female partners of male patients, must take extreme care to avoid pregnancy during and for 6 months after treatment has been stopped. Two forms of effective contraception must be used.

Breastfeeding: It is not known if ribavirin appears in breast milk. Consult your doctor before you begin breastfeeding.

Children: Safety and effectiveness of ribavirin capsules have not been established.

Elderly: Use ribavirin capsules with caution in elderly patients. Dosage adjustments may be necessary.

Lab tests will be required to monitor therapy with ribavirin capsules. Tests include pregnancy tests, blood counts, and liver and thyroid function tests.

Drug Interactions:

Tell your doctor or pharmacist if you are taking or planning to take any over-the-counter or prescription medications or dietary supplements with ribavirin. Doses of one or both drugs may be modified or a different drug may need to be prescribed. Antacids (eg *Mylanta*) interact with ribavirin.

Side Effects:

Every drug is capable of producing side effects. Many ribavirin users experience no, or minor, side effects. The frequency and severity of side effects depend on many factors including dose, duration of therapy, and individual susceptibility. Possible side effects include:

Aerosol only –

Respiratory System: Difficulty breathing; worsening of breathing status; collapse of lung; bacterial pneumonia; fluid in the lungs.

Other: Abnormal blood tests; anemia; rash; eye redness and inflammation; decrease in blood pressure; changes in heart rate.

Capsules only –

Nervous System: Dizziness; sleeplessness; irritability; depression; nervousness; emotional lability.

Digestive Tract: Nausea; appetite loss; indigestion; abnormal taste sensation.

Other: Rash; itching; difficulty breathing; sinus inflammation; fatigue; rigors; weakness; muscle and joint pain; anemia.

Guidelines for Use:

- *Capsules* — Review Medication Guide before using and after each refill of medication.
  Dosage is individualized. Take exactly as prescribed.
  Do not change the dose or stop taking unless directed by your doctor.
  Intron A injection must be used in conjunction with ribavarin capsules in order to provide the most effective therapy. Use of ribavirin without *Intron A* is not effective.
  Drink plenty of water while taking ribavirin.
  It is not known if ribavirin reduces the risk of transmitting hepatitis virus to others through sexual contact or blood transfusion.
  Appropriate precautions to prevent transmitting hepatitis C virus to others should be taken.
  Ribavirin is contraindicated in pregnant women, including partners of male patients. Therapy should not be started until a negative pregnancy test has been obtained.
  Women of child-bearing potential, including female partners of male patients, must use 2 forms of reliable contraception during treatment and for 6 months after treatment has been stopped.
  If a dose is missed, take it as soon as possible. If several hours have passed or it is nearing time for the next dose, do not double the dose to catch up, unless advised to do so by your doctor. If more than one dose is missed or it is necessary to establish a new dosage schedule, contact your doctor or pharmacist.
  Do not take any OTC or prescription medications or dietary supplements unless advised to do so by your doctor.
  Lab tests will be required to monitor therapy. Be sure to keep appointments.
  Store at room temperature (59° to 86°F).
- *Aerosol* — Ribavirin will be prepared and administered by your health care provider in a hospital setting.
  Hospital personnel will closely monitor the patient's status and responses to treatment.
  Ribavirin will be administered by a specially designed machine.
  Ribavirin treatment will be administered over 12 to 18 hours a day for 3 to 7 days.
  Ribavirin is not indicated for use by adults. It is never to be used in pregnant women or during times when pregnancy might occur.
  Avoid direct care of patient if you are a mother or health care provider who is pregnant or planning to become pregnant. Aerosol ribavirin is given in rooms with special ventilation. Wear appropriate respirator masks. The aerosol machine should be turned off 5 to 10 minutes before prolonged patient contact.

	Generic Name *Brand Name Example*	Supplied As	Generic Available
Rx	**Rimantadine HCl**		
	Flumadine	**Tablets**: 100 mg	No
	Flumadine	**Syrup**: 50 mg/5 mL	No

Type of Drug:

Antiviral drug for influenza A virus.

How the Drug Works:

It is not fully understood how rimantadine acts to inhibit the growth and spread of the influenza A virus.

Uses:

To prevent the symptoms of infection caused by the influenza A virus in adults and children younger than 1 year of age.

To treat adults with illness caused by strains of the influenza A virus.

Precautions:

Do not use in the following situations: Allergy to rimantadine or amantadine (eg, *Symmetrel*) or any of their ingredients.

Use with caution in the following situations:

- epilepsy
- kidney disease
- liver disease
- patients whose contacts are at high risk for influenza A illness

Flu vaccine: A yearly vaccination with the influenza vaccine ("flu shot") is still the best way to prevent influenza.

Seizures: Seizure-like activity has been reported in a small number of patients with a history of seizures who were not taking anticoagulant medication.

Pregnancy: There are no adequate and well-controlled studies in pregnant women. Use only if clearly needed and the potential benefits to the mother outweigh the possible hazards to the fetus.

Breastfeeding: It is not known if rimantadine appears in breast milk. Consult your doctor before you begin breastfeeding.

Children: The safety and effectiveness in the treatment of influenza symptoms have not been established in children. Prophylaxis studies have not been performed in children younger than 1 year of age.

Elderly: An increase in adverse reactions in persons older than 64 years of age has been shown. May need lower doses than other individuals.

Drug Interactions:

Tell your doctor if you are taking or planning to take any over-the-counter or prescription medications or dietary supplements with rimantadine. Doses of one or both drugs may need to be modified or a different drug may need to be prescribed. The following drugs and drug classes interact with rimantadine:

acetaminophen (eg, *Tylenol*)
aspirin
cimetidine (eg, *Tagamet*)

Side Effects:

Every drug is capable of producing side effects. Many rimantadine users experience no, or minor, side effects. The frequency and severity of side effects depend on many factors including dose, duration of therapy, and individual susceptibility. Possible side effects include:

Digestive Tract: Nausea; vomiting; stomach pain; appetite loss.

Nervous System: Sleeplessness; dizziness; headache; nervousness; fatigue.

Other: Weakness; dry mouth.

Guidelines for Use:

- Dosage is individualized. Take exactly as prescribed.
- Do not change the dose or stop taking unless directed by your doctor.
- May be taken without regard to meals.
- Children 10 years of age and older should receive the adult dose.
- *For treatment in adults* — Start as soon as possible after onset of symptoms and continue for 7 days. Rimantadine is most effective when started 48 hours or less after the onset of "flu" symptoms.
- Stop taking and immediately contact your health care provider if you experience seizures.
- May cause dizziness. Use caution while driving or performing other tasks requiring alertness, coordination, or physical dexterity.
- Contact your doctor if you develop persistent sleeplessness, dizziness, nausea, or vomiting.
- Store at room temperature (59° to 86°F).

If you have any questions, consult your doctor, pharmacist, or health care provider.

	Generic Name *Brand Name Example*	Supplied As	Generic Available
Rx	**Zanamivir**		
	Relenza	**Powder for inhalation:** 5 mg/blister	No

Type of Drug:

Antiviral drug used to treat influenza A and B virus.

How the Drug Works:

Zanamivir interferes with viral enzymes (neuramindase) that allow respiratory viruses to grow and spread.

Uses:

Indicated for the treatment of uncomplicated acute illness (flu symptoms) due to influenza virus A and B in adults and adolescents 7 years of age and older who have been symptomatic for 2 days or less.

Precautions:

Do not use in the following situations: Allergy to zanamivir or any of its ingredients.

Use with caution in the following situations:

asthma
lung disease, chronic obstructive

Pregnancy: There are no adequate and well-controlled studies in pregnant women. Use only if clearly needed and the potential benefits to the mother outweigh the possible hazards to the fetus.

Breastfeeding: It is not known if zanamivir appears in breast milk. Consult your doctor before you begin breastfeeding.

Children: Safety and effectiveness in patients younger than 12 years of age have not been established.

Drug Interactions:

Tell your doctor or pharmacist if you are taking or planning to take any over-the-counter or prescription medications or dietary supplements while taking zanamivir. Doses of one or both drugs may need to be modified or a different drug may need to be prescribed.

Side Effects:

Every drug is capable of producing side effects. Many zanamivir users experience no, or minor, side effects. The frequency and severity of side effects depend on many factors including dose, duration of therapy, and individual susceptibility. Possible side effects include:

Digestive Tract: Diarrhea; nausea; vomiting; stomach pain.

Nervous System: Headache; dizziness; general body discomfort; fatigue; fever.

Respiratory System: Nasal signs and symptoms; bronchitis; bronchospasm; difficulty breathing; cough; sinus infection; ear, nose, or throat infections.

Other: Muscle pain; joint pain; rash; hives.

Guidelines for Use:

- Read and carefully follow the patient instructions for use provided with zanamivir. Safe and effective use of zanamivir requires proper use of the *Diskhaler* to inhale the drug.
- This medicine is for administration to the respiratory tract by inhalation through the mouth only, using the *Diskhaler* provided.
- The recommended dose for patients 7 years of age and older is 2 inhalations (one 5 mg blister per inhalation for a total dose of 10 mg) 2 times daily (approximately 12 hours apart) for 5 days. Take 2 doses on the first day of treatment whenever possible, provided there are at least 2 hours between doses. On subsequent days, take doses about 12 hours apart (eg, morning and evening) at approximately the same time each day.
- Complete the entire 5-day course of treatment even if you begin to feel better.
- If you are scheduled to take an inhaled bronchodilator at the same time as this medicine, take the bronchodilator first.
- There is no evidence of zanamivir's effectiveness when started less than 2 days after the onset of signs or symptoms of influenza, or in the treatment of any other illness caused by agents other than influenza virus A or B.
- Use of this medicine has not been shown to reduce the risk of transmission of influenza to others.
- Zanamivir does not cure patients of influenza. It reduces time for improvement by 1 to 1.5 days.
- Zanamivir does not eliminate the need for an annual influenza vaccine in high-risk patients (eg, patients with asthma, diabetes, or heart disease; elderly patients).
- If you have asthma or chronic lung disease, you must have a fast-acting bronchodilator available. Stop this medicine and notify your doctor if you experience worsening of respiratory symptoms.
- Do not puncture any blister until immediately before taking a dose with the *Diskhaler*.
- Store at room temperature (59° to 86°F). Keep out of the reach of children.

If you have any questions, consult your doctor, pharmacist, or health care provider.

	Generic Name *Brand Name Example*	Supplied As	Generic Available
Rx	**Oseltamivir Phosphate**		
	Tamiflu	**Capsules**: 75 mg	No
	Tamiflu	**Suspension, oral**: 12 mg/mL	No

Type of Drug:

Antiviral drug for influenza A and B virus.

How the Drug Works:

Oseltamivir interferes with viral enzymes (neuramidase) that allow respiratory flu viruses to grow and spread. Oseltamivir is not active until after it has been absorbed into the body.

Uses:

For the treatment of uncomplicated acute illness due to influenza A or B infection in adults and pediatric patients 1 year of age and older who have had flu symptoms for no more than 2 days, and for the prevention of influenza A or B in adults and adolescents 13 years of age and older.

Precautions:

Do not use in the following situations: Allergy to oseltamivir phosphate or any of its ingredients.

Use with caution in the following situations:

kidney disease, severe
liver disease

Flu vaccine: A yearly vaccination with the influenza vaccine ("flu shot") is still the best way to prevent influenza.

Pregnancy: There are no adequate and well-controlled studies in pregnant women. Use only if clearly needed and the potential benefits to the mother outweigh the possible hazards to the fetus.

Breastfeeding: It is not known if oseltamivir appears in breast milk. Consult your doctor before you begin breastfeeding.

Children: Safety and effectiveness in children younger than 1 year of age have not been established.

Drug Interactions:

Tell your doctor or pharmacist if you are taking or planning to take any over-the-counter or prescription medications or dietary supplements while taking oseltamivir phosphate. Doses of one or both drugs may need to be modified or a different drug may need to be prescribed.

Side Effects:

Every drug is capable of producing side effects. Many oseltamivir phosphate users experience no, or minor, side effects. The frequency and severity of side effects depend on many factors including dose, duration of therapy, and individual susceptibility. Possible side effects include:

Digestive Tract: Nausea; vomiting; diarrhea; stomach pain.

Other: Cough; dizziness; headache; fatigue; bronchitis; sleeplessness; vertigo (feeling of whirling motion).

Guidelines for Use:

- Dosage is individualized. Take exactly as prescribed.
- Do not stop taking or change the dose, unless directed by your doctor.
- Patients should begin treatment as soon as possible following the first appearance of flu symptoms or following close contact with an infected individual. This medicine is not beneficial if started more than 2 days after flu symptoms are first noticed or after 2 days following close contact with an infected individual.
- May be taken without regard to meals or snacks. Take with food if stomach upset occurs.
- Patients should take missed doses as soon as they remember, except within 2 hours of next scheduled dose, and then continue normal dosage intervals.
- May cause dizziness. Use caution while driving or performing other tasks requiring alertness, coordination, or physical dexterity.
- Store at room temperature (59° to 86°F).

If you have any questions, consult your doctor, pharmacist, or health care provider.

	Generic Name *Brand Name Examples*	Supplied As	Generic Available
Rx	**Amprenavir**		
	Agenerase	**Capsules**: 50 mg, 150 mg	No
	Agenerase[1]	**Solution, oral**: 15 mg/mL	No
Rx	**Indinavir Sulfate**		
	Crixivan	**Capsules**: 100 mg, 200 mg, 333 mg, 400 mg	No
Rx	**Nelfinavir Mesylate**		
	Viracept	**Tablets**: 250 mg	No
	Viracept[2]	**Powder, oral**: 50 mg/g	No
Rx	**Ritonavir**		
	Norvir	**Capsules**: 100 mg	No
	Norvir[3]	**Solution, oral**: 80 mg/mL	No
Rx	**Saquinavir**		
	Invirase	**Capsules**: 200 mg (as mesylate)	No
	Fortovase	**Capsules, soft gelatin**: 200 mg	No
Rx	**Lopinavir/Ritonavir**		
	Kaletra	**Capsules**: 133.3 mg/33.3 mg	No
	Kaletra	**Solution, oral**: 80 mg/ 20 mg/mL	No

[1] Contains propylene glycol.
[2] Contains phenylalanine.
[3] Contains alcohol.

Type of Drug:

Antiviral; protease inhibitor; AIDS drug.

How the Drug Works:

Protease inhibitors inhibit the growth of the human immunodeficiency virus type 1 (HIV-1), the virus that causes acquired immunodeficiency syndrome (AIDS).

Uses:

Used alone or in combination with other antiretroviral agents for treatment of HIV-1 infection.

Precautions:

Do not use in the following situations:

allergy to the protease inhibitor or any of its ingredients
amiodarone therapy, concurrent (nelfinavir, ritonavir only)
bepridil therapy, concurrent
dihydroergotamine therapy, concurrent
ergotamine therapy, concurrent

HMG-CoA reductase inhibitor therapy, concurrent (nelfinavir, ritonavir, lopinavir/ritonavir only)
midazolam therapy, concurrent
pregnancy (amprenavir oral solution only)
quinidine therapy, concurrent (nelfinavir, ritonavir only)
rifampin therapy, concurrent (nelfinavir, saquinavir, lopinavir/ritonavir only)
St. John's wort use, concurrent
triazolam therapy, concurrent

Use with caution in the following situations:

allergy to sulfonamides (amprenavir only)
diabetes
hemophilia A or B
liver disease, moderate to severe

Diabetes: Exacerbation of preexisting diabetes mellitus and of hyperglycemia (high blood sugar) have been reported with protease inhibitor use. Some patients require initiation or dosage adjustments of insulin or hypoglycemic (blood sugar-lowering) agents.

Fat redistribution: Changes in body fat including central (stomach and chest) obesity, dorsocervical fat enlargement (buffalo hump), peripheral wasting (skinny arms and legs), and breast enlargement have occurred in patients receiving antiretrovial therapy. The cause of this and the long-term consequences of these changes are not known at this time.

Phenylketonuria patients: Nelfinavir powder contains phenylalanine. Consult your doctor or pharmacist.

Vitamin E: Amprenavir capsules and oral solution contain large amounts of vitamin E, exceeding the Reference Daily Intake. Adults and pediatric patients taking amprenavir should not take supplemental vitamin E.

Pregnancy: There are no adequate and well-controlled studies in pregnant women. Use only if clearly needed and the potential benefits to the mother outweigh the possible hazards to the fetus. Amprenavir oral solution is contraindicated in pregnant women.

Breastfeeding: The Centers for Disease Control and Prevention (CDC) recommends that HIV-infected mothers not breastfeed their infants to avoid risking postnatal transmission of HIV. It is not known if protease inhibitors appear in breast milk. Consult your doctor before you begin breastfeeding.

Children: Safety and effectiveness of amprenavir have not been established in patients younger than 4 years of age. Safety and effectiveness of indinavir have not been established in pediatric patients. Safety and effectiveness of nelfinavir and ritonavir have not been established in patients younger than 2 years of age. Safety and effectiveness of saquinavir have not been established in patients younger than 16 years of age. Safety and effectiveness of lopinavir/ritonavir have not been established in patients younger than 6 months of age.

Elderly: Administer with caution in elderly patients.

Lab tests will be required to monitor therapy. Tests include cholesterol and triglyceride levels, liver enzymes, and blood sugar levels.

Drug Interactions:

Tell your doctor or pharmacist if you are taking or planning to take any over-the-counter or prescription medications or dietary supplements while taking a protease inhibitor. Doses of one or both drugs may need to be modified or a different drug may need to be prescribed. The following drugs and drug classes interact with protease inhibitors:

- amiodarone (eg, *Cordarone*) (amprenavir only)
- antacids (eg, *Maalox*) (amprenavir only)
- anticoagulants (eg, warfarin)
- anticonvulsants (eg, carbamazepine)
- azole antifungals (eg, ketoconazole)
- benzodiazepines (eg, midazolam, triazolam)
- bepridil (*Vascor*)
- contraceptives, oral (eg, *Ortho-Novum*)
- didanosine (*Videx*) (amprenavir only)
- ergot alkaloids (eg, ergotamine)
- HMG-CoA reductase inhibitors (eg, lovastatin)
- immunosuppressants (eg, cyclosporine)
- lidocaine (eg, *Xylocaine*) (amprenavir only)
- quinidine (eg, *Quinora*) (amprenavir only)
- rifamycins (eg, rifampin)
- sildenafil (*Viagra*)
- St. John's wort
- tricyclic antidepressants (eg, amitriptyline) (amprenavir only)
- vitamin E

Side Effects:

Every drug is capable of producing side effects. Many protease inhibitor users experience no, or minor, side effects. The frequency and severity of side effects depend on many factors including dose, duration of therapy, and individual susceptibility. Possible side effects include:

Nervous System: Depression; headache; sleeplessness; anxiety; sex drive changes; drowsiness; dizziness.

Digestive Tract: Nausea; vomiting; diarrhea; loose stools; stomach pain; taste disorders; acid regurgitation; dry mouth; indigestion; gas; constipation; appetite changes.

Skin: Severe and life-threatening skin reactions (eg, Stevens-Johnson syndrome); rash, itching; abnormal skin sensations; tingling or numb sensation around the mouth (amprenavir only); eczema; warts.

Other: Lab test abnormalities; new onset of diabetes mellitus; exacerbation of preexisting diabetes mellitus; high blood sugar; redistribution or accumulation of body fat; numbness in the arms or legs; fatigue; pain; weakness; back, muscle, or bone pain; kidney stones (indinavir only); weakness; general body discomfort.

Guidelines for Use:

- Read the patient information handout provided with your medicine.
- Dosage is individualized. Take exactly as prescribed.
- Do not change the dose or stop taking, unless directed by your doctor. Continuous therapy and strict compliance is necessary to obtain the maximum benefit from therapy.
- Amprenavir may be taken with or without food, but avoid taking with high-fat meals, which decrease absorption into the body.
- Take indinavir without food, but with water 1 hour before or 2 hours after a meal, or take with other liquids (eg, skim milk, juice) or a light meal (eg, cereal and skim milk, toast with jelly).
- Take nelfinavir with a meal or light snack. The oral powder may be mixed with a small amount of water, milk, formula, soy formula, soy milk, or dietary supplement (eg, *Ensure*). Once mixed, consume the entire contents within 6 hours to obtain the full dose. Acidic food or juice (eg, orange juice, apple juice, apple sauce) are not recommended because of the bitter taste. Do not mix in the original container.
- Take ritonavir with food, if possible. The taste of the oral solution may be improved by mixing it with 8 oz of chocolate milk, *Ensure*, or *Advera* and taking it within 1 hour of mixing.
- Saquinavir should be taken with a meal or up to 2 hours after a meal.
- Take lopinavir/ritonavir with food.
- *Indinavir* — To reduce the risk of kidney stones, drink at least 48 oz (6 to 8 oz glasses) of liquids daily.
- If a dose is missed by less than 4 hours (2 hours for indinavir), take it as soon as possible and then return to the normal schedule. If a dose is missed by greater than 4 hours (2 hours for indinavir), wait and take the next dose at the regularly scheduled time. Do not double the next dose to catch up.
- If you are taking estrogen-based oral contraceptives (eg, *Ortho-Novum*), you must use alternate or additional forms of contraception during amprenavir, nelfinavir, ritonavir, or lopinavir/ritonavir therapy.
- Amprenavir capsules and oral solution are not interchangeable on a mg-per-mg basis.
- Remain under the care of your doctor while taking a protease inhibitor.
- Protease inhibitors are not a cure for HIV infection. You may continue to develop opportunistic infections and other complications associated with HIV.
- Protease inhibitors do not reduce the risk of transmitting HIV to others through sexual contact or blood contamination.
- HIV-infected mothers should not breastfeed because of the risk of transmitting the HIV infection.
- Do not share this medication with anyone else.
- May cause drowsiness or dizziness. Use caution while driving or performing other tasks requiring alertness, coordination, and physical dexterity.
- Inform your doctor if you are pregnant, plan on becoming pregnant, or become pregnant while taking this medicine.

Guidelines for Use (cont.):

- *Saquinavir* — *Invirase* and *Fortovase* are not bioequivalent and cannot be used interchangeably.
- Long-term effects of protease inhibitors are not known at this time.
- Lab tests will be required to monitor therapy. Be sure to keep appointments.
- Store as directed by the package labeling.

If you have any questions, consult your doctor, pharmacist, or health care provider.

	Generic Name *Brand Name Example*	Supplied As	Generic Available
Rx	**Tenofovir Disoproxil Fumarate**		
	Viread	**Tablets**: 300 mg (245 mg tenofovir disoproxil)	No

Type of Drug:

Antiretroviral; AIDS drug.

How the Drug Works:

Tenofovir inhibits the growth of the human immunodeficiency virus type 1 (HIV-1), the virus that causes acquired immunodeficiency syndrome (AIDS).

Uses:

Used in combination with other antiretroviral agents for the treatment of HIV-1 infection.

Precautions:

Do not use in the following situations: Allergy to tenofovir or any of its ingredients.

Use with caution in the following situations:

kidney disease
liver disease

Fat redistribution: Changes in body fat including central (stomach and chest) obesity, dorsocervical fat enlargement (buffalo hump), peripheral wasting (skinny arms and legs), and breast enlargement have occurred in patients receiving antiretrovial therapy. The cause of this and the long-term consequences of these changes are not known at this time.

Lactic acidosis: Lactic acidosis (excessive acid in blood) and severe hepatomegaly (enlarged liver) with steatosis (fat deposits in liver) have been associated with nucleoside analog therapy. If lactic acidosis or hepatoxicity are suspected or confirmed, therapy will be stopped.

Pregnancy: There are no adequate and well-controlled studies in pregnant women. Use only if clearly needed and the potential benefits to the mother outweigh the possible hazards to the fetus.

Breastfeeding: The Centers for Disease Control and Prevention (CDC) recommends that HIV-infected mothers not breastfeed their infants to avoid risking postnatal transmission of HIV. It is not known if tenofovir appears in breast milk. Consult your doctor before you begin breastfeeding.

Children: Safety and effectiveness have not been established.

Lab tests may be required to monitor therapy. Tests include kidney and liver function.

Drug Interactions:

Tell your doctor or pharmacist if you are taking or planning to take any over-the-counter or prescription medications or dietary supplements while taking tenofovir. Doses of one or both drugs may need to be modified or a different drug may need to be prescribed. The following drugs and drug classes interact with tenofovir:

acyclovir (*Zovirax*)
cidofovir (*Vistide*)
didanosine (*Videx*)
ganciclovir (*Cytovene*)
valciclovir (*Valtrex*)
valganciclovir (*Valcyte*)

Side Effects:

Every drug is capable of producing side effects. Many tenofovir users experience no, or minor, side effects. The frequency and severity of side effects depend on many factors including dose, duration of therapy, and individual susceptibility. Possible side effects include:

Digestive Tract: Nausea; diarrhea; vomiting; gas; stomach pain; appetite loss.

Other: Redistribution and accumulation of body fat; abnormal lab tests; headache; weakness.

Guidelines for Use:

- Read the patient information handout provided with this medicine.
- Dosage is individualized. Take exactly as prescribed.
- Do not change the dose or stop taking, unless directed by your doctor.
- Take with meals to increase effectiveness.
- If taking with didanosine (*Videx*), take tenofovir 2 hours before or 1 hour after didanosine.
- If a dose is missed, take it as soon as possible. If several hours have passed or it is nearing time for the next dose, do not double the dose to catch up, unless advised to do so by your doctor. If more than one dose is missed or it is necessary to establish a new dosage schedule, contact your doctor or pharmacist.
- Notify your health care provider immediately if you experience difficulty breathing, unexplained rapid breathing or shortness of breath, muscle pain, general body discomfort, unusual drowsiness, or swelling or pain in the upper right stomach area. These could be symptoms of a serious side effect such as lactic acidosis or an enlarged liver.
- Notify your health care provider if you experience intolerable gastrointestinal problems or changes in body fat distribution.
- Tenofovir is not a cure for HIV infection. You may continue to develop opportunistic infections and other complications associated with HIV.
- Tenofovir does not reduce the risk of transmitting HIV to others through sexual contact or blood contamination.
- To be effective, this medicine must be taken with other HIV medications.
- HIV-infected mothers should not breastfeed because of the risk of transmitting the HIV infection.
- Do not share your medicine with anyone else.
- The long-term effects of tenofovir are unknown at this time.
- Lab tests will be required to monitor therapy. Be sure to keep appointments.
- Store at room temperature (59° to 86°F).

If you have any questions, consult your doctor, pharmacist, or health care provider.

	Generic Name *Brand Name Examples*	Supplied As	Generic Available
Rx	**Abacavir**		
	Ziagen	**Tablets**: 300 mg	No
	Ziagen	**Solution, oral**: 20 mg/mL	No
Rx	**Didanosine**		
	Videx[1]	**Tablets, buffered, chewable/ dispersible**: 25 mg, 50 mg, 100 mg, 150 mg, 200 mg	No
	Videx EC	**Capsules, delayed-release (with enteric-coated beadlets)**: 125 mg, 200 mg, 250 mg, 400 mg	No
	Videx	**Powder for oral solution, buffered**: 100 mg, 167 mg, 250 mg/packet	No
	Videx[2]	**Powder for oral solution, pediatric**: 2 g, 4 g/bottle	No
Rx	**Lamivudine**		
	Epivir-HBV	**Tablets**: 100 mg	No
	Epivir	**Tablets**: 150 mg	No
	Epivir-HBV	**Solution, oral**: 5 mg/mL	No
	Epivir	**Solution, oral**: 10 mg/mL	No
Rx	**Stavudine**		
	Zerit	**Capsules**: 15 mg, 20 mg, 30 mg, 40 mg	No
	Zerit	**Powder for oral solution**: 1 mg/mL	No
Rx	**Zalcitabine**		
	Hivid	**Tablets**: 0.375 mg, 0.75 mg	No
Rx	**Zidovudine**[3]		
	Retrovir	**Tablets**: 300 mg	No
	Retrovir	**Capsules**: 100 mg	No
	Retrovir	**Syrup**: 50 mg/5 mL	No
Rx	**Lamivudine/Zidovudine**		
	Combivir	**Tablets**: 150 mg/300 mg	No
Rx	**Abacavir Sulfate/Lamivudine/Zidovudine**		
	Trizivir	**Tablets**: 300 mg/150 mg/ 300 mg	No

[1] Contains phenylalanine.
[2] Contains 1380 mg sodium/packet.
[3] Also available as an intravenous injection.

Type of Drug:

Antiretroviral agents for use in the treatment of human immunodeficiency virus type 1 (HIV-1) infection; nucleoside reverse transcriptase inhibitors (NRTIs).

How the Drug Works:

NRTIs inhibit the growth of HIV-1, the virus that causes acquired immunodeficiency syndrome (AIDS) and hepatitis B virus (HBV).

Uses:

Used in combination with other antiretroviral agents for the treatment of HIV-1 infection.

Epivir-HBV: For the treatment of chronic hepatitis B infection associated with evidence of hopatitis B viral replication and active liver inflammation.

Precautions:

Do not use in the following situations: Allergy to the NRTI or any of its ingredients.

Use with caution in the following situations:

bone marrow suppression (zidovudine only)
cardiomyopathy (zalcitabine only)
concurrent hepatitis B and HIV infection (*Epivir-HBV* only)
congestive heart failure (zalcitabine only)
kidney disease
liver disease, current or risk factors for
pancreatitis in children, history or risk of
peripheral neuropathy, history or risk of
prolonged nucleoside (NRTI) exposure

Epivir/Epivir-HBV interchangeability: Epivir tablets and oral solution contain a higher dose of the same active ingredient (lamivudine) than *Epivir-HBV* tablets and solution. Therefore, *Epivir* and *Epivir-HBV* are not interchangeable.

Fatal hypersensitivity reactions: Fatal hypersensitivity (allergic) reactions have been associated with NRTI therapy. NRTIs must be stopped immediately in patients who develop signs or symptoms of hypersensitivity (eg, fever; rash; fatigue; dizziness; fainting; gastrointestinal symptoms such as nausea, vomiting, diarrhea, stomach pain; respiratory symptoms such as sore throat, shortness of breath, cough). Do not restart taking the NRTI because a more severe reaction could occur.

Lactic acidosis: Lactic acidosis (acid in the blood) and severe hepatomegaly (liver enlargement) with steatosis (fatty changes in the liver) have been associated with NRTI therapy. Symptoms include feeling very weak or tired, unusual or unexpected stomach discomfort, unexplained shortness of breath or rapid breathing, feeling cold, dizzy, or lightheaded, and slow or irregular heartbeat. If lactic acidosis or hepatoxicity are suspected or confirmed, NRTI therapy should be stopped.

Pancreatitis: Didanosine, lamivudine, stavudine, and zalcitabine have been associated with pancreatitis (inflammation of pancreas gland). Stop taking and notify your doctor immediately if you experience nausea, vomiting, or stomach pain or tenderness.

Peripheral neuropathy: Didanosine, lamivudine, stavudine, and zalcitabine have been associated with peripheral neuropathy (numbness, tingling, burning, or pain in the hands of feet). Stop using and notify your doctor immediately if symptoms develop.

Phenylketonuria: Some of these products contain phenylalanine. Consult your doctor or pharmacist.

Pregnancy: There are no adequate and well-controlled studies in pregnant women. Use only if clearly needed and the potential benefits to the mother outweigh the possible hazards to the fetus.

Breastfeeding: The Centers for Disease Control and Prevention (CDC) recommends that HIV-infected mothers not breastfeed their infants to avoid risking postnatal transmission of HIV. It is not known if NRTIs appear in breast milk. Consult your doctor before you begin breastfeeding.

Children: Safety and effectiveness of abacavir in patients 3 months to 13 years of age have been established. Didanosine delayed-release capsules have not been studied in children. Safety of *Epivir-HBV* has not been established in children younger than 2 years of age. Safety of lamivudine and zidovudine has been established in patients 3 months of age and older. Didanosine and stavudine use in children is supported by adequate and well-controlled studies. Safety of zalcitabine has not been established in children younger than 13 years of age. Abacavir/lamivudine/zidovudine is not intended for pediatric use.

Elderly: Use with caution in elderly patients. Dosage adjustments may be necessary.

Lab tests may be required to monitor therapy. Tests include liver, kidney, and pancreas function tests, blood counts, and eye exams.

Drug Interactions:

Tell your doctor or pharmacist if you are taking or planning to take any over-the-counter or prescription medications while taking an NRTI. Doses of one or both drugs may need to be modified or a different drug may need to be prescribed. The following drugs and drug classes interact with NRTIs:

- allopurinol (eg, *Zyloprim*) (didanosine only)
- antacids (zalcitabine only)
- atovaquone (*Mepron*) (zidovudine only)
- azole antifungals (eg, ketoconazole) (didanosine only)
- cimetidine (eg, *Tagamet*) (zalcitabine only)
- doxorubicin (eg, *Adriamycin RDF*) (zidovudine only)
- ethanol (abacavir only)
- ganciclovir (*Cytovene*) (zidovudine only)
- indinavir (*Crixivan*) (didanosine only)
- methadone (eg, *Dolophine*) (abacavir, zidovudine only)
- phenytoin (eg, *Dilantin*) (zidovudine only)
- probenecid (zalcitabine, zidovudine only)
- quinolones (eg, ciprofloxacin) (didanosine only)

stavudine (*Zerit*) (zidovudine only)
zalcitabine (*Hivid*) (lamivudine only)
zidovudine (*Retrovir*) (stavudine only)

Side Effects:

Every drug is capable of producing side effects. Many NRTI users experience no, or minor, side effects. The frequency and severity of side effects depend on many factors including dose, duration of therapy, and individual susceptibility. Possible side effects include:

Nervous System: Dizziness; headache; depression; sleeplessness and other sleep disorders; convulsions.

Digestive Tract: Nausea; vomiting; diarrhea; appetite loss; stomach pain or cramps; indigestion; constipation.

Skin: Rash; itching; hives.

Respiratory System: Difficulty breathing; cough; nasal signs and symptoms (eg, discharge, congestion); wheezing.

Other: Numbness, tingling, or pain in the hands or feet; retinal changes; optic neuritis; abnormal lab tests; pancreatitis; liver damage; severe allergic reactions (eg, rash, low blood pressure, difficulty breathing); lactic acidosis; fever; muscle pain or weakness; bone pain; joint pain or swelling; sweating; chills; general body discomfort; fatigue; ear, nose, or throat infection; ear pain, discharge, redness, or swelling; taste sensation changes; sore throat; sores in mouth or esophagus (food pipe); redistribution or accumulation of body fat.

Guidelines for Use:

- Review the Patient Package Insert each time you fill your prescription. There may be new information added since your last refill.
- Dosage is individualized. Take exactly as prescribed.
- Do not change the dose or stop taking unless directed by your doctor. Strict compliance is crucial to prevent the virus from becoming resistant to the medicine.
- Take didanosine and zalcitabine on an empty stomach, at least 30 minutes before or 2 hours after a meal. All other NRTIs may be taken with or without food.
- *Didanosine chewable/buffered tablets* — Do not swallow whole. Take at least 2, but no more than 4 tablets per dose. Thoroughly chew or disperse in 2 or more tablespoons of water prior to taking. Stir until a uniform dispersion forms and drink the entire mixture immediately. If additional flavoring is desired, the mixture may be diluted with 2 tablespoons of clear apple juice. Do not use any other type of juice. Stir just before taking. The dispersion may be stored at room temperature for up to 1 hour.
- *Didanosine delayed-release capsules* — Do not open, crush, or chew capsules. Swallow whole.

Guidelines for Use (cont.):

- *Didanosine buffered powder for oral solution* — Open packet and pour into approximately 4 ounces of water. Do not mix with fruit juice or other acid-containing liquid. Stir until the powder dissolves completely (approximately 2 to 3 minutes). Drink entire solution right away.
- *Didanosine pediatric oral solution* — Shake well before each use. Throw away any unused solution after 30 days.
- If a dose is missed, take it as soon as possible. If several hours have passed or it is nearing time for the next dose, do not double the dose to catch up, unless advised by your doctor. If more than one dose is missed or it is necessary to establish a new dosage schedule, contact your doctor or pharmacist.
- Abacavir tablets and oral solution can be used interchangeably.
- Zidovudine tablets, capsules, and syrup can be used interchangeably.
- Stop using and notify your doctor immediately if you experience fever, rash, fatigue, dizziness, fainting, gastrointestinal symptoms (eg, nausea, vomiting, diarrhea, stomach pain), respiratory symptoms (eg, sore throat, shortness of breath, unexplained rapid breathing, cough), slow or irregular heartbeat, or changes in vision (eg, blurring, color changes). These could be symptoms of a potentially fatal allergic reaction or toxic reaction.
- Women of childbearing age should use effective contraception while taking zalcitabine.
- NRTIs are not cures for HIV infection. You may continue to develop opportunistic infections and other complications associated with HIV.
- NRTIs do not reduce the risk of transmitting HIV to others through sexual contact or blood contamination.
- NRTIs must be used in combination with other HIV drugs to prevent the virus from becoming resistant.
- *Epivir-HBV* is not a cure for hepatitis B infection. It does not reduce the risk of transmitting hepatitis B to others through sexual contact or blood transfusions.
- Do not share this medicine with anyone else.
- The long-term effects of NRTIs are unknown at this time.
- Lab tests may be required to monitor therapy. Be sure to keep appointments.
- Store as directed by the package labeling.

If you have any questions, consult your doctor, pharmacist, or health care provider.

	Generic Name *Brand Name Examples*	Supplied As	Generic Available
Rx	**Delavirdine Mesylate**		
	Rescriptor	**Tablets**: 100 mg, 200 mg	No
Rx	**Efavirenz**		
	Sustiva	**Capsules**: 50 mg, 100 mg, 200 mg	No
	Sustiva	**Tablets**: 600 mg	No
Rx	**Nevirapine**		
	Viramune	**Tablets**: 200 mg	No
	Viramune	**Suspension, oral**: 50 mg (as nevirapine hemihydrate)/5 mL	No

Type of Drug:

Antiretrovirals; NNRTIs; AIDS drugs.

How the Drug Works:

These non-nucleoside reverse transcriptase inhibitors (NNRTIs) inhibit the growth of the human immunodeficiency virus type 1 (HIV-1), the virus that causes acquired immunodeficiency syndrome (AIDS).

Uses:

For use in combination with other appropriate antiretroviral agents, including nucleoside analogs (eg, zidovudine) to treat HIV-1-infected adults when therapy is warranted (eg, deterioration of health).

Precautions:

Do not use in the following situations:

- allergy to the NNRTI or any of its ingredients
- alprazolam therapy, concurrent
- ergot-derivative therapy, concurrent
- midazolam therapy, concurrent
- St. John's wort use, concurrent
- triazolam therapy, concurrent

Use with caution in the following situations:

- kidney disease
- liver disease
- mental illness, history of (efavirenz only)
- rash
- substance abuse, history of (efavirenz only)

Pregnancy: There are no adequate and well-controlled studies in pregnant women. Use only if clearly needed and the potential benefits to the mother outweigh the possible hazards to the fetus.

Breastfeeding: The Centers for Disease Control and Prevention (CDC) recommends that HIV-infected mothers not breastfeed their infants to avoid risking postnatal transmission of HIV. NNRTIs may appear in breast milk. Consult your doctor before you begin breastfeeding.

Children: Safety and effectiveness of delavirdine mesylate in children younger than 16 years of age have not been established. Safety and effectiveness of efavirenz in children younger 3 years of age or children who weigh less than 29 pounds have not been established. Nevirapine has been used in infants as young as 2 months of age.

Elderly: Use with caution. Safety and effectiveness of delavirdine mesylate and efavirenz have not been extensively studied in patients older than 65 years of age. Safety and effectiveness of nevirapine have not been extensively studied in patients older than 55 years of age.

Lab tests will be required to monitor therapy. Tests include kidney and liver function, blood counts, and cholesterol and triglyceride levels.

Drug Interactions:

Tell your doctor or pharmacist if you are taking or planning to take any over-the-counter or prescription medications or dietary supplements while taking an NNRTI. Doses of one or both drugs may need to be modified or a different drug may need to be prescribed. The following drugs and drug classes interact with NNRTIs:

- antacids (eg, *Maalox*) (delavirdine only)
- antiarrythmics (eg, amiodarone)
- benzodiazepines (eg, triazolam)
- calcium channel blockers (eg, nifedipine)
- carbamazepine (eg, *Tegretol*)
- clarithromycin (*Biaxin*)
- corticosteroids (eg, dexamethasone) (delavirdine only)
- dapsone (delavirdine only)
- ergot derivatives (eg, ergotamine)
- fluoxetine (eg, *Prozac*) (delavirdine only)
- H_2 receptor antagonists (eg, cimetidine) (delavirdine only)
- HMG-CoA reductase inhibitors (eg, lovastatin)
- hormonal contraceptives (eg, ethinyl estradiol) (efavirenz, nevirapine only)
- ketoconazole (eg, *Nizoral*) (delavirdine only)
- methadone (eg, *Dolophine*)
- nucleoside reverse transcriptase inhibitors (eg, didanosine)
- phenobarbital (eg, *Solfoton*)
- phenytoin (eg, dilantin) (efavirenz, delavirdine only)
- protease inhibitors (eg, ritonavir)
- proton pump inhibitors (eg, omeprazole)
- quinidine (eg, *Quinora*)
- rifamycins (eg, rifabutin)
- sildenafil (*Viagra*)
- St. John's wort
- warfarin (eg, *Coumadin*)

Side Effects:

Every drug is capable of producing side effects. Many NNRTI users experience no, or minor, side effects. The frequency and severity of side effects depend on many factors including dose, duration of therapy, and individual susceptibility. Possible side effects include:

Nervous System: Headache; dizziness; sleeplessness; impaired concentration; drowsiness; abnormal dreams; hallucinations; euphoria; confusion; agitation; memory loss; stupor; abnormal thinking; depersonalization; depression; anxiety; nervousness; diminished sensitivity to stimulation.

Digestive Tract: Nausea; diarrhea; stomach pain; vomiting; indigestion; gas; appetite loss.

Other: Rash; itching; fever; fatigue; numbness or tingling in the arms or legs; abnormal skin sensations; weakness; muscle pain; abnormal lab tests; hepatitis; increased sweating; flu-like symptoms; bronchitis; cough; sore throat; sinus inflammation; yellowing of skin or eyes; joint pain.

Guidelines for Use:

- Read the patient information handout provided with your medication.
- Dosage is individualized. Take exactly as prescribed.
- Do not change the dose or stop taking, unless directed by your doctor.
- Take efavirenz on an empty stomach, preferably at bedtime, to reduce side effects.
- Take delavirdine or nevirapine without regard to food. Take delavirdine and antacids at least 1 hour apart.
- Take delavirdine tablets whole. Delavirdine 100 mg tablets may be dispersed in water prior to taking. To disperse, add four 100 mg tablets to at least 3 ounces of water, allow to stand for a few minutes and then stir gently. Take immediately after mixing. Rinse glass with water and swallow rinse to ensure entire dose is taken.
- Gently shake nevirapine suspension before taking. Use oral dosage syringe or dosing cup to measure the correct dose. Rinse the dosing cup with water and swallow the rinse to ensure entire dose is taken.
- If a dose is missed, take it as soon as possible. If several hours have passed or it is nearing time for the next dose, do not double the dose to catch up, unless advised to do so by your doctor. If more than one dose is missed or it is necessary to establish a new dosage schedule, contact your doctor or pharmacist.
- Severe and life-threatening skin reactions have occurred in patients using NNRTIs. Notify your doctor if you experience severe rash, rash with fever, blistering, peeling, scaling, mouth sores, eye infection, muscle or joint aches, or general body discomfort.
- May cause dizziness, drowsiness, or impaired concentration. Use caution while driving or performing other tasks that require alertness, coordination, and physical dexterity.
- *Efavirenz* — Inform your doctor immediately if you experience serious psychiatric symptoms (eg, depression, behavior or personality changes).

Guidelines for Use (cont.):

- *Nevirapine* — Inform your doctor if you experience persistent fatigue, appetite loss, nausea, right upper stomach pain, tenderness, or swelling, or if you notice yellowing of the skin or eyes.
- NNRTIs are not cures for HIV infection. You may continue to develop opportunistic infections and other complications associated with HIV.
- NNRTIs do not reduce the risk of transmitting HIV to others through sexual contact or blood contamination.
- Women of childbearing potential should not become pregnant while taking an NNRTI. Use nonestrogen-based contraceptives (eg, condoms) to prevent pregnancy.
- HIV-infected mothers should not breastfeed because of the risk of transmitting the HIV infection.
- Do not share your medicine with anyone else.
- To be effective, this medicine must be taken with other HIV medications.
- The duration of effectiveness of these agents is variable and unpredictable.
- Lab tests will be required to monitor therapy. Be sure to keep appointments.
- Store at room temperature in a tightly closed container. Protect from high humidity.

If you have any questions, consult your doctor, pharmacist, or health care provider.

	Generic Name *Brand Name Example*	Supplied As	Generic Available
Rx	**Albendazole**		
	Albenza	**Tablets**: 200 mg	No

Type of Drug:
Drug for tapeworm infections.

How the Drug Works:
Albendazole kills parasites (tapeworms) by interfering with their metabolism.

Uses:
To treat parenchymal neurocysticercosis (cysts in the brain tissue) caused by larval forms of the pork tapeworm, *Taenia solium*.

To treat cystic hydatid disease of the liver, lung, and peritoneum (lining of abdominal cavity) caused by the larval form of the dog tapeworm, *Echinococcus granulosus*.

Surgery is considered the treatment of choice for hydatid disease if medically feasible. When administering albendazole in the pre- or postsurgical setting, optimal killing of cyst contents is achieved when 3 courses of therapy have been given.

Precautions:
Do not use in the following situations: Allergy to albendazole, benzimidazoles (eg, mebendazole), or any of their ingredients.

Use with caution in the following situations: Liver disease.

Pregnancy: There are no adequate and well-controlled studies in pregnant women. Use in pregnant women only when no alternative therapy is available. If a patient becomes pregnant during therapy, discontinue albendazole immediately. Patients should not become pregnant for at least 1 month after stopping albendazole therapy.

Breastfeeding: It is not known if albendazole appears in breast milk. Consult your doctor before you begin breastfeeding.

Children: Safety and effectiveness in children younger than 6 years of age have not been established. Albendazole has been used safely and effectively in a small number of infants and children.

Lab tests will be required periodically during treatment. Tests may include white blood cell counts, liver function tests, and theophylline blood levels.

Drug Interactions:

Tell your doctor or pharmacist if you are taking or planning to take any over-the-counter or prescription medications or dietary supplements with albendazole. Doses of one or both drugs may need to be modified or a different drug may need to be prescribed. The following drugs or drug classes interact with albendazole:

cimetidine (eg, *Tagamet*)
dexamethasone (eg, *Decadron*)
praziquantel (*Biltricide*)

Side Effects:

Every drug is capable of producing side effects. Many albendazole users experience no, or minor, side effects. The frequency and severity of side effects depend on many factors including dose, duration of therapy, and individual susceptibility. Possible side effects include:

Nervous System: Headache; dizziness; vertigo (feeling of whirling motion).

Digestive Tract: Stomach pain; nausea; vomiting.

Other: Fever; hair loss (temporary); decreased white blood cell count; abnormal liver function tests; meningeal signs (eg, headache, stiff neck).

Guidelines for Use:

- Dosage is individualized. Take exactly as prescribed.
- Do not change the dose or stop taking unless directed by your doctor.
- Usual dose is twice daily. Take with food to increase absorption and effectiveness.
- If a dose is missed, take it as soon as possible. If several hours have passed or it is nearing time for the next dose, do not double the dose to catch up, unless advised to do so by your doctor. If more than one dose is missed or it is necessary to establish a new dosage schedule, contact your doctor or pharmacist.
- Inform your doctor if you are pregnant, become pregnant, plan on becoming pregnant, or are breastfeeding before beginning therapy. Albendazole may cause fetal harm. Begin treatment only after a negative pregnancy test has been conducted in women of child-bearing age. Patients should not become pregnant for at least 1 month following cessation of albendazole.
- Women of childbearing age should use effective contraception during therapy.
- May cause dizziness. Use caution while driving or performing other tasks requiring alertness, coordination, or physical dexterity.
- Patients being treated for neurocysticercosis may require oral or injectable steroid and anticonvulsant therapy.
- Lab tests will be required to monitor therapy. Blood counts and liver function tests will be performed at the start of each 28-day treatment cycle and every 2 weeks during each 28-day cycle. Be sure to keep appointments.
- Store at a controlled room temperature (68° to 77°F).

If you have any questions, consult your doctor, pharmacist, or health care provider.

	Generic Name *Brand Name Examples*	Supplied As	Generic Available
Rx	**Mebendazole**		
	Vermox	**Tablets, chewable:** 100 mg	Yes

Type of Drug:

Drug for intestinal worms.

How the Drug Works:

Mebendazole kills parasitic worms by blocking glucose (sugar uptake), thus depleting glycogen stored in the parasite. Without glycogen as an energy source, the parasite cannot reproduce or survive.

Uses:

To treat parasitic infections such as pinworm (Enterobiasis), common roundworm (Ascariasis), common hookworm (*Ancyclostoma duodenale*), American hookworm (*Necator americanus*) and whipworm (Trichuriasis).

Effectiveness depends on pre-existing diarrhea, gastrointestinal transit time, degree of infection and type of parasite.

Precautions:

Do not use in the following situations: Allergy to this medicine.

Pregnancy: Adequate studies have not been done in pregnant women, or animal studies may have shown a risk to the fetus. This drug is not recommended for use in pregnant women, especially during the first trimester. Use only if clearly needed and potential benefits outweigh the possible hazards to the fetus.

Breastfeeding: It is not known if mebendazole appears in breast milk. Contact your doctor before beginning breastfeeding.

Children: Safety and effectiveness is not established for children under 2 years of age.

Drug Interactions:

Tell your doctor or pharmacist if you are taking or if you are planning to take any over-the-counter or prescription medications. Doses of one or both drugs may need to be modified or a different drug may need to be prescribed. The following drugs and drug classes may interact with this medicine.

carbamazepine (eg, *Tegretol*)
cimetidine (eg, *Tagamet*)
hydantoins (eg, phenytoin)

Side Effects:

Every drug is capable of producing side effects. Many patients experience no, or minor, side effects. The frequency and severity of side effects depend on many factors including dose, duration of therapy and individual susceptibility. Possible side effects include stomach pain and diarrhea.

Guidelines for Use:

- Use exactly as prescribed. Doses vary according to type of parasite.
- The tablets may be chewed, swallowed or crushed and mixed with food.
- Parasite death may be slow. Removal from digestive tract may take up to 3 days after treatment. Effectiveness depends of factors such as degree of infection or resistance of parasites to treatment, presence of diarrhea and how quickly things pass through the digestive system.
- Laxative therapy and fasting are not necessary.
- *Adults and children* — One tablet morning and evening for 3 consecutive days when treating hookworm, roundworm, and whipworm. The pinworm dose is a single table given once.
- If a dose is missed, take it as soon as possible. If several hours have passed or if it is nearing time for the next dose, do not double the dose in order to "catch up" (unless advised to do so by your doctor). If more than one dose is missed or it is necessary to establish a new dosage schedule, contact your doctor or pharmacist.
- If not cured in 3 weeks, a second treatment is recommended.
- Inform your doctor if you are pregnant, become pregnant, are planning to become pregnant, or if you are breastfeeding.
- Pinworm infections are easily spread to others. If one family member has a pinworm infection, treat all family members in close contact with the patient. This decreases the chance of spreading the infection.
- Strict hygiene is essential to prevent reinfection. Disinfect toilets daily. Change and wash underwear, bed linens, towels and nightclothes daily. Wash hands before eating.
- Store at controlled room temperature (59° to 86°F).

If you have any questions, consult your doctor, pharmacist, or health care provider.

Generic Name / *Brand Name Examples*	How Supplied	Generic Available
otc **Pyrantel**		
Pin-Rid, Reese's Pinworm	**Capsules, soft gel:** 180 mg	No
Antiminth	**Oral Suspension:** 50 mg/mL	No
Pin-Rid, Pin-X, Reese's Pinworm	**Liquid:** 50 mg/mL	No

Type of Drug:

Drug for intestinal worms.

How the Drug Works:

Pyrantel paralyzes the nervous system of the intestinal parasites (worms). Muscles of the worm do not function properly and the worms separate from the intestine. The worms are then eliminated from the body during bowel movements.

Uses:

To treat pinworm infection (enterobiasis).

Precautions:

Do not use in the following situations:

allergy to this medicine
liver disease
pregnancy

Pregnancy: Do not use during pregnancy unless otherwise directed by your doctor.

Children: Safety and effectiveness is not established for children under 2 years of age.

Drug Interactions:

Tell your doctor or pharmacist if you are taking or are planning to take any over-the-counter or prescription medications while taking this medicine. Doses of one or both drugs may need to be modified or a different drug may need to be prescribed. Theophylline (eg, *Theo-Dur*) may interact with this medicine.

Side Effects:

Every drug is capable of producing side effects. Many patients experience no, or minor, side effects. The frequency and severity of side effects depend on many factors including dose, duration of therapy and individual susceptibility. Possible side effects include:

Digestive Tract: Nausea; vomiting; diarrhea; stomach ache and cramps; appetite loss.

Nervous System: Headache; dizziness; drowsiness; sleeplessness.

Other: Rash; fever.

Guidelines for Use:

- Use exactly as prescribed. Follow the guidelines in the patient information available with this medicine.
- A single dose is required. The dose is based on body weight.
- May be taken with food, milk, juice or on an empty stomach anytime during the day. Be certain to take the entire dose.
- Using a laxative after taking the drug to facilitate removal of the parasites is not necessary.
- Pinworm infections are easily spread to others. If one family member has a pinworm infection, treat all family member in close contact with the patient. This deceases the chance of spreading the infection.
- Strict hygiene is essential to prevent reinfection. Disinfect toilet seats and bath tubs daily. Change and wash underwear, bed linens, towels and nightclothes at the time of treatment.
- Children should take morning showers to remove any pinworm eggs deposited at night.
- Trim an infected child's nails and wash hands frequently, especially before meals and after using the toilet.
- Store at controlled room temperature (59° to 86°F).

If you have any questions, consult your doctor, pharmacist, or health care provider.

Generic Name *Brand Name Examples*	Supplied As	Generic Available
Rx **Thiabendazole**		
Mintezol	**Tablets, chewable:** 500 mg	No
Mintezol	**Oral Suspension:** 500 mg/tsp	No

Type of Drug:

Drug for intestinal worms.

How the Drug Works:

The exact mechanism of thiabendazole is not known, but it kills intestinal parasites, suppresses egg or larvae production and may inhibit the subsequent development of those eggs or larvae that are passed in the stools.

Uses:

To treat parasitic worms including pinworm (enterobiasis), threadworm (strongyloidiasis), large roundworm (ascariasis), hookworm (uncinariasis), whipworm (trichuriasis), creeping eruption (cutaneous larva migrans) and visceral larva migrans.

To alleviate symptoms of trichinosis during the invasion phase.

Precautions:

Do not use in the following situations: Allergy to this medicine.

Use with caution in the following situations:

anemia
dehydration (fluid loss)
kidney disease
liver disease
malnutrition

Pregnancy: Adequate studies have not been done in pregnant women. Use only if clearly needed and potential benefits outweigh the possible hazards to the fetus.

Breastfeeding: It is not known if thiabendazole appears in breast milk. Contact your doctor before you begin breastfeeding.

Children: Safety and effectiveness are not established in children weighing less than 30 pounds.

Lab tests may be required. Lab tests may include liver function tests.

Drug Interactions:

Xanthines (eg, theophylline) interact with this medicine.

Side Effects:

Every drug can produce side effects. The frequency or severity of side effects depend on dose, duration of therapy and individual susceptibility. Side effects may include:

Digestive Tract: Nausea; vomiting; diarrhea; stomach pain; appetite loss.

Nervous System: Dizziness; tiredness; drowsiness; giddiness; headache; numbness; irritability; convulsions; collapse; psychic disturbances.

Skin: Itching; rectal rash; hives; redness; facial flushing; yellowing of skin or eyes.

Other: Blood or crystals in urine; bedwetting; asparagus-like odor of urine; fever; chills; eye irritation; blurred vision; vision changes (objects appearing yellow); dry mouth and eyes; ringing in the ears; difficulty breathing; low blood pressure; high blood sugar levels.

Guidelines for Use:

- Use exactly as prescribed.
- May cause stomach upset; take with food.
- Usual dose is twice daily. Dosage is determined by the patient's weight.
- *Tablets* — Chew thoroughly before swallowing.
- *Oral Suspension* — Shake well before use.
- Dietary restrictions or cleansing enemas are not needed.
- Duration of therapy varies from 2 or more days depending upon the condition being treated.
- If a dose is missed, take it as soon as possible. If several hours have passed or if it is nearing time for the next dose, do not double the dose in order to "catch up" (unless advised to do so by your doctor). If more than one dose is missed or it is necessary to establish a new dosage schedule, contact your doctor or pharmacist.
- Strict hygiene is essential to prevent reinfection. Disinfect toilets daily. Change and wash underwear, bed linens, towels and nightclothes daily.
- Pinworm infections are easily spread to others. If one family member has a pinworm infection, treat all family members in close contact with the patient. This decreases the chance of spreading the infection.
- *Pinworm infections* — Repeat therapy in 7 days to prevent reinfection.
- May produce drowsiness or dizziness. Use caution when driving or performing other tasks requiring alertness, coordination or physical dexterity.
- Store tablets and suspension in well closed containers at room temperature.

If you have any questions, consult your doctor, pharmacist, or health care provider.

	Generic Name *Brand Name Examples*	Supplied As	Generic Available
	Ivermectin		
Rx	*Stromectol*	**Tablets:** 6 mg	No

Type of Drug:
Anthelmintic (antiparasitic) agent.

How the Drug Works:
Ivermectin causes paralysis of the nerve and muscle cells of certain parasitic worms.

Uses:
To treat strongyloidiasis of the intestinal tract and to treat onchocerciasis.

Precautions:
Do not use in the following situations: allergy to drug or any ingredients

Use with caution in the following situations: immunocompromised hosts

Pregnancy: Adequate studies have not been done in pregnant women; animal studies may have shown a risk to the fetus. Use only if clearly needed and potential benefits outweigh the possible hazards to the fetus.

Breastfeeding: Ivermectin appears in breast milk. Consult your doctor before breastfeeding.

Children: Safety and effectiveness in children weighing less than 33 lbs is not established.

Drug Interactions:
Tell your doctor or pharmacist if you are taking or planning to take any over-the-counter or prescription medications while taking this medicine. Doses of one or both drugs may need to be modified or a different drug may need to be prescribed.

Side Effects:
Every drug is capable of producing side effects. Many patients experience no, or minor, side effects. The frequency and severity of side effects depend on many factors including dose, duration of therapy and individual susceptibility. Side effects may include: Fast heartbeat; itching; rash; skin disorder; abnormal sensation in eyes; swelling of eyelids; eye inflammation/redness; enlarged and tender lymph nodes; joint pain and swelling; fever; facial swelling; swelling of arms and legs; headache; muscle pain; diarrhea; nausea; dizziness; dizziness or lightheadedness when rising quickly from a sitting or lying position.

Guidelines for Use:

- Take as a single oral dose with a full glass of water.
- The dose is based on body weight. Take the prescribed number of tablets.
- *Strongyloidiasis* — Repeated stool examinations are recommended.
- *Onchocerciasis* — Treatment with ivermectin does not kill adult onchocerca parasites and repeated follow-up and retreatment is usually required.
- Lab tests will be required to monitor treatment. Be sure to keep appointments.
- Store at temperatures below 86°F.

If you have any questions, consult your doctor, pharmacist, or health care provider.

	Generic Name *Brand Name Examples*	Supplied As	Generic Available
Rx	**Methenamine Hippurate**		
	Hiprex,[1] *Urex*	**Tablets:** 1 g	No
Rx	**Methenamine Mandelate**		
	Mandelamine	**Tablets, film coated:** 0.5 g, 1 g	Yes

[1] Contains the dye tartrazine.

Type of Drug:

Urinary anti-infective drugs.

How the Drug Works:

Methenamine is broken down in acid urine to produce ammonia and formaldehyde. Formaldehyde kills certain bacteria in the urine. The salt forms of methenamine (mandelate and hippurate) are acid salts and help keep the urine acidic. An acid urine increases the effectiveness of methenamine.

Uses:

For long-term therapy to suppress or eliminate bacteria in the urine that cause certain urinary tract infections after the use of other antimicrobial drugs.

Precautions:

Do not use in the following situations:

allergy to the drug
concurrent use of sulfonamides
dehydration, severe (fluid loss)
kidney disease
liver disease

Use with caution in the following situations:

acid urine cannot be maintained
elderly, debilitated or people susceptible to lipid pneumonia

Active infection: Methenamine does not treat urinary tract infections; it only prevents recurrent infections. Use only after a urinary tract infection has been treated with other antibiotics.

Pregnancy: Adequate studies have not been done in pregnant women. Use only if clearly needed and potential benefits outweigh the possible hazards to the fetus.

Breastfeeding: Methenamine appears in breast milk. Consult your doctor before you begin breastfeeding.

Lab tests are required during therapy. Be sure to keep appointments. Tests will include liver function studies and repeated urine cultures.

Tartrazine: Some of these products may contain the dye tartrazine (FD & C Yellow No. 5) which can cause allergic reactions in certain individuals. Check package label when available or consult your doctor or pharmacist.

Drug Interactions:

Tell your doctor or pharmacist if you are taking or if you are planning to take any over-the-counter or prescription medications with methenamine. Doses of one or both drugs may need to be modified or a different drug may need to be prescribed. The following drugs and drug classes interact with methenamine:

- potassium citrate (eg, *Urocit-K*)
- sodium acetate
- sodium bicarbonate
- sodium citrate
- sodium lactate
- sulfonamides (eg, sulfamethizole)
- tromethamine (eg, *Tham*)

Side Effects:

Every drug is capable of producing side effects. Many methenamine users experience no, or minor, side effects. The frequency and severity of side effects depend on many factors including dose, duration of therapy and individual susceptibility. Possible side effects include:

Urinary and Reproductive Tract: Urination problems; blood or protein in urine.

Digestive Tract: Nausea; upset stomach; vomiting; stomach cramps.

Skin: Rash; itching.

Guidelines for Use:

- Take as directed by your doctor. The daily dose varies depending on individual needs. Do not adjust the dose without consulting your pharmacist or doctor.
- Take the full course of therapy to ensure best results. Do not stop the drug without consulting your doctor.
- It may be necessary to attempt to acidify the urine in order to get the best clinical response. Ascorbic acid (vitamin C) at doses of 2 g/day or administration of 8 to 12 g of ammonium chloride per day may acidify the urine. Intake of cranberries, plums, prunes, or cranberry juice may help slightly in producing an acid urine.
- Avoid heavy intake of medications such as bicarbonate and acetazolamide. They may change the urine from acid to alkaline.
- Large doses (up to 8 g/day for 3 to 4 weeks) may cause bladder irritation, painful and frequent urination, and protein or blood in the urine.
- Notify your doctor if rash, urination problems or severe stomach upset occurs.
- Lab tests will be required and may include urine cultures and liver enzymes. Keep appointments.
- Store at controlled room temperature (59° to 86°F). Protect from light.

If you have any questions, consult your doctor, pharmacist, or health care provider.

	Generic Name *Brand Name Examples*	Supplied As	Generic Available
Rx	**Fosfomycin Tromethamine**		
	Monurol	**Single-dose sachet:** 3 g	No

Type of Drug:

Urinary tract anti-infective.

How the Drug Works:

Fosfomycin inhibits bacterial cell wall reproduction and reduces bacteria from adhering to cells lining the urinary tract.

Uses:

To treat uncomplicated urinary tract infections in women caused by susceptible bacteria.

Precautions:

Do not use in the following situations:
allergy to the drug

Use with caution in the following situations:
acute cystitis
kidney disease

Pregnancy: Fosfomycin does cross the placenta. Studies in pregnant women or in animals have been judged not to show a risk to the fetus. However, no drug should be used during pregnancy unless clearly needed.

Breastfeeding: It is not known if fosfomycin tromethamine appears in breast milk. Consult your doctor before you begin breastfeeding.

Children: Safety and effectiveness in children less than 12 years of age have not been established.

Drug Interactions:

Tell your doctor or pharmacist if you are taking or planning to take any over-the-counter or prescription medications while taking this medicine. Doses of one or both drugs may need to be modified or a different drug may need to be prescribed. Metoclopramide (eg, *Reglan*) may interact with this medicine.

Side Effects:

Every drug is capable of producing side effects. Many patients experience no, or minor, side effects. The frequency and severity of side effects depend on many factors including dose, duration of therapy and individual susceptibility. Possible side effects include: Diarrhea; nausea; indigestion; sore throat; abdominal pain; dizziness; nasal congestion; runny nose; inflammation of the vagina; painful menstruation; rash; headache; weakness; back pain; pain.

Guidelines for Use:

- May be taken with or without food.
- Recommended dosage is 1 packet.
- The packet should not be taken in its dry form. Mix with 3 to 4 oz of cold water before ingesting. (Do not use hot water.) Take immediately after dissolving in water.
- If symptoms do not improve 2 to 3 days after taking fosfomycin tromethamine, contact the healthcare provider.
- Do not use more than one single dose to treat a single occurrence of minor urinary tract infection. Repeated daily doses did not improve clinical success, but did increase the incidence of side effects.
- Store at controlled room temperature (59° to 86°F).

If you have any questions, consult your doctor, pharmacist, or health care provider.

	Generic Name *Brand Name Examples*	Supplied As	Generic Available
Rx	**Nalidixic Acid**		
	NegGram	**Caplets:** 250 mg, 500 mg, 1 g	No
		Suspension: 250 mg/5 mL	No

Type of Drug:

Urinary tract anti-infection drug.

How the Drug Works:

Nalidixic acid interferes with DNA formation in certain bacteria.

Uses:

To treat urinary tract infections caused by susceptible bacteria.

Precautions:

Do not use in the following situations:

allergy to nalidixic acid
seizures, history of

Use with caution in the following situations:

cerebral arteriosclerosis (hardening of the arteries)
epilepsy
glucose-6-phosphate dehydrogenase (G-6-PD) deficiency
insufficient blood flow to brain
kidney disease
liver disease
parkinsonism
photosensitivity to drugs, history (light sensitivity)

Lab Tests: Blood counts and liver and kidney function tests may be required periodically if treatment continues for more than 2 weeks.

Pregnancy: Adequate studies have not been done in pregnant women; animal studies may have shown a risk to the fetus. Use only if clearly needed and potential benefits outweigh possible hazards to the fetus.

Breastfeeding: It is not known if nalidixic acid appears in breast milk. Consult your doctor before you begin breastfeeding.

Children: Use with caution. Not recommended for children under 3 months of age.

Drug Interactions:

Tell your doctor or pharmacist if you are taking or if you are planning to take any over-the-counter or prescription medications with nalidixic acid. Doses of one or both drugs may need to be modified or a different drug may need to be prescribed. Drugs that interact with nalidixic acid include:

antacids (eg, *Maalox*)
caffeine (eg, *NoDoz*)
iron (eg, *Feosol*)
nitrofurantoin (eg, *Macrodantin*)
oral anticoagulants (eg, *Coumadin*)
sucralfate (eg, *Carafate*)
theophylline (eg, *TheoDur*)
zinc

Side Effects:

Every drug is capable of producing side effects. Many nalidixic acid users experience no, or minor, side effects. The frequency and severity of side effects depend on many factors including dose, duration of therapy and individual susceptibility. Possible side effects include:

Digestive Tract: Nausea; vomiting; diarrhea; stomachache; infectious colitis.

Nervous System: Drowsiness; weakness; dizziness; headache; feeling of whirling motion; convulsions.

Skin: Itching; rash; hives.

Other: Joint pain, swelling and stiffness; eye and skin sensitivity to light; difficulty focusing; double vision; decreased visual acuity; yellowing of skin or eyes; change in color perception; blood disorder.

Guidelines for Use:

- May be taken with or without food. Take with food if GI upset occurs.
- Drink fluids liberally. Do not take with antacids.
- Administer to adults and children in 4 equally divided doses per-day.
- May cause drowsiness, dizziness or lightheadedness, or blurred vision. Use caution when driving or performing other tasks requiring alertness, coordination, or physical dexterity.
- *Sensitivity to sunlight* — Nalidixic acid may cause sensitivity to the sun and other sources of ultraviolet light. Avoid prolonged exposure to the sun and artificial ultraviolet lights. Use sunscreens and wear protective clothing if exposure cannot be avoided. Discontinue therapy if phototoxicity occurs.
- If seizures, diarrhea (possible pseudomembranous colitis), skin rash or other signs of allergic reaction occur while taking nalidixic acid, contact your doctor immediately.
- Use OTC caffeine-containing products and caffeinated beverages cautiously while taking nalidixic acid. Increased caffeine effects (eg, tremors, rapid heartbeat, sleeplessness) may occur.
- Store at room temperature. While the suspension does not need to be refrigerated, it may be chilled to improve the taste. Avoid freezing the suspension.

If you have any questions, consult your doctor, pharmacist, or health care provider.

	Generic Name *Brand Name Examples*	Suplied As	Generic Available
Rx	**Nitrofurantoin**		
	Macrobid	**Capsules:** 25 mg	No
	Furadantin	**Oral Suspension:** 25 mg/tsp	No
Rx	**Nitrofurantoin Macro-crystals**		
	Macrodantin	**Capsules:** 25 mg, 50 mg, 100 mg	Yes

Type of Drug:

Urinary anti-infective.

How the Drug Works:

Nitrofurantoin interferes with metabolism and protein synthesis, and may also disrupt cell wall formation in susceptible bacteria.

Uses:

To treat urinary tract infections caused by susceptible bacteria.

Precautions:

Do not use in the following situations:

- allergy to nitrofurantoin
- infants under 1 month of age
- labor and delivery, during
- kidney disease
- pregnant women at term

Use with caution in the following situations:

- anemia
- diabetes
- electrolyte imbalance
- glucose-6-phosphate dehydrogenase (G-6-PD) deficiency
- vitamin B deficiency

Superinfection – Use of antibiotics (especially prolonged or repeated therapy) may result in bacterial or fungal overgrowth. Such overgrowth may lead to a second infection. Nitrofurantoin may need to be stopped and another antibiotic prescribed for the second infection.

Lab tests: Lab tests may be required to monitor therapy. Be sure to keep appointments.

Pregnancy: Studies in pregnant woman or in animals have been judged not to show a risk to the fetus, except late in pregnancy. However, no drug should be used during pregnancy unless clearly needed. Do not use in pregnant women at term, or during labor and delivery.

Breastfeeding: Nitrofurantoin appears in breast milk. Consult your doctor before you begin breastfeeding.

Children: Safety and effectiveness have not been established for children under 12 years of age. Do not use in children less than 1 month old.

Drug Interactions:

Tell your doctor or pharmacist if you are taking or if you are planning to take any over-the-counter or prescription medications while taking this medicine. Doses of one or both drugs may need to be modified or a different drug may need to be prescribed. The following drugs and drug classes interact with this medicine.

anticholinergics (eg, atropine)
magnesium salts (eg, antacids)
probenecid (eg, *Benemid*)
sulfinpyrazone (eg, *Anturane*)

Side Effects:

Every drug is capable of producing side effects. Many patients experience no, or minor, side effects. The frequency and severity of side effects depend on many factors including dose, duration of therapy and individual susceptibility. Possible side effects include:

Digestive Tract: Nausea; vomiting; gas; appetite loss; stomach ache; indigestion; constipation; diarrhea; inflammation of the salivary glands or the mouth.

Nervous System: Headache; dizziness; drowsiness; weakness; vertigo (feeling of whirling motion); tingling or numbness in hands or feet; confusion; depression.

Skin: Rash; redness; itching; hives; temporary hair loss; light sensitivity.

Other: Asthma; difficult breathing; cough; fever; chills; muscle or joint pain; swelling; changes in heartbeat; vision problems; rapid eye movement; yellowing of eyes or skin; general body discomfort; anemia; abnormal lab and blood values.

Guidelines for Use:

- *Macrodantin Capsules, Furadantin Oral Solution* - Usual dose is 4 times a day, with meals and at bedtime.
- *Macrobid Macrocrystals* - Usual dose is 1 capsule every 12 hours for 7 days.
- May cause stomach upset; take with food or milk.
- Shake suspension well before use.
- Many patients who cannot tolerate the macrocrystals *(Macrobid)* are able to take *Macrodantin* without nausea.
- Avoid antacids containing magnesium (eg, *Maalox*) while taking this medicine.
- If a dose is missed, take it as soon as possible. If several hours have passed or it is nearing time for the next dose, do not double the dose in order to "catch up," unless advised by your doctor. If more than one dose is missed, contact your doctor or pharmacist.
- Continue use until all of the prescribed medicine has been taken, even if fever or other symptoms of infection have disappeared. Failure to take all of the medicine may prevent complete elimination of bacteria, allowing the infection to return.
- Use of antibiotics (especially prolonged or repeated therapy) may result in bacterial or fungal overgrowth. Such overgrowth may lead to a second infection. Nitrofurantoin may need to be stopped and another antibiotic prescribed for the second infection.
- If severe diarrhea, stomach pain/cramps or bloody stools occur, contact your doctor immediately. This could be a sign of a serious side effect requiring immediate medical attention. Do not treat diarrhea without consulting your doctor.
- Contact your doctor immediately if numbness or tingling in feet or hands, fever, chills, cough, chest pain, difficulty breathing, skin rash, general body discomfort, or severe stomach upset occurs.
- A brownish discoloration of the urine may occur. This is normal.
- This medicine may cause a false-positive reaction for glucose in the urine.
- Lab tests may be required to monitor therapy. Be sure to keep appointments.
- Exposure to strong light may darken the oral solution. Protect from light.
- Store at room temperature (59° to 86°F), away from light.

If you have any questions, consult your doctor, pharmacist, or health care provider.

Generic Name *Brand Name Examples*	Supplied As	Generic Available
Rx **Sulfonamide Combinations**		
Urobiotic-250	**Capsules:** 250 mg sulfamethizole, 250 mg oxytetracycline, 50 mg phenazopyridine HCl	No
Azo-Sulfisoxazole	**Tablets:** 500 mg sulfisoxazole, 50 mg phenazopyridine HCl	Yes
Bactrim[1], *Cotrim, Septra*[1]	**Tablets:** 400 mg sulfamethoxazole, 80 mg trimethoprim	Yes
Bactrim DS, Cotrim D.S., Septra DS	**Tablets, double strength:** 800 mg sulfamethoxazole, 160 mg trimethoprim	Yes
Bactrim Pediatric, Cotrim Pediatric, Septra, Sulfatrim	**Oral Suspension:** 200 mg sulfamethoxazole, 40 mg trimethoprim/tsp	Yes
Rx **Methenamine Combinations**		
Trac Tabs 2X	**Tablets:** 120 mg methenamine, 30 mg phenyl salicylate, 0.06 mg atropine sulfate, 0.03 mg hyoscyamine sulfate, 7.5 mg benzoic acid, 6 mg methylene blue	No
Prosed/DS	**Tablets:** 81.6 mg methenamine, 36.2 mg phenyl salicylate, 10.8 mg methylene blue, 9 mg benzoic acid, 0.06 mg atropine sulfate, 0.06 mg hyoscyamine sulfate	No
Urimar-T, Urogesic Blue	**Tablets:** 81.6 mg methenamine, 40.8 mg sodium biphosphate, 36.2 mg phenyl salicylate, 10.8 mg methylene blue, 0.12 mg hyoscyamine sulfate	No
Uro-Phosphate	**Tablets:** 300 mg methenamine, 434.78 mg sodium biphosphate	No
Uroquid-Acid No. 2	**Tablets:** 500 mg methenamine mandelate, 500 mg sodium acid phosphate monohydrate	No
Urisedamine	**Tablets:** 500 mg methenamine mandelate, 0.15 mg hyoscyamine	No

Generic Name *Brand Name Examples*	Supplied As	Generic Available
Atrosept, Dolsed, UAA, Uridon Modified, Urinary Abtiseptic No. 2, Urised, Uritin	**Tablets:** 40.8 mg methenamine, 18.1 mg phenyl salicylate, 0.03 mg atropine sulfate, 0.03 mg hyoscyamine (as sulfate), 4.5 mg benzoic acid, 5.4 mg methylene blue	Yes
otc Cystex	**Tablets:** 162 mg methenamine, 162.5 mg sodium salicylate, benzoic acid	No

[1] Also available as an injection.

For further information, see methenamine and methenamine salts; sulfonamides; tetracycline and oxytetracycline; trimethoprim (TMP); sulfamethoxazole and trimethoprim combinations (TMP-SMZ).

Type of Drug:

Urinary anti-infective combinations.

Uses:

For relief of frequent, painful, or burning urination. To treat urinary tract infections caused by susceptible bacteria.

Methenamine is an anti-infective and acidifies the urine.

Phenazopyridine HCl, sodium salicylate, and phenyl salicylate are pain relievers.

Belladonna alkaloids (eg, atropine, hyoscyamine) relieve urinary tract spasms.

Sodium biphosphate (sodium acid phosphate) and benzoic acid acidify the urine.

Guidelines for Use:

- Use exactly as prescribed.
- Take each dose with a full glass of water. Drink plenty of fluids while taking these drugs.
- *OTC Products* – Do not use without first talking to your doctor if you are pregnant or breastfeeding or if this is the first time you have had urinary tract infection symptoms (eg, frequent or burning urination).
  Discontinue use when symptoms subside. If symptoms do not get better in 5 days, discontinue use and consult your doctor.
- *Oral Suspension* – Shake well before use.
- If a dose is missed, take it as soon as possible. If several hours have passed or if it is nearing time for the next dose, do not double the dose in order to catch up, unless advised by your doctor. If more than one dose is missed, contact your doctor or pharmacist.
- Continue use until all of the prescribed medicine has been taken, even if fever or other symptoms have disappeared. Failure to take all of the medicine may prevent complete elimination of bacteria, allowing the infection to return.
- Notify your doctor if rash, hives, sore throat, fever, chills, pale skin, yellowing of skin or eyes, rash, or unusual bleeding or bruising occurs.
- *Superinfection* – Use of antibiotics (especially prolonged or repeated therapy) may result in bacterial or fungal overgrowth (secondary infections). This medicine may need to be stopped and another antibiotic prescribed for the second infection.
- Some of these products may cause sensitivity to sunlight. Avoid prolonged exposure to the sun or other forms of ultraviolet (UV) light (eg, tanning beds). Use sunscreens and wear protective clothing until tolerance is determined.
- Some of these products contain sulfonamides. Consult your doctor or pharmacist if you are allergic to sulfonamides.
- Lab tests may be required to monitor treatment. Be sure to keep appointments.
- Store at room temperature (59° to 86°F); protect from moisture and light.

If you have any questions, consult your doctor, pharmacist, or health care provider.

	Generic Name *Brand Name Examples*	Supplied As	Generic Available
Rx	**Capreomycin**		
	Capastat Sulfate	**Powder for Injection:** 1 g/vial	No
Rx	**Cycloserine**		
	Seromycin Pulvules	**Capsules:** 250 mg	No
Rx	**Ethambutol Hydrochloride**		
	Myambutol	**Tablets:** 100 mg, 400 mg	No
Rx	**Ethionamide**		
	Trecator-SC	**Tablets:** 250 mg	No
Rx	**Isoniazid (INH)**	**Tablets:** 100 mg, 300 mg	Yes
		Syrup: 50 mg/5 mL	Yes
	Nydrazid	**Injection:** 100 mg/mL	Yes
Rx	**Isoniazid w/Rifampin**		
	Rifamate	**Capsules:** 150 mg isoniazid and 300 mg rifampin	No
Rx	**Pyrazinamide**	**Tablets:** 500 mg	Yes
Rx	**Rifabutin**		
	Mycobutin	**Capsules:** 150 mg	No
Rx	**Rifampin**		
	Rifadin	**Capsules:** 150 mg, 300 mg	No
	Rimactane	**Capsules:** 300 mg	No
	Rifadin	**Injection:** 600 mg/vial	No
Rx	**Rifampin w/Isoniazid and Pyrazinamide**		
	Rifater	**Tablets:** 120 mg rifampin, 50 mg isoniazid, 300 mg pyrazinamide	No
Rx	**Rifapentine**		
	Priftin	**Tablets:**150 mg	No

Type of Drug:

Drugs for treating tuberculosis (TB).

How the Drug Works:

Antituberculosis agents kill or stop the growth of tuberculosis organisms. Many of these drugs must be used in combination with other antituberculosis drugs during therapy. Therapy with these agents is usually long-term.

Uses:

All (except Rifabutin): To treat tuberculosis infections caused by susceptible organisms.

Cycloserine: To treat urinary tract infections caused by susceptible organisms when more conventional antibiotic therapy has failed.

Isoniazid: To prevent and to treat tuberculosis.

Rifabutin: To prevent spreading of *Mycobacterium avium* complex (MAC) disease in patients with advanced HIV infection.

Rifampin: To treat asymptomatic carriers of *Neisseria meningitidis.*

Unlabeled Use(s): Occasionally doctors may prescribe rifampin to treat certain infections (eg, Legionnaires' disease, leprosy, and to prevent meningitis due to *Haemophilus influenzae*). Isoniazid may be used to improve severe tremors in patients with multiple sclerosis.

Precautions:

Do not use in the following situations:

All — allergy to the drug or any of its ingredients
Cycloserine — epilepsy; depression; severe anxiety; psychosis; severe kidney disease; excessive concurrent alcohol use
Ethambutol — optic neuritis (inflammation of optic nerve)
Ethionamide — severe liver disease and impairment
Isoniazid — previous isoniazid-associated liver damage; other severe reactions to isoniazid (eg, fever, chills, arthritis); or liver disease of any etiology or cause
Pyrazinamide — acute gout; severe liver damage
Rifabutin — allergy to any other rifamycin; active tuberculosis
Rifapentine and Rifampin — allergy to any other rifamycin

Use with caution in the following situations:

Capreomycin – kidney disease; hearing impairment
Ethambutol — kidney disease; cataracts, diabetic retinopathy, or other vision problems
Ethionamide — diabetes mellitus
Isoniazid — kidney or liver disease; daily users of alcohol; older than 35 years of age; chronically administered medicines, concurrent use; history of previous discontinuation of isoniazid; peripheral neuropathy, existence or conditions of; pregnancy; injectable drug abusers; post-partum women of minority groups; HIV-seropositive patients.
Pyrazinamide — diabetes mellitus; liver disease; kidney disease; history of gout; increased risk of liver disease; elderly; daily users of alcohol
Rifampin — liver disease
Rifapentine — liver disease

Hypersensitivity Reaction: Allergic-type reactions may occur with the use of these drugs. Symptoms may include fever, rash, hives, swollen lymph nodes, itching, difficulty breathing, yellowing of the eyes or skin, and false blood or liver tests.

Capreomycin: Audiometric (hearing) measurements and assessments of vestibular function (balance) should be performed prior to initiation of therapy and at regular intervals during treatment.

Cycloserine: Patients receiving greater than 500 mg daily should be closely monitored. Anticonvulsant drugs or sedatives may be effective in controlling symptoms of CNS toxicity, such as convulsions, anxiety, and tremor. Toxicity is closely related to excessive blood levels. Risk of convulsions is increased in chronic alcoholics. Cycloserine blood level tests should be determined at least weekly for patients with kidney disease, individuals receiving daily dosage greater than 500 mg, and for those showing signs and symptoms of toxicity.

Vitamin B_{12} and folic acid deficiencies and anemia have been associated with the use of cycloserine. Contact your doctor to determine if supplementation is required.

Ethambutol: Adverse effects on vision may occur with the use of ethambutol. Physical exams should include ophthalmoscopy, finger perimetry, and testing of color discrimination. Tests should be repeated periodically during therapy. Changes in visual activity may be in one or both eyes; therefore each eye must be tested separately and both eyes together. Any drug-induced changes in vision are generally reversible when the drug is discontinued. Changes in color perception are the first signs of toxicity. Contact your doctor if you experience any changes in vision. Renal function monitoring is encouraged.

Ethionamide: Diabetics may experience an increased difficulty in the management of diabetes. Adverse effects on vision may occur with use of ethionamide. Ophthalmic examinations should be performed before and periodically during therapy. Contact your doctor if you experience any changes in vision.

Isoniazid: Pyridoxine (vitamin B_6) deficiency is sometimes seen during treatment with isoniazid. Contact your doctor to determine if vitamin B_6 supplements are required. Ophthalmic examinations should be performed before and periodically during therapy. Contact your doctor if you experience any changes in vision.

Pyrazinamide: If high blood uric acid levels are accompanied by acute gouty arthritis, pyrazinamide should be discontinued. Diabetics may experience an increased difficulty in the management of diabetes.

Rifabutin: Rifabutin prophylaxis of MAC must not be used in patients with active tuberculosis. If active TB symptoms develop, contact your doctor immediately.

Rifampin and Rifapentine: If diarrhea develops during rifampin or rifapentine use, consider pseudomembranous colitis. This inflammatory condition of the colon is due to overgrowth of bacteria that are not killed by rifampin or rifapentine. The primary cause is a toxin produced by a bacteria known as *Clostridia difficile*. Colitis symptoms may range from mild to life-threatening. Mild cases usually respond by stopping the antibiotic. In more serious cases, another antibiotic may need to be prescribed.

Rifapentine, rifabutin, and rifampin: Urine, stool, saliva, sputum, sweat, and tears may be colored red-orange or reddish brown. This is not harmful. Soft contact lenses may be permanently stained.

Pregnancy: Safety for use during pregnancy has not been established for many of these medications. Therefore, routine use of these medications during pregnancy is not appropriate.

Breastfeeding: Isoniazid, pyrazinamide, and rifampin appear in breast milk. It is not known if other antituberculosis drugs appear in breast milk. Consult your doctor before you begin breastfeeding.

Children: Safety and effectiveness of capreomycin, cycloserine, and rifabutin have not been established. Rifampin with isoniazid and pyrazinamide is not recommended for use in children under 15 years of age. Ethambutol is not recommended for use in children under 13 years of age. Ethionamide and rifapentine is not recommended for use in children under 12 years of age. Isoniazid may be used in infants and children. Rifampin dosing is available for infants and children. Pyrazinamide appears to be well tolerated in children. Rifabutin has been used in a limited number of children (1 to 16 years of age) with HIV.

Elderly: Safety and dosage have not been sufficiently determined. However, in general, dose selection for elderly patients should be cautious, starting with the lowest effective dose.

Lab tests and periodic doctor visits may be required during treatment with these drugs. Tests may include eye examinations, liver and kidney function tests, blood counts, urine tests, blood electrolytes, uric acid tests, blood drug levels, and hearing and eye tests.

Drug Interactions:

Tell your doctor or pharmacist if you are taking or if you are planning to take any over-the-counter or prescription medications with antituberculosis drugs. Doses of one or both drugs may need to be modified or a different drug may need to be prescribed. The following drugs and drug classes interact with antituberculosis drugs.

All antituberculosis drugs — alcohol

Capreomycin — injectable antituberculosis agents (eg, streptomycin, viomycin), nonantituberculosis antibiotics (eg, gentamicin)

Cycloserine — isoniazid (eg, *Nydrazid*), ethionamide

Ethionamide – isoniazid (eg, *Nydrazid*), cycloserine, excessive ethanol

Isoniazid —

- acetaminophen (eg, *Tylenol*)
- aluminum salts (eg, some antacids)
- anticoagulants, oral (eg, warfarin)
- benzodiazepines (eg, clonazepam)
- carbamazepine (eg, *Tegretol*)
- disulfiram (*Antabuse*)
- enflurane (*Enthrane*)
- hydantoins (eg, phenytoin)
- ketoconazole *(Nizoral)*
- meperidine (eg, *Demerol*)
- primidone (eg, *Mysoline*)
- rifampin (eg, *Rifadin*)
- theophylline (eg, *Slo-Bid*)
- valproate sodium (eg, *Depakote*)

Pyrazinamide — *Acetest* and *Ketostix* urine tests

Rifabutin —

cardiac glycosides (eg, digoxin)
narcotics (eg, methadone)
zidovudine (*Retrovir*)

Because of similarities between rifabutin, rifapentine, and rifampin, similar interactions may be expected. See rifampin interactions.

Rifampin —

analgesics, narcotics (eg, methadone)
antacids (eg, *Maalox*)
antiarrhythmics (eg, disopyramide)
anticoagulants, oral (eg, warfarin)
anticonvulsants (eg, phenytoin)
azole antifungals (eg, fluconazole)
barbiturates (eg, phenobarbital)
benzodiazepines, (eg, diazepam)
beta blockers (eg, propranolol)
cardiac glycosides (eg, digoxin)
calcium channel blockers (eg, diltiazem)
chloramphenicol (*Chloromycetin*)
clarithromycin (*Biaxin*)
clofibrate (eg, *Atromid-S*)
contraceptives, oral (eg, *Ortho-Novum*)
corticosteroids (eg, prednisone)
co-trimoxazole (eg, *Bactrim*)
cyclosporine (eg, *Sandimmune*)
digitoxin (*Crystodigin*)
doxycycline (eg, *Vibramycin*)
enalapril (*Vasotec*)
estrogens (eg, estrone)
fluoroquinolones (eg, ciprofloxacin)
haloperidol (eg, *Haldol*)
halothane (eg, *Fluothane*)
hydantoins (eg, phenytoin)
isoniazid (eg, *Nydrazid*)
mexiletine *(Mexitil)*
probenecid
progestins (eg, *Provera*)
propafenone (*Rythmol*)
quinidine (eg, *Quinora*)
sulfasalazine (eg, *Azulfidine*)
sulfones (eg, dapsone)
sulfonylureas (eg, tolbutamide)
tacrolimus (*Prograf*)
theophylline (eg, *Theo-Dur*)
thyroid drugs (eg, levothyroxine)
tocainide *(Tonocard)*
tricyclic antidepressants (eg, nortriptyline)
zidovudine (*Retrovir*)

Rifapentine —

contraceptives, oral (eg, *Ortho-Novum*)
itraconazole (*Sporanox*)
nifidipine (eg, *Procardia*)
protease inhibitors (eg, indinavir)

Because of similarities between rifabutin, rifapentine, and rifampin, similar interactions may be expected. See rifampin interactions.

Side Effects:

Every drug is capable of producing side effects. Many antituberculosis drug users experience no, or minor, side effects. The frequency and severity of side effects depend on many factors including dose, duration of therapy, and individual susceptibility. Possible side effects include:

Digestive Tract: Nausea; vomiting; appetite loss; diarrhea; stomach pain; upset stomach.

Nervous System: Dizziness; unusual tiredness; weakness; drowsiness; confusion; headache.

Skin: Rash; itching; hives.

Other: Muscle or joint pain; vision problems; fever; abnormal lab tests (eg, liver function, blood count); numbness, pain, or tingling in hands or feet; general body discomfort. In addition to the side effects listed, many of the drugs have specific side effects:

Capreomycin – Damage to kidney cells; hearing loss; ringing in ears; feeling of whirling motion; excessive bleeding at injection site; increased or decreased white blood counts; pain, hardness, or abscess at injection site; nerve damage; blood disorders.

Cycloserine – Slurred speech; tremor; sudden development of congestive heart failure; convulsions; behavioral changes; vitamin B_{12} or folic acid deficiency; partial or complete paralysis; exaggerated reflexes; feeling of a whirling motion; disorientation with memory loss; psychosis (possibly with suicidal tendencies); hyperirritability; aggression; allergy; skin rash; coma; drowsiness; sleepiness; depression; confusion; headache; abnormal skin sensations; anemia; seizures; allergic reaction.

Ethambutol – Changes in vision (see Precautions); disorientation; hallucinations; gout; joint pain; elevated blood uric acid levels; liver impairment; allergic reactions; skin inflammation; headache; abnormal lung x-rays.

Ethionamide – Metallic taste; excessive salivation; yellowing of the eyes or skin; hepatitis; depression; difficulty managing diabetes; fainting; restlessness; sensitivity to light; low blood sugar levels; breast growth; impotence; acne; weight loss; decreased blood platelets; pellagra syndrome.

Isoniazid – Numbness, pain, or tingling in hands or feet; yellowing of the eyes or skin; increased blood sugar; breast enlargement; vitamin B_6 or pyridoxine deficiency; vision problems; swollen lymph nodes; inflammation of blood vessels; abnormal blood cell counts; general ill feeling; hepatitis; agranulocytosis; skin eruptions; niacin deficiency; rheumatic syndrome; peripheral neuropathy; pellagra; anemia; fever; blood disorders; convulsions; memory impairment; high blood sugar.

Pyrazinamide – Dark urine; gout; yellowing of the eyes or skin; joint pain; anemia; low platelet count; muscle pain or tenderness; difficult or painful urination; acne; porphyria; sensitivity to light; blood disorders.

Rifabutin – Chest pain; indigestion; belching; gas; sleeplessness; taste perversion; reddish discoloration of body fluids; muscle pain or tenderness; low white blood cell counts; lab test abnormalities.

Rifampin – Menstrual irregularities; reddish orange discoloration of body fluids; heartburn; gas; cramps; sore mouth and tongue; flushing; inability to concentrate; generalized numbness; behavioral changes; fluid retention; shortness of breath; wheezing; low blood pressure; liver dysfunction; yellowing of the eyes or skin; decreased platelets; blood cell disorders; hepatitis; conjunctivitis; anemia; leukopenia; decreased hemoglobin; clumsiness; allergic reaction; muscular weakness; flu-syndrome; myopathy; shock; visual disturbances; pain in hands or feet; injection site reaction; pemphigoid reaction; fever.

Rifapentine – Abnormal liver tests; pus in urine; excess protein in urine; blood in urine; acne; anemia; decreased white blood counts; joint pain; pain; high blood pressure; decreased platelet count; vomiting blood; abnormal urine tests; reddish orange discoloration of body fluids.

Guidelines for Use:

- Generally two or more antituberculosis drugs are prescribed to treat active TB. All prescribed drugs must be taken as prescribed to reduce the chance of a resistant TB organism developing and to increase the chance of effectively treating the infection.
- Take as directed. Avoid missing doses. Do not stop taking this medicine before consulting your doctor. Failure to adhere to the drug regimen for the full duration of treatment can result in treatment failure and lead to other serious health risks. Treatment is often long-term.
- If a dose is missed, take it as soon as possible. If several hours have passed or if it is nearing time for the next dose, do not double the dose in order to catch up (unless advised to do so by your doctor). If more than one dose is missed, or if it is necessary to establish a new dosage schedule, contact your doctor or pharmacist. Use exactly as prescribed.
- Contact your doctor if any of the following occurs: Fever; rash; hives; swollen lymph nodes; itching; difficulty breathing; yellowing of skin or eyes.
- Lab tests will be required to monitor therapy. Be sure to keep appointments.
- *Capreomycin* —
  Usual dosage is 1 g/day (not to exceed 20 mg/kg day) given intramuscularly or by infusion intravenously for 60 to 120 days, followed by 1 g, 2 to 3 times weekly.
  Reduced dosage should be used for patients with known or suspected kidney impairment.
  Therapy for tuberculosis should be maintained for 12 to 24 months.
  If facilities for administering injectable medication are not available, change to appropriate oral therapy as indicated on patient's release from hospital.
  The solution may turn pale yellow and darken. After reconstitution, all solutions may be stored in a refrigerator up to 24 hours.
  Store at room temperature (59° to 86°F) before reconstitution.
- *Cycloserine* —
  Initial adult dosage is 250 mg twice daily at 12-hour intervals for the first 2 weeks. Usual dosage is 500 mg to 1 g daily in divided doses monitored by blood levels. Daily dose of 1 g should not be exceeded.
  May cause drowsiness. Use caution when driving or performing other tasks requiring alertness, coordination, or physical dexterity.
  Avoid excessive alcohol consumption.

Guidelines for Use (cont.):

- *Cycloserine* — (cont.)
  Contact your doctor if any of these symptoms occur: Convulsions; psychosis; excessive drowsiness; depression; confusion; exaggerated reflexes; headache; tremor; feeling of a whirling motion; partial or complete paralysis; slurred speech. These may be signs or symptoms of CNS toxicity. Cycloserine should be discontinued or the dosage reduced. Patients receiving more than 500 mg daily should be closely monitored.
  Store at room temperature (59° to 86°F).
- *Ethambutol* —
  For initial treatment, usual dose is 7 mg per pound of body weight taken as a single oral dose once every 24 hours. For retreatment, the dose is 11 mg per pound of body weight, taken as a single oral dose once every 24 hours. After 60 days, the dose is decreased to 7 mg per pound of body weight taken as a single oral dose once every 24 hours.
  Proper dose may require combination of different sized tablets taken at the same time. Be sure to check tablets before each dose to make sure the proper number and strength are being taken.
  May cause stomach upset. Take with food if this occurs.
  Notify your doctor if changes in vision (eg, blurring, red-green color blindness) or skin rash occurs.
  Store at room temperature (59° to 86°F).
- *Ethionamide* —
  Usual adult dosage is 7 mg to 9 mg per pound of body weight taken once-daily. If stomach upset occurs with once daily administration, then divide into 2 to 3 doses. Concomitant administration of pyridoxine is recommended. Duration of treatment should be based on individual response.
  Avoid excessive alcohol consumption. Psychotic reactions have been reported.
  Take with food to reduce stomach upset.
  May cause stomach upset, appetite loss, metallic taste, or salivation. Notify your doctor if these effects persist or are severe.
  Notify your doctor of any changes in vision or eye pain during treatment.
  Store at room temperature (77°F) in a tight container.
- *Isoniazid* —
  Take on an empty stomach, at least 1 hour before or 2 hours after meals. Studies have shown the absorption of isoniazid is reduced significantly when administered with food. However, isoniazid may be taken with food if stomach upset occurs.
  Minimize alcohol use. Alcohol may increase the risk of hepatitis.
  Discontinue the drug and notify your doctor if any of the following occurs: Weakness; numbness or tingling of hands or feet; right upper quandrant discomfort; persistent fatigue or fever lasting longer than 3 days; general body discomfort; appetite loss; nausea; vomiting; yellowing of skin or eyes; dark urine; abdominal tenderness. Isoniazid should be discontinued promptly since continued use may cause more liver damage.

Guidelines for Use (cont.):

- *Isoniazid* — (cont.)
  Concomitant administration of vitamin B_6 (pyridoxine) is recommended in malnourished patients, patients at risk of developing neuropathy (eg, alcoholics, diabetics), and children.
  Store at room temperature (59° to 86°F) and protect from light. Injection may crystallize at low temperatures. If this occurs, warm the vial to room temperature before use to dissolve crystals.
- *Isoniazid w/ Rifampin* —
  Usual dosage is 2 capsules (600 mg rifampin, 300 mg isoniazid) once daily, 1 hour before or 2 hours after a meal. Concomitant administration of pyridoxine (B_6) is recommended in malnourished patients, those predisposed to neuropathy (eg, alcoholics, diabetics), and children.
  Also see isoniazid and rifampin.
- *Pyrazinamide* —
  Administer orally, 7 mg to 14 mg per pound of body weight, once daily. Do not exceed 3 g (6 tablets) per day. Alternatively, a twice-weekly dosage regimen has been developed on an outpatient basis.
  In patients with concomitant HIV infection, a longer course of treatment may be required.
  Notify your doctor if fever, appetite loss, general body discomfort, nausea, vomiting, dark urine, yellowing of the skin or eyes, or pain or swelling of the joints occurs.
  Store at room temperature (59° to 86°F) in a tightly sealed container.
- *Rifabutin* —
  Usual dosage is 300 mg once daily. If stomach upset occurs, taking 150 mg twice daily with food may help.
  Contact your doctor if you develop symptoms or signs of either tuberculosis or *M. avium* complex (MAC). These may include persisent fever, weight loss, night sweats, or productive cough.
  May cause a reddish orange discoloration of urine, stools, saliva, tears, sweat, sputum, and skin. This is not harmful. May also permanently discolor soft contact lenses.
  Oral contraceptives may not be as effective while taking this medicine. Patients should use nonhormonal methods of birth control.
  Store at room temperature (59° to 86°F) in a tightly sealed container.
- *Rifampin* —
  A 3-drug regimen consisting of rifampin, isoniazid, and pyrazinamide is recommended in the initial phase of short–course therapy which is usually continued for 2 months. Treatment should be continued with rifampin and isoniazid for at least 4 months. Injection is indicated for initial treatment when oral dosage is not possible. Injection is for intravenous infusion only. Do not administer by intramuscular or subcutaneous route.
  Usual adult dosage to treat TB is 10 mg per kg of body weight (not to exceed 600 mg) taken as a single daily dose.
  Usual adult dosage to treat meningococcal carriers is 600 mg twice daily for 2 days.

Guidelines for Use (cont.):

- *Rifampin* — (cont.)
  Take on an empty stomach, at least 1 hour before or 2 hours after meals with a full glass of water. Food reduces absorption of rifampin.
  Take rifampin at least 1 hour before any antacid.
  May cause a reddish orange discoloration of urine, stools, saliva, tears, sweat, and sputum. This is not harmful. May also permanently discolor soft contact lenses.
  Notify your doctor if fever, general body discomfort, nausea, vomiting, appetite loss, yellowing of the skin or eyes, dark urine, or pain or swelling of the joints occurs.
  Oral contraceptives may not be as effective while taking this medicine. Patients should use nonhormonal methods of birth control.
  Store capsules in a tightly closed container in a dry place. Avoid excessive heat. Do not store capsules above 86°F. Protect injection from light and do not store above 104°F.
- *Rifampin w/Isoniazid and Pyrazinamide* —
  Usual dose (based on weight) is given once daily, 1 hour before or 2 hours after a meal with a full glass of water: 4 tablets if less than 98 pounds; 5 tablets if 99 to 120 pounds; 6 tablets if more than 120 pounds. Initial phase therapy is usually continued for 2 months, followed by rifampin and isoniazid for at least 4 months.
  Concomitant administration of vitamin B_6 (pyridoxine) is recommended in malnourished patients, patients at risk of developing neuropathy (eg, alcoholics, diabetics), and children.
  Store at room temperature (59° to 86°F). Protect from excessive moisture.
  Also see isoniazid, pyrazinamide, and rifampin.
- *Rifapentine* —
  Intensive phase therapy lasts 2 months. Dosage is 600 mg (4 tablets) given twice weekly with intervals of 3 or more days (more than 72 hours) between doses. Following the intensive phase, treatment is usually continued at 600 mg once weekly for 4 or more months combined with other TB drugs.
  Take on an empty stomach at least 1 hour before or 2 hours after meals. May be taken with food if stomach upset occurs.
  May cause a reddish orange discoloration of urine, stools, saliva, tears, sweat, and sputum. This is not harmful. May also permanently discolor soft contact lenses.
  Oral contraceptives may not be as effective while taking this medicine. Patients should use nonhormonal methods of birth control.
  Notify your doctor if fever, appetite loss, general body discomfort, nausea, vomiting, dark urine, yellowing of skin or eyes, or pain or swelling of the joints occurs.
  Concomitant administration of vitamin B_6 (pyridoxine) is recommended in malnourished patients, patients at risk of developing neuropathy (eg, alcoholics, diabetics), and children.
  Store at room temperature (59° to 86°F). Protect from heat and humidity.

If you have any questions, consult your doctor, pharmacist, or health care provider.

	Generic Name *Brand Name Examples*	Supplied As	Generic Available
Rx	**Atovaquone**		
	Mepron[1]	**Suspension:** 750 mg/5 mL	No

[1] Contains benzyl alcohol.

Type of Drug:

Antiprotozoal agent to treat *Pneumocystis carinii* pneumonia (PCP), a serious respiratory infection.

How the Drug Works:

The mechanism of action is not fully known. Studies indicate that it may inhibit enzymes necessary for the organism to grow and reproduce.

Uses:

To treat mild to moderate PCP infection in patients who cannot tolerate trimethoprim-sulfamethoxazole (TMP-SMZ) (eg, *Septra*). Atovaquone is not used to prevent PCP infection.

Precautions:

Do not use in the following situations:
allergy to atovaquone or any of its ingredients

Use with caution in the following situations:
elderly
presence of other respiratory infections
stomach and intestinal disorders

Pregnancy: Adequate studies have not been done in pregnant women. Use only if clearly needed and potential benefits outweigh the possible hazards to the fetus.

Breastfeeding: It is not known if atovaquone appears in breast milk. Consult your doctor before you begin breastfeeding.

Children: Safety and effectiveness in children have not been established.

Elderly: Use with caution in the elderly.

Lab tests may be required to monitor therapy. Tests may include blood cell counts, liver and kidney function tests, x-rays, and blood gases.

Drug Interactions:

Tell your doctor or pharmacist if you are taking or if you are planning to take any over-the-counter or prescription medications while taking atovaquone. Doses of one or both drugs may need to be modified or a different drug may need to be prescribed. The following drugs may interact with atovaquone:

rifabutin (*Mycobutin*)
rifampin (eg, *Rifadin*)

Side Effects:

Every drug is capable of producing side effects. Many atovaquone users experience no, or minor, side effects. The frequency and severity of side effects depend on many factors including dose, duration of therapy, and individual susceptibility. Possible side effects include:

Digestive Tract: Nausea; diarrhea; vomiting; mouth sores; stomach pain; constipation; appetite loss; indigestion; taste changes; mouth infections; inflammation of the pancreas.

Nervous System: Headache; sleeplessness; dizziness; anxiety.

Respiratory System: Cough; sinus inflammation; runny nose.

Other: Pain; weakness; rash; itching; sweating; fever; low blood sugar; low blood pressure; abnormal liver function tests; abnormal blood cell counts; eye problems; sudden kidney failure.

Guidelines for Use:

- Use exactly as prescribed.
- Shake gently before use.
- Recommended dose is 750 mg (1 teaspoonful) with meals twice daily for 21 days (total daily dose 1500 mg).
- Administration with meals enhances atovaquone's absorption. Failure to take with food may result in therapeutic failure.
- Continue to use medicine until all of it is gone. Failure to take all of the medicine may allow the infection to worsen or recur.
- If a dose is missed, take it as soon as possible. If several hours have passed or if it is nearing time for the next dose, do not double the dose to catch up. If more than one dose is missed, contact your doctor or pharmacist.
- Do not share your medication with anyone else.
- Atovaquone is not effective for existing pulmonary (lung) conditions such as bacterial, viral, or fungal pneumonia or mycobacterial (eg, tuberculosis) diseases. Another medicine may need to be prescribed to treat other lung conditions that are present.
- Stomach and intestinal disorders may limit absorption of atovaquone.
- Lab tests will be required to monitor therapy. Be sure to keep appointments.
- Store at room temperature (59° to 77°F) in a tightly sealed container. Do not freeze.

If you have any questions, consult your doctor, pharmacist, or health care provider.

	Generic Name *Brand Name Example*	Supplied As	Generic Available
Rx	**Pentamidine Isethionate**[1]		
	NebuPent	**Aerosol:** 300 mg	No

[1] This product is also available as an injection.

Type of Drug:

Aerosolized pentamidine. Drug for prevention of *Pneumocystis carinii* pneumonia (PCP). Drug for HIV-infected patients.

How the Drug Works:

The mechanism of action is not fully understood. Studies indicate that the drug interferes with the production of DNA, RNA, phospholipids and protein.

Uses:

To prevent *Pneumocystis carinii* pneumonia (PCP) infection in high-risk HIV-infected patients who either have had a previous episode of PCP infection or whose T4 cell count is equal to or less than 200 cells/mm^3.

Unlabeled Use(s): Occasionally, doctors may prescribe pentamidine IV to treat trypanosomiasis and visceral leishmaniasis (serious infections caused by protozoa).

Precautions:

Do not use in the following situations:
anaphylactic allergy to pentamidine isethionate in any dosage form

Use with caution in the following situations:
abnormal ECG
anemia
asthma
blood count disorders
diabetes
heart rhythm disturbance
high blood potassium levels
hives
kidney disease
liver disease
low blood pressure (hypotension)
low blood sugar levels
low calcium levels
lung infection
pancreatitis
smoking
Stevens-Johnson syndrome

Pregnancy: Adequate studies have not been done in pregnant women, or animal studies may have shown a risk to the fetus. Use only if clearly needed and potential benefits outweigh the possible hazards to the fetus.

Breastfeeding: It is not known if pentamidine isethionate appears in breast milk. Consult your doctor before you begin breastfeeding.

Children: Safety and effectiveness in children less than 16 years of age have not been established.

Lab tests may be required because of limited experience with chronic (long-term) aerosolized pentamidine use. Tests that may be required include: Electrocardiogram; blood sugar; calcium; complete blood count and liver, kidney and pancreas function tests.

Drug Interactions:

Tell your doctor or pharmacist if you are taking or planning to take any over-the-counter or prescription medications while taking pentamidine isethionate. Doses of one or both drugs may need to be modified or a different drug may need to be prescribed. The following drugs and drug classes interact with pentamidine isethionate:

aminoglycosides (eg, neomycin sulfate)
amphotericin B (eg, *Albecet*)
cisplatin (*Platinol-AQ*)
foscarnet (*Foscavir*)
vancomycin (eg, *Vancocin*)

Side Effects:

Every drug is capable of producing side effects. Many pentamidine isethionate aerosol users experience no, or minor, side effects. The frequency and severity of side effects depend on many factors including dose, duration of therapy and individual susceptibility. Possible side effects include:

Digestive Tract: Nausea; vomiting; appetite loss; diarrhea; stomach ache; colon inflammation; sore throat.

Nervous System: Dizziness; fatigue; headache; lightheadedness.

Respiratory System: Shortness of breath; chest pain; congestion; cough; bronchitis; wheezing; difficulty breathing; upper respiratory infection; sinus infection.

Other: Night sweats; bad taste; anemia; inflammation of pancreas; diabetes; throat irritation; herpes; flu; fever; infection; allergic reaction; rash; chills; blood in stool; abnormal blood counts; fast heartbeat; mouth infection; abnormal heart rhythms.

The injection product may cause additional and more severe side effects.

Guidelines for Use:

- Prepare and administer pentamidine aerosol solution as instructed by your healthcare provider.
- Administer 300 mg pentamidine isethionate only by the *Respigard* II nebulizer with a high-pressure compressor air or oxygen source at a flow rate of 5 to 7 L/min. Treatment usually takes 30 to 45 minutes and is given once every 4 weeks.
- Do not use more than once a month. Do not increase dose.
- Freshly prepared solutions for aerosol use are recommended. Reconstitute only with Sterile Water for Injection.
- Do not mix the pentamidine solution with any other drugs. Do not use the *Respigard* II nebulizer to administer a bronchodilator.
- If severe sudden abdominal pain, nausea or fever occur, contact your doctor immediately.
- If difficulty breathing, cough or fever develop, contact your doctor. This could indicate the presence of PCP.
- Use of a bronchodilator drug prior to treatment may reduce breathing side effects (bronchospasm, cough).
- Lab tests will be required. Be sure to keep appointments.
- Store at room temperature and protect from light. The reconstituted solution is stable for 48 hours if stored at room temperature and protected from light. Discard unused portion after this time.

If you have any questions, consult your doctor, pharmacist, or health care provider.

	Generic Name *Brand Name Example*	Supplied As	Generic Available
Rx	**Interferon alfa-n3 (Human leukocyte derived)**		
	Alferon N	**Injection**: 5 million IU/mL	No

Type of Drug:

Miscellaneous anti-infective; drug used to treat genital warts.

How the Drug Works:

The specific mechanism of action is unknown. Interferon alfa-n3 binds to membranes on cell surfaces, which initiates a series of responses, including inhibition of virus replication, suppression of cell proliferation, and immunomodulation.

Uses:

To treat refractory or recurring external condylomata acuminata (genital warts) in patients at least 18 years of age who have not satisfactorily responded to other treatments (eg, podophyllin resin, surgery, laser or cryo therapy).

Precautions:

Do not use in the following situations: Allergy to interferon alfa-n3, other human interferon alpha proteins, mouse immunoglobulin (IgG), egg protein, neomycin, or any other ingredients.

Use with caution in the following situations:

- cardiovascular disease (eg, CHF, angina)
- coagulation disorders
- diabetes mellitus with ketoacidosis
- fever
- myelosuppression, severe
- pulmonary disease, severe
- seizure disorders

Fertility impairment: Interferon alpha has been shown to affect the menstrual cycle and decrease serum estradiol and progesterone levels in adult females. Use interferon alfa-n3 with caution in fertile men.

Pregnancy: Abortions have occured in nonhuman primates receiving high doses of recombinant interferon alpha. There are no adaquate and well-controlled studies that determine whether interferon alfa-n3 can cause fetal harm or affect reproductive capacity. Fertile women should use effective contraception during therapy. Use only if clearly needed and the potential benefits to the mother outweigh possible hazards to the fetus.

Breastfeeding: It is not known if interferon alfa-n3 appears in breast milk. Consult your doctor before you begin breastfeeding.

Children: Safety and effectiveness have not been established in children under 18 years of age.

Lab tests may be required to monitor therapy. Tests may include white blood cell and platelet counts; hemoglobin, alkaline phosphatase, and bilirubin levels; and certain enzyme levels.

Drug Interactions:

Tell your doctor or pharmacist if you are taking or planning to take any over-the-counter or prescription medications or dietary supplements with interferon alfa-n3. Doses of one or both drugs may need to be modified or a different drug may need to be prescribed. The following drugs and drug classes interact with interferon alfa-n3:

corticosteroids (eg, prednisone)
melphalan (*Alkeran*)
theophyllines (eg, aminophylline)
zidovudine (AZT; *Retrovir*)

Side Effects:

Every drug is capable of producing side effects. Many interferon alfa-n3 users experience no, or minor, side effects. The frequency and severity of side effects depend on many factors including dose, duration of therapy, and individual susceptibility. Possible side effects include:

Digestive Tract: Nausea; vomiting; heartburn; indigestion; diarrhea; appetite loss.

Nervous System: Headache; dizziness; light-headedness; numbness; stiffness; general body discomfort; insomnia; fatigue; depression; confusion.

Other: Fever; sweating; chills; muscle, chest, joint, or back pain; rash; hives; itching; runny nose; sinus congestion; blurred vision; sore mouth; low blood pressure; soreness at the injection site; abnormal blood counts.

Guidelines for Use:

- This medicine will be prepared and administered by your health care provider in a medical setting. The dose is injected into the base of each wart.
- Interferon will be administered twice weekly for up to, but no more than, 8 weeks.
- Inform your doctor if you are pregnant, become pregnant, plan on becoming pregnant, or are breastfeeding.
- Female patients should use effective contraception during therapy.
- Inform your doctor if you experience any new symptoms or begin taking any other prescription or nonprescription medication.
- Contact your doctor immediately if you experience any signs of allergic reactions (eg, hives, itching, redness, rash, tightness of the chest, wheezing, hypotension).
- Lab tests may be required to monitor therapy. Be sure to keep appointments.

If you have any questions, consult your doctor, pharmacist, or health care provider.

	Generic Name Brand Name Examples	Supplied As	Generic Available
Rx	**Interferon alfacon-1**		
	Infergen[1]	**Injection**: 9 mcg/0.3 mL; 15 mcg/0.5 mL	No

[1] Preservative free.

Type of Drug:

Miscellaneous anti-infective.

How the Drug Works:

The exact mechanism of action of interferon alfacon-1 is unknown. It may directly destroy the virus, prevent viral reproduction or alter the body's natural defense against the virus.

Uses:

To treat long-term (chronic) hepatitis C virus (HCV) infection in patients greater than 18 years of age with compensated (normal liver function) liver disease who have anti-HCV serum antibodies or the presence of HCV RNA.

Unlabeled Use(s): Doctors may occasionally prescribe interferon alfacon-1, along with other agents, for the treatment of hairy-cell leukemia. Further investigation is needed.

Precautions:

Do not use in the following situations:

allergy to alpha interferons
allergy to any ingredient of the product
allergy to *E. coli*-derived products
autoimmune (active) liver disease
severe mental disorders, history of

Use with caution in the following situations:

autoimmune disorders (eg, systemic lupus erythematosis)
bone marrow suppression agents, use with
depression, history of
diabetes
endocrine disorders, history of (eg, low thyroid)
heart disease, pre-existing
high blood pressure
high triglycerides
immunosuppressive use (eg, azathioprine)
long-term illness
low blood cell counts
transplantation patients

Postadministration reaction: Flu-like symptoms, such as headache, fatigue, rigors, muscle discomfort, sweating and joint pain, often occur shortly after the drug is given. These symptoms are usually mild and can be treated with acetaminophen.

Pregnancy: Adequate studies have not been done in pregnant women or animal studies may have shown a risk to the fetus. Use only if clearly needed and potential benefits outweigh the possible hazards to the fetus.

Breastfeeding: It is not known if interferon alfacon-1 appears in breast milk. Consult your doctor before you begin breastfeeding.

Children: Safety and effectiveness have not been established in patients less than 18 years of age. Not recommended in pediatric patients.

Lab tests will be required to monitor therapy. Be sure to keep appointments. Tests may include: Complete blood counts; blood cell differential; liver, kidney and thyroid function tests and blood lipids (or fats).

Drug Interactions:

Tell your doctor or pharmacist if you are taking or planning to take any over-the-counter or prescription medications while taking interferon alfacon-1. Doses of one or both drugs may need to be modified or a different drug may need to be prescribed. The following drug classes interact with interferon alfacon-1:

agents known to cause bone marrow suppression (eg, azathioprine, immunosuppressant drugs)
agents metabolized by cytochrome P450 pathway (eg, theophylline, warfarin, diazepam, phenytoin)

Side Effects:

Every drug is capable of producing side effects. Many patients experience side effects. The frequency and severity of side effects depend on many factors including dose, duration of therapy and individual susceptibility. Possible side effects include:

Digestive Tract: Stomach pain; nausea; diarrhea; appetite loss; indigestion; vomiting; constipation; gas; toothache; hemorrhoids; dry mouth.

Nervous System: Depression; sleeplessness; dizziness; abnormal skin sensations; memory loss; decreased sensitivity to touch; tense muscles; confusion; drowsiness; nervousness; anxiety; unstable emotions; abnormal thinking; agitation.

Circulatory System: High blood pressure; pounding in chest (palpitations); fast heartbeat.

Respiratory System: Upper respiratory infection; cough; sinus discomfort; nasal congestion; chest congestion; runny nose; nosebleed; difficulty breathing; bronchitis.

Urinary and Reproductive Tract: Painful menstruation; inflammation of the vagina; menstrual disorder; yeast infection.

Skin: Hair loss; itching; rash; redness; dry skin; wound; unusual bruising.

Senses: Earache; ear infection; ringing in the ears; taste perversion; eye pain; eye infection; abnormal vision.

Other: Flu-like symptoms (eg, headache, tiredness, fever, chills, increased sweating, muscle and joint pain); injection site reactions (redness, pain, bruising); body pain; hot flushes; general body discomfort; weakness; swelling of arms and legs; allergic reaction; weight loss; abnormal blood cell counts; back, chest, limb, neck and bone pain; muscle-bone disorder; decreased sex drive; sore throat; swollen lymph glands; liver tenderness/enlargement; infection; abnormal thyroid tests.

Guidelines for Use:

- Follow the injection procedure taught to you by your health care provider. This drug must be given subcutaneously (SC) (beneath the skin).
- Inject this medicine as a single dose 3 times a week. At least 48 hours should elapse between doses. The dose varies depending on individual needs.
- Flu-like side effects may be treated with nonnarcotic analgesics (eg, ibuprofen).
- If flu-like side effects are bothersome, administration at bedtime may lessen the problem.
- Follow proper disposal procedure for used syringes and needles.
- May be warmed to room temperature before injecting.
- Do not use if contents of the vial are discolored or have particulate matter.
- Use each vial only once. Discard any unused solution. Do not save unused solution for later use.
- Do not stop taking this medicine or change the dose unless advised by your doctor.
- Do not use other forms of interferon without consulting your pharmacist or doctor. Products manufactured by different companies may not be equally effective.
- Temporarily discontinue the dosage if severe adverse reactions occur. If the reaction does not become tolerable, the dosage may be reduced or discontinued as recommended by your doctor.
- Notify your doctor immediately if you experience depression, unusual bleeding or bruising, fever, or infection.
- Lab tests are recommended to monitor treatment. Be sure to keep appointments.
- Visual exams are recommended before therapy begins in patients with diabetes mellitus or hypertension.
- Store in the refrigerator (36° to 46°F). Do not freeze. Avoid vigorous shaking.

If you have any questions, consult your doctor, pharmacist, or health care provider.

	Generic Name *Brand Name Example*	Supplied As	Generic Available
Rx	**Interferon gamma-1b**		
	Actimmune[1]	**Injection:** 100 mcg (2 million IU)/0.5 mL	No

[1] Contains mannitol, sodium succinate, and polysorbate 20.

Type of Drug:

Miscellaneous anti-infective; biologic response modifier.

How the Drug Works:

Interferon gamma-1b appears to alter the body's natural defense against the causes of certain diseases.

Uses:

For reducing the frequency and severity of serious infections associated with chronic granulomatous disease.

For delaying time to disease progression in patients with severe, malignant osteopetrosis (bone overgrowth).

Precautions:

Do not use in the following situations: Allergy to interferon-gamma, *E. coli*-derived products, or any component of this medicine.

Use with caution in the following situations:

bone marrow suppression
central nervous system disorders
heart disease
seizure disorder

Pregnancy: There are no adequate and well-controlled studies in pregnant women. Use only if clearly needed and the potential benefits to the mother outweigh the possible hazards to the fetus.

Breastfeeding: It is not known if interferon gamma-1b appears in breast milk. Consult your doctor before you begin breastfeeding.

Children: Safety and effectiveness for use in children under 1 year of age have not been established.

Lab tests will be required during treatment. Tests may include blood cell counts, liver and kidney function tests, and urinalysis.

Drug Interactions:

Tell your doctor or pharmacist if you are taking or if you are planning to take any over-the-counter or prescription medications or dietary supplements while taking interferon gamma-1b. Doses of one or both drugs may need to be modified or a different drug may need to be prescribed. The following drugs and drug classes interact with interferon gamma-1b:

agents metabolized by cytochrome P450 pathway (eg, theophylline)
bone marrow suppressants (eg, azathioprine)

Side Effects:

Every drug is capable of producing side effects. Many interferon gamma-1b users experience no, or minor, side effects. The frequency and severity of side effects depend on many factors including dose, duration of therapy, and individual susceptibility. Possible side effects include:

Digestive Tract: Vomiting; nausea; diarrhea; stomach pain.

Nervous System: Depression; headache.

Other: Flu-like symptoms; fever; chills; rash; redness, tenderness, or pain at injection site; fatigue; joint or muscle pain.

Guidelines for Use:

- Dosage is individualized. Take exactly as prescribed.
- For subcutaneous (beneath the skin) injection only.
- Visually inspect the solution for discoloration or particles. Do not use the solution if particles or discoloration are seen.
- Follow the preparation and injection procedures taught to you by your health care provider.
- If flu-like side effects are bothersome, administering your dose at bedtime may lessen the problem.
- Acetaminophen (eg, *Tylenol*) can be used before the injection to prevent or partially alleviate the fever and headache associated with therapy.
- Follow proper disposal procedures for used syringes and needles.
- Use each vial only once. Discard any unused solution. Do not save unused solution for later use.
- Lab tests will be required to monitor treatment. Be sure to keep appointments.
- Refrigerate immediately (36° to 46°F). Do not freeze or shake. If left at room temperature for more than 12 hours, discard the vial. Do not use after the expiration date stamped on the vial.

If you have any questions, consult your doctor, pharmacist, or health care provider.

	Generic Name *Brand Name Examples*	Supplied As	Generic Available
Rx	**Crotamiton**		
	Eurax	**Cream:** 10%	No
	Eurax	**Lotion:** 10%	No
Rx	**Lindane (Gamma Benzene Hexachloride)**	**Lotion:** 1%	Yes
		Shampoo: 1%	Yes
Rx	**Malathion**		
	Ovide	**Lotion:** 0.5%	No
Rx/ *otc*[1]	**Permethrin**[2]	**Lotion:** 1%	Yes
Rx	*Acticin, Elimite*	**Cream:** 5%	Yes
otc	*Nix*[2]	**Liquid (cream rinse):** 1%	No
otc	**Pyrethrins**[3]		
	Tisit	**Liquid:** 0.3%	No
	Tisit[4]	**Shampoo:** 0.3%	No
	A-200,[4] *Clear Total Lice Elimination System,*[5] *Pronto,*[6] *Pyrinyl Plus,*[2] *R&C,*[2] *RID*[7]	**Shampoo:** 0.33%	No
	A-200[2]	**Gel:** 0.33%	No
	RID	**Mousse:** 0.33%	No

[1] This product is available *Rx* or *otc*, depending on package labeling.
[2] In kit containing removal comb.
[3] Available only in combination with piperonyl butoxide.
[4] Available in kits containing comb or spray.
[5] In kit containing lice egg remover and comb.
[6] Available in kits containing comb, creme rinse, spray, disposable gloves, magnifying glass, or hair separators.
[7] Available in kits containing spray or gel.

Type of Drug:

Scabicides; pediculicides; drugs for lice, crabs, and scabies.

How the Drug Works:

It is not clear how these drugs kill lice. They may attack the nervous system of the adult parasite and the developing nervous system of the egg. Pyrethrins are used only in combination with piperonyl butoxide, a product that enhances the effectiveness.

Uses:

Crotamiton: To treat scabies and relieve nonspecific itching of skin.

Lindane: To treat head lice and crab (pubic) lice and their eggs. The lotion is also indicated for scabies.

Malathion: To treat head lice and their eggs.

Permethrin: The cream is used to treat scabies. The lotion and liquid are used to treat head lice and their eggs.

Pyrethrins: To treat head, body, and crab (pubic) lice and their eggs.

Precautions:

Do not use in the following situations:

- allergy to any ingredient in the product
- primary irritation to topical medicines
- skin irritation, skin infection

Use with caution in the following situations:

- allergy to ragweed (pyrethrins only)
- asthma or breathing difficulty

Pregnancy: Adequate studies have not been done in pregnant women. Potential effects on the fetus are unknown. Studies in pregnant women or in animals have been judged not to show a risk to the fetus in individuals using permethrin. However, use during pregnancy only if clearly needed.

Breastfeeding: It is not known if these products appear in breast milk. Consult your doctor before you begin breastfeeding.

Children: Crotamiton - Safety and effectiveness in children have not been established.

Permethrin – Safety and effectiveness in children under 2 months have not been established.

Drug Interactions:

Tell your doctor or pharmacist if you are using or if you are planning to use any over-the-counter or prescription medications. One or both drugs may need to be modified or a different drug may need to be prescribed.

Side Effects:

Every drug is capable of producing side effects. Many scabicide/pediculicide users experience no, or minor, side effects. The frequency and severity of side effects depend on many factors including dose, duration of therapy, and individual susceptibility. Possible side effects include:

Skin: Allergic skin irritation; burning; itching; stinging; redness; tingling; numbness; swelling; rash; discomfort.

Guidelines for Use:

- For external use only.
- Patient instructions and information are available with the product. Do not exceed the prescribed dosage.
- Avoid contact with open cuts, eyes, nose, mouth or other mucous membranes, acutely inflamed skin, or raw skin oozing a liquid.
- If contact occurs between the eye and the drug, flush the eye thoroughly with tap water for several minutes.
- Contact your doctor if the condition being treated worsens or if itching, stinging, redness, burning, swelling, or skin rash occurs.
- Discontinue use if severe irritation or sensitization develops.
- Consult a doctor if infestation of eyebrows or eyelashes occurs.
- Shake liquids and shampoos well before use.
- Change clothing and bed linens the morning following application. Patients should maintain proper hygiene (eg, routine bathing).
- Sexual partners of infected individuals should be treated to avoid infection.
- Frequency of application and length of treatment depends on the condition being treated, drug utilized, strength of the drug and dosage form employed. For assistance in product selection and dosage guidelines, consult your pharmacist or doctor.

If you have any questions, consult your doctor, pharmacist, or health care provider.

Immune Globulins, 1249

Monoclonal Antibody
Palivizumab, 1256

Agents for Active Immunization, 1258

Vaccines
Rabies, 1262
Diphtheria/Tetanus/Pertussis, 1264
Hemophilus b, 1268
Diphtheria/Tetanus/Pertussis/Hemophilus b, 1271
Polio, 1273
Measles, Mumps and Rubella Virus, 1277
Varicella, 1280
Influenza, 1282
Hepatitis A, 1286
Hepatitis B, 1289
Hepatitis A/Hepatitis B, 1293
Pneumococcal, 1296
Lyme Disease, 1299
Pneumococcal 7-Valent Conjugate, 1302

Tuberculin Tests, 1304

	Generic Name *Brand Name Examples*	**Uses**
Rx	**Antithymocyte Globulin (Rabbit) (ATG Rabbit)** *Thymoglobulin*	*Kidney transplant rejection:* For treatment in conjunction with other immunosuppressant therapy.
Rx	**Cytomegalovirus Immune Globulin Intravenous (Human) (CMV-IGIV)** *CytoGam*	*Cytomegalovirus (CMV):* To prevent CMV disease associated with kidney, lung, liver, pancreas, or heart transplantation.
Rx	**Hepatitis B Immune Globulin (Human) (HBIG)** *BayHep B,* *Nabi-HB*	*For postexposure:* Prevention of hepatitis B infection following exposure (eg, by accidental "needle-stick", splash, sexual exposure, oral ingestion) to hepatitis B-positive materials such as blood. *For infants* born to hepatitis B-positive mothers. *For individuals who are at high risk of hepatitis B infection:* Protection is achieved when HBIG is given before, or at the same time as, active immunization for hepatitis B with hepatitis B vaccine.
Rx	**Immune Globulin (Human) (IG; IGIM; Gamma Globulin; IgG)** *BayGam*	*Hepatitis A:* To prevent hepatitis A when given before or within 2 weeks after exposure. Not for patients with symptoms of hepatitis or those exposed more than 2 weeks previously. *Measles (Rubeola):* To prevent measles in patients (who have not been vaccinated or had measles previously) exposed < 6 days previously. *Immunoglobulin deficiency:* May prevent serious infection in patients who are unable to produce sufficient amounts of protective antibodies (IgG antibodies). *Varicella (chickenpox) in immunosuppressed patients:* If varicella-zoster immune globulin is unavailable, IGIM may be used for passive immunization.

	Generic Name *Brand Name Examples*	Uses
	Immune Globulin (Human) (IG; IGIM; Gamma Globulin; IgG) (cont.)	*Rubella:* Some studies suggest use in susceptible pregnant women exposed to rubella can lessen the likelihood of infection and fetal damage.
Rx	**Immune Globulin Intravenous (Human) (IGIV)** *Gamimune N, Gammagard S/D, Gammar-P I.V., Iveegam, Panglobulin, Polygam S/D, Sandoglobulin, Venoglobulin-S*	*Immunodeficiency syndrome:* For maintenance treatment of patients who are unable to produce sufficient amounts of protective antibodies (IgG antibodies) to prevent infection. *Idiopathic thrombocytopenic purpura (ITP), acute and chronic (Gamimune N, Gammagard S/D, Panglobulin, Polygam S/D, Sandoglobulin, Venoglobulin-S):* To create a rapid but temporary rise in the platelet count (platelets aid in clotting blood), to prevent or control bleeding, and to allow a patient with ITP to undergo surgery. Not all patients will respond. *B-cell chronic lymphocytic leukemia (CLL) (Gammagard S/D, Polygam S/D):* For prevention of bacterial infections in patients with hypogammaglobulinemia and/or recurrent bacterial infections associated with B-cell CLL. *Kawasaki syndrome (Gammagard S/D, Iveegam, Polygam S/D, Venoglobulin-S):* In conjunction with high dose aspirin for the prevention of coronary artery aneurysms associated with Kawasaki syndrome. *Bone marrow transplantation (Gamimune N):* Prevention of septicemia (blood poisoning), pneumonia, and acute graft-vs-host disease in transplant patients ≥ 20 years of age.

	Generic Name *Brand Name Examples*	Uses
	Immune Globulin Intravenous (Human) (IGIV) (cont.)	*Pediatric HIV infection (Gamimune N):* To decrease the frequency of serious and minor bacterial infections, the frequency of hospitalization, and to increase the time free of serious bacterial infections in children with evidence of HIV disease.
Rx	**Lymphocyte Immune Globulin, Antithymocyte Globulin (Equine), (LIG, ATG)** *Atgam*	*Kidney transplant rejection:* To manage allograft rejection or as an adjunct to other immunosuppressive therapy to delay onset of allograft rejection. *Aplastic anemia:* To treat moderate to severe cases in patients who are unsuitable for bone marrow transplantation.
Rx	**Rabies Immune Globulin (Human) (RIG)** *BayRab,* *Imogam Rabies-HT*	*Rabies exposure:* In conjunction with rabies vaccine to treat patients suspected of exposure to rabies, particularly severe exposure (but not people who have previously been immunized with HDCY rabies vaccine in a pre- or postexposure treatment series).
Rx	**Respiratory Syncytial Virus Immune Globulin Intravenous (Human) (RSV-IGIV)** *RespiGam*	*Respiratory Syncytial Virus (RSV):* To prevent serious lower respiratory tract infection caused by RSV in children < 24 months of age with bronchopulmonary dysplasia (BPD) or a history of premature birth (≤ 35 weeks gestation).
Rx	**Rh_o(D) Immune Globulin (Human)** *BayRho-D Full Dose,* *RhoGAM*	*Full-term delivery:* To prevent hemolytic disease of the newborn. Used within 72 hours of birth in a Rh_o(D)-negative mother not previously exposed to the Rh_o(D)-positive factor who has delivered a Rh_o(D)-positive baby. Also used in certain Rh_o(D)-negative patients after incomplete pregnancy or transfusions of Rh incompatible blood or blood products.

	Generic Name *Brand Name Examples*	Uses
Rx	**Rh_o(D) Immune Globulin Micro-Dose (Rh_o[D] IG Micro-dose)** *BayRho-D Mini Dose, MICRhoGAM*	*Incomplete pregnancy (of ≤ 12 weeks gestation) or transfusions:* Prevents isoimmunization of Rh_o(D)-negative women when the father is not known to be Rh_o(D) negative.
Rx	**Rh_o(D) Immune Globulin IV (Human)** *WinRho SDF*	*Full-term delivery:* To prevent Rh isoimmunization of the mother when a Rh_o(D)-negative mother not previously exposed to the Rh_o(D)-positive factor has a Rh_o(D)-positive baby. Also used in certain Rh_o(D)-negative women after incomplete pregnancy or transfusions with Rh_o(D)-positive blood or blood products. *Immune Thrombocytopenic Purpura (ITP):* To increase platelet count and to control excessive bleeding in Rh_o(D)-positive children with chronic or acute ITP, adults with chronic ITP, or anyone with ITP secondary to HIV.
Rx	**Tetanus Immune Globulin (Human) (TIG)** *BayTet*	*Tetanus:* Prevention of tetanus following injury in patients whose tetanus immunization is incomplete or uncertain. Also indicated in the regimen of treatment of active cases of tetanus.
Rx	**Varicella-Zoster Immune Globulin (Human) (VZIG)**	*Varicella-Zoster:* For passive immunization of exposed, susceptible patients who are at greater risk of complications from varicella (chickenpox or zoster) than healthy individuals (eg, immunocompromised patients, newborns of mothers with varicella shortly before or after delivery, premature infants, normal, susceptible adults, susceptible high-risk infants < 1 year of age).

Type of Drug:

Immune globulins; antibodies.

How the Drug Works:

Passive immunization: Most immune globulins contain antibodies from plasma obtained from human blood donors. LIG, ATG contains antibodies derived from horse (equine) serum and ATG rabbit contains antibodies derived from rabbit serum. Administration of immune serums temporarily increases the antibody concentration in the person receiving the serum. Protection derived from these products will be of rapid onset, but will only protect for a short period of time (1 week to 3 months).

Precautions:

Do not use in the following situations:

allergic response to antithymocyte globulin (equine) or other equine immunoglobulin preparations (LIG, ATG equine only)
allergic response to gamma globulin or anti-immunoglobulin A (IgA) antibodies
allergic response to human immunoglobulin preparation
allergic response to rabbit proteins (ATG rabbit only)
immunoglobulin A (IgA) deficiency
pregnancy after 12 weeks gestation (Rh_o(D) IG micro-dose only)
viral illness, acute (ATG rabbit only)

Use with caution in the following situations:

bleeding disorder (IM administration only)
cardiovascular disease, history of (IGIV products only)
diabetes mellitus (IGIV products only)
kidney disease, pre-existing (IGIV products only)
nephrotoxic drug therapy (IGIV products only)
older than 65 years of age (IGIV products only)
paraproteinemia (IGIV products only)
sepsis (IGIV products only)
thrombocytopenia (IGIV products only)
thrombotic episodes (IGIV products only)
volume depletion (IGIV products only)

Infectious agents: Products made from human plasma may contain infectious agents, such as viruses that can cause disease. Multiple steps are taken to remove all infectious agents from these products but there is a very small possibility that unknown infectious agents may still be present. Discuss the risks and benefits with your health care provider.

Pregnancy: There are no adequate and well-controlled studies in pregnant women. Use only if clearly needed and the potential benefits to the mother outweigh the possible hazards to the fetus. *BayRho-D Mini-Dose* is not indicated for use during pregnancy and it should be administered only postabortion or postmiscarriage of 12 weeks or less gestation.

Breastfeeding: It is not known if immune globulins appear in breast milk. Safety has not been established. Consult your doctor before you begin breastfeeding.

Children: Safety and effectiveness have not been established in children. Do not inject infants with Rh_o(D) IGIV, Rh_o(D) IGIM, or Rh_o(D) IG micro-dose. RSV-IGIV is indicated for use in children < 24 months of age; however, safety and effectiveness in children with congenital heart disease have not been established.

Lab tests may be required to monitor therapy. Tests include kidney function, urine output, and blood counts.

Drug Interactions:

Live virus vaccines are typically recommended for administration at least 2 weeks before or 3 months after administration of immune serums. The immune serum may reduce the effectiveness of the vaccine. It may be necessary to revaccinate people who received immune serums shortly after live virus vaccination. Consult the specific product information on guidelines for administering vaccines before or after use of an immune globulin.

Side Effects:

Modern immune sera and immune globulins are generally safe and effective. Many immune globulin recipients experience no, or minor, local side effects. The severity of side effects depends on many factors including dose and individual susceptibility. Possible side effects include:

Local: Hives; swelling; itching; muscle stiffness; tenderness, pain, redness, heat, burning, ache, or irritation at injection site.

Nervous System: Headache; dizziness; anxiety; night sweats; lightheadedness; fatigue; shaking; agitation; lethargy; listlessness.

Digestive Tract: Vomiting; nausea; diarrhea; stomach pain; inflammation of the mouth; sore mouth or throat; mouth sores.

Circulatory System: Irregular heartbeat; inflammation of muscular walls of the heart; congestive heart failure; chest tightness; abnormal blood counts; clotted A/V fistula; change in blood pressure; change in heart rate; low oxygen concentration in blood.

Other: General body discomfort; enlarged liver or spleen; seizures; difficulty breathing; sweating; wheezing; pounding in the chest; joint stiffness; burning soles or palms; foot sole pain; abnormal liver or kidney function tests; serum sickness-like symptoms; nosebleed; tender or swollen lymph nodes; rash; pneumonia; fluid retention; urinary tract infection; vaginal infection; bluish discoloration of the skin; herpes simplex infection; weakness; fever; chills; flushing; swelling of feet and ankles; muscle cramps; back, joint, muscle, chest, hip, neck, flank, or leg pain.

Guidelines for Use:

- These immune globulins will be prepared and administered by your health care provider in a medical setting.
- Live virus vaccines are not typically recommended for administration within 3 months of immune globulin administration. In some cases, this period may be longer. Consult the specific product information for administration guidelines. It may be necessary to revaccinate persons who received immune globulin shortly after live virus vaccination.
- Protection received from these immunizations will be of rapid onset, but short duration (generally 1 week to 3 months).
- Immediate allergic reactions (eg, anaphylaxis) are a possibility. If an allergic reaction occurs, your health care provider will discontinue the immune globulin and provide emergency treatment as indicated.
- Serum sickness-like reactions (skin rashes with inflammation, pain in the joints, and fever) have been reported in aplastic anemia patients administered *Atgam*. Resolution of symptoms is generally prompt and long-term sequelae have not been observed. Administration of corticosteroids may decrease the frequency of this reaction.
- Aseptic meningitis syndrome (AMS) has been reported to occur infrequently in association with Immune Globulin Intravenous (IGIV) treatment. The syndrome usually begins within several hours to 2 days following treatment. It is characterized by severe headache, neck stiffness, drowsiness, fever, eye sensitivity to light, painful eye movements, nausea, and vomiting. Contact your doctor immediately if you notice any of these symptoms. AMS may occur more frequently in association with high-dose treatment. Discontinuation of IGIV treatment has resulted in remission of AMS within several days.
- Kidney dysfunction has been reported in association with treatment with IGIV products. Notify your doctor immediately if you experience decreased urination, sudden weight gain, fluid retention or swelling, or shortness of breath.
- Local reactions to injections may occur (eg, tenderness, pain, burning, irritation). Application of a warm compress may alleviate symptoms. If these persist or become bothersome, contact your doctor.
- *LIG, ATG* — A skin test is usually performed before the first dose to check for possible allergy to serum.
- Lab tests will be required to monitor therapy. Be sure to keep appointments.

If you have any questions, consult your doctor, pharmacist, or health care provider.

	Generic Name *Brand Name Examples*	How Supplied	Generic Available
Rx	**Palivizumab**		
	Synagis	**Powder for injection:** 100 mg[1]	No

[1] Lyophilized.

Type of Drug:

Antiviral drug for treatment of respiratory syncytial virus (RSV) infection.

How the Drug Works:

Palivizumab is an immune system protein which is designed to be highly specific for the RSV virus to inhibit viral replication.

Uses:

For the prevention of serious lower respiratory tract disease caused by respiratory syncytial virus (RSV) in pediatric patients at high risk.

Safety and effectiveness were established in infants with bronchopulmonary dysplasia (BPD) and in infants with a history of prematurity (≤ 35 weeks gestational age).

Precautions:

Do not use in the following situations:
allergy to this product or its components

Use with caution in the following situations:
abnormal blood clotting
low blood platelets

Pregnancy: It is not known if palivizumab causes fetal harm. Palivizumab is not indicated for use in adults.

Drug Interactions:

Tell your doctor or pharmacist if you are giving or plan to give your baby any over-the-counter or prescription medications while giving palivizumab. Doses of one or both drugs may need to be modified or a different drug may need to be prescribed.

Side Effects:

Every drug is capable of producing side effects. Many palivizumab users experience no, or minor, side effects. The frequency and severity of side effects depend on many factors including dose, duration of therapy, and individual susceptibility. Possible side effects include:

Digestive Tract: Diarrhea; stomach irritation; vomiting.

Respiratory System: Upper respiratory tract infection due to other organisms; runny nose; asthma; sore throat; bronchitis; cough; wheezing; croup; pneumonia; difficulty breathing; sinus infection.

Skin: Fungal skin inflammation; itching; oily skin; rash; injection site redness and pain.

Other: Ear infection; hernia; failure to thrive; nervousness; abnormal liver function tests; eye redness or inflammation; other viral infections; mouth infection; anemia; flu-like syndrome; mouth sores.

Guidelines for Use:

- Palivizumab is not indicated for adult use.
- Palivizumab will be administered by a health care professional and should be administered exactly as prescribed. It is for IM use only.
- *Preparation of solution* — Slowly add 1 mL Sterile Water for Injection to 100 mg vial. Gently swirl for 30 seconds; avoid foaming. Do not shake. Allow reconstituted solution to stand at room temperature for a minimum of 20 minutes until the solution becomes clear. Administer within 6 hours of reconstitution.
- This drug is for IM administration only, preferably injected in the front part of the thigh. The buttocks (gluteal region) should not be used as a regular injection site because of the risk of damage to the sciatic nerve.
- The recommended dose is 15 mg/kg body weight. The first dose should be administered IM prior to the beginning of the RSV season (November through April in the northern hemisphere). Patients, including those who develop an RSV infection, should receive monthly doses throughout the RSV season.
- This medication is designed to prevent RSV infection. It is not used to treat an established RSV infection.
- Store unreconstituted vial at 35° to 46°F. Do not freeze. Do not use after expiration date.

If you have any questions, consult your doctor, pharmacist, or health care provider.

Recommended childhood vaccination schedule – United States, 2002

Range of recommended ages for vaccination	Vaccines to be assessed and administered if necessary to catch-up	Preadolescent assessment

Vaccine	Birth	1 Mo.	2 Mos.	4 Mos.	6 Mos.	12 Mos.	15 Mos.	18 Mos.	24 Mos.	4-6 Yrs.	11-12 Yrs.	13-18 Yrs.
Hepatitis B[1]	Hep B #1											
		Hep B #2			Hep B #3				Hep B series			
Diphtheria Tetanus, Pertussis[2]			DTaP	DTaP	DTaP		DTaP			DTaP	Td	
Haemophilus influenzae type b[3]			Hib	Hib	Hib	Hib						
Inactivated Polio[4]			IPV	IPV	IPV					IPV		
Measles, Mumps, Rubella[5]						MMR #1				MMR #2	MMR #2	
Varicella[6]						Varicella			Varicella			
Pneumococcal[7]			PCV	PCV	PCV	PCV			PCV		PPV	
Hepatitis A[8]									Hep A series			
Influenza[9]					Influenza (yearly)							

This schedule indicates the recommended ages for routine administration of currently licensed childhood vaccines as of December 1, 2001, for children through 18 years of age. Any dose not given at the recommended age should be given at any subsequent visit when indicated and feasible. Additional vaccines may be licensed and recommended during the year. Licensed combination vaccines may be used whenever any components of the combination are indicated and its other components are not contraindicated. Providers should consult the manufacturers' package inserts for detailed recommendations.

Approved by the Advisory Committee on Immunization Practices (www.cdc.gov/nip/acip), the American Academy of Pediatrics (www.aap.org), and the American Academy of Family Physicians (www.aafp.org).

[1] **Hepatitis B vaccine (Hep B):** All infants should receive the first dose of Hep B soon after birth and before hospital discharge; the first dose may also be given by 2 months of age if the infant's mother is HBsAg-negative. Only monovalent Hep B can be used for the birth dose. Monovalent or combination vaccine containing Hep B may be used to complete the series; 4 doses of vaccine may be administered if combination vaccine is used. The second dose should be given at least 4 weeks after the first dose, except for Hib-containing vaccine, which cannot be administered before 6 weeks of age. The third dose should be given at least 16 weeks after the first dose and at least 8 weeks after the second dose. The last dose in the vaccination series (third or fourth dose) should not be administered before 6 months of age.

Infants born to HBsAg-positive mothers should receive Hep B and 0.5 mL hepatitis B immune globulin (HBIG) at separate sites within 12 hours of birth. The second dose is recommended at 1 to 2 months of age and the vaccination series should be completed (third or fourth dose) at 6 months of age.

Infants born to mothers whose HBsAg status is unknown should receive the first dose of Hep B within 12 hours of birth. Maternal blood should be drawn at the time of delivery to determine the mother's HBsAg status; if the HBsAg test is positive, the infant should receive HBIG as soon as possible (no later than 1 week of age).

[2] **Diphtheria and tetanus toxoids and acellular pertussis vaccine (DTaP):** The fourth dose of DTaP may be administered as early as 12 months of age, provided 6 months have elapsed since the third dose and if the child is unlikely to return at 15 to 18 months of age. Tetanus and diphtheria toxoids (Td) is recommended at 11 to 12 years of age if at least 5 years have elapsed since the last dose of tetanus and diptheria toxoid-containing vaccine. Subsequent routine Td boosters are recommended every 10 years.

[3] ***Haemophilus influenzae* type b (Hib) conjugate vaccine:** Three Hib conjugate vaccines are licensed for infant use. If PRP-OMP (*PedvaxHIB* or *ComVax* [Merck]) is administered at 2 to 4 months of age, a dose at 6 months of age is not required. DTaP/Hib combination products should not be used for primary immunization in infants at 2, 4, or 6 months of age, but can be used as boosters following any Hib vaccine.

[4] **Inactivated polio vaccine (IPV):** An all-IPV schedule is recommended for routine childhood polio vaccination in the US. All children should receive 4 doses of IPV at 2, 4, 6 to 18 months, and 4 to 6 years of age.

[5] **Measles, mumps, and rubella vaccine (MMR):** The second dose of MMR is recommended routinely at 4 to 6 years of age but may be administered during any visit, provided at least 4 weeks have elapsed since the first dose and that both doses are administered beginning at or after 12 months of age. Those who have not previously received the second dose should complete the schedule by 11 to 12 years of age visit.

[6] **Varicella vaccine:** Varicella vaccine is recommended at any visit at or after 12 months of age for susceptible children (ie, those who lack a reliable history of chickenpox). Susceptible patients > 13 years of age should receive 2 doses, given at least 4 weeks apart.

[7] **Pneumococcal vaccine:** The heptavalent pneumococcal conjugate vaccine (PCV) is recommended for all children 2 to 23 months of age. It also is recommended for certain children 24 to 59 months of age. Pneumoccocal polysaccharide vaccine (PPV) is recommended in additon to PCV for cerain high-risk groups. See *MMWR.* 2000:49(RR-9);1-35.

[8] **Hepatitis A vaccine:** Hepatitis A vaccine is recommended for use in selected states and regions, and for certain high-risk groups; consult the local public health authority. See *MMWR.* 1999:48(RR-12);1-37.

[9] **Influenza vaccine:** Influenza vaccine is recommended annually for children > 6 months of age with certain risk factors (eg, asthma, cardiac disease, sickle cell disease, HIV, diabetes) and can be administered to all others wishing to obtain immunity; see *MMWR.* 2001:50(RR-4);1-44. Children ≤ 12 years of age should receive vaccine in a dosage appropriate for their age (0.25 mL if 6 to 35 months of age or 0.5 mL if ≥ 3 years of age). Children ≤ 8 years who are receiving influenza vaccine for the first time should receive 2 doses separated by at least 4 weeks.

Type of Drug:

Bacterial and viral vaccines and toxoid injections; immunizations.

How the Drug Works:

Vaccines contain either killed or weakened viruses or bacteria that cause recipients to make their own protective antibodies against infection. Either partial or whole viruses and bacteria may be used. These viral or bacterial vaccines do not themselves cause disease, but are used to prevent disease. Toxoids are a kind of vaccine made by inactivating bacterial toxins. Toxoids are not toxic. Vaccines usually cause ≈ 80% to 99% of recipients to make protective antibodies. Vaccines usually lower the risk of infection 60% to 99%, depending on the type.

Active immunization with bacterial and viral vaccines and toxoids provides long-term protection (immunity) against various infections.

Uses:

See individual product descriptions.

Precautions:

Immune system diseases: Do not give live, weakened virus vaccines to people with immune deficiency diseases (reduced ability to produce antibodies and fight infection), and those with decreased ability for immune response (eg, leukemia, lymphoma, cancer, or therapy with corticosteroids, cancer drugs, or radiation).

Children with symptomatic AIDS: Do not give live-virus and live-bacterial vaccines to children or young adults with AIDS unless specifically recommended by the Advisory Committee on Immunization Practices (ACIP). After exposure to measles or chicken pox, these patients may receive passive immunization with immune globulin or varicella-zoster immune globulin.

Immunization with DTP, inactivated polio vaccine (IPV), *Haemophilus influenzae* type b, pneumococcal, and influenza (flu) vaccines is recommended, although immunization may be less effective than it would be for children with a normal immune system. Immunization with influenza and pneumococcal vaccines for children > 2 years of age is recommended.

Children with previously diagnosed with asymptomatic AIDS: Children with previously diagnosed AIDS, but without symptoms, have received live-virus vaccines without side effects. However, observe for possible side effects and for occurrence of vaccine-preventable diseases, because immunization may be less effective than for children with a normal immune system.

Do not use oral polio vaccine (OPV). Use IPV routinely to immunize these children or members of a household in which there is an HIV-positive patient. DTP, *Haemophilus influenzae* type b, and hepatitis B vaccines may be given in accordance with ACIP recommendations.

Simultaneous vaccinations: Most vaccines can be administered simultaneously at separate injection sites.

Illnesses with fever: Delay immunization of people with severe acute illness until the illness is treated.

Vaccination during pregnancy: Live, weakened virus vaccines are not generally given to pregnant women or to those likely to become pregnant within 3 months after receiving the vaccine(s). Do not give some of these vaccines during pregnancy, particularly rubella, measles, mumps, and varicella. When a vaccine is to be given during pregnancy, waiting until the second or third trimester to minimize any link to coincidental miscarriage is a reasonable precaution. However, there has been no evidence of congenital rubella syndrome in infants born to mothers who received rubella vaccine during pregnancy. Experience to date has not revealed any risks of other vaccines to the fetus.

Any vaccine may be given safely to children and other contacts of pregnant women.

Give vaccines against influenza, hepatitis B, meningococcal disease, tetanus, and diphtheria to pregnant women to adequately protect against these diseases in the mother or child.

Allergy to vaccine components: Vaccines produced in allergenic substances (eg, eggs) may cause allergic reactions. Therefore, do not give such vaccines (eg, influenza, yellow fever vaccines) to people with known allergy to these components. These vaccines are only rarely associated with serious allergic reactions.

Live virus vaccines prepared by growing viruses in cell cultures usually do not contain allergenic substances. On very rare occasions, allergic reactions to measles vaccine have been reported in persons with allergy to eggs. However, measles vaccine can be given safely to egg-allergic individuals provided the symptoms of the allergy are not severe. The same precautions apply to mumps vaccine.

Some vaccines contain preservatives (eg, thimerosal) or small amounts of antibiotics (eg, neomycin) to which patients may rarely be allergic.

Immunization for other diseases: Immunization for other diseases is recommended for people with a risk of exposure. Specific immunization requirements and recommendations for international travel can be obtained from the Superintendent of Documents, US Government Printing Office, Washington, DC, 20402 in the publication *Health Information for International Travel.*

Centers for Disease Control and Prevention (CDC):

Information Hotline	800–232–2522
International Travel Hotline	877–394–8747
Spanish Hotline	800–232–0233
CDC Web site	www.cdc.gov

Refer to the Immunization Gateway: Your Vaccine Fact-Finder at www.immunofacts.com for direct links to all the best vaccine resources on the Internet.

Side Effects:

Modern vaccines are extremely safe and effective. Side effects following immunization have been reported with all vaccines. These range from frequent, minor, local reactions to extremely rare, severe, bodily illness such as paralysis associated with oral polio vaccine. See individual product descriptions for details.

If you have any questions, consult your doctor, pharmacist, or health care provider.

	Generic Name *Brand Name Examples*	Uses
Rx	**Rabies Vaccine** *RabAvert*	For pre- and postexposure immunization against rabies. Preexposure immunization should be boosted periodically to provide continuous protection.

Individuals at high risk include: Veterinarians; animal handlers; wildlife officers; laboratory workers; travelers to high-risk areas; people whose activities bring them into contact with potentially rabid dogs, cats, foxes, skunks, bats or other species at risk of having rabies.

Carnivorous wild animals (especially skunks, raccoons, foxes and coyotes) and bats are the animals most commonly infected with rabies. Unless an animal is tested and shown not to be rabid, initiate postexposure vaccination.

The likelihood that a domestic dog or cat is infected with rabies varies from region to region; therefore so does the need for postexposure prophylaxis.

Rodents (eg, squirrels, hamsters, guinea pigs, gerbils, chipmunks, rats, mice) and lagomorphs (eg, rabbits, hares) are rarely infected with rabies and have not been shown to cause human rabies in the US. Contact the state and local health department before initiating postexposure antirabies prophylaxis.

An unprovoked attack is more likely than a provoked attack to indicate an animal is rabid. Consider bites inflicted when a person is attempting to feed or handle an apparently healthy animal to be "provoked."

Rabies is transmitted by introducing the virus into open cuts or wounds in skin or through mucous membranes. The likelihood of rabies infection varies with nature and extent of exposure. Consider two categories of exposure: 1) Bites, any penetration of the skin by teesth, to the face and hands have the highest risk, but the site of the bite should not influence the decision to begin treatment; 2) a non-bite can be scratches, abrasions, open wounds or mucous membranes contaminated with saliva or other potentially infectious material. Casual contact, such as petting, does not indicate prophylaxis.

Post-bite exposure may require use of both vaccine and immune globulin treatment.

Type of Drug:

Active immunization for rabies virus.

How the Drug Works:

Rabies vaccine provides long-term protection against rabies by stimulating the body to produce antibodies against the virus.

Precautions:

Do not use in the following situations: Allergy to egg, immediate reaction

Use with caution in the following situations:

- allergy to bovine gelatin, chicken protein, neomycin, chlortetracycline and amphotericin B
- convalescent
- infectious disease, active stage
- sick
- immunosuppressive illness

Pregnancy: Adequate studies have not been done pregnant women. Use only if clearly needed and potential benefits outweigh the possible risks.

Drug Interactions:

Tell your doctor or pharmacist if you are taking or if you are planning to take any over-the-counter or prescription medications with the rabies vaccine. Doses of one or both drugs may need to be modified or a different drug may need to be prescribed. The following drugs and drug classes interact with the rabies vaccine.

- antimalarials (eg, chloroquin)
- corticosteroids (eg, prednisone)
- immunosuppressive agents (eg, azathioprine, cyclosporine)

Side Effects:

Every drug is capable of producing side effects. Many patients experience no, or minor, side effects. The frequency and severity of side effects depend on many factors including dose, duration of therapy and individual susceptibility. Possible side effects include:

Local: Swelling; reddening; hardening; pain at the injection site; swollen lymph nodes.

Other: Headache; dizziness; general body discomfort; muscle pain; fever; swollen lymph nodes; GI problems.

Guidelines for Use:

- *Recommended vaccination schedule* —
  Preexposure: Usual regimen consists of three injections. The second and third doses are given 7 days and 21 or 28 days after the inital injection, respectively.
  Postexposure: Begin immunization as soon as possible after exposure. Usual regimen consists of five injections. The last four doses are given 3, 7, 14 and 28 days after the initial injection.
  Postexposure therapy of previously immunized people: Usual regimen consists of two injections, one immediately and one 3 days later.
- It is not guaranteed that the vaccine will protect everyone from rabies.
- *Booster doses:* Certain individuals who are at high risk of contracting rabies will need booster doses. Blood tests determine when the booster dose is due.
- The vaccine will be prepared and administered by a healthcare provider.

If you have any questions, consult your doctor, pharmacist, or health care provider.

	Generic Name *Brand Name Examples*	Uses
Rx	**Tetanus Toxoid Adsorbed**	For active immunization against tetanus in adults and children 2 months of age or older.
Rx	**Diphtheria and Tetanus Toxoids, Adsorbed Combined** *Pediatric (DT)*	For active immunization against diphtheria and tetanus in infants and children between 6 weeks and 7 years of age.
	Adult (Td)	For active immunization against diphtheria and tetanus in adults and children 7 years and older.
Rx	**Diphtheria and Tetanus Toxoids and Pertussis Vaccine (DTP, DPT, DTwP)** *Tri-Immunol*	For active immunization of infants and children between 6 weeks and 7 years of age against diphtheria, tetanus and pertussis (whooping cough).
Rx	**Diphtheria and Tetanus Toxoids and Acellular Pertussis Vaccine Adsorbed (DTaP)** *Acel-Imune* *Tripedia*	For active immunization of infants and children between 6 weeks and 7 years of age against diphtheria, tetanus and pertussis (whooping cough). *Unlabeled uses:* To immunize adults against pertussis.

Type of Drug:

Diphtheria, tetanus, pertussis vaccines (shots). Active immunization.

How the Drug Works:

These vaccines provide long-term protection against diphtheria, tetanus and pertussis by stimulating the body to produce antibodies against the organisms causing these infections.

Precautions:

Do not use in the following situations:

- allergy to thimerosal
- allergy to the vaccine or its components
- chemotherapy (cancer drugs)
- children over 7 years old (DT, DPT, DTaP)
- corticosteroids (eg, prednisone)
- illness, acute
- pertussis, history (DTaP, DTP, DPT, DTwP)
- polio outbreak
- radiation
- seizures or unconsciousness after a previous dose

Use with caution in the following situations:

- coagulation disorder
- convulsions (within 3 days of prior vaccine)
- fever, high (within 48 hours of prior vaccine)
- immune deficiency disorder
- infection, active
- nervous system disorder
- persistent crying, over 3 hours (within 48 hours of prior vaccine)
- seizures, family history
- shock (within 48 hours of prior vaccine)

Toxoids: Never use tetanus, pertussis or diphtheria toxoids to treat actual infections, nor for immediate protection of unimmunized people.

Fluid tetanus toxoid: Use fluid tetanus toxoid to immunize patients who are allergic to the adsorbed tetanus toxoid.

Immunodeficiency: People receiving corticosteroids, chemotherapy, radiation or with an immunodeficiency disorder (eg, AIDS) may not respond well to these vaccines. Defer vaccination until immunosuppressive therapy has ended, or give another dose 1 month after therapy has ended. However, vaccination of AIDS patients is recommended.

Nervous system complications, such as convulsions, degenerative diseases of the brain and diseases affecting the nerves, including Guillain-Barre Syndrome, and Sudden Infant Death Syndrome have been reported following administration of preparations containing diphtheria, tetanus and/or pertussis antigens. No cause and effect relationships have been established.

Pregnancy: Adequate studies have not been done in pregnant women, or animal studies may have shown a risk to the fetus. Tetanus toxoid is the preferred vaccine for pregnant women. It has been administered safely to thousands of pregnant women in an effort to prevent tetanus in newborns considered to be at high risk. Avoid unnecessary drugs and biologics in pregnant women, especially in the first trimester. Use tetanus toxoid only if clearly needed.

Breastfeeding: It is not known if these vaccines appear in breast milk. Consult your doctor before you begin breastfeeding.

Children: DTwP or DTaP is the recommended immunization for most children under 7 years of age. Safety and effectiveness of DTaP in children under 6 weeks of age has not been established. Tetanus toxoid may be used in children. However, for children 6 years of age and younger, DT (For Pediatric Use) is preferred to tetanus toxoid alone if pertussis vaccine is not indicated. For children 7 years of age and older, tetanus and diphtheria toxoids (Td) (For Adult Use) is preferred to tetanus toxoid alone.

Drug Interactions:

Tell your doctor or pharmacist if you are taking or if you are planning to take any over-the-counter or prescription medications while taking this medicine. Doses of one or both drugs may need to be modified or a different drug may need to be prescribed. The following drugs and drug classes interact with the medicine.

anticoagulants (eg, warfarin)
chloramphenicol (eg, *Chloromycetin)*
cimetidine (eg, *Tagamet)*
immunosuppressants (eg, cancer drugs)

Side Effects:

Every vaccine is capable of producing side effects. Many patients experience no, or minor, side effects. The frequency and severity of side effects depend on many factors including dose and individual susceptibility. Possible side effects include:

Local: Redness; warmth; hardening of skin; tenderness; swelling; nodules; abscess.

Other (moderate) – Fever; chills; appetite loss; drowsiness; vomiting; diarrhea; fussiness; general body discomfort; aches and pains; headache; flushing; rash; hives; itching; irritability; rapid heartbeat; low blood pressure; nasal congestion; muscle pain; degenerative brain disease; loss of consciousness; neurological problems.

Other (severe) – Fever of 105°F or higher; persistent crying lasting 3 hours or more; unusual high-pitched crying; collapse; shock-like state; seizures; convulsions with or without fever.

Guidelines for Use:

- *Primary immunization (DTaP, and DPT):* For children 6 weeks through 7 years (ideally beginning at age 6 weeks to 2 months). Given on three occasions at 4 to 8 week intervals with a fourth injection 6 to 12 months after the third injection.
- *Booster doses* are given when the child is 4 to 6 years of age (preferably prior to entering kindergarten or elementary school). However, if the fourth dose of the basic series was administered after the fourth birthday, a recall (booster) of DTaP, DT or DTP prior to school entry is not necessary.
- *Tetanus boosters:* After complete primary tetanus immunization, boosters — even for wound management — need to be given only every 10 years when wounds are minor and uncontaminated. For other wounds, a booster is appropriate if the patient has not received tetanus toxoid within the preceding 5 years. Administering booster doses more frequently than recommended may cause increased incidence and severity of reactions.
- Before the administration of any dose of vaccine, the parent, guardian or adult patient will be asked about the recent health status and immunization history of the patient being immunized in order to determine whether any problems may exist that would prevent vaccination.

Guidelines for Use (cont.):

- *Tetanus boosters:* (cont.)
- When the patient returns for the next dose in a series, he or she should be questioned concerning the occurrence of any symptoms or side effects after the previous dose.
- *Tetanus and Diphtheria Toxoids Adsorbed For Adult Use* is the preferred preparation for active tetanus immunization in wound management of patients 7 years of age or older. This is to enhance diphtheria protection. Given on two occasions at 4- to 8-week intervals with a third injection 6 to 12 months after the second injection.
- Delay vaccination when infections are present. Only healthy individuals should be injected. Delay voluntary immunization of patients during a polio outbreak.
- Never use diphtheria, pertussis or tetanus toxoids to treat actual tetanus, diphtheria or pertussis (whooping cough) infections.
- Tetanus or diphtheria infection does not ensure immunity; initiation or completion of vaccination is required at the time of recovery from these infections. However, children who have recovered from pertussis do not need further pertussis vaccination.
- Patients receiving corticosteroids, chemotherapy or radiation, and those with a recent injection of immune globulin or an immunodeficiency disorder (eg, AIDS) may not respond well to active immunization. When possible, interrupt treatment of these conditions when immunization is considered due to a tetanus-prone wound.
- If any of the following occurs after administration, contact your doctor immediately and avoid further use of this product: Allergy to any component of the vaccine including thimerosal, fever of 105°F or greater within 48 hours of injection, collapse or shock, crying lasting 3 hours or more, unusual high-pitched crying occurring within 48 hours, seizures with or without fever within 3 days or nervous system symptoms including unconsciousness occurring within 7 days.
- *DPT* — Not recommended for use in adults or in children over 7 years of age.
- Fever, chills, crying, aching and redness and tenderness at the injection site may occur following vaccination. Contact your doctor if these symptoms persist or become bothersome.
- Vaccination may not result in development of antibodies in all individuals.
- Do not give a pertussis-containing vaccine within 3 days of the influenza vaccine.
- Acetaminophen *(Tylenol)* may be given at time of vaccination and every 4 to 6 hours to reduce post-vaccination fever.

If you have any questions, consult your doctor, pharmacist, or health care provider.

	Generic Name Brand NameExamples	Uses
Rx	**Haemophilus b Conjugate Vaccine** *ActHIB*, *Hib TITER*, *OmniHIB*, *PedvaxHIB*, *ProHIBiT*	*ActHIB and OmniHIB:* for the routine immunization of children 2 months to 5 years of age. *Hib TITER and PedvaxHIB:*For the routine immunization of children 2 to 71 months of age. *ProHIBiT:* For the routine immunization of children 15 months to 5 years of age or as a booster vaccination of children 12 to 15 months of age. These vaccines will not protect against *Haemophilus influenzae* other than type b or other bacteria or viruses that cause meningitis or other infections.

Haemophilus influenzae type b (Haemophilus b) is a leading cause of serious bacterial infections in the US. Most cases of H. *influenzae* meningitis among children are caused by type b. In addition to meningitis, Haemophilus b is responsible for other diseases, including epiglottitis, sepsis, septic arthritis, osteomyelitis, pericarditis and pneumonia.

Approximately 17% of all cases of Haemophilus b disease occur in infants less than 6 months of age, 47% by 1 year of age and the remaining 53% over the next 4 years. Peak incidence occurs between 6 and 11 months of age. Incidence rates of Hib disease are increased in high risk groups, such as Native Americans, blacks, low-income individuals, household contacts of cases, caucasians who lack the G2m (n or 23) immunoglobulin allotype and patients with asplenia, sickle cell disease, Hodgkin's disease and immune deficiency syndromes. Recent studies suggest that risk for children under 5 acquiring Hib disease appears greater for those who attend daycare facilities than for those who do not.

Type of Drug:

Active immunization for *Haemophilus influenzae* type b infections.

How the Drug Works:

Hemophilus b vaccine provides long-term protection against *H. influenzae* type b by stimulating the body to produce antibodies to the organism.

Precautions:

Do not use in the following situations:

allergy to components of vaccine (eg, diphtheria and tetanus toxoids, meningococcal proteins, pertussis vaccine)
allergy to thimerosal (eg, *Mercurochrome*)

Use with caution in the following situations:

- blood clotting disorders
- chemotherapy (cancer drugs)
- fever
- immune deficiency disorders (decreased antibody production)
- immunosuppressive therapy
- infection, active
- radiation therapy

Pregnancy: Adequate studies have not been done in pregnant women, or animal studies may have shown a risk to the fetus. Use is not recommended. Use only if clearly needed and potential benefits outweigh the possible hazards to the fetus.

Children: Hib TITER and *PedvaxHIB* are not recommended in children younger than 2 months of age; however, the vaccine may sometimes be given as early as 6 weeks of age. *ProHIBiT* is not recommended for use in children younger than 12 months of age. *ActHIB* and *OmniHIB* are not recommended in children younger than 6 weeks of age.

Drug Interactions:

Tell your doctor or pharmacist if you are taking or planning to take any over-the-counter or prescription medication while receiving this vaccine. The following drugs and drug classes interact with this vaccine:

- anticoagulants (eg, warfarin)
- immunosuppressive agents (eg, corticosteroids)

Side Effects:

Every vaccine is capable of producing side effects. Many patients experience no, or minor, side effects. The frequency and severity of side effects depend on many factors including dose and individual susceptibility. Possible side effects include:

Local: Redness; rash; swelling; tenderness; hardening of skin.

Other: Fever; crying; irritability; drowsiness; diarrhea; vomiting; appetite loss; respiratory infection; difficulty breathing; cough; ear infection.

Guidelines for Use:

- Delay the vaccine when there is fever or infection present.
- *Haemophilus b disease* may be contracted during the week after vaccination, prior to the onset of the protective effects of the vaccine.
- For recommended immunization schedules, see page 1258.
- Fever, crying and redness, hardness and tenderness at the injection site may occur following vaccination. Contact your doctor if these symptoms persist or become bothersome.
- These vaccines may not work for everybody.
- *Recommended vaccination schedule* —
  ActHIB and *OmniHIB:* In children 2 to 6 months of age, 3 doses; in children 7 to 11 months of age, 2 doses; in children 12 to 14 months of age, 1 dose. These doses will be followed by a booster. Previously unvaccinated children 15 to 60 months of age should receive 1 dose; a booster is not required.
  Hib TITER: In children 2 to 6 months of age, 3 doses; in children 7 to 11 months of age, 2 doses; in children 12 to 14 months of age, 1 dose. These doses will be followed by a booster. Previously unvaccinated children 15 to 71 months of age should receive 1 dose; a booster is not required.
  PedvaxHIB: In children 2 to 10 months of age, two doses followed by a booster.
  In children 11 to 14 months of age, 2 doses; previously unvaccinated children 15 to 71 months of age should receive 1 dose; a booster is not required.
  ProHIBiT: A booster dose of *ProHIBiT* should be given to children 12 to 15 months of age previously immunized with any licensed Hib conjugate vaccine.
  In children 15 months to 5 years of age, one dose. A booster is not necessary.

If you have any questions, consult your doctor, pharmacist, or health care provider.

Generic Name *Brand Name Examples*	Uses
Diphtheria and Tetanus Toxoids and Pertussis Vaccine Adsorbed and Haemophilus b Conjugate Vaccine	
Tetramune	For active immunization against diphtheria, tetanus, pertussis and Haemophilus b in children between 2 months and 5 years of age.

Type of Drug:

Active immunization against diphtheria, tetanus, pertussis and Haemophilus b.

How the Drug Works:

This vaccine provides long-term protection against diphtheria, tetanus, pertussis and Haemophilus b by stimulating the body to produce antibodies against the organisms causing these infections.

Precautions:

Do not use in the following situations:

- allergy to thimerosal
- allergy to the vaccine or its components
- fever
- infection, acute or active
- pertussis, history
- polio outbreak
- previous nervous system reactions tovaccine (eg, seizures)
- seizures, history

Use with caution in the following situations:

- blood clotting disorder
- chemotherapy (cancer drugs)
- children over 5
- corticosteroid therapy (eg, prednisone)
- immune deficiency disorders
- nervous system disorders, history
- radiation

Pregnancy: Adequate studies have not been done in pregnant women. Use is not recommended in individuals 7 years of age or older. The proper agent for immunization in adults is diphtheria and tetanus toxoids (Td).

Children: Safety and effectiveness in children less than 6 weeks of age have not been determined.

Drug Interactions:

Tell your doctor or pharmacist if you are taking or if you are planning to take any over-the-counter or prescription medications while receiving this vaccine. Doses of one or both drugs may need to be modified or a different drug may need to be prescribed. The following drugs and drug classes interact with this vaccine:

- anticoagulants (eg, warfarin)
- immunosuppressive agents (eg, corticosteroids)

Side Effects:

Every drug is capable of producing side effects. Many patients experience no, or minor, side effects. The frequency and severity of side effects depend on many factors including dose, duration of therapy and individual susceptibility. Possible side effects include:

Consider side effects from Diphtheria/Tetanus/Pertussis and Haemophilus b vaccines as well.

Local: Redness; pain/tenderness; swelling; warmth.

Other: Fever; irritability; drowsiness; restless sleep; appetite loss; vomiting; diarrhea; rash; crying.

Guidelines for Use:

- It is important that the patient complete the immunization series.
- Report any serious adverse reaction to your doctor.
- This vaccine may not work for everybody.
- Delay vaccination when fever or infection are present.
- Doses of the vaccine are generally given at 2 months, 4 months, 6 months and between 15 to 18 months.
- In certain circumstances, this vaccine may be used beyond 5 years of age. Use is not recommended in individuals 7 years of age or older.

If you have any questions, consult your doctor, pharmacist, or health care provider.

	Generic Name *Brand Name Examples*	Uses
Rx	**Poliovirus Vaccine, Live, Oral, Trivalent (TOPV; OPV; Sabin)** *Orimune*	To prevent poliomyelitis caused by Poliovirus 1, 2 and 3.
Rx	**Poliovirus Vaccine, Inactivated (PIV; Salk)** *IPOL, Poliovax*	To prevent poliomyelitis caused by Poliovirus 1, 2 and 3.

Immunization is recommended for certain adults who are at greater risk of poliomyelitis (polio) than the general population, including: Travelers to areas or countries where polio immunization is needed, members of communities or specific population groups with disease caused by wild polioviruses, laboratory workers handling specimens which may contain poliovirus, healthcare workers in close contact with patients who may be excreting polioviruses and incompletely or unvaccinated adults in contact with children receiving OPV.

Persons with immune-deficiency diseases such as agammaglobulinemia, acquired immune deficiency syndrome (AIDS), or immune diseases or immunosuppressive therapy (eg, corticosteroids) as well as persons with close contacts or household members who have such conditions, should receive Poliovirus Vaccine Inactivated if immunization is indicated.

It is recommended that routine immunization of children against polio be accomplished using Poliovirus Vaccine Live Oral. However, Poliovirus Vaccine Inactivated is preferred in children with immunodeficiency or who have siblings with immunodeficiency until the immune status of the family can be documented.

Type of Drug:

Active immunization against polio.

How the Drug Works:

Poliovirus vaccine provides long-term protection against poliomyelitis by stimulating the body to produce antibodies against the virus causing the disease.

Precautions:

Do not use in the following situations:

- allergy to vaccine or any of its components, including streptomycin, poliomyxin B or neomycin (IPV only)
- diarrhea (OPV only)
- fever, severe
- illness, acute
- vomiting (OPV only)

Use with caution in the following situations:

- immune globulin (IG) vaccine (OPV only)

Immune diseases: The oral vaccine (OPV) must not be given to people with immune deficiency diseases or those with altered immune states (eg, leukemia, lymphoma or generalized malignancy, HIV) or with immune systems compromised by therapy with corticosteroids, cancer chemotherapy or radiation. Because the vaccine virus may be spread by the vaccinated person (through feces), OPV should not be given to family members of people with altered immune status. IPV is the preferred method for immunizing these individuals.

Vaccine-associated paralysis: When the vaccine is introduced into a household with adults who have never been vaccinated or whose immune status cannot be determined, risk may be minimized by giving them 2 doses of IPV a month apart before the children receive OPV. The children may receive the first dose of OPV at the same time as the adults receiving the second dose of IPV. The adults should also take precautions, such as handwashing after diaper changes.

The Centers for Disease Control report that during the years 1973 through 1984 approximately 274 million doses of OPV were distributed in the US. During this same period, 105 vaccine-associated cases were reported. Of these, 35 "vaccine-associated" and 50 "contact vaccine-associated" paralytic cases were reported. Fourteen other "vaccine-associated" cases have been reported in persons (recipients or contacts) with immune deficiency conditions and 6 other cases occurred in persons with no history of vaccine exposure.

Recipients of the OPV should avoid close contact with all persons with altered immune status for 6 to 8 weeks.

Pregnancy: Safety for use during pregnancy has not been established, or animal studies may have shown a risk to the fetus. Use only when clearly needed and when potential benefits outweigh the possible hazards to the fetus. However, if immediate protection against poliomyelitis is needed, OPV is recommended.

Breastfeeding: Women should avoid breastfeeding for 2 to 3 hours before and after the infant is vaccinated so that it does not interfere with the vaccine.

Children: Safety and effectiveness for use in children under 6 weeks have not been established.

Drug Interactions:

Tell your doctor or pharmacist if you are taking or planning to take any over-the-counter or prescription medications while taking this medicine. Doses of one or both drugs may need to be modified or a different drug may need to be prescribed. The following drugs and drug classes interact with this medicine.

cholera vaccine
immunosuppressants (eg, corticosteroids)

Side Effects:

Every vaccine is capable of producing side effects. Many patients experience no, or minor, side effects. The frequency and severity of side effects depend on many factors including dose and individual susceptibility. Possible side effects include:

Oral – Vaccine-associated paralysis: Paralysis following the use of live poliovirus vaccines have been reported in individuals given the vaccine and in persons who were in close contact with people who have recently been vaccinated.
The risk of vaccine-associated paralysis is extremely small for those vaccinated, susceptible family members and other close personal contacts.

Injection – Redness, hardness and pain or discomfort at injection site (within 6-12 hours of vaccination and lasting 1-3 days); fever; sleepiness; fussiness; reduced appetite; crying; spitting up feedings.

Guidelines for Use:

- The polio vaccine series is three doses.
  OPV — The ACIP and the American Academy of Pediatrics recommend that the series be started at 6 to 12 weeks of age. The second dose should be given not less than 6, and preferably 8, weeks later. The third dose is given 8 to 12 months after the second dose. An optional dose may be given at 6 months.
  IPV — The first two doses are given at 2 and 4 months of age with an interval of not less than 4, and preferably 8, weeks, commonly with the first DTP immunization at 2 months of age. The third dose is given not less than 6, and preferably 12, months later.
  School entrance - When entering elementary school, all children who have completed the primary series should receive a single followup dose of OPV, unless they received the third dose on or after their fourth birthday. All others should complete the primary series. The ACIP does not recommend routine booster doses of vaccine beyond those given when entering school.
  Older children, adolescents and adults: Two doses of OPV, given not less than 6, and preferably 8, weeks apart and the third dose 6 to 12 months after the second dose. An optional third dose may be given 6 to 8 weeks after the second dose.
- Delay vaccination when vomiting, diarrhea, fever or infection are present.
- People allergic to neomycin, polymyxin B or streptomycin should not receive IPV vaccine.
- The vaccine will not change or prevent cases of existing or incubating poliomyelitis.
- *Vaccine-associated paralysis* — Paralytic disease following OPV vaccination has been reported in individuals receiving the vaccine and in persons who were in close contact with vaccines. The risk is greater in those with immune-deficiency diseases.
- *Guillain-Barre syndrome (GBS),* characterized by paralysis, has occurred rarely after the administration of the OPV vaccine. No cause and effect relationship has been established. Evaluate the possible risk of GBS against the risk of polio and its complications.
- Redness, hardness and tenderness at the injection site, sleepiness, fussiness, reduced appetite and crying may occur beginning 6 to 12 hours following vaccination. They will begin to disappear in 1 to 3 days. Contact your doctor if any of these symptoms persist or become bothersome.
- Vaccination may not work in everybody.

If you have any questions, consult your doctor, pharmacist, or health care provider.

	Generic Name *Brand Name Examples*	Uses
Rx	**Measles (Rubeola) Virus Vaccine, Live, Attenuated** *Attenuvax*	For immunization against measles (rubeola) in children 15 months or older and adults.
Rx	**Rubella Virus Vaccine, Live** *Meruvax II*	For immunization against rubella in children 12 months or older and adults.
Rx	**Mumps Virus Vaccine, Live** *Mumpsvex*	For immunization against mumps in children 12 months or older and adults.
Rx	**Rubella and Mumps Virus Vaccine, Live** *Biavax II*	For simultaneous immunization against rubella and mumps in children 12 months or older and adults.
Rx	**Measles (Rubeola) and Rubella Virus Vaccine, Live** *M-R-Vax II*	For simultaneous immunization against measles and rubella in children 15 months or older and adults.
Rx	**Measles, Mumps and Rubella Virus Vaccine, Live** *M-M-R II*	For simultaneous immunization against measles, mumps and rubella in children 15 months or older and adults.

Children in kindergarten and the first grades of elementary school may be required to have measles, mumps and rubella vaccinations because they are often the major source of infection in the community.

A two-dose schedule for MMR vaccination is now recommended to improve control of measles. When rubella vaccine is part of a combination that includes measles, give the combination to children at 15 months of age or older to maximize protection. A second dose of MMR is recommended at school entry. Vaccinate older children who have not received rubella vaccine promptly.

Strongly recommended for: Children living in schools, orphanages and similar institutions; malnourished children; those with inactive or active tuberculosis under treatment; those with chronic diseases such as cystic fibrosis, heart disease, asthma and other chronic lung diseases.

Type of Drug:

Active immunization against measles, mumps and rubella.

How the Drug Works:

Measles, mumps and rubella vaccines provide long-term protection against measles (rubeola), mumps or rubella by stimulating the body to produce antibodies to organisms causing these illnesses.

Precautions:

Do not use in the following situations:

AIDS
allergy to eggs, severe
allergy to neomycin
blood diseases (eg, leukemia)
infection, with fever
immune deficiency disorders (decreased antibody production), including family history
immunosuppressive therapy (eg,chemotherapy)
infection with fever
pregnancy
tuberculosis, active, untreated

Use with caution in the following situations:

brain injury, history
conditions where stress due to fever should be avoided
seizures, individual or family history

Pregnancy: Do not use during pregnancy. Avoid pregnancy for 3 months following vaccination. Adequate studies of the vaccine strain of the measles virus have not been done in pregnant women. Contracting measles during pregnancy increases the possibility of fetal harm. Increased rates of miscarriage, stillbirth, congenital defects and prematurity have been reported after contracting natural measles. The vaccine may also be capable of inducing harm to the fetus for up to 3 months following vaccination. If measles exposure occurs during pregnancy, consider providing temporary protection with immune serum globulin (ISG).

Breastfeeding: It is not known if these vaccines appear in breast milk. Consult your doctor before you begin breastfeeding.

Children: Use with caution in children with a history of fever convulsions, head injury or conditions in which stress due to fever should be avoided. Fever may occur following vaccination. Children infected with immune deficiency disorders but without manifestations of the disorders should be monitored closely. Mumps and rubella vaccines are not recommended for children under 1.

Side Effects:

Every vaccine is capable of producing side effects. Many patients experience no, or minor, local side effects. The frequency and severity of side effects depend on many factors including dose and individual susceptibility. Possible side effects include fever (up to 103° F for up to 1 month); rash (between 5th and 12th days); hives; swelling, redness, hardness, tenderness, burning or stinging at injection site; swollen glands; muscle and joint aches; general body discomfort; cough; nasal congestion; sore throat; headache; dizziness; nausea; vomiting; diarrhea; nerve inflammation; inflammation of the eye.

Guidelines for Use:

- *MMR* is given after 15 months of age followed by a second dose at school entry.
- Children vaccinated when younger than 12 months of age should be revaccinated at 15 months of age.
- Do not administer within one month of DTaP, DTP or OPV.
- Delay vaccination when fever or infection is present.
- People who have had severe allergic reactions to eggs or neomycin should not receive these vaccines.
- Vaccination should be deferred for at least 3 months following blood or plasma transfusions, or administration of ISG.
- Fever (up to 103° F) may occur for up to 1 month following vaccination. A rash may appear between the 5th and 12th day following vaccination. Swelling, redness, burning or stinging at the injection site, swollen glands and muscle and joint aches may also occur. Contact your doctor if any of these symptoms persist or become bothersome.
- *Tuberculin skin test:* Measles, mumps and rubella vaccines may temporarily depress tuberculin skin reaction. Administer the test before or at the same time as the vaccine.
- *Measles —*
  If immediate protection against measles is required for persons in whom the vaccine is not recommended, passive immunization with ISG is recommended. (See page 1258). Do not give ISG with measles vaccination.
- Giving the live virus vaccine immediately after exposure to natural measles may prevent illness. When in doubt, vaccination is recommended.
- The mumps vaccine does not give protection when given after exposure to natural mumps.
- *Guillain-Barre syndrome (GBS),* characterized by paralysis, has occurred rarely after administration of the live measles virus. No cause and effect relationship has been established. Evaluate the possible risk of GBS as compared with the risk of measles and its complications.
- These vaccinations may not result in development of antibodies in all individuals.

If you have any questions, consult your doctor, pharmacist, or health care provider.

	Generic Name *Brand Name Examples*	Uses
Rx	**Varicella Virus Vaccine, Live** *Varivax*	For immunization of persons over 12 months of age who have not yet had the varicella virus (chickenpox).

Type of Drug:

Active immunization against varicella.

How the Drug Works:

The varicella vaccine provides protection against varicella (chickenpox) by stimulating the body to produce antibodies to the virus causing this illness.

Precautions:

Do not use in the following situations:

allergy to the vaccine or its ingredients, including gelatin
allergy to neomycin
acquired immunodeficiency syndrome (AIDS)
blood, bone marrow or lymph system diseases
immune deficiency disorders (deceased antibody production), including family history
immunosuppressive therapy
infection, active with fever
pregnancy (or those attempting to become pregnant)
respiratory illness, with fever
tuberculosis, active, untreated

Pregnancy: Adequate studies have not been done in women, or animal studies may have shown a risk to the fetus. It is recommended that the vaccine not be administered during pregnancy. Contracting varicella during pregnancy (via the live vaccine) increases the possibility of fetal harm. Avoid pregnancy for 3 months following vaccination.

Breastfeeding: It is not known if this vaccine virus appears in breast milk. Consult your doctor before you begin breastfeeding.

Children: Safety and effectiveness in children younger than 1 year of age have not been established.

Drug Interactions:

Tell your doctor or pharmacist if you are taking or if you are planning to take any over-the-counter or prescription medications while taking this medicine. Doses of one or both drugs may need to be modified or a different drug may need to be prescribed. Immunosuppressants and salicylates (eg, aspirin) interact with this medicine.

Side Effects:

Every drug is capable of producing side effects. Many patients experience no, or minor, side effects. The frequency and severity of side effects depend on many factors including dose, duration of therapy and individual susceptibility. Possible side effects include:

Local: Pain, swelling, rash, itching, stiffness, hardness, redness, numbness, bruising at injection site.

Digestive Tract: Diarrhea; appetite changes; vomiting; nausea; constipation; stomach pain.

Nervous System: Irritability; nervousness; tiredness; sleep disorders; headache.

Respiratory System: Runny nose; upper or lower respiratory illness; cough.

Other: Fever; chills; ear infection; teething; general body discomfort; eye problems; muscle or joint pain; stiff neck; dry skin; cold/canker sores.

Guidelines for Use:

- *Recommended vaccination schedule* —Ages 1-12 years: one dose; Ages 12+ years: two doses given 1-2 months apart.
- Contact your doctor if any of the following occurs: itching, rash, fever, difficulty breathing.
- Female patients should avoid becoming pregnant for 3 months after receiving this vaccine.
- Do not use salicylates (eg, aspirin) for 6 weeks after receiving this vaccine.
- Persons given this vaccine could pass the active vaccine virus to others. Therefore, avoid close contact with pregnant women, infants and people with low immune systems.
- Wait at least 5 months to receive this vaccine after blood/plasma transfusions, immune globulin or varicella zoster immune globulin (VZIG) therapy.
- Any immune globulin, including VZIG, should not be given for 2 months after administration of this vaccine.
- This vaccine may be given at the same time as the measles, mumps, rubella, diptheria, tetanus and pertussis vaccines.
- The length of protection from the virus is not known, nor is it a guarantee that the vaccine will protect everyone from the chickenpox virus.

If you have any questions, consult your doctor, pharmacist, or health care provider.

	Generic Name *Brand Name Examples*	Uses
Rx	**Influenza Virus Vaccine**[1] *Fluogen*; *FluShield*; *Fluvirin*; *Fluzone (subvirion and whole virion)*	For high-risk persons ≥ 6 months of age; medical care personnel and primary providers of care in the home; children and teenagers (6 months to 18 years of age) receiving long-term aspirin therapy; persons infected with human immunodeficiency virus (HIV); and other persons who wish to reduce their chances for acquiring influenza.

[1] Contains 0.01% thimerosal and sulfites.

Groups at increased risk for influenza complications include: Adults and children with chronic lung and heart disorders, including children with asthma; residents of nursing homes and other chronic care facilities housing patients of any age with chronic medical conditions; persons ≥ 65 years of age; adults and children who have required regular medical follow-up or hospitalization during the preceding year because of chronic metabolic diseases (including diabetes mellitus), kidney disease, blood disorders, or immunosuppression; children and teenagers (6 months to 18 years of age) who are receiving long-term aspirin therapy and therefore may be at risk of developing Reye's syndrome after influenza; and women who will be in the second or third trimester of pregnancy during the influenza season.

Groups capable of transmitting influenza to high-risk persons include: Doctors, nurses, and others in both hospital and outpatient care; employees of nursing homes and chronic care facilities who have contact with patients or residents; providers of home care to high-risk persons (eg, health care workers); and household members (including children) of high-risk persons.

General population: Any person who wishes to reduce the chance of acquiring influenza should be vaccinated. Persons who provide essential community services (eg, the military) and students or others in institutional settings (eg, those who reside in dormitories) may consider vaccination to prevent the disruption of routine activities during outbreaks.

Pregnant women who have other medical conditions that increase their risks for complications from influenza should be vaccinated. Although the vaccine is considered safe for pregnant women, the clinical judgement of the attending doctor should prevail at all times in determining whether to administer the vaccine to a pregnant woman.

Persons infected with HIV: Little information exists regarding the frequency and severity of influenza illness or benefits among persons infected with HIV. Because influenza may result in serious illness and complications, vaccination is recommended. However, response to the vaccine may be low in persons with advanced HIV-related illnesses and a second dose has not been shown to improve response.

Travelers: The risk of exposure to influenza during travel depends on the time of year and destination. Persons at high risk for complications of influenza should consider influenza vaccination before travel if they were not vaccinated with the influenza vaccine during the preceding fall or winter and they plan to travel to the Tropics, travel with large, organized tourist groups at any time of year, or travel to the Southern Hemisphere from April through September. Persons at high risk who received the previous season's vaccine before travel should be revaccinated with the current vaccine in the following fall or winter. Because the influenza vaccine might not be available during the summer in North America, persons ≥ 65 years of age and others at high risk should consult their doctors regarding symptoms and risks of influenza before embarking on travel during the summer.

Type of Drug:

Flu vaccine (flu shot).

How the Drug Works:

Injection of material from inactivated influenza virus stimulates the production of specific antibodies. Protection from this injection is only against those strains from which the vaccine is prepared, or against closely related strains. Having received a vaccination for one flu season does not prevent the need to be revaccinated for subsequent flu seasons to provide ideal protection.

Precautions:

Do not use in the following situations:

allergy to any component of the vaccine
allergy to chicken eggs, chicken, chicken feathers, or chicken dander
allergy to thimerosal (eg, mercury)
children < 6 months of age
febrile illness, acute
Guillain-Barré syndrome, history
neurologic disorder, active

Use with caution in the following situations:

anticoagulant therapy, concurrent
children 6 to 35 months of age
coagulation disorder (eg, thrombocytopenia)
impaired immune response

Other vaccinations: Because children are accessible when pediatric vaccines are given, the influenza vaccine may be given with other routine pediatric vaccines, but at a different injection site.

Pneumococcal, measles-mumps-rubella, oral polio, and *Haemophilus* b vaccines can be given at the same time as the influenza vaccine. Vaccines should be given at different injection sites. Influenza vaccine is given annually; pneumococcal vaccine should be given only once.

Guillain-Barré syndrome (GBS), which causes paralysis, has occurred within 10 weeks following influenza vaccine. However, it is usually self-limited and reversible. Most persons recover without permanent weakness, although about 5% of cases are fatal. Current vaccines (since 1980) have not been associated with an increased frequency of GBS. Nonetheless, be aware of the possible risk as compared with the risk of influenza and its complications.

Immunosuppressed patients (eg, persons with leukemia, lymphoma, cancer, or persons undergoing therapy with corticosteroids, cancer drugs, or radiation) may experience a lower than expected response to the vaccine. Oral amantadine may be given to supplement vaccination in high-risk patients.

Pregnancy: Pregnancy has not been demonstrated to be a risk factor for severe influenza infection. However, pregnant women with medical conditions that increase the risk of complications from influenza should be vaccinated. Influenza vaccine is considered safe for pregnant women without a severe egg allergy. Vaccination should be given after the first trimester. However, it may be undesirable to delay vaccinating a pregnant woman who has a high-risk condition and will still be in the first trimester of pregnancy when the influenza season usually begins. Influenza vaccine should be given to a pregnant woman only if clearly needed. The clinical judgement of the attending doctor should prevail at all times in determining whether to administer the vaccine to a pregnant woman.

Breastfeeding: Influenza vaccine does not affect the safety of mothers who are breastfeeding or their infants. Breastfeeding does not adversely affect immune response and is not a contraindication for vaccination.

Children: Influenza split virus vaccines (*Fluogen*, *FluShield*, *Fluzone*, *Fluvirin*) are not approved for infants < 6 months of age. The likelihood of fever-induced convulsions is greater in children 6 months through 35 months of age. Therefore, special care should be taken in weighing the risks and benefits of vaccination. The whole virus vaccine (*Fluzone*) should not be given to children < 13 years of age. The safety and effectiveness of *Fluvirin* in children between 6 months and 4 years of age has not been established. However, vaccination for children ≥ 6 months of age is strongly recommended because of the increased risk of complications from influenza.

Drug Interactions:

Tell your doctor or pharmacist if you are taking or planning to take any over-the-counter or prescription medications or dietary supplements before being vaccinated against the influenza virus. Doses of one or both drugs may need to be modified or a different drug may need to be prescribed. The following drugs and drug classes interact with influenza virus vaccine:

- carbamazepine (eg, *Tegretol*) (*Fluzone* only)
- theophylline (eg, *Theo-Dur*)
- warfarin (eg, *Coumadin*)

Side Effects:

Every vaccine is capable of producing side effects. Many patients experience no, or minor, side effects. The frequency and severity of side effects depend on many factors including dose and individual susceptibility. Possible side effects include soreness at the injection site (1 to 2 days), fever, general body discomfort, and muscle aches.

Guidelines for Use:

- This vaccine will be prepared and administered by your health care provider in a medical setting.
- *Recommended vaccination schedule* — Beginning each September, influenza vaccine should be offered to persons at high risk when they are seen by health care providers for routine care or as a result of hospitalization. For organized vaccination campaigns, the optimal time to vaccinate persons in high-risk groups is usually from October through mid-November because influenza activity in the United States generally peaks between late December and early March. Administering vaccine too far in advance of the influenza season should be avoided in certain facilities (eg, nursing homes) because antibody levels may begin to decline within a few months following vaccination. Children < 9 years of age not previously vaccinated require 2 doses administered at least 1 month apart. The second dose should be given before December, if possible.
- People allergic to chicken eggs, chicken, chicken feathers, or chicken dander should not receive this vaccine. In addition, administer vaccine with caution in patients with latex sensitivity since packaging includes some dry natural rubber.
- In persons suspected of having an allergy to chicken eggs, chicken, chicken feathers, or chicken dander, a scratch test should be performed prior to immunization. The scratch test will determine sensitivity to the vaccine. If the reaction is positive, the vaccine is not recommended.
- Delay the vaccine in acute illness with fever.
- *Children* — Because children are accessible when pediatric vaccines are given, it may be desirable to give the influenza vaccine at the same time as routine pediatric vaccines, but at a different injection site.
- Talk to your doctor about the risks of developing Guillain-Barré syndrome.
- Soreness at the injection site, fever, and muscle aches may occur following vaccination. Consult your doctor if these persist or become bothersome.
- Vaccination may not result in development of antibodies in all individuals.
- Contact your doctor if you experience rash, hives, itching, difficulty breathing, or redness or swelling at the injection site.

If you have any questions, consult your doctor, pharmacist, or health care provider.

	Generic Name *Brand Name Examples*	Uses
Rx	**Hepatitis A Vaccine, Inactivated**	
	Havrix, VAQTA	For active immunization of people ≥ 2 years of age against infection caused by the hepatitis A virus (HAV). This vaccine will not prevent infections caused by other hepatitis viruses or other infectious agents that can infect the liver.

Individuals at high risk include:

Travelers: People living in or traveling to areas where hepatitis A is common. These areas include, but are not limited to, Africa, Asia (except Japan), the Mediterranean basin, Eastern Europe, the Middle East, Central and South America, Mexico, and parts of the Caribbean. Consult current Centers for Disease Control and Prevention (CDC) advisories with regard to specific locales.

Certain ethnic and geographic populations that experience cyclic hepatitis A epidemics: Native peoples of Alaska and the Americas.

Certain institutional workers: Caretakers for the developmentally challenged, employees of child daycare centers, laboratory workers who handle live HAV, and handlers of primates that may be harboring the HAV.

Others: Military personnel, persons involved in high-risk sexual activity (eg, homosexual males), users of illicit injectable drugs, residents of a community experiencing an outbreak of hepatitis A, people with chronic liver disease (eg, alcoholic cirrhosis, hepatitis B, hepatitis C) or clotting-factor disorders, hemophiliacs and other recipients of therapeutic blood products, and certain food handlers.

For persons requiring postexposure prophylaxis or needing immediate protection (eg, travel on short notice to endemic areas), the vaccine may be supplemented with an injection of immune globulin (IG).

Type of Drug:

Vaccine to immunize against HAV infection.

How the Drug Works:

Hepatitis A vaccine provides active protection (immunization) against HAV by stimulating the body to produce antibodies against the virus causing this illness.

Primary immunization should be completed ≥ 2 weeks prior to expected exposure to HAV.

Precautions:

Do not use in the following situations: Allergy to hepatitis A vaccine or any of its ingredients.

Use with caution in the following situations:

anticoagulant (eg, warfarin) therapy, concurrent
bleeding disorders
fever
immune deficiency disorders (eg, HIV-positive patients)
immunosuppression (due to illness or drug therapy)
infection, acute
low platelet count

Pregnancy: There are no adequate or well-controlled studies in pregnant women. Use only if clearly needed and potential benefits to the mother outweigh the possible hazards to the fetus.

Breastfeeding: It is not known if hepatitis A vaccine appears in breast milk. Consult your doctor before you begin breastfeeding.

Children: Safety and effectiveness in children < 2 years of age have not been established.

Drug Interactions:

Tell your doctor or pharmacist if you are taking or planning to take any over-the-counter or prescription medications or dietary supplements while receiving hepatitis A vaccine. Doses of one or both drugs may need to be modified or a different drug may need to be prescribed. Anticoagulants (eg, warfarin) may increase bleeding at the injection site.

Side Effects:

Every vaccine is capable of producing side effects. Many patients experience no, or minor, side effects. The frequency and severity of side effects depend on many factors including dose and individual susceptibility. Most side effects are mild and do not last for > 24 hours. Possible side effects include:

Local: Soreness; swelling; redness; warmth; pain; tenderness; unusual bruising or swelling at injection site.

Digestive Tract: Stomach pain; appetite loss; nausea; diarrhea; vomiting.

Other: Headache; sleeplessness; fatigue; fever; general body discomfort; itching; rash; hives; congestion; sore throat; upper respiratory infection; back, arm, joint, or muscle pain; stiffness; menstruation disorder; weakness; dizziness; sensitivity to light.

Guidelines for Use:

- This medicine will be prepared and administered by your health care provider in a medical setting. The vaccine must be administered intramuscularly (IM; into a muscle) in the deltoid region of the shoulder.
- *Recommended vaccination schedule* — People who wish to be protected against HAV should complete the primary immunization schedule at least 2 weeks before exposure to HAV if possible. Booster doses result in prolonged protection. Dosing regimens depend on the agent selected and the age of the patient.
- The vaccination may not be effective for several days (15 to 30), and it may not prevent unrecognized HAV infection that exists at the time of vaccination. Immune globulin, which is used to provide rapid but temporary protection against HAV, can be administered at the same time.
- Contact your doctor if you experience rash, hives, itching, or difficulty breathing.
- Inform you doctor if you are pregnant, become pregnant, plan on becoming pregnant, or are breastfeeding.
- This vaccine should not be given when a fever is present.
- Immunosuppressed people or those receiving immunosuppressive therapy may not be fully protected and acquire the virus even after vaccination.
- Travelers to areas where HAV is common should take all necessary precautions to avoid contact and ingestion of HAV-contaminated food and water. Contact the CDC for specific travel destination information.
- The length of protection from the virus following complete immunization is not known, but may persist for at least 10 years. There is no guarantee that the vaccine will protect everyone from the hepatitis A virus.

If you have any questions, consult your doctor, pharmacist, or health care provider.

	Generic Name *Brand Name Examples*	Uses
Rx	**Hepatitis B Vaccine**[1] *Engerix-B,* *Recombivax HB*[2]	For immunization of adults, infants, and children at high risk against infection caused by all known types of the hepatitis B virus (HBV). Immunity to HBV also protects against the hepatitis D virus; hepatitis D can only infect and cause illness in people with HBV. This vaccine will not prevent infections caused by other hepatitis viruses or other diseases which can infect the liver.

[1] Contains 0.005% thimerosal (mercury).
[2] Also available in dialysis formulation.

Individuals at high risk include:

Health care personnel: Doctors; podiatrists; surgeons; dentists; dental hygienists; oral surgeons; nurses; paramedics; blood bank and plasma fractionation workers; laboratory personnel who handle blood, blood products, and patient specimens; custodial staff who may be exposed to blood or patient specimens; dental, medical, and nursing students.

Selected patients and patient contacts: Patients and staff in hemodialysis and hematology/oncology units; patients requiring frequent or large-volume blood transfusions (eg, hemophiliacs); hemodialysis patients and patients with early renal failure before they require hemodialysis; residents and staff of institutions for the mentally handicapped; classroom contacts of deinstitutionalized mentally handicapped persons who exhibit aggressive behavior or have persistent HBV antigenemia; infants born to HBsAg-positive mothers; household and other intimate contacts with persons with persistent HBV type infections.

Adolescents: The Advisory Committee on Immunization Practices (ACIP) and the Committee on Infectious Diseases of the American Academy of Pediatrics (AAP) have endorsed universal infant immunization to lower the incidence of HBV. These advisory committees recommend vaccination of all adolescents at 11 to 12 years of age if previously unvaccinated. High-risk adolescents at older ages should also be vaccinated.

Populations with high incidence of the disease: Alaskan natives; Pacific islanders; Indochinese immigrants; Haitian or other immigrants from areas where there is a high rate of HBV; infants born in areas where HBV is prevalent.

Persons at increased risk due to their sexual practices: Homosexual males; prostitutes; persons who repeatedly contract sexually transmitted diseases; persons with multiple sex partners (eg, > 1 partner in a 6-month period).

Persons with chronic hepatitis C virus: Risk factors for hepatitis C are similar to those for HBV. Immunization with hepatitis B vaccine is recommended for patients with chronic hepatitis C.

Travelers to high-risk areas: Contact the Centers for Disease Control and Prevention (CDC) with regard to such locales.

Others: Military personnel; international travelers; police and fire department personnel who render first aid or medical assistance; morticians; embalmers; prisoners; IV drug abusers; any others who may be exposed to HBV through work or personal lifestyle.

Type of Drug:

Vaccine to prevent hepatitis B viral infection.

How the Drug Works:

Hepatitis B vaccine provides active protection (immunization) against HBV by stimulating the body to produce antibodies against the virus causing the illness.

Precautions:

Do not use in the following situations: Allergy to hepatitis B vaccine, thimerosal, yeast, or any other hepatitis B vaccine ingredients.

Use with caution in the following situations:

anticoagulant (eg, warfarin) therapy, concurrent
fever
immune deficiency disorders (eg, HIV-positive patients)
infection, active
radiation therapy, concurrent

Pregnancy: There are no adequate or well-controlled studies in pregnant women. Use only if clearly needed and potential benefits to the mother outweigh the possible hazards to the fetus.

Breastfeeding: It is not known if hepatitis B vaccine appears in breast milk. Empirical evidence suggests no harm. Consult your doctor before you begin breastfeeding.

Children: Hepatitis B vaccine is well-tolerated in infants and children of all ages. Newborns also respond well. However, the safety and effectiveness of the dialysis formulation in children have not been established.

Elderly: HBV immunity is somewhat reduced in patients ≥ 65 years of age.

Drug Interactions:

Tell your doctor or pharmacist if you are taking or planning to take any over-the-counter or prescription medications or dietary supplements while receiving hepatitis B vaccine. Doses of one or both drugs may need to be modified or a different drug may need to be prescribed. Anticoagulants (eg, warfarin) and interleukin-2 (*Leuvectin*) interact with hepatitis B vaccine.

Side Effects:

Every vaccine is capable of producing side effects. Many patients experience no, or minor, side effects. The frequency and severity of side effects depend on many factors including dose and individual susceptibility. Possible side effects include:

Local: Itching, pain, soreness, tenderness, redness, swelling, bruising, warmth, or nodule formation at injection site.

Nervous System: Headache; weakness; fatigue; dizziness; lightheadedness; feeling of whirling motion; fainting; sleeplessness; drowsiness.

Digestive Tract: Nausea; vomiting; appetite loss; stomach pain or cramps; indigestion; diarrhea.

Respiratory System: Sore throat; upper respiratory tract infection; asthma-like symptoms; cough.

Skin: Rash; hives; flushing; hair loss; unusual bleeding or bruising; flushing; abnormal skin sensations (eg, burning, prickling, tingling).

Other: General body discomfort; achiness; fatigue; joint, muscle, back, arm, or shoulder pain; neck stiffness or pain; facial swelling; low blood pressure; flu-like symptoms; fever; warmth; sweating; chills; earache; painful or difficult urination; abnormal liver function tests.

Guidelines for Use:

- This medicine will be prepared and administered by your health care provider in a medical setting. For adults and adolescents, the preferred intramuscular (IM; into a muscle) injection site is the deltoid muscle of the shoulder. For infants and young children, the anterolateral thigh is the preferred site for injection. Patients at high risk of bleeding following an IM injection may receive the vaccine subcutaneously (SC; beneath the skin) but the response may be less than optimal.
- *Recommended vaccination schedule* – Usual regimen consists of 3 consecutive doses. The second and third doses are given at 1 month and 6 months after the initial vaccine, respectively. Alternate schedules may also be used.
- This vaccine should not be given when a fever is present, unless recommended by a doctor.
- The vaccination may not be effective for several days, and it may not prevent unrecognized HBV infections that exist at the time of vaccination.
- Soreness, tenderness, redness, and warmth at injection site, fever, or nausea may occur following vaccination. Contact your doctor if these symptoms persist or become bothersome.
- Contact your doctor if you experience rash, hives, itching, or difficulty breathing.
- Inform you doctor if you are pregnant, become pregnant, plan on becoming pregnant, or are breastfeeding.
- Immunosuppressed patients or those receiving immunosuppressive therapy may not be fully protected and acquire the virus even after vaccination.
- The length of protection against the virus following complete immunization is not known, nor is it a guarantee that the vaccine will protect everyone from HBV.
- Lab tests may be required to monitor therapy. Be sure to keep appointments.

If you have any questions, consult your doctor, pharmacist, or health care provider.

	Generic Name *Brand Name Example*	Uses
Rx	**Hepatitis A, Inactivated and Hepatitis B, Recombinant Vaccine** *Twinrix*[1]	For immunization of people ≥ 18 years of age against infection caused by hepatitis A virus (HAV) and all known subtypes of hepatitis B virus (HBV). Immunity to HBV also protects against hepatitis D virus; hepatitis D can only infect and cause illness in people with HBV. This vaccine will not prevent infections caused by other hepatitis viruses or other diseases that can infect the liver.

[1] Contains thimerosol (less than 1 mcg mercury per mL).

Individuals at high risk:

See the Hepatitis A and Hepatitis B monographs in this chapter for a complete listing of people at high risk of HAV and HBV infections.

Type of Drug:

Vaccine to immunize against HAV and HBV-type infections.

How the Drug Works:

Hepatitis A and hepatitis B vaccine provides protection against HAV and HBV by stimulating the body to produce antibodies against the virus causing the illness.

Precautions:

Do not use in the following situations: Allergy to hepatitis A vaccine, hepatitis B vaccine, thimerosol, yeast, or any other ingredients within the vaccine.

Use with caution in the following situations:

anticoagulant (eg, warfarin) therapy, concurrent
Bell palsy
fever
immune deficiency disorders (eg, HIV-positive patients)
immunosuppressive therapy, concurrent
infection, acute, moderate to severe
low platelet count

Patients 40 years of age and older: Hepatitis B vaccine may not be as effective if given to patients 40 years of age and older. Consult you doctor.

Pregnancy: There are no adequate or well-controlled studies in pregnant women. Use only if clearly needed and the potential benefits to the mother outweigh the possible hazards to the fetus.

Breastfeeding: It is not known if hepatitis A and hepatitis B vaccine appears in breast milk. Consult your doctor before you begin breastfeeding.

Children: Safety and effectiveness in people under 18 years of age have not been established.

Elderly: There are no sufficient studies in patients 65 years of age and older. Use with caution in elderly patients.

Drug Interactions:

Tell your doctor or pharmacist if you are taking or planning to take any over-the-counter or prescription medications or dietary supplements while receiving hepatitis A and hepatitis B vaccine. Doses of one or both drugs may need to be modified or a different drug may need to be prescribed. The following drugs or drug classes interact with hepatitis A and hepatitis B vaccine:

anticoagulants (eg, warfarin)
corticosteroids (eg, prednisone)
immunosuppressants (eg, cyclosporine)
interleukin-2 (*Leuvectin*)
yellow fever vaccine (*YF-Vax*)

Side Effects:

Every vaccine is capable of producing side effects. Many patients experience no, or minor, side effects. The frequency and severity of side effects depend on many factors including dose and individual susceptibility. Possible side effects include:

Local: Soreness; tenderness; pain; redness; swelling; hardening; warmth; itching.

Other: Headache; fever; fatigue; diarrhea; nausea; vomiting; upper respiratory infection.

Guidelines for Use:

- This medicine will be prepared and administered by your health care provider in a medical setting.
- *Recommended vaccination schedule* — Primary immunization for adults consists of 3 doses given at 1 month and 6 months after the initial vaccination. Alternate schedules may also be used.
- The vaccination may not be effective for several days, and it may not prevent unrecognized HAV or HBV infections that exist at the time of vaccination.
- This vaccine should not be administered when a fever is present, unless recommended by a doctor.
- Contact your doctor if you experience rash, hives, itching, or difficulty breathing.
- Inform your doctor if you are pregnant, become pregnant, plan on becoming pregnant, or are breastfeeding.
- Immunosuppressed people or those receiving immunosuppressive therapy may not be fully protected and acquire the virus even after vaccination.
- The length of protection against HAV and HBV following complete immunization is not known, nor is there a guarantee that the vaccine will protect everyone.
- Contact the Centers for Disease Control and Prevention for specific travel destination information concerning the prevalence of HAV and HBV if you are a world traveler.

If you have any questions, consult your doctor, pharmacist, or health care provider.

	Generic Name *Brand Name Examples*	Uses
Rx	**Pneumococcal Vaccine** *Pneumovax 23*[1], *Pnu-Imune 23*[2]	For high-risk people ≥ 2 years of age, certain population groups (eg, Native Americans), people in closed institutions (eg, residential schools, nursing homes), and during a general pneumonia outbreak.

[1] Contains 0.25% phenol.
[2] Contains 0.01% thimerosal (mercury).

Individuals at high risk include:

Adults over 50 years of age; people 2 years of age or younger at high risk due to chronic illnesses (eg, cardiovascular or pulmonary disease, diabetes, alcoholism, cirrhosis, CSF leaks) or compromised immune systems (eg, spleen, kidney, or liver disorders, organ transplantations, sickle cell disease, cancers, HIV infection); Hodgkin disease (if the vaccine can be given 10 days before treatment).

Type of Drug:

Pneumococcal vaccine (pneumonia).

How the Drug Works:

Injection of material from inactivated pneumococcal bacteria stimulates the production of specific antibodies. Protection from this injection is only against those strains from which the vaccine is prepared.

Precautions:

Do not use in the following situations:

allergy to pneumococcal vaccine or any of its ingredients
fever
Hodgkin disease patients less than 14 days prior to immunosuppressive therapy
Hodgkin disease patients who have received chemotherapy or nodal irradiation
infection, acute respiratory or other

Use with caution in the following situations:

heart disease, severe
impaired immune responsiveness
lung disease, severe

Revaccination: Do not give a repeat (booster) injection to previously vaccinated patients, except for those at highest risk of pneumococcal infection. Revaccination may result in more frequent and severe local reactions at the injection site.

Children at highest risk: Children with asplenia, sickle cell disease, or splenectomy should be revaccinated after 3 to 5 years if they will be ≤ 10 years of age.

Antibiotic therapy: Patients who require antibiotic therapy against possible pneumococcal infection should continue the antibiotic therapy after vaccination.

Chemotherapy or immunosuppresion: The interval between immunization and initiation of chemotherapy or immunosuppression should be ≥ 2 weeks.

Pregnancy: There are no adequate or well-controlled studies in pregnant women. Use only if clearly needed and the potential benefits to the mother outweigh the possible hazards to the fetus.

Breastfeeding: It is not known if this drug appears in breast milk. Consult your doctor before you begin breastfeeding.

Children: Safety and effectiveness have not been established for children < 2 years of age.

Drug Interactions:

Tell your doctor or pharmacist if you are taking or planning to take any over-the-counter or prescription medications while taking this medicine. Doses of one or both drugs may need to be modified or a different drug may need to be prescribed. Immunosuppressants (eg, corticosteroids) interact with this vaccine.

Side Effects:

Every vaccine is capable of producing side effects. Many patients experience no, or minor, side effects. The frequency and severity of side effects depend on many factors including dose, duration of therapy, and individual susceptibility. Possible side effects include: Soreness, hardness, warmth, redness, or swelling at the injection site (within 2 days of vaccination); fever; rash; muscle or joint pain; headache; nausea; vomiting; general body discomfort; weakness.

Guidelines for Use:

- Delay the vaccine when respiratory illness with fever or infection is present.
- This vaccination may not work for everyone.
- Patients who require antibiotic therapy against possible pneumococcal infection should continue the antibiotic therapy after vaccination.
- *Guillain-Barré syndrome (GBS):* This syndrome, characterized by paralysis, has occurred rarely after the administration of the pneumococcal vaccination. No cause and effect relationship has been established. Evaluate the possible risk of GBS as compared with the risk of pneumonia and its complications.
- A single administration of the pneumoncoccal vaccine is generally adequate for a lifetime. The exception is those adults at highest risk for acquiring a pneumococcal infection (eg, splenic dysfunction, Hodgkin's disease, lymphoma, multiple myeloma, nephrotic syndrome, organ transplant recipients).
- This vaccine may be given at the same time as the flu vaccine.
- Store at 36° to 46°F. Do not freeze.

If you have any questions, consult your doctor, pharmacist, or health care provider.

Generic Name *Brand Name Example*		Uses
Rx	**Lyme Disease Vaccine** *LYMErix*	For active immunization against Lyme disease in individuals 15 to 70 years of age

Individuals most at risk for Lyme disease may be those who live or work in *Borrelia burgdorferi*-infected tick-infested grassy or wooded areas (eg, those who work in landscaping, brush clearing, forestry, or wildlife and parks management) and those who plan to travel or pursue recreational activities (eg, hiking, camping, fishing, hunting) in such areas. Most cases of Lyme disease in the US are thought to be acquired in the periresidential environment through routine activities of property maintenance, recreation, or exercise of pets.

Type of Drug:

Bacterial vaccine; agent for active immunization.

How the Drug Works:

Lyme disease vaccine stimulates the body to produce antibodies against the bacterial spirochete, which causes Lyme disease in North America.

Precautions:

Do not use in the following situations:

- allergy to the vaccine or any of its ingredients
- fever, moderate-to-severe
- Lyme arthritis, treatment resistant (antibiotic refractory)
- patients under 15 or over 70 years of age

Use with caution in the following situations:

- allergy to rubber (prefilled syringe only)
- anticoagulant therapy, concurrent
- blood clotting disorder
- immunosuppressive therapy, concurrent

Previous Lyme disease infection: Previous infection with *B. burgdorferi* may not confer protective immunity. Therefore, people with a history of Lyme disease may benefit from vaccination with Lyme disease vaccine.

Immunosuppression: Patients who are immunosuppressed or are receiving immunosuppressive therapy may not obtain the expected immune response. For patients receiving immunosuppressive therapy, defer vaccination for 3 months after therapy has been completed.

Pregnancy: It is not known whether Lyme disease vaccine can cause fetal harm when administered to a pregnant woman. Use only if clearly needed and the potential benefits to the mother outweigh the possible risks to the fetus. Health care providers are encouraged to register pregnant women who receive Lyme disease vaccine in the SmithKline Beecham Pharmaceuticals vaccination pregnancy registry by calling (800)366–8900, ext. 5231.

Breastfeeding: It is not known if Lyme disease vaccine appears in breast milk. Use caution when administered to a nursing woman. Consult your doctor before you begin breastfeeding.

Children: Safety and efficacy in patients < 15 years of age have not been established.

Drug Interactions:

Tell your doctor or pharmacist if you are taking or planning to take any over-the-counter or prescription medications or dietary supplements while receiving Lyme disease vaccine. Doses of one or both drugs may need to be modified or a different drug may need to be prescribed. Anticoagulants (eg, heparin) may increase bleeding at the Lyme disease vaccine site.

Side Effects:

Every drug is capable of producing side effects. Many patients experience no, or minor, side effects. The frequency and severity of side effects depend on many factors including dose, duration of therapy, and individual susceptibility. Possible side effects include:

Digestive Tract: Nausea; diarrhea.

Nervous System: Dizziness; headache; depression; fatigue.

Respiratory System: Bronchitis; coughing; sore throat; runny nose; sinus infection; upper respiratory tract infection.

Skin: Pain, redness, or soreness at injection site; rash; abnormal skin sensations (burning, prickling, tingling); skin inflammation; diminished skin sensitivity to stimulation.

Other: Tendon inflammation; joint, muscle, or back pain; achiness; chills or rigors; fever; viral infection; flu-like symptoms; arthritis; stiffness; joint deterioration; false positive test result for *B. burgdorferi.*

Guidelines for Use:

- This vaccine will be prepared and administered intramuscularly (into a muscle) by your health care provider in a medical setting.
- It is important to return for the subsequent dose(s) in any vaccination series. Three doses of Lyme disease vaccine, administered over a 12–month period, are required to achieve maximum benefit.
- In addition to vaccination with the Lyme disease vaccine, people can further decrease their risk of acquiring tick-borne infections by taking standard preventative measures such as wearing long-sleeved shirts and long pants rather than shorts, tucking pants into socks, treating clothing with tick repellant (preferably DEET), checking for and removing attached ticks.
- Lyme disease vaccine is not a treatment for Lyme disease.
- As with any vaccine, Lyme disease vaccine may not protect 100% of individuals. The duration of immunity following a complete schedule of immunization with Lyme disease has not been established.
- Inform your doctor if you have ever experienced a vaccine-related adverse reaction or if you experience any reaction following any of the 3 Lyme disease vaccine doses.
- Lyme disease vaccine does not provide protection against other tick-borne diseases such as babesiosis or ehrlichiosis.
- Lyme disease vaccine will not prevent Lyme disease in those who have an unrecognized Lyme disease infection at the time of vaccination.
- Patients with a history of *B. burgdorferi* infection may not have protection against subsequent disease or asymptomatic infection.

If you have any questions, consult your doctor, pharmacist, or health care provider.

	Generic Name *Brand Name Example*	Supplied As	Generic Available
Rx	**Pneumococcal 7-Valent Conjugate Vaccine**		
	Prevnar	**Injection:** 2 mcg each of 6 polysaccharide isolates; 4 mcg of 1 polysaccharide isolate per 0.5 mL dose	No

Type of Drug:

Bacterial vaccines.

How the Drug Works:

Pneumococcal 7–valent conjugate vaccine provides long-term protection to infants and toddlers against 7 of the most common forms of serious bacterial infections caused by *Streptoccoccus pneumoniae*. Protection from this vaccine is only against those strains contained in the vaccine and not all causes of bacterial infection.

Approximately 80% of serious infections in children (eg, pneumonia, middle ear infections, meningitis, sinus infections, blood infections) are caused by these 7 types of *S. pneumoniae*.

Uses:

To immunize infants and toddlers against bacterial infections caused by the 7 most common types of *S. pneumoniae*. This vaccine is not intended to be used for treatment of active infection.

Precautions:

Do not use in the following situations:

allergy to any component of the vaccine, including diphtheria toxoid
fever, moderate to severe

Use with caution in the following situations:

bleeding disorder (eg, thrombocytopenia)
latex sensitivity, history of

Impaired immune responsiveness: Children with an impaired immune system (eg, immunosuppressive therapy, chemotherapy, HIV infection) may have a reduced response to the vaccine.

Pregnancy: It is not known whether pneumococcal 7–valent conjugate vaccine can cause fetal harm when administered to a pregant women or whether it can affect reproductive capacity. Pneumococcal 7–valent conjugate vaccine is not recommended for use in pregnant women.

Breastfeeding: It is not known whether vaccine antigens or antibodies are excreted in breast milk. This vaccine is not recommended for use in nursing mothers.

Children: The safety and efficacy of pneumococcal 7–valent conjugate vaccine in children < 6 weeks of age have not been established. Immune responses elicited by pneumococcal 7–valent conjugate vaccine among infants born prematurely have not been studied.

Elderly: This vaccine is not recommended for use in adult patients. Do not use as a substitute for the 23–valent pneumococcal polysaccharide vaccine used in elderly patients.

Drug Interactions:

Tell your doctor or pharmacist if you are taking or if you are planning to take any over-the-counter or prescription medications or dietary supplements with pneumococcal 7–valent conjugated vaccine. Doses of one or both drugs may need to be modified or a different drug may need to be prescribed. The following drugs and drug classes interact with pneumococcal 7–valent conjugated vaccine:

anticoagulants (eg, heparin)
immunosuppressive agents (eg, corticosteroids)

Side Effects:

Every drug is capable of producing side effects. Many pneumococcal 7–valent conjugate vaccine users experience no, or minor, side effects. The frequency and severity of side effects depend on many factors including dose, duration of therapy, and individual susceptibility. Possible side effects include:

Digestive Tract: Decreased appetite; vomiting; diarrhea.

Other: Fever; drowsiness; rash; hives; irritability; restless sleep; redness, swelling, or tenderness at injection site.

Guidelines for Use:

- This medicine will be prepared and administered by your health care provider in a medical setting.
- Contact your doctor if any side effect becomes bothersome.

If you have any questions, consult your doctor, pharmacist, or health care provider.

	Generic Name *Brand Name Examples*	Supplied As	Generic Available
Rx	**Tuberculin Purified Protein Derivative**		
	Tubersol	1 TU (tuberculin unit)/0.1 mL	No
	Aplisol, Tubersol	5 TU/0.1 mL	No
	Tubersol	250 TU/0.1 mL	No
Rx	**Tuberculin PPD Multiple Puncture Device**		
	Aplitest, Tine Test PPD	5 TU/test	No
Rx	**Old Tuberculin, Multiple Puncture Devices**		
	Mono-Vacc Test (O.T.); Tuberculin, Old, Tine Test	5 TU/test	No

Type of Drug:

Skin test for tuberculosis (TB); Mantoux; Tine Test.

How the Drug Works:

The test involves injecting inactive material from the tuberculosis organism just under the skin. People previously exposed to TB infection will develop a local skin reaction 2 to 3 days after the skin test is given.

Uses:

To aid in diagnosing TB infection.

To determine risk of TB exposure in high-risk health care workers or institutionalized persons (eg, long-term hospital patients, prisoners, military personnel).

Precautions:

Repeated testing: Repeated testing of the uninfected individual does not cause sensitivity to tuberculin.

Tuberculin-positive reactors: Not to be given to known tuberculin-positive reactors because of the severe reactions that may occur at the test site.

Altered reactivity: Reactivity to tuberculin may be reduced for as long as 4 weeks by bacterial or viral infections; live virus vaccines (eg, measles, smallpox, polio, rubella, mumps); severe fever, sarcoidosis, or cancer; overwhelming tuberculosis; use of corticosteroids or immunosuppressive drugs; immunosuppressive infections (eg, HIV); old age; and malnutrition. In most patients who are very sick with tuberculosis, the previously negative tuberculin test becomes positive after a few weeks of treatment. A positive reaction does not necessarily signify active disease. Further diagnostic procedures such as chest x-ray and bacteriologic examinations of sputum must be done before there is a diagnosis of tuberculosis.

Pregnancy: The risk of unrecognized tuberculosis and the close postpartum contact between a mother with active disease and her infant leaves the infant in grave danger of tuberculosis and complications such as tuberculous meningitis. No adverse effects upon the fetus recognized as being due to tuberculosis skin testing have been reported.

Breastfeeding: It is unlikely that tuberculin is excreted in breast milk. Consult your doctor before you begin breastfeeding.

Children: A child who has been exposed to a tuberculosis adult must not be judged free of infection until there is a negative tuberculin reaction at least 10 weeks after exposure to the tuberculosis person.

Side Effects:

Every vaccine is capable of producing side effects. Many patients experience no, or minor, side effects. The frequency and severity of side effects depend on many factors including dose and individual susceptibility. Possible side effects include redness, swelling; ulceration; bleeding; pain, itching at injection site; dead skin organs;
scarring.

Guidelines for Use:

- *"Positive" skin test* — A blister or hardness develops at the site 48 to 72 (96 hours for Mono-Vacc) hours after it is given. The size of the affected area is also important in deciding test results.
- *"Positive" skin test* does not mean you have an active TB infection. Further tests will be needed.
- TB skin tests should not be given on areas affected by acne or hair.
- TB tests may be given first at 1 year of age before measles vaccination and every year or two thereafter.
- TB tests should not be given to persons who are known to have active TB, prior positive test reactions or known severe allergic reactions to it.
- Current infections, recent vaccination, certain drug use, serious illness or pregnancy may interfere with test results.

If you have any questions, consult your doctor, pharmacist, or health care provider.

General Guidelines for Topical Ophthalmic Drug Therapy, 1309

Agents for Glaucoma
- Alpha-2 Adrenergic Agonists, 1311
- Beta-Blockers, 1313
- Miotics, Cholinesterase Inhibitors, 1316
- Miotics, Direct-Acting, 1319
- Prostaglandin Agonists, 1322
- Sympathomimetics, 1325
- Apraclonidine HCl, 1328
- Carbonic Anhydrase Inhibitors – Dorzolamide HCl/Brinzolamide, 1330
- Dorzolamide HCl/Timolol Maleate, 1332
- Combinations, 1335

Alpha-Adrenergic Blocking Agents, 1337

Ophthalmic Vasoconstrictors
- Decongestants, 1339
- Decongestant Combinations, 1343

Cycloplegic Mydriatics, 1345

Ophthalmic Anti-inflammatory Agents
- Corticosteroids, 1348
- Loteprednol, 1351
- Mast Cell Stabilizers, 1353
- Nonsteroidal Anti-inflammatory Agents, 1356

Levocabastine HCl, 1358

Antihistamines
- Azelastine, 1360

Olopatadine, 1362

Ketotifen Fumarate, 1364

Ophthalmic Anti-infectives
- Antibiotics, 1366
- Steroid and Antibiotic Combinations, 1370
- Natamycin, 1374
- Antiviral Agents, 1376
- Fomivirsen Sodium, 1378

Ophthalmic Phototherapy
- Verteporfin, 1380

Artificial Tears, 1383

Ocular Lubricants, 1386

Contact Lens Products
- Hard Contact Lens Products, 1387
- Rigid Gas Permeable Contact Lens Products, 1390
- Soft (Hydrogel) Contact Lens Products, 1393

Otic Antibiotics, 1397

Otic Preparations
- Miscellaneous, 1400

Topical (surface) application is the most common way to administer ophthalmic drugs. Advantages of topical administration include convenience, simplicity, noninvasive nature, and the ability of the patient to self-administer the medication. Topical medications do not typically penetrate in useful concentrations into the internal eye structures. Therefore, they are of no therapeutic benefit for diseases of the retina, optic nerve, and other internal structures of the eye.

Medications:

Solutions and Suspensions – Most topical eye preparations are commercially available as solutions or suspensions that are applied directly to the eye from the bottle, which serves as the eye dropper. Avoid touching the dropper tip to the eye because this can lead to contamination of the medication and also may cause injury to the eye.

Recommended Procedure for Administration of Solutions or Suspensions
1. Wash hands thoroughly before use.
2. Shake suspensions well before using.
3. Tilt head backward or lie down and gaze upward.
4. Gently grasp lower eyelid below eyelashes and pull the eyelid away from the eye to form a pouch.
5. Place dropper directly over eye. Avoid contact of the dropper tip with the eye, finger, or any surface.
6. Look upward just before applying a drop.
7. After instilling (applying) the drop, look downward for several seconds.
8. Release the lid slowly and close eyes gently.
9. With eyes closed, apply gentle pressure with fingers to the inside corner of the eye (next to the bridge of the nose) for 3 to 5 minutes. This prevents drainage of solution from the intended area.
10. Do not rub the eye or squeeze the eyelid. Minimize blinking.
11. Do not rinse the dropper.
12. Do not use eye drops that have changed color or contain particles.
13. If more than one drop or type of eye drop is used, wait at least 5 minutes before using the second drop or drug.
14. When the instillation of eye drops is difficult (eg, children, adults with particularly strong blink reflex), the closed-eye method may be used. This involves lying down, placing the prescribed number of drops on the eyelid in the inner corner of the eye, then opening the eye so that drops will fall into the eye by gravity.
15. Temporary blurring of vision or irritation may occur after use. Contact your doctor or pharmacist with any concerns.

Lid Scrubs – Commercially available eyelid cleansers or antibiotic solutions or ointments can be directly applied to the lid. This is best accomplished by applying the drug to the end of a cotton-tipped applicator and then scrubbing the eyelid margin several times daily. The gauze pads supplied with commercially available eyelid cleansers are also convenient.

Ointments – The primary purpose for an eye ointment is to prolong drug contact time with the surface of the eye. This is particularly useful for treating children, who may "cry out" topically applied solutions, and for medicating eye injuries, such as corneal abrasions, when the eye is to be patched.

Recommended Procedures for Administration of Ointments	
1.	Wash hands thoroughly before using.
2.	Tilt head backward or lie down and gaze upward.
3.	Gently pull down the lower lid to form a pouch.
4.	Place 0.25 to 0.5 (¼ to ½) inch of ointment with a sweeping motion inside the lower lid by squeezing the tube gently and then slowly release the eyelid.
5.	Close the eye for 1 to 2 minutes and roll the eyeball in all directions.
6.	Temporary blurring of vision may occur. Avoid activities requiring clear vision until blurring clears.
7.	Remove excessive ointment around the eye or ointment tube tip with a tissue.
8.	If using more than one kind of ointment, wait about 10 minutes before applying the second drug.
9.	If using eye drops and ointments, instill the drops first. Ointments prevent entry of drops.

Gels – Ophthalmic gels are similar in thickness and clinical usage to eye ointments. Pilocarpine (*Pilopine HS*) and timolol maleate (*Timoptic-XE*) are currently the only eye preparations available in gel form. They are intended to serve as "sustained-release preparations," requiring only once-daily use (at bedtime).

Sprays – Although not commercially available, some practitioners use mydriatics or cycloplegics, alone or in combination, administered as a spray to the eye to dilate (open) the pupil or for cycloplegic examination. This is most often used for pediatric patients, and the solution is administered using a sterile atomizer or spray bottle.

Ophthalmic products contain a variety of preservatives, antioxidants, buffers, and other nontherapeutic formulation ingredients. Patients may be hypersensitive (allergic) to one or more of these agents. Any unexpected or discomforting itching, irritation, watering from the eye, redness, or sensitivity should be reported to a doctor or pharmacist.

If you have any questions, consult your doctor, pharmacist, or health care provider.

Generic Name *Brand Name Example*	Supplied As	Generic Available
Rx **Brimonidine Tartrate**		
Alphagan	**Solution:** 0.2% in 5 mL, 10 mL	No

Type of Drug:

Alpha-adrenergic receptor stimulator.

How the Drug Works:

Ophthalmic receptor stimulators decrease fluid production and increases the outflow. They lower pressure in the eye.

Uses:

To lower intraocular (fluid) pressure in open-angle glaucoma or ocular hypertension (pressure in the eye).

Precautions:

Do not use in the following situations:

- allergy to the drug
- monoamine oxidase (MAOI) inhibitor therapy

Use with caution in the following situations:

- cardiovascular disease, severe
- cerebral insufficiency
- contact lens wear
- coronary insufficiency
- depression
- kidney impairment
- liver impairment
- orthostatic hypotension
- Raynaud's phenomenon
- thromboangitis obliterans

Pregnancy: Studies in women or in animals have been judged not to show a risk to the fetus. However, no drug should be used during pregnancy unless clearly needed.

Breastfeeding: It is not known if brimonidine tartrate appears in breast milk. Consult your doctor before you begin breastfeeding.

Children: Safety and effectiveness in children have not been established.

Drug Interactions:

Tell your doctor or pharmacist if you are taking or planning to take any over-the-counter or prescription medications or dietary supplements while taking this medicine. Doses of one or both drugs may need to be modified or a different drug may need to be prescribed. The following drugs and drug classes interact with this medicine.

- antihypertensives (eg, *hydrochlorothiazide)*
- beta-blockers, ophthalmic and systemic (eg, *timolol, propranolol)*
- cardiac glycosides (eg, *digoxin)*
- CNS depressants (alcohol, barbiturates, opiates, sedatives, anesthetics)
- IOP-lowering medication (eg, *pilocarpine)*
- tricyclic antidepressants (eg, *amitriptyline)*

Side Effects:

Every drug is capable of producing side effects. Many patients experience no, or minor, side effects. The frequency and severity of side effects depend on many factors including dose, duration of therapy, and individual susceptibility. Possible side effects include the following:

Nervous System: Headache; fatigue/drowsiness; dizziness; depression; anxiety; sleeplessness.

Circulatory System: High blood pressure; pounding in the chest.

Eyes or Ocular: Red or blood shot eyes; burning/stinging; blurring; allergic reactions; itching; sensitive to light; redness of the eyelid; ache/pain; dryness; tearing; eyelid swelling; conjunctival edema; irritation; whitening; abnormal or change in vision; lid crusting; bleeding; discharge; conjunctival follicles.

Other: Muscular pain; abnormal taste; nasal dryness; fainting; weakness; dry mouth.

Guidelines for Use:

- Usual dose is 1 drop 3 times daily, 8 hours apart.
- Soft contact wearers should wait 15 minutes after using this medication before inserting lenses.
- This medicine may cause drowsiness. Use caution while driving or performing other tasks requiring mental alertness, coordination, or physical dexterity.
- Store below 77°F.

If you have any questions, consult your doctor, pharmacist, or health care provider.

	Generic Name *Brand Name Examples*	Supplied As	Generic Available
Rx	**Betaxolol HCl**	**Solution**: 0.5%	Yes
	Betoptic S	**Suspension**: 0.25%	No
Rx	**Carteolol HCl**		
	Ocupress	**Solution**: 1%	Yes
Rx	**Levobetaxolol HCl**		
	Betaxon	**Suspension**: 0.5%	No
Rx	**Levobunolol HCl**		
	Betagan Liquifilm[1]	**Solution**: 0.25%, 0.5%	Yes
Rx	**Metipranolol HCl**		
	OptiPranolol	**Solution**: 0.3%	No
Rx	**Timolol Maleate**		
	Timoptic[1], *Timoptic in Ocudose*	**Solution**: 0.25%, 0.5%	Yes
	Timoptic-XE	**Gel**: 0.25%, 0.5%	Yes

[1] Contains sulfites.

Type of Drug:

Nonselective beta-adrenergic blocking agents for the eye.

How the Drug Works:

Ophthalmic beta-blockers decrease the fluid pressure in the eye. They may be used alone or in combination with other drugs.

Uses:

To help lower intraocular (fluid) pressure (IOP) in chronic open-angle glaucoma. Also used to help manage ocular hypertension (high intraocular pressure).

Precautions:

Do not use in the following situations:

- allergy to the beta-blocker or any of its ingredients
- bronchial asthma
- cardiogenic shock
- chronic obstructive pulmonary disease, severe
- heart failure
- slowed heart rate/heart block

Use with caution in the following situations:

- decreased blood flow to brain
- diabetes
- heart disease
- hyperthyroidism (overactive thyroid)
- lung disease or breathing difficulties (eg, bronchitis, emphysema)
- myasthenia gravis
- surgery, with anesthesia

Diabetes: Diabetic patients and patients subject to hypoglycemia (low blood sugar) should use caution. Beta-blockers may mask the signs of hypoglycemia.

Pregnancy: There are no adequate and well-controlled studies in pregnant women. Use only if clearly needed and the potential benefits to the mother outweigh the possible hazards to the fetus.

Breastfeeding: Timolol maleate appears in breast milk. It is not known if betaxolol, carteolol, levobetaxolol, levobunolol, or metipranolol appear in breast milk. Consult your doctor before you begin breastfeeding.

Children: Safety and effectiveness in children have not been established.

Sulfites: Some of these products may contain sulfite preservatives, which can cause allergic reactions in certain individuals. Check package label when available or consult your doctor or pharmacist.

Drug Interactions:

Tell your doctor or pharmacist if you are taking or if you are planning to take any over-the-counter or prescription medications or dietary supplements while taking a beta-blocker. Doses of one or both drugs may need to be modified or a different drug may need to be prescribed. The following drugs and drug classes interact with beta-blockers:

beta-blockers, oral (eg, propranolol)
calcium antagonists (eg, verapamil)
catecholamine-depleting drugs (eg, reserpine)
digitalis (eg, *Lanoxin)*
epinephrine, topical and ophthalmic (eg, *Epifrin)*
phenothiazines (eg, promethazine)
quinidine (eg, *Quinora)*

Also consider all drug interactions reported for oral beta-blockers (eg, propranolol). (See the monograph in the Cardiovascular Drugs chapter.)

Side Effects:

Every drug is capable of producing side effects. Many beta-blocker users experience no, or minor, side effects. The frequency and severity of side effects depend on many factors including dose, duration of therapy, and individual susceptibility. Possible side effects include the following:

Eyes or Ocular: Temporary stinging or pain when instilling drops; double vision; swelling; crusting; visual problems; irritation; blurred vision; burning; inflammation; tearing; dry eyes; foreign body sensation; itching eyes; cataracts; light sensitivity; drooping of upper eyelid; red eyes.

Digestive Tract: Appetite loss; taste changes; dry mouth; nausea; diarrhea; stomachache; constipation.

Nervous System: Depression; confusion; dizziness; headache; drowsiness; nervousness; nightmares; memory loss; hallucinations; sleeplessness; anxiety; vertigo (feeling of whirling motion).

Circulatory System: Abnormal heart rhythm; palpitations (pounding in the chest); congestive heart failure; chest pain; changes in blood pressure; worsening of angina.

Respiratory System: Difficulty breathing; cough; runny nose.

Skin: Rash; itching; hives; abnormal skin sensations; worsening of psoriasis.

Other: Weakness; fatigue; muscle pain; fainting; hair loss; nasal congestion; inflammation of the tongue; gout; increased blood lipids; arthritis; nosebleed; changes in sense of smell; sexual dysfuction (male); masked symptoms of hypoglycemia (low blood sugar); cold hands and feet; incoordination. Also consider the side effects associated with oral beta-blockers (eg, propranolol).

Guidelines for Use:

- Dosage is indvidualized. Use exactly as prescribed. Do not skip doses.
- If a dose is missed, instill it as soon as possible. If several hours have passed or it is nearing time for the next dose, do not double the dose to catch up, unless advised by your doctor. If more than one dose is missed, contact your doctor or pharmacist.
- Take contact lenses out of your eyes prior to instilling this medicine. You may reinsert contact lenses 15 minutes following instillation.
- Avoid allowing the tip of the dispensing container to contact the eye or surrounding area to avoid contamination. Replace cap immediately after use.
- May cause stinging or pain when first instilled in the eye.
- Temporary blurred vision may occur for up to 5 minutes, impairing your ability to perform hazardous tasks. Use caution before operating machinery or driving a motor vehicle.
- Intraocular pressure will have to be monitored periodically by your doctor. Be sure to keep appointments.
- Notify your doctor if you plan to have eye surgery or if you experience an eye infection or trauma. You may have to stop using the drops.
- *Betaxolol, levobetaxolol* — Shake well before using.
- *Timolol maleate gel* — Invert the closed container and shake once before each use. Other eye medications should be used 10 minutes before the gel.
- Wait at least 5 minutes before using any other eye medications.
- Store upright at room temperature (59° to 86°F). Avoid freezing. Protect from light.

If you have any questions, consult your doctor, pharmacist, or health care provider.

AGENTS FOR GLAUCOMA — MIOTICS, CHOLINESTERASE INHIBITOR

	Generic Name *Brand Name Examples*	Supplied As	Generic Available
Rx	**Demecarium Bromide**		
	Humorsol	**Solution:** 0.125%, 0.25%	No
Rx	**Echothiophate Iodide**		
	Phospholine Iodide	**Powder for Reconstitution:** 1.5 mg (to make 0.03%); 3 mg (0.06%); 6.25 mg (0.125%); 12.5 mg (0.25%)	No
Rx	**Physostigmine**		
	Eserine Sulfate	**Ointment:** 0.25%	No

Type of Drug:

Drugs that cause the pupil to constrict (decrease in size); glaucoma drugs.

How the Drug Works:

Cholinesterase inhibitor miotics decrease the fluid pressure inside the eye by increasing the outflow of fluid (aqueous humor) from the eye. They cause the pupils to get smaller (miosis) and cause the ciliary muscle of the eye to contract.

Uses:

To treat open-angle glaucoma.

Demecarium also is used after iridectomy (surgical removal of a portion of the iris) or to treat accommodative esotropia or certain conditions affecting aqueous (fluid) outflow.

Echothiophate also is used to treat some types of angle-closure glaucoma after iridectomy (surgical removal of a portion of the iris), strabismus, and esotropia.

Precautions:

Do not use in the following situations:

allergy to these drugs or their ingredients
glaucoma, angle-closure (echothiophate only)
inflammation of the iris, choroid or ciliary body, with or without glaucoma
pregnancy (demecarium only)

Use with caution in the following situations:

asthma
epilepsy
heart attack, recent
low blood pressure, severe
myasthenia gravis (muscle weakness)
narrow-angle glaucoma, chronic
eye conditions/problems, other
parkinsonism
peptic ulcer
slow heart rate, severe
surgery, prior to
spastic GI conditions (stomach cramping)
vagotonia (irritability of the vagal nerve)

Eye exams will be required to monitor treatment. Be sure to keep appointments.

Pregnancy:

Demecarium – Do not use during pregnancy. The risk of use in a pregnant woman clearly outweighs any possible benefit.

All others – Adequate studies have not been done in pregnant women, or animal studies may have shown a risk to the fetus. Use only if clearly needed and potential benefits outweigh the possible hazards to the fetus.

Breastfeeding: It is not known if these drugs appear in breast milk. Because of the risk of serious reactions in infants, consult your doctor before breastfeeding.

Children: Safety and effectiveness of physostigmine have not been established. Use demecarium with extreme caution in children who may require general anesthesia.

Drug Interactions:

Tell your doctor or pharmacist if you are taking or if you are planning to take any over-the-counter or prescription medications or dietary supplements while taking these medicines. Doses of one or both drugs may need to be modified or a different drug may need to be prescribed. Anticholinesterases (eg, ambenonium), insecticides/pesticides (carbamate or organophosphate) and succinylcholine (eg, *Sucostrin*) interact with these medicines.

Side Effects:

Every drug is capable of producing side effects. Many patients experience no, or minor, side effects. The frequency and severity of side effects depend on many factors including dose, duration of therapy and individual susceptibility. Possible side effects include the following:

Eyes or Ocular: Tearing; burning; redness; lid twitching; nearsightedness; blurred vision; browache/headache; inflammation of iris; retinal detachment; cloudy lens; increase in intraocular pressure; cysts.

Other: Nausea; vomiting; stomach cramps; diarrhea; loss of bladder control; excessive salivation or sweating; fainting; muscle weakness; difficulty breathing; irregular heartbeat.

Guidelines for Use:

- Use exactly as prescribed. Do not use more often than directed.
- Follow Administration Guidelines found at the beginning of this chapter.
- Wash hands before and immediately after instilling these drugs.
- If a dose is missed, instill it as soon as possible. If several hours have passed or if it is nearing time for the next dose, do not the double the dose in order to "catch up" (unless advised to do so by your doctor). If more than one dose is missed, contact your doctor or pharmacist.
- Local irritation and headache may occur when you first start using these drugs.
- May cause vision problems in poor light. Use caution while driving at night or performing tasks in poor lighting.
- Discontinue this medication and consult your doctor if any of the following occur: Excess sweating or mouth watering, loss of bladder control, stomach cramps, diarrhea, muscle weakness, difficulty breathing, or irregular heartbeat.
- Eye ointments may slow corneal healing.
- *Echothiophate* — Tolerance may develop after prolonged use; a rest period usually restores response to the medication.
- *Storage* — Store demecarium and physostigmine between 59° to 86° F, away from heat and cold. Keep tightly closed. After mixing echothiophate, store in refrigerator and use within 6 months. Use solution within 1 month if it is stored at room temperature (59° to 86° F).

If you have any questions, consult your doctor, pharmacist, or health care provider.

	Generic Name *Brand Name Examples*	Supplied As	Generic Available
Rx	**Acetylcholine Chloride, Intraocular**		
	Miochol-E	**Solution**: 1%	No
Rx	**Carbachol, Intraocular**		
	Carbastat, Miostat	**Solution**: 0.01%	No
Rx	**Carbachol, Topical**		
	Carboptic, Isopto Carbachol	**Solution**: 0.75%, 1.5%, 2.25%, 3%	Yes
Rx	**Pilocarpine HCl**		
	Adsorbocarpine, Akarpine, Isopto Carpine, Pilocar, Piloptic, Pilopto-Carpine, Pilostat, Storzine 2	**Solution**: 0.25%, 0.5%, 1%, 2%, 3%, 4%, 5%, 6%, 8%, 10%	Yes
	Pilopine HS	**Gel**: 4%	No
	Ocusert Pilo	**Ocular therapeutic system**: 20 mcg/hr, 40 mcg/hr	No
Rx	**Pilocarpine Nitrate**		
	Pilagan	**Solution**: 1%, 2%, 4%	No

Type of Drug:

Drugs that cause the pupil to constrict (decrease in size); glaucoma drugs.

How the Drug Works:

Direct-acting miotics decrease the fluid pressure inside the eye by increasing the outflow of fluid (aqueous humor) from the eye. They cause the pupils to get smaller (miosis) and cause the ciliary muscle of the eye to contract.

Uses:

To decrease elevated intraocular (fluid) pressure in glaucoma.

Acetylcholine, carbachol (intraocular): To induce miosis (pupil constriction) during surgery.

Pilocarpine HCl and nitrate: To reverse mydriasis (pupil dilation).

Precautions:

Do not use in the following situations:

- allergy to any of these drugs
- glaucoma, pupillary block or secondary
- inflammation of eye interior or iris, severe

Use with caution in the following situations:

- asthma
- blood pressure, high or low
- corneal abrasion (carbachol only)
- GI spasm (cramping)
- heart problems
- hyperthyroidism
- Parkinson's disease
- peptic ulcer
- retinal disease, history
- urinary tract obstruction

Pregnancy: Adequate studies have not been done in pregnant women, or animal studies may have shown a risk to the fetus. Use only if clearly needed and potential benefits outweigh the possible hazards to the fetus.

Breastfeeding: It is not known if these agents appear in breast milk. Consult your doctor before you begin breastfeeding.

Children: Safety and effectiveness have not been established.

Drug Interactions:

Tell your doctor or pharmacist if you are taking or if you are planning to take any over-the-counter or prescription medications or dietary supplements while taking these medicines. Doses of one or both drugs may need to be modified or a different drug may need to be prescribed. Topical nonsteroidal anti-inflammatory drugs (NSAIDs, eg, suprofen, flurbiprofen) interact with these medicines.

Side Effects:

Every drug is capable of producing side effects. Many patients experience no, or minor, side effects. The frequency and severity of side effects depend on many factors including dose, duration of therapy, and individual susceptibility. Possible side effects include the following:

Eyes or Ocular: Burning; stinging; tearing; blurring; redness; inflammation of cornea and conjunctiva (white of eyes); reduced vision in poor light; nearsightedness; detached retina (floaters, flashes of light).

Other: Stomach cramps; nausea; vomiting; diarrhea; flushing; fainting; excess salivation; sweating; headache; changes in blood pressure; bladder tightness; frequent urination; bronchial spasms; asthma; difficulty breathing; irregular heartbeat.

Guidelines for Use:

- Use exactly as prescribed.
- Follow Administration Guidelines found at the beginning of this chapter.
- If a dose is missed, instill it as soon as possible. If several hours have passed or if it is nearing time for the next dose, do not double the dose in order to "catch up." If more than one dose is missed, contact your doctor or pharmacist.
- If accidental overdosage occurs, flush eyes with water and contact your doctor.
- Report any changes in vision to your doctor immediately.
- May sting when used, especially the first few times. May also cause headache, browache, or decreased night vision. Use caution while driving at night or performing tasks in poor lighting.
- *Solution* — To avoid contamination, do not touch tip of container to any surface, including the eye. Wash hands before and immediately after use. Keep bottle tightly closed when not in use. Discard solution after expiration date. Store at room temperature. Do not freeze. Keep out of reach of children.
- *Gel* — Apply once daily at bedtime. If other glaucoma medications (drops) are also being used, use drops at least 5 minutes before the gel. Store at room temperature. Do not freeze.
- *Pilocarpine ocular systems (Ocusert Pilo)* —
  Follow the patient instructions provided in the package.
  Wash hands with soap and water before touching or manipulating the system.
  If a displaced system contacts unclean surfaces, rinse with cool tap water before replacing. Discard contaminated systems and replace with a fresh unit.
  Check for the presence of the system before retiring at night and upon arising. If keeping the unit in the eye is a problem, contact your doctor.
  Damaged or deformed systems should not be placed or retained in the eye.
  Store in the refrigerator (36° to 46°F).

If you have any questions, consult your doctor, pharmacist, or health care provider.

	Generic Name *Brand Name Examples*	Supplied As	Generic Available
Rx	**Bimatoprost**		
	Lumigan	**Solution**: 0.03%	No
Rx	**Latanoprost**		
	Xalatan	**Solution**: 0.005%	No
Rx	**Travoprost**		
	Travatan	**Solution**: 0.004%	No
Rx	**Unoprostone Isopropyl**		
	Rescula	**Solution**: 0.15%	No

Type of Drug:

Agents for glaucoma.

How the Drug Works:

Prostaglandin agonists reduce pressure on the eye by increasing the outflow of aqueous humor (fluid) in the eye.

Uses:

For the reduction of elevated intraocular pressure (IOP) in patients with open-angle glaucoma or ocular hypertension who are intolerant of other IOP-lowering medications or insufficiently responsive to another IOP-lowering medication.

Precautions:

Do not use in the following situations: Allergy to the prostaglandin agonist, benzalkonium chloride (a preservative in the eye drop), or any other ingredients.

Use with caution in the following situations:

absence of lens of the eye
contact lens wear
intraocular inflammation, active (eg, uveitis)
kidney impairment
liver impairment
macular edema, risk factors for
pseudophakic patients with a torn posterior lens capsule

Eye changes: Prostaglandin agonists may gradually change eye color, causing the irises to become more brown. This is more noticeable in green-brown, blue/gray-brown, or yellow-brown eyes. Eyelid skin darkening and gradual changes in the eyelashes (eg, length, thickness, pigmentation, number of lashes) also have been reported. These changes may be permanent. The long-term effects are currently unknown.

Pregnancy: There are no adequate and well-controlled studies in pregnant women. Use only if clearly needed and the potential benefits to the mother outweigh the possible hazards to the fetus. Travoprost may interfere with the maintenance of pregnancy and should not be used by women during pregnancy or by women attempting to become pregnant.

Breastfeeding: It is not known if prostaglandin agonists appear in breast milk. Consult your doctor before you begin breastfeeding.

Children: Safety and effectiveness in children have not been established.

Drug Interactions:

Tell your doctor or pharmacist if you are taking or planning to take any over-the-counter or prescription medications or dietary supplements while using a prostaglandin agonist. Doses of one or both drugs may need to be modified or a different drug may need to be prescribed. Eye drops containing thimerosal may interact with prostaglandin agonists.

Side Effects:

Every drug is capable of producing side effects. Many prostaglandin agonist users experience no, or minor, side effects. The frequency and severity of side effects depend on many factors including dose, duration of therapy, and individual susceptibility. Possible side effects include the following:

Eyes or Ocular: Changes in vision (eg, blurred vision, double vision); burning or stinging; red eyes; eye color change; dry eye; excessive tearing; eye pain; lid crusting; lid swelling; lid discomfort or pain; light sensitivity; foreign body sensation; eyelid itching; eyelash changes (eg, length, thickness, number of lashes, pigmentation); eye discharge.

Nervous System: Anxiety; depression; headache; weakness; dizziness.

Respiratory System: Upper respiratory tract infection; cold; flu; sinus inflammation; runny nose.

Skin: Rash; itching; excessive hair growth; eyelid skin darkening.

Other: Muscle, joint, back, or chest pain; indigestion; high cholesterol levels; changes in blood pressure; infection; pain; prostate disorder; urinary incontinence; urinary tract infection; abnormal liver function tests; diabetes mellitus; sore throat.

Guidelines for Use:

- The recommended dose of bimatoprost, latanoprost, and travoprost is 1 drop in the affected eye(s) once daily in the evening. The recommended dose of unoprostone is 1 drop in the affected eye(s) twice daily.
- Wait at least 5 minutes between use of other eye drops or eye products.
- Do not use while wearing contact lenses; they may be reinserted 15 minutes after administration.
- Changes in eye or eyelid color and eyelash changes may occur in the treated eye(s). These changes may be permanent.
- To prevent contamination of the solution or dropper tip of the bottle, do not touch the eyelids or surrounding areas with the dropper tip.
- Contact your doctor if you experience eye trauma, infection, or surgery during treatment. Also contact your doctor if you experience eye inflammation, irritation, discharge, or lid reactions.
- Store as directed on the container. Protect from light.

If you have any questions, consult your doctor, pharmacist, or health care provider.

	Generic Name *Brand Name Examples*	Supplied As	Generic Available
Rx	**Dipivefrin**		
	AKPro, Propine	**Solution**: 0.1%	Yes
Rx	**Epinephrine (as HCl)**		
	Epifrin, Glaucon[1]	**Solution**: 0.1%, 0.5%, 1%, 2%	Yes
Rx	**Epinephrine (as Borate)**		
	Epinal	**Solution**: 0.5%, 1%	No

[1] Contains sulfites.

Type of Drug:

Vasoconstrictors. Drugs that cause the pupil to dilate (widen) and intraocular pressure to decrease.

How the Drug Works:

Sympathomimetics decrease the intraocular (fluid) pressure in the eye by decreasing formation of fluid (aqueous humor). They also relax the ciliary muscle, dilate the pupil, and increase aqueous humor flow out of the eye. May be used alone or in combination with other drugs.

Uses:

To help manage open-angle (chronic simple) glaucoma.

Precautions:

Do not use in the following situations:

absence of lens in the eye (epinephrine only)
allergy to these medicines or their ingredients
narrow-angle glaucoma
narrow-angles (but no glaucoma)
shallow-angle glaucoma
soft contact lens wear

Use with caution in the following situations:

anesthesia
absence of lens in the eye (dipivefrin only)
asthma
cerebral arteriosclerosis (hardening of the arteries)
diabetes
heart disease
high blood pressure
hyperthyroidism (overactive thyroid), untreated

Pregnancy:

Epinephrine – Adequate studies have not been done in pregnant women, or animal studies may have shown a risk to the fetus. Safety for use has not been established. Use only when clearly needed and potential benefits outweigh possible hazards to the fetus.

Dipivefrin – Studies in pregnant women or in animals have been judged not to show a risk to the fetus. However, no drug should be used during pregnancy unless clearly needed.

Breastfeeding: It is not known if these drugs appear in breast milk. Consult your doctor before you begin breastfeeding.

Children: Safety and effectiveness have not been established.

Elderly: Use with caution in elderly patients.

Sulfites: Some of these products contain sulfite preservatives, which can cause allergic reactions in certain individuals. Check package label when available or consult your doctor or pharmacist.

Drug Interactions:

Tell your doctor or pharmacist if you are taking or if you are planning to take any over-the-counter or prescription medications or dietary supplements while taking these medicines. Doses of one or both drugs may need to be modified or a different drug may need to be prescribed. The following drugs and drug classes interact with these medicines.

- anesthetics (eg, halothane)
- beta-blockers (eg, propranolol)
- bretylium (*Bretylol*)
- ergotrate
- guanethidine (*Ismelin*)
- methylergonovine (*Methergine*)
- oxytocin (eg, *Pitocin*)
- tricyclic antidepressants (eg, amitriptyline)

Side Effects:

Every drug is capable of producing side effects. Many patients experience no, or minor, side effects. The frequency and severity of side effects depend on many factors including dose, duration of therapy, and individual susceptibility. Possible side effects include:

Eyes or Ocular: Eyeache; stinging; burning; redness or irritation of eyelid; sensitivity to light; glare; changes in eye color.

Nervous System: Fainting; headache; browache.

Circulatory System: Heart pounding (palpitations); increased heart rate; abnormal heart rhythm; high blood pressure.

Guidelines for Use:

- For use in eyes only.
- Do not use if solution is brown or contains particles.
- Follow Administration Guidelines found at the beginning of this chapter.
- To avoid contamination, do not touch tip of container to any surface. Replace cap after use.
- If a dose is missed, instill it as soon as possible. If several hours have passed or if it is nearing time for the next dose, do not double the dose to "catch up" (unless advised to do so by your doctor). If more than one dose is missed or it is necessary to establish a new dosage schedule, contact your doctor or pharmacist.
- Do not use while wearing soft contact lenses. Discoloration of lenses may occur.
- If overdosage occurs, flush eye(s) with water or normal saline.
- May cause stinging or burning when you first instill drops into the eyes. Headache or browache may occur.
- May cause a sensitivity to bright light. Protect eyes and wear sunglasses.
- Report any changes in vision to your doctor immediately.
- *Epinephrine* may cause temporary blurred or unstable vision after instillation. Use caution while driving, operating machinery, or performing other tasks requiring clear vision.
- *Storage* — Store in a cool place (36° to 75° F), away from light. Do not freeze. Keep container tightly sealed.

If you have any questions, consult your doctor, pharmacist, or health care provider.

	Generic Name *Brand Name Examples*	Supplied As	Generic Available
Rx	**Apraclonidine HCl**		
	Iopidine	**Solution**: 0.5%	No

Type of Drug:

Vasoconstrictor. A drug that causes the pupil to dilate (widen).

How the Drug Works:

Apraclonidine reduces intraocular (fluid) pressure, IOP, in the eye by decreasing the rate of fluid production.

Uses:

For short-term therapy to lower intraocular (fluid) pressure in adults who are on the highest tolerated medical therapy.

Precautions:

Do not use in the following situations:

allergy to apraclonidine or clonidine
monoamine oxidase inhibitor (MAOI) use

Use with caution in the following situations:

depression
heart attack, recent
heart disease
hypertension (high blood pressure)
kidney disease
liver disease
vascular disease (eg, Raynaud's disease, thromboangiitis obliterans, cerebrovascular disease)

Pregnancy: Adequate studies have not been done in pregnant women, or animal studies may have shown a risk to the fetus. Use only if clearly needed and potential benefits outweigh possible hazards to the fetus.

Breastfeeding: It is not known if apraclonidine appears in breast milk. Consult your doctor before you begin breastfeeding.

Children: Safety and effectiveness in children have not been established.

Lab tests will be required periodically.

Drug Interactions:

Tell your doctor or pharmacist if you are taking or if you are planning to take any over-the-counter or prescription medications or dietary supplements while taking this medicine. Doses of one or both drugs may need to be modified or a different drug may need to be prescribed. The following drugs and drug classes interact with this medicine.

alcohol
anesthetics (eg, halothane)
antihypertensives (eg, methyldopa)
barbiturates (eg, phenobarbital
beta-blockers (eg, propranolol)
cardiac glycosides (eg, digoxin)
MAO inhibitors (eg, phenelzine)
opiates (eg, morphine)
sedatives (eg, diazepam)
tricyclic antidepressants (eg, amitriptyline)

Side Effects:

Every drug is capable of producing side effects. Many patients experience no, or minor, side effects. The frequency or severity depend on many factors, including dose, duration of therapy and individual susceptibility. Possible side effects include the following:

Eyes or Ocular: Blood-shot eyes; discomfort; tearing; itching; swelling of eyelid; feeling of a foreign body in the eye; dry eyes; blurred vision; discharge from the eyes; paleness of inner lining of eyelid.

Other: Dry mouth; dry nose; headache; weakness; changes in taste; dizziness; drowsiness.

Guidelines for Use:

- Place 1 to 2 drops in the affected eye(s) 3 times daily. Wait 5 minutes before using any other eye medications.
- Do not touch the dropper tip to any surface, including your eye, because this may contaminate the contents or cause damage/infect the eye.
- *Soft contact lenses* — Do not wear during treatment.
- Do not increase or decrease this medicine without your doctor's approval. If a dose is missed, instill it as soon as possible. If several hours have passed or if it is within 2 hours of the next dose, do not double the dose to "catch up" unless advised to do so by your doctor). If more than one dose is missed or it is necessary to establish a new dosage schedule, contact your doctor or pharmacist. Use exactly as prescribed.
- Contact your doctor immediately if any of the following occurs: Blood-shot eyes; itching; discomfort; tearing; feeling of a foreign body in the eye; swelling of the eyelid. You may need to stop using the medicine.
- This medicine may cause drowsiness or dizziness. Avoid driving or performing other tasks requiring alertness or coordination until effects are known, then use caution.
- Lab and visual tests (especially for glaucoma patients) may be required to monitor therapy. Be sure to keep appointments.
- Do not share this medicine with anyone else.
- Store between 36 to 80°F. Protect from freezing and light.

If you have any questions, consult your doctor, pharmacist, or health care provider.

	Generic Name *Brand Name Examples*	Supplied As	Generic Available
Rx	**Brinzolamide**		
	Azopt	**Suspension**: 1%	No
	Dorzolamide HCl		
	Trusopt [1]	**Solution**: 2%	No

[1] Contains benzalkonium chloride.

Type of Drug:

Carbonic anhydrase inhibitor.

How the Drug Works:

Brinzolamide and dorzolamide reduce fluid pressure in the eye by decreasing the rate of fluid production.

Uses:

Brinzolamide and dorzolamide lower fluid pressure in the eyeball in patients with ocular hypertension or open-angle glaucoma. Dorzolamide may be used in combination with other medications.

Precautions:

Do not use in the following situations:

- allergy to brinzolamide or dorzolamide, to any of its ingredients, or its relatives (eg, sulfa drugs)
- kidney function, severely impaired
- soft contact lens wear (dorzolamide)

Use with caution in the following situations:

- oral carbonic anhydrase inhibitor use
- soft contact lens wear (brinzolamide)
- kidney function, reduced
- liver disease

Pregnancy: Adequate studies have not been done in pregnant women, or animal studies may have shown a risk to the fetus. Use only if clearly needed and potential benefits outweight possible hazards to the fetus.

Breastfeeding: It is not known if brinzolamide and dorzolamide appear in breast milk. Consult your doctor before you begin breastfeeding.

Children: Safety and effectiveness in children have not been established.

Drug Interactions:

Tell your doctor or pharmacist if you are taking or if you are planning to take any over-the-counter or prescription medications or dietary supplements while taking these medicines. Doses of one or both drugs may need to be modified or a different drug may need to be prescribed. High dose salicylates (eg, aspirin) and oral carbonic anhydrase inhibitors (acetazolamide, dichlorphenamide, methazolamide) may interact with brinzolamide and dorzolamide.

Side Effects:

Every drug is capable of producing side effects. Many patients experience no, or minor, side effects. The frequency and severity of side effects depend on many factors including dose, duration of therapy, and individual susceptibility. Possible side effects include the following:

Eyes or Ocular: Burning, stinging or discomfort immediately following use; tearing; blurred vision; dryness; light sensitivity; skin or eyelid inflammation; dry eye; foreign body sensation; cornea inflammation; eye discharge, pain and itching.

Other: Bitter, sour or unusual taste; sinus infection; headache.

Guidelines for Use:

- Shake brinzolamide suspension well before use.
- Place one drop in the affected eye(s) 3 times daily. Do not increase or decrease this medicine without your doctor's approval. Wait at least 10 minutes before using any other eye medications. Use exactly as prescribed
- Brief stinging or burning of the eye may occur after administration. This is normal. Contact your doctor if the symptom(s) continue or worsen.
- Do not touch the dropper tip to any surface, including your eye, because this may contaminate the contents or damage/infect the eye.
- Dorzolamide contains benzalkonium chloride, a preservative that may be absorbed by soft contact lenses.
- Soft contact lenses — Do not wear during treatment with dorzolamide. May be reinserted 15 minutes after brinzolamide use.
- Dorzolamide may cause sensitivity to bright light. Protect your eyes and wear sunglasses if this occurs.
- Temporary blurred vision is possible following use. Use caution when operating machinery or driving a motor vehicle.
- Contact your doctor if you receive an eye injury or undergo eye surgery; your medication may need to be changed.
- Discontinue this medicine immediately and contact your doctor if any of the following occurs: Swelling of the eyelids; redness; itching; discharge; tearing or any other signs of an infection or eye irritation.
- Brinzolamide and dorzolamide are sulfonamides and although administered topically, can be absorbed into the body. Therefore, the same types of side effects that can occur with sulfonamides can also occur with this drugs.
- Do not use either of these drugs if you are allergic to sulfonamides. Do not use with other carbonic anhydrase inhibitors.
- Store brinzolamide at controlled room temperature (36° to 86°F). Store dorzolamide at room temperature (59° to 86°F). Protect from light.

If you have any questions, consult your doctor, pharmacist, or health care provider.

	Generic Name *Brand Name Examples*	Supplied As	Generic Available
Rx	**Dorzolamide HCl/Timolol Maleate**		
	Cosopt	**Solution**: 2% dorzolamide, 0.5% timolol	No

Type of Drug:

A combination of two drugs, a carbonic anhydrase inhibitor (dorzolamide HCl) and a beta–adrenergic receptor blocker (timolol maleate), each of which lowers pressure within the eye (intraocular). Antiglaucoma medicines.

How the Drug Works:

Reduces fluid formation within eyeball resulting in lowering of intraocular pressure.

Uses:

Reduction of elevated intraocular pressure (IOP) in patients with open-angle glaucoma or ocular hypertension who have not responded to beta blockers alone.

Precautions:

Do not use in the following situations:

- allergy to dorzolamide HCl or sulfa drugs
- allergy to timolol maleate
- bronchial asthma, current or history
- heart conduction problems
- heart failure, overt
- sudden decreased heart function
- chronic obstructive lung disease, severe
- kidney impairment, severe
- sinus bradycardia (slow heart rate)

Use with caution in the following situations:

- bronchitis, chronic
- chronic obstructive lung disease, mild to moderate
- diabetes mellitus
- emphysema, chronic
- heart failure, history
- hypoglycemia, spontaneous
- liver impairment
- major surgery
- myasthenia gravis
- surgical anesthesia
- thyroid disorder

Pregnancy: Adequate studies have not been done in pregnant women. Use only if clearly needed and potential benefits outweigh the possible hazards to the fetus.

Breastfeeding: It is not known if dorzolamide appears in breast milk. Timolol appears in breast milk. Consult your doctor before you begin breastfeeding. A decision should be made whether to discontinue nursing or discontinue the drug, taking into account the importance of the drug to the mother.

Children: Safety and effectiveness in children have not been established.

Lab tests and eye examinations may be required during therapy.

Drug Interactions:

Tell your doctor or pharmacist if you are taking or planning to take any over-the-counter or prescription medications or dietary supplements while taking this medicine. Doses of one or both drugs may need to be modified or a different drug may need to be prescribed. The following drugs and drug classes interact with this medicine:

- beta-adrenergic blocking agents, oral or topical (eg, propranolol)
- calcium antagonists, oral or intravenous (eg, verapamil)
- carbonic anhydrase inhibitors, oral (eg, acetazolamide)
- catecholamine-depleting drugs (eg, reserpine)
- digitalis (eg, digoxin)
- quinidine (eg, *Quinora*)

Side Effects:

Every drug is capable of producing side effects. Many dorzolamide HCl/timolol maleate users experience no, or minor, side effects. The frequency and severity of side effects depend on many factors including dose, duration of therapy, and individual susceptibility. Possible side effects include the following:

Eyes or Ocular: Stinging, itching, or burning eyes; blurred vision; cloudy vision; dry eyes; eye debris; eye discharge; eye pain; eye tearing; eye swelling; eyelid pain, discomfort, or swelling; eyelid redness; eyelid discharge or scales; cataract; corneal staining; conjunctivitis; corneal erosion; lens opacity; decreased corneal sensitivity; visual disturbances including refractive changes and double vision; foreign body sensation.

Digestive Tract: Taste changes; stomach pain; indigestion; nausea; sore throat.

Nervous System: Bronchitis; cough; upper respiratory tract infection; sinus infection; bronchospasm.

Other: Back pain; urinary tract infection; influenza; dizziness; headache; high blood pressure.

Guidelines for Use:

- Recommended dose is 1 drop in the affected eye(s) 2 times daily.
- Do not allow the tip of the dispensing container to contact the eye as it may become contaminated with bacteria known to cause eye infections. Serious eye damage and loss of vision can result.
- If more than 1 topical ophthalmic drug is being used, the drugs should be administered at least 10 minutes apart.
- Contact lenses should be removed prior to administration of the solution. Lenses may be reinserted 15 minutes following administration.
- Discontinue the drug and notify your doctor immediately if any of the following occurs: Hives; itching; rash; difficulty breathing; shortness of breath; swelling in feet or ankles; inflammation of eye or eyelids; changes in vision; muscle weakness.
- This drug may mask certain signs (eg, fast heartbeat) of hyperthyroidism. Hyperthyroid patients should be managed carefully by their doctor.
- Patients using this medication with a history of allergies or severe anaphylactic reactions to a variety of allergens may be unresponsive to the usual doses of epinephrine used to treat reactions.
- Your doctor may have you gradually stop this drug before elective surgery.
- Store between 59° and 77°F. Protect from light.

If you have any questions, consult your doctor, pharmacist, or health care provider.

Generic Name *Brand Name Examples*	Supplied As	Generic Available
Rx **Pilocarpine and Epinephrine**[1]		
E-Pilo-1, P_1E_1	**Solution**: 1% pilocarpine HCl and 1% epinephrine bitartrate	No
E-Pilo-2, P_2E_1	**Solution**: 2% pilocarpine HCl and 1% epinephrine bitartrate	No
E-Pilo-3, P_3E_1	**Solution**: 3% pilocarpine HCl and 1% epinephrine bitartrate	No
E-Pilo-4, P_4E_1	**Solution**: 4% pilocarpine HCl and 1% epinephrine bitartrate	No
E-Pilo-6, P_6E_1	**Solution**: 4% pilocarpine HCl and 1% epinephrine bitartrate	No
Rx **Pilocarpine and Physostigmine**		
Isopto P-ES	**Solution**: 2% pilocarpine HCl and 0.25% physotigmine salicylate	No

[1] These products contain sulfites.

Type of Drug:

Combination products to lower intraocular (fluid) pressure in the eye.

How the Drug Works:

Epinephrine reduces pressure in the eye by decreasing the rate of fluid production. Improved fluid outflow has also been reported.

Physostigmine increases outflow of aqueous humor.

Pilocarpine lowers pressure in the eye by improving fluid (aqueous humor) outflow and, to a lesser extent, by decreasing aqueous humor production.

Combinations of pilocarpine and physostigmine have been used on the theory that improved response may result. Studies do not show that additive pressure lowering effects are achieved over either agent used alone. The combination of pilocarpine and epinephrine provides additive effects in lowering intraocular pressure. These fixed combinations do not permit the flexibility needed to adjust the dosage of each agent.

Uses:

To lower intraocular (fluid) pressure in glaucoma.

Guidelines for Use:

- May cause temporary blurred or unstable vision. Use caution while driving or performing other hazardous tasks.
- Do not use while wearing soft contact lenses. Lenses may become discolored.
- Report any vision changes to your doctor immediately.
- *Storage* — Store in a cool, dark place. Discard if solution becomes brown or discolors, becomes cloudy, or contains particles.

If you have any questions, consult your doctor, pharmacist, or health care provider.

	Generic Name *Brand Name Example*	Supplied As	Generic Available
Rx	**Dapiprazole HCl**		
	Rēv-Eyes	**Ophthalmic powder for reconstitution**: 5 mg/mL	No

Type of Drug:

Pupil constrictor.

How the Drug Works:

Dapiprazole produces pupil constriction by blocking the alpha-adrenergic receptors in the dilator muscle of the iris.

Uses:

To reverse mydriasis (extreme dilation of the pupil) due to treatment with phenylephrine or tropicamide during eye examinations or surgery.

Precautions:

Do not use in the following situations:

- acute iritis
- allergy to any component of the product
- open-angle glaucoma, treatment of reduction of intraocular pressure

Pregnancy: Adequate studies have not been done in pregnant women. Use only if clearly needed and potential benefits outweigh the possible hazards to the fetus.

Breastfeeding: It is not known if dapiprazole appears in the breast milk. Consult your doctor before you begin breastfeeding.

Children: Safety and effectiveness for use in children have not been established.

Side Effects:

Every drug is capable of producing side effects. Many dapiprazole users experience no, or minor, side effects. The frequency and severity of side effects depend on many factors including dose, duration of therapy and individual susceptibility. Possible side effects include the following:

Eyes or Ocular: Burning when first instilled; drooping eyelids; eyelid redness; eyelid inflammation; edema (fluid retention) of eyelids; itching; inflammation and formation of deposits on cornea; conjunctival congestion and edema; sensitivity to light; dry eyes; tearing; blurred vision.

Other: Headache; browache.

Guidelines for Use:

- For use in eyes only.
- Shake container for several minutes to ensure mixing.
- Instill 2 drops into each eye, followed 5 minutes later by an additional 2 drops.
- Do not touch dropper to lids or any surface, as this may contaminate the solution. Recap container after use.
- If a dose is missed, instill it as soon as possible. If several hours have passed or if it is nearing time for the next dose, do not double the dose in order to "catch up" (unless advised to do so by your doctor). If more than one dose is missed or it is necessary to establish a new dosage schedule, contact your doctor or pharmacist. Use exactly as prescribed.
- Do not use more than once a week.
- May cause stinging or burning when you first instill drops into the eyes.
- May cause vision problems in poor light. Use caution when driving at night or performing other tasks in poor lighting.
- May cause sensitivity to light. This may be reduced by wearing sunglasses.
- Store at room temperature (59° to 86°F) for 21 days after reconstitution. Discard any solution that is not clear and colorless.

If you have any questions, consult your doctor, pharmacist, or health care provider.

	Generic Name *Brand Name Examples*	Supplied As	Generic Available
	Naphazoline HCl		
otc	*Allerest Eye Drops, Allergy Drops, Clear Eyes, Clear Eyes ACR*[1], *Comfort Eye Drops, Degest 2, Maximum Strength Allergy Drops, Naphcon, Vaso-Clear*	**Solution**: 0.012%, 0.02%, 0.03%	Yes
Rx	*AK-Con, Albalon, Nafazair, Naphcon Forte, Vasocon Regular*	**Solution**: 0.1%	Yes
	Oxymetazoline HCl		
otc	*OcuClear, Visine L.R.*	**Solution**: 0.025%	No
	Phenylephrine HCl		
otc	*AK-Nefrin, Prefrin Liquifilm, Relief*	**Solution**: 0.12%	Yes
Rx	*AK-Dilate, Mydfrin 2.5%* [1], *Neo-Synephrine, Neo-Synephrine Viscous, Phenoptic*	**Solution**: 2.5%, 10%	Yes
	Tetrahydrozoline HCl		
otc	*AR Eye Drops - Astringent Redness Reliever*[1], *Collyrium Fresh, Eye Drops, Eye Drops Extra, Eyesine, Geneye, Geneye Extra, Mallazine Eye Drops, Murine Plus, Optigene 3, Tetrasine, Tetrasine Extra, Visine, Visine Moisturizing*	**Solution**: 0.05%	Yes

[1] Contains sulfites.

Type of Drug:

Ophthalmic vasoconstrictors; drugs that reduce redness and cause the pupil to dilate (widen).

How the Drug Works:

The effects of these agents on the eye include the following: Pupil dilation (widening), increase in outflow of fluid (aqueous humor) and vasoconstriction (narrowing of blood vessels).

The strong vasoconstrictors (phenylephrine 2.5% and 10%) are used to prepare the eye for diagnostic exams, during surgery, and to prevent scarring. Intermediate strength solutions (epinephrine 0.5% to 2%) are used in open-angle glaucoma, alone, or with other drugs. Weak solutions (phenylephrine 0.12%, naphazoline, tetrahydrozoline) are used as ophthalmic decongestants (that narrow conjunctival blood vessels) to relieve redness due to minor eye irritations.

Uses:

To dilate the pupils (phenylephrine 2.5%, 10% only).

To temporarily reduce irritation and redness caused by minor eye irritations, such as smoke, smog, sunglare, contact lens wear, allergies, swimming, or wind.

Precautions:

Do not use in the following situations:

- allergy to any of these medicines
- aneurysm (phenylephrine 10% only)
- infants (phenylephrine 10% only)
- iridectomy (surgical removal of a portion of the iris), prior to
- narrow-angle glaucoma
- narrow angles (but no glaucoma)

Use with caution in the following situations:

- anesthetics (general), use
- anesthetics, local (prior to use of phenylephrine)
- arteriosclerosis (hardening of the arteries)
- children, low body weight
- diabetes
- elderly
- glaucoma, narrow-angle (to free adhesions)
- heart disease, history (phenylephrine 10% only)
- high blood pressure
- hyperthyroidism (overactive thyroid), untreated

Pigment floaters: Phenylephrine may cause temporary pigment floaters ("black spots") in the visual field of older individuals.

Rebound congestion (redness or swelling of the eye surface) may occur with frequent or extended use of ophthalmic vasoconstrictors.

Rebound miosis (decrease in size of pupil) may occur in some patients 1 day after using phenylephrine.

Pregnancy: Adequate studies have not been done in pregnant women, or animal studies may have shown a risk to the fetus. Use only if clearly needed and potential benefits outweigh the possible hazards to the fetus.

Breastfeeding: Safety and effectiveness have not been established. Consult your doctor before you begin breastfeeding.

Children: Safety and effectiveness have not been established. Do not use phenylephrine 10% in infants. Use with caution in children of low body weight.

Elderly: Those with a history of heart problems should use caution when using phenylephrine 10%.

Sulfites: Some of these products may contain sulfite preservatives, which can cause allergic reactions in certain individuals. Check package label when available or consult your doctor or pharmacist.

Drug Interactions:

Tell your doctor or pharmacist if you are taking or if you are planning to take any over-the-counter or prescription medications or dietary supplements while taking these medicines. Doses of one or both drugs may need to be modified or a different drug may need to be prescribed. The following drugs and drug classes interact with these medicines.

anesthetics (eg, cyclopropane, halothane)
beta-blockers (eg, propranolol)
monoamine oxidase inhibitors (MAOIs, eg, phenelzine)

Also consider drug interactions that may occur with systemic sympathomimetics.

Side Effects:

Every drug is capable of producing side effects. Many patients experience no, or minor, side effects. The frequency and severity of side effects depend on many factors including dose, duration of therapy and individual susceptibility. Possible side effects include the following:

Eyes or Ocular: Stinging; blurring; redness; eye discomfort; allergic reactions; inflammation of cornea; tearing; glaucoma; decrease in pupil size (phenylephrine).

Circulatory System: Palpitations (pounding in the chest); collapse; blood clots; high blood pressure; heart attack; stroke; irregular heartbeat.

Other: Pale skin; sweating; dizziness; nausea; nervousness; drowsiness; weakness; high blood sugar; headache; browache.

Guidelines for Use:

- Use exactly as prescribed.
- Follow Administration Guidelines found at the beginning of this chapter.
- If a dose is missed, instill it as soon as possible. If several hours have passed or if it is nearing time for the next dose, do not double the dose in order to "catch up" (unless advised to do so by your doctor). If more than one dose is missed or it is necessary to establish a new dosage schedule, contact your doctor or pharmacist.
- Do not use for more than 48 to 72 hours (2 to 3 days) without contacting your doctor.
- Overuse may produce increased eye redness.
- *Phenylephrine* — May cause temporary blurred or unstable vision. Use caution when driving, operating machinery, or performing other tasks requiring clear vision.
- Discontinue use and contact your doctor if any of the following occur: Severe eye pain, headache, vision changes, floating spots, dizziness, decrease in body temperature, drowsiness, acute eye redness, or pain when exposed to light.
- Discontinue use and contact your doctor if any of the following persist: Irritation, blurring, redness.
- Do not use if you have glaucoma unless advised by your doctor.
- Some of these products may contain sulfite preservatives, which can cause allergic reactions in certain individuals. Check package label when available or consult your doctor or pharmacist.
- Do not use if solution changes color, becomes cloudy, or contains particles.
- Store in a cool place (36° to 75°F) away from light. Keep container tightly sealed. Avoid freezing.

If you have any questions, consult your doctor, pharmacist, or health care provider.

	Generic Name *Brand Name Examples*	Supplied As	Generic Available
otc	**Phenylephrine-containing Solutions**		
	Zincfrin	**Solution**: 0.12% phenylephrine HCl and 0.25% zinc sulfate	No
	Naphazoline containing Solutions		
otc	*Vasocon-A*	**Solution**: 0.05% naphazoline HCl and 0.5% antazoline phosphate	Yes
otc	*Naphazoline Plus, Naphcon-A*	**Solution**: 0.025% naphazoline HCl and 0.3% pheniramine maleate	Yes
Rx	*Naphoptic-A*	**Solution**: 0.025% naphazoline HCl and 0.3% pheniramine maleate	Yes
otc	*Opcon-A*	**Solution**: 0.027% naphazoline HCl and 0.315% pheniramine maleate	No
otc	*Clear Eyes ACR*	**Solution**: 0.012% naphazoline HCl and 0.25% zinc sulfate	No
otc	*VasoClear A*	**Solution**: 0.02% naphazoline HCl and 0.25% zinc sulfate	No
	Tetrahydrozoline-containing Solutions		
otc	*Geneye AC Allergy Formula, Visine Allergy Relief*	**Solution**: 0.05% tetrahydrozoline HCl and 0.25% zinc sulfate	Yes

Type of Drug:

Ophthalmic decongestants; agents to reduce eye redness.

How the Drug Works:

In these combinations:

Phenylephrine HCl, naphazoline HCl, and tetrahydrozoline are used for their decongestant actions. (See phenylephrine monograph for complete information.)

Hydroxypropylmethylcellulose and polyvinyl alcohol are used to increase the thickness of the solution, increasing contact time with the eye.

Zinc sulfate is used as an astringent (agent that tightens the tissues).

Pheniramine maleate and antazoline are antihistamines.

Uses:

Temporary relief of minor eye symptoms of itching and redness caused by pollen, animal hair, smoke, smog, contact lens wear, wind, sunglare, swimming, etc.

Precautions:

Use with caution in the following situations:

narrow-angle glaucoma or a history of glaucoma

Also see precautions for ophthalmic decongestants.

Guidelines for Use:

- Use exactly as prescribed.
- Follow Administration Guidelines found at the beginning of this chapter.
- If a dose is missed, instill it as soon as possible. If several hours have passed or if it is nearing time for the next dose, do not double the dose in order to "catch up" (unless advised to do so by your doctor). If more than one dose is missed or it is necessary to establish a new dosage schedule, contact your doctor or pharmacist.
- Do not use longer than 48 to 72 hours (2 to 3 days) without contacting your doctor.
- May cause temporary blurred or unstable vision. Use caution when driving, operating machinery, or performing other tasks requiring clear vision.
- Discontinue use and consult your doctor if any of the following occurs: Severe eye pain, headache, vision changes, floating spots, dizziness, decrease in body temperature, drowsiness, swelling, acute eye redness, pain when exposed to light.
- Discontinue use and consult your doctor if any of the following persist: Irritation, blurring, redness, or swelling.
- Do not use if solution changes color, becomes cloudy, or contains particles.
- Store in a cool place (36° to 75°F), away from light. Keep container tightly sealed. Avoid freezing.

If you have any questions, consult your doctor, pharmacist, or health care provider.

	Generic Name *Brand Name Examples*	Supplied As	Generic Available
Rx	**Atropine Sulfate**		
	Atropine Sulfate	**Ointment**: 1%	Yes
	Atropine Care, Atropine-1, Atropisol, Isopto Atropine	**Solution**: 0.5%, 1%, 2%	Yes
Rx	**Cyclopentolate HCl**		
	AK-Pentolate, Cyclogyl, Pentolair	**Solution**: 0.5%, 1%, 2%	Yes
Rx	**Homatropine HBr**		
	AK-Homatropine, Isopto Homatropine	**Solution**: 2%, 5%	Yes
Rx	**Scopolamine HBr (Hyoscine HBr)**		
	Isopto Hyoscine	**Solution**: 0.25%	No
Rx	**Tropicamide**		
	Mydriacyl, Opticyl, Tropicacyl	**Solution**: 0.5%, 1%	Yes
Rx	**Mydriatic Combinations**		
	Cyclomydril	**Solution**: 0.2% Cyclopentolate HCl and 1% phenylephrine HCl	No
	Murocoll-2[1]	**Drops**: 0.3% scopolamine HBr and 10% phenylephrine HCl	No
	Paremyd	**Solution**: 0.25% tropicamide and 1% hydroxyamphetamine HBr	No

[1] Contains sulfites.

Type of Drug:

Pupil dilators.

How the Drug Works:

Cycloplegic mydriatics relax the muscles of the eye to cause the pupil to dilate (widen) and prevent the eye from focusing (cycloplegia) on near objects.

Uses:

To dilate the pupil when there is eye inflammation or when an eye exam is performed.

Precautions:

Do not use in the following situations:

adhesions (scarring) between iris and lens
allergy to belladonna alkaloids or any component of the formulation
children, previous severe reaction to atropine
glaucoma, active or tendency toward

Use with caution in the following situations:

brain damage, children	nursing women
Down's syndrome	small children, infants
elderly	

Pregnancy: Adequate studies have not been done in pregnant women, or animal studies may have shown a risk to the fetus. Use only if clearly needed and potential benefits outweigh the possible hazards to the fetus.

Breastfeeding: Atropine and homatropine appear in breast milk. It is not known if cyclopentolate appears in breast milk. Consult your doctor before you begin breastfeeding.

Children: Tropicamide and cyclopentolate may cause dangerous nervous system disturbances in infants and children. Infants, young children, and children with spastic paralysis or brain damage may be more susceptible to cyclopentolate. Feeding intolerance may follow use of cyclopentolate in newborns. Withhold feeding for 4 hours after examination.

Sulfites: Some of these products may contain sulfite preservatives, which can cause allergic reactions in certain individuals. Check package label when available or consult your doctor or pharmacist.

Side Effects:

Every drug is capable of producing side effects. Many patients experience no, or minor, side effects. The frequency and severity of side effects depend on many factors including dose, duration of therapy, and individual susceptibility. Possible side effects include the following:

Eyes or Ocular: Increased intraocular (fluid) pressure; stinging; burning; irritation; sensitivity to light; blurred vision.

Nervous System: Headache; drowsiness; hallucinations; psychotic reaction or behavioral disturbance, usually in children (cyclopentolate and tropicamide).

Other: Flushing; rash; decreased sweating or salivation; dryness of mouth, sinuses and skin; stomach bloating (in infants); urinary retention; constipation; rapid heart rate; fever.

Guidelines for Use:

- For use in eyes only. Use exactly as prescribed.
- Follow Administration Guidelines found at the beginning of this chapter.
- To avoid contamination, do not touch dropper tip to any surface. Replace cap after using.
- If instilling this medicine for someone else, wash your hands and theirs following administration.
- Avoid excessive systemic absorption by using your fingers to press on the corner of the eye next to the nose during use and for 2 to 3 minutes after use.
- Do not exceed recommended dosages. If overdosage occurs, flush eyes with water or normal saline.
- If a dose is missed, instill it as soon as possible. If several hours have passed or if it is nearing time for the next dose, do not double the dose in order to "catch up." If more than one dose is missed, contact your doctor or pharmacist.
- May cause drowsiness, blurred vision, or sensitivity to light (due to dilated pupils). Use caution while driving, operating machinery, or performing other tasks requiring clear vision and alertness. Protect eyes in bright sunlight or illumination.
- If eye pain occurs, discontinue use and contact your doctor immediately.
- Store at room temperature (46° to 75°F) away from heat and light.

If you have any questions, consult your doctor, pharmacist, or health care provider.

	Generic Name *Brand Name Examples*	Supplied As	Generic Available
Rx	**Dexamethasone**		
	Maxidex	**Suspension**: 0.1%	Yes
Rx	**Dexamethasone Sodium Phosphate**		
	AK-Dex, Decadron Phosphate[1]	**Solution**: 0.1%	Yes
	AK-Dex, Decadron Phosphate, Maxidex	**Ointment**: 0.05%	Yes
Rx	**Fluorometholone**		
	Flarex, Fluor-Op, FML, FML Forte	**Suspension**: 0.1%, 0.25%	No
	FML S.O.P.	**Ointment**: 0.1%	No
Rx	**Medrysone**		
	HMS	**Suspension**: 1%	No
Rx	**Prednisolone Acetate**		
	Pred Mild[1], *Econopred, Econopred Plus, Pred Forte*[1]	**Suspension**: 0.12%, 0.125%, 1%	Yes
Rx	**Prednisolone Sodium Phosphate**		
	AK-Pred[1], *Inflamase Forte, Inflamase Mild*	**Solution**: 0.125%, 1%	Yes
Rx	**Rimexolone**		
	Vexol	**Suspension**: 1%	No

[1] Contains sulfites

Type of Drug:

Anti-inflammatory agents for the eye.

How the Drug Works:

Corticosteroids inhibit the inflammatory response (redness, swelling, warmth, etc) of tissues to mechanical, chemical, or allergy-causing agents. Prostaglandins are chemicals produced by the body in response to irritating substances. The mechanism of action of corticosteroids, in part, is thought to be inhibition of the production of prostaglandins.

Uses:

To treat inflammatory conditions of the eye, injuries to the cornea, anterior uveitis, and graft rejection after keratoplasty (corneal graft).

Precautions:

Do not use in the following situations:

- after removal of a minor corneal foreign body
- allergy to the drug
- fungal eye infections
- herpes simplex inflammation of the cornea
- inflammation of the iris (medrysone only)
- inflammation of the uvea (medrysone only)
- mustard gas keratitis
- mycobacterial diseases of the eye
- Sjogren's keratoconjunctivitis (dry eye, etc)
- tuberculosis of the eye
- viral infections of the eye

Pregnancy: Adequate studies have not been done in pregnant women, or animal studies may have shown a potential risk to the fetus. Use only if clearly needed and potential benefits outweigh the possible hazards to the fetus.

Breastfeeding: It is not known if topical steroids appear in breast milk. Consult your doctor before you begin breastfeeding.

Children: Safety and effectiveness have not been established.

Sulfites: Some of these products may contain sulfite preservatives, which can cause allergic reactions in certain individuals. Check package label when available or consult your doctor or pharmacist.

Side Effects:

Every drug is capable of producing side effects. Many patients experience no, or minor, side effects. The frequency and severity of side effects depend on many factors including dose, duration of therapy, and individual susceptibility. Possible side effects include the following:

Note: Also consider all side effects reported for systemic corticosteroids (see Hormones chapter) when using ophthalmic corticosteroids.

Eyes or Ocular: Glaucoma with optic nerve damage; blurring; cataracts; eye infections; perforation of the eye; stinging; burning; discharge; discomfort; pain; foreign body sensation; engorgement of blood; itching (rimexolone only).

Other: Headache; low blood pressure; runny nose; sore throat; taste changes.

Guidelines for Use:

- Use exactly as prescribed.
- Follow Administrative Guidelines found at the beginning of this chapter.
- To avoid contamination, do not touch applicator tip to any surface. Replace cap after use.
- If a dose is missed, instill it as soon as possible. If several hours have passed or if it is nearing time for the next dose, do not double the dose in order to "catch up" (unless advised to do so by your doctor). If more than one dose is missed or it is necessary to establish a new dosage schedule, contact your doctor or pharmacist.
- Prolonged use may result in glaucoma, optic nerve damage, blurred vision, cataracts or infections. Frequent eye exams are required to monitor treatment. Be sure to keep appointments.
- If improvement does not occur within several days or if pain, itching or swelling of the eye occurs, contact your doctor. Do not stop using this drug without consulting your doctor.
- Store upright at room temperature (46° to 77° F). Do not freeze.

If you have any questions, consult your doctor, pharmacist, or health care provider.

	Generic Name / *Brand Name Example*	Supplied As	Generic Available
Rx	**Loteprednol Etabonate**		
	Alrex	**Suspension**: 0.2%	No
	Lotemax	**Suspension**: 0.5%	No

Type of Drug:

Topical anti-inflammatory drug for treating symptoms involving the eye.

How the Drug Works:

Corticosteroids inhibit the inflammatory response (swelling, redness, etc) of tissues to irritating agents. The mechanism of action of corticosteroids is thought to be due, in part, to the inhibition of the body's chemical response to irritating substances.

Uses:

Alrex: For temporary relief of seasonal allergy eye symptoms.

Lotemax: To treat inflammatory conditions of the eye due to allergies, bacteria or virus (eg, iritis, acne rosacea, herpes zoster keratitis) and post-operative eye surgery inflammation.

Precautions:

Do not use in the following situations:

- allergy to this drug or to corticosteroids
- fungal eye infections
- mycobacterial eye infections
- ocular herpes simplex, history
- ocular viral infections
- soft contact lens (*Lotemax* only)

Use with caution in the following situations:

- contact lens use (*Alrex* only)
- corneal thinning
- eye discharge
- eye infections (not included above)
- glaucoma
- post cataract surgery (*Lotemax* only) (may delay wound healing)

Pregnancy: Adequate studies have not been done in pregnant women, or animal studies may have shown a risk to the fetus. Use only if clearly needed and potential benefits outweigh the possible hazards to the fetus.

Breastfeeding: It is not known if topical corticosteroids appear in breast milk. Consult your doctor before you begin breastfeeding.

Children: Safety and effectiveness in children have not been established.

Lab tests may be required with long-term steroid use. Tests may include fungal cultures and intraocular (fluid) pressure.

Drug Interactions:

Tell your doctor or pharmacist if you are planning to take any over-the-counter or prescription medications or dietary supplements while taking loteprednol. Doses of one or both drugs may need to be modified or a different drug may need to be prescribed.

Side Effects:

Every drug is capable of producing side effects. Many loteprednol users experience no, or minor, side effects. The frequency and severity of side effects depend on many factors including dose, duration of therapy, and individual susceptibility. Possible side effects include the following:

Note: Also consider all side effects reported for systemic corticosteroids (see Hormones chapter) when using ophthalmic corticosteroids.

Eyes or Ocular: Optic nerve damage; blurred vision; elevated intraocular pressure; cataracts; eye infections; secondary ocular infections (eg, herpes simplex); perforation of the eye; eyelid swelling; burning; discharge; dry eyes; foreign body sensation; itching; discomfort; pain; tearing; light sensitivity; redness; irritation; abnormal vision.

Other: Headache; rhinitis; sore or inflamed throat.

Guidelines for Use:

- For ophthalmic use only.
- Shake well before using.
- *Lotemax* — Eye disease inflammation/allergies: Place 1 drop into the affected eye(s) 4 times daily. During first week of treatment, dosage may be increased up to 1 drop per hour if needed. Effectiveness depends on consistency of use.
- *Lotemax* — For postoperative inflammation apply 1 to 2 drops 4 times daily beginning 24 hours after surgery. Continue using regularly for 14 days after surgery.
- *Lotemax* – Do not wear soft contact lenses when using *Lotemax*.
- *Alrex* — Dosage is 1 drop 4 times daily.
- *Alrex* — Patients should be advised not to wear a contact lens if their eye is red.
- *Alrex* — Do not use this product to treat contact lens related irritations. The preservative benzalkonium chloride may be absorbed by soft contact lenses. Patients who wear soft contact lenses and whose eyes are not red, should wait 10 minutes after applying before inserting contact lenses.
- To avoid contamination do not touch dropper tip to any surface.
- Prolonged use may result in glaucoma, optic nerve damage, blurred vision, and cataracts or infections. Eye exams may be required to monitor treatment. Be sure to keep appointments.
- If improvements do not occur after 2 days, or eye redness or itching increases, contact your doctor.
- Store upright between 59° to 77°F. Do not freeze.

If you have any questions, consult your doctor, pharmacist, or health care provider.

	Generic Name *Brand Name Examples*	Supplied As	Generic Available
Rx	**Cromolyn Sodium**		
	Crolom	**Solution, ophthalmic**: 4%	Yes
Rx	**Lodoxamide Tromethamine**		
	Alomide	**Solution, ophthalmic**: 0.1%	No
Rx	**Nedocromil Sodium**		
	Alocril	**Solution, ophthalmic**: 2%	No
Rx	**Pemirolast Potassium**		
	Alamast	**Solution, ophthalmic**: 0.1%	No

Type of Drug:

Mast cell stabilizer; antiallergy agent for the eye.

How the Drug Works:

Mast cell stabilizers prevent allergy symptoms (eg, itching, redness, tearing) that involve the eye by preventing the local release of histamine and other chemicals that cause allergic symptoms from mast cells.

Uses:

For the prevention and treatment of eye itching caused by allergic reactions (allergic conjunctivitis).

Lodoxamide tromethamine and cromolyn sodium — For the treatment of vernal (occuring in the springtime) keratoconjunctivitis, vernal conjunctivitis, and vernal keratitis.

Precautions:

Do not use in the following situations:

allergy to the mast cell stabilizer or any of its ingredients
soft contact lens wear (cromolyn sodium only)

Pregnancy: There are no adequate and well-controlled studies in pregnant women. Use only if clearly needed and the potential benefits to the mother outweigh the possible hazards to the fetus.

Breastfeeding: It is not known if mast cell stabilizers are excreted in breast milk. Consult your doctor before you begin breastfeeding.

Children: Safety and effectiveness of use of lodoxamide in children less than 2 years of age are not established. Safety and effectiveness of use of nedocromil and pemirolast in children less than 3 years of age are not established. Safety and effectiveness of use of cromolyn sodium in children less than 4 years of age are not established.

Drug Interactions:

Tell your doctor or pharmacist if you are taking or if you are planning to take any over-the-counter or prescription medications or dietary supplements while using a mast cell stabilizer. Doses of one or both drugs may need to be modified or a different drug may need to be prescribed.

Side Effects:

Every drug is capable of producing side effects. Many mast cell stabilizer users experience no, or minor, side effects. The frequency or severity of side effects depend on many factors including dose, duration of therapy, and individual susceptibility. Possible side effects include the following:

Eyes or Ocular: Burning; stinging; dry eye; foreign body sensation; redness; discomfort or irritation; tearing; discharge; styes; itching; watery eyes; puffy eyes; sensitivity to light; blurred vision.

Respiratory System: Runny nose; cold or flu symptoms; cough; bronchitis; sinus inflammation; sneezing; nasal congestion; asthma.

Other: Headache; allergy; back pain; painful menstruation; fever; unpleasant taste sensation.

Guidelines for Use:

- Dosage is individualized. Use exactly as prescribed.
- Effectiveness of mast cell stabilizers is dependent on administration at regular intervals. They are not effective when used sporadically or "as needed."
- For topical ophthalmic use only. Not for injection or oral use.
- Review guidelines at the beginning of this chapter for proper technique for instilling eye drops.
- Temporary stinging or burning sensations may occur following application. Inform your doctor if this becomes bothersome or intolerable.
- If a dose is missed, take it as soon as possible. If several hours have passed or it is nearing time for the next dose, do not double the dose to catch up, unless advised to do so by your doctor. If more than one dose is missed or it is necessary to establish a new dosage schedule, contact your doctor or pharmacist.
- To prevent contamination of the dropper tip and solution, do not touch the eyelids or surrounding areas with the dropper tip.
- *Contact lens wearers* — Do not wear contact lenses while you have signs and symptoms of allergic conjunctivitis. Do not wear soft contact lenses during treatment with cromolyn sodium, nedocromil, or lodoxamide. The preservative in pemirolast potassium, lauralkonium chloride, may be absorbed by soft contact lenses. If you wear soft contact lenses and your eyes are not red, wait at least 10 minutes after instilling pemirolast potassium before inserting contact lenses. Do not wear contact lens if your eye is red. Do not use to treat a contact lens-related irritation.
- Symptoms usually respond to therapy within a few days, but it may take up to 6 weeks. Once relief of symptoms has occurred, continue the medicine on a regular basis to prevent return of symptoms.
- Store at room temperature. Keep the bottle tightly closed. Replace cap immediately after use.

If you have any questions, consult your doctor, pharmacist, or health care provider.

	Generic Name *Brand Name Examples*	Supplied As	Generic Available
Rx	**Diclofenac Sodium**		
	Voltaren	**Solution**: 0.1%	No
Rx	**Flurbiprofen Sodium**		
	Ocufen	**Solution**: 0.03%	No
Rx	**Ketorolac Tromethamine**		
	Acular	**Solution**: 0.5%	No
Rx	**Suprofen**		
	Profenal	**Solution**: 1%	No

Type of Drug:

Nonsteroidal anti-inflammatory drugs for the eye; NSAIDs.

How the Drug Works:

NSAIDs for the eye are thought to inhibit the inflammatory response (redness, itching, swelling, warmth, etc) of tissues to mechanical, chemical, or allergy-causing agents. Prostaglandins are chemicals produced by the body that respond to irritating substances and cause constriction (narrowing) of the pupil of the eye during cataract surgery. NSAIDs inhibit the production of prostaglandins.

Uses:

Diclofenac — To treat eye inflammation after cataract surgery.

Flurbiprofen and Suprofen — To prevent pupil constriction (miosis) during surgery.

Ketorolac — For the relief of ocular itching due to seasonal allergic conjunctivitis.

Unlabeled Use(s): Occasionally doctors may prescribe flurbiprofen for eye inflammation after surgery, cystoid macular edema or uveitis (inflammation of the uvea) syndromes.

Precautions:

Do not use in the following situations:

allergy to any component of the formulation
herpes simplex infection of the eye (flurbiprofen and suprofen only)
soft contact lens wearers (diclofenac and ketorolac only)

Use with caution in the following situations:

allergy to aspirin
allergy to other NSAIDs
bleeding tendency (ocular surgical patients)
prolonged bleeding time or known bleeding tendencies

Pregnancy: Adequate studies have not been done in pregnant women. Use only if clearly needed and potential benefits outweigh the possible hazards to the fetus. Diclofenac use should be avoided in late stages of pregnancy.

Breastfeeding: Suprofen appears in breast milk after oral use. Eye drops may be absorbed into the body. It is not known if flurbiprofen or ketorolac appears in breast milk. Because of the potential for adverse effects, a decision should be made whether to discontinue nursing or the drug, taking into account the importance of the drug to the mother. Consult your doctor.

Children: Safety and effectiveness have not been established.

Side Effects:

Every drug is capable of producing side effects. Many ophthalmic NSAID users experience no, or minor, side effects. The frequency and severity of side effects depend on many factors including dose, duration of therapy and individual susceptibility. Possible side effects include the following:

Other:

Most frequent – Temporary burning or stinging; irritation; redness/burning (contact lens wearers).

Diclofenac and ketorolac – Inflammation of cornea; ocular allergy.

Diclofenac – Nausea; vomiting; viral infections.

Guidelines for Use:

- Consult your doctor if you have experienced bleeding tendencies, are on drugs that prolong bleeding time (eg, "blood thinners"), or have herpes simplex infection of the eye.
- *Flurbiprofen* — May delay wound healing.
- Use proper administration technique.
- Mild burning or stinging after instillation is no cause for alarm unless symptoms persist or worsen.

If you have any questions, consult your doctor, pharmacist, or health care provider.

Generic Name / *Brand Name Example*	Supplied As	Generic Available
Rx **Levocabastine Hydrochloride**		
Livostin	**Suspension**: 2.5 mL, 5 mL, 10 mL	No

Type of Drug:

Antiallergy (antihistamine) for the eye.

How the Drug Works:

Levocabastine is systemically absorbed and reduces itching in the eye due to seasonal allergies.

Uses:

To relieve the symptoms of seasonal conjunctivitis.

Precautions:

Do not use in the following situations:
allergy to levocabastine
soft contact lens use

Pregnancy: Adequate studies have not been done in pregnant women. Use only if clearly needed and potential benefits outweigh the possible hazards to the fetus.

Breastfeeding: Levocabastine appears in breast milk. Consult your doctor before you begin breastfeeding.

Children: Safety and effectiveness in children below the age of 12 have not been established.

Drug Interactions:

Tell your doctor or pharmacist if you are taking or if you are planning to take any over-the-counter or prescription medications or dietary supplements with levocabastine. Doses of one or both drugs may need to be modified or a different drug may need to be prescribed.

Side Effects:

Every drug is capable of producing side effects. Many levocabastine users experience no, or minor, side effects. The frequency and severity of side effects depend on many factors including dose, duration of therapy, and individual susceptibility. Possible side effects include the following:

Nervous System: Headache; sleepiness; fatigue.

Respiratory System: Difficulty breathing; cough; pharyngitis.

Other: Rash; nausea; dry mouth.

Eyes or Ocular: Visual disturbances; fluid retention in the eyelids; mild, transient stinging and burning; eye pain; dryness; red eyes; discharge from the eye.

Guidelines for Use:

- For topical use only. Not for injection.
- Do not touch eyelids or surrounding areas with the dropper tip of the bottle.
- Do not use if the suspension has discolored.
- Store at room temperature. Protect from freezing.
- Shake well before using.

If you have any questions, consult your doctor, pharmacist, or health care provider.

	Generic Name *Brand Name Example*	Supplied As	Generic Available
Rx	**Azelastine**		
	Optivar	**Solution, ophthalmic**: 0.05%	No

Type of Drug:

Antihistamine.

How the Drug Works:

Azelastine inhibits the release of histamine and other chemicals from cells involved in the allergic response. It also antagonizes the effect of histamine.

Uses:

For the treatment of itching of the eye associated with allergic conjunctivitis.

Precautions:

Do not use in the following situations: Allergy to azelastine or any of its ingredients.

Pregnancy: There are no adequate and well-controlled studies in pregnant women. Use only if clearly needed and the potential benefits to the mother outweigh the possible hazards to the fetus.

Breastfeeding: It is not known if azelastine appears in breast milk. Consult your doctor before you begin breastfeeding.

Children: Safety and effectiveness in children less than 3 years of age have not been established.

Drug Interactions:

Tell your doctor or pharmacist if you are taking or planning to take any over-the-counter or prescription medications or dietary supplements while using azelastine. Doses of one or both drugs may need to be modified or a different drug may need to be prescribed.

Side Effects:

Every drug is capable of producing side effects. Many azelastine users experience no, or minor, side effects. The frequency or severity of side effects depend on many factors including dose, duration of therapy, and individual susceptibility. Possible side effects include the following:

Eyes or Ocular: Burning; stinging; pain; blurred vision.

Other: Headache; bitter taste sensation; asthma; runny nose; itching; sore throat; flu-like symptoms; fatigue; difficulty breathing.

Guidelines for Use:

- The usual dose is 1 drop in the affected eye(s) twice daily.
- Do not change the dose or stop taking this medicine, unless advised to do so by your doctor.
- For topical ophthalmic use only; not for injection or oral use.
- To avoid contaminating the dropper tip and solution, do not touch any surface, the eyelids, or surrounding areas with the dropper tip of the bottle.
- *Contact lens wearers* — Do not wear a contact lens if your eye is red. Do not use azelastine to treat contact lens-related irritation. The preservative, benzalkonium chloride, may be absorbed by soft contact lenses. Wait at least 10 minutes after instilling azelastine before you insert a contact lens.
- Store upright between 30° and 77°F. Keep container tightly closed.

If you have any questions, consult your doctor, pharmacist, or health care provider.

Generic Name *Brand Name Example*	Supplied As	Generic Available
Rx **Olopatadine**		
Patanol	**Solution:** 0.1%	No

Type of Drug:

Topical antihistamine.

How the Drug Works:

Olopatadine is an antihistamine that blocks the release of histamine.

Uses:

To prevent itching of the eye due to allergic conjunctivitis or allergies.

Precautions:

Do not use in the following situations:

allergy to the drug
soft contact lens wear

Pregnancy: Adequate studies have not been done in pregnant women, or animal studies may have shown a risk to the fetus. Use only if clearly needed and potential benefits outweigh the possible hazards to the fetus.

Breastfeeding: It is not known if olopatadine appears in breast milk. Consult your doctor before you begin breastfeeding.

Children: Safety and effectiveness in children under 3 years of age have not been established.

Drug Interactions:

Tell your doctor or pharmacist if you are taking or planning to take any over-the-counter or prescription medications or dietary supplements while taking this medicine. Doses of one or both drugs may need to be modified or a different drug may need to be prescribed.

Side Effects:

Every drug is capable of producing side effects. Many patients experience no, or minor, side effects. The frequency and severity of side effects depend on many factors including dose, duration of therapy, and individual susceptibility. Possible side effects include the following:

Eyes or Ocular: Burning/stinging; dry eye; foreign body sensation; congestion; irritation; swelling of the lid; itching.

Other: Headaches; weakness; cold syndrome; sore throat; nasal congestion; sinus infection; change in taste.

Guidelines for Use:

- The recommended dose is 1 to 2 drops in the affected eye(s) twice daily every 6 to 8 hours.
- Olopatadine is for topical use only. Do not use as an injection.
- Do not use while wearing contact lenses.
- Do not touch the eyelids or surrounding areas with the dropper tip of the bottle to prevent contamination of the solution/dropper tip.
- Store at 39° to 86°F. Keep bottle tightly closed.

If you have any questions, consult your doctor, pharmacist, or health care provider.

	Generic Name *Brand Name Example*	Supplied As	Generic Available
Rx	**Ketotifen Fumarate**		
	Zaditor	**Solution**: 0.025%	No

Type of Drug:

Antiallergy (antihistamine) for the eye.

How the Drug Works:

Ketotifen prevents allergy symptoms (eg, itching, redness) that involve the eye by preventing the local release of histamine and other chemicals that cause allergic symptoms.

Uses:

For the temporary prevention of itching of the eye due to allergic conjunctivitis.

Precautions:

Do not use in the following situations:
allergy to ketotifen or any of its ingredients

Pregnancy: There are no adequate and well-controlled studies in pregnant women. Use only if clearly needed and the potential benefits to the mother outweigh the possible hazards to the fetus.

Breastfeeding: It is not known if ketotifen appears in breast milk. Consult your doctor before you begin breastfeeding.

Children: Safety and effectiveness in patients less than 3 years of age have not been established.

Drug Interactions:

Tell your doctor or pharmacist if you are taking or planning to take any over-the-counter or prescription medications or dietary supplements while taking ketotifen. Doses of one or both drugs may need to be modified or a different drug may need to be prescribed.

Side Effects:

Every drug is capable of producing side effects. Many ketotifen users experience no, or minor, side effects. The frequency and severity of side effects depend on many factors including dose, duration of therapy, and individual susceptibility. Possible side effects include the following:

Eyes or Ocular: Conjunctivitis; eye burning, stinging, discharge, pain, or rash; dry or itchy eyes; eyelid disorder; keratitis; lacrimation disorder; enlarged pupils; sensitivity to light; tearing.

Other: Headaches; runny nose; flu-like symptoms; sore throat; allergic reaction.

Guidelines for Use:

- The recommended dosage is 1 drop in the affected eye(s) every 8 to 12 hours.
- For topical ophthalmic use only. Do not take by mouth or place in the ear.
- To prevent contamination of the dropper tip and solution, care should be taken not to touch the eyelids or surrounding area with the dropper tip of the bottle.
- Temporary burning or stinging of the eye may occur when instilled into the eye. If symptoms persist or are bothersome, contact your doctor.
- Do not wear contact lenses if your eyes are red.
- Do not use to treat contact lens irritation.
- Benzalkonium chloride, the preservative in ketotifen solution, may be absorbed by soft contact lenses. If you wear soft contact lenses and your eyes are not red, wait at least 10 minutes after instilling ketotifen before you insert your lenses.
- Store at 39° to 77°F. Keep bottle tightly closed when not in use.

If you have any questions, consult your doctor, pharmacist, or health care provider.

	Generic Name *Brand Name Examples*	Supplied As	Generic Available
Rx	**Bacitracin**		
	AK-Tracin	**Ointment**: 500 units/g	Yes
Rx	**Chloramphenicol**		
	Chloromycetin, *Chloroptic*	**Ointment**: 1%	Yes
	Chloromycetin	**Powder for solution**: 25 mg/vial	No
	Chloroptic	**Solution**: 0.5%	Yes
Rx	**Ciprofloxacin HCl**		
	Ciloxan	**Ointment**: 0.3%	No
	Ciloxan[1]	**Solution**: 3.5 mg/mL	No
Rx	**Erythromycin**	**Ointment**: 0.5%	Yes
Rx	**Gentamicin**		
	Garamycin, *Genoptic*, *Gentacidin*, *Gentak*	**Ointment**: 0.3%	Yes
	Garamycin[1], *Genoptic*[1], *Gentacidin*[1], *Gentak*[1]	**Solution**: 0.3%	Yes
Rx	**Levofloxacin**		
	Quixin[1]	**Solution**: 0.5%	No
Rx	**Ofloxacin**		
	Ocuflox[1]	**Solution**: 0.3%	No
Rx	**Polymyxin B Sulfate Sterile**	**Powder for solution**: 6000 units/mg	Yes
Rx	**Sulfacetamide Sodium**		
	AK-Sulf[1], *Bleph-10*, *Sodium Sulamyd*[1]	**Ointment**: 10%	Yes
	AK-Sulf[2], *Bleph-10*[1], *Ocusulf-10*[2], *Sodium Sulamyd*[2], *Sulf-10*[1,2]	**Solution**: 10%, 30%	Yes
Rx	**Tobramycin**		
	Tobrex	**Ointment**: 0.3%	No
	AK-Tob[1], *Tobrex*[1]	**Solution**: 0.3%	Yes

[1] Contains benzalkonium chloride.
[2] Contains sulfites.

Type of Drug:

Topical antibiotics for use in treating or preventing bacterial infections of the eye.

How the Drug Works:

Ophthalmic antibiotics stop or prevent susceptible bacteria infections of the eyeball and eyelid by either killing or inhibiting the growth of susceptible bacteria.

Uses:

To treat superficial eye infections caused by susceptible bacteria. The spectrum of antibacterial activity of the ophthalmic anti-infectives is variable. Consult specific product information to determine potential antibacterial susceptibility.

Chloramphenicol — Only for serious infections for which less potentially dangerous drugs are ineffective or not recommended.

Erythromycin — For the prevention of ophthalmia neonatorum (eye infection in newborn) due to *Neisseria gonorrhoeae* or *Chlamydia trachomatis.*

Precautions:

Do not use in the following situations: Allergy to the antibiotic or any of its ingredients.

Use with caution in the following situations:
- corneal lesions
- pus in eye (sulfacetamide sodium only)

Superinfection: Use of antibiotics (especially prolonged or repeated therapy) may result in bacterial or fungal overgrowth. Such overgrowth may lead to a second infection. The first antibiotic may need to be stopped and another antibiotic may need to be prescribed for the second infection.

Pregnancy: Safety for use during pregnancy has not been established. Use only if clearly needed and if the potential benefits to the mother outweigh the possible hazards to the fetus.

Breastfeeding: Chloramphenicol and tobramycin appear in breast milk. It is not known if topical ciprofloxacin, levofloxacin, or ofloxacin appears in breast milk. Because of the potential for side effects in breastfed infants, decide whether to discontinue nursing or discontinue the drug, taking into account the importance of the drug to the mother. Consult your doctor before you begin breastfeeding.

Children: Gentamicin and tobramycin are safe and effective in children. Erythromycin is safe and effective in newborns and children. Safety and effectiveness of sulfacetamide sodium in infants less than 2 months of age have not been established. Safety and effectiveness of chloramphenicol, ciprofloxacin solution, levofloxacin, and ofloxacin in children less than 1 year of age have not been established. Safety and effectiveness of ciprofloxacin ointment in children less than 2 years of age have not been established.

Lab tests may be required during treatment. Tests may include bacterial culture and susceptibility testing.

Sulfites: Some of these products contain sulfite preservatives, which can cause allergic reactions in certain individuals. Check package label when available or consult your doctor or pharmacist.

Drug Interactions:

Tell your doctor or pharmacist if you are taking or if you are planning to take any over-the-counter or prescription medications or dietary supplements with ophthalmic antibiotics. Doses of one or both drugs may need to be modified or a different drug may need to be prescribed. Silver preparations interact with sulfacetamide sodium.

Consider all drug interactions reported for oral anti-infectives when using ophthalmic anti-infectives. Refer to the individual drug monographs in the Anti-infectives chapter.

Side Effects:

Every drug is capable of producing side effects. Many ophthalmic antibiotic uses experience no, or minor, side effects. The frequency and severity of side effects depend on many factors including dose, duration of therapy, and individual susceptibility. Possible side effects include the following:

Eyes or Ocular: Lid crusting, crystals/scales, foreign body sensation, corneal staining, decreased vision, tearing, sensitivity to light (ciprofloxacin, levofloxacin, and ofloxacin only); irritation; burning; stinging; pain; itching; lid swelling; redness; dryness; watering; blurred vision.

Other: Bad or abnormal taste sensation (ciprofloxacin, levofloxacin, and ofloxacin only); sore throat (ciprofloxacin, levofloxacin, and ofloxacin only); aplastic anemia (chloramphenicol only); rash; headache.

Oral anti-infective-associated side effects should be considered when using these agents in the eye. Refer to the individual drug monographs in the Anti-infectives chapter.

Guidelines for Use:

- Dosage is individualized. Use exactly as prescribed.
- Do not change the dose or stop taking this medicine, unless advised to do so by your doctor.
- Review guidelines at the beginning of this chapter for proper technique for instilling eye drops or eye ointments.
- To avoid contamination, do not touch tip of container to any surface. Replace cap after using.
- May cause temporary stinging or blurring of vision following administration.
- Contact your doctor if stinging, burning, or itching becomes pronounced or if redness, irritation, swelling, decreasing vision, or pain persists or worsens.
- In general, patients being treated for bacterial conjunctivitis should not wear contact lenses; however, if your doctor considers contact lens use appropriate, wait at least 15 minutes after using any solutions containing benzalkonium chloride before inserting the lens, as it may be absorbed by the lens.
- *Ciprofloxacin, levofloxacin, and ofloxacin* — Discontinue use and notify your doctor if you experience skin rash or other signs of allergic reactions.
- Lab tests may be required to monitor therapy. Be sure to keep appointments.
- Store at controlled room temperature (59° to 86°F). Keep bottles and tubes tightly closed. Protect from light.
- Polymyxin B ophthalmic solution must be stored in a refrigerator (36° to 46°F). Discard unused solution after 72 hours.

If you have any questions, consult your doctor, pharmacist, or health care provider.

	Generic Name *Brand Name Examples*	Steroid	Antibiotic	Generic Available
Rx	**Steroid and Antibiotic Suspensions and Solutions**			
	Chloromycetin/ Hydrocortisone for Suspension	0.5% hydrocortisone acetate	0.25% chloramphenicol	Yes
	AK-Spore H.C. Ophthalmic Suspension, Cortisporin Suspension	1% hydrocortisone	Neomycin sulfate equivalent to 0.35% neomycin base and 10,000 units polymyxin B sulfate/mL	Yes
	Terra-Cortril Suspension	1.5% hydrocortisone acetate	0.5% oxytetracycline	No
	Poly-Pred Suspension	0.5% prednisolone acetate	Neomycin sulfate equivalent to 0.35% neomycin base and 10,000 units polymyxin B sulfate/mL	No
	Pred-G Suspension	1% prednisolone acetate	Gentamycin sulfate equivalent to 0.3% gentamicin base	No
	AK-Neo-Dex Solution, Neo-Dexameth, Neodecadron Solution	0.1% dexamethasone phosphate	Neomycin sulfate equivalent to 0.35% neomycin base	Yes
	TobraDex Suspension	0.1% dexamethasone	0.3% tobramycin	No

	Generic Name *Brand Name Examples*	Steroid	Antibiotic	Generic Available
	AK-Trol Suspension, Dexacidin Suspension, Maxitrol Suspension	0.1% dexamethasone	Neomycin sulfate equivalent to 0.35% neomycin base and 10,000 units polymyxin B sulfate/mL	Yes
Rx	**Steroid and Antibiotic Ointments**			
	Ophthocort[1]	0.5% hydrocortisone acetate	1% chloramphenicol, 10,000 units polymyxin B/g	No
	AK-Spore H.C.[1], *Cortisporin*	1% hydrocortisone	Neomycin sulfate equivalent to 0.35% neomycin base, 400 units bacitracin zinc, 10,000 units polymyxin B sulfate/g	Yes
	Neotricin HC	1% hydrocortisone acetate	Neomycin sulfate equivalent to 0.35% neomycin base, 400 units bacitracin zinc, 10,000 units polymyxin B sulfate/g	No
	Pred-G S.O.P.	0.6% prednisolone acetate	Gentamicin sulfate equivalent to 0.3% gentamicin base	No
	NeoDecadron	0.05% dexamethasone phosphate	Neomycin sulfate equivalent to 0.35% neomycin base	No
	TobraDex	0.1% dexamethasone	0.3% tobramycin	No

	Generic Name *Brand Name Examples*	Steroid	Antibiotic	Generic Available
	AK-Trol, Dexacidin, Dexasporin, Maxitrol	0.1% dexamethasone	Neomycin sulfate equivalent to 0.35% neomycin base, 10,000 units polymyxin B sulfate/g	Yes
Rx	**Steroid and Sulfonamide, Suspensions and Solutions**			
	FML-S Suspension	0.1% fluorometholone	10% sodium sulfacetamide	No
	Blephamide Suspension	0.2% prednisolone acetate	10% sodium sulfacetamide	No
	Isopto Cetapred Suspension	0.25% prednisolone acetate	10% sodium sulfacetamide	No
	AK-Cide Suspension, Metimyd Suspension	0.5% prednisolone acetate	10% sodium sulfacetamide	No
	Sulster Solution, Vasocidin Solution	0.25% prednisolone sodium phosphate	10% sodium sulfacetamide	Yes
Rx	**Steroid and Sulfonamide, Ointments**			
	Blephamide	0.2% prednisolone acetate	10% sodium sulfacetamide	No
	Cetapred	0.25% prednisolone acetate	10% sodium sulfacetamide	No
	AK-Cide, Metimyd, Vasocidin	0.5% prednisolone acetate	10% sodium sulfacetamide	No

[1] Preservative free.

For more information, see the ophthalmic antibiotic monograph and steroid monograph.

Type of Drug:

Antibiotic/anti-inflammatory combinations for use in the eye.

Uses:

To treat eye infections or inflammatory conditions of the eye in which bacterial infection or risk of infection exists.

To treat chronic anterior uveitis and corneal injury from chemical, radiation or heat burns, or from penetration of foreign bodies.

Guidelines for Use:

- Use exactly as prescribed.
- Follow the Administration Guidelines found at the beginning of this chapter.
- Shake suspensions well before use.
- If a dose is missed, instill it as soon as possible. If several hours have passed or if it is nearing time for the next dose, do not double the dose in order to "catch up" (unless advised to do so by your doctor). If more than one dose is missed or it is necessary to establish a new dosage schedule, contact your doctor or pharmacist.
- May cause temporary blurring of vision or stinging following administration.
- Contact your doctor if stinging, burning, itching, redness, irritation, swelling, decreasing vision, or pain persists or worsens.
- Continue use until all of the prescribed medicine has been used, even if redness or other symptoms have disappeared. Failure to use all of the medicine may prevent complete elimination of bacteria, allowing the infection to return.
- *Superinfection* – Use of antibiotics (especially prolonged or repeated therapy) may result in bacterial or fungal overgrowth. Such overgrowth may lead to a second infection. This medicine may need to be stopped and another antibiotic may need to be prescribed for the second infection.
- Some of these products may contain sulfite preservatives, which can cause allergic reactions in certain individuals (eg, asthmatics). Check package label when available or consult your doctor or pharmacist.
- Do not use with contact lenses unless advised to do so by your eye doctor.
- Do not use if solution has particles or discoloration.
- Store at room temperature (59° to 86°F), away from heat and light. Do not freeze.

If you have any questions, consult your doctor, pharmacist, or health care provider.

	Generic Name *Brand Name Examples*	Supplied As	Generic Available
Rx	**Natamycin**		
	Natacyn	**Suspension**: 5%	No

Type of Drug:

Topical antifungal.

How the Drug Works:

Natamycin appears to bind to the cell membrane of susceptible fungi. This alters the cell wall and allows essential elements of the fungus to leak out of the cell. This results in cell death.

Uses:

To treat fungal eye infections caused by susceptible fungi.

Precautions:

Do not use in the following situations:
allergy to natamycin or any component of the product

Pregnancy: Adequate studies have not been done in pregnant women, or animal studies may have shown a risk to the fetus. Use only if clearly needed and the potential benefits outweigh the possible hazards to the fetus.

Breastfeeding: It is not known if natamycin appears in breast milk. Consult your doctor before you begin breastfeeding.

Children: Safety and effectiveness in children have not been established.

Lab tests may be required to monitor therapy. Be sure to keep appointments.

Side Effects:

Every drug is capable of producing side effects. Many natamycin users experience no, or minor, side effects. The frequency and severity of side effects depend on many factors including dose, duration of therapy, and individual susceptibility. Possible side effects include redness and swelling.

Guidelines for Use:

- Follow Administration Guidelines found at the beginning of this chapter.
- Shake well before mixing.
- For topical use only. Not for injection.
- Continue therapy for 14 to 21 days or until the fungal infection disappears.
- Notify your doctor if improvement does not occur within 7 to 10 days.
- Do not use with contact lenses without first consulting with your eye doctor.
- Lab tests or exams may be required to monitor therapy. Be sure to keep appointments.
- Store at room temperature (46° to 75° F) or in the refrigerator (36° to 46° F). Do not freeze. Avoid exposure to sunlight and excessive heat.

If you have any questions, consult your doctor, pharmacist, or health care provider.

	Generic Name *Brand Name Examples*	Supplied As	Generic Available
Rx	**Trifluridine (Trifluorothymidine)**		
	Viroptic	**Solution**: 1%	No
Rx	**Vidarabine (Adenine Arabinoside; Ara-A)**		
	Vira-A	**Ointment**: 3%	No

Type of Drug:

Topical ophthalmic antiviral.

How the Drug Works:

Ophthalmic antivirals kill susceptible viruses by preventing viral cell reproduction that may result in eye infections.

Uses:

To treat herpes simplex keratitis (viral inflammation of the cornea of the eye).

Precautions:

Do not use in the following situations: Allergy to this medicine or any of its ingredients.

Corticosteroids may accelerate the spread of viral infections and are usually not to be used in herpes simplex infections. If corticosteroid (eg, prednisolone) therapy is used with this medicine, corticosteroid-induced side effects (eg, glaucoma, cataract formation, worsening of bacterial or viral infection) also may occur.

Pregnancy: Adequate studies have not been done in pregnant women. Use only if clearly needed and the potential benefits outweigh the possible hazards to the fetus.

Breastfeeding: It is not known if these medicines appear in breast milk. Consult your doctor before you begin breastfeeding.

Children: Safety and effectiveness have not been established for children less than 2 years of age for vidarabine and for children less than 6 years of age for trifluridine.

Drug Interactions:

Tell your doctor or pharmacist if you are taking or if you are planning to take any over-the-counter or prescription medications or dietary supplements while taking an ophthalmic antiviral agent. Doses of one or both drugs may need to be modified or a different drug may need to be prescribed.

Side Effects:

Every drug is capable of producing side effects. Many ophthalmic antiviral agent users experience no, or minor, side effects. The frequency and severity of side effects depend on many factors including dose, duration of therapy, and individual susceptibility. Possible side effects include the following: Irritation; pain; swelling of the eye or lids; increased tearing; sensitivity to light; clouding of vision; allergic reaction; foreign body sensation; increased fluid pressure in the eye; inflammation; red eye; dry eye; corneal changes; mild transient burning or stinging upon instillation.

Guidelines for Use:

- Use exactly as prescribed. Follow administration and dosing guidelines provided by your doctor or pharmacist.
- *Trifluridine* — Instill 1 drop onto cornea of affected eye(s) every 2 hours while awake for a maximum daily dose of 9 drops. After apparent healing, instill 1 drop every 4 hours while awake for a minimum daily dose of 5 drops for an additional 7 days to prevent recurrence. Temporary burning or stinging may occur upon administration.
- *Vidarabine* — Administer approximately ½ inch of ointment into the lower conjunctival sac of the affected eye(s) 5 times daily at 3-hour intervals. After apparent healing, administer twice daily for an additional 7 days to prevent recurrence.
- If both eye drops and eye ointment are used, instill eye drops at least 10 minutes before instilling the ointment.
- A temporary visual haze may occur upon administration.
- Other forms of therapy may be needed if there are no signs of improvement after 7 to 14 days or complete healing has not occurred by 14 days for trifluridine or 21 days for vidarabine. Some severe cases may require longer treatment. Continued use of trifluridine for more than 21 days is not recommended due to potential toxicity to the eye.
- May cause sensitivity to light. This may be minimized by wearing sunglasses.
- Do not stop using this medicine unless instructed to do so by your doctor. Use for the full course of therapy as directed by your doctor.
- Do not use more often or for a longer period of time than prescribed.
- Do not use with contact lenses without first consulting your eye doctor.
- If used with a corticosteroid (eg, prednisolone), corticosteroid-induced side effects (eg, glaucoma, cataract formation, worsening of bacterial or viral infections) may occur.
- Notify your doctor if condition worsens or if decreased vision, pain, itching, or swelling of the eye occurs.
- Recurrence of infection may be seen if medication is not used exactly as prescribed.
- *Trifluridine* — Store in the refrigerator (36° to 46°F).
- *Vidarabine* — Store at room temperature (59° to 86°F).

If you have any questions, consult your doctor, pharmacist, or health care provider.

	Generic Name *Brand Name Examples*	Supplied As	Generic Available
Rx	**Fomivirsen Sodium**		
	Vitravene	**Intravitreal injection**: 6.6 mg/mL	No

Type of Drug:

Injectable ophthalmic antiviral.

How the Drug Works:

Ophthalmic antivirals kill susceptible viruses by preventing viral cell reproduction that may result in eye infections.

Uses:

Fomivirsen sodium is indicated for the local treatment of cytomegalovirus (CMV) retinitis in patients with acquired immunodeficiency syndrome (AIDS) who are intolerant of or have a contraindication to other treatment(s) for CMV retinitis or who were insufficiently responsive to previous treatment(s) for CMV retinitis.

Precautions:

Do not use in the following situations: Allergy to this medicine or any of its ingredients.

Corticosteroids may accelerate the spread of viral infections and are usually not to be used in herpes simplex infections. If corticosteroid (eg, prednisolone) therapy is used with this medicine, corticosteroid-induced side effects (eg, glaucoma, cataract formation, worsening of bacterial or viral infection) also may occur.

Pregnancy: Adequate studies have not been done in pregnant women. Use only if clearly needed and the potential benefits to the mother outweigh the possible hazards to the fetus.

Breastfeeding: It is not known if these medicines appear in breast milk. Consult your doctor before you begin breastfeeding.

Children: Safety and effectiveness in children have not been established.

Drug Interactions:

Tell your doctor of pharmacist if you are taking or if you are planning to take any over-the-counter or prescription medications or dietary supplements with fomivirsen. Doses of one or both drugs may need to be modified or a different drug may need to be prescribed.

Side Effects:

Every drug is capable of producing side effects. Many fomivirsen users experience no, or minor, side effects. The frequency and severity of side effects depend on many factors including dose, duration of therapy, and individual susceptibility. Possible side effects include the following:

Eyes or Ocular: Abnormal vision; blurred vision; cataract; vision changes; pain; floaters; increased fluid pressure in eye; sensitivity to light; retinal detachment; bleeding in eye; eye inflammation; application site reaction; bloodshot eye; eye swelling; eye irritation; low fluid pressure in eye; retinal edema; retinal pigment changes.

Other: Stomach pain; weakness; diarrhea; fever; headache; nausea; pneumonia; rash; infection; vomiting; sinus infection; abnormal thinking; allergic reactions; appetite loss; back pain; chest pain; weight loss; dehydration; depression; dizziness; difficulty breathing; flu syndrome; increased cough; abnormal nerve sensations; sweating; abnormal blood cell count; anemia; abnormal liver tests; infection; systemic CMV; bronchitis; catheter infection; kidney failure; pain; pancreas infection; oral fungus.

Guidelines for Use:

- Use exactly as prescribed. Follow administration and dosage guidelines provided by your doctor or pharmacist.
- The diagnosis and evaluation of CMV rotinitis is ophthalmologic and should be made by comprehensive retinal examination by a physician.
- Fomivirsen is for direct injection into the eye by a medical professional. It is not for topical administration.
- Other forms of therapy may be needed if there are no signs of improvement after 7 to 14 days or complete healing has not occurred by 14 to 21 days. Severe cases may require longer treatment.
- May cause sensitivity to light. This may be minimized by wearing sunglasses.
- Do not use with contact lenses without first consulting your eye doctor.
- If used with a corticosteroid (eg, prednisolone), corticosteroid-induced side effects (eg, glaucoma, cataract formation, worsening of bacterial or viral infections) may occur.
- Notify your doctor if condition worsens or if decreased vision, pain, itching, or swelling of the eye occurs.

If you have any questions, consult your doctor, pharmacist, or health care provider.

OPHTHALMIC PHOTOTHERAPY — VERTEPORFIN

	Generic Name *Brand Name Example*	Supplied As	Generic Available
Rx	**Verteporfin**		
	Visudyne	**Lyophilized cake**: 15 mg (reconstituted to 2 mg/mL)	No

Type of Drug:

Photosensitizing agent; light-activated drug used in photodynamic therapy.

How the Drug Works:

Verteporfin therapy is a 2-step process requiring administration of drug and light. The first step is an IV infusion of verteporfin; the second is the activation of verteporfin with light from a nonthermal diode laser.

Verteporfin accumulates in abnormal blood vessels in the eye. In the presence of light, verteporfin produces short-lived radicals, which damage the blood vessels, temporarily blocking them.

Uses:

For the treatment of age-related macular degeneration in patients with predominantly classic subfoveal choroidal neovascularization (CNV).

During clinical studies, older patients (≈ 75 years of age), patients with dark irides, patients with occult lesions, or patients with < 50% classic CNV were less likely to benefit from verteporfin therapy.

Precautions:

Do not use in the following situations:
- allergy to verteporfin or any component of the preparation
- porphyria

Use with caution in the following situations:
- liver disease, moderate to severe

Pregnancy: There are no adequate and well-controlled studies in pregnant women. Use during pregnancy only if clearly needed and the potential benefits outweigh the possible hazards to the fetus.

Breastfeeding: It is not known whether verteporfin is excreted in breast milk. Use caution when verteporfin is administered to a woman who is breastfeeding. Consult your doctor.

Children: Safety and efficacy of verteporfin in children have not been established.

Elderly: A reduced treatment effect was seen with increasing age.

Lab tests will be required periodically during treatment with verteporfin. Liver function tests will be conducted.

Drug Interactions:

Tell your doctor or pharmacist if you are taking or if you are planning to take any over-the-counter or prescription medications or dietary supplements with verteporfin. Doses of one or both drugs may need to be modified or a different drug may need to be prescribed. The following drugs and drug classes interact with verteporfin:

β-carotene
calcium channel blockers (eg, nifedipine)
dimethyl sulfoxide (eg, *Rimso 50*)
diuretics (eg, hydrochlorothiazide)
ethanol
griseofulvin (*Fulvicin*)
hypoglycemic agents (eg, sulfonylureas)
mannitol (*Resectisol*)
phenothiazines (eg, cholorpromazine)
polymyxin B
sulfonamides (eg, sulfanilamide)
tetracyclines (eg, oxytetracycline)
thromboxane A_2 inhibitors (eg, dipyridamole)

Side Effects:

Every drug is capable of producing side effects. Many verteporfin users experience no, or minor, side effects. The frequency and severity of side effects depend on many factors including dose, duration of therapy, and individual susceptibility. Possible side effects include the following:

Digestive Tract: Constipation; gastrointestinal cancer; nausea.

Nervous System: Headache; diminished sensitivity to stimuli; sleep disorder; feeling of whirling motion.

Circulatory System: Abnormal heart rhythms; high blood pressure; blood vessel disorders; varicose veins; anemia; decreased white blood count; increased white blood count.

Respiratory System: Sore throat; pneumonia.

Skin: Rash; injection site reactions; itching; skin inflammation; eczema; sunburn.

Eyes or Ocular: Severe vision decrease; blurred vision; decreased visual acuity; visual field defects; cataracts; eye inflammation; double vision; dry eyes; ocular itching; eye muscle spasms; excessive tearing of eyes; bleeding.

Other: Protein in the urine; increased creatinine; decreased hearing; joint pain or dysfunction; muscle weakness; back pain; fever; flu syndrome; sensitivity to light; prostatic disorder; abnormal liver function tests.

Guidelines for Use:

- This medicine will be prepared and administered by your health care provider in a medical setting.
- Treatment is a 2-step process. The first step is the intravenous (into a vein) administration of verteporfin. The second step is the activation of verteporfin with light from a laser. Therapy may be repeated depending on the results.
- Avoid exposure of unprotected skin, eyes, or other body organs to direct sunlight or bright indoor light (eg, tanning beds, bright halogen lighting) for 5 days after treatment.
- Wear protective clothing and dark sunglasses if you must go outdoors in daylight during the first 5 days after treatment. Ultraviolet (UV) sunscreens are not effective in protecting the skin.
- Expose skin to ambient indoor light. Do not stay in the dark. This will help inactivate the drug in the skin.

If you have any questions, consult your doctor, pharmacist, or health care provider.

	Generic Name *Brand Name Examples*	Supplied As	Generic Available
otc	**Artificial Tear Solutions**		
	Akwa Tears, Aquasite[1]*, Artificial Tears, Artificial Tears Plus, Celluvisc*[1]*, Dry Eyes, Dry Eye Therapy, Duratears Naturale, GenTeal Multidose, HypoTears, Hypo Tears PF*[1]*, Isopto Plain, Isopto Tears, Just Tears, Liquifilm Tears, Moisture Eyes, Murocel, Muro 128 2%, Muro 128 5%, Preservative Free Moisture Eyes*[1]*, Puralube, Refresh*[1]*, Refresh Plus*[1]*, Refresh Tears, Teargen, Teargen II, Tearisol, Tears Naturale, Tears Naturale II, Tears Naturale Free*[1]*, Tears Plus, Tears Renewed, Ultra Tears*	**Solution**	Yes
Rx	**Artificial Tear Insert**		
	Lacrisert[1]	**Insert:** 5 mg hydroxypropyl cellulose	No

[1] Preservative free.

Type of Drug:

Artificial tear solutions and device.

The artificial tear solutions contain a diverse group of chemicals. This monograph does not follow the typical format due to the lack of consistency of information from product to product. Also, products may not share the same inactive ingredients. For additional information about a specific product, consult the product package labeling or your doctor or pharmacist.

How the Drug Works:

Provide tear-like lubrication for relief of dry eyes and eye irritation. Components of these products include:

Boric acid is a buffering agent that adjusts pH.

Methylcellulose, hydroxyethylcellulose, hydroxypropyl methylcellulose, hydroxypropyl cellulose, propylene glycol, gelatin, dextran, povidone, polyvinyl alcohol, and polyethylene glycol are thickening agents that prolong eye contact time.

Benzalkonium chloride, methyl- and propylparabens, chlorobutanol, and thimerosal are preservatives that maintain sterility.

Balanced amounts of salts help to maintain isotonicity (0.9% NaCl equivalent).

Uses:

Solution — For relief of dry eyes and eye irritation that are generally associated with reduced tear production. Also used as lubricants for artificial eyes. Some of these products can be used with hard contact lenses.

Insert — To treat moderate to severe dry eye syndromes including keratoconjunctivitis sicca (inflammation of the cornea and conjunctiva), exposure keratitis (inflammation of the cornea), decreased corneal sensitivity, and recurrent corneal erosions.

Precautions:

Do not use in the following situations: Allergy to any ingredient of the medicine.

Side Effects:

Every drug is capable of producing side effects. Many artificial tears solution and device users experience no, or minor, side effects. The frequency and severity of side effects depend on many factors including dose, duration of therapy, and individual susceptibility. Possible side effects include the following:

Other: Inserts — Transient blurring of vision; eye discomfort or irritation; matting or stickiness of eyelashes; sensitivity to light; allergic reaction; swelling of eyelids; red eyes.

Guidelines for Use:

- For use in eyes only.
- May produce temporary blurring of vision. Use caution while driving or performing other hazardous tasks.
- Remove contact lenses before use.

Solutions —

- Wash hands thoroughly before use.
- Pull down the lower lid of the affected eye, forming a "V" pocket.
- Instill 1 to 2 drops into eye(s) 3 to 4 times daily. Repeat as needed or as advised by your doctor.
- Do not use if solution changes color or becomes cloudy.
- Do not use *Liquifilm Tears*, *Teargen II*, or *Tearisol* on or with soft contact lenses.
- If headache, eye pain, changes in vision, continued redness, or irritation occurs, or if condition worsens or persists for more than 72 hours, discontinue use and consult your doctor.
- For single-dose applications, use immediately after opening. Do not store open containers. Discard single-dose applicator/container after installation of solution.
- To avoid contamination, do not touch the tip of the container or dropper to any surface. Close multi-use container immediately after each use.
- Store at room temperature (59° to 86°F) and keep tightly closed and out of the reach of children.

Inserts —

- Wash hands thoroughly before use.
- Use 1 insert daily.
- If insert is placed improperly in the eye, a corneal abrasion (scrape) may result. Practice insertion and removal of insert while in your doctor's office until the technique is mastered. Illustrated instructions are included in each package. Follow instructions carefully.
- Occasionally, the insert is expelled from the eye. To avoid displacement of insert, do not rub the eye(s), especially when awakening. Another insert may be used if the initial insert is expelled.
- To avoid transient blurred vision, the insert may be removed a few hours after insertion. Another insert may be used if needed.
- If symptoms worsen or persist, remove insert and notify your doctor.
- Store at room temperature (59° to 86°F) and out of the reach of children. Do not remove from storage blister until just prior to insertion.

If you have any questions, consult your doctor, pharmacist, or health care provider.

Generic Name / *Brand Name Examples*	Supplied As	Generic Available
otc **Ocular Lubricants**		
Akwa Tears[1], *Artificial Tears, Dry Eyes, Duratears Naturale*[1], *HypoTears, Lacri-Lube S.O.P., Moisture Eyes PM, Refresh PM*	**Ointment**	Yes
Tears Naturale II[1], *Dry Eyes*[1]	**Drops**	Yes

[1] Preservative free.

Type of Drug:

Ocular lubricants. Most products contain white petrolatum and mineral oil to lubricate the eye.

How the Drug Works:

Forms a smooth, comfortable protective film to protect and lubricate the cornea and conjunctiva (eye).

Precautions:

Do not use in the following situations: If you are allergic to the medicine or any of its ingredients.

Guidelines for Use:

- For use in eyes only.
- Remove contact lenses before using.
- Pull down the lower lid of the affected eye forming a "V" pocket. Apply 1 drop of solution or a small amount (¼ inch) of ointment to the inside of the eyelid, 1 or more times daily, or as directed by your doctor. Look downward before closing the eye(s).
- Generally, tear substitute drops are used during the day and ointments at nighttime.
- To avoid contamination, do not touch tip to any surface. Replace the cap immediately after each use.
- If eye pain, change in vision, continued redness, or irritation occurs, or if condition worsens or persists for more than 72 hours, discontinue use and consult your doctor.
- Ointment may cause a visual "haze" or blurring of vision. Use caution while driving or performing hazardous tasks.
- Store at room temperature (59° to 86°F), and keep tightly closed and out of the reach of children.

If you have any questions, consult your doctor, pharmacist, or health care provider.

	Generic Name *Brand Name Examples*	Uses
otc	**Wetting Solutions**	
	Liquifilm Wetting[1], *Sereine*[1]	Wetting solutions contain surfactants to maintain the water content of the hard lens surface. These solutions include methylcellulose and derivatives, polyvinyl alcohol, povidone, some newer polymers, preservatives, and buffering agents. These agents increase solution thickness and act as a physical cushioning agent between the lens and cornea.
otc	**Wetting/Soaking Solutions**	
	Soac-Lens, *Wetting & Soaking*, *Wet-N-Soak Plus*	These solutions, in addition to wetting the lens surface, also can be used as soaking solutions.
otc	**Cleaning, Soaking, and Wetting Solution**	
	Total[1]	This solution, in addition to wetting and soaking, also can be used as a cleaning solution.
otc	**Rewetting Solutions**	
	Boston Rewetting Drops, *Clerz 2*[1], *Lens Drops*[1], *Opti-Tears Soothing Drops*[1]	Rewetting solutions are intended for use directly in the eye with a contact lens. These products improve wearing time by rewetting the eye and the lens, which may become dry and contaminated during wear.
otc	**Cleaning Solutions and Gels**	
	LC-65, *MiraFlow Extra Strength*[2], *Opti-Clean Daily Cleaner*, *Opti-Clean II*[1], *Opti-Free Daily Cleaner*	Cleaning solutions and gels contain surfactant cleaners to ease removal of debris from lens surface. To adequately clean, physically rub lens with solution or gel and rinse with water or sterile saline solution.
otc	**Cleaning and Soaking Solution**	
	Clean-N-Soak[1]	This solution eases removal of debris from the lens surface.

	Generic Name *Brand Name Examples*	Uses
otc	**Enzymatic Cleaner**	
	Opti-Free Enzymatic Cleaner Especially for Sensitive Eyes	Enzymatic cleaning, by soaking the lens in a solution prepared from enzyme tablets, is recommended once weekly. This is intended to remove protein and other lens deposits. Contact lens must be rinsed and disinfected before wearing.

[1] Thimerosal free.
[2] Preservative free.

For optimum comfort and to minimize problems, conventional hard lenses require care with separate wetting, cleaning, and soaking solutions.

Type of Drug:

Hard contact lens products.

How the Drug Works:

Contact lens products are sterile, isotonic, and free of particulate matter. They contain various chemical ingredients to achieve specific goals of contact lens care.

Precautions:

Do not use in the following situations: Allergy to the product or any of its ingredients.

Side Effects:

These products are capable of producing side effects. Many contact lens users experience no, or minor side effects. The frequency and severity of side effects depend on many factors including individual susceptibility and adherence to instructions for proper lens care. Possible side effects include the following:

Eyes or Ocular: Stinging, burning, or itching of eye(s); excessive tearing; unusual eye secretions; redness of eye(s); reduced sharpness of vision; blurred vision; sensitivity to light; dry eyes; infection.

Guidelines for Use:

- Proper contact lens care will increase success and decrease complications.
- See individual product information for detailed directions and safety information. Problems with contact lens and lens care products could result in serious injury to the eye. Always follow label directions and your doctor's recommendations.
- Cleaning does not disinfect lenses. Disinfecting does not clean lenses.
- Wash and rinse hands thoroughly before handling contact lenses.
- Do not take enzymatic tablets internally.
- Do not use enzymatic tablets that are soft and sticky or irregular in appearance.
- Weekly enzymatic/disinfection cycle is not a substitute for daily cleaning and disinfecting.
- Do not insert contact lenses if eyes are red or irritated.
- Do not wear contact lenses while sleeping.
- For hard contact lens care, use only products designed for hard contact lenses. Because many of these products can only be used with certain lens types, consult your eye doctor before using any product if you are uncertain which type of lens you wear.
- If cleaner or disinfectant gets in eye(s), remove lens immediately and flush eye(s) with water or saline for several minutes.
- Do not change or substitute products from a different manufacturer without consulting your doctor.
- Do not store lenses in tap water.
- Never use saliva to wet contact lenses.
- Never reuse the solution in your lens case.
- To avoid contamination, do not touch tip of container to any surface. Replace cap and keep tightly closed when not in use.
- Do not instill topical medications while contact lenses are being worn unless directed to do so by your doctor.
- Eye problems, including corneal ulcers, can develop rapidly and lead to loss of vision. If eye discomfort; excessive tearing; vision changes; or eye redness, burning, or irritation occur, immediately remove your lenses. If the problem stops and the lenses appear to be undamaged, thoroughly clean, rinse, and disinfect the lenses and reinsert them. If the problem continues or a lens appears damaged, remove the lens and contact your eye care practitioner immediately.
- It is recommended that contact lens wearers see their eye doctor twice a year, or more frequently if directed.
- Use before the expiration date marked on the carton and bottle, or within the time indicated on the package (usually within 60 to 90 days).
- Keep contact lens care products out of the reach of children.
- Store tablets in a dry place. Do not remove from foil pouch until just prior to use.
- Do not use solution if it becomes cloudy or discolored.
- Store at room temperature.

If you have any questions, consult your doctor, pharmacist, or health care provider.

	Generic Name *Brand Name Examples*	Uses
otc	**Disinfecting/Wetting/ Soaking Solutions**	
	Boston Advance Comfort[1], *Boston Advance Comfort Formula Convenience Pack*, *Boston Conditioning*[1], *Boston Simplicity Multi-Action*, *Wet-N-Soak*, *Wet-N-Soak Plus*[1]	These solutions are used for disinfecting and help to maintain the water content of the lens.
otc	**Cleaning/Soaking Solution**	
	Boston Reconditioning Drops	This solution eases removal of debris from the lens surface. For use with the *Boston Lens.*
otc	**Cleaning Solutions**	
	Boston Advance Cleaner[1], *Boston Cleaner (original formula)*, *LC-65 Daily Cleaner*[1], *Opti-Clean Daily Cleaner*, *Opti-Clean II*[1], *Opti-Free Daily Cleaner*, *Opti-Free Supra Clens Daily Protein Remover*[2]	These solutions are used for daily cleaning to prevent the accumulation of deposits and to remove other debris.
otc	**Enzymatic Cleaners**	
	Boston One Step Liquid, *Opti-Zyme Enzymatic Cleaner*, *Opti-Zyme Especially for Sensitive Eyes*, *ProFree/GP Weekly Enzymatic Cleaner Tablets*	Enzymatic cleaning, by soaking in a solution prepared from enzyme tablets, is recommended once weekly. This is intended to remove protein and other lens deposits. Contact lenses must be rinsed and disinfected before wearing.
otc	**Rewetting Solutions**	
	Wet-N-Soak[1], *Opti-Tears Soothing Drops*[1], *Lens Drops*[1], *Boston Rewetting Drops*[1]	Rewetting solutions may be used directly in the eye to wet and improve lens comfort.

[1] Thimerosal free.
[2] Preservative free.

Rigid gas (oxygen) permeable contact lens (RGP) care regimens include use of a surfactant cleaner and storage in a chemical disinfecting solution. Follow the lens care procedure provided by the lens manufacturer. The advantages of RGP lenses are that they maintain the natural state of the cornea, preventing complications. However, they are predisposed to drying and accumulating protein and lipid deposits.

Type of Drug:

Rigid gas permeable contact lens products.

How the Drug Works:

Contact lens products are sterile, isotonic, and free of particulate matter. They contain various chemical ingredients to achieve specific goals of contact lens care.

Precautions:

Do not use in the following situations: Allergy to the product or any of its ingredients.

Side Effects:

These products are capable of producing side effects. Many contact lens users experience no, or minor side effects. The frequency and severity of side effects depend on many factors including individual susceptibility and adherence to instructions for proper lens care. Possible side effects include the following:

Eyes or Ocular: Stinging, burning, or itching of eye(s); excessive tearing; unusual eye secretions; redness of eye(s); reduced sharpness of vision; blurred vision; sensitivity to light; dry eyes; infection.

Guidelines for Use:

- Proper contact lens care will increase success and decrease complications.
- See individual product information for detailed directions and safety information. Problems with contact lens and lens care products could result in serious injury to the eye. Always follow label directions and your doctor's recommendations.
- Cleaning does not disinfect lenses. Disinfecting does not clean lenses.
- Wash and rinse hands thoroughly before handling contact lenses.
- Do not take enzymatic tablets internally.
- Do not use enzymatic tablets that are soft and sticky or irregular in appearance.
- Weekly enzymatic/disinfection cycle is not a substitute for daily cleaning and disinfecting.
- Do not insert contact lenses if eyes are red or irritated.
- Do not wear contact lenses while sleeping.
- For rigid gas permeable lens care, use only products designed for rigid gas permeable lenses. Because many of these products can only be used with certain lens types, consult your eye doctor before using any product if you are uncertain of which type of lens you wear.
- If cleaner or disinfectant gets in eye(s), remove lens immediately and flush eye(s) with water or saline for several minutes.
- Do not change or substitute products from a different manufacturer without consulting your doctor.
- Do not store lenses in tap water.
- Never use saliva to wet contact lenses.
- Never reuse the solution in your lens case.
- To avoid contamination, do not touch tip of container to any surface. Replace cap and keep tightly closed when not in use.
- Do not instill topical medications while contact lenses are being worn unless directed by your doctor.
- Eye problems, including corneal ulcers, can develop rapidly and lead to loss of vision. If eye discomfort; excessive tearing; vision changes; eye redness, burning, or irritation occur, immediately remove your lenses. If the problem stops and the lenses appear to be undamaged, thoroughly clean, rinse, and disinfect the lenses and reinsert them. If the problem continues or a lens appears damaged, remove the lens and contact your eye care practitioner immediately.
- It is recommended that contact lens wearers see their eye doctor twice a year, or more frequently if directed.
- Use before the expiration date marked on the carton and bottle, or within the time indicated on the package (usually within 60 to 90 days).
- Keep contact lens care products out of the reach of children.
- Store tablets in a dry place. Do not remove from foil packet until just prior to use.
- Do not use solution if it becomes cloudy or discolored.
- Store at room temperature.

If you have any questions, consult your doctor, pharmacist, or health care provider.

	Generic Name *Brand Name Examples*	Uses
otc	**Preserved Saline Solutions**	
	Opti-Soft[1], *Saline Solution*[1], *Sensitive Eyes Saline*[1], *Sensitive Eyes Plus Saline*	These solutions are for rinsing and storage of soft lenses in conjunction with heat disinfection. Thimerosal-free preserved saline solutions may be used by patients sensitive to thimerosal or mercury-containing compounds.
otc	**Preservative Free Saline Solutions**[2]	
	Blairex Sterile Saline, *Ciba Vision Saline*, *Lens Plus*, *Sensitive Eyes Sterile Saline Spray*, *Unisol*, *Unisol 4*	These solutions are for patients intolerant to preservatives. Use them for rinsing or storage and to help minimize mucus accumulation.
otc	**Surfactant Cleaning Solutions**	
	Ciba Vision Daily Cleaner[1], *Daily Cleaner*[1], *LC-65*, *Lens Plus Daily Cleaner*[2], *MiraFlow Extra Strength*[2], *Opti-Clean II*[1], *Opti-Clean Daily Cleaner*, *Opti-Free Daily Cleaner*[1], *Opti-Free Supra Clens Daily Protein Remover*[1], *Pliagel*[1], *Pure Eyes Cleaner/Rinse*[1,2], *Pure Eyes Disinfecting/Soaking*[1,2], *Sensitive Eyes Daily Cleaner*[1], *Sensitive Eyes Saline/Cleaning Solution*[1]	Cleaning solutions are used for daily cleaning to prevent the accumulation of deposits and to remove other debris.
otc	**Enzymatic Tablet Cleaners**	
	Allergan Enzymatic, *Opti-Free Enzymatic Cleaner*, *Opti-Zyme Enzymatic Cleaner Especiallyfor Sensitive Eyes*[2], *ReNu 1 Step*, *ReNu Effervescent*, *Sensitive Eyes Enzymatic Cleaner*, *Ultrazyme*	Enzymatic cleaning, by soaking in a solution prepared from enzyme tablets, is recommended once weekly. This is intended to remove protein and other deposits from the lens. Contact lens must be rinsed and disinfected before wearing.

SOFT (HYDROGEL) CONTACT LENS PRODUCTS

	Generic Name *Brand Name Examples*	Uses
otc	**Rewetting Solutions**	
	Clerz 2 Lubricating and Rewetting Drops, Lens Drops, Lens Plus Rewetting Drops[2], *Opti-Free Rewetting Drops*[1], *Opti-Tears Soothing Drops*[1], *ReNu Lubricating and Rewetting Drops*[1], *Sensitive Eyes Drops*[1]	Rewetting solutions may be used directly in the eye to wet and improve comfort of soft lenses.
otc	**Chemical Disinfection Systems**	
	One-solution systems	
	AOSept[1], *Disinfecting Solution, Opti-Free, Opti-Free Express, Opti-Soft Disinfecting*[1], *ReNu Multi-Purpose*[1], *ReNu MultiPlus*[1]	Chemical disinfection is an alternative to heat. One-solution systems use the same solution for rinsing and storing. Two-solution systems use separate disinfecting and rinsing solutions.
	Two-solution systems	
	AOSept Disinfecting, Oxysept Disinfection System, Quick Care Starting Solution[1,2]	**Warning:** Lenses must not be disinfected by heating when using most of these solutions. See individual label for restrictions.

[1] Thimerosal free.
[2] Preservative free.

Soft (hydrogel) contact lenses must be maintained in a wet state in saline to prevent them from becoming brittle. Soft lenses will absorb many substances; therefore, use only solutions specifically formulated for soft lenses. In addition, these lenses must be disinfected either by heating or by soaking in a chemical solution. *Heating lenses in solutions used for chemical disinfection may cause them to become opaque.*

Soft lens solutions are especially made to be compatible with, and to meet the particular needs of, soft contact lenses. Of particular importance to soft lens care is the need for thorough cleaning to remove deposits that coat and may discolor the lens, especially when subjected to disinfection by heating.

WARNING: DO NOT use conventional (hard) lens solutions on soft contact lenses. Consult your eye doctor for product selection. Not all products are intended for use in all types of soft lenses.

Type of Drug:

Soft contact lens products.

How the Drug Works:

Contact lens products are sterile, isotonic, and free of particulate matter. They contain various chemical ingredients to achieve specific goals of contact lens care.

Precautions:

Do not use in the following situations: If you are allergic to the product or any of its ingredients

Side Effects:

These products are capable of producing side effects. Many contact lens users experience no, or minor side effects. The frequency and severity of side effects depend on many factors including individual susceptibility, length of wear, and adherence to instructions for proper lens care. Possible side effects include the following:

Eyes or Ocular: Stinging, burning, or itching of eye(s), excessive tearing; unusual eye secretions; redness of eye(s); reduced sharpness of vision; blurred vision; sensitivity to light; dry eyes; infection.

Guidelines for Use:

- Proper contact lens care will increase success and decrease complications.
- See individual product information for detailed direction and safety information. Always follow label directions and your doctor's recommendations. Problems with contact lens and lens care products could result in serious injury to the eye.
- Cleaning does not disinfect lenses. Disinfecting does not clean lenses.
- Wash and rinse hands thoroughly before handling contact lenses.
- Do not take enzymatic tablets internally.
- Do not use enzymatic tablets that are soft and sticky or irregular in appearance.
- Weekly enzymatic/disinfection cycle is not a substitute for cleaning and disinfecting.
- Do not insert contact lenses if eyes are red or irritated.
- Do not wear contact lenses while sleeping unless they have been prescribed for extended wear. Daily wear lenses are not indicated for overnight wear and should not be worn while sleeping because this may cause serious side effects.
- Remove extended-wear lenses regularly for cleaning and disinfecting or for disposal and replacement on the schedule prescribed by your doctor to avoid serious side effects. The risk of serious side effects increases the longer extended-wear lenses are worn before removal for cleaning and disinfecting or for disposal and replacement. Smokers have a higher incidence of side effects.
- For soft lens care, use only products designed for soft lenses. Because many of these products can only be used with certain lens types, consult your eye doctor before using any product if you are uncertain which type of lens you wear.

Guidelines for Use (cont.):

- *Homemade saline solution* — Soft contact lens wearers who use homemade saline (salt) solutions are at risk of developing *Acanthamoeba keratitis*, a serious and painful corneal infection. This infection may cause impaired vision or blindness. Homemade saline solution is not recommended. Use commercial sterile saline solutions.
- If cleaner or disinfectant gets in eye(s), remove lens immediately and flush eye(s) with water or saline for several minutes.
- Do not put lens in eye(s) until rinsed with a neutralizer or saline unless it is a one-solution system.
- Do not change or substitute products from a different manufacturer without consulting your doctor.
- Do not store lenses in tap water.
- Never use saliva to wet contact lenses.
- Never reuse the solution in your lens case. To prevent contamination and to avoid eye injury, always empty and rinse lens case with fresh rinsing solution and allow to air dry. Do not use tap water, soap, or detergent.
- To avoid contamination, do not touch tip of container to any surface. Replace cap and keep tightly closed when not in use.
- Do not transfer saline to another container since the packaged container keeps the saline sterile.
- *Perservative Free Salines* — Discard bottle and contents 30 days after opening. Because the preservative free salines have no strong preservatives, they will not remain sterile indefinitely after opening and therefore should not be used as an eye drop.
- Do not instill topical medications while contact lenses are being worn unless directed to do so by your doctor.
- Eye problems, including corneal ulcers, can develop rapidly and lead to loss of vision. If eye discomfort; excessive tearing; vision changes; eye redness, burning, or irritation occur, immediately remove your lenses. If the problem stops and the lenses appear to be undamaged, thoroughly clean, rinse, and disinfect the lenses and reinsert them. If the problem continues or a lens appears damaged, remove the lenses and contact your eye care practitioner immediately.
- It is recommended that contact lens wearers see their eye doctor twice a year, or more frequently if directed.
- Use before the expiration date marked on the carton and bottle, or within the time indicated on the package (usually within 60 to 90 days).
- Keep contact lens care products out of the reach of children.
- Do not use solution if it becomes cloudy or discolored.
- Store tablets in a dry place. Do not open foil packets until just prior to use.
- Store tablets and solutions at room temperature.

If you have any questions, consult your doctor, pharmacist, or health care provider.

	Brand Name Examples	Antibiotic	Steroid
Rx	*Chloromycetin Otic*	**Solution**: 0.5% chloramphenicol/mL	
Rx	*Otobiotic Otic*[1]	**Solution**: 10,000 units polymyxin B sulfate/mL	0.5% hydrocortisone per mL
Rx	*AK-Spore H.C. Otic*[1], *Cortisporin Otic*[1]	**Solution**: 3.5 mg neomycin sulfate, 10,000 units polymyxin B sulfate/mL	1% hydrocortisone per mL
Rx	*AK-Spore H.C. Otic, Cortisporin Otic*	**Suspension**: 3.5 mg neomycin sulfate, 10,000 units polymyxin B sulfate/mL	1% hydrocortisone per mL
Rx	*Coly-Mycin S Otic, Cortisporin-TC*	**Suspension**: 3.3 mg neomycin sulfate, 3 mg colistin, 0.05% thonzonium bromide/mL	1% hydrocortisone per mL

[1] Contains sulfites.

Type of Drug:

Antibiotic and antibiotic-steroid combinations for the ear. Used to treat superficial bacterial infections of the outer ear.

How the Drug Works:

Antibiotics interfere with protein production and cellular activity of susceptible bacteria. This interference may impair reproductive ability or kill the bacteria. Steroids inhibit the inflammatory response (eg, redness, swelling) of tissues due to mechanical, chemical, or allergy-causing agents, and infectious processes.

Uses:

To treat susceptible bacterial infections of the outer ear. The steroid ingredient (usually hydrocortisone) has an anti-inflammatory effect.

Precautions:

Do not use in the following situations:

allergy to these drugs or any of their ingredients
fungal infections of the ear
perforated eardrum (solutions only)
viral infections of the ear (eg, herpes simplex, varicella-zoster)

Use with caution in the following situations:

chronic otitis media (middle ear infection)
perforated eardrum (suspensions only)

Superinfection: Use of antibiotics (especially prolonged or repeated therapy) may result in resistant bacterial or fungal overgrowth. Such overgrowth may lead to a second infection. The medication may need to be stopped and another antibiotic may need to be prescribed for the second infection.

Neomycin sensitization: When using neomycin-containing products to control secondary infection in the chronic dermatoses (eg, chronic otitis externa, stasis dermatitis), keep in mind that the skin in these conditions is more liable than healthy skin to become sensitized to many substances, including neomycin.

Pregnancy: No adequate and well-controlled studies have been done in pregnant women. Use only if clearly needed and potential benefits to the mother outweigh the possible hazards to the fetus.

Breastfeeding: Otic antibiotics and hydrocortisone appear in breast milk. Consult your doctor before you begin breastfeeding.

Children: Contact your doctor or pharmacist before using in children less than 12 years of age.

Lab tests may be required to verify the identification of the organism. Tests include cultures and susceptibility tests.

Sulfites: Some of these products may contain sulfite preservatives that can cause allergic reactions in certain individuals. Check package label when available or consult your doctor or pharmacist.

Side Effects:

Every drug is capable of producing side effects. Many users of topical antibiotic combinations for the ear experience no, or minor, side effects. The frequency and severity of side effects depend on many factors including dose, duration of therapy, and individual susceptibility. Possible side effects include the following:

Skin: Irritation; itching; burning; redness; rash; hives; stinging; dryness; allergic skin reaction; tearing of skin.

Other: Secondary infection.

Guidelines for Use:

- *Suspension* — Shake the container for 10 seconds before using.
- *Suspension and Solution* — To warm the medication before use, hold the container in the hand for a few minutes. To avoid loss of potency, do not heat above body temperature .
- *AK-Spore H.C., Cortisporin, and Otobiotic* — Instill 4 drops in the affected ear(s) 3 to 4 times daily. Instill 3 drops 3 to 4 times daily for infants and children.
- *Coly-Mycin S and Cortisporin-TC* — Instill 5 drops in the affected ear(s) 3 times daily. Instill 4 drops 3 times daily for infants and children.
- *Chloromycetin* — Instill 2 to 3 drops in the affected ear(s) 3 times daily.
- *Drops* — Administer the prescribed number of drops using the calibrated dropper included with each bottle of drops.
- Do not use in eyes.
- Clean the outer ear canal thoroughly and dry with a sterile cotton applicator before using the medicine.
- Avoid touching the dropper to the ear, fingers, counter top, or other surfaces.
- Lie on your side or tilt the affected ear up prior to administering the drug.
- Keep the ear tilted for about 5 minutes after administration. To assist the drops in running into the external ear canal, hold the earlobe up and back in adults and down and back in children.
- If preferred, insert a cotton wick into the ear canal and saturate it with solution. Keep wick moist by adding solution every 4 hours. Replace the wick at least once every 24 hours.
- If reddening with swelling, dry scaling, burning, or itching occurs or persists after use, contact your doctor.
- Duration of therapy should be limited to no more than 10 consecutive days.
- If infection is not improved after 1 week, your doctor will repeat the cultures and susceptibility tests to verify the identity of the infecting organism and to determine whether therapy should be changed.
- Allergic cross-reactions may occur with neomycin which could prevent the use of any or all of the following antibiotics for the treatment of future infections: Kanamycin, paromomycin, streptomycin, and possibly gentamicin.
- Store between 59° to 86°F. Store *Cortisporin* between 59° and 77°F. Store *Otobiotic* between 36° and 86°F.

If you have any questions, consult your doctor, pharmacist, or health care provider.

	Brand Name Examples	Supplied As	Generic Available
Rx	*Acetasol, Borofair Otic, VōSol Otic*	**Solution**: 2% acetic acid	Yes
Rx	*Americaine Otic, Otocain*	**Solution**: 20% benzocaine	No
Rx	*Tympagesic*[1]	**Solution**: 5% benzocaine, 5% antipyrine, 0.25% phenylephrine HCl	No
Rx	*Allergen Ear Drops, Auralgan Otic, Auroto Otic*	**Solution**: 1.4% benzocaine, 5.4% antipyrine, glycerin	Yes
otc	*Aurocaine 2*	**Solution**: 2.75% boric acid, 97.25% isopropyl alcohol	No
otc	*Auro Ear Drops, Aurocaine Ear Drops, Debrox Drops, E•R•O Ear Drops, Mollifene Ear Wax Removal Aid, Murine Ear Drops, Murine Ear Wax Removal System*	**Solution**: 6.5% carbamide peroxide	No
Rx	*Cortic Ear Drops, Zōtō-HC Ear Drops*	**Solution**: 0.1% chloroxylenol, 1% hydrocortisone, 1% pramoxine HCl	No
Rx	*Cresylate*	**Solution**: 25% m-cresyl acetate, 0.5% acetic acid	No
Rx	*EarSol-HC*	**Solution**: 1% hydrocortisone	No
Rx	*Acetasol-HC, VōSol HC Otic*	**Solution**: 1% hydrocortisone, 2% acetic acid	No
otc	*Auro-Dri, Dri/Ear, Ear-Dry, Swim Ear*	**Solution**: 95% isopropyl alcohol, 5% anhydrous glycerin	No
otc	*Star-Otic*	**Solution**: Modified Burow's solution (aluminum acetate), acetic acid, boric acid	No
Rx	*Cerumenex Drops*	**Solution**: 10% triethanolamine polypeptide oleate-condensate	No

[1] Contains metabisulfite.

Type of Drug:

Drugs used to treat various external ear conditions.

Uses:

In these combinations:

Acetic acid, aluminum acetate, boric acid, chloroxylenol, and *m-cresyl acetate* provide antibacterial or antifungal action.

Antipyrine is a pain reliever with local anesthetic action.

Benzocaine and pramoxine HCl are local anesthetics that provide relief from pain or itching.

Carbamide peroxide and triethanolamine dissolve ear wax.

Glycerin is a solvent.

Hydrocortisone is a steroid used for its anti-inflammatory and antipruritic (anti-itch) effects.

Isopropyl alcohol is an antiseptic in topical anti-infective products.

Phenylephrine HCl is a vasoconstrictor, which may be a decongestant, and is used to decrease swelling.

Precautions:

Do not use in the following situations:

- allergy to the medicine or any of its ingredients
- chickenpox (steroid only)
- ear discharge (benzocaine, antipyrine, phenylephrine only)
- herpes simplex (steroid only)
- perforated eardrum
- vaccine (steroid only)

Use with caution in the following situations:

- dizziness
- ear pain, severe
- otitis media, severe

Pregnancy: There are no adequate and well-controlled studies in pregnant women. Use only if clearly needed and potential benefits to the mother outweigh the possible risks to the fetus.

Breastfeeding: It is not known if these otic preparations appear in breast milk. Consult your doctor before you begin breastfeeding.

Children: Consult your doctor about dosing and safety in children. Safety and effectiveness have not been established for *Cerumenex*. Do not use *Americaine Otic* in children less than 1 year of age. Do not use *Earsol-HC* in children less than 2 years of age except under the advice and supervision of your doctor. Safety and effectiveness have not been established for children less than 3 years of age for *Acetasol*, , *Acetasol-HC*, *VōSol* and *VōSol HC*. Safety and effectiveness have not been established for children less than 12 years of age for *Tympagesic*.

Sulfites: Some of these products may contain sulfite preservatives, which can cause allergic reactions in certain individuals (eg, asthmatics). Check package label when available or consult your doctor or pharmacist.

Drug Interactions:

Tell your doctor or pharmacist if you are taking or if you are planning to take any over-the-counter or prescription medications or dietary supplements with otic preparations. Doses of one or both drugs may need to be modified or a different drug may need to be prescribed.

Side Effects:

Every drug is capable of producing side effects. Many otic preparation users experience no, or minor, side effects. The frequency and severity of side effects depend on many factors including dose, duration of therapy, and individual susceptibility. Possible side effects include the following:

Local: Stinging; burning; irritation; skin inflammation; swelling; flushing; redness of the outer ear canal; itching; pain; rash; hives; dryness; inflammation of the hair follicles; excess hair growth; acne-like eruptions; decrease in skin or tissue coloration; tenderness.

Other: Headache; dizziness; restlessness; anxiety.

Guidelines for Use:

- For use in the ear only. Avoid contact with eyes. Do not use in eyes or take internally.
- To properly administer ear drops, observe the following steps: Avoid touching the dropper to the ear. Hold the container in the hand for a few minutes to warm it if it has been refrigerated.
  Lie on your side or tilt the affected ear(s) up prior to administering the drug. Administer the prescribed number of drops. Keep the ear(s) tilted up for about 2 minutes. To assist the drops in running into the outer ear canal, hold the earlobe up and back in adults and down and back in children. Cotton may be placed in the ear to prevent drops from escaping.
- If problem persists or worsens after recommended treatment period, consult your doctor.
- Discontinue use and contact your doctor promptly if sensitization or irritation occurs after use.
- *Allergen*, *Auralgan*, and *Tympagesic* — Do not rinse dropper after use. Discard the solution 6 months after the dropper is first placed into the solution. Do not use if solution is brown or contains solid particles floating in the solution.
- Do not use wax-removing solutions if you have ear drainage or discharge, ear pain, irritation, rash in the ear, or if you are dizzy.
- Indiscriminate use of anesthetic ear drops may mask symptoms of an infection in the middle ear.
- *Debrox Drops* foam on contact with ear wax due to release of oxygen. There may be an associated crackling sound.
- Store at room temperature (59° to 86°F). Protect from freezing, direct sunlight, and excessive heat. Keep container tightly closed and out of the reach of children. Store *VōSol*, *VōSol-HC*, and *Acetasol HC* between 68° and 77°F.

If you have any questions, consult your doctor, pharmacist, or health care provider.

Mouth and Throat Products
- Carbamide Peroxide, 1405
- Chlorhexidine, 1407
- Saliva Substitutes, 1409
- Tetracycline HCl, 1412
- Amlexanox, 1414
- Benzyl Alcohol, 1416
- Mouth and Throat Products, 1417

Vaginal Preparations
- Douche Products, 1425
- Spermicides, 1428

Anorectal Preparations, 1430

Acne Products
- Benzoyl Peroxide, 1435
- Azelaic Acid, 1438
- Sulfur, 1440
- Tretinoin, 1441
- Miscellaneous Combinations, 1444

Agents for Psoriasis
- Anthralin, 1450
- Calcipotriene, 1452
- Acitretin, 1454
- Methotrexate, 1457
- Psoralens, 1460

Antiacne, Antipsoriatic
- Tazarotene, 1464

Diabetic Ulcer Agent
- Becaplermin, 1467

Burn Preparations
- Mafenide, 1469
- Silver Sulfadiazine, 1471

Antiseborrheics
- Selenium Sulfide, 1473
- Miscellaneous, 1475
- Combinations, 1479

Anesthetics
- For Mucous Membranes, 1481
- For Skin Disorders, 1485

Keratolytics
- Cantharidin, 1489
- Podofilox, 1491
- Salicylic Acid, Topical, 1493

Emollients, 1496
- Miscellaneous, 1498

Analgesics
- Capsaicin, 1500

Antihistamines, 1502

Antiseptics and Germicides, 1505

Diaper Rash Products, 1507

Minoxidil, 1509

Poison Ivy Treatment Products, 1512

Rubs and Liniments, 1514

Sunscreens, 1516

Skin Cleansers, 1525

Astringents
- Aluminum Acetate, 1526

Miscellaneous Topical Agents, 1527

Eflornithine HCl, 1533

	Generic Name *Brand Name Examples*	Supplied As	Generic Available
otc	**Carbamide Peroxide**		
	Orajel Perioseptic	**Liquid**: 15%	No
	Cankaid, Gly-Oxide Liquid	**Solution**: 10%	No
	Proxigel	**Gel**: 10%	No

Type of Drug:

Antiseptic mouth-cleansing agent for irritated and inflamed areas.

How the Drug Works:

Carbamide peroxide releases oxygen into irritated mouth tissue to provide a cleansing effect. This helps reduce inflammation, relieve pain and inhibit growth of odor-forming bacteria so that healing can begin.

Uses:

To treat and prevent minor mouth and gum irritation or inflammation (eg, canker sores, accidental injuries, dentures, orthodontic appliances, postdental procedures).

Aid to oral hygiene when normal cleansing measures are inadequate or impossible (eg, total care geriatrics or when patient wears orthodontic or dental appliances).

Precautions:

Use with caution in the following situations:

dental irritation or oral inflammation, severe or persistant gingivitis

Children: Do not use in children under 2 years of age (*Cankaid* — under 3 years of age) unless directed by a doctor or dentist.

Side Effects:

Every drug is capable of producing side effects. Most carbamide peroxide users experience no, or minor, side effects. Possible side effects include irritation; rash; inflammation; gingivitis; swelling; fever.

Guidelines for Use:

- Do not swallow.
- *Liquid and Solution* — No not dilute. Apply 4 times daily after meals and at bedtime or as directed. Place several drops directly on the affected area; expectorate (spit out) after 2 to 3 minutes or place 10 drops on the tongue, mix with saliva, swish thoroughly and expectorate (spit out).
- *Gel* — Do not dilute. Use 4 times daily or as directed. Massage gently on the affected area. Allow medicine to remain in place for 1 minute then spit out. Do not drink or rinse mouth for 5 minutes after use. Replace bottle tip after each use.
- Avoid contact with eyes.
- Do not use for more than 7 days.
- Severe or persistant oral inflammation, dental irritation or gingivitis may be serious. Consult your doctor or dentist immediately.
- If condition persists or worsens, or if irritation, redness, swelling or fever occurs, stop using this medication and contact your doctor or dentist.
- Do not use for children under 2 years of age (*Cankaid* — under 3 years of age) unless directed by a doctor or dentist.
- Cap tightly. Protect from heat and light.

If you have any questions, consult your doctor, pharmacist, or health care provider.

Generic Name *Brand Name Examples*	Supplied As	Generic Available
Rx **Chlorhexidine Gluconate**		
Peridex[1]	**Oral rinse**: 0.12%	No

[1] Contains alcohol.

Type of Drug:

Antibacterial oral rinse for treating inflamed gingiva (gums).

How the Drug Works:

Chlorhexidine gluconate is an oral rinse that decreases bacteria in the mouth.

Uses:

To treat gingivitis (redness and swelling of the gums) characterized by redness, swelling, and bleeding of the gums upon probing.

Precautions:

Do not use in the following situations:
allergy to the drug or any ingredient

Staining of oral surfaces (eg, teeth, restorations, tongue) may occur. Stains will be more pronounced in patients with heavy plaque accumulations.

Stains resulting from use does not adversely affect health of the gums or other oral tissues. Stains can be removed from most tooth surfaces by conventional dental cleaning techniques (make take longer). Patients who have restorations with rough surfaces or margins should use with caution; stains in these areas may be difficult to remove.

Changes in taste perception may occur while undergoing treatment. Most patients indicate it is less noticeable with continued use.

Pregnancy: Studies in pregnant women have not shown a risk to the fetus. However, no drug should be used during pregnancy unless clearly needed.

Breastfeeding: It is not known if chlorhexidine gluconate appears in breast milk. Consult your doctor before you begin breastfeeding.

Children: Safety and effectiveness in children under 18 years of age have not been established.

Side Effects:

Every drug is capable of producing side effects. Many chlorhexidine gluconate users experience no, or minor, side effects. Possible side effects include:

Mouth – Staining of teeth and other oral surfaces (eg, restorations, tongue); tartar increase; altered taste perception; minor sloughing of the oral mucosa (especially in children); dry mouth; mouth inflammation; gingivitis; red, inflamed tongue; mouth ulcers; diminished sensitivity; swelling; abnormal sensations in the mouth.

Other: Stomach upset or nausea (if swallowed); allergy symptoms.

Guidelines for Use:

- Begin therapy after a thorough cleaning of teeth by a dentist or dental hygienist.
- Usual dose is 15 mL (undiluted) twice daily, morning and evening, after brushing the teeth.
- Do not dilute.
- Do not rinse mouth with water or other mouthwash, brush teeth or eat immediately after rinsing with *Peridex*.
- To minimize discoloration, brush and floss daily emphasizing areas that begin to stain.
- To avoid taste interference, rinse with *Peridex* after meals.
- Tooth staining may occur.
- Taste changes may occur during use.
- Do not swallow the drug. Spit out after rinsing.
- Dental checkups are necessary every 6 months.
- Store above freezing.

If you have any questions, consult your doctor, pharmacist, or health care provider.

	Generic Name *Brand Name Example*	Supplied As	Generic Available
otc	*Entertainer's Secret, Moi-Stir, Moi-Stir 10, Mouthkote,*[1] *Optimoist, Saliva Substitute*[2]	**Solution**: Contains a variety of lubricants	No
otc	*Moi-Stir Swabsticks*	**Swabsticks**: Contains a variety of lubricants	No
otc	*Salivart*[1,2]	**Aerosol spray**: Contains a variety of lubricants	No
otc	*Salix*	**Tablets**: Contains a variety of lubricants	No

[1] Sugar free.
[2] Dye free.

Type of Drug:

Saliva substitute.

Uses:

To relieve dry mouth and throat caused by xerostomia (dry mouth) after surgery or from some illnesses (eg, Sjögren's syndrome, Bell's Palsy), some medications (eg, antidepressants, tranquilizers, antihistamines) and aging.

To aid healing after medical or surgical procedures (eg, chemotherapy, radiation, tracheotomy) that adversely affect the throat.

Guidelines for Use:

- Dosing varies. Be sure to read package insert for instructions.
- *Solution* — Squirt or spray a small quantity into the mouth as often as needed to moisten and lubricate.
- Solution may be swallowed or expectorated (spit out).
- *Tablets* — Allow to move around and slowly dissolve in mouth. Repeat one tablet per hour as necessary.
- *Entertainer's Secret* — Can spray into each nostril while inhaling to apply drug to upper throat.
- Do not drink water immediately after use.
- *Solutions* — Close container between uses.
- Store at room temperature.

If you have any questions, consult your doctor, pharmacist, or health care provider.

	Generic Name *Brand Name Examples*	Supplied As	Generic Available
Rx	**Pilocarpine HCl**		
	Salagen	**Tablets**: 5 mg	No

Type of Drug:

Salivary gland stimulator.

How the Drug Works:

Pilocarpine increases the production of saliva by stimulating muscles found in salivary glands.

Uses:

To treat xerostomia (dry mouth) in patients with malfunctioning salivary glands due to cancer radiotherapy of the head and neck.

To treat the symptoms of dry mouth caused by Sjögren's syndrome.

Precautions:

Do not use in the following situations:

allergy to pilocarpine
asthma, uncontrolled
glaucoma, narrow-angle
iritis, acute

Use with caution in the following situations:

asthma, controlled
bronchitis, chronic
chronic obstructive lung disease, requiring drug therapy
gall bladder disease
heart disease, significant
high blood pressure
kidney disease
liver disease
mental illness
nephrolithiasis
retinal disease
visual problems (eg, night blindness)

Pregnancy: Adequate studies have not been done in pregnant women. Use only if potential benefits outweigh possible hazards to the fetus.

Breastfeeding: It is not known if pilocarpine appears in breast milk. Consult your doctor before you begin breastfeeding.

Children: Safety and effectiveness in children have not been established.

Drug Interactions:

Tell your doctor or pharmacist if you are taking or if you are planning to take any over-the-counter or prescription medications or dietary supplements with pilocarpine. Doses of one or both drugs may need to be modified or a different drug may need to be prescribed. The following drugs and drug classes interact with pilocarpine:

anticholinergic agents (eg, atropine, inhaled ipratropium bromide)
beta-adrenergic blockers (eg, propranolol)

Side Effects:

Every drug is capable of producing side effects. Many pilocarpine users experience no, or minor, side effects. The frequency and severity of side effects depend on many factors including dose, duration of therapy and individual susceptibility. Possible side effects include:

Digestive Tract: Nausea; vomiting; diarrhea; gas; indigestion; stomach ache; difficulty swallowing; taste distortion.

Nervous System: Dizziness; headache; tremor.

Circulatory System: Edema (fluid retention); high blood pressure; rapid or slow heart beat; flushing; low blood pressure.

Respiratory System: Nasal congestion; sore throat; runny nose; sinus pain.

Skin: Sweating; chills; rash; itching.

Other: Urinary frequency; vaginitis (itching, inflammation or abnormal discharge); weakness; abnormal vision; eye inflammation; excess tears; nosebleed; ringing in ears; voice alteration; back pain; blurred vision; impaired depth perception.

Guidelines for Use:

- Take 1 tablet 3 times daily.
- *Sjögren's syndrome:* Take 1 tablet 4 times daily.
- If a dose is missed, take it as soon as possible. If several hours have passed or if it is nearing time for the next dose, do not double the dose in order to "catch up" (unless advised to do so by your doctor). If more than one dose is missed or it is necessary to establish a new dosage schedule, contact your doctor or pharmacist. Use exactly as prescribed.
- Maximum benefit may not be reached for several weeks.
- The lowest tolerable yet effective dose should be used for maintenance as adverse effects may increase with higher doses.
- Patients should have eye examinations before beginning treatment with pilocarpine.
- May cause visual problems. Use caution while driving, especially at night or when performing hazardous activities in reduced lighting.
- Notify your doctor if any of the following occurs: Headache, visual problems, tearing, excessive sweating, difficulty breathing, stomach cramps, nausea, vomiting, diarrhea, fast or slow pulse, blood pressure changes, confusion, tremor or irregular heartbeat.
- Store at room temperature (59° to 86°F).

If you have any questions, consult your doctor, pharmacist, or health care provider.

	Generic Name *Brand Name Examples*	Supplied As	Generic Available
Rx	**Tetracycline HCl**		
	Actisite	**Fiber**: 12.7 mg/23 cm	No

Type of Drug:

Topical antibiotic.

How the Drug Works:

Tetracycline reduces bacterial infections by inhibiting protein synthesis.

Uses:

Topical treatment for gum disease (periodontitis) in adults. It is used in combination with good hygiene, scaling, and root planing.

Precautions:

Do not use in the following situations:

allergy to any tetracyclines

Use with caution in the following situations:

abscess, acute
candidiasis, oral
kidney disease
medical disorders, contributing

Superinfection – Use of antibiotics (especially prolonged or repeated therapy) may result in bacterial or fungal overgrowth. Such overgrowth may lead to a second infection. Tetracycline may need to be stopped and another antibiotic may need to be prescribed for the second infection.

Photosensitivity – May cause photosensitivity (tendency to sunburn). Avoid prolonged exposure to the sun or other forms of ultraviolet light (eg, tanning beds). Use sunscreens and wear protective clothing until tolerance is determined. Discontinue use at the first sign of redness of the skin.

Pregnancy: Adequate studies have not been done in pregnant women, or studies in animals may have shown a risk to the fetus. Use only if clearly needed and the potential benefits outweigh the possible hazards to the fetus (See Children).

Breastfeeding: Tetracycline appears in breast milk. Because of the potential for serious side effects in nursing infants, use in a nursing woman only if clearly needed. Consult your doctor before you begin breastfeeding.

Children: Safety and effectiveness in children have not been established. The use of tetracycline class drugs during tooth development (last half of pregnancy, infancy and childhood to 8 years of age) may cause permanent discoloration of the teeth. Tetracycline drugs should not be used in these age groups unless other treatment is not likely to be effective or if alternative therapy is contraindicated.

Side Effects:

Every drug is capable of producing side effects. Many patients experience no, or minor, side effects. The frequency and severity of side effects depend on many factors including dose, duration of therapy and individual susceptibility. Possible side effects include discomfort on fiber placement and redness following removal.

Guidelines for Use:

- Avoid actions which may dislodge the fiber. Do not chew hard, crusty or sticky foods; do not brush or floss near any treated areas (continue to clean other teeth); do not engage in any other hygienic practices that could dislodge the fibers and do not probe at the treated area with tongue or fingers.
- The antibiotic-containing fiber provides continuous release of tetracycline for 10 days. At the end of 10 days of treatment, all fibers must removed by the dentist. Any fibers lost before the end of 7 days must be replaced by the dentist.
- Notify the dentist promptly if the fiber is dislodged or falls out before the scheduled visit, or if pain, swelling or other problems occur.
- May cause photosensitivity (tendency to sunburn). Avoid prolonged exposure to the sun or other forms of ultraviolet light (eg, tanning beds). Use sunscreen and wear protective clothing until tolerance is determined. Discontinue use at first sign of redness of the skin.
- Store at room temperature (59° to 86° F).

If you have any questions, consult your doctor, pharmacist, or health care provider.

	Generic Name *Brand Name Example*	Supplied As	Generic Available
Rx	**Amlexanox**		
	Aphthasol	**Paste, oral**: 5%	No

Type of Drug:

Mouth ulcer ("canker sore") treatment.

How the Drug Works:

The mechanism of action is unknown. The drug seems to inhibit inflammatory reactions.

Uses:

For the treatment of mouth ulcers ("canker sores") in patients with normal immune systems.

Precautions:

Do not use in the following situations: Allergy to amlexanox or any of its ingredients.

Pregnancy: Studies in pregnant women or in animals have been judged not to show a risk to the fetus. However, no drug should be used during pregnancy unless clearly needed.

Breastfeeding: It is not known if amlexanox appears in breast milk. Consult your doctor before you begin breastfeeding.

Children: Safety and effectiveness of amlexanox in children have not been established.

Drug Interactions:

Tell your doctor or pharmacist if you are taking or planning to take any over-the-counter or prescription medications or dietary supplements while taking amlexanox. Doses of one or both drugs may need to be modified or a different drug may need to be prescribed.

Side Effects:

Every drug is capable of producing side effects. Many amlexanox users experience no, or minor, side effects. The frequency and severity of side effects depend on many factors including dose, duration of therapy, and individual susceptibility. Possible side effects include: Transient pain; stinging or burning at the application site.

Guidelines for Use:

- Apply the paste 4 times a day following oral hygiene after breakfast, lunch, dinner, and at bedtime as directed by your doctor. Begin therapy as soon as you notice symptoms of a mouth ulcer.
- Squeeze a dab (¼ inch) of paste onto fingertip. Dab the paste onto each ulcer in the mouth using gentle pressure.
- Wash hands immediately after applying amlexanox. In the event of rash or contact irritation, discontinue use and contact your doctor.
- Wash eyes promptly if there is contact with the paste.
- Use the paste until the ulcers heal. If significant healing or pain reduction has not occurred in 10 days, consult your dentist or doctor.
- Keep out of the reach of children.
- Store at controlled room temperature (59° to 86°F).

If you have any questions, consult your doctor, pharmacist, or health care provider.

	Generic Name *Brand Name Examples*	Supplied As	Generic Available
otc	**Benzyl Alcohol**		
	Zilactin[1]	**Gel**: 10%	No

[1] Contains tannic acid.

Type of Drug:

Soft tissue protectant.

How the Drug Works:

Benzyl alcohol reduces sensory stimulation to relieve pain, burning, and itching.

Uses:

To provide temporary relief of pain, burning and itching in cold sores, canker sores, and fever blisters.

Side Effects:

Every drug is capable of producing side effects. Most benzyl alcohol users experience no, or minor, side effects. Possible side effects include temporary burning upon application (short duration) and allergic reactions.

Guidelines for Use:

- Apply this product 4 times daily for a minimum of 2 days. Use every 4 to 6 hours as needed. Wipe the affected area dry before applying the gel. Hold the affected area away from the other elements of the oral cavity for 30 to 60 seconds after application to maximize tissue binding.
- Do not use in or around eyes. If contact with eyes occurs, flush the eye(s) immediately and continuously with clean tap water for 10 minutes. Consult your doctor if pain or irritation persists.
- Burning of a temporary nature when applied to an open sore or blister is normal and no cause for concern.
- Do not peel off protective film. Attempting to peel off film may result in skin irritation or tenderness. To remove film, first apply another coat of *Zilactin* to film, then immediately wipe the area with a gauze pad or tissue.
- If inflammation persists beyond 10 days or worsens, stop using and consult your doctor.

If you have any questions, consult your doctor, pharmacist, or health care provider.

	Generic Name *Brand Name Examples*	Supplied As
otc	**Lozenges**	
	Cēpastat Fast-Acting[5]	**Lozenges**: 14.5% phenol, menthol
	Cēpacol ColdCare (Peppermint)[1,2]	**Lozenges**: 9 mg zinc
	Cēpacol [3] (Cherry)	**Lozenges**: 3.6 mg menthol, cetylpyridinium chloride
	Cēpacol[3] (Mint)	**Lozenges**: 2 mg menthol, cetylpyridinium chloride
	Cēpacol Maximum Strength[3] (Mint)	**Lozenges**: 10 mg benzocaine, 2 mg menthol, cetylpyridinium chloride
	Cēpacol Maximum Strength[3] (Cherry)	**Lozenges**: 10 mg benzocaine, 3.6 mg menthol, cetylpyridinium chloride
	Cēpacol Sugar Free,[4] *Maximum Strength* (Cherry)	**Lozenges**: 10 mg benzocaine, 4.5 mg menthol, cetylpyridinium chloride
	Cēpacol Sugar Free,[4] *Maximum Strength* (Mint)	**Lozenges**: 10 mg benzocaine, 2.5 mg menthol, cetylpyridinium chloride
	Cēpastat Cherry[4,5]	**Lozenges**: 14.5 mg phenol, menthol
	Cēpastat Extra Strength[4,5]	**Lozenges**: 29 mg phenol, menthol
	Vicks Chloraseptic	**Lozenges**: 6 mg benzocaine, 10 mg menthol
	Hall's Mentho-Lyptus[6]	**Lozenges**: 7 mg menthol and eucalyptus oil
	Mycinettes[4,5]	**Lozenges**: 15 mg benzocaine, cetylpyridinium chloride
	N'ice[4,5]	**Lozenges**: 5 mg menthol
	Spec-T [1,3,7] (Rasping Coughs)	**Lozenges**: 10 mg benzocaine, 10 mg dextromethorphan HCl
	Spec-T [1,3,7] (Nasal Congestion)	**Lozenges**: 10 mg benzocaine, 5 mg phenylephrine HCl, 10.5 mg phenylpropanolamine HCl
	Spec-T [3] (Sore Throat)	**Lozenges**: 10 mg benzocaine
	Sucrets (Wild Cherry)	**Lozenges**: 2 mg dyclonine HCl
	Sucrets (Original Mint)	**Lozenges** : 2 mg dyclonine HCl
	Sucrets (Assorted Flavors)	**Lozenges**: 2 mg dyclonine HCl
	Sucrets (Vapor Lemon)[6]	**Lozenges**: 2 mg dyclonine HCl
	Sucrets, Children's (Cherry)	**Lozenges**: 1.2 mg dyclonine HCl

	Generic Name *Brand Name Examples*	Supplied As
	Sucrets Maximum Strength[6] (Cherry)	**Lozenges**: 3 mg dyclonine HCl, menthol
	Sucrets Maximum Strength[6] (Wintergreen)	**Lozenges**: 2 mg dyclonine HCl
	Trocaine[7]	**Lozenges**: 10 mg benzocaine
otc	**Mouthwashes and Sprays**	
	Cēpacol[7,8,9]	**Mouthwash/Gargle**: 0.05% cetylpyridinium chloride
	Cēpacol Maximum Strength[4]	**Throat spray**: 0.1% dyclonine HCl, cetylpyridinium chloride
	Listerine[8]	**Mouthwash**: 0.064% thymol, 0.092% eucalyptol, 0.060% methyl salicylate, 0.042% menthol
	Scope[8]	**Mouthwash**: cetylpyridinium chloride
otc	**Preparations for Sensitive Teeth**	
	Aquafresh Sensitive Teeth	**Toothpaste**: 0.243% sodium fluoride, 5% potassium nitrate
	De-Sensitize Plus[5]	**Toothpaste**: 5% potassium nitrate, sodium fluoride
	Oral-B Sensitive with Fluoride	**Toothpaste**: 5% potassium nitrate, 0.225% sodium fluoride
	Promise Sensitive	**Toothpaste**: Potassium nitrate
	Crest Sensitivity Protection,[5] *Sensodyne Cool Gel for Sensitive Teeth and Cavity Prevention,*[5] *Sensodyne w/ Baking Soda for Sensitive Teeth and Cavity Prevention,*[5] *Sensodyne-SC Original Formula for Sensitive Teeth,*[5] *Sensodyne Extra Whitening for Sensitive Teeth*[4]	**Toothpaste**: Potassium nitrate, sodium fluoride

[1] Contains dextrose.
[2] Dietary supplement to promote general well being during cold season.
[3] Contains glucose, sucrose.
[4] Sugar free.
[5] Contains sorbitol.
[6] Contains sucrose.
[7] Contains the dye tartrazine.
[8] Contains alcohol.
[9] Contains edetate disodium, polysorbate 80, saccharin.

Type of Drug:

Mouth and throat products used to treat a variety of product specific conditions.

Uses:

In these combinations:

Benzocaine is a local anesthetic.

Cetylpyridinium chloride, eucalyptus oil, thymol, benzalkonium chloride, and hexylresorcinol have mild antiseptic activity.

Menthol, dyclonine, clove oil, phenol and methylsalicylate are used for their anti-itch, mild local anesthetic and counterirritant activities.

Sodium fluoride is used to prevent cavities and *potassium nitrate* is a desensitizing agent.

Zinc is considered a dietary supplement and is not approved by the FDA for any other uses.

Precautions:

Tartrazine: Some of these products may contain the dye tartrazine (FD&C Yellow No. 5), which can cause allergic reactions in certain individuals. Check package label when available or consult your pharmacist or doctor.

Guidelines for Use:

- Do not exceed recommended dosage.
- Dosing and symptoms treated by these products vary. Please read the instructions on the packaging carefully before using any of these products.
- *Lozenges* — Allow lozenge to dissolve slowly in mouth.
- If sore mouth or throat is severe, if irritation, redness or pain persists or worsens or it is accompanied by high fever, headache, swelling, rash, nausea or vomiting, contact your doctor or dentist promptly.
- Do not use products containing benzocaine if you are allergic to procaine, butacaine, benzocaine or other "-caine" anesthetics.
- Do not take throat lozenges for ongoing cough such as occurs with smoking, asthma or emphysema, or if cough is accompanied by a lot of mucous unless directed by your doctor.
- Sensitive teeth may mean that there is a serious problem that requires care by a dentist. See your dentist if the problem is ongoing or worsens. Do not use toothpaste for sensitive teeth longer than 4 weeks unless recommended by a dentist or doctor.
- A persistent cough could be a sign of a serious condition. If cough persists greater than 1 week, tends to recur or is accompanied by rash, fever or persistent headache, contact your doctor.

If you have any questions, consult your doctor, pharmacist, or health care provider.

	Brand Name Examples	Supplied As	Use
otc	*Amosan*	**Powder**: Sodium peroxyborate monohydrate	Soothes sore gums, canker sore pain, denture and orthodontic irritation and oral injuries after dental procedures
otc	*Anbesol*[2]	**Liquid**: 6.3% benzocaine, 0.5% phenol, menthol, camphor **Gel:** 6.3% benzocaine, 0.5% phenol, camphor	For relief of denture or orthodontic appliance irritation, toothache, sore gums, cold sores, fever blisters, braces, canker sores and minor dental procedure pain
otc	*Anbesol Cool Mint*	**Gel**: 10% benzocaine	
otc	*Anbesol Maximum Strength*	**Gel**[3,4] and **Liquid**:[2,3] 20% benzocaine	
otc	*Babee Teething*[1,2]	**Lotion**: 2.5% benzocaine, 0.02% cetalkonium chloride, thymol, urea, eucaplyptol, menthol, camphor	For teething discomfort or the pain of children's braces
otc	*Baby Numz•it*[3]	**Gel**: 7.5% benzocaine, clove and peppermint oil	For temporary relief of sore gums due to teething in children at least 4 months of age
otc	*Baby Orajel* [3,9] (Cherry Flavored)	**Gel**: 7.5% benzocaine	For the relief of teething pain in children at least 4 months of age
otc	*Benzodent*	**Cream**: 20% benzocaine, petrolatum	For relief of denture pain or discomfort
otc	*Blistex Lip*[2]	**Ointment**: 1% allantoin, 0.6% menthol, 0.5% phenol, 0.5% camphor	For dry, chapped lips, pain and itching caused by cold sores and fever blisters
otc	*Blistex Lip Medex*	**Ointment**: Petrolatum, 1% camphor, 1% menthol, 0.5% phenol, cocoa butter, lanolin, oil of cloves	For treatment of fever blisters and sore, dry and cracked lips

	Brand Name Examples	**Supplied As**	**Use**
otc	*Kanka*[2,3]	**Liquid**: 20% benzocaine, cetylpyridinium chloride, benzyl alcohol tincture compound, tannic acid	To relieve pain of mouth and canker sores and brace irritation
Rx	*Kenalog in Orabase*	**Paste**: 0.1% triamcinolone acetonide, mineral oil gel base	To aid in treating and relieving inflamed mouth sores and ulcers resulting from trauma
otc	*Orabase-B*	**Gel**: 20% benzocaine in plasticized hydrocarbon gel	For fast, temporary relief of canker sore pain, denture and orthodontic appliance irritations and mouth and gum sores
otc	*OrabaseGel*[3,6]	**Gel**: 15% benzocaine, salicylic acid	To relieve pain, itching and burning associated with canker sores, cold sores and fever blisters
otc	*Orabase-Plain*	**Paste**: Plasticized hydrocarbon gel	For temporary relief from minor irritations of the mouth and gums and denture discomfort, mouth sores, orthodontic appliance irritations, toothbrush abrasions and minor mouth surgery
otc	*Orajel*[3]	**Gel**: 10% benzocaine	For temporary relief of toothache pain until dentist is consulted
otc	*Orajel Denture*[3]	**Gel**: 20% benzocaine, menthol	To relieve pain and discomfort from dentures and minor irritation from orthodontic appliances
otc	*Orajel, Maximum Strength*	**Gel**,[3] **Liquid**:[2,3,5] 20% benzocaine	For temporary relief of toothache until medical attention is available

	Brand Name Examples	Supplied As	Use
otc	*Orajel Mouth-Aid*	**Liquid**:[3,5,6] 20% benzocaine **Gel**:[3,7] 20% benzocaine, 0.02% benzalkonium chloride, 0.1% zinc chloride, peppermint oil	To relieve pain and inflammation of cold sores, fever blisters, canker sores, mouth and gum sores and other minor mouth irritations
otc	*Peroxyl*	**Gel**: 1.5% hydrogen peroxide in mint flavored gel base	For canker sores and cleaning minor wounds or gum inflammation from minor dental procedures, braces, dentures, mouth and gum irritations
otc	*Peroxyl* [3,6,9]	**Solution**: 1.5% hydrogen peroxide, menthol	To cleanse canker sores, gum irritations, dental and mouth sores, orthodontic irritations, mouth burns and cheek bites and toothbrush abrasions
otc	*Pfeiffer's Cold Sore*[2]	**Lotion**: 7% gum benzoin, camphor, menthol, thymol and eucalyptol	For cold sores, fever blisters and cracked lips
otc	*Rid-A-Pain Dental*[2]	**Drops**: 6.3% benzocaine, 0.5% phenol, camphor, menthol	For temporary relief of toothache, brace and denture pain, orthodontic device irritation, sore gums, cold and canker sores and fever blisters
otc	*Tanac*[3]	**Liquid**: 10% benzocaine, 0.12% benzalkonium chloride and tannic acid	For the pain relief of mouth sores, canker sores, gum irritations and fever blisters

[1] Sugar free.
[2] Contains alcohol.
[3] Contains saccharin.
[4] Contains methylparaben.
[5] Contains tartrazine.
[6] Contains ethyl alcohol.
[7] Contains edetate disodium.
[8] Contains sorbitol.

Type of Drug:

Mouth and throat products. Ingredient(s) determine use.

Uses:

In these products:

Benzocaine is a local anesthetic.

Cetylpyridinium chloride, hydrogen peroxide and *eucalyptus oil* have mild antiseptic activity.

Menthol, camphor and *phenol* are used for their antipruritic, mild local anesthetic and counterirritant activities.

Eugenol is a mild pain reliever.

Tannic acid protects oral tissue and possesses astringent (drying) properties.

Triamcinolone acetonide and *hydrocortisone acetate* have anti-inflammatory action.

Precautions:

Do not use in the following situations:

- allergy to any ingredient of the drug
- fungal, viral or bacterial infections of mouth or throat (*Kenalog in Orabase* only)

Use with caution in the following situations:

- diabetes
- peptic ulcer
- pregnancy (*Kenalog in Orabase* only)
- tuberculosis

Tartrazine: Some of these products many contain the dye tartrazine (FD&C Yellow No. 5), which can cause allergic reactions in certain individuals. Check package label when available or consult your pharmacist or doctor.

Guidelines for Use:

- Dosing and uses for products vary. Carefully read the instructions on the packaging before using any of these medications.
- Do not exceed recommended dosage.
- Do not swallow products.
- Do not use benzocaine-containing products if there is a history of allergy to local anesthetics such as procaine, butacaine, benzocaine or other "-caine" anesthetics. Do not use if there is an allergy to any other ingredients.
- Do not use for fungal, viral or bacterial infections of the mouth or throat.
- If sore mouth conditions last for more than 7 days; if irritation, pain and redness persists or worsens; or if swelling, rash or fever develops, see your doctor or dentist.
- Do not use for longer than 5 to 7 days unless directed by your doctor or dentist. Do not use *Tanac* for longer than 5 consecutive days.
- Fever and nasal congestion are not symptoms of teething and may indicate an infection.
- Mild burning may occur at application site.
- Allergic reactions at place of application may occur after prolonged or repeated use; discontinue use and contact your doctor if this occurs.
- Benzocaine products may make swallowing difficult or inhibit gag reflexes in infants and children.
- Avoid contact with eyes.
- Keep away from flame.
- Do not apply over large areas of the body or cover with a bandage.
- Inform your doctor if you are pregnant, become pregnant, are planning to become pregnant or if you are breasfeeding.
- Do not use in young children (ages are specified on packaging).

If you have any questions, consult your doctor, pharmacist, or health care provider.

	Brand Name Examples	Supplied As
otc	*Massengill Douche*	**Powder**: Sodium chloride, ammonium alum, phenol, methyl salicylate, eucalyptus oil, menthol, thymol
otc	*Trichotine Douche*	**Powder**: Sodium lauryl sulfate, sodium perborate monohydrate, silica
	Trichotine Liquid Douche Concentrate[1]	**Liquid concentrate**: Sodium lauryl sulfate
otc	*Massengill Disposable Douche, Summer's Eve Disposable Douche, Summer's Eve Post-Menstrual Disposable Douche*	**Solution**: Contents of these products vary by manufacturer. See package labels for complete product contents.
otc	*Massengill Extra Mild Disposable Douche, Summer's Eve Douche*[2]	**Solution**: Purified water, vinegar
otc	*Massengill Extra Cleansing Disposable Douche*[1]	**Solution**: Purified water, vinegar, cetylpyridinium chloride, diazolidinyl urea
otc	*Massengill Baking Soda and Water Disposable Douche*	**Solution**: Sanitized water, sodium bicarbonate
otc	*Massengill "Scented" Disposable Douches*[1,3]	**Solution**: Water, SD alcohol 40, lactic acid, sodium lactate, octoxynol-9, cetylpyridinium chloride, propylene glycol, diazolidinyl urea
otc	*Zonite Douche*[1]	**Liquid concentrate**: Benzalkonium chloride, menthol, thymol, acetic acid
otc	*Massengill Douche*	**Liquid concentrate**: Lactic acid, sodium bicarbonate, SD alcohol 40 and octoxynol 9, eucalyptol, menthol, thymol
otc	*Massengill Medicated Disposable Douche*	**Solution**: Povidone-iodine
otc	*Betadine Medicated Disposable Douche, Summer's Eve Medicated Disposable Douche*	**Solution**: 0.3% povidone-iodine

[1] Contains EDTA.
[2] Contains benzoic acid.
[3] Contains parabens, fragrance, coloring.

Type of Drug:

Vaginal cleansing agents; douches.

How the Drug Works:

Povidine-iodine, eucalyptol, menthol, phenol, sodium perborate and thymol may have antiseptic or germicidal activity.

Povidine-iodine also relieves minor irritation. It may be absorbed from the vagina. Patients with thyroid disorders and pregnant patients should avoid iodine-containing douches.

Eucalyptol, menthol, phenol, methyl salicylate and thymol are counterirritants used for their anesthetic or antipruritic effects.

Ammonium alum is an astringent that reduces local edema and inflammation; high concentrations can be irritating.

Octoxynol 9, sodium lauryl sulfate and benzalkonium chloride are surfactants that facilitate douche spread over vaginal mucosa.

Sodium perborate and lactic acid affect pH.

Uses:

For general cleansing of the vaginal and genital area.

For deodorizing vaginal area.

To relieve minor vaginal itching and irritation.

To remove vaginal discharge, secretions and mucus.

To alter vaginal acidity.

Guidelines for Use:

- For external use only. See packaging for instructions.
- Consult manufacturer's recommendations for proper dilution and use of these products. Follow instructions carefully.
- Avoid contact with eyes.
- *Iodine-containing products* — Do not use if allergic to iodine, or if you are pregnant or breastfeeding.
- Vaginal douches are not contraceptive agents. Also, do not use for the treatment or prevention of pelvic inflammatory disease or sexually transmitted diseases. Do no use as a contraceptive or to self-treat or prevent sexually transmitted diseases or pelvic inflammatory disease.
- Do not douche for at least 6 hours after use of a vaginal spermicide.
- Do not use douche products during pregnancy unless instructed to do so by your doctor.
- If you have pelvic or stomach pain, fever, chills, nausea, vomiting, pus-like yellow cervical discharge with an odor, painful or frequent urination, genital sores or vaginal bleeding, contact your doctor immediately.
- If pain, soreness, swelling, redness, itching, excessive dryness, irritation, odor or discharge occurs or persists, or if symptoms continue after 7 days, discontinue use and call your doctor.
- An association has been reported between excessive douching and pelvic inflammatory disease, ectopic pregnancy and infertility.

If you have any questions, consult your doctor, pharmacist, or health care provider.

	Brand Name Examples	Supplied As
otc	*Conceptrol*	**Vaginal gel**: 100 mg nonoxynol-9
otc	*Conceptrol Contraceptive Inserts*	**Vaginal suppositories** :100 mg nonoxynol-9
otc	*Delfen Contraceptive*	**Vaginal foam**: 100 mg nonoxynol-9
otc	*Encare*	**Vaginal insert**: 100 mg nonoxynol-9
otc	*Gynol II Original Formula*	**Vaginal jelly**: 2% nonoxynol-9
otc	*Gynol II Extra Strength, Koromex*	**Vaginal jelly**: 3% nonoxynol-9
otc	*Koromex Clear*	**Vaginal gel**: 30% nonoxynol-9
otc	*Ortho-Gynol Contraceptive*	**Vaginal jelly**: 100 mg octoxynol 9
otc	*Semicid* [1]	**Vaginal suppositories**: 100 mg nonoxynol-9
otc	*Milex Shur-Seal*	**Vaginal gel**: 2% nonoxynol-9
otc	*Durex*	**Spermicide-containing condom**: 5% nonoxynol-9

[1] Contains methylparaben.

Topical contraceptive agents provide spermicidal action that is generally reliable when properly used either with a vaginal diaphragm or as the sole method of contraception. These agents are generally less effective than oral contraceptives. To reduce the potential for conception (pregnancy), follow directions for use carefully.

Type of Drug:

Vaginal contraceptive.

How the Drug Works:

Spermicides (nonoxynol-9, octoxynol) are agents that immobilize and inactivate sperm cells by rupturing or removing their outer membrane. The gel, cream, foam or jelly vehicle which carries the spermicide also serves as a partial barrier to the union of sperm with an egg by adhering to the opening of the cervix.

Uses:

To prevent pregnancy. Can be used alone (at high concentrations [eg, at least 8%] or in large amounts) or with other contraceptive methods (eg, diaphragm, cervical cap, contraceptive sponge, condoms).

Precautions:

Do not use in the following situations:

allergy to the active drug or any ingredient of the formulation

Use with caution in the following situations:

burning or irritation of vagina, penis or genital area following use
inability to understand directions for proper use

Condom use and sexually transmitted diseases (STDs): The CDC advises using condoms to prevent STDs. If used properly, condoms may help prevent infection by *Chlamydia trachomatis*, *Ureaplasma urealyticum*, *Trichomonas vaginalis*, *Candida albicans*, herpes simplex 1 and 2 (when lesions are on penis or female genital area), human papilloma virus, *Treponema pallidum*, *Haemophilus ducreyi* and AIDS.

Nonoxynol-9 has been shown to inhibit or reduce the risk of chlamydia and, to a lesser degree, gonorrhea. Use of nonoxynol-9 has been shown to increase the risk of developing a yeast infection.

Side Effects:

Every drug is capable of producing side effects. Most spermicide users experience no. or minor, side effects. Possible side effects include burning, irritation and itching.

Guidelines for Use:

- Strictly follow manufacturer's instructions for proper use of these products in order to achieve maximum protection.
- *Contraceptive foam* — Thoroughly shake the aerosol canister before use.
- *Vaginal spermicides* — Apply at least 10 minutes (but no more than 1 hour) before intercourse to ensure effectiveness. Products provide 1 hour of protection and should be reapplied for repeated intercourse.
- Apply high in the vagina, near the cervix.
- One applicatorful of spermicide is enough for only one act of intercourse. A new dose is required prior to each act of intercourse.
- Do not douche for 6 or more hours after intercourse. Premature douching may dilute the spermicide and may propel sperm into the uterus.
- *Diaphragm* — For contraceptive effectiveness, leave the diaphragm in place for 6 hours after intercourse, but remove it as soon as possible thereafter. Toxic shock syndrome, which can be fatal, has been reported with the use of diaphragms.
- *Vaginal suppositories* must melt and be dispersed before intercourse. Suppositories may not be as effective a mechanical barrier over the cervical opening as foams, creams, jellies and gels. Do not insert suppositories into the urinary opening.
- Contact your doctor if vaginal, penile, or genital burning, itching, irritation or painful urination follows use.
- These agents are not as effective as oral contraceptives or certain combination methods of contraception (eg, condom plus spermicide).
- These products are inserted into the vagina only, not into the urethra or rectum.
- If pregnancy is medically contraindicated, consult your doctor for a contraception program.
- These products have not been shown to protect against STDs.

If you have any questions, consult your doctor, pharmacist, or health care provider.

	Generic Name *Brand Name Examples*	Supplied As
Rx	**Steroid-Containing Products**	
	Carmol HC	**Cream**: 1% hydrocortisone acetate, 10% urea, sodium bisulfite, propylene glycol, alcohol, EDTA
	Proctocort	**Cream**: 1% hydrocortisone, propylene glycol, benzyl alcohol
		Suppositories: 30 mg hydrocortisone acetate
	ProctoFoam-HC	**Aerosol foam**: 1% hydrocortisone acetate, 1% pramoxine HCl, propylene glycol, parabens, alcohol
	Anucort-HC, Anumed-HC, Hemorrhoidal HC	**Suppositories**: 25 mg hydrocortisone acetate
otc	*Nupercainal*	**Cream**: 1% hydrocortisone cream, white petrolatum, propylene glycol, alcohol
otc	*Corticaine*	**Cream**: 0.5% hydrocortisone acetate, propylene glycol, methylparaben
otc	*Anusol HC-1*	**Ointment**: 1% hydrocortisone, mineral oil, propylene glycol, white petrolatum, parabens
otc	**Local Anesthetic-Containing Products**	
	Medicone	**Ointment**: 20% benzocaine, methylparaben
	Nupercainal	**Ointment**: Dibucaine
	Anusol	**Ointment**: 1% pramoxine HCl, benzyl benzoate, Peruvian balsam, 12.5% zinc oxide with mineral oil, cocoa butter
	Tronolane	**Cream**: 1% pramoxine HCl in zinc oxide, glycerin, parabens, beeswax, alcohol
	ProctoFoam	**Aerosol foam**: 1% pramoxine HCl, propylene glycol, parabens, alcohol

	Generic Name *Brand Name Examples*	Supplied As
otc	**Local Vasoconstrictor-Containing Products**	
	Pazo Hemorrhoid	**Ointment**: 0.2% ephedrine sulfate, 2% camphor and 5% zinc oxide with lanolin and petrolatum
	Preparation H	**Ointment**: 71.9% petrolatum, 14% mineral oil, 3% shark liver oil and 0.25% phenylephrine HCl, glycerin, parabens, beeswax, lanolin
		Suppositories: 85.5% cocoa butter, 0.25% phenylephrine HCl, 3% shark liver oil, parabens
	Tronolane	**Suppositories**: 5% zinc oxide, 95% hard fat
	Medicone	**Suppositories**: 0.25% phenylephrine HCl, 88.7% hard fat, mineral oil, white petrolatum, propylene glycol, parabens
	Hem-Prep	**Suppositories**: 0.25% phenylephrine HCl, 11% zinc oxide, hard fat
otc	**Miscellaneous Combinations**	
	Rectagene Medicated Rectal Balm	**Ointment**: Live yeast cell derivative that suppplies 2000 units of skin respiratory factor per ounce, 3% shark liver oil, 1:10,000 phenylmerconic nitrate, white petrolatum, lanolin
	Calmol 4	**Suppositories**: 80% cocoa butter, 10% zinc oxide, parabens
	Nupercainal	**Suppositories**: 2.1 g cocoa butter, 0.25 g zinc oxide, bismuth subgallate and sodium bisulfite
	Anusol	**Suppositories**: 51% topical starch, benzyl alcohol
otc	**Perianal Hygiene Products**	
	Tucks, Tucks Take-Alongs	**Pads**: 50% witch hazel, glycerin, propylene glycol, parabens, alcohol
	Balneol Perianal Cleansing	**Lotion**: Mineral oil, propylene glycol, glyceryl stearate, lanolin oil, sodium acetate and acetic acid, methylparaben
	ConvaTec Aloe Vesta Perineal	**Solution**: Sodium C_{12-14} olefin sulfonate, disodium cocoamphodiacetate, propylene glycol, aloe vera, sorbitol, DMDM hydantoin, cetethyl morpholinium ethosulfate and citric acid

The anorectal (anus and rectum) preparations are used primarily for the symptomatic relief of the discomfort associated with hemorrhoids and perianal itching or irritation. In addition to the products listed in this section, many of the Topical Local Anesthetics and Topical Corticosteroids may also be used in anorectal therapy.

Type of Drug:

Preparations used for minor disorders of the anus and rectum region.

Uses:

The various components of these products are briefly discussed below. For complete information on these ingredients, refer to the appropriate monographs.

Hydrocortisone reduces inflammation, itching and swelling. Steroids are not recommended in fungal and most viral infections of the skin, including herpes, vaccinia, and varicella.

Local anesthetics (eg, benzocaine, dibucaine, pramoxine) temporarily relieve pain, itching and irritation. The most frequent side effects of topical local anesthetic use are allergic reactions (eg, burning, rash, itching).

Vasoconstrictors (eg, ephedrine or phenylephrine) reduce swelling and congestion of anorectal tissues. They relieve local itching by a slight anesthetic effect. These agents are not effective in stopping bleeding from tissues.

Astringents (eg, witch hazel, zinc oxide) shrink skin cells, protecting the underlying tissue and decreasing the cell volume. They lessen mucus and other secretions and relieve anorectal irritation and inflammation.

Antiseptics (eg, phenylmercuric nitrate, zinc oxide) are not of value when applied to the anorectal area. There is no convincing evidence that they prevent infection in the anorectal area. Many are present as preservatives.

Emollients/protectants (eg, cod liver oil, hard fat, glycerin, lanolin, mineral oil, petrolatum, zinc oxide, cocoa butter, shark liver oil, bismuth salts) form a physical barrier on the skin and lubricate tissues, preventing irritation of the anorectal area and water loss from the tissues. Many of these substances are used as bases and carriers of active ingredients.

Humectants (eg, propylene glycol) are water absorbing to blot and dry moisture from affected tissue.

Counterirritants (eg, menthol, camphor) evoke a feeling of comfort, cooling, tingling or warmth and diminish the perception of pain and itching.

Keratolytics (eg, resorcinol) cause shedding and sloughing of surface cells and may help to expose underlying tissue to therapeutic agents.

Wound-healing agents (eg, balsam Peru, skin respiratory factor [SRF]), yeast-cell derivative) are claimed to promote wound healing or tissue repair. Effectiveness of these compounds has not been demonstrated.

Precautions:

Do not use in the following situations:

allergy to any ingredient in the preparations
diabetes
enlarged prostate gland
heart disease
high blood pressure
thyroid disease

Use with caution in the following situations:

children
infections, dermatological
occlusive dressings

Pregnancy: Adequate studies have not been done in pregnant women. Use only if clearly needed and potential benefits outweigh the possible hazards to the fetus.

Breastfeeding: It is not known if topical administration of corticosteroids subsequently appears in breast milk. Consult your doctor before you begin breastfeeding.

Children: Use steroid-containing agents with caution as children may demonstrate greater susceptibility to topical corticosteroid-induced HPA axis suppression due to a larger skin surface area-to-body weight ratio. Chronic cortiosteroid therapy may interfere with growth development.

Side Effects:

Every drug is capable of producing side effects. Many anorectal preparations users experience no, or minor side effects. The frequency and severity of side effects depend on many factors including dose, duration of therapy and individual susceptibility. Possible side effects include:

Skin: Burning; itching; irritation; dryness; inflammation of follicles or skin; acne; allergic contact dermatitis; skin disorder; loss of pigmentation; allergic reaction; flaking of the skin; secondary infection.

Guidelines for Use:

- Avoid contact with eyes.
- Dosage and uses vary. Please read the instructions for use on the packaging before using any of these medications.
- Creams, ointments and foams are for external use only.
- Do not use if you are allergic to any ingredient in these products.
- Do not use in young children (ages vary depending on product) unless instructed by your doctor.
- Maintain normal bowel movements by proper diet, adequate fluid intake and regular exercise.
- Avoid excessive laxative use.
- Stool softeners or bulk laxatives may be useful as an aid to some therapies.
- Avoid scratching or rubbing area; washing with strong or scented soaps; or eating spicy foods, peppers or tomatoes.
- Notify your doctor if symptoms do not improve in 7 days, or if bleeding, protrusion or seepage occurs. *Hydrocortisone-containing products* may cause the following side effects: Burning; itching; irritation; dryness; flaking of the skin; loss of pigment; allergic reaction; infection; blistering; abnormal hair growth; swelling of skin; skin disorder.
- Tell your doctor if you are pregnant, become pregnant, planning to become pregnant or are breastfeeding.
- *Hydrocortisone-containing products* — Do not bandage or cover with plastic dressings unless directed by your doctor. Do not use with tight-fitting diapers or plastic pants.
- *Products containing vasoconstrictors (eg, ephedrine, phenylephrine)* — Do not use if you have heart disease, high blood pressure, thyroid disease, diabetes or enlarged prostate with difficulty urinating unless directed by your doctor. Also, do not use if currently taking medications for high blood pressure or depression unless directed by your doctor.

If you have any questions, consult your doctor, pharmacist, or health care provider.

	Generic Name *Brand Name Examples*	Supplied As	Generic Available
	Benzoyl Peroxide, Cleansers		
Rx	*Benzac W Wash 5 and 10, Desquam-X Wash*	**Liquid**: 5%, 10%	No
otc	*Fostex 10% Wash*	**Liquid**: 10%	No
otc	*Panoxyl*	**Bar**: 5%, 10%	No
otc	**Benzoyl Peroxide, Lotions**		
	Benoxyl 5,[3,4] Benoxyl 10,[3,4] Clearasil 10%, Loroxide	**Lotion**: 5%, 5.5%, 10%	Yes
otc	**Benzoyl Peroxide, Creams**		
	Clearasil Maximum Strength,[3,4] Fostex[5]	**Cream**: 5%, 10%	No
	Benzoyl Peroxide, Gels		
otc	*Del Aqua-5, Del Aqua-10, Fostex, OxyBalance, Oxy 10 Balance, Persa-Gel W*	**Gel**: 5%, 10%	No
Rx	*Benzac 5 and 10,[1] Benzac W 2.5, 5 and 10, Benzagel,[1] Desquam-E, Desquam-X 5 and 10, PanOxyl 5 and 10,[1] PanOxyl AQ 2.5, 5 and 10[3]*	**Gel**: 2.5%, 5%, 10%	Yes
Rx	**Benzoyl Peroxide Combinations**		
	Benzamycin[1,2]	**Gel**: 5% benzoyl peroxide and 3% erythromycin	No
	Sulfoxyl Regular	**Lotion**: 5% benzoyl peroxide and 2% sulfur, propylene glycol	No
	Sulfoxyl Strong	**Lotion**: 10% benzoyl peroxide and 5% sulfur, propylene glycol	No
	Vanoxide-HC	**Lotion**: 5% benzyl peroxide, 0.5% hydrocortisone, mineral oil, lanolin, propylene glycol, parabens	No

[1] Contains alcohol.
[2] For more information, see Erythromycin monograph.
[3] Contains methylparaben.
[4] Contains propylparaben.
[5] Contains salicylic acid.

Type of Drug:

Acne products.

How the Drug Works:

The effectiveness of benzoyl peroxide is related primarily to its keratolytic (skin sloughing) and antibacterial action, especially against *Propionibacterium acnes,* which is the predominant bacteria in sebaceous follicles and comedones (blackheads). The antibacterial activity is most likely related to its effects on bacterial proteins. Benzoyl peroxide's action is also aided by a drying action, removal of excess sebum (oil) and decreased sebum formation.

Uses:

To treat mild to moderate acne vulgaris and oily skin. These medications can be used alone or in combination with other acne medications, including antibiotics. These agents should not be used to treat acne rosacea.

Precautions:

Do not use in the following situations:

allergy to benzoyl peroxide, benzoic acid, cinnamon or any ingredients of the medications
hypersensitive skin

Pseudomembranous colitis may occur with the long-term use of *Benzamycin*. If severe diarrhea, stomach pain/cramps or bloody stools occur, contact your doctor immediately. This could be a symptom of a serious side effect requiring immediate medical attention. Do not treat diarrhea associated with *Benzamycin* use without consulting your doctor.

Pregnancy: Adequate studies have not been done in pregnant women. Use only if clearly needed and potential benefits outweigh the possible hazards to the fetus.

Breastfeeding: It is not known if benzoyl peroxide appears in breast milk. Consult your doctor before you begin breastfeeding.

Children: Safety and effectiveness in children under 12 years of age have not been established.

Drug Interactions:

Tell your doctor or pharmacist if you are taking or if you are planning to take any over-the-counter or prescription medications or dietary supplements with benzoyl peroxide.

Side Effects:

Every drug is capable of producing side effects. Many benzoyl peroxide users experience no, or minor, side effects. The frequency and severity of side effects depend on many factors including dose, duration of therapy and individual susceptibility. Possible side effects include: Excessive dryness, peeling, facial swelling, oiliness, redness, tenderness of skin; sloughing of skin; local irritation; edema (fluid accumulation in the treated area); stinging and burning on application; itching; blistering; excessive hair growth; loss of skin pigment; skin disorder; photosensitivity to sunlight or tanning beds.

Guidelines for Use:

- Directions for use vary. Read instructions for medications carefully.
- For external use only. Keep away from eyes, eyelids, mouth, lips, inside the nose, any mucous membrane, and highly inflamed or damaged skin. If contact with eyes occurs, flush with water.
- May produce a temporary feeling of warmth or slight stinging. Expect dryness and peeling.
- If dryness, itching, swelling, redness, or peeling becomes excessive, reduce the frequency of application or discontinue use temporarily and contact your doctor.
- Adjust applications on a given day from no application to 2 applications. Eventually a routine schedule can be established.
- If irritation continues or becomes severe, discontinue use and consult your doctor.
- Use of other topical acne medications at the same time or following each other may increase dryness and irritation of the skin. If this occurs, use one medicine at a time unless directed by your doctor.
- Use moisturizers, cool compresses, or topical steroids (eg, hydrocortisone) to treat the side effects of excessive sensitivity, drying, redness, or peeling.
- Use a sunscreen and avoid sunlight, sunlamps, or other topical acne medications and sources of skin irritation unless directed by your doctor.
- Concurrent use of some of these products and PABA-containing sunscreens may result in temporary skin discoloration.
- May bleach hair or colored fabric. Avoid contact with hair and fabric if possible.
- Water-based cosmetics may be used after benzoyl peroxide use. Thoroughly remove prior to application of benzoyl peroxide.
- *Cleansers* (washes and bar soaps) — Use once or twice daily on the affected skin. Wet area prior to application and thoroughly rinse after application.
- *Creams, lotions, gels* — Apply once daily for the first few days. If dryness, redness, or peeling does not occur, increase frequency of application to 2 to 3 times daily.

If you have any questions, consult your doctor, pharmacist, or health care provider.

	Generic Name *Brand Name Examples*	Supplied As	Generic Available
Rx	**Azelaic Acid**		
	Azelex, Finevin	**Cream**: 20%	No

Type of Drug:
Acne product.

How the Drug Works:
The exact mechanism of action is not known. This medicine has been shown to have antibacterial action against certain bacteria when applied to the skin.

Uses:
A skin cream used to treat mild to moderate acne in patients older than 12 years of age.

Precautions:
Do not use in the following situations: Allergy to azelaic acid or any of its ingredients.

Use with caution in the following situations: Persons with dark complexions.

Pregnancy: Studies in pregnant women or in animals have been judged not to show a risk to the fetus. However, no drug should be used during pregnancy unless clearly needed.

Breastfeeding: Azelaic acid may appear in breast milk. Consult your doctor before you begin breastfeeding.

Children: Safety and effectiveness in children under 12 years of age have not been established.

Side Effects:
Every drug is capable of producing side effects. Many azelaic acid users experience no, or minor, side effects. The frequency and severity of side effects depend on many factors including dose, duration of therapy, and individual susceptibility. Possible side effects include:

Skin: Itching; burning; stinging; tingling; rash; irritation; redness; dryness; peeling; skin color changes.

Guidelines for Use:

- Dosage is individualized. Use exactly as prescribed.
- Continue use until all of the prescribed medicine has been used. Failure to use a full course of therapy may prevent complete elimination of bacteria.
- For use on the skin only. Do not use in eyes.
- Wash skin thoroughly and pat dry. Gently, but thoroughly, massage a thin film of the medicine into the affected area twice a day (morning and evening). Wash hands following use. Length of treatment may vary depending upon the severity of the acne. Improvement usually occurs within 4 weeks.
- If a dose is missed, apply it as soon as possible. If several hours have passed or if it is nearing time for the next dose, do not double the dose to catch up, unless advised to do so by your doctor. Of more than one dose is missed or it is necessary to establish a new dosage schedule, contact your doctor or pharmacist.
- If sensitivity or severe irritation develops with the use of this medicine, discontinue use and contact your doctor.
- Do not use tight dressings or wrappings on the affected areas.
- Do not use near mouth, eyes, or other mucous membranes (eg, nose). If this medicine does come into contact with eyes, wash eyes with large amounts of tap water. Contact your doctor if eye irritation persists.
- If you have a dark complexion, contact your doctor if you have any changes in skin color (eg, light spots).
- Temporary skin irritation (ie, itching, burning, stinging) may occur when this medicine is applied to broken or inflamed skin, usually at the beginning of treatment. This irritation usually subsides with continued use. If irritation continues, use only once-a-day, or stop using this medicine until the side effects have subsided. If irritation persists, stop using this medicine and contact your doctor.
- Store at room temperature (59° to 86°F). Do not freeze.

If you have any questions, consult your doctor, pharmacist, or health care provider.

	Generic Name *Brand Name Examples*	Supplied As	Generic Available
	Sulfur Preparations		
otc	*Fostex Medicated Cover-Up*	**Cream**: 2% sulfur	No
otc	*Transact*	**Gel**: 2% sulfur, 40% alcohol and laureth-4	No
otc	*Xerac*	**Gel**: 4% microcrystalline sulfur and 44% isopropyl alcohol	No
otc	*Liquimat*	**Lotion**: 5% sulfur and 22% alcohol	No
otc	*Sulpho-Lac*	**Soap**: 5% sulfur	No
Rx	*Bensulfoid*[1]	**Powder**: Highly reactive sulfur on colloidal bentonite	No

[1] For compounding prescriptions.

Type of Drug:

Acne product.

How the Drug Works:

Sulfur provides antibacterial, peeling and drying actions. Although it may help to clear up comedones ("blackheads"), it may also promote the development of new ones.

Uses:

To aid in the treatment of mild acne and oily skin.

Guidelines for Use:

- For external use only.
- Apply a thin film 1 to 3 times daily. Cleanse skin thoroughly with a mild cleanser prior to use.
- Avoid overuse and contact with the eyes. Certain people may be allergic to one or more ingredients. If skin irritation develops or becomes excessive, discontinue use and consult your doctor.

If you have any questions, consult your doctor, pharmacist, or health care provider.

	Generic Name *Brand Name Examples*	Supplied As	Generic Available
Rx	**Tretinoin**		
	Retin-A	**Cream**: 0.025%, 0.05%, 0.1%	No
	Retin-A,[1] *Avita*[1]	**Gel**: 0.025%,	No
	Retin-A[1]	**Gel**: 0.01%	No
	Retin-A[1]	**Liquid**: 0.05%	No

[1] Contains alcohol.

Type of Drug:

Acne agent. Trans-retinoic acid, vitamin A acid. Also used as a "wrinkle remover," but this use is not approved

How the Drug Works:

The exact mechanism of action is not known. Tretinoin appears to increase skin-cell turnover and to reduce the tendency for skin cells to stick together. This reduces the formation of pimples and allows quicker healing of pimples that do develop.

Uses:

To treat mild to moderate acne vulgaris.

Unlabeled Use(s): Occasionally doctors may prescribe tretinoin to treat several different forms of skin cancer, lamellar ichthyosis, mollusca contagiosa, verrucae plantaris, verrucae planae juveniles, ichthyosis vulgaris, bullous congenital ichthyosiform, pityriasis rubra pilaris. Tretinoin has also been used to reduce the smaller, finer wrinkles and liver spots associated with aging, and to enhance the absorption of topical minoxidil.

Precautions:

Do not use in the following situations:

- allergy to any ingredient of the drug
- near heat or flame
- sunburn
- skin irritation, severe or persistant
- UV tanning booths

Use with caution in the following situations:

- eczema
- skin irritation, redness or dryness
- sun or extreme weather exposure

Photosensitivity: Minimize exposure to sunlight and sunlamps. Use effective sunscreen any time you are outside, even on hazy days. For extended sun exposure, wear protective clothing. Do not use artificial sunlamps while using *Retin-A*. If sunburn occurs, stop therapy until skin has recovered.

Pregnancy: Adequate studies have not been done in pregnant women. Use only if clearly needed and potential benefits outweigh the possible hazards to the fetus.

Breastfeeding: It is not known if tretinoin appears in breast milk. Consult your doctor before you begin breastfeeding.

Drug Interactions:

Tell your doctor or pharmacist if you are taking or if you are planning to take any over-the-counter or prescription medications or dietary supplements with tretinoin. Doses of one or both drugs may need to be modified or a different drug may need to be prescribed. Topical keratolylic (peeling) agents (eg, sulfur, resorcinol, benzoyl peroxide, salicylic acid), use of another topical medication at the same time, medicated or abrasive soaps and cleansers with a strong drying effect (eg, alcohol, astringents, spices, lime) interact with tretinoin.

Side Effects:

Every drug is capable of producing side effects. Many tretinoin users experience no, or minor, side effects. The frequency and severity of side effects depend on many factors including dose, duration of therapy and individual susceptibility. Possible side effects include: Red, swollen, irritated skin; blistered or crusted skin; increased or decreased skin pigmentation (color); increased sensitivity to sunlight.

Guidelines for Use:

- Use exactly as prescribed.
- For external use only.
- Read patient instructions provided with product.
- Wash with a mild soap to cleanse area to be treated thoroughly before use and dry skin gently. Wait 20 to 30 minutes before applying medication to let skin dry thoroughly.
- Lightly apply to affected area once a day at bedtime. Wash hands immediately after use.
- Keep away from the eyes, mouth, angles of nose, mucous membranes and open wounds.
- *Liquid* — Apply with fingertip, gauze pad or cotton swab. Do not overwet. Liquid may run into unaffected areas.
- *Gel* — Excessive application results in "pilling" of the gel.
- Application may cause a feeling of warmth and slight stinging. This is normal.
- Use may cause severe redness and peeling at the site of application. If these symptoms persist, use the medication less frequently, stop use temporarily or stop use altogether if recommended by your doctor.
- *Sensitivity to sunlight* — Tretinoin may cause sensitivity to sunlight and other sources of ultraviolet light. Avoid prolonged exposure to the sun. Use sunscreens and wear protective clothing.
- May cause an unusual sensitivity to wind and cold. Avoid when possible.
- Use of other agents to promote sloughing of skin (eg, sulfur, resorcinol, salicylic acid) is not recommended. "Rest" the skin for a few days before beginning tretinoin.
- If excessive medication is applied, redness, peeling and pain may occur. Excessive application does not improve results.
- Apply a moisturizer with sunscreen that will not aggravate your acne every morning after washing the affected area.
- Cosmetics may be used. However, thoroughly remove cosmetics before applying tretinoin.
- Early in treatment, acne may appear worse due to the action of the drug. Do not stop therapy. Positive effects should be seen in 2 to 3 weeks, but may not be optimal for 6 weeks or more. Many users see improvement by 12 weeks.
- Once tolerance is determined, the frequency of application may be increased. Application procedures, drug concentration and dose frequency will be closely monitored by your doctor.
- Once a good response is seen, therapy may be maintained with less frequent application or lower concentrations.
- Do not allow anyone else to use this medication.
- Store the liquid and gel below 86°F and the cream below 80°F. Avoid freezing. The gel is flammable. Keep away from heat and flame.

If you have any questions, consult your doctor, pharmacist, or health care provider.

ACNE PRODUCTS – MISCELLANEOUS COMBINATIONS

Brand Name Examples	Sulfur	Salicylic Acid	Other Content
Creams, Lotions and Gels			
otc Acno Lotion	3%		
otc Acnomel Cream	8%		11% alcohol, 2% resorcinol
otc Acnotex Lotion	8%		20% isopropyl alcohol, 2% resorcinol
Rx Bensulfoid Cream	8%[1]		12% alcohol, 2% resorcinol
otc Clearasil Adult Care Cream	†		Resorcinol, 10 % alcohol, parabens
otc Clearasil Clearstick Maximum Strength		2%	39% alcohol, menthol, EDTA
otc Clearasil Clearstick Regular Strength		1.25%	39% alcohol, aloe vera gel, menthol, disodium, EDTA
otc Clearasil Double Clear Maximum Strength Pads		2%	40% alcohol, witch hazel distillate, menthol
otc Clearasil Double Clear Regular Strength Pads		1.25%	40% alcohol, witch hazel distillate, menthol
otc Cuticura Ointment	0.5%[2]		0.1% phenol, 0.05% oxyquinoline
otc Finac Lotion		2%	22.5% isopropyl alcohol, propylene glycol, acetone
otc Fostex Acne Cleansing Cream		2%	Stearyl alcohol, EDTA
otc Fostril Lotion	†		Zinc oxide, parabens, EDTA
otc Medicated Acne Cleanser	4%		2% resorcinol
otc Neutrogena Drying Gel			Isopropyl alcohol, witch hazel, EDTA, parabens, tartrazine
Rx Novacet Lotion	5%		10% sodium sulfacetamide, cetyl alcohol, benzyl alcohol, EDTA, sodium thiosulfate

Brand Name Examples	**Sulfur**	**Salicylic Acid**	**Other Content**
otc Oxy Night Watch Maximum Strength Lotion		2%	Cetyl alcohol, EDTA, parabens, stearyl alcohol
otc Oxy Night Watch Sensitive Skin Lotion		1%	Cetyl alcohol, EDTA, stearyl alcohol, parabens
otc PROPApH Acne Maximum Strength Cream		2%	Lanolin alcohol, cetearyl alcohol, stearyl alcohol, menthol, EDTA
otc PROPApH Cleansing Lotion for Normal/ Combination Skin		0.5%	SD alcohol 40, menthol, EDTA
otc PROPApH Cleansing Pads			
otc PROPApH Cleansing for Oily Skin Lotion		0.6%	SD alcohol 40, EDTA, menthol
otc RA Lotion			43% alcohol, 3% resorcinol
otc Rezamid Lotion	5%		28% alcohol, 2% resorcinol
otc R/S Lotion			
otc Sal-Clens Acne Cleanser Gel		2%	
otc Seale's Lotion Modified	6.4%		
otc Sebasorb Lotion		2%	10% attapulgite
Rx Sodium Sulfacetamide 10% and Sulfur 5%	5%		10% sodium sulfacetamide, cetyl alcohol, benzyl alcohol, EDTA
otc Stridex Clear Gel		2%	9.3% SD alcohol
Rx Sulfacet-R Lotion	5%		10% sodium sulfacetamide, parabens
otc Sulforcin Lotion	5%		11.65% SD alcohol, 2% resorcinol, methylparaben
otc Therac Lotion	10%[1]		

Brand Name Examples	Sulfur	Salicylic Acid	Other Content
Medicated Bar Cleansers			
otc Aveeno Cleansing for Acne-Prone Skin[3]		†	Colliodal oatmeal, glycerin, titanium dioxide
otc Buf-Puf Acne Cleansing		2%	Vitamin E acetate, EDTA
otc Clearasil Antibacterial Soap			triclosan
otc Fostex Acne Medication Cleansing Bar		2%	EDTA
otc Oxy Medicated Soap			1% triclosan, EDTA
otc Salicylic Acid Cleansing Bar		2%	EDTA
otc Salicylic Acid and Sulfur Soap	10%	3%	
otc SAStid Soap	10%		EDTA
otc Sulfur Soap			
otc Stri-Dex Cleansing Bar			1% triclosan, lanolin, alcohol, EDTA
Abrasive Cleansers			
otc Brasivol			Aluminum oxide in a surfactant cleansing base
otc Ionax			Benzalkonium Cl, SD alcohol 40
otc Listerex Scrub		2%	Methylparaben, tartrazine
otc Pernox Lathering Abradant Scrub Lotion	†	†	
otc Pernox Scrub for Oily Skin	†	†	EDTA
otc PROPApH Peel-Off Acne Mask		2%	Polyvinyl alcohol, parabens, SD alcohol 40, vitamin E acetate

Brand Name Examples	Sulfur	Salicylic Acid	Other Content
otc Seba-Nil Cleansing Mask			SD alcohol 40, castor oil, methylparaben
Liquid Cleansers			
otc Acno Cleanser			60% isopropyl alcohol, EDTA
otc Clearasil Double Textured Pads Maximum Strength		2%	40% alcohol, aloe vera gel, menthol, EDTA
otc Clearasil Double Textured Pads Regular Strength		2%	40% alcohol, glycerin, aloe vera gel, EDTA
otc Clearasil Medicated Deep Cleaner		0.5%	42% alcohol, menthol, EDTA, aloe vera gel, castor oil
otc Drytex Lotion		†	40% isopropyl alcohol, 10% acetone, tartrazine
otc Exact		2%	Propylene glycol, parabens, aloe vera gel, EDTA, menthol, glycerin, diazolidinyl urea
otc Ionax Astringent Cleanser		†	EDTA, isopropyl alcohol
otc Ionax Foam			Benzalkonium Cl, propylene glycol
otc Neutrogena Antiseptic Cleanser for Acne-Prone Skin			Benzethonium chloride, butylene glycol, menthol, methylparaben, witch hazel, camphor, peppermint oil, eucalyptus oil, cornmint oil
otc Neutrogena Oil-Free Acne Wash		2%	EDTA, propylene glycol, aloe, tartrazine
otc Oil of Olay Foaming Face Wash Liquid			Potassium cocoyl, collagen, glycerin, EDTA
otc Oxy Medicated Cleanser & Pads Regular Strength		0.5%	40% alcohol, citric acid, menthol, propylene glycol

ACNE PRODUCTS – MISCELLANEOUS COMBINATIONS

Brand Name Examples	Sulfur	Salicylic Acid	Other Content
otc *Oxy Medicated Pads Maximum Strength*		2%	50% alcohol, propylene glycol, citric acid, menthol
otc *Oxy Medicated Pads Sensitive Skin*		0.5%	22% alcohol, disodium lauryl sulfosuccinate, menthol, trisodium EDTA
otc *Oxy ResiDON'T Medicated Face Wash*			Cocamidopropyl betaine, sodium laureth sulfate, sodium cocoyl isethionate, triclosan, diazolidinyl urea
otc *PROPApH Cleansing Maximum Strength Pads*		2%	SD alcohol 40, EDTA, propylene glycol, menthol, aloe vera gel
otc *PROPApH Cleansing for Sensitive Skin Pads*		0.5%	SD alcohol 40, EDTA, menthol, aloe vera gel
otc *PROPApH Foaming Face Wash*		2%	EDTA, menthol, aloe vera gel
otc *SalAc Cleanser*	2%		Benzyl alcohol, glyceryl cocoate
otc *Seba-Nil Oily Skin Cleanser*			SD alcohol 40, acetone
otc *Stri-Dex Pads Oil Fighting Formula*		2%	citric acid, 54% SD alcohol, menthol
otc *Stri-Dex Pads Maximum Strength*		2%	44% SD alcohol, citric acid, menthol
otc *Stri-Dex Pads Regular Strength*		0.5%	28% SD alcohol, citric acid, menthol
otc *Stri-Dex Pads Sensitive Skin*		0.5%	Citric acid, menthol, aloe vera gel, 28% SD alcohol
otc *Tyrosum Cleanser Liquid and Packets*			50% isopropanol, 2% polysorbate 80, 10% acetone

Brand Name Examples	Sulfur	Salicylic Acid	Other Content
Rx Xerac AC			6.25% aluminum chloride hexahydrate in 96% anhydrous ethyl alcohol

[1] As colloidal sulfur.
[2] As precipitated sulfur.
[3] Soap free.
† Percentage not listed in manufacturer insert.

Type of Drug:

Acne products.

How the Drug Works:

These products contain keratolytics (peeling agents) and astringents (shrinking agents) to aid in removing keratin and to dry the skin. Many products also contain water, alcohol or organic solvent bases to aid in the removal of sebum (oil).

Uses:

Parachlorometaxylenol, sodium thiosulfate and *sodium sulfacetamide* have antimicrobial activity (treat or prevent infection).

Benzalkonium chloride, oxyquinoline, methylbenethzonium chloride, ethanol, isopropyl alcohol, phenol, triclosan, thymol and *sulfur* are antiseptics (prevent infection).

Zinc oxide and *calamine* are astringents.

Methylsalicylate is a local anesthetic and counterirritant.

Salicylic acid, resorcinol and *sulfur* are keratolytics.

Titanium dioxide and *zinc oxide* are protectives and absorbants.

Guidelines for Use:

- Use exactly as prescribed or directed.
- For external use only.
- *Lotions* — Shake well before using.
- Apply a thin film 1 to 3 times daily. Cleanse the skin thoroughly with a mild cleanser and dry the skin before applying the medication.
- Avoid overuse.
- Avoid contact with eyes, mouth, nose or other mucous membranes. If contact occurs, bathe the area with large amounts of tap water for several minutes.
- Certain people may be sensitive to one or more ingredients. If skin irritation develops or becomes excessive, discontinue use and consult your doctor.

	Generic Name *Brand Name Examples*	Supplied As	Generic Available
Rx	**Anthralin** *Anthra-Derm* *Drithocreme, Drithocreme HP 1%,* *Dritho-Scalp*	**Ointment**: 0.1, 0.25, 0.5, 1% **Cream:** 0.1, 0.25, 0.5, 1%	No No

Type of Drug:

Agent for psoriasis.

How the Drug Works:

Anthralin apparently slows the rate of skin cell growth by inhibiting formation of DNA.

Uses:

To treat psoriasis.

Precautions:

Do not use in the following situations: Allergy to anthralin, acute or inflamed psoriasis, or use on face.

Use with caution in the following situations: Kidney disease or long-term anthralin use.

Pregnancy: Adequate studies have not been done in pregnant women, or animal studies may have shown a risk to the fetus. Use only if clearly needed and potential benefits outweigh the possible hazards to the fetus.

Breastfeeding: It is not known if anthralin appears in breast milk. Consult your doctor before you begin breastfeeding.

Children: Safety and effectiveness have not been established.

Lab tests or exams may be required to monitor therapy. Keep appointments.

Side Effects:

Every drug is capable of producing side effects. Many patients experience no, or minor, side effects. The frequency and severity of side effects depend on many factors including dose, duration of therapy and individual susceptibility. Possible side effects include: Irritation of normal skin, discoloration of fingernails and hair.

Guidelines for Use:

- Use exactly as prescribed.
- For external use only. Remove by washing. Rinse tub with hot water after use.
- Apply with plastic gloves. Wash hands after use. May stain fabrics, skin or hair.
- Apply a thin layer as directed to psoriatic lesions only. Rub gently until absorbed.
- Therapy may be gradually increased. High concentrations may cause irritation.
- Keep away from eyes. Do not use on face, genitalia, folds or creases of skin. Remove any residue from behind ears. Stop use if allergic reactions or if skin irritation develops. If excessive soreness occurs or lesions spread, reduce application frequency; if severe, stop using and consult your doctor.
- Wait at least 1 week between discontinuing topical steroids and starting anthralin therapy. Continue treatment until skin is entirely clear.
- Store at room temperature (59° to 88° F) in a tightly sealed container.

If you have any questions, consult your doctor, pharmacist, or health care provider.

	Generic Name *Brand Name Example*	Supplied As	Generic Available
Rx	**Calcipotriene**		
	Dovonex	**Ointment**: 0.005%	No

Type of Drug:
Agent for psoriasis.

How the Drug Works:
Calcipotriene is a synthetic vitamin D_3 derivative.

Uses:
To treat psoriasis.

Precautions:
Do not use in the following situations:
allergy to calcipotriene or any of its components
evidence of vitamin D poisoning
excess calcium in the blood

Use with caution in the following situations:
elevated calcium levels in the blood.
irritation of psoriasis lesions and surrounding skin.

Pregnancy: Adequate studies have not been done in pregnant women. Use only if clearly needed and potential benefits outweigh the possible hazards to the fetus.

Breastfeeding: It is not known if calcipotriene appears in breast milk. Consult your doctor before you begin breastfeeding.

Children: Safety and effectiveness have not been established.

Elderly: Side effects may be more severe.

Side Effects:
Every drug is capable of producing side effects. Many calcipotriene users experience no, or minor, side effects. The frequency and severity of side effects depend on many factors including dose, duration of therapy and individual susceptibility. Possible side effects include: Burning; itching; irritation; redness; inflammation; dry skin; peeling; rash and worsening of psoriasis; including development of facial or scalp psoriasis.

Guidelines for Use:

- For external use only.
- Use only as directed by your physician. Keep away from eyes; do not apply to face. Wash hands after using.
- Apply a thin layer to the affected skin twice daily and rub in gently and completely.
- Do not use this medication for any disorder other than that for which it was prescribed.
- Report to your physician any signs of local adverse reactions. If irritation develops, discontinue use.

If you have any questions, consult your doctor, pharmacist, or health care provider.

Generic Name *Brand Name Examples*	Supplied As	Generic Available
Rx **Acitretin**		
Soriatane[1]	**Capsules**: 10 mg, 25 mg	No

[1] Contains gelatin, methyl- and propylparabens, benzyl alcohol and edetate calcium disodium.

Type of Drug:

A retinoid. Related to retinoic acid and retinol (vitamin A).

How the Drug Works:

The mechanism of action is unknown.

Uses:

To treat severe psoriasis unresponsive to other therapies or when other treatments are contraindicated in adults.

Precautions:

Do not use in the following situations:

- alcohol consumption
- allergy to any ingredient in the product
- benign intracranial hypertension
- blood donor
- breastfeeding
- paraben sensitivity
- pregnancy
- visual difficulties

Use with caution in the following situations:

- diabetes
- kidney disease, severe
- lipid disturbance, family history
- liver disease, severe
- obesity
- spine, bone, joint problems
- triglyceride increases
- vitamin A use
- women of childbearing potential

Pseudotumor cerebri (benign intracranial hypertension) has occurred with acitretin. Early signs and symptoms include pain behind the eyes, headache, nausea, vomiting and visual disturbances. If present, discontinue the drug immediately and consult your doctor.

Pregnancy: Women who are pregnant or who may become pregnant must not use acitretin. There is an extremely high risk that a deformed infant will result if pregnancy occurs while taking this drug in any amount, even for short periods. Potentially all exposed fetuses can be affected.

Breastfeeding: It is not known if acetretin appears in breast milk. However, nursing mothers should not take acitretin because of the potential for excretion in milk and the serious adverse reactions that may have on the infant.

Children: Safety and effectiveness in children have not been established.

Lab tests are required to monitor treatment. Tests may include blood lipid, triglycerides, cholesterol, liver function and pregnancy. Be sure to keep appointments.

Drug Interactions:

Tell your doctor or pharmacist if you are taking or planning to take any over-the-counter or prescription medications or dietary supplements while taking acitretin. Doses of one or both drugs may need to be modified or a different drug may need to be prescribed. The following drugs and drug classes interact with acitretin:

- alcohol
- methotrexate (*Rheumatrex*)
- progestin microdosed "minipill"
- vitamin A

Side Effects:

Every drug is capable of producing side effects. Most acitretin users experience side effects. The frequency and severity of side effects depend on many factors including dose, duration of therapy and individual susceptibility. Possible side effects include:

Digestive Tract: Nausea; vomiting; swollen and bleeding gums; increased saliva; bloating; stomach ulcer/pain; diarrhea; tongue disorder; increased/decreased appetite.

Nervous System: Depression; sleeplessness; drowsiness; tiredness.

Skin: Peeling skin; dry skin; itching; nail disorder; red rash; diminished sensitivity to stimulation; abnormal skin sensation; sticky skin; loss of skin elasticity (atrophy); abnormal skin odor; abnormal hair texture; blisters; cold, clammy skin; swollen skin; increased sweating; infection; psoriasis-like rash; red/purple spots; pus-filled sores; excessively oily skin; cracking of skin; sunburn; flushing.

Senses: Dry eyes; eye irritation; brow and lash loss; Bell's Palsy; swollen and crusting eyelids; blurred vision; eye infection; cataracts; decreased night vision; double vision; itchy eyes or eyelids; sore eyes; visual disturbance; sensitivity to light; earache; taste perversion; ringing in the ears.

Other: Flushing; congested or runny nose; headache; bone abnormality; swollen lips; nosebleed; dry mouth; hair loss; joint, back, muscle or bone pain/disorder; chills; thirst; pain; muscle stiffness; swelling; hot flashes; arthritis.

Guidelines for Use:

- Individualize dosage. Initial dosage is 25 or 50 mg/day as a single dose given with the main meal.
- Therapy should be terminated when sores have healed and when directed by your doctor.
- If a dose is missed, take it as soon as possible. If several hours have passed or it is nearing time for the next dose, do not double the dose to "catch up" (unless advised by your doctor). If more than one dose is missed or it is necessary to establish a new dosage schedule, contact your doctor or pharmacist. Use exactly as prescribed.
- A prescription will not be given until a report of a negative pregnancy test has been received by your doctor. Pregnancy testing and counseling will be done on a regular basis.
- Sexually active women of childbearing potential should practice contraception 1 month before starting therapy, during therapy and for at least 3 years after therapy has been stopped.
- Two reliable forms of contraception should be used at the same time unless abstinence is the chosen method.
- Contact your doctor immediately if pregnancy is suspected during therapy. Major birth defects have been associated with acitretin use. Discuss continuation of the pregnancy with your doctor.
- Discontinue the drug and contact your doctor immediately if pain behind the eyes, headache, nausea, vomiting, visual disturbances and decreased tolerance of contact lens wear occurs.
- Women of childbearing potential should be advised to not drink beverages or take products containing alcohol while taking acetretin and for 2 months after treatment has been stopped.
- Most patients experience a relapse of psoriasis after stopping therapy. Other courses of therapy have produced similar results to the first course.
- Do not take vitamin A supplements while taking acitretin.
- Worsening of psoriasis may be seen during initial treatment and it may be 2 to 3 months before the full benefit of acitretin is seen.
- If you experience visual difficulties, discontinue use and contact your doctor.
- Do not donate blood during and for 3 years following therapy.
- Avoid the use of sun lamps and excessive exposure to sunlight. Use appropriate sunscreen and wear protective clothing.
- Regularly scheduled appointments will be made to check your response to the medication and lab tests are required. Tests include: Blood lipid, triglycerides, cholesterol, liver function and pregnancy. Be sure to keep appointments.
- Store between 59° and 77°F. Protect from light, high temperatures and moisture.

Generic Name *Brand Name Examples*	Supplied As	Generic Available
Rx **Methotrexate (MTX)**		
Rheumatrex Dose Pack[1]	**Tablets**: 2.5 mg	Yes
Methotrexate Sodium Injection,[2] *Methotrexate LPF Sodium*[3]	**Injection**: 25 mg/mL	Yes
Methotrexate Sodium For Injection[3]	**Powder for injection**: 20 mg/vial, 1 g/vial	Yes

[1] Contains lactose.
[2] Contains benzyl alcohol.
[3] Preservative free.

Type of Drug:

Agent for psoriasis, rheumatoid arthritis, and certain types of cancer.

How the Drug Works:

Methotrexate (MTX) is an antimetabolite which interferes with folic acid production, DNA production, and cellular reproduction. It is used in conditions involving rapidly growing tissue (eg, psoriasis, cancer). Methotrexate inhibits cell production.

Uses:

To treat severe, disabling psoriasis when other therapy fails.

To treat certain types of cancer, alone or with other anticancer agents (see Antimetabolites monograph).

To treat severe, disabling rheumatoid arthritis when other therapy fails.

Unlabeled Use(s): Occasionally doctors may prescribe methotrexate for Reiter disease.

Precautions:

Do not use in the following situations:

- abnormal blood counts (eg, low platelet and white-cell count)
- alcoholism
- allergy to the drug or any ingredients
- anemia
- blood disorders before MTX therapy
- breastfeeding
- immunodeficiency syndrome
- liver disease
- pregnancy
- women of childbearing potential

Use with caution in the following situations:

- bone marrow depression
- infection, active
- kidney disease
- liver damage
- peptic ulcer, active
- poor health and debility
- ulcerative colitis

Liver: Methotrexate may be highly toxic to the liver, particularly at high doses or with prolonged therapy. Liver atrophy, necrosis, cirrhosis, fatty liver and liver fibrosis may occur. Liver function should be determined before methotrexate therapy begins and monitored regularly.

Pregnancy: Methotrexate has caused fetal death and severe birth defects. Defective egg (ovum) or sperm formation caused by methotrexate has been reported. Women of childbearing potential should not use MTX unless benefits outweigh the risks. Not generally recommended for pregnant psoriasis or rheumatoid arthritis patients.

Breastfeeding: Methotrexate appears in breast milk. Since the drug may accumulate in the newborn, breastfeeding is not recommended. Decide whether to discontinue breastfeeding or to discontinue the drug, taking into account the importance of the drug to the mother.

Children: Safety and effectiveness in children have not been established other than in cancer chemotherapy.

Lab tests will be required during treatment with MTX. Tests will include: Blood counts, urine tests, kidney, liver and pulmonary function tests and chest x-rays. When high dose or long-term therapy is used, a liver biopsy or bone marrow sample may be needed.

Drug Interactions:

Tell your doctor or pharmacist if you are taking or if you are planning to take any over-the-counter or prescription medications or dietary supplements with methotrexate. Doses of one or both drugs may need to be modified or a different drug may need to be prescribed. The following drugs and drug classes interact with methotrexate:

bismuth subsalicylate
charcoal
chloramphenicol (eg, *Chloromycetin Kapseals)*
cisplatin (*Platinol-AQ)*
digoxin (eg, *Lanoxin)*
folic acid (eg, *Folvite)*
nonsteroidal anti-inflammatory agents (eg, indomethacin, ketoprofen, naproxen)
penicillins
phenylbutazone (eg, *Azolid)*
phenytoin (eg, *Dilantin)*
probenecid (eg, *Benemid)*
salicylates (eg, aspirin)
sulfonamides (eg, *Sulfisoxazole)*
tetracycline (eg, *Achromycin V)*
theophylline (eg, *Slo-Phyllin)*
trimethoprim-sulfamethoxazole (eg, *Bactrim)*

Side Effects:

Every drug is capable of producing side effects. Many methotrexate users experience no, or minor, side effects. The frequency and severity of side effects depend on many factors including dose, duration of therapy and individual susceptibility. Possible side effects include:

Digestive Tract: Nausea; vomiting; appetite loss; diarrhea; mouth ulcers.

Hematologic: Decreased platelet count; decreased white blood count; decreased other cell count.

Nervous System: Dizziness; headache.

Respiratory System: Lung disease; cough; nasal congestion; nosebleed.

Skin: Rash; itching; sensitivity to sunlight and tanning lamps; "burning" of skin lesions; sweating.

Urinary and Reproductive Tract: Vaginal discharge; painful urination.

Other: Fever; joint pain; decreased resistance to infection; liver disease; chest pain; hair loss; eye discomfort.

Guidelines for Use:

- Dosing and administration vary depending on disease; follow the directions given to you by your doctor and read all package insert materials before taking this drug.
- Deaths have been reported from MTX use for treating psoriasis and rheumatoid arthritis. Patients given MTX must receive close medical supervision. Risks of therapy must be fully understood.
- Avoid alcohol, aspirin, other salicylates, NSAIDs and prolonged exposure to sunlight or sunlamps.
- Contact your doctor if nausea, vomiting, appetite loss, infection, hair loss, skin rash, boils or acne occurs or persists.
- Discontinue the drug and contact your doctor if any of the following symptoms occur: Diarrhea, abdominal pain, black sticky stools, fever, chills, sore throat, unusual bruising or bleeding, sores in or around the mouth, cough, shortness of breath, yellow discoloration of the skin or eyes, dark urine, bloody urine, swelling of the feet or legs, or joint pain.
- Rule out pregnancy at least 2 weeks before beginning therapy with MTX. Use contraceptive measures for at least 8 weeks after stopping therapy to decrease the risk of severe birth defects or fetal death if pregnancy should occur.
- Avoid pregnancy if either partner is using methotrexate.
- *Conception* — Men should wait at least 3 months and women should wait at least 1 ovulatory cycle after stopping use of MTX before attempting conception.
- Prior to therapy, a complete blood workup, urinalysis, chest x-ray and kidney and liver function tests are required. Follow-up tests will also be required.

If you have any questions, consult your doctor, pharmacist, or health care provider.

	Generic Name *Brand Name Examples*	Supplied As	Generic Available
Rx	**Methoxsalen (8-Methoxypsoralen)**		
	Oxsoralen-Ultra[1]	**Capsules**: 10 mg	No
Rx	**Methoxsalen**		
	Oxsoralen[2,3]	**Lotion**: 1%	No
Rx	**Trioxsalen**		
	Trisoralen[1]	**Tablets**: 5 mg	No

[1] Contains the dye tartrazine.
[2] For office use only; never dispensed to a patient.
[3] Contains alcohol.

Type of Drug:

Photosensitizing drugs used in combination with ultraviolet (UV) light for the treatment of psoriasis, vitiligo and other skin disorders.

How the Drug Works:

Psoralens act as "photosensitizers." Oral psoralens reach the skin by the bloodstream. When the skin is exposed to UV light, an inflammatory reaction occurs. The inflammation is followed over several days to weeks by repair which is seen as increased darkening and thickening of the skin layers.

Uses:

Oxsoralen-Ultra: To control symptoms of severe resistant disabling psoriasis not responsive to other therapy when the diagnosis has been supported by biopsy. Used only with long wave UV radiation. *Oxsoralen-Ultra* should not be interchanged with *Oxsoralen* lotion.

Oxsoralen (topical), trioxsalen: Used with long wave UV radiation or sunlight. For repigmentation (darkening) of idiopathic vitiligo.

Trioxsalen: For increasing tolerance to sunlight and for enhancing pigmentation.

Precautions:

Do not use in the following situations:

absence of lens of eye (aphakia)
adverse reaction to psoralen compounds, history
albinism
allergy to psoralens
children under 12 years of age (*Oxsoralen* lotion and trioxsalen)
diseases associated with light sensitivity (porphyria, acute lupus erythematosus, leukoderma)
melanoma, history
squamous cell cancer
use of other photosensitizing drugs
xeroderma pigmentosum

Use with caution in the following situations:

- arsenic therapy, history
- basal cell carcinoma, history
- cataracts
- fair-skinned individuals
- grenz or x-ray therapy, history
- heart disease
- liver disease
- tar or UVB treatment, prolonged

Photosensitizing (light sensitizing) agents: Exercise special care in treating patients who are receiving therapy (either topically or systemically) with other known photosensitizing agents such as:

- anthralin
- bacteriostatic soaps
- coal tar (and derivatives)
- dyes (methylene blue, toluidine blue, rose bengal, methyl orange)
- griseofulvin
- nalidixic acid
- phenothiazines
- sulfonamides
- tetracycline
- thiazide diuretics

Furocoumarin-containing foods: No clinical reports or tests show that serious reactions may result, but eating the following while on psoralen therapy may be dangerous: Limes, figs, parsley, parsnips, mustard, carrots and celery.

Skin cancer: Studies have shown an increased risk of squamous cell and basal cell carcinoma among patients receiving psoralens and (UV) radiation.

Cataracts: Like the skin, psoralens reach the lens of the eye by the bloodstream. If the eye is exposed to UVA while methoxsalen is in the lens, cataracts may appear. However, if the lens is shielded from UVA, the methoxsalen will leave the eye in 24 hours. Wear UVA-absorbing, wraparound sunglasses for the 24 hours following oral use of methoxsalen, whether exposed to direct or indirect sunlight in the open, or through window glass.

Oxsoralen-Ultra should not be substituted for regular *Oxsoralen.*

Pregnancy: Adequate studies have not been done in pregnant women. Use only if clearly needed and potential benefits outweigh the possible hazards to the fetus.

Breastfeeding: It is not known if psoralens appear in breast milk. Consult your doctor before you begin breastfeeding.

Children: Safety of methoxsalen use in children has not been established. Potential hazards include possible cancer, cataracts and premature aging of skin. Oral trioxsalen and methoxsalen lotion are not recommended in children under 12 years of age.

Lab tests are required before and at regular intervals during therapy with psoralens. Tests may include: Blood counts, antinuclear antibodies, liver and kidney function tests and eye exams.

Tartrazine: Some of these products may contain the dye tartrazine (FD&C Yellow No. 5) which can cause allergic reactions in certain individuals. Check package label when available or consult your pharmacist or doctor.

Drug Interactions:

Tell your doctor or pharmacist if you are taking or planning to take any over-the-counter or prescription medications or dietary supplements while taking this medicine. Doses of one or both drugs may need to be modified or a different drug may need to be prescribed. Photosensitizing agents (see Precautions) interact with psoriasis agents.

Side Effects:

Every drug is capable of producing side effects. Many psoralen users experience side effects. The frequency and severity of side effects depend on many factors including dose, duration of therapy and individual susceptibility. Possible side effects include:

Skin: Burns (from excessive sunlight or sunlamp UV exposure); skin cancer; decreased pigmentation; skin rash; herpes simplex; hives; itching; redness; swelling; blisters.

Nervous System: Nervousness; sleeplessness; depression; lethargy; dizziness; headache.

Other: Fluid retention (edema); leg cramps; general body discomfort; low blood pressure; spread of psoriasis; tenderness or aging of the skin; herpes simplex eruptions; nausea.

Combined methoxsalen/UVA therapy – Itching may be lessened with frequent application of bland emollients or other topical agents. Severe itching may require oral treatment. If itching is unresponsive, shield itching areas from further UVA exposure until the condition improves. If itching is "all over," discontinue UVA treatment until itching disappears. Mild, transient redness 24 to 48 hours after PUVA therapy is expected. It indicates a therapeutic interaction between methoxsalen and UVA. Shield any area showing moderate redness during future UVA exposures until the redness is gone. Discuss all symptoms with your doctor.

Serious burns from either UVA or sunlight (even through window glass) may occur if recommended dosage of the drug or exposure schedules are exceeded.

Guidelines for Use:

- Individualize treatment. Take self-administered products exactly as prescribed.
- Do not stop taking this medicine or change the dose without checking with your doctor; this could have serious adverse effects.
- *Use topical methoxsalen* only on small, well defined lesions which can be protected by clothing from exposure to sunlight. If used to treat vitiligo of face or hands, keep the treated area protected from sunlight or other UV light exposure by use of protective clothing or sunscreens. The area of application may be highly photosensitive (light-sensitive) for several days and may result in severe burns if exposed to additional UV or sunlight. This medicine is only applied by a doctor under controlled lighting conditions.

Guidelines for Use (cont.):

- Treatment frequency is generally once a week or less, depending on the results, but should never be given more than once every other day. Significant repigmentation may require 6 to 9 months of treatment. Retreatment may be required. Repigmentation occurs less rapidly over less fleshy areas such as the back of the hands or tops of the feet.
- *Before use* — Do not sunbathe during the 24 hours prior to methoxsalen ingestion and UV exposure. Sunburn may prevent an accurate evaluation of the patient's response to photochemotherapy.
- *After use* — Wear UVA-absorbing, wraparound sunglasses during daylight for 24 hours to prevent cataracts (see Precautions). The protective eyewear must prevent entry of stray radiation to the eyes, including that which may enter from the sides of the eyewear.
- *Avoid sun exposure,* even through window glass or cloud cover, for at least 8 hours after use. If sun exposure cannot be avoided, wear protective devices such as a hat and gloves, or apply sunscreens that filter out UVA radiation (eg, sunscreens with SPF 15 or more). Apply sunscreens to all areas that might be exposed to the sun (including lips). Do not apply sunscreens to areas affected by psoriasis until after treatment in the UVA chamber.
- *During PUVA therapy,* wear total UVA-absorbing/blocking goggles mechanically designed to give maximal protection. Failure to do so may increase the risk of cataract formation. A radiometer can verify elimination of UVA transmission through the goggles. Protect lips with light-screening lipstick.
- Protect abdominal skin, breasts, genital organs and other sensitive areas for approximately one-third of the initial exposure time until tanning occurs. Unless affected by disease, shield male genital organs.
- *After combined methoxsalen/UVA therapy:* Wear UVA-absorbing, wraparound sunglasses during the daylight for 24 hours after therapy. Do not sunbathe for 48 hours after therapy. Redness or burning due to photochemotherapy and sunburn are additive.
- Minimize or avoid nausea by taking the drug with milk or food, or by dividing into two doses, taken 1/2 hour apart.
- Do not exceed prescribed dosage or exposure time. Serious burns may result.
- Avoid furocoumarin-containing foods (eg, limes, figs, parsley, parsnips, mustard, carrots, celery).
- *Oxsoralen-Ultra* should not be substituted for regular *Oxsoralen.*
- Use of methoxsalen with UV light should only occur when a doctor experienced in diagnosis and treatment of psoriasis and vitiligo is involved.
- UVA therapy may cause ocular damage, skin aging and skin cancer. The safe total dose of UVA given over a long period of time has not been established.
- Eye exams are recommended before the start of therapy and then every year. Periodic lab tests are required, as well. Be sure to keep appointments.

If you have any questions, consult your doctor, pharmacist, or health care provider.

	Generic Name *Brand Name Examples*	Supplied As	Generic Available
Rx	**Tazarotene**		
	Tazorac[1]	**Gel, topical**: 0.05%; 0.1%	No

[1] Contains benzyl alcohol as a preservative.

Type of Drug:

Topical psoriasis drug; antiacne medicine.

How the Drug Works:

The exact mechanism of drug action is unknown. The drug reduces skin inflammation and changes associated with the development of psoriasis and acne.

Uses:

For the topical treatment of psoriasis of up to 20% of the body surface.
For the topical treatment of mild-to-moderate acne.

Precautions:

Do not use in the following situations:

allergy to the drug or any of its ingredients
application to eyes, eyelids and mouth
eczema
itching, burning, redness or peeling of the skin
pregnancy
skin medications causing strong drying effects

Use with caution in the following situations:

concurrent administration of other photosensitizing drugs (eg, tetracyclines, thiazides, quinolones, sulfonamides)
exposure to sunlight or sun lamps
extreme weather conditions (wind or cold)

Pregnancy: Do not use during pregnancy. The risk of use in a pregnant woman clearly outweighs any possible benefit.

Breastfeeding: It is not known if tazarotene appears in breast milk. Consult your doctor before you begin breastfeeding.

Children: Safety and effectiveness have not been established in children under 12 years of age.

Drug Interactions:

Tell your doctor or pharmacist if you are taking or planning to take any over-the-counter or prescription medications or dietary supplements while taking tazarotene. Doses of one or both drugs may need to be modified or a different drug may need to be prescribed. The following drugs and drug classes interact with tazarotene:

thiazides (eg, chlorthalidone, hydrochlorothiazide)
tetracyclines (eg, doxycycline)
fluoroquinolones (eg, ciprofloxacin)

phenothiazines (eg, promethazine)
sulfonamides (eg, sulfamethoxazole)

Side Effects:

Every drug is capable of producing side effects. Many tazarotene users experience no, or minor, side effects. The frequency and severity of side effects depend on many factors including dose, duration of therapy and individual susceptibility. Possible side effects include:

Skin: Itching; burning; stinging; redness; worsening of psoriasis; irritation; skin pain; rash; peeling of skin; contact skin inflammation; cracking, splitting of skin; bleeding; dry skin; localized swelling; skin discoloration.

Guidelines for Use:

- For external use only. Keep away from eyes, mouth and nose.
- Apply this medication as directed by your doctor. Contact your doctor if the psoriasis or acne becomes worse.
- If itching, burning, redness, peeling or stinging occurs, discontinue use and contact your doctor immediately. If irritation is excessive, application should be discontinued.
- *For psoriasis:*
  - Apply once a day in the evening to lesions on no more than 20% of the body surface using enough to cover only the lesion with a thin film.
  - Skin should be clean and dry before applying gel.
  - Avoid application to unaffected skin, because it may be more susceptible to irritation. Avoid eyes and mouth.
- *For acne:*
  - Cleanse face gently.
  - After the skin is dry, apply a thin film once a day in the evening where lesions appear.
  - Use enough to cover the entire affected area.
- If you become pregnant while using tazarotene, immediately discontinue use and contact your doctor.
- Women of child-bearing potential who use tazarotene should use contraceptive measures while using this medicine.
- If you use a cream or lotion to soften or lubricate your skin, remove the cream or lotion first and then apply tazarotene after ensuring that there is no more cream or lotion on the skin.
- Do not cover the treated areas with dressings or bandages.
- Wash hands after applying the medication unless you are treating your hands for psoriasis. If the gel accidently gets on areas you do not need to treat, wash it off.
- If tazarotene comes in contact with your eyes, wash your eyes with large amounts of cool water and contact a doctor if eye irritation persists.
- If a dose is missed, apply it as soon as possible. If several hours have passed or it is nearing time for the next application, do not double the application to "catch up" (unless advised by your doctor). If more than one application is missed or it is necessary to establish a new application schedule, contact your doctor or pharmacist. Use exactly as prescribed.
- Use with caution on eczema (dry scaly skin).
- Avoid, if possible, any topical medication or cosmetic that has a strong drying effect.
- May cause photosensitivity (sensitivity to sunlight). Avoid prolonged exposure to the sun or other forms of ultraviolet light (eg, tanning beds). Use sunscreens and wear protective clothing.
- Store at 59° to 86°F.

If you have any questions, consult your doctor, pharmacist, or health care provider.

Generic Name *Brand Name Examples*	Supplied As	Generic Available
Rx **Becaplermin**		
Regranex	**Gel**: 100 mcg/g	No

Type of Drug:

Biologic; human platelet-derived growth factor.

How the Drug Works:

Stimulates the body to grow new tissue in areas of tissue damage (ulcer site) where it is applied.

Uses:

For the treatment of lower-extremity (limb) diabetic neuropathic ulcers that extend under the skin or deeper and have adequate blood supply. It is used along with proper ulcer care and infection treatment.

Precautions:

Do not use in the following situations:

allergy to drug or any of its ingredients
tumors at site of application
wounds that are likely to heal by themselves

Pregnancy: Adequate studies have not been done in pregnant women. Use only if clearly needed and potential benefits outweigh the possible hazard to the fetus.

Breastfeeding: It is not known if becaplermin appears in breast milk. Consult your doctor before you begin breastfeeding.

Children: Safety and effectiveness in children less than 16 years of age have not been established.

Drug Interactions:

Tell your doctor or pharmacist if you are taking or planning to take any over-the-counter or prescription medications or dietary supplements while taking becaplermin. Doses of one or both drugs may need to be modified or a different drug may need to be prescribed.

Side Effects:

Every drug is capable of producing side effects. Many becaplermin users experience no, or minor, side effects. The frequency and severity of side effects depend on many factors including dose, duration of therapy and individual susceptibility. Possible side effects include:

Other: Infection; inflammation of tissue; bone infection; red rash; tissue irritation.

Guidelines for Use:

- For external use only.
- Apply amount once a day as prescribed by your doctor. The amount varies depending on individual needs and should be re-evaluated periodically by a doctor.
- Directions for use:
  - Wash hands thoroughly before applying.
  - Squeeze gel on to a clean, firm, non-absorbable surface (eg, wax paper).
  - With a clean cotton swab, tongue depressor or similar application aid, spread measured gel over ulcer surface in an even layer.
  - Cover with a saline-moistened gauze dressing.
  - After about 12 hours, rinse the ulcer with saline or water to remove residual gel and cover with a saline-moistened gauze dressing without the gel.
- The tip of the tube should not come into contact with the ulcer or any other surface. Recap tube tightly after each use.
- Use the gel with a strict non-weight-bearing program.
- Applying more gel than prescribed does not increase healing rate.
- Do not apply other topical products to the ulcer site.
- Becaplermin does not replace good ulcer care practices. It is used in addition to good ulcer care practices.
- If a dose is missed, apply it as soon as possible. If several hours have passed or if it is nearing time for the next dose, do not double the dose to "catch up" (unless advised by your doctor). If more than one dose is missed or it is necessary to adjust the dosage schedule, contact your doctor or pharmacist.
- Do not stop applying this medicine without consulting your doctor.
- Notify your doctor if a reaction at the ulcer site occurs while applying becaplermin.
- Store in refrigerator (36° to 46°F). Do not freeze.
- Use this medication by the expiration date noted on bottom of tube.

If you have any questions, consult your doctor, pharmacist, or health care provider.

	Generic Name *Brand Name Example*	Supplied As	Generic Available
Rx	**Mafenide**		
	Sulfamylon[1]	**Cream** : 85 mg/g	No

[1] Contains sulfites and parabens.

Type of Drug:

Antibacterial burn agent.

How the Drug Works:

Mafenide reduces the number of bacteria in second- and third-degree burn wounds. This permits healing. It is active even when pus and blood serum are present.

Uses:

To treat and prevent bacterial infection in second- and third-degree burns. Used in combination with other treatments.

Precautions:

Do not use in the following situations:

allergy to mafenide
sulfite sensitivity
G6PD deficiency

Use with caution in the following situations:

kidney or lung disease

Superinfection: Use of antibiotics (especially prolonged or repeated therapy) may result in overgrowth of nonsusceptible bacteria or fungi. Such overgrowth may lead to a second infection. Mafenide may need to be stopped and another antibiotic prescribed for the nonsusceptible secondary infection.

Pregnancy: Adequate studies have not been done in pregnant women. Use only if clearly needed and potential benefits outweigh the possible hazards to the fetus.

Breastfeeding: It is not known if mafenide appears in breast milk. Because of the potential for serious side effects in nursing infants, decide whether to discontinue the drug or discontinue breastfeeding. Consult your doctor.

Children: Use for children is the same as for adults.

Lab tests will be required to monitor therapy. Tests may include acid base balance.

Sulfites: This product may contain sulfite preservatives which can cause allergic reactions in certain individuals. Check package label when available or consult your doctor or pharmacist.

Drug Interactions:

Tell your doctor or pharmacist if you are taking or if you are planning to take any over-the-counter or prescription medications or dietary supplements with mafenide. Doses of one or both drugs may need to be modified or a different drug may need to be prescribed.

Side Effects:

Every drug is capable of producing side effects. Many mafenide users experience no, or minor, side effects. The frequency and severity of side effects depend on many factors including dose, duration of therapy and individual susceptibility. Possible side effects include:

Skin: Pain or burning sensation on application; rash; itching; hives; blisters; redness of skin.

Other: Fluid retention (edema); facial swelling; rapid breathing; swelling; increase in serum chloride.

Guidelines for Use:

- For external use only. Use exactly as prescribed.
- Using a sterile glove, apply once or twice daily to burned areas to a thickness of about 1/16 inch. Whenever necessary, reapply the cream to any areas from which it has been removed (eg, by patient activity).
- The treated area may be covered by a dressing, but this is not required.
- Bathe the burned area daily. A whirlpool bath is particularly helpful.
- Continue treatment until healing occurs or until the site is ready for grafting. Treatment may have to be discontinued if significant side effects occur.
- Do not stop using while there is the possibility of infection.
- Contact your doctor if hyperventilation (rapid breathing) or burn irritation occurs or if condition worsens.

If you have any questions, consult your doctor, pharmacist, or health care provider.

	Generic Name *Brand Name Examples*	Supplied As	Generic Available
Rx	**Silver sulfadiazine**		
	SSD,[1] *SSD AF,*[1] *Silvadene*[1]	**Cream**: 1%	No

[1] Contains petrolatum and methylparaben

Type of Drug:

Antibacterial burn agent.

How the Drug Works:

Silver sulfadiazine reduces the number of bacteria in second-and third-degree burn wounds.

Uses:

To help prevent and treat bacterial burn wound infections in second- and third-degree burns. Also used in combination with other medicines.

Precautions:

Do not use in the following situations:

allergy to silver sulfadiazine or any ingredient in the preparation
allergy to sulfonamides (sulfa drugs)
infants less than 2 months old
pregnant women at or near delivery date
premature infants

Use with caution in the following situations:

fungal growth in burn
glucose-6-phosphate dehydrogenase (G-6-PD) deficiency
kidney disease
liver disease
topical proteolytic enzyme use

Superinfection: Use of antibiotics (especially prolonged or repeated therapy) may result in bacterial or fungal overgrowth. Such overgrowth may lead to a second infection. Silver sulfadiazine may need to be stopped and another antibiotic may need to be prescribed for the second infection.

Pregnancy: Safety for use during pregnancy has not been established. Use during pregnancy only if clearly justified, especially in women approaching or at delivery date.

Breastfeeding: It is not known if silver sulfadiazine cream appears in breast milk. Sulfonamides are known to be excreted in breast milk and since all sulfonamide derivatives have the potential to cause problems in the nursing infant, consult your doctor before you begin breastfeeding.

Children: Safety and effectiveness in children have not been established.

Lab tests are recommended during treatment. Tests may include blood drug concentrations, kidney function tests (blood and urine) and white blood cell counts. Be sure to keep appointments.

Drug Interactions:

Tell your doctor or pharmacist if you are taking or if you are planning to take any over-the-counter or prescription medications or dietary supplements with silver sulfadiazine cream. Doses of one or both drugs may need to be modified or a different drug may need to be prescribed. Topical proteolytic enzymes interact with silver sulfadiazine cream.

Side Effects:

Every drug is capable of producing side effects. Many silver sulfadiazine users experience no, or minor, side effects. The frequency and severity of side effects depend on many factors including dose, duration of therapy and individual susceptibility. Possible side effects include:

Other: Burning; rash; itching; dead skin; hives, redness; skin discoloration; decrease in white blood cell count. Because sulfadiazine may be absorbed, it is possible that any of the side effects of sulfonamides may occur (see sulfonamide monograph).

Use of Silvadene – may delay the separation of the dead skin from the new skin, requiring a procedure involving scraping of the wound (escharotomy) in order to prevent abnormal skin development.

Guidelines for Use:

- For external use only. Use exactly as prescribed.
- Apply once or twice daily to a thickness of about 1/16th of an inch. Apply using a sterile glove. Wash hands before and after application.
- Burn areas should be covered with silver sulfadiazine cream at all times.
- Reapply immediately after bathing and to any areas from which it has been removed by activity.
- May be covered by a dressing, but this is not required.
- Bathe the burned area daily. A whirlpool bath is particularly helpful.
- Continue treatment until healing occurs, until the site is ready for grafting or unless a significant side effect occurs.
- *Sulfonamide allergy* — If you are allergic to other sulfa drugs, you may react to silver sulfadiazine.
- If burn wounds involve extensive areas of the body, the sulfa drug may be absorbed to a significant extent. This could lead to systemic side effects.

If you have any questions, consult your doctor, pharmacist, or health care provider.

	Generic Name *Brand Name Examples*	Supplied As	Generic Available
	Selenium Sulfide		
otc	*Selsun Blue (Regular, pH Balanced,[1] Medicated[1]), Head and Shoulders Intensive Treatment*	**Lotion shampoo**: 1%	Yes
Rx	*Selsun*	**Lotion shampoo**: 2.5%	Yes

[1] Contains menthol.

Type of Drug:

Controls dandruff flaking and itching.

How the Drug Works:

Selenium sulfide reduces growth and multiplication of skin cells.

Uses:

For treatment of dandruff, seborrheic dermatitis of the scalp and tinea versicolor (a fungal infection, *2.5% selenium sulfide only*).

Precautions:

Do not use in the following situations:

allergy to any ingredient of the product
inflamed, broken skin

Pregnancy: Adequate studies have not been done in pregnant women. Use only if clearly needed and potential benefits outweigh the possible hazards to the fetus.

Children: Safety and effectiveness in infants have not been established.

Side Effects:

Every drug is capable of producing side effects. Many selenium sulfide users experience no, or minor, side effects. The frequency and severity of side effects depend on many factors including dose, duration of therapy and individual susceptibility. Possible side effects include: Skin irritation; hair discoloration (minimize by thorough rinsing); oiliness or dryness of hair and scalp; hair loss.

Guidelines for Use:

- *For dandruff, seborrheic dermatitis* — Shake well. Shampoo and rinse thoroughly. Use regularly for best results, at least twice a week as directed by your doctor.
- *For fungal infection* — Apply to affected areas and lather with a small amount of water. Allow to remain on skin for 10 minutes. Rinse thoroughly. Repeat daily for 7 days.
- For external use only.
- Avoid contact with the eyes. If contact occurs, rinse eye(s) thoroughly with water.
- If irritation occurs, discontinue use.
- Thoroughly rinse after application.
- Wash hands thoroughly after treatment.
- If condition worsens or does not improve after regular use of this product as directed, contact your doctor or pharmacist.
- Do not use on broken or inflamed skin.
- If using on bleached, tinted, gray or permed hair, rinse hair for at least 5 minutes.
- May damage jewelry; remove before using.
- Avoid contact of the shampoo in the genital area and skin folds as it may cause irritation and burning. Thoroughly rinse these areas after use.

If you have any questions, consult your doctor, pharmacist, or health care provider.

	Generic Name *Brand Name Examples*	Supplied As	Generic Available
Rx	**Chloroxine**		
	Capitrol[2,7]	**Shampoo**: 2%	No
otc	**Pyrithione Zinc**		
	DHS Zinc, Head and Shoulders Dandruff, Sebulon, Zincon	**Shampoo**: 1%, 2%	Yes
Rx	**Sulfacetamide Sodium**		
	Sebizon	**Lotion**: 10%	No
otc	**Tar Derivatives, Shampoos**		
	DHS Tar	**Shampoo**: 0.5% coal tar	No
	Neutrogena T/Gel[5]	**Shampoo**: 0.5% coal tar	Yes
	Polytar[2,3]	**Shampoo**: 0.5% coal tar	
	Neutrogena T/Gel Extra Strength[5]	**Shampoo**: 1% coal tar	
	Zetar[6]	**Shampoo**: 1% coal tar	Yes
	Tegrin Medicated Advanced Formula[1,5]	**Shampoo**: 1.1% coal tar	No
	Denorex Medicated[1]	**Shampoo**: 1.8% coal tar	No
	Denorex Medicated	**Shampoo and Conditioner**: 1.8% coal tar	No
	Duplex T	**Shampoo**: 2% coal tar	Yes
	Pentrax Gold[5]	**Shampoo**: 2% coal tar	
	Duplex T[1]	**Shampoo and Conditioner**: 2% coal tar	No
	Denorex Extra Strength[1,4]	**Shampoo**: 2.5% coal tar	No
	Denorex Extra Strength	**Shampoo and Conditioner**: 2.5% coal tar	No
	MG217	**Shampoo**: 3% coal tar	No
	Pentrax	**Shampoo**: 4.3% coal tar	No
	Tar Derivatives, Bath Products		
otc	*Balnetar*	**Oil**: 0.5% coal tar	No
otc	*Polytar*[2]	**Soap**: 0.5% coal tar	No
otc	*Cutar Bath Oil*[5]	**Emulsion**: 1.5% coal tar	No
Rx	*Zetar*[8]	**Emulsion**: 30% coal tar	No
	Tar Derivatives, Emollients		
otc	*Tegrin*[1]	**Cream**: 0.8% coal tar	No

otc Medotar	**Ointment**: 1% coal tar	No
otc T/Derm	**Emollient**: 1.2% coal tar	No
otc PsoriGel	**Gel**: 1.75% coal tar	No
otc Fototar[1]	**Cream**: 2% coal tar	No
otc MG217 Medicated Intensive Strength	**Ointment**: 2% coal tar	No
otc Oxipor VHC[1]	**Lotion**: 5% coal tar	No
otc Estar[1,7]	**Gel**: 5% coal tar	No

[1] Contains alcohol.
[2] Contains edetate disodium.
[3] Contains lanolin.
[4] Contains menthol.
[5] Contains parabens.
[6] Contains parachlorometaxylenol 0.5%.
[7] Contains benzyl alcohol.
[8] Requires dilution prior to use.

Type of Drug:

Antiseborrheic products.

How the Drug Works:

Chloroxine reduces excess scaling and inhibits growth of bacteria and some fungi.

Pyrithione zinc reduces skin cell growth, flaking, itching and inhibits fungal growth.

Selenium sulfide reduces skin cell growth and inhibits growth of organisms associated with chronic flaking and itching.

Sulfacetamide sodium inhibits bacterial growth and reproduction.

Tar derivatives help correct abnormalities in the formation of keratin. Keratin is a protein found in skin (epidermis), hair and nails. Inhibits bacterial and fungal growth and helps control itching, flaking, scaling, irritation and redness.

Uses:

Shampoos: To treat chronic scalp psoriasis, seborrhea, dandruff, eczema, cradle cap and other oily conditions of the scalp.

Bath products, solutions, lotions, gels, creams: To treat psoriasis, seborrheic dermatitis, atopic dermatitis, eczema and other chronic skin disorders.

Precautions:

Do not use in the following situations:

allergy to any of ingredients in product
allergy to sulfonamides (sulfacetamide sodium only)
open, inflamed or infected lesions (chloroxine and tar derivatives)
photosensitive (light sensitive) people (tar derivatives only)

Use with caution in the following situations:
sun or ultraviolet light exposure (tar derivatives only)

Superinfection: Use of antibiotics (especially prolonged or repeated therapy) may result in bacterial or fungal overgrowth. Such overgrowth may lead to a second infection. Antiseborrheic products may need to be stopped and another antibiotic prescribed for the second infection.

Pregnancy: Adequate studies of these products have not been done in pregnant women. Use only if clearly needed and potential benefits outweigh the possible hazards to the fetus.

Breastfeeding: Safety for use of these products while breastfeeding has not been established. Consult your doctor before you begin breastfeeding.

Children: Safety and effectiveness of sulfacetamido sodium in children under 12 have not been established.

Drug Interactions:

Tell your doctor or pharmacist if you are using or if you are planning to use any over-the-counter or prescription medications or dietary supplements with these medicines. Silver preparations interact with sulfacetamide sodium. Tetracyclines, psoralens and topical retinoic acid may interact with tar.

Side Effects:

Every drug is capable of producing side effects. Many antiseborrheic product users experience no, or minor, side effects. The frequency and severity of side effects depend on many factors including dose, duration of therapy and individual susceptibility. Possible side effects include: Minor irritation; inflammation of follicles (after long-term use); allergic rash; sensitivity to light; blisters, swelling of skin.

Guidelines for Use:

- For external use only.
- Directions for use vary from product to product. Read and follow instructions for use carefully.
- Avoid contact with eyes. If contact occurs, rinse thoroughly with water.
- *Chloroxine* — May discolor blond, gray or bleached hair.If irritation, burning or rash occurs, discontinue use and contact your doctor.Massage thoroughly into wet scalp. Allow lather to remain on scalp for 3 minutes; rinse. Repeat. Two treatments per week are usually sufficient.
- *Pyrithione zinc* — If condition worsens or does not improve with regular use as directed, see your doctor. May temporarily discolor blond, gray, bleached or tinted hair.
- *Selenium sulfide* — May discolor bleached, tinted, gray or permed hair; rinse for 5 minutes.
  If condition worsens or does not improve after regular use, discontinue use and notify your doctor.
- *Sulfacetamide sodium* — If irritation occurs or continues, or if rash develops, discontinue use and notify your doctor. Discontinue promptly if any arthritis, fever or sores in the mouth develop.
  Do not use with silver-containing medications (eg, *Silvadene*).
- *Tar derivatives* — If condition covers a large area of the body, worsens or does not improve, or if irritation develops after regular use as directed, consult your doctor. Do not use for prolonged periods or with other psoriasis therapy such as ultraviolet light or prescription drugs unless directed by your doctor.
  May stain clothing or temporarily discolor white, blond, gray, bleached or tinted hair. Skin may tingle during treatment.
  Sensitivity to sunlight — Avoid prolonged exposure to direct sunlight. Topical tar plus ultraviolet light may increase tendency to sunburn for 24 to 72 hours. Do not apply to genital or rectal area.
- *Seborrheic dermatitis* — In mild cases involving the scalp and skin, apply at bedtime and allow to remain overnight. Shampoo first if the hair and scalp are oily or greasy or if there is considerable debris. In severe cases, apply twice daily. Initially, and as frequently as needed thereafter, clean the hair and scalp with a nonirritating shampoo before using the medication.
- Contact your doctor if you notice any unusual side effects after using any of these medications.

	Generic Name *Brand Name Examples*	Supplied As
	Antiseborrheic Shampoos	
otc	*Sebulex, Sebulex with Conditioners*	**Shampoo**: 2% sulfur and 2% salicylic acid
	Ionil	**Shampoo**: 2% salicylic acid, benzalkonium chloride and 12% SD alcohol 40
	Ionil T	**Shampoo**: 5% coal tar solution, benzalkonium chloride, 4% isopropyl alcohol and 12% alcohol
	Meted, Maximum Strength	**Shampoo**: 5% sulfur and 3% salicylic acid
	P & S	**Shampoo**: 2% salicylic acid
	Sebex	**Shampoo**: 2% salicylic acid, 2% colloidal sulfur
	SLT Lotion	**Lotion**: 2.5% coal tar solution, isopropyl alcohol, benzalkonium chloride
	Tarsum	**Shampoo/Gel**: 10% coal tar solution
	X-Seb T Plus,, X-Seb T Pearl	**Shampoo**: 10% coal tar solution
otc	**Medicated Hair Dressings**	
	P & S	**Liquid**: Phenol, mineral oil and glycerin
	Sebucare	**Lotion**: 1.8% salicylic acid with 61% alcohol

Type of Drug:

Drugs used to treat seborrhea, dandruff, psoriasis and related skin conditions.

Uses:

In these combinations:

Salicylic acid and sulfur: Used for sebum (oil)-reducing and skin-sloughing actions.

Tar preparations: Used for their anti-itch, antibacterial and antiseborrheic actions.

Benzalkonium chloride and *phenol:* Used as antiseptics.

Guidelines for Use:

- For external use only.
- Avoid contact with eyes or mucous membranes. Flush with water if contact occurs.
- Discontinue use and consult your doctor if skin irritation develops or worsens.
- Tar increases sensitivity to the sun and may increase tendency to sunburn for up to 24 hours after use.
- Do not use for prolonged periods without consulting a doctor.
- Do not use on large areas of the body.
- If condition does not improve or worsens, see your doctor.
- Do not use these products with other psoriasis therapy such as ultraviolet light or prescription drugs unless directed by your doctor.
- Do not use on broken skin or around the genital area unless directed by your doctor.
- Do not use on children under 2 years of age.
- Products containing tar may temporarily discolor blond, gray, bleached or tinted hair, or cause slight staining of clothing.

If you have any questions, consult your doctor, pharmacist, or health care provider.

	Generic Name *Brand Name Examples*	Supplied As	Generic Available
	Benzocaine		
otc	*Anbesol, Hurricaine,*[6] *Maximum Strength Anbesol,*[6] *Orabase-B Gel,*[3] *Orajel Mouth-Aid*[5]	**Gel**: 6.3%, 10%, 15%, 20%	Yes
	Anbesol, Hurricaine, Maximum Strength Anbesol , Orajel Mouth-Aid[3,4]	**Liquid**: 6.3%, 20%	Yes
	Hurricaine	**Spray**: 20%	No
c-II	**Cocaine HCl**	**Solution**: 4% 10%	Yes
		Powder[1]	Yes
Rx	**Dyclonine HCl**		
	Dyclone	**Solution**: 0.5%, 1%	No
Rx	**Lidocaine HCl**		
	Xylocaine	**Ointment**: 2.5%, 5%	No
	Anestacon, Xylocaine	**Jelly**: 2%	No
	Xylocaine	**Liquid**: 5%	No
	Xylocaine, Xylocaine Viscous, Xylocaine-MPF	**Solution**: 2%, 4%	Yes
	Xylocaine 10% Oral	**Spray**: 10%	No
Rx	**Tetracaine HCl**		
	Pontocaine HCl	**Solution**: 0.5%	No
otc	**Topical Anesthetic Combinations**		
	Vagisil, New Improved[2]	**Cream**: 5% benzocaine and 1% dimethicone	No
	Vagisil, Maximum Strength	**Cream**: 20% benzocaine, 1% dimethicone	No

1 Amount of anesthetic in the product is unknown.
2 Contains methyl- and propylparabens.
3 Contains ethyl alcohol.
4 Contains tartrazine.
5 Contains edetate disodium.
6 Contains methylparaben and saccharin.

Type of Drug:

Topical anesthetics for mucous membrane pain and discomfort.

How the Drug Works:

Topical anesthetics applied externally inhibit conduction of nerve impulses from sensory nerves, thereby producing anesthesia (lack of feeling, numbness). Abrasions or ulcers of the membrane increase absorption and thus increase the effectiveness of the drug (however, side effects could be increased).

Uses:

Local anesthesia for the examination of mucous membranes including: Oral, nasal and throat membranes; respiratory tract; digestive tract; and urinary tract.

To treat itching due to hemorrhoids or an inflamed anal or vaginal area.

Cocaine: Should only be used for office and surgical procedures.

Precautions:

Do not use in the following situations:

allergy to any component of the product
eyes, use in or around

Use with caution in the following situations:

allergy to externally applied drugs
blood disorder (eg, methoglobinemia)
children
ear problems
elderly
illness, acute
infants less than 1 year of age
infection at site of use
liver disease, severe
severely injured or damaged skin
shock or heart block (lidocaine and dyclonine only)

Chronic use: – Do not apply to large areas of the body or use for prolonged periods of time. Chronic use may result in tissue irritation, breathing difficulties, seizures, low blood pressure, mental confusion, ringing in the ears and blurred or poor vision.

Dependence: – Cocaine is addicting. Continual use of cocaine creates an excessively strong dependence and, sometimes, depression. Chronic use may cause progression from euphoria to paranoid psychosis; included may be perceptual changes (halo lights) and intense itching ("cocaine bugs"). This drug produces the highest degree of dependence seen among abused drugs.

Pregnancy:

Lidocaine – Studies in pregnant women or in animals have been judged not to show a risk to the fetus. However, no drug should be used during pregnancy unless clearly needed.

Cocaine – Adequate studies have not been done in pregnant women, or animal studies may have shown a risk to the fetus. Use only if clearly needed and potential benefits outweigh the possible hazards to the fetus. Women who use cocaine during pregnancy are at significant risk for complications such as shorter gestation, premature delivery and spontaneous abortion.

Other Anesthetics – Adequate studies have not been done in pregnant women, or animal studie may have shown a risk to the fetus. Use only if clearly needed and potential benefits outweigh the possible hazards to the fetus.

Breastfeeding: Lidocaine appears in breast milk. Safety for use of any of these medicines during breastfeeding has not been established. The

American Academy of Pediatrics recommends that cocaine never be used during breastfeeding. Consult your doctor.

Children: Safety and effectiveness for use of cocaine in children have not been established. Safety and effectiveness for use of dyclonine and tetracaine in children less than 12 years of age have not been established. Safety and effectiveness of other topical anesthetics have not been established in children less than 1 year of age.

Elderly: Dosage adjustments may be necessary for elderly patients.

Tartrazine: Some of these products may contain the dye tartrazine (FD&C Yellow No. 5) which can cause allergic reactions in certain individuals. Check package label when available or consult your doctor or pharmacist.

Sulfites: Some of these products may contain sulfite preservatives which can cause allergic reactions in certain individuals. Check package labels when available or consult your doctor or pharmacist.

Drug Interactions:

Tell your doctor or pharmacist if you are taking or if you are planning to take any over-the-counter or prescription medications or dietary supplements while using these medicines. One or both drugs may need to be modified or a different drug may need to be prescribed. The following drugs and drug classes interact with these medicines: Class I antiarrhythmic agents (eg, tocainide, mexiletine).

Side Effects:

Every drug is capable of producing side effects. Many patients experience no, or minor, side effects. The frequency and severity of side effects depend on many factors including dose, duration of therapy and individual susceptibility. Possible side effects include:

Cocaine –

Nervous System: Nervousness; restlessness; exaggerated sense of well-being; excitement; tremor; seizures; shock; depression; paranoia.

Circulatory System: Changes in heart rate; increased blood pressure.

Other: Damage to nasal tissues and to nasal septum (abuse); withdrawal symptoms.

Other Topical Anesthetics –

Skin: Allergic contact dermatitis; hives; redness; rash; swelling; burning; stinging; irritation; tenderness; skin sloughing; lesions; bluish discoloration.

Other: Difficulty breathing; painful urination; blood in urine; seizures.

Guidelines for Use:

- For external use only. Do not use in or around eyes.
- Do not eat, drink or chew gum for at least 1 hour after use in mouth or throat, or if the mouth or throat area still feels numb. This is especially important for children who eat more frequently.
- Topical anesthetics can impair the ability to swallow and increase risk of choking (especially when eating or drinking), injury (eg, biting tongue), or vocal damage in singers who use these products to mask vocal discomfort during performances.
- Use lowest dose possible that still provides adequate pain relief.
- Doses and frequency of use depend on the condition, area being treated, blood supply in the area, individual tolerance and dosage form. Individual products should be reviewed for their use and dosage guidelines. Consult your pharmacist or doctor for product-specific information.
- A thin layer of solution, cream, lotion or ointment is all that is necessary. Additional doses can cause severe side effects. Do not use for an extended period of time.
- Stop therapy if irritation, rash or redness develops. Consult your doctor.
- Dosage adjustments may be necessary for the elderly, severely ill patients or children.
- When lidocaine is used, all feeling in the treated skin may be blocked. Avoid accidental injury to the skin by not scratching, rubbing or exposing the skin to extreme hot or cold temperatures until all feeling has returned.
- Store these products at room temperature unless otherwise instructed by specific product label guidelines. Avoid extreme heat, cold, sunlight or moisture.

If you have any questions, consult your doctor, pharmacist, or health care provider.

	Generic Name *Brand Name Examples*	Supplied As	Generic Available
otc	**Benzocaine**		
	Bicozene, Lanacane	**Cream**: 5%, 6%	Yes
	Detane	**Gel**: 7.5%	No
	Americaine First Aid, Boil-Ease, Foille Medicated First Aid, Chiggerex[1]	**Ointment**: 5%, 20%	No
	Dermoplast, Solarcaine	**Lotion**: 8%, 20%	No
	Chigger-Tox,[1] *Sting-Kill*	**Liquid**: 20%	No
	Aerocaine, Aerotherm, Dermacoat, Dermoplast, FoillePlus, Foille Medicated FirstAid, Lanacane, Solarcaine	**Aerosol/Spray**: 4.5%, 5%, 13.6%, 20%	No
otc	**Butamben Picrate**		
	Butesin Picrate	**Ointment:** 1%	No
otc	**Dibucaine**		
	Nupercainal	**Cream**: 0.5%	No
	Nupercainal	**Ointment**: 1%	Yes
otc	**Lidocaine HCl**		
	Dr. Scholl's Cracked Heel Relief, Solarcaine Aloe Extra Burn Relief, Unguentine Plus	**Cream**: 0.5%, 2%	No
	Solarcaine Aloe Extra Burn Relief, DermaFlex	**Gel**: 0.5%, 2.5%	No
	Xylocaine	**Ointment:** 2.5%, 5%	Yes
	Bactine Antiseptic Anesthetic, ProTech First-Aid Stik, SkeeterStik, Zilactin-L	**Liquid**: 2.5%, 4%	No
	Bactine Antiseptic Anesthetic, Medi-Quik, Solarcaine Aloe ExtraBurn Relief	**Spray**: 0.5%, 2%, 2.5%	No
otc	**Pramoxine HCl**		
	Prax, Tronothane HCl	**Cream**: 1%	No
	Itch-X, PrameGel	**Gel**: 1%	No
	Prax	**Lotion**: 1%	No
	Itch-X	**Spray**: 1%	No

	Generic Name *Brand Name Examples*	Supplied As	Generic Available
otc	**Tetracaine**		
	Pontocaine	**Cream**: 1%	No
	Pontocaine	**Ointment**: 0.5%	No
	Topical Anesthetic Combinations		
Rx	*Cetacaine*	**Aerosol, Gel, Liquid, Ointment**:14% benzocaine, 2% tetracaine	No
Rx	*EMLA*	**Cream**: 2.5% lidocaine, 2.5% prilocaine	No

[1] Amount of anesthetic in the product is unknown.

Similar products of equal strengths are listed together in this table. However, they may not share the same inactive ingredients. For further information about the ingredients in these products, check individual package labels.

Type of Drug:

Topical anesthetics for skin discomfort and pain.

How the Drug Works:

Topical local anesthetics applied externally inhibit conduction of nerve impulses from sensory nerves, thereby producing anesthesia (lack of feeling, numbness). Abrasions or skin ulcers increase the absorption of the drug and therefore increase its effectiveness; however, side effects can also be increased.

Uses:

To relieve skin pain, itching and discomfort associated with minor burns, scalds, prickly heat, abrasions, sunburn, allergy to certain plants (such as poison ivy), insect bites, eczema and other skin conditions.

Lidocaine/Prilocaine: To ease the pain of some injections.

Precautions:

Do not use in the following situations:

allergy to any component of the product
bacterial infection
eyes, use in or around

Use with caution in the following situations:

allergy to externally applied drugs
children
elderly
illness, acute
infection or damaged skin at siteof use
liver disease
blood disorders (eg,methemoglobinemia)

Chronic use – Do not apply to large areas of the body or use for prolonged periods of time. Chronic use may result in tissue irritation, breathing difficulties, seizures, low blood pressure, mental confusion, ringing in the ears and blurred or poor vision.

Pregnancy:

Lidocaine – Studies in pregnant women or in animals have been judged not to show a risk to the fetus. However, no drug should be used during pregnancy unless clearly needed.

Other anesthetics – Adequate studies have not been done in pregnant women, or animal studies may have shown a risk to the fetus. Use only if clearly needed and potential benefits outweigh the possible hazards to the fetus.

Breastfeeding: Lidocaine appears in breast milk. It is not known if other anesthetics appear in breast milk. Consult your doctor before breastfeeding.

Children: Safety and effectiveness of tetracaine have not been established in children less than 12 years of age. Safety and effectiveness of the other anesthetics have not been established in children less than 1 year of age.

Elderly: Dosages may need to be adjusted according to age, size and physical condition.

Tartrazine: Some of these products may contain the dye tartrazine (FD&C Yellow No. 5) which can cause allergic reactions in certain individuals. Check package label when available or consult your doctor or pharmacist.

Sulfites: Some of these products may contain sulfite preservatives which can cause allergic reactions in certain individuals. Check package label when available or consult your doctor or pharmacist.

Drug Interactions:

Tell your doctor or pharmacist if you are taking or if you are planning to take any over-the-counter or prescription medications or dietary supplements while taking this medicine. Doses of one or both drugs may need to be modified or a different drug may need to be prescribed. Class I antiarrhythmic drugs (eg, tocainide and mexiletine) interact with this medicine.

Side Effects:

Every drug is capable of producing side effects. Many patients experience no, or minor, side effects. The frequency and severity of side effects depend on many factors including dose, duration of therapy and individual susceptibility. Possible side effects include: Allergic contact dermatitis; redness; rash; swelling; burning; stinging; irritation; lesions; sloughing of skin.

Guidelines for Use:

- For external use only. Do not use in or around the eyes.
- Topical anesthetics only relieve pain. They do not promote healing or prevent infection.
- Stop therapy and contact your doctor if irritation, rash, redness, blisters or swelling develop.
- Use the minimal effective dose. Doses and frequency of use depend on thecondition, area being treated, blood supply in the area, individual tolerance anddosage form. Individual products should be reviewed for their use and dosageguidelines. Consult your pharmacist or doctor for product-specific information.
- A thin layer of solution, cream, lotion or ointment is all that is necessary.Additional benefit will not be achieved with larger amounts.
- Apply to the affected area as needed. Ointments and creams may be applied togauze or a bandage before applying to skin.
- When lidocaine/prilocaine is used, all feeling in the treated skin may be blocked.Avoid accidental injury to the skin by not scratching, rubbing or exposing the skinto extreme hot or cold temperatures until all feeling has returned.
- Store at room temperature.

If you have any questions, consult your doctor, pharmacist, or health care provider.

Generic Name *Brand Name Examples*	Supplied As	Generic Available
Rx **Cantharidin**		
Verr-Canth	**Liquid**: 0.7%	No

Type of Drug:

An agent that promotes sloughinglpeeling of skin; skin softening dissolving agent; wart remover.

How the Drug Works:

Cantharidin causes a sloughing of benign skin growths (eg, warts) by destroying cells in the epidermal layer (outer layer of skin). It does not attack deeper tissue at prescribed doses; therefore, there is no scarring from external application.

Uses:

To treat warts.

To treat molluscum contagiosum (a disease which causes soft rounded tumors on the skin).

Precautions:

Do not use in the following situations:

- ano-genital area (anus, genitals)
- birthmarks
- diabetics
- eyes
- inflamed or irritated tissue
- lesions treated with other agents
- moles
- mucous membranes
- poor circulation
- skin folds (eg, between fingers and toes)
- warts with hair growing from them

Use with caution in the following situations:

- eyelid warts
- fair complexion (eg, blond hair, blue eyes)

Pregnancy: Adequate studies have not been done in pregnant women, or animal studies may have shown a risk to the fetus. Use only if clearly needed and potential benefits outweigh the possible hazards to the fetus.

Breastfeeding: It is not known if cantharidin appears in breast milk. Use is not recommended while breastfeeding. Consult your doctor.

Side Effects:

Every drug is capable of producing side effects. Many patients experience no, or minor, side effects. The frequency and severity of side effects depend on many factors including dose, duration of therapy and individual susceptibility. Possible side effects include: Itching; inflammation; pain; ring-shaped warts; skin color changes.

Guidelines for Use:

- For external use only.
- May produce blisters on normal skin or mucous membranes. If it is spilled on skin, wipe it off at once with alcohol, acetone or tape remover. Then wash with warm, soapy water and rinse well.
- If spilled on mucous membranes or in the eyes, flush with water, remove the residue and flush with water again for an additional 15 minutes. Contact your doctor.
- If burning or tenderness occurs, soak the area in cool water for 10 to 15 minutes. Repeat as required. If soreness and blisters persist, contact your doctor.
- Patients with fair skin and blue eyes should expect a more intense reaction to the drug.
- Do *not* apply to the same lesion more than once per week. Delay a second application if inflammation is too severe.
- Do *not* use in the ano-genital area.
- Tingling, burning and itching may occur within a few hours after application. This is not cause for alarm unless symptoms persist or worsen.
- The application site is usually tender for 2 to 6 days.
- Antibiotic ointment or cream is recommended until new skin grows back in the treated area.
- Preparation of the area for drug use depends on the nature of the growth. Such preparation and frequency of treatment must be discussed with and directed by a doctor experienced in using the drug.

If you have any questions, consult your doctor, pharmacist, or health care provider.

	Generic Name *Brand Name Example*	Supplied As	Generic Available
Rx	**Podofilox**		
	Condylox	**Gel**: 0.5%	No
	Condylox	**Solution**: 0.5%	No

Type of Drug:

An agent that promotes cell death of ano-genital wart tissue.

How the Drug Works:

The exact mechanism of action is unknown. Podofilox prevents cell growth resulting in the destruction of the visible wart tissue.

Uses:

To treat external warts of the genital area; the gel is also used to treat external warts of the anal area (perianal).

Precautions:

Do not use in the following situations:

allergy or intolerance to any ingredient of the formulation
warts on mucous membranes
perianal warts (solution only)

Correct diagnosis of warts is essential. Certain types of genital warts are not to be treated with podofilox.

Pregnancy: Adequate studies have not been done in pregnant women. Use only if clearly needed and potential benefits outweigh the possible hazards to the fetus.

Breastfeeding: It is not known if podofilox appears in breast milk. Consult your doctor before you begin breastfeeding.

Children: Safety and effectiveness for use in children have not been established.

Drug Interactions:

Tell your doctor or pharmacist if you are taking or if you are planning to take any over-the-counter or prescription medications or dietary supplements with podofilox. Doses of one or both drugs may need to be modified or a different drug may need to be prescribed.

Side Effects:

Every drug is capable of producing side effects. Many podofilox users experience no, or minor, side effects. The frequency and severity of side effects depend on many factors including dose, duration of therapy and individual susceptibility. Possible side effects include:

Skin: Burning; pain; inflammation; stinging; scabbing; discoloration; rash; skin splitting; ulceration; itching; chafing; blistering; crusting; dryness; peeling; tingling; bleeding; tenderness; erosion; scarring.

Other: Headache; pain with intercourse; sleeplessness; offensive odor; dizziness; blood in the urine; vomiting.

Guidelines for Use:

- External use only. Use exactly as prescribed.
- Patient package insert available with product.
- Apply twice daily morning and evening (every 12 hours) for 3 consecutive days, then withhold use for 4 consecutive days. This 1-week treatment cycle may be repeated up to 4 times until there is no visible wart tissue. If the response is incomplete after 4 treatment weeks, stop using and consider an alternative treatment. Safety and effectiveness of more than 4 treatment weeks have not been established. There is no evidence to suggest that more frequent applications will increase effectiveness.
- Wash hands thoroughly before each application. Apply podofilox with the applicator tip (supplied with the drug). Use the minimum amount of medicine necessary to cover the wart. The gel may also be applied with the finger.
- Allow the solution to dry before returning skin surfaces to their normal positions.
- After each treatment, the used applicator should be carefully disposed of and patients should wash their hands.
- Do not alter recommended method of application, frequency of application and duration of usage.
- Podofilox is not indicated in the treatment of internal mucous membrane warts (including those of the urethra, rectum and vagina).
- If you miss a dose of this drug, wait until the next scheduled dose and extend treatment accordingly.
- Avoid contact with the eyes. If contact occurs, immediately flush the eye(s) thoroughly with water and contact your doctor.
- *Storage* — Avoid excessive heat. Keep product away from open flame. Store at controlled room temperature between 59° to 86°F. Do not freeze.

If you have any questions, consult your doctor, pharmacist, or health care provider.

	Brand Name Examples	Supplied As
otc	*Calicylic Creme*[2,3,4]	**Cream**: 5%, 10%
otc	*Compound W,*[1,9] *Duoplant Gel*	**Gel**: 17%
otc	*Hydrisalic* [1]	**Gel**: 5%
otc	*Compound W,*[1,5,8,9] *Off-Ezy Wart Remover,*[1,8,9] *Wart-Off Maximum Strength,*[1,7] *Occlusal-HP, Duofilm*[1,7]	**Liquid**: 17%
otc	*Gordofilm*	**Liquid**: 16.7%
otc	*Compound W, Compound W Wart Remover for Kids*	**Pad**: 40%
otc	*Salactic Film*[5,8]	**Film**: 17%
otc	*Mediplast*	**Plaster**: 40%
Rx	*Trans-Ver-Sal*	**Transdermal patch**: 15%
otc	*Gets-It* [6]	**Liquid**: 12%

[1] Contains alcohol.
[2] Contains cetyl alcohol.
[3] Contains urea.
[4] Contains methyl- and propylparabens.
[5] Contains isopropyl alcohol.
[6] Collodion base contains ether.
[7] Flexible collodion.
[8] Contains ether.
[9] Collodion.

Type of Drug:

An agent that promotes sloughing or peeling of skin; skin softening or dissolving.

How the Drug Works:

Salicylic acid produces sloughing of the horny layer of skin (keratin) by dissolving the "cement" between skin cells. This causes the thickened epithelium to swell, soften and slough off.

Uses:

To treat common warts and dry, scaly or calloused skin. Some products (not all) are approved for use in treating plantar warts. Read individual product labels carefully. Common warts have a rough, "cauliflower-like" appearance on the surface. Plantar warts are tender and located on the bottom of the foot.

Precautions:

Do not use in the following situations:

- allergy to salicylic acid or its ingredients
- birthmarks
- diabetes
- irritated, infected, reddened skin
- genital warts
- large areas, especially children
- moles
- breastfeeding
- open wounds
- poor circulation
- pregnancy
- warts on face or mucous membranes (inside mouth, nose, lips, anus, genitals)

warts with hair growing from them, red edges or unusual color

Use with caution in the following situations:

kidney disease
liver disease

Salicylic poisoning: Prolonged use over large areas has caused salicylic poisoning. Symptoms include nausea; vomiting; dizziness; ringing in ears; hearing loss; diarrhea. For additional information on salicylate side effects, see the salicylate monograph.

Pregnancy: Adequate studies have not been done in pregnant women. Do not use during pregnancy without consulting your doctor.

Breastfeeding: Salicylic acid appears in breast milk. Because of the potential for serious side effects in breastfed infants, decide whether to discontinue breastfeeding or discontinue the drug. Consult your doctor.

Children: Do not use in young children (ages are specified in the product packaging).

Drug Interactions:

Tell your doctor or pharmacist if you are using or if you are planning to use any topical over-the-counter or prescription medications or dietary supplements with salicylic acid (including bismuth subsalicylate). One or both drugs may need to be modified or a different drug may need to be prescribed. Tretinoin (eg, *Retin-A*) interacts with topical salicylic acid.

Consider all drug interactions reported for salicylates (see monograph) when using this drug.

Side Effects:

Every drug is capable of producing side effects. Many topical salicylic acid users experience no, or minor, side effects. The frequency and severity of side effects depend on many factors including dose, duration of therapy and individual susceptibility. Possible side effects include:

Skin: Excessive redness; excessive sloughing and scaling; localized irritation.

Guidelines for Use:

- For external use only. Use exactly as instructed.
- Apply once or twice daily as needed for 12 weeks.
- *Hydrisalic Gel* and *Trans-Ver-Sal* — Apply medicine at night and cover area. Wash off in the morning.
- Avoid contact with eyes, face, genitals, rectum, mucous membranes (eg, mouth, nose, genitals, lips) and normal skin.
- May produce reddening or scaling of skin when used on open skin lesions.
- Wash affected area. Soak skin in warm water 5 minutes before applying salicylic acid to enhance the effect. Remove loose tissue with brush, wash cloth or emery board and dry skin thoroughly.
- Wash hands thoroughly after use.
- Discontinue treatment if excessive irritation or discomfort persists and consult your doctor.
- Do not use on irritated, infected or reddened skin, if you are a diabetic, or if you have poor blood circulation.
- Do not use on moles, birthmarks, warts with hair growing from them, genital warts, warts on face or mucous membranes.
- If contact with eyes or mucous membranes occurs, flush thoroughly with water for 15 minutes and contact your doctor.
- Avoid inhaling the vapors of the medicine.
- Prolonged use over large areas may cause salicylism. This is most likely in children and in patients with liver or kidney damage.
- Medicine should not come into contact with normal skin surrounding warts.
- Keep away from fire and flame. Contents are flammable.

If you have any questions, consult your doctor, pharmacist, or health care provider.

	Generic Name *Brand Name Examples*	Supplied As	Use
otc	**Dexpanthenol**		
	Panthoderm[1]	**Cream**: 2%	To relieve itching and aid healing of skin in mild eczemas, minor wounds, insect bites, poison ivy, poison oak, minor skin irritations, diaper rash and chafing
	Urea		
Rx	*Carmol 40*	**Cream**: 40%	To slough off dead skin or scabbed from burns and promote healing of infected skin sores
otc	*Nutraplus,*[1] *Rea-Lo,*[2,5] *Ureacin-20,*[1,4] *Carmol 20*	**Cream**: 10%, 20%, 30%	To moisturize skin in dry skin conditions and to treat very dry, rough, cracked, hardened or calloused skin
	Aquacare,[5] *Carmol 10, Rea-Lo, Ultra Mide 25, Ureacin-10*[1,4,5]	**Lotion**: 10%, 15%, 25%	
otc	**Petrolatum and Lanolin**		
	A and D[3]	**Ointment**	To treat and prevent diaper rash; heal dry, flaky and chafed skin; protects and soothes minor cuts and burns
otc	**Vitamin A and D**		
	Lobana Derm-Ade[1,5]	**Cream**	To provide relief of discomfort due to minor skin irritations including burns, sunburn, windburn, cuts and scrapes, bed sores and chapped skin; to treat and prevent diaper rash; ointment protects skin against wetness from urine, feces and other skin irritants
	Lobana Peri-Garde[5]	**Ointment**	
otc	**Vitamin E**		
	Vite E,[1] *Vitec*	**Cream, Lotion**	For control of dry or chapped skin. Also for temporary relief of minor skin disorders such as burns, sunburn and irritated skin

	Generic Name *Brand Name Examples*	Supplied As	Use
otc	**Zinc Oxide**		
	Balmex, Desitin[1,2,3]	**Ointment**	To treat and prevent diaper rash; protects against wetness from urine, feces and other skin irritants

[1] Contains parabens.
[2] Contains talc.
[3] Contains lanolin.
[4] Contains EDTA.
[5] Contains alcohol.

The emollients contain a diverse group of chemicals. This monograph does not follow the typical format due to the lack of consistency of information from product to product. Primary ingredients and their uses are listed. However, they may not share the same inactive ingredients. For additional information about a particular product, consult your pharmacist or doctor.

Type of Drug:

A variety of agents with differing primary uses (eg, skin softening, moisturizing, healing, soothing).

Uses:

Uses are indicated in the preceding table.

Guidelines for Use:

- For external use only.
- Do not use in eyes or allow to come in contact with the eye(s).
- Do not use if you are allergic to any ingredient of the products.
- Do not use on irritated or broken skin without consulting your doctor or pharmacist.
- If the condition for which these preparations is used persists or worsens or if irritation, develops, discontinue use and consult your doctor.
- Apply locally to affected skin with gentle massage. For minor burns and other minor skin irritations, the affected area may be covered with a loose layer of gauze or other suitable dressing. This is not required.
- These products do not contain antibiotic ingredients. Do not use to treat infection.
- *Vitamin A & D* — Do not apply over deep or puncture wounds, infections or lacerations.
- Stinging, burning, itching or irritation may develop with the use of these products.

If you have any questions, consult your doctor, pharmacist, or health care provider.

	Generic Name *Brand Name Examples*	Supplied As	Other
	Emollients		Uses: To lubricate and moisturize skin. To reduce dryness and itching.
Rx	*Lac-Hydrin*	**Lotion**:	
otc	*Allercreme Ultra, Aveeno, Catrix, Complex 15, Curel Moisturizing, Cutemol, Hydrisinol, Keri Creme, Lubriderm, Masse Breast, Neutrogena Norwegian Formula, Nivea Moisturizing, Nutraderm, Pedi-Vit A, Pen-Kera, Purpose DrySkin, Shepard's Skin*	**Cream**:	Guidelines for Use: •For external use only. •Do not use in eyes. •If the condition for which these preparations are used persists, or if irritation develops, discontinue use and consult your doctor.
	Balmex	**Ointment**:	
	Neutrogena Body, NiveaMoisturizing, Nivea Skin	**Oil**:	•Apply locally to affected skin with gentle massage.
	Allercreme Skin, Aveeno, Balmex, Complex 15, Corn Huskers, Curel, Derma Viva, DML, Epilyt,Esoterica, Eucerin, Keri, Keri-Light, Lac-Hydrin Five, LactiCare, LobanaBody, Lubriderm, Moisturel, Neutrogena Body, Nivea, Moisturizing, Nutraderm, Pro-Cute, Ultra Derm, Wondra	**Lotion**:	For minor burns and other minor skin irritations, cover affected area with a layer of gauze or other suitable dressing.
otc	**Skin Protectants**		Uses: To protect skin against contact irritants and to coat minor sores.
	Covicone, Kerodex	**Cream**:	
	BlisterGard, New-Skin	**Liquid**:	
	Hydropel, Silicone No. 2, White Cloverine Salve	**Ointment**:	Guidelines for Use: •For external use only.
	New-Skin Antiseptic	**Spray liquid**:	•Do not use silicone-containing preparations on rash or wet, oozing lesions.
	Aerozoin	**Spray**:	

	Generic Name *Brand Name Examples*	Supplied As	Other
	Benzoin, TinBen, TinCo-Ben	**Tincture**:	
otc	**Bath Oils**		Uses: To relieve minor skin irritations and itching of common skin problems and dry skin.
	Alpha Keri Therapeutic, AveenoOilated Bath, Aveeno Regular, Cameo, Domol Bath and Shower, Lubriderm, LubraSol, Nutraderm, Nutra-Soothe, Therapeutic Bath, *Ultra Derm*	**Oil**:	
	Pedi-Bath Salts	**Salts**:	Guidelines for Use: •For external use only. •Use caution to avoid slipping in the tub.
	Alpha Keri	**Spray**:	•Do not use on raw skin. •Avoid contact with the eyes; flush with clear water.

If you have any questions, consult your doctor, pharmacist, or health care provider.

Generic Name *Brand Name Examples*	Supplied As	Generic Available
otc **Capsaicin**		
Zostrix	**Cream**: 0.025%	No
Zostrix-HP	**Cream**: 0.075%	No

Type of Drug:

Topical analgesic (pain relieving) cream.

How the Drug Works:

Capsaicin is a natural chemical derived from plants. It is believed that capsaicin causes the skin to become insensitive to pain by causing the removal of substance P, a pain-transmitting compound from the nerve endings. With the lowered amount of substance P at the nerve endings, pain impulses cannot be transmitted to the brain. The active ingredient is found in red chili peppers.

Uses:

For temporary relief of pain from rheumatoid arthritis, osteoarthritis, painful diabetic neuropathy or following shingles (herpes zoster).

Precautions:

Do not use in the following situations:

- allergy to any ingredient in the products
- in or around the eyes or other mucous membranes
- open wounds or damaged skin

Children: Do not use in children under 2 except with the supervision of a doctor.

Side Effects:

Every drug is capable of producing side effects. Many capsaicin users experience no, or minor, side effects. The frequency and severity of side effects depend on many factors including dose, duration of therapy and individual susceptibility. Possible side effects include a burning sensation upon application (usually temporary).

Guidelines for Use:

- For external use only.
- Onset of relief may take several weeks.
- Apply to affected area 3 to 4 times daily to achieve maximum pain relief. Thoroughly rub into the area so no residue is left on the skin surface. Wash hands after application.
- Avoid contact with eyes or other mucous membranes. If contact occurs, flush the affected area thoroughly with water.
- Do not use on children under 2 unless directed by a doctor.
- Do not apply to open wounds, damaged or irritated skin.
- Do not bandage tightly.
- Discontinue use if condition worsens or does not improve after 28 days. Consult a doctor.
- Warm water or excessive sweating may intensify burning sensation.
- Keep this and all medications out of the reach of children.

If you have any questions, consult your doctor, pharmacist, or health care provider.

	Brand Name Examples	Supplied As
otc	*Benadryl, Maximum Strength Benadryl 2%*	**Cream or spray**: 1% or 2% diphenhydramine HCl
otc	*Cala-gen*	**Lotion**: 1% diphenhydramine HCl, camphor, 2% alcohol
otc	*Calamycin*	**Lotion**: Pyrilamine maleate, 10% zinc oxide, 10%calamine, benzocaine, chloroxylenol, zirconium oxide
otc	*Clearly Cala-gel*	**Gel**: Diphenhydramine HCl, menthol, zinc acetate, benzethonium chloride
otc	*Dermamycin*	**Cream**: 2% diphenhydramine HCl
otc	*Derma-Pax*	**Lotion**: 0.22% pyrilamine maleate, 0.22% pheniramine maleate, 0.06% chlorpheniramine maleate
otc	*Dermarest*	**Gel**: 2% diphenhydramine HCl, 2% resorcinol
otc	*Dermarest Plus*	**Gel or spray**: 2% diphenhydramine HCl, 1% menthol
otc	*Di-Delamine*	**Gel or spray**: 1% diphenhydramine HCl, 0.5% tripelennamine HCl, 0.12% benzalkonium chloride and 1% menthol
otc	*Sting-Eze*	**Concentrate**: Diphenhydramine HCl, camphor, phenol, benzocaine and eucalyptol
otc	*Ziradryl*	**Lotion**: 2% diphenhydramine HCl and 2% zinc oxide
otc	*Zonalon*	**Cream**: 5% doxepin HCl

Type of Drug:

Topical antihistamines.

How the Drug Works:

The topical antihistamines counteract the effects of histamine. Histamine is the chemical in the body which causes blood vessels to dilate (widen), smooth muscle to contract, and heart rate and stomach secretions to increase. These effects play a role in allergic reactions.

Topical antihistamines have some local anesthetic activity and relieve itching.

Other ingredients which may be combined with the antihistamines include benzocaine (local anesthetic); camphor, menthol or phenol (anti-itching and anesthetic action); and calamine, titanium dioxide, zirconium oxide and zinc oxide (astringents).

Uses:

To treat hives, insect bites or stings, and itching due to minor skin disorders, poison ivy, poison oak or sumac; mild sunburn.

Precautions:

Do not use in the following situations:

allergy to this medicine or any of its ingredients
narrow angle glaucoma, untreated (doxepin only)
history of urinary retention, history of (doxepin only)

Use with caution in the following situations: Redness, swelling, inflammation, or pain.

Pregnancy: There are no adequate and well-controlled studies of doxepin in pregnant women. Use during pregnancy only if clearly needed.

Breastfeeding: It is not known if topical doxepin appears in breastmilk. Consult your doctor before you begin breastfeeding.

Children: Do not use on children less than 2 years of age. Safety and effectiveness of doxepin in children have not been established. Consult a doctor before treating chlidren less than 12 years of age with *Benadryl.*

Drug Interactions:

Tell your doctor or pharmacist if you are taking or planning to take any over-the-counter or prescription medications or dietary supplements while using topical antihistamines. Doses of one or both drugs may need to be modified or a different drug may need to be prescribed. The following drugs and drug classes interact with doxepin only:

alcohol
antiarrhythmic drugs (eg, *Quinidine)*
carbamazepine (eg, *Tegretol)*
cimetidine (eg, *Tagamet)*
MAO inhibitors (eg, *Parnate)*
phenothiazines (eg, *Thorazine)*

Side Effects:

Every drug is capable of producing side effects. Many topical antihistamine users experience no, or minor, side effects. The frequency and severity of side effects depend on many factors including dose, duration of therapy, and individual susceptibility. Possible side effects include:

Doxepin only – Drowsiness; headache; fatigue; dizziness; emotional changes; dry mouth or lips; fluid retention; thirst; taste changes.

Skin: Dry skin; abnormal skin sensation; burning and stinging; increased itching or aggravation of skin disorder; local irritation; rash; redness.

Guidelines for Use:

- For external use only. Do not use in or near eyes.
- Do not apply to mucous membranes or to skin which is blistered, raw, or oozing a liquid.
- Do not use occlusive dressings unless directed by your doctor.
- If rash, burning, or irritation develops or worsens where the medicine is applied, stop using the medicine. Wash area with soap and water and contact your doctor.
- Avoid prolonged use or use on extensive skin areas, especially in infants.
- Do not use on chickenpox or measles unless supervised by your doctor.
- *Doxepin* — Allow an interval of 3 to 4 hours between applications. Do not bandage area being treated. May cause drowsiness. Use caution while driving or performing other tasks requiring alertness, coordination, or physical dexterity. Alcohol may cause added drowsiness. Do not use for more than 8 days.

If you have any questions, consult your doctor, pharmacist, or health care provider.

	Generic Name *Brand Name Examples*	Use(s)
otc	**Iodine** *Iodex*	For external use against bacteria, fungi, viruses, spores, protozoa, and yeasts. Available as an ointment, solution, and tincture.
otc	**Povidone-Iodine** *ACU-dyne*, Betadine, *Iodex*, *Operand*, *Pharmadine*, *Polydine*	Povidone-iodine liberates about 9% to 12% free iodine. It is bactericidal but does not irritate skin and mucous membranes (unless one is allergic to iodine). Also cleanses and deodorizes. Available as an ointment, solution, liquid, gauze pads, swabs, swabsticks, skin cleanser, surgical scrub solution, spray, cream, shampoo, perineal wash, mouthwash, vaginal suppositories, foil, douche, foam, pad, and stick.
otc	**Thimerosal**	To treat contaminated wounds and disinfect healthy skin prior to surgery. Contains 49% mercury and has activity against bacteria and fungus. Available as a tincture, solution, and swabs.
Rx	**Hexachlorophene** *pHisoHex*, *Septi-Soft*	For use as a surgical scrub and skin cleanser. Hexachlorophene is an antibacterial agent with activity against bacteria. Available as a foam, liquid skin cleanser, detergent cleaner, wash, shampoo, and sponge.
otc	**Chlorhexidine Gluconate** *Chlorostat*, *Hibiclens Antiseptic/Antimicrobial Skin*, *Hibiclens*, *Hibistat Germicidal Hand*	For use as a surgical scrub, preoperative skin cleanser, skin wound cleanser, and hand rinse. Chlorhexidine gluconate is an antibacterial agent effective against a wide range of bacteria (including *Pseudomonas aeruginosa*). Available as a skin cleanser, sponge, liquid, towlettes, and rinse.
otc	**Benzalkonium Chloride** *Benza*, *Benz-all*, *Zephiran*	For disinfection of skin, mucous membranes, and small wounds; preoperative preparation of skin; surgeons' hand and arm soaks; treatment of wounds; preservation of ophthalmic solutions; irrigations of the eye, body cavities, bladder, and urethra; and vaginal douching.An anti-rust factor in this agent has been shown to be effective in the chemical disinfection of professional and hospital instruments and equipment. Benzalkonium chloride is a rapidly-acting anti-infective with a long duration of action. It is active against bacteria, some viruses, fungi, and protozoa. Available as a solution, tincture, and spray.

	Generic Name *Brand Name Examples*	Use(s)
otc	**Glutaraldehyde** *Cidex, Cidex Formula-7, Cidex Plus*	To disinfect and sterilize certain types of plastic, metal, or rubber respiratory or anesthesia equipment against vegetative bacteria (eg, *Pseudomonas aeruginosa*, pathogenic fungi, and certain viruses). Glutaraldehyde is mildly acidic. Do not use on skin or mucous membranes. Available as a 2.4% and 3.4% solution and test strips.
otc	**Peracetic Acid** *Cidex PA*	To disinfect and sterilize metals (stainless steel and aluminium alloy), plastics, and elastomers. Do not use with brass or copper. Avoid contact with eyes. Available as a 0.08% solution.
otc	**Sodium Hypochlorite** *Dakin's Solution Half Strength, Dakin's Solution Full Strength*	To disinfect skin against vegetative bacteria and viruses and, to some degree, against spores and fungi. It has germicidal, deodorizing, and bleaching properties. Sodium hypochlorite is bleach and is not to be used on skin or wounds. Sodium hypochlorite may produce chemical burns if it comes in contact with skin or eyes.Available as a solution.
otc	**Oxychlorosene Sodium** *Clorpactin WCS-90*	To treat localized infections, remove dead tissue, counteract odorous discharges; for use as a pre- and postoperative irrigant; and for cleansing and disinfecting fistulas, the sinus tract, empyemas, and wounds.Available as a powder for solution or a concentrate.

Type of Drug:

Antiseptics and germicides (topical); agents that prevent or arrest the spread of disease-causing microorganisms.

Uses:

Selected products and their primary use(s) are included in the table above.

Guidelines for Use:

- Doses and frequency of use depend on the condition, area to be treated, individual tolerance, and dosage form. Individual products should be reviewed for their use and dosage guidelines. Consult your pharmacist or doctor for product-specific information.
- Discontinue use and consult your doctor if redness, irritation, swelling, or pain increases.
- *Sodium hypochlorite* is toxic to fish. Do not dispose product where it will drain into lakes, streams, or public water.
- *Benzalkonium chloride's* effects are deactivated by soap.

If you have any questions, consult your doctor, pharmacist, or health care provider.

	Generic Name *Brand Name Examples*	Supplied As	Generic Available
otc	**Methionine**	**Tablets**: 500 mg	Yes
		Powder: 200 mg/tsp	Yes
	Pedameth, Uracid	**Capsules**: 200 mg	No
	Pedameth	**Liquid**: 75 mg/5 mL	No
otc	**Miscellaneous Diaper Rash Products**		
	Balmex Diaper Rash	**Ointment**: 11.3% zinc oxide, aloe vera gel, balsam peru	No
	Desitin	**Ointment**: 40% zinc oxide, cod liver oil, talc, petrolatum, lanolin	No
	Desitin Creamy	**Ointment**: 10% zinc oxide	No
	Desitin with Zinc Oxide	**Powder**: 88.2% corn starch, 10% zinc oxide	No
	Diaparene	**Powder**: Methylbenzethonium chloride, corn starch	No
	Diaparene Medicated	**Cream**: 0.1% methylbenzethonium chloride, white petrolatum, glycerin	No
	Diaparene Peri-Anal Medicated	**Ointment**: 0.1% methylbenzethonium chloride, zinc oxide, cod liver oil, white petrolatum, starch, lanolin calcium caseinate	No
	Flanders Buttocks	**Ointment**: Zinc oxide, balsam peru	No
	Mexsana Medicated	**Powder**: Corn starch, zinc oxide, kaolin, benzethonium chloride	No

Type of Drug:

Diaper rash products.

How the Drug Works:

Methionine (for oral ingestion) creates an acid condition in the urine that results in an ammonia-free urine, and therefore, less diaper rash, odor, skin inflammation, and ulceration by urine.

The agents applied externally as ointment, cream, or powder contain a variety of ingredients:

Antimicrobial agents (benzethonium chloride, methylbenzethonium chloride) minimize bacterial growth.

Balsam peru is claimed to promote wound healing and tissue repair but its effectiveness has not been documented.

Corn starch, kaolin, and talc absorb moisture.

Protectants (petrolatum, lanolin) and lubricants (glycerin, cod liver oil) minimize chafing and irritation.

Zinc oxide is an astringent that dries the skin.

Uses:

Methionine —

To prevent or treat diaper rash, urine odor, ammonia dermatitis (inflammation), and skin ulcers caused by excess ammonia in urine.

Topical products —

To provide a protective barrier against wetness and soothe and moisturize skin.

Precautions:

Do not use in the following situations:

liver disease, active (methionine only)
liver disease, history of (methionine only)

Side Effects:

Every drug is capable of producing side effects. Many diaper rash product users experience no, or minor, side effects. The frequency and severity of side effects depend on many factors including dose, duration of therapy, and individual susceptibility. Possible side effects related to topical diaper rash products include: Rash; irritation; itching; burning.

Guidelines for Use:

- *Methionine* —
  Dosage will be individualized. Do not exceed recommended dosage.
  Take with meals.
  Do not take with dairy products.
  Capsules may be opened and the contents mixed with food, formula, juice, or water.
  Adequate protein intake must be maintained during therapy to prevent below normal weight gain.
- *Ointments, creams, or powders* —
  For external use only.
  Apply to the affected area several times daily as needed, especially at bedtime or any time when exposure to wet diapers may be prolonged.
  Cleanse the affected area and allow it to dry before application.
  Do not use on broken skin.
  Avoid contact with the eyes.
  Keep powder away from child's face to avoid inhalation, which can cause breathing problems.
  Consult a doctor if condition worsens or symptoms do not improve within 7 days.

If you have any questions, consult your doctor, pharmacist, or health care provider.

	Generic Name *Brand Name Examples*	Supplied As	Generic Available
otc	**Minoxidil**		
	Rogaine for Men,[1] *Rogaine for Women*[1]	**Solution**: 2%	Yes
	Rogaine Extra Strength for Men[1]	**Solution**: 5%	No

[1] Contains alcohol.

Type of Drug:

Topical scalp agent. Promotes hair growth.

How the Drug Works:

It is not known how minoxidil stimulates scalp hair growth. It is possible that it dilates blood vessels in the scalp, which may improve hair follicle function and stimulate scalp hair growth.

Uses:

To treat male pattern baldness in men and diffuse hair loss or thinnning of hair on forehead or temples in females. There is no effect in men with predominantly frontal hair loss.

Unlabeled Use(s): Occasionally, doctors may prescribe minoxidil for alopecia areata (a disease in which patches of hair fall out over a period of a few days on any part of the body).

Precautions:

Do not use in the following situations:

- allergy to minoxidil or any of its ingredients
- childbirth-associated hair loss
- no family history of hair loss
- patients less than 18 years of age
- red, inflamed, infected, irritated, or painful scalp
- sudden or patchy hair loss
- undergoing therapy with another topical scalp medication
- unknown reason for hair loss
- women (*Rogaine Extra Strength* only)

Use with caution in the following situations:

- heart disease
- inflamed or diseased scalp

Results: At least 4 months of continuous use is generally required before evidence of hair growth can be expected. Further growth continues through 1 year of treatment. The new growth of hair is not permanent. Continued use is necessary to increase and keep hair growth or hair loss will begin again.

Pregnancy: Adequate studies have not been conducted in pregnant women. Do not use if you are pregnant.

Breastfeeding: Because of the potential for adverse effects, do not use when breastfeeding.

Children: Safety and effectiveness in patients less than 18 years of age have not been established. Do not use on babies and children.

Side Effects:

Every drug is capable of producing side effects. Many minoxidil users experience no, or minor, side effects. The frequency and severity of side effects depend upon many factors including dose, duration of therapy, and individual susceptibility. Possible side effects include:

Digestive Tract: Nausea; vomiting; diarrhea.

Nervous System: Headache; dizziness; faintness; lightheadedness; feeling of whirling motion.

Circulatory System: Blood pressure changes; changes in heart rate; chest pain; pounding in chest.

Other: Aches or pain; fluid retention; ear infections; weight gain; sinus infection; skin irritation or inflammation; hives.

Guidelines for Use:

- For external use only.
- Minoxidil is indicated for patients who have a general thinning of hair on the top of the scalp. It is not intended for frontal baldness or a receding hairline.
- *Rogaine Extra Strength* is not for use by women. It may cause facial hair growth and be harmful during pregnancy or breastfeeding.
- Dry hair and scalp prior to application.
- Apply 1 mL (or 6 sprays if using *Extra Strength for Men*) 2 times a day directly onto the scalp in the hair loss area. Do not apply to other parts of the body.
- Do not exceed 2 mL daily. Larger or more frequent doses do not speed up or increase hair growth, but do increase the chance of side effects.
- If applied with fingertips, wash hands afterwards.
- First hair growth may be soft, downy, colorless, and barely visible. After further treatment, the new hair should be the color and thickness of other scalp hair.
- Apply to a healthy scalp only. Inflammation or disease of the scalp (eg, abrasions, severe sunburn, psoriasis, dermatitis) may increase absorption of the drug and increase the risk of side effects. Be alert for a rapid heart rate, weight gain, edema (fluid retention), and other side effects.
- *Contains alcohol* — May cause burning or irritation of sensitive skin, eyes, and mucous membranes. If the drug comes in contact with the eyes, mucous membranes, or sensitive skin areas, bathe the area with large amounts of cool tap water. Consult your doctor if irritation continues.
- Do not use with other topical scalp medications.
- Discontinue use and consult your doctor if you experience chest pain, rapid heartbeat, faintness, dizziness, sudden unexplained weight gain, swollen hands or feet, redness, or irritation at application site.
- Evidence of hair growth usually takes at least 4 months. If you do not see hair regrowth in 4 months with *Extra Strength for Men*, 8 months with *Rogaine for Women*, or 12 months with *Rogaine for Men*, stop treatment and contact your doctor.
- Use continuously to increase and keep your hair regrowth. If treatment is stopped, new hair will probably be shed within a few months.
- If a treatment is missed, do not attempt to make it up. Apply next treatment at regularly scheduled time.
- *Caution* — Accidental oral ingestion could produce significant side effects. Avoid inhalation of the spray mist.
- Store at controlled room temperature (68° to 77°F).

If you have any questions, consult your doctor, pharmacist, or health care provider.

	Brand Name Examples	Supplied As	Generic Available
otc	*Aveeno*	**Cream, Lotion, Powder**: Colloidal oatmeal	No
otc	*Cala-gen, Calagesic*	**Lotion**: 8% calamine, 1% pramoxine HCl	No
otc	*Calaclear*	**Lotion**: 1% pramoxine HCl, 0.1% zinc acetate	No
otc	*Calamine*	**Lotion**: 6.97% calamine, 6.97% zinc oxide, glycerin, bentonite magma in calcium hydroxide solution	Yes
otc	*Ivy-Rid*	**Spray**: Isobutane, methylene chloride, benzalkonium chloride, alcohol, isopropyl myristate	No
otc	*Phenolated Calamine*	**Lotion**: 8% calamine, 8% zinc oxide, 2% glycerin, bentonite magma, 1% phenol in calcium hydroxide solution	Yes
otc	*RhuliAerosol*	**Solution**: 0.67% phenylcarbinol, 4.7% calamine, 0.025% menthol, 0.25% camphor, 1.15% benzocaine, 28.8% alcohol	No
otc	*RhuliGel*	**Gel**: 2% phenylcarbinol, 0.3% menthol, 0.3% camphor, 31% SD alcohol	No
otc	*RhuliSpray*	**Spray**: 0.67% phenylcarbinol, 4.7% calamine, 0.025% menthol, 0.25% camphor, 1.15% benzocaine, 28.8% alcohol	No

Type of Drug:

Poison ivy treatment products.

Uses:

To relieve itching, pain, and discomfort due to ivy, oak, and sumac poisoning. Some products are also recommended for nonpoisonous insect bites, sunburn, prickly heat, and other minor skin irritations.

In these products:

Benzalkonium chloride is used for its antimicrobial activity.

Benzocaine, phenylcarbinol, and pramoxine HCl are local anesthetics that temporarily relieve pain, itching, and irritation.

Calamine, zinc oxide, and zirconium oxide are used to shrink skin cells, thereby tightening skin.

Camphor, menthol, and methyl salicylate are counterirritants.

Colloidal oatmeal is a demulcent (soothing agent).

Isopropyl alcohol, phenol, and phenylcarbinol are antiseptics.

Precautions:

Children: Do not use on children less than 2 years of age without consulting your doctor.

Guidelines for Use:

- For external use only.
- Shake well before use.
- Before each use cleanse the skin with soap and water and dry the affected area.
- Apply to affected area 3 to 4 times daily.
- A cotton pledget or soft cloth may be used for ease of application.
- Avoid contact with the eyes and mucous membranes.
- If the condition for which these products are used worsens or does not improve within 7 days, or if rash, irritation, or allergy develops, discontinue use and consult your doctor.
- Store at room temperature (59° to 86°F).

If you have any questions, consult your doctor, pharmacist, or health care provider.

	Generic Name *Brand Name Examples*	Supplied As
otc	**Menthol**	
	Absorbine Jr., Cool'n Hot Gel, Cool Hot Gel, Eucalyptamint	**Gel, cream, ointment**
otc	**Methyl Salicylate**	
	Exocaine Plus Rub, Gordogesic Creme	**Gel, cream, ointment**
otc	**Methyl Salicylate** and **Menthol**	
	Analgesic Balm, Ben Gay, Icy Hot, Pain Bust-R II Cream, Podiacin Soak'n Massage Gel, Thera-gesic	**Gel, cream, ointment**
	Banalg Hospital Strength Lotion	**Lotion, liniment**
otc	**Methyl Salicylate**, **Menthol**, and **Camphor**	
	Ben Gay Ultra Strength Cream, Panalgesic Gold Cream	**Gel, cream, ointment**
	Banalg Muscle Pain Reliever	**Lotion, liniment**
otc	**Methyl Salicylate**, **Methyl Nicotinate**, and **Menthol**	
	ArthriCare Rub	**Gel, cream, ointment**
otc	**Methyl Salicylate**, **Methyl Nicotinate**, **Camphor**, and **Menthol**	
	Deep-Down Rub	**Gel, cream, ointment**
otc	**Triethanolamine Salicylate**	
	Aspercreme, Exocaine Odor Free Creme, Mobisyl Creme, Sportscreme	**Gel, cream, ointment**
	Aspercreme Rub	**Lotion, liniment**
otc	**Miscellaneous Combinations**	
	Heet Spray	**Aerosol**

Generic Name *Brand Name Examples*	**Supplied As**
Argesic Cream, Arthro-Therapy Gel, Eucalypta-mint 2000 Gel, Iodex w/Methyl Salicylate Ointment, Methagual, Myoflex Creme, Pain Relief Cream, Rid-a-Pain Cream, Rid-a-Pain HP Cream, Soltice Quick-Rub, Vicks Vapo Rub	**Gel, cream, ointment**
Arth-Rx Lotion, ArthriCare Lotion, ArthriCare Ultra Rub, Capsin Lotion, Sloan's Liniment	**Lotion, liniment**

Rubs and liniments contain a diverse group of chemicals. This monograph does not follow the usual format seen in this book due to the lack of consistency of information from product to product. For additional information about a particular product, consult your pharmacist or doctor.

Uses:

To relieve pain of muscular aches, nerve pain, rheumatism, arthritis, sprains, and similar conditions when skin is intact.

Precautions:

Do not use in the following situations:

allergy to any ingredient in the formulation
allergy to salicylates (eg, aspirin)

Tartrazine: Some of these products may contain the dye tartrazine (FD&C Yellow No. 5), which can cause allergic reactions in certain individuals. Check package label when available or consult your pharmacist or doctor.

Guidelines for Use:

- For external use only.
- Avoid contact with eyes and mucous membranes.
- Apply only to affected areas. Do not apply to irritated skin. Discontinue use if excessive irritation occurs.
- Consult your doctor if pain persists for more than 7 to 10 days, if redness is present, or if the condition affects a child younger than 12 years of age.
- If applied to large skin areas, salicylate side effects (eg, ringing in the ears, nausea, vomiting) may occur. May be toxic if ingested.
- May cause local irritation in patients with sensitive skin.

If you have any questions, consult your doctor, pharmacist, or health care provider.

	Generic Name *Brand Name Examples*	Supplied As	SPF
otc	**Creams, Foams, Gels, Lotions, Oils, and Sprays**		
	SolBar PF	**Cream**: Oxybenzone, octyl methoxycinnamate, octocrylene	50
	Banana Boat Baby, Banana Boat Maximum, Banana Boat Sport	**Lotion**: Octocrylene, octyl methoxycinnamate, oxybenzone, octyl salicylate	
	Hawaiian Tropic Baby Faces	**Lotion**: Octyl methoxycinnamate, octyl salicylate, titanium dioxide	
	Coppertone Sport	**Lotion**: Octyl methoxycinnamate, oxybenzone, homosalate, octyl salicylate	48
	Biosun Professional Sun Protection	**Lotion**: Octyl methoxycinnamate, octocrylene, oxybenzone, octyl salicylate	45
	Bullfrog for Babies	**Lotion**: Octocrylene, octyl methoxycinnamate, benzophenone-3, titanium dioxide, menthyl anthranilate, octyl salicylate	
	Bullfrog SuperBlock	**Lotion**: Octocrylene, octyl methoxycinnamate, oxybenzone, menthyl anthranilate, octyl salicylate, titanium dioxide	
	Coppertone All Day, Coppertone Oil-Free, Coppertone Shade	**Lotion**: Ethylhexyl p-methoxycinnamate, 2-ethylhexyl salicylate, oxybenzone, homosalate	
	Coppertone Water Babies	**Lotion**: Octyl methoxycinnamate, oxybenzone, octyl salicylate, homosalate	
	Hawaiian Tropic 45 Plus	**Lotion**: Octyl methoxycinnamate, octyl salicylate, titanium dioxide	
	Neutrogena Sunblock	**Lotion**: Homosalate, octyl methoxycinnamate, benzophenone-3, octyl salicylate	
	Coppertone Water Babies Lotion	**Spray**: Octyl methoxycinnamate, oxybenzone, octyl salicylate, homosalate	
	Coppertone Kids Wacky Foam	**Foam**: Octyl methoxycinnamate, oxybenzone, octyl salicylate, octocrylene	40

Coppertone Kids, Coppertone Kids Colorblock	**Lotion**: Octyl methoxycinnamate, octyl salicylate, oxybenzone, homosalate	40
Bullfrog Body Gel	**Gel**: Octocrylene, octyl methoxycinnamate, oxybenzone	36
Bullfrog for Kids	**Gel**: Benzophenone-3, octocrylene, octyl methoxycinnamate	
Bullfrog Quik Stick	**Stick**: Octyl methoxycinnamate, octocrylene, oxybenzone, octyl salicylate	
Elta Block	**Cream**: Octyl methoxycinnamate, octyl salicylate, zinc oxide, titanium dioxide	32
PreSun Ultra	**Cream**: Avobenzone, octyl methoxycinnamate, octyl salicylate, oxybenzone	30
Coppertone Shade	**Gel**: Ethylhexyl p-methoxycinnamate, homosalate, oxybenzone	
Kiss My Face	**Gel**: Titanium dioxide, octyl methoxycinnamate	
Fisher-Price Sunscreen for Kids, PreSun Ultra	**Gel**: Avobenzone, octyl methoxycinnamate, octyl salicylate, oxybenzone	
SolBar PF	**Liquid**: Octocrylene	
Bain de Soleil All Day Extended Protection, Bain de Soleil GentleBlock, Bain de Soleil Kids	**Lotion**: Octyl methoxycinnamate, octocrylene, oxybenzone, titanium dioxide	
Banana Boat Kids, Banana Boat Ultra	**Lotion**: Octyl methoxycinnamate, oxybenzone, octyl salicylate	
Bullfrog Body Lotion, Bullfrog Magic Block, Bullfrog Sport Lotion	**Lotion**: Octocrylene, octyl methoxycinnamate, oxybenzone, octyl salicylate	
Coppertone All Day, Coppertone Kids, Coppertone Kids Colorblock, Coppertone Oil-Free	**Lotion**: Ethylhexyl p-methoxycinnamate, 2-ethylexyl salicylate, homosalate, oxybenzone	
Coppertone Bug & Sun	**Lotion**: Octocrylene, ethylhexyl p-methoxycinnamate, oxybenzone, n,n-diethyl m-toluamide	

Coppertone Shade UVA Guard	**Lotion**: Ethylhexyl p-methoxycinnamate, oxybenzone, 2-ethylhexyl salicylate, homosalate, avobenzone	30
Coppertone Sport, *Coppertone Water Babies*	**Lotion**: Octyl methoxycinnamate, oxybenzone, homosalate, octyl salicylate	
DuraScreen	**Lotion**: Octyl methoxycinnamate, octyl salicylate, benzophenone-3, phenylbenzimidazole sulfonic acid, titanium dioxide	
Hawaiian Tropic 30 Plus, *Hawaiian Tropic Super Waterproof*	**Lotion**: Octyl salicylate, octyl methoxycinnamate, titanium dioxide	
Neutrogena Sunblock	**Lotion**: Octyl methoxycinnamate, homosalate, octyl salicylate, benzolphenone-3, avobenzone	
Neutrogena Kids, *Neutrogena Oil-Free*	**Lotion**: Homosalate, octyl methoxycinnamate, benzophenone-3, octyl salicylate	
Ti•Screen	**Lotion**: Octocrylene, octyl methoxycinnamate, benzophenone-3, octyl salicylate, avobenzone	
Coppertone Kids Spray 'n Splash	**Spray**: Ethylhexyl p-methoxycinnamate, oxybenzone, 2-ethylhexyl salicylate, homosalate	
Coppertone Shade	**Spray**: Octyl methoxycinnamate, octyl salicylate, homosalate, oxybenzone, avobenzone	
Coppertone Sport, *Coppertone to Go*, *Coppertone Water Babies*	**Spray**: Octyl methoxycinnamate, octyl salicylate, homosalate, oxybenzone	
Kiss My Face, *Sun Splash*	**Spray**: Octyl methoxycinnamate, octyl salicylate, benzophenone-3	
Coppertone Kids, *Coppertone Shade*	**Stick**: Ethylhexyl p-methoxycinnamate, oxybenzone, 2-ethylhexyl salicylate, homosalate	
Coppertone Sport	**Stick**: Octyl methoxycinnamate, oxybenzone, octyl salicylate, homosalate	

Fisher-Price Sensitive Skin Sunblock for Kids, PreSun Sensitive	**Cream**: Titanium dioxide	28
Fisher-Price Spray Mist Sunscreen for Kids, PreSun Ultra	**Spray**: Avobenzone, octyl methoxycinnamate, octyl salicylate, oxybenzone	27
Biosun Faces	**Lotion**: Octyl methoxycinnamate, oxybenzone, octyl salicylate	25
Banana Boat Action Sport	**Spray**: Octyl methoxycinnamate, octyl salicylate, homosalate, oxybenzone	
RVPaque	**Cream**: Red petrolatum, zinc oxide, cinoxate	24
Banana Boat Faces Plus	**Lotion**: Octyl methoxycinnamate, oxybenzone, octyl salicylate	23
Ti•Screen	**Spray**: Octyl mathoxycinnamate, octocrylene, menthyl anthranilate, benzophenone-3	
Ti•Screen Sports Gel	**Gel**: Octyl methoxycinnamate, benzophenone-3, octyl salicylate, avobenzone	20
Neutrogena Oil-Free	**Spray**: Homosalate, octyl methoxycinnamate, octyl salicylate, menthyl anthranilate	
Bullfrog Quik Gel	**Gel**: Benzophenone-3, octyl methoxycinnamate, octyl salicylate	18
Kiss My Face	**Gel**: Titanium dioxide	
Neutrogena Sensitive Skin	**Lotion**: Titanium dioxide	17
Ti•Baby Natural, Ti•Screen Natural	**Lotion**: Titanium dioxide	16
PreSun Ultra	**Cream**: Avobenzone, octyl methoxycinnamate, octyl salicylate, oxybenzone	15
Bain de Soleil Orange Gelee	**Gel**: Octyl methoxycinnamate, octocrylene, octyl salicylate, oxybenzone	
PreSun Ultra	**Gel**: Avobenzone, octyl methoxycinnamate, octyl salicylate, oxybenzone	
Abuval Sport	**Lotion**: Octyl methoxycinnamate, octyl salicylate	

Bain de Soleil All Day Extended Protection, Bain de Soleil Mademoiselle	**Lotion**: Octyl methoxycinnamate, octocrylene, titanium dioxide, oxybenzone	
Banana Boat Sport, Coppertone Sport	**Lotion**: Octyl methoxycinnamate, oxybenzone, octyl salicylate	
Coppertone All Day, Coppertone Oil-Free	**Lotion**: Ethylhexyl p-methoxycinnamate, oxybenzone	
Coppertone Bug & Sun	**Lotion**: Ethylhexyl p-methoxycinnamate, oxybenzone, 2-ethylhexyl salicylate, homosalate, n,n diethyl m-toluamide	
DuraScreen	**Lotion**: Octyl methoxycinnamate, octyl salicylate, benzophenone-3, titanium dioxide	
Hawaiian Tropic 15 Plus, Hawaiian Tropic Super Waterproof	**Lotion**: Octyl methoxycinnamate, octyl salicylate, titanium dioxide	
Neutrogena Moisture	**Lotion**: Octyl methoxycinnamate, octyl salicylate, benzophenone-3	
Neutrogena Sunblock	**Lotion**: Octyl methoxycinnamate	
Ray Block	**Lotion**: Octyl dimethyl PABA, benzophenone-3	
Ti•Screen	**Lotion**: Octyl methoxycinnamate, benzophenone-3	
Abuval Sport	**Spray**: Octyl methoxycinnamate, oxybenzone, octyl salicylate	
Coppertone Sport, Coppertone to Go	**Spray**: Octyl methoxycinnamate, octyl salicylate, homosalate, oxybenzone	
Bain de Soleil Orange Gelee	**Gel**: Octyl methoxycinnamate, octocrylene, octyl salicylate, oxybenzone	8
Bain de Soleil Mademoiselle	**Lotion**: Octyl methoxycinnamate, octocrylene, titanium dioxide	
Coppertone All Day,Coppertone Oil-Free	**Lotion**: Ethylhexyl p-methoxycinnamate, oxybenzone	
Coppertone Sport	**Lotion**: Octyl methoxycinnamate, oxybenzone	

	Product	Formulation	SPF
	Panama Jack	**Lotion**: Ethylhexyl p-methoxycinnamate, 2-ethylhexyl salicylate	8
	Bain de Soleil Tanning Mist	**Spray**: Octyl methoxycinnamate, octocrylene, oxybenzone	
	Bain de Soleil Orange Gelee	**Gel**: Octyl methoxycinnamate, octyl salicylate	4
	Bain de Soleil Mega Tan	**Lotion**: Octyl methoxycinnamate, octocrylene	
	Bain de Soleil Tropical Deluxe	**Lotion**: Octyl methoxycinnamate, octyl salicylate	
	Banana Boat Dark Tannning	**Lotion**: Padimate O	
	Coppertone Moisturizing Suntan	**Lotion**: Ethylhexyl p-methoxycinnamate, oxybenzone	
	Hawaiian Tropic Dark Tanning	**Lotion**: 2-ethylhexyl p-methoxycinnamate, menthyl anthranilate	
	Panama Jack Dark Tanning	**Lotion**: Octyl methoxycinnamate	
	Coppertone Gold Dark Tanning	**Oil**: Homosalate, oxybenzone	
	Panama Jack Dark Tanning	**Oil**: Octyl dimethyl PABA	
	Banana Boat Dark Tanning	**Oil**: Padimate O, octyl methoxycinnamate	
	Bain de Soleil Tanning Mist	**Spray**: Octyl methoxycinnamate, octocrylene	
	Banana Boat Dark Tanning	**Oil**: Padimate O, octyl methoxycinnamate	2
	Coppertone Gold Tan Magnifier	**Oil**: Triethanolamine salicylate	
	Coppertone Gold Dark Tanning Dry Oil	**Spray**: Homosalate	
otc	**Lip Protectants**		
	Coppertone Water Babies Little Licks	**Lip Balm**: Ethylhexyl p-methoxycinnamate, oxybenzone, 2-ethylhexyl salicylate	30
	Chapstick Ultra	**Lip Balm**: Octocrylene, octyl methoxycinnamate, octyl salicylate, oxybenzone	
	Blistex DCT	**Lip Balm**: Octyl methoxycinnamate, oxybenzone	20

Chapstick Flava-Craze	**Lip Balm**: Octyl methoxycinnamate, oxybenzone	15
Coppertone Aloe and Vitamin E, Coppertone Natural Fruit Flavor, Ti•Screen	**Lip Balm**: Ethylhexyl p-methoxycinnamate, oxybenzone	
Blistex	**Lip Balm**: Padimate O, oxybenzone	

Type of Drug:

Suntan and sunscreen topical agents.

How the Drug Works:

Sunscreens provide either a chemical or physical barrier to sunlight by absorbing or reflecting harmful ultraviolet (UV) radiation (UVA and UVB rays). UVB rays cause sunburn and UVA and UVB rays both cause photoaging. Sunscreens help prevent sunburn, premature aging, actinic keratosis, and reduce incidences of skin cancer. Chemical sunscreens act by absorbing UV light rays responsible for sunburning and suntanning. Physical sunscreens reflect or scatter light, preventing penetration of the skin.

Sunscreen effectiveness is dependent on UV absorption, concentration, vehicle, and ability to withstand swimming or sweating.

Examples of chemical barrier and physical barrier sunscreens are listed below:

Chemical Barriers:

Benzophenones (avobenzone, oxybenzone, benzophenone-3)
P-amino benzoic acid (PABA) and PABA esters (padimate O)
Cinnamates (cinoxate, ethylhexyl p-methoxycinnamate, octocrylene, octyl methoxycinnamate)
Salicylates (2–ethylhexyl salicylate, octyl salicylate, homosalate, triethanolamine salicylate)
Miscellaneous (menthyl anthranilate, phenylbenzimidazole sulfonic acid)

Physical Barriers:

Titanium dioxide, red petrolatum, zinc oxide

Uses:

To prevent sunburn. Overexposure to the sun may cause premature skin aging and skin cancer. The liberal and regular use of these products may help reduce the occurrence of these harmful effects.

For persons with conditions such as systemic lupus erythematosus, solar urticaria (hives), erythropoietic protoporphyria, or those taking photosensitizing drugs. A brief list of drugs that may cause photosensitivity includes:

antidepressants (eg, amitriptyline, doxepin, trazodone)

antihistamines (eg, diphenhydramine)

antihypertensives (eg, captopril, diltiazem)
anti-infectives (eg, tetracyclines)
antineoplastic agents (eg, fluorouracil)
antipsychotic agents (eg, phenothiazines)
diuretics (eg, thiazides)
hypoglycemic agents (eg, sulfonylureas)
nonsteroidal anti-inflammatory drugs (eg, naproxen)
miscellaneous (eg, cosmetics, coal tar, psoralens, amiodarone, oral contraceptives, quinidine, disopyramide, gold salts, isotretinoin, carbamazepine)

Precautions:

Do not use in the following situations: Allergy to the sunscreen or any of its ingredients.

Use with caution in the following situations:

diseased or inflamed skin
rash, itching, burning, or irritation during or after application of the sunscreen
sensitivity to benzocaine, procaine, sulfonamides, thiazide diuretics, aniline dyes, paraphenylenediamine (an ingredient in hair dyes), PABA, or PABA esters

SPF (Sun Protection Factor): SPF reveals the amount of protection from sunburn the product provides compared to unprotected skin. For example, use of a product with an SPF value of 6 would permit 6 times more sun exposure before burning when compared to unprotected skin of the same type. Determine your skin type (see chart) and then select a product with the appropriate SPF factor.

Skin Type	Skin Characteristics[1]	Suggested Product SPF
I	Always burns easily; never tans (sensitive)	15+
II	Always burns easily; tans minimally (sensitive)	15+
III	Burns moderately; tans gradually (light brown, normal)	10 to 15
IV	Burns minimally; always tans well (moderate brown, normal)	6 to 10
V	Rarely burns; tans easily (dark brown, insensitive)	4 to 6
VI	Never burns; dark skin (insensitive)	None indicated

[1] Based on first 45 to 60 minutes of sun exposure after winter season or no sun exposure.

The value of an SPF greater than 15 is unknown. An SPF of 15 or more is recommended for most individuals by the Skin Cancer Foundation.

Children: Consult your doctor when using sunscreens on children less than 6 months of age.

Elderly: Vitamin D deficiency may occur in the elderly. Sunscreens that block certain types of UV light may block the synthesis of vitamin D by the skin.

Tartrazine: Some of these products may contain the dye tartrazine (FD&C Yellow No. 5), which can cause allergic reactions in certain individuals. Check package label when available or consult your pharmacist or doctor.

Side Effects:

Every drug is capable of producing side effects. Many sunscreen users experience no, or minor, side effects. The frequency and severity of side effects depend on many factors including dose, duration of therapy, and individual susceptibility. Possible side effects include: Burning; rash; itching; inflammation; unexpected sensitivity to UV light (photosensitivity).

Guidelines for Use:

- *Regular sunscreens* may need to be reapplied after swimming or excessive perspiration. *Water-resistant* formulas maintain sunburn protection after being in the water up to 40 minutes. *Waterproof* formulas are designed to maintain sunburn protection after being in the water up to 80 minutes. Check individual package labeling for instructions.
- Apply liberally to exposed areas at least 30 minutes prior to sun exposure (up to 2 hours for PABA and its esters) to allow for penetration into the skin. Reapply every 1 to 2 hours after swimming or excessive sweating. Reapplication does not extend the protection period.
- Reapply sun protection every 2 hours, even on cloudy days.
- Consult your doctor when using sunscreens on children less than 6 months of age.
- For external use only. Do not swallow. Avoid contact with the eyes.
- Avoid prolonged exposure to sun and to tanning lamps. Sun-sensitive persons in particular should exercise caution.
- If signs of irritation or rash occur, wash off the sunscreen and do not use again.
- PABA may produce a permanent yellow stain on clothing.
- Do not use sunscreens that contain alcohol on skin that is inflamed or eczematous.
- Be aware of the following facts related to sun exposure:
  The sun's rays are strongest and most direct between 10 am and 2 pm daily.
  Each 1000-foot increase in altitude adds 4% to light intensity.
  Reflection of light off water is almost 100% when the sun is directly overhead.
  Fresh snow reflects approximately 85% of light.
  Sand reflects approximately 20% to 25% of light.

If you have any questions, consult your doctor, pharmacist, or health care provider.

	Generic Name *Brand Name Examples*	Supplied As
otc	**Soap-Free Cleansers**	
	Aquanil, Cetaphil, Nivea Visage	**Cream, lotion**
	Basis Cleaner Clean Face Wash, Basis Comfortably Clean Face Wash, Cetaphil, Cetaphil Oily Skin, Formula 405 AHA, Neutrogena, Neutrogena Oil-Free Acne Wash, Neutrogena Antiseptic Cleanser for Acne-Prone Skin, pHisoDerm Acne, pHisoDerm Baby, pHisoDerm Normal to Dry, pHisoDerm Normal to Oily, pHisoDerm Sensitive Skin, Spectro-Jel	**Liquid**
	Ceta Cleanser, Neutrogena Non-Drying, Oilatum-AD, SFC	**Lotion**
	Sulfoil, Teraseptic	**Shampoo/Liquid**
	Lowila Cake	**Cleanser**
otc	**Modified Bar Soaps**	
	Alpha Keri Shower and Bath, Aveeno Acne Treatment, Aveeno Combination Skin, Aveeno Dry Skin, Basis All Clear, Basis Sensitive Skin, Cuticura Medicated Antibacterial, Formula 405 Mois- turizing, Lubiderm, Neutrogena, Neutrogena Acne-Prone Skin, Neutrogena Dry Skin, Neutrogena Oily Skin, Nivea Creme, Oilatum, Purpose, Teraseptic	**Bar**

Type of Drug:

Therapeutic skin cleansers. Soap-free and modified bar soap products.

How the Drug Works:

Soap-free therapeutic cleansers are less irritating to sensitive skin than regular soap-containing cleansing products. Modified bar soap products contain emollient components or are adjusted to a neutral or slightly acidic PH.

Uses:

For patients with sensitive, dry, or irritated skin who may react to soap products.

Guidelines for Use:

- For external use only.
- Follow package instructions exactly.
- Avoid overuse and contact with the eyes.
- Certain people may be sensitive to one or more ingredients. If skin irritation develops or becomes excessive, discontinue use and consult your doctor.

If you have any questions, consult your doctor, pharmacist, or health care provider.

	Generic Name *Brand Name Examples*	Supplied As	Generic Available
otc	**Aluminum Acetate Solution (Burow's or Modified Burow's Solution)**		
	Burow's Solution	**Solution**: Aluminum acetate	Yes
	Bluboro Powder, Boropak, Buro-Sol, Domeboro Powder Packets, Pedi-Boro Soak Paks	**Powder packets**: Aluminum sulfate, calcium acetate	No
	Domeboro Tablets	**Tablets, effervescent**: Aluminum sulfate, calcium acetate	No

Type of Drug:

Astringent.

Uses:

To aid in the relief of inflammation and irritation of the skin due to allergies, contact dermatitis, insect bites, poison ivy, poison oak, poison sumac, or athlete's foot. Also aids in the relief of swelling associated with minor bruises.

Drug Interactions:

The activity of the topical enzyme collagenase may be inhibited by Burow's solution. Cleanse the site with repeated washings of normal saline between applications of Burow's solution and the collagenase ointment.

Guidelines for Use:

- For external use only. Keep away from eyes.
- Follow individual product instructions.
- *Powder Packets* - Dissolve packets in required amount of cool or warm water. Stir solution until fully dissolved. Do not strain or filter. Discard used solution after each use. Prepare fresh solution daily.
- *Effervescent Tablets* - Dissolve 1 or 2 tablets in required amount of cool or warm water. Stir solution until fully dissolved. Do not strain or filter the solution. Discard used solution after each use. Unused solution may be stored at room temperature in a clean, capped container for up to 7 days.
- Discontinue use and contact your doctor if symptoms persist for more than 7 days or if irritation or worsening of condition occurs.
- Do not cover wet dressing with plastic or other materials that prevent evaporation.
- Remove, remoisten, and reapply dressing every 15 to 30 minutes for 4 to 8 hours or as directed by your doctor.
- Do not allow dressing to dry out.
- Do not use over a large area of the body.
- Store at room temperature.

	Generic Name *Brand Name Examples*	Supplied As	Uses
Rx	**Aluminum Chloride Hexahydrate**		
	Drysol	**Solution:** 20%	To aid in the management of excessive sweating.
otc	**Arnica**	**Tincture:** 20%	To relieve pain from sprains and bruises (of doubtful value)
otc	**Boric Acid Ointment**		
	Boric Acid, Borofax	**Ointment:** 5%, 10%	To soothe chafed skin, abrasions, burns and other skin irritations.
otc	**Chlorophyll Derivatives**		
	Chloresium	**Ointment:** 0.5%	To treat various skin ulcers, malignant lesions, traumatic injuries, skin grafting, skin defects and other skin disorders.
	Chloresiom	**Solution:** 0.2%	
otc	**Dihydroxyacetone**		
	Chromelin Complexion Blender	5%	To treat vitiligo and hyperpigmented skin
otc	**Hamamelis Water (Witch Hazel)**	**Liquid**	For temporary relief of anal or vaginal irritation and itching, hemorrhoids, postepisiotomy discomfort and anorectal surgical discomfort
	Tucks Hemorrhoidal	**Cream:** 50%	
	A•E•R	**Pads:** 50%	

	Generic Name *Brand Name Examples*	Supplied As	Uses
Rx	**Masoprocol**		
	Actinex	**Cream:** 10%	To treat actinic (solar) keratoses (sun induced skin growths that may develop into skin cancer).
Rx	**Monobenzone**		
	Benoquin	**Cream:** 20%	To treat light patches of the skin caused by extensive vitiligo
otc	**Zinc Oxide**	**Ointment:** 20%	To treat minor skin irritations, abrasions, chafed skin and diaper rash
	Combinations		
otc	*Aluminum Paste*	**Ointment:** 10% metallic aluminum	An occlusive skin protectant.
otc	*Boil-Ease*	**Salve**: 5% benzocaine, 0.44% sulfur, 1.86% ichthammol, camphor, anhydrous lanolin, eucalyptus oil, liquified phenol, juniper tar, menthol, paraffin, petrolatum, rosin, sexadecyl alcohol, thymol, yellow wax and zinc oxide	
otc	*Campho-Phenique*	**Liquid**: 10.8% camphor, 4.7% phenol, eucalyptus oil and light mineral oil	For relief of pain and to combat minor infections.
otc	*Dome-Paste*	**Wound dressing**: Zinc oxide, calamine and gelatin	For conditions of the arms and legs (eg, varicose ulcers) requiring protection and support.

	Generic Name *Brand Name Examples*	Supplied As	Uses
otc	*Dr. Dermi-Heal*	**Ointment**: 1% allantoin, zinc oxide, balsam Peru, castor oil and petrolatum	For relief of diaper rash, chafing, minor burns, bed sores, external vaginal itching and irritation, ostomy irritation and heat rash
otc	*Mammol*	**Ointment**: 40% bismuth subnitrate, 30% castor oil, 22% anhydrous lanolin, 7% ceresin wax and 1% balsam Peru	For prevention of sore, cracked nipples during breastfeeding.
otc	*Ostiderm*	**Lotion**: 14.5 mg aluminum sulfate, 10 mg phenol per g, glycerin, zinc oxide, bentonite, silica, propylene glycol alginate, camphor and iron oxides	For the relief of bromhidrosis and hyperhidrosis, dermatitis, itching and poison ivy.
otc	*Outgro*	**Solution**: 25% tannic acid, 5% chlorbutanol and 83% isopropyl alcohol	For temporary pain relief of ingrown toenails
otc	*Oxyzal Wet Dressing*	**Liquid**: Oxyquinolone sulfate and benzalkonium chloride 1:2000	For minor infections
otc	*Proderm Topical*	**Dressing**: 650 mg castor oil and 72.5 mg balsam Peru per 0.82 mL	For prevention and management of decubitus ulvers.
otc	*ProTech First-Aid Stick*	**Liquid**: 10% povidone iodine, 2.5% lidocaine	For cleaning and pain relief of cuts, scrapes and burns.

	Generic Name *Brand Name Examples*	Supplied As	Uses
otc	*Saratoga*	**Ointment**: Zinc oxide, boric acid, eucalyptol, acetylated lanolin alcohols, white petrolatum and white beeswax	For temporary relief of itching and minor skin irritations, chapped and chafed skin, diaper rash, bed sores and mild burns.
otc	*Sarna Anti-Itch*	**Lotion and Foam**: 0.5% camphor, 0.5% menthol, carbomer 940, DMDM hydantoin, glyceryl stearate, PEG-8 and PEG-100 stearate and petrolatum	For relief of dry, itching skin.
Rx	*Scarlet Red Ointment Dressings*	**Wound dressings**: 5% scarlet red, lanolin, olive oil and petrolatum in fine mesh absorbent gauze	For healing of donor sites, burns and wounds
otc	*Schamberg*	**Lotion**: 8.25% zinc oxide, 0.25% menthol, 1.5% phenol, 30% cottonseed oil, 15% olive oil and lime water	For itchy eczema.
otc	*Schamberg's*	**Lotion**: Zinc oxide, 0.15% menthol, 1% phenol, peanut oil and lime water	For temporary relief of itching.
otc	*Soothaderm*	**Lotion**: 2.07 mg pyrilamine maleate, 2.08 mg benzocaine and 41.35 mg zinc oxide per mL with simethicone, parabens, propylene glycol, wysteria oil, apple blossom oil, camphor and menthol	For relief of itching.

	Generic Name *Brand Name Examples*	Supplied As	Uses
otc	*Stypto-Caine*	**Solution**: 250 mg aluminum chloride, 2.5 mg tetracaine HCl and 1 mg oxy-quinolone sulfate per g with glycerin	To stop bleeding in minor cuts.
otc	*Topic*	**Gel**: 5% benzyl alcohol, camphor, menthol and 30% isopropyl alcohol	For temporary relief of itching.
otc	*Unguentine*	**Solution**: Benzo-caine in alcohol	For pain relief in minor burns.
		Ointment: 1% phe-nol petrolatum, oleostearine, zinc oxide, eucalyptus oil and thyme oil	

Type of Drug:
Miscellaneous topical agents.

Guidelines for Use:

- For external use only. Avoid contact with eyes.
- Cleanse affected area before application.
- Apply to affected area as directed. Check individual package labels for directions.
- Do not use tight-fitting dressings.
- Hands should be washed after use.
- May stain clothing or fabrics.

If you have any questions, consult your doctor, pharmacist, or health care provider.

	Generic Name *Brand Name Examples*	Supplied As	Generic Availabl
otc	**Nit Removal System** *Step 2*	**Creme rinse**: Benzyl alcohol, cetyl alcohol, 8% formic acid, glyceryl stearate, PEG-100 staerate, polyquaternium-10	No

Type of Drug:

Adjunctive treatment for use with pediculicides.

How the Drug Works:

It appears to loosen the bond that continues to hold both live and dead lice eggs to the hair shaft after pediculicide treatment. Surviving eggs can cause reinfestation if not removed. It does not kill head lice or its eggs.

Uses:

For use following a pediculicide to aid in cleansing lice eggs from the hair shaft.

Side Effects:

Every drug is capable of producing side effects. Many nit removal system users experience no, or minor, side effects. The frequency and severity of side effects depend on many factors including dose, duration of therapy and individual susceptibility. Possible side effects include itching, redness and swelling of the scalp.

Guidelines for Use:

- For external use only. Avoid contact with eyes. If contact occurs, immediately fluch with water.
- Shake well before using.
- Protect eyes with a dry towel.
- Apply to wet hair after rinsing out the pediculicide. Apply enough to saturate each hair shaft and cover the entire scalp, making sure to cover the area around the ears and back of neck. Do not apply to eyelashes or eyebrows. Leave on the hair for approximately 10 minutes. Rinse with lukewarm water and dry with a hair dryer.
- May cause itching, redness or swelling of the scalp. Notify your doctor if these symptoms persist.
- In order to prevent accidental ingestion by children, the remaining contents should be discarded after use.

If you have any questions, consult your doctor, pharmacist, or health care provider.

Generic Name *Brand Name Example*	Supplied As	Generic Available
Rx **Eflornithine HCl**		
Vaniqa	**Cream**: 13.9%	No

Type of Drug:

Agent for reducing facial hair.

How the Drug Works:

Eflornithine irreversibly inhibits ornithine decarboxylase with an enzyme found in the hair follicle of the skin needed for hair growth.

Uses:

To retard growth of unwanted facial hair in women.

Precautions:

Do not use in the following situations: Allergy to eflornithine or any of its ingredients.

Use with caution in the following situations: Irritated or broken skin.

Pregnancy: There are no adequate and well-controlled studies in pregnant women. Use only if clearly needed and the potential benefits to the mother outweigh the possible hazards to the fetus.

Breastfeeding: It is not known if eflornithine appears in breast milk. Consult your doctor before you begin breastfeeding.

Children: Safety and effectiveness in children less than 12 years of age have not been established.

Drug Interactions:

Tell your doctor or pharmacist if you are taking or if you are planning to take any over-the-counter or prescription medications or dietary supplements with eflornithine. Doses of one or both drugs may need to be modified or a different drug may need to be prescribed. It is not known if eflornithine interacts with other topically applied drugs.

Side Effects:

Every drug is capable of producing side effects. Many eflornithine users experience no, or minor, side effects. The frequency and severity of side effects depend on many factors including dose, duration of therapy, and individual susceptibility. Possible side effects include:

Digestive Tract: Indigestion; appetite loss; nausea.

Nervous System: Headache; dizziness; weakness.

Skin: Acne; ingrown hair; hair bumps; inflamed hair follicles; rosacea; tingling, stinging, or burning skin; rash; dry, red, or itchy skin; skin irritation; facial swelling; activation of herpes simplex.

Guidelines for Use:

- Dosage is individualized. Use exactly as prescribed.
- Apply a thin layer of eflornithine to the affected areas of the face and adjacent involved areas under the chin. Rub in thoroughly. You should not wash the treated areas for at least 4 hours after application.
- For external use only. Avoid getting this medicine in your eyes or inside your nose or mouth. If it gets in your eyes, rinse thoroughly with water and contact your doctor.
- Wait a few minutes after applying eflornithine before you apply cosmetics or sunscreen.
- If you miss a dose, apply it as soon as possible. If several hours have passed, or if it is nearing time for the next application, do not double the dose to catch up, unless advised by your doctor.
- Eflornithine may cause temporary redness, rash, burning, stinging, or tingling, especially when the skin is damaged. If irritation continues, stop taking this medicine and contact your doctor.
- Improvement in the condition occurs gradually, taking 4 to 8 weeks. You will need to continue your normal procedures for hair removal until desired results have been achieved.
- Check with your doctor before using any facial or skin creams, or before taking any over-the-counter medicines, prescription medicines, or dietary supplements.
- This medicine is not a depilatory. It does not permanently remove hair or "cure" unwanted hair.
- Inform your doctor is you are pregnant, become pregnant, are planning to become pregnant, or if you are breastfeeding.
- Store at controlled room temperature (59° to 86°F). Do not freeze.

If you have any questions, consult your doctor, pharmacist, or health care provider.

General Information, 1537

Antimetabolites, 1541
Capecitabine, 1546

Camptothecins, 1549

Busulfan, 1552

Etoposide, 1554

Miotic Inhibitors
Vinorelbine Tartrate, 1556

Anthracyclines
Daunorubicin, 1558
Doxorubicin, 1560
Epirubicin, 1563
Idarubicin, 1565
Valrubicin, 1567

Hormones
Androgens, 1569
Antiandrogens, 1571
Progestins, 1574
Estrogens, 1576
Antiestrogens, 1578
Estrogen/Nitrogen Mustard, 1581
Anastrozole, 1583
Letrozole, 1585
Goserelin Acetate, 1587

Biological Response Modifier
Levamisole, 1591

Alkylating Agents
Carmustine, 1593
Lomustine, 1596
Streptozocin, 1598
Estrogen/Nitrogen Mustard, 1600
Nitrogen Mustards, 1602

Antibiotics
Plicamycin, 1606

Immunologic Agents
Interferons, 1608

Retinoids
Tretinoin, 1612

Miscellaneous Preparations, 1615

Enzymes
Pegaspargase, 1621

Porfirmer Sodium, 1624

Monoclonal Antibody
Rituximab, 1627
Trastuzumab, 1629

Type of Drug:

Chemotherapy, "chemo," cancer drugs.

How the Drug Works:

Cancer drugs include a wide range of drugs that work by various mechanisms. Although development has been directed toward agents that work only on cancer cells, those presently available cause significant toxicity in normal tissues.

Combinations of cancer drugs are superior to single drug therapy in the management of many diseases, leading to higher response rates and increased length of remissions. Improved response may be due to the use of agents that work by differing mechanisms. Cancer cells that acquire rapid resistance to a single agent develop resistance less rapidly when treated with a combination of agents.

Selection of agents for combination cancer drug therapy is based on: Mechanism of drug action; specificity of action; responsiveness to dosage schedules; and drug toxicity. Increased responsiveness to combination therapy may permit reduction in dose and, therefore, decreased toxicity.

The mechanism of action by which these agents slow the growth of cancer cells is not fully understood. Generally, they affect one or more stages of cell growth or reproduction. Major side effects on normal tissues include bone marrow, blood, hair follicles and mucous membranes of the digestive tract.

Alkylating agents alter DNA. The defective DNA molecules are unable to carry out normal cell reproduction. Alkylating agents include: Busulfan, carboplatin, carmustine, chlorambucil, cisplatin, cyclophosphamide, dacarbazine, estramustine, ifosfamide, lomustine, mechlorethamine, melphalan, pipobroman, streptozocin, thiotepa and uracil mustard.

Antimetabolites include a group of compounds that interfere with various metabolic processes, thereby disrupting normal cellular functions. These agents may act by: Incorporating the drug into an essential chemical compound; or inhibiting a key enzyme from functioning normally. Antimetabolites include: Cytarabine, floxuridine, 5-fluorouracil, fludarabine, gemcitabine, hydroxyurea, mercaptopurine, methotrexate and thioguanine.

Hormones have been used to treat several types of cancer cells. Hormonal therapy interferes at the cell membrane. The mechanism of action, however, is still unclear. Corticosteroids are used primarily for their effects on blood cells in leukemia and lymphomas (tumors in lymph glands) and as a component in many combination regimens. The effect of androgens, estrogens and progestins has been used in the therapy of cancer of tissues dependent upon these sex-related hormones (eg, tumors of the breast, endometrium and prostate). These agents have the advantage of being more specific for tissues responsive to their effects, thus inhibiting cell growth without a direct toxic action. Hormones include: Aminoglutethimide, anastrozole, bicalutamide, diethylstilbestrol, estramustine, flutamide, goserelin, leuprolide, medroxyprogesterone, megestrol, mitotane, polyestradiol, tamoxifen and testolactone.

Antibiotic type agents are capable of disrupting cellular functions of tissues. Their primary mechanisms of action are to delay or inhibit cell division. Antibiotics include: Bleomycin, dactinomycin, daunorubicin, doxorubicin, idarubicin, mitomycin, mitoxantrone, pentostatin and plicamycin.

Mitotic inhibitors prevent cell division. These agents are derived from plants, eg, the periwinkle plant (vincristine, vinblastine and vinoreletoposide) or the May-apple plant (etoposide and teniposide). Another class of mitotic inhibitors called taxanes include paclitaxel and docetaxel.

Radioactive molecules (chromic phosphate, sodium iodide and strontium-89) exert a direct effect on exposed tissue via radiation. Use is restricted to doctors licensed by the Nuclear Regulatory Commission.

Biological response modifiers have complex antineoplastic, antiviral and immunomodulating activities. It is believed that direct action against tumor cells and modification of immune response (ability to produce antibodies) play important roles in the antitumor activity of interferon alfa-2a, recombinant and interferon alfa-2b, recombinant. Examples of biological agents are: Aldesleukin (human interleukin-2), interferon alfa-2a (recombinant DNA), interferon alfa-2b (recombinant DNA), interferon alfa-n3 (human leukocyte) and interferon gamma-1B (recombinant DNA).

Miscellaneous: Metabolism of altretamine is required for cytotoxicity, although the mechanisms are not clear. L-asparaginase is an enzyme that inhibits protein production in cancer cells. BCG promotes a local inflammatory reaction in the urinary bladder and reduces cancerous lesion. Cladribine inhibits DNA synthesis and repair through a complex mechanism. Levamisole is an immunomodulator with complex effects. Porfimer is a photsensitivity agent. Procarbazine produces toxic metabolites that cause chromosomal breakage. Topotecan and irinotecan are topoisomerase inhibitors. Tretinoin is related to vitamin A which induces cytodifferentiation.

Side Effects:

Extravasation (loss of drug from blood vessel) occurs when IV fluid and medication leak into tissue. Damage resulting from extravasation of certain cancer drugs can range from painful red swelling to deep lesions, requiring surgical removal of dead and contaminated tissue and skin grafting.

Prevention of extravasation injury is based on careful and accurate administration of IV drugs. Areas of previous radiation (x-ray) therapy and arms and legs with poor circulation for IV placement must be avoided.

Treatment of extravasation includes stopping the drug immediately and appropriate use of an antidote. Goals of treatment are prevention of tissue damage. Immediate removal of the IV followed by application of ice has been recommended for all agents except etoposide, vinblastine and vincristine (warm compresses are recommended for these agents).

Hydrocortisone sodium succinate or dexamethasone sodium phosphate have been used for their anti-inflammatory activity. However, the use of these agents as well as other drugs such as sodium bicarbonate and dimethyl sulfoxide (DMSO) is unproven for antidote use.

The following drugs are associated with severe local tissue damage and cell death when extravasation occurs:

dacarbazine
dactinomycin
daunorubicin
doxorubicin
idarubicin
mechlorethamine
mitomycin
streptozocin
vinblastine
vincristine
vinorelbine

Nausea and vomiting may be the most prominent side effects of cancer treatment from the patient's perspective, with 30% or more of patients experiencing some degree of vomiting. The cancer drugs with the highest potential to cause vomiting are:

carboplatin
carmustine
cisplatin
cyclophosphamide
cytarabine
dacarbazine
dactinomycin
doxorubicin
mechlorethamine
methotrexate
procarbazine
streptozocin

The agents with moderate ability to cause vomiting are:

asparaginase
daunorubicin
etoposide
fluorouracil
hexamethylmelamine
idarubicin
ifosfamide
lomustine
mitomycin
mitoxantrone
paclitaxel
plicamycin
vinblastine
vinorelbine

The incidence of vomiting with these and other agents varies greatly among individuals. Dose, schedule, other medications, other medical complications and psychological conditions may affect the incidence as well.

Treatment of nausea and vomiting should include measures such as dietary adjustment, restriction of activity and positive support. However, if drug management is necessary, several agents or groups of agents may prove useful. Some drugs that have been used with varying degrees of success, either alone or in combination, include phenothiazines, butyrophenones, cannabinoids, corticosteroids, antihistamines, benzodiazepines, metoclopramide, ACTH, selective 5–HT_3 receptor antagonist and scopolamine, see pages 379 to 392a. Since only 30% to 40% of patients are effectively treated with a single agent, studies using combination therapy have increased.

Guidelines for Use:

- Because of the complexities and dangers in cancer chemotherapy, use should be restricted to, or under the direct supervision of, doctors experienced in their use. In addition to drug therapy, surgery and radiation are also employed when appropriate.
- *Handling of Antineoplastic Agents* — Direct contact may cause irritation of the skin, eyes and mucous membranes. Safe handling of parenteral (intravenous, IV; intramuscular, IM) cancer drugs by medical personnel involved in preparation and administration of these agents is mandatory. Potential risks from repeated contact with cancer drugs can be controlled by a combination of special equipment and proper work techniques.

If you have any questions, consult your doctor, pharmacist, or health care provider.

	Generic Name *Brand Name Examples*	Supplied As	Generic Available
Rx	**Fluorouracil**		
	Efudex, Fluoroplex	**Solution:** 1%, 2%, 5%	No
	Efudex, Fluoroplex	**Cream:** 1%, 5%	No
Rx	**Mercaptopurine (6-MP)**		
	Purinethol	**Tablets:** 50 mg	No
Rx	**Methotrexate (MTX)**		
	Rheumatrex Dose Pack	**Tablets:** 2.5 mg	Yes
	Methotrexate	**Injection:** 25 mg/mL	Yes
Rx	**Thioguanine**	**Tablets:** 40 mg	Yes

Cytarabine and floxuridine, antimetabolites available as injections, are not included in this monograph. For more information on chemotherapy treatment, see the introduction to this chapter.

Type of Drug:

Chemotherapy drugs; anticancer drugs; antitumor drugs.

How the Drug Works:

Antimetabolites are similar to naturally occurring nutrients such as amino acids and vitamins. Cells use the antimetabolites instead of the naturally occuring nutrients. Once inside the cell, antimetabolites work by inhibiting nucleic acid synthesis needed for cell growth and reproduction.

Uses:

Topical Fluorourcil: To treat solar keratoses (precancerous skin growths) and superficial basal cell carcinomas.

Mercaptopurine: To treat acute lymphatic leukemia.

Methotrexate: To treat cancer of the breast, cervix, head and neck, lung, colon, ovary, prostate, stomach and pancreas, sarcomas, acute lymphocytic leukemia, lymphoma and choriocarcinoma. To control severe and disabling psoriasis and rheumatoid arthritis unresponsive to other drug therapy.

Thioguanine: To treat chronic myelogenous leukemia, acute nonlymphocytic leukemias.

Unlabeled Use(s): Occasionally doctors may prescribe methotrexate as additional therapy in the treatment of bone cancer and to reduce corticosteroid needs in patients with severe corticosteroid-dependent asthma. Fluorouracil has been used in the treatment of condylomata acuminata.

Precautions:

Do not use in the following situations: Allergy to the antimetabolite or any of its ingredients.

mercaptopurine only—

CNS leukemia
chronic lymphatic leukemia
lymphomas (including Hodgkin)
prior resistance to this drug or thioguanine
solid tumors

methotrexate only—

blood disorders
immunodeficiency
nursing mothers
pregnant women with psoriasis or rheumatoid arthritis

thioguanine only—

prior resistance to this drug or to mercaptopurine

fluorouracil only—

depressed bone marrow function
infections, serious
pregnancy

Use with caution in the following situations:

anemia
decreased blood cell count
fever, severe
immunosuppression
infection
kidney disease
liver disease

fluorouracil only—

alkylating agent therapy
combination therapy
coronary artery disease
radiation of the pelvis
spreading tumors of bone marrow

methotrexate only—

blood disorders
debility
diabetes
immunodeficiency syndromes
kidney disease
liver disease, active
lung disease
obesity
peptic ulcer
spinal cord injection
ulcerative colitis
vaccines

Sensitivity to light: Antimetabolites may cause sensitivity to light. Avoid prolonged exposure to the sun. Use sunscreens and wear protective clothing until tolerance is determined.

Pregnancy: Studies have shown that antimetabolites can harm the fetus. Do not use during pregnancy unless the potential benefits to the mother outweigh the possible hazards to the fetus. Women of childbearing potential should avoid becoming pregnant during antimetabolite therapy. Do not administer methotrexate to pregnant psoriatic or rheumatoid arthritis patients.

Breastfeeding: Methotrexate appears in breast milk. It is not known if fluorouracil, mercaptopurine or thioguanine appears in breast milk. Because of the potential for serious side effects, decide whether to discontinue breastfeeding or discontinue the drug, taking into account the importance of the drug to the mother.

Children: Methotrexate, mercaptopurine and thioguanine have been given to children with leukemia. Safety and effectiveness of methotrexate, other than in cancer chemotherapy, have not been established. Safety and effectiveness of fluorouracil have not been established.

Elderly: Due to poor liver and kidney function in the elderly, lower doses of antimetabolites may be used.

Lab tests will be required frequently during treatment with the antimetabolites. Tests include: Complete blood and platelet counts, liver, lung and kidney function tests, chest x-rays, drug levels in the blood and platelet count.

Drug Interactions:

Tell your doctor or pharmacist if you are taking or planning to take any over-the-counter or prescription medications or dietary supplements with antimetabolites. Doses of one or both drugs may need to be modified or a different drug may need to be prescribed. The following drugs and drug classes interact with antimetabolites:

fluorouracil — leucovorin calcium

methotrexate —

alcohol
aminoglycosides, oral (eg, neomycin sulfate)
antibiotics, oral
azathioprine (eg, *Imuran)*
charcoal
cisplatin
digoxin (eg, *Lanoxin)*
etretinate (*Tegison)*
folic acid
mercaptopurine (eg, *Purinethol)*
nonsteroidal anti-inflammatory drugs (eg, ketoprofen)
penicillin phenylbutasone
phenytoin (eg, *Dilantin)*
probenecid (eg, *Benemid)*
procarbazine (*Matulane)*
salicylates (*Aspirin)*

mercaptopurine —

allopurinol (eg, *Zyloprim)*
trimethoprim/sulfamethoxazole (eg, *Septra)*

thioguanine —

busulfan (*Myleran)*
salicylates (eg, aspirin)
sulfonamides (eg, sulfisoxazole)
trimethoprim/sulfamethoxazole (eg, *Septra)*

Side Effects:

Most antimetabolite users experience side effects. The frequency and severity of side effects depend on many factors including dose, duration of therapy, and individual susceptibility. Possible side effects include:

Topical fluorouracil: Pain; itching; excess pigmentation; irritation; inflammation; burning; tenderness; scaling; soreness; sensitivity to light; swelling; hair loss; insomnia; irritability; medicinal taste; watery eyes.

Oral doseforms —

Digestive Tract: Nausea; vomiting; stomach ache; appetite loss; diarrhea.

Nervous System: Fatigue; drowsiness; dizziness; headache; seizures; paralysis.

Respiratory System: Difficulty breathing; lung inflammation; lung disease.

Skin: Boils; acne; rash; hives; hair loss; itching; sensitivity to sunlight and tanning lamps; excessive pigmentation; yellowing of skin or eyes; unusual bleeding or bruising; chills.

Other: Fever; painful mouth sores; sore throat; infection; joint pain; liver disease; kidney damage; swelling of feet and legs due to fluid retention; excess uric acid in blood; cough; chest pain; blurred vision; difficulty speaking; abnormal blood counts.

Guidelines for Use:

- Contraceptive (birth control) measures are recommended for men and women during therapy.
- Notify your doctor if any of the following occurs: Fever; sore throat; chills; nausea; vomiting; unusual bleeding or bruising; black, tarry stools; diarrhea; cough or shortness of breath; darkened urine; bloody urine; yellow discoloration of the skin or eyes; abdominal pain; mouth sores or swelling; flank or joint pain; swelling of the feet or legs.
- May cause diarrhea, fever and weakness. Notify your doctor if these become pronounced.
- Drink plenty of liquids while taking this drug.
- If a dose is missed, take it as soon as possible. If several hours have passed or it is nearing time for the next dose, do not double the dose to catch up, unless advised to do so by your doctor. If more than one dose is missed, or it is necessary to establish a new dosage schedule, contact your doctor or pharmacist. Use exactly as prescribed.
- *Infections* — These drugs may lower your body's ability to fight infection. Notify your doctor of any signs of infection including fever, sore throat, rashes or chills.
- *Methotrexate* — Avoid alcohol, salicylates (eg, aspirin) and prolonged exposure to sunlight or sunlamps (particularly patients with psoriasis).
  May cause appetite loss, hair loss, skin rash, boils or acne. Notify your doctor if these effects persist.
  Pharmacists should give no more than a 7-day supply of the drug at a time. Refills should only be by direct order (written or oral) of the physician.
- *Fluorouracil (topical)* — Use nonmetal applicator or gloves when applying.
  Wash hands immediately after applying. Use caution near the eyes, nose and mouth.
  Reaction in the treated area may be unsightly during therapy and, in some cases, for several weeks after therapy has ended. Avoid airtight bandages.
  May cause temporary hair loss.
  Avoid prolonged exposure to ultraviolet light (eg, sunlight, tanning beds).

If you have any questions, consult your doctor, pharmacist, or health care provider.

	Generic Name *Brand Name Example*	Supplied As	Generic Available
Rx	**Capecitabine**		
	Xeloda	Tablets: 150 mg, 500 mg	No

For more information on chemotherapy treatment, see the introduction to this chapter.

Type of Drug:

Anticancer drug; antitumor drug.

How the Drug Works:

Capecitabine is converted in the body to the anticancer drug 5-fluorouracil which kills certain types of cancer cells and decreases the size of some tumors.

Uses:

Capecitabine is an oral medication for the treatment of advanced breast cancer resistant to treatment with paclitaxel and an anthracycline-containing chemotherapy regimen, and for patients for whom further anthracycline therapy is not indicated.

Precautions:

Do not use in the following situations: Allergy to 5-fluorouracil, or capecitabine or any of its ingredients.

Use with caution in the following situations:
coronary artery disease
kidney disease
liver dysfunction due to cancer in the liver
pregnancy

Diarrhea: Capecitabine can cause severe diarrhea. Fluid and mineral replacement may be needed.

Pregnancy: There are no adequate or well controlled studies in pregnant women. Be aware of the potential hazard to the fetus if you become pregnant while taking this medicine. Women of childbearing potential should avoid becoming pregnant while taking capecitabine.

Breastfeeding: It is not known if capecitabine appears in breast milk. Consult your doctor before you begin breastfeeding.

Children: Safety and efficacy in children have not been established.

Elderly: Patients older than 80 years of age may experience gastrointestinal side effects (eg, diarhea, nausea, vomiting) more frequently than younger patients.

Lab tests will be required to monitor therapy. Be sure to keep appointments. Tests may include: Kidney function, liver function, blood counts, toxicity monitoring.

Drug Interactions:

Tell your doctor if you are taking or planning to take any over-the-counter or prescription medications or dietary supplements with capecitabine. Doses of one or both drugs may need to be modified or a different drug may need to be prescribed. The following drugs and drug classes interact with capecitabine:

aluminum hydroxide- and magnesium hydroxide-containing antacids (eg, *Maalox*)
folic acid
leucovorin (eg, *Wellcovorin*)

Side Effects:

Every drug is capable of producing side effects. Many capecitabine users may experience side effects. The frequency and severity of side effects depend on many factors including dose, duration of therapy, and individual susceptibility. Possible side effects include:

Digestive Tract: Diarrhea; nausea; vomiting; mouth or throat sores; stomach pain; constipation; indigestion; intestinal obstruction.

Nervous System: Abnormal skin sensations; dizziness; sleeplessness.

Circulatory System: Decreased white blood cells; decreased blood platelets; anemia; increased bilirubin; chest pain; irregular heartbeat; electrocardiograph changes.

Skin: Nail disorder; hand-and-foot syndrome (palms of the hands or soles of the feet become numb, painful, swollen, or red); rash; dry or itchy skin.

Other: Fatigue; fever; appetite loss or decreased appetite; dehydration; eye irritation; weakness; pain in limbs or muscles; edema.

Guidelines for Use:

- Take each dose within 30 minutes after the end of a meal (breakfast and dinner).
- Specific dosage will be determined by your doctor. Take in 2 divided doses daily (morning and evening) with food for 2 weeks, followed by a 1-week rest period, given as 3-week cycles.
- Tablets should be swallowed with water.
- Take as directed by your doctor. The dose varies depending on individual needs. Do not adjust the dose without consulting your doctor. Specific dosage changes may be necessary during therapy.
- Your doctor may want you to take a combination of 150 mg and 500 mg tablets for each dose. If a combination is prescribed, it is very important to correctly identify the tablets. Taking the wrong tablets could result in an overdose or underdose.
- If you miss a dose, do not take the missed dose and do not double the dose to catch up. Continue your regular dosing schedule and contact your doctor.
- If you are taking the vitamin folic acid, inform your doctor.
- May cause photosensitivity (sensitivity to sunlight). Avoid prolonged exposure to the sun or other forms of ultraviolet (UV) light (eg, tanning beds). Use sunscreens and wear protective clothing until tolerance is determined.
- Notify your doctor immediately if you experience severe diarrhea (more than 4 bowel movements each day or any diarrhea at night); vomiting more than once per day; loss of appetite; pain, redness, swelling, or sores in the mouth; pain, swelling, or redness of the hands or feet; or a temperature of 100.5°F or greater, or other evidence of infection.
- Do not take aluminum hydroxide- and magnesium hydroxide-containing antacids (eg, *Maalox*) while undergoing therapy with this medicine.
- Lab tests may be required. Be sure to keep appointments.
- Store at room temperature (about 65° to 85°F) in a tightly sealed container.

If you have any questions, consult your doctor, pharmacist, or health care provider.

	Generic Name *Brand Name Examples*	Supplied As	Generic Available
Rx	**Topotecan**		
	Hycamtin	**Injection:** 1 mg/mL after reconstitution in 4 mg vials	No
Rx	**Irinotecan**		
	Camptosar	**Injection:** 20 mg/mL in 5 mL vials	No

For more information on chemotherapy treatment, see the introduction to this chapter.

Type of Drug:

Chemotherapy agents; anticancer drugs.

How the Drug Works:

Works on an enzyme affecting DNA synthesis in cells by causing small breaks in DNA. The agents then bind to the DNA and prevent the closing of these breaks. Human and tumor cells are affected by this action.

Uses:

Irinotecan: To treat cancer of the colon or rectum when disease has recurred or progressed following 5–FU therapy.

Topotecan: To treat cancer of the ovary after failure of initial or subsequent chemotherapy.

Precautions:

Do not use in the following situations:

allergy to camptothecins or any of their ingredients
nursing mothers
pregnancy
severe bone marrow depression (topotecan only)

Use with caution in the following situations:

irinotecan only —

decreased ability to fight infection
diarrhea
elderly
pelvic/abdominal irradiation

topotecan only —

anemia
blood disorder
bone marrow suppression
decreased blood platelets
inadequate bone marrow reserves

Diarrhea: Irinotecan can induce diarrhea, possibly preceded by stomach cramps and profuse sweating. Patients with severe diarrhea should be carefully watched and given fluids to avoid dehydration. Late diarrhea (developing 24 hours or more after administration) should be treated promptly with loperamide.

Pregnancy: Studies have shown a potential adverse effect on the fetus. Use only if clearly needed and potential benefits outweigh the possible risks.

Breastfeeding: Irinotecan appears in breast milk. Because of the potential for serious adverse reactions in nursing infants, it is recommended that nursing be discontinued when receiving therapy with irinotecan. It is not known if topotecan appears in breast milk. Consult your doctor before you begin breastfeeding.

Children: Safety and effectiveness in children under 16 years of age have not been established.

Elderly: No change in dosage and administration is recommended for elderly patients, other than adjustments related to renal function.

Lab tests are recommended before each dose of irinotecan. Be sure to keep appointments. Tests may include white blood cell count with differential, hemoglobin, and platelet count.

Drug Interactions:

Tell your doctor or pharmacist if you are taking or planning to take any over-the-counter or prescription medications or dietary supplements while taking this medicine. Doses of one or both drugs may need to be modified or a different drug may need to be prescribed. The following drugs and drug classes interact with this medicine:

- cisplatin (*Platinol*) (topotecan only)
- dexamethasone (eg, *Decadron*) (irinotecan only)
- diuretics (irinotecan only)
- filgrastim (*Neupogen*) (topotecan only)
- prochlorperazine (*Compazine*) (irinotecan only)

Side Effects:

Every drug is capable of producing side effects. Many patients experience no, or minor, side effects. The frequency and severity of side effects depend on many factors including dose, duration of therapy, and individual susceptibility. Possible side effects include:

Irinotecan only —

Gastrointestinal: Diarrhea; nausea; vomiting; appetite loss; constipation; gas; inflammation of the mouth; indigestion.

Circulatory System: Abnormal blood counts; anemia; blood disorder; flushing.

Body As A Whole: Weakness, stomach cramping or pain; fever; pain; headache; back pain; chills; minor infection; fluid retention; swelling of the stomach.

Skin: Hair loss; sweating; rash.

Respiratory: Difficulty breathing; increased coughing; sinus infection or congestion.

Nervous System: Sleeplessness; dizziness.

Topotecan only —

Gastrointestinal: Nausea; vomiting; diarrhea; constipation; stomach pain; inflammation of the mouth; appetite loss.

Circulatory System: Blood disorder; abnormal blood counts: decreased platelets; anemia.

Body As A Whole: Fatigue; fever; infection; weakness.

Skin: Hair loss.

Respiratory: Difficulty breathing.

Nervous System: Headache; abnormal skin sensations (eg, burning, prickling).

Guidelines for Use:

- These drugs may lower your body's ability to fight infection. Notify your doctor of signs of infection including fever, sore throat, rashes or chills.
- Patients should be informed of the expected toxic effects of these drugs, especially nausea, vomiting and diarrhea.
- The use of laxatives should be avoided, discuss any laxative use with your doctor.
- Patients should be alerted to the possibility of hair loss.
- These medications will be prepared and administered by your health care provider.
- Appointments for lab tests to monitor treatment are required.
- Store at room temperature in the original carton. Keep protected from light.

If you have any questions, consult your doctor, pharmacist, or health care provider.

Generic Name *Brand Name Example*	Supplied As	Generic Available
Rx **Busulfan**		
Myleran	**Tablets:** 2 mg	No

For more information on chemotherapy treatment, see the introduction to this chapter.

Type of Drug:

Chemotherapy drug; anticancer drug; alkylating agent.

How the Drug Works:

Busulfan slows down reproduction and growth of certain white blood cells. It is used to control, not cure, certain types of leukemia. Leukemia is a disease in which the body makes too many white blood cells.

Uses:

To control, not cure, chronic myelogenous leukemia.

Precautions:

Do not use in the following situations:

acute leukemia
chronic lymphocytic leukemia
chronic myelogenous leukemia ("blastic crisis")
prior resistance to therapy

Use with caution in the following situations:

history of seizures or head trauma
bone marrow depression from radiation or chemotherapy

Lung dysplasia: A rare but serious complication of busulfan therapy. Symptoms have occurred within 8 months to 10 years after beginning therapy. Symptoms include: Harmful cough, difficulty breathing and low-grade fever.

Pregnancy: Studies have shown busulfan may cause harm to the fetus. Avoid use during pregnancy if possible.

Breastfeeding: It is not known if busulfan appears in breast milk. Consult your doctor before you begin breastfeeding.

Lab tests including blood and platelet counts are necessary and should be performed weekly to monitor for toxicity.

Drug Interactions:

Tell your doctor or pharmacist if you are taking or planning to take any over-the-counter or prescription medications or dietary supplements with busulfan. Doses of one or both drugs may need to be modified or a different drug may need to be prescribed. Thioguanine interacts with busulfan.

Side Effects:

Most busulfan users experience side effects. The frequency and severity of side effects depend on many factors including dose, duration of therapy, and individual susceptibility. Possible side effects include:

Blood: Severely decreased blood and platelet counts.

Digestive Tract: Diarrhea; appetite loss; nausea; vomiting.

Nervous System: Weakness; dizziness; confusion; fatigue; seizures.

Respiratory System: Shortness of breath; cough.

Skin: Unusual bleeding or bruising; hair loss; darkening of the skin; redness; hives; dry skin and mucous membranes.

Other: Fever; sore throat; lower back pain; joint pain; stomach ache; cataracts (long term use); weight loss.

Guidelines for Use:

- Take this medication at the same time every day.
- Drink plenty of fluids while taking this drug.
- If a dose is missed, take it as soon as possible. If several hours have passed or it is nearing time for the next dose, do not double the dose to catch up, unless advised to do so by your doctor. If more than one dose is missed or it is necessary to establish a new dosage schedule, contact your doctor or pharmacist. Use exactly as prescribed.
- If nausea or vomiting occurs, it may help to take the drug on an empty stomach.
- Contraception (birth control) is recommended while taking this drug.
- Notify your doctor if unusual bleeding or bruising, fever, seizures, cough, shortness of breath, flank, stomach or joint pain occurs.
- May cause darkening of skin, diarrhea, dizziness, fatigue, appetite loss, mental confusion, nausea and vomiting. Notify your doctor if these become pronounced.
- These drugs may lower your body's ability to fight infection. Notify your doctor of any signs of infection including fever, sore throat, rashes or chills.

If you have any questions, consult your doctor, pharmacist, or health care provider.

	Generic Name *Brand Name Example*	Supplied As	Generic Available
Rx	**Etoposide**		
	VePesid[1]	**Capsules:** 50 mg	No

[1] Also available as an injection.

Vincristine sulfate and vinblastine sulfate, mitotic inhibitors available only as injections, are not incuded in this monograph. For more information on chemotherapy treatment, see the introduction to this chapter.

Type of Drug:

Chemotherapy agent; anticancer drug; mitotic inhibitor.

How the Drug Works:

Etoposide inhibits tumor cells from dividing (mitosis), thereby preventing the spread of certain types of cancer. Often used with other anticancer drugs.

Uses:

To treat cancer of the testicles when other treatments are not working.

To treat small cell lung cancer.

Unlabeled Use(s): Occasionally doctors may prescribe etoposide to treat certain types of lymphomas and leukemias, including Hodgkin disease and Kaposi sarcoma.

Precautions:

Do not use in the following situations:
allergy to etoposide or any of its ingredients
allergy to podophyllum

Pregnancy: Studies have shown a potential adverse effect to the fetus. Use only if clearly needed and potential benefits outweigh the possible risks.

Breastfeeding: It is not known if etoposide appears in breast milk. Consult your doctor before you begin breastfeeding.

Children: Safety and effectiveness have not been established.

Lab tests may be required during treatment with etoposide. Tests may include complete blood counts and platelet counts.

Drug Interactions:

Tell your doctor or pharmacist if you are taking or planning to take any over-the-counter or prescription medications or dietary supplements with etoposide. Doses of one or both drugs may need to be modified or a different drug may need to be prescribed. Warfarin (eg, *Coumadin*) interacts with etoposide.

Side Effects:

Every drug is capable of producing side effects. Most etoposide users experience no, or minor, side effects. The frequency and severity of side effects depend on many factors including dose, duration of therapy, and individual susceptibility. Possible side effects include:

Allergic Reactions: Chills; fever; rapid heart rate; painful or difficult breathing; decreased blood pressure.

Digestive Tract: Nausea; vomiting; appetite loss; diarrhea; constipation; stomach ache; difficulty swallowing.

Skin: Hair loss; rash; itching; skin discoloration.

Other: Short-term blindness; changes in blood pressure; aftertaste; fever; inflammation of the mouth; decrease in blood counts.

Guidelines for Use:

- If a dose is missed, take it as soon as possible. If several hours have passed or it is nearing time for the next dose, do not double the dose to catch up, unless advised to do so by your doctor. If more than one dose is missed, or it is necessary to establish a new dosage schedule, contact your doctor or pharmacist. Use exactly as prescribed.
- Consult your doctor if chills, fever, rapid heartbeat, lightheadedness, flushing or difficult breathing occurs.
- Contraceptive measures (birth control) are recommended during treatment with etoposide.
- *Infections* — These drugs may lower your body's ability to fight infection. Notify your doctor of any signs of infection including fever, sore throat, rashes, or chills.
- Lab tests may be required to monitor therapy. Be sure to keep appointments.
- Capsules must be stored at 36° to 46°F. They will retain their effectiveness for 2 years under refrigeration, 3 months at room temperature. Do not freeze.

If you have any questions, consult your doctor, pharmacist, or health care provider.

	Generic Name *Brand Name Example*	Supplied As	Generic Available
Rx	**Vinorelbine Tartrate**		
	Navelbine[1]	**Injection:** 10 mg/mL	No

[1] Preservative free.

For more information on chemotherapy treatment, see the introduction to this chapter.

Type of Drug:

Chemotherapy agent; anticancer drug; mitotic inhibitor.

How the Drug Works:

Vinorelbine prevents tumor cells from dividing (mitosis), which slows or stops tumor growth.

Uses:

To treat advanced non-small-cell lung cancer that cannot be surgically removed. May be used in combination with cisplatin.

Unlabeled Use(s): Occasionally doctors may prescribe vinorelbine for other forms of cancer, desmoid tumors and fibromatosis, advanced Kaposi sarcoma, and and Hodgkin disease.

Precautions:

Do not use in the following situations:

- allergy to vinorelbine or any of its ingredients
- low blood (granulocyte) counts (less than 1000 cells/mm^3)

Use with caution in the following situations:

- bone marrow, compromised
- bronchospasm
- chemotherapy, recovery from
- constipation
- infection
- intestinal disorder (eg, ileus, obstruction, perforation)
- liver disease
- lung disease
- neuropathy, active or history of
- radiation therapy, prior

Pregnancy: Studies have shown a potential adverse effect to the fetus. Use only if clearly needed and the potential benefits to the mother outweigh the possible hazards to the fetus. Women of childbearing potential should avoid becoming pregnant during vinorelbine treatment.

Breastfeeding: It is not known if vinorelbine appears in breast milk. Consult your doctor before you begin breastfeeding.

Children: Safety and effectiveness in children have not been established.

Lab tests may be required to monitor therapy. Tests include frequent blood counts.

Drug Interactions:

Tell your doctor or pharmacist if you are taking or if you are planning to take any over-the-counter or prescription medications or dietary supplements while taking vinorelbine. Doses of one or both drugs may need to be modified or a different drug may need to be prescribed. The Following drugs or drug classes interact with vinorelbine:

cisplatin (*Platinol*)
mitomycin (*Mutamycin*)
P450 (CYP 3A) isoenzyme inhibitors (eg, zafirlukast)
paclitaxel (eg, *Taxol*)

Side Effects:

Every drug is capable of producing side effects. Many vinorelbine users experience no, or minor, side effects. The frequency and severity of side effects depend on many factors including dose, duration of therapy, and individual susceptibility. Possible side effects include:

Digestive Tract: Nausea; vomiting; mild to severe constipation; diarrhea; appetite loss; mouth soreness; stomach pain; bowel obstruction or disorder.

Skin: Hair loss; vein discoloration; pain or reactions at injection site; flushing; rash; itching; decreased sensitivity to touch; asbnormal sensitivity to touch, pain, or other stimuli; blisters; hives; skin sloughing; abnormal skin sensations (eg, burning, tingling, prickling).

Other: Headache; weakness; fatigue; back, jaw, joint, or muscle pain; fever; infection; incoordination; abnormal blood counts; difficulty breathing; abnormal liver function tests; chills; anemia; low white blood cell counts; decreased blood platelets; loss of tendon reflexes; abnormal gait; bladder inflammation; nerve damage; chest pain.

Guidelines for Use:

- This medicine will be prepared and administered by your health care provider in a medical setting.
- For intravenous (IV; into a vein) use only.
- Avoid contact with skin and eyes. If the solution contacts the skin, wash immediately with soap and water. If the solution contacts the eyes, immediately and thoroughly flush with water.
- *Infections* — These drugs reduce your body's ability to fight infection. Notify your doctor of any signs of infection including fever, sore throat, rashes, or chills.
- Contraceptive measures (birth control) are recommended during treatment with vinorelbine in patients who are sexually active.
- Notify your doctor immediately if you experience chills, fever, difficulty breathing, cough, chest or stomach pain, hives, rash, or constipation.
- Lab tests will be required to monitor therapy. Be sure to keep appointments.

If you have any questions, consult your doctor, pharmacist, or health care provider.

	Generic Name *Brand Name Example*	Supplied As	Generic Available
Rx	**Daunorubicin HCl**	**Injection**: 5 mg/mL (= to 5.34 mg daunorubicin HCl)[1]	Yes
Rx	**Daunorubicin Citrate Liposome**		
	DaunoXome	**Injection**: 2 mg/mL (= to 50 mg daunorubicin base)	No

[1] Contains sodium chloride.

For more information on chemotherapy treatment, see the introduction to this chapter.

Type of Drug:

Antineoplastic; anticancer drug; antitumor drug.

How the Drug Works:

Daunorubicin interferes with cancer cell division and can produce cancer cell death, primarily by interfering with the normal functioning of the genetic material (eg, DNA) of cancer cells.

Uses:

Daunorubicin HCl — In combination with other approved anticancer drugs, for remission induction in acute nonlymphocytic (myelogenous, monocytic, erythroid) of adults and for remission induction in acute lymphocytic leukemia in children and adults.

Daunorubicin citrate liposome — First-line cytotoxic therapy for advanced HIV-associated Kaposi sarcoma.

Precautions:

Do not use in the following situations:

allergy to daunorubicin or any of its ingredients
bone marrow suppression, drug-induced preexisting
previously received the highest cumulative dose of either doxorubicin or daunorubicin

Use with caution in the following situations:

doxorubicin therapy, previous
heart disease, preexisting
kidney disease
liver disease
myelosuppression
systemic infection, uncontrolled

Secondary leukemias: There have been reports of secondary leukemias in patients exposed to topoisomerase II inhibitors when used in combination with other antineoplastic agents or radiation therapy.

Pregnancy: There are no adequate and well-controlled studies in pregnant women. Use only if clearly needed and the potential benefits to the mother outweigh the possible hazards to the fetus.

Breastfeeding: It is not known if daunorubicin appears in breast milk. However, mothers should be advised to discontinue breastfeeding during therapy. Consult your doctor before breastfeeding is resumed.

Children: Safety and effectiveness in children have not been established. Cardiac toxicity may be more frequent and occur at lower doses in children.

Elderly: Safety and effectiveness in elderly patients have not been established. Cardiac toxicity may be more frequent in the elderly. Use caution in patients who have inadequate bone marrow reserves or kidney function impaiment because of age.

Lab tests will be required to monitor therapy. Tests include blood, heart, kidney, and liver function.

Drug Interactions:

Tell your doctor or pharmacist if you are taking or planning to take any over-the-counter or prescription medicines or dietary supplements while taking daunorubicin. Doses of one or both drugs may need to be modified or a different drug may need to be prescribed. The following drugs and drug classes interact with daunorubicin:

cyclophosphamide (eg, *Cytoxan*)
hepatoxic medications (eg, methotrexate)
myelosuppressive agents (eg, mitomycin)

Side Effects:

Every drug is capable of producing side effects. Many daunorubicin users experience side effects. The frequency and severity of side effects depend on many factors including dose, duration of therapy, and individual susceptibility. Possible side effects include:

Daunorubicin HCl — Acute nausea and vomiting (usually mild); diarrhea; stomach pain; injection site reaction; reversible hair loss; rash; hives; itching; fever; chills; bone marrow suppression; secondary leukemia.

Daunorubicin citrate liposomal — Stomach pain; appetite loss; constipation; diarrhea; nausea; vomiting; depression; dizziness; fatigue; headache; sleeplessness; general body discomfort; nerve disease; chest tightness; flushing; hair loss; itching; back, joint, or muscle pain; rigors; cough; difficulty breathing; runny nose; sinus irritation.

Guidelines for Use:

- This medicine will be prepared and administered by your health care provider in a medical setting.
- Dosage is individualized.
- Your urine may become reddish-colored while you are undergoing therapy. This is not cause for concern.
- Lab tests will be required to monitor therapy. Be sure to keep appointments.

If you have any questions, consult your doctor, pharmacist, or health care provider.

	Generic Name *Brand Name Examples*	Supplied As	Generic Available
Rx	**Doxorubicin, conventional**		
	Adriamycin RDF	**Powder for injection (lyophilized)**: 10 mg, 20 mg, 50 mg, 150 mg	Yes
	Rubex	**Powder for injection (lyophilized)**: 50 mg, 100 mg	No
	Adriamycin PFS	**Injection**: 10 mg, 20 mg, 50 mg, 75 mg	No
Rx	**Doxorubicin, liposome**		
	Doxil	**Injection**: 20 mg	No

Type of Drug:

Antineoplastic; anticancer drug; antitumor drug.

How the Drug Works:

This drug is toxic to cells, particularly rapidly-dividing cancer cells, by a variety of mechanisms.

Uses:

Doxorubicin, conventional — To produce regression in disseminated neoplastic conditions such as the following: Acute lymphoblastic leukemia, acute myeloblastic leukemia, Wilms' tumor, neuroblastoma, soft tissue and bone sarcomas, breast carcinoma, ovarian carcinoma, transitional cell bladder carcinoma, thyroid carcinoma, Hodgkin and non-Hodgkin lymphomas, bronchogenic carcinoma (the small-cell histologic type is the most responsive), and gastric carcinoma.

Doxorubicin, liposome — For treatment of AIDS-related Kaposi sarcoma in patients with disease that has progressed on prior combination chemotherapy or in patients who are intolerant to such therapy.

Precautions:

Do not use in the following situations:

- allergy to doxorubicin or any of its ingredients
- myelosuppression, marked and induced by previous treatment with other antitumor agents or by radiotherapy (conventional only)
- nonresponsive neoplastic conditions (eg, malignant melanoma, kidney carcinoma, large bowel carcinoma, brain tumors, metastases to the central nervous system)
- previous treatment with the complete cumulative doses of doxorubicin, daunorubicin, idarubicin, or other anthracyclines and anthracenes

Use with caution in the following situations:

- elderly
- heart disease, history of
- high blood pressure
- liver disease

Pregnancy: Safety for use during pregnancy has not been established. Fetal harm can occur if used in a pregnant woman. Use only if clearly needed and the potential benefits to the mother outweigh the possible hazards to the fetus.

Breastfeeding: Conventional doxorubicin appears in breast milk. It is not known if liposomal doxorubicin appears in breast milk. Mothers should, however, be advised to discontinue breastfeeding during therapy. Consult your doctor before breastfeeding is resumed.

Children: Doxorubicin may contribute to delayed cardiac toxicity, prepubertal growth failure, and gonadal impairment. Use with extreme caution in pediatric patients.

Elderly: Elderly patients may have an increased risk for cardiac toxicity.

Lab tests will be required to monitor therapy. Tests include blood counts, heart and liver function, and blood uric acid level.

Drug Interactions:

Tell your doctor or pharmacist if you are taking or planning to take any over-the-counter or prescription medicines or dietary supplements while taking doxorubicin. Doses of one or both drugs may need to be modified or a different drug may need to be prescribed. The following drugs and drug classes interact with doxorubicin:

actinomycin-D
cyclophosphamide (eg, *Cytoxan*)
cyclosporine (eg, *Neoral*)
digoxin (eg, *Lanoxin*)
mercaptopurine (*Purinethol*)
paclitaxel (eg, *Taxol*)
phenobarbital (eg, *Solfoton*)
phenytoin (eg, *Dilantin*)
progesterone (eg, *Prometrium*)
radiation therapy
streptozocin (*Zanosar*)
verapamil (eg, *Calan*)

Side Effects:

Every drug is capable of producing side effects. Many doxorubicin users experience side effects. The frequency and severity of side effects depend on many factors including dose, duration of therapy, and individual susceptibility. Possible side effects include:

Doxorubicin, conventional — Nausea; vomiting; sensory or motor disturbances; appetite loss; diarrhea; fever; chills; reversible, complete hair loss; hyperpigmentation of nail beds and skin creases (primarily in children); loosening of the nails; skin reaction; hives; injection site reaction; facial flushing; myelosuppression; abnormal blood counts; eye inflammation; infection (eg, candidiasis, cytomegalovirus, herpes simplex, Pneumocystis carinii pneumonia, mycobacterium avium).

Doxorubicin, liposome — Skin flushing; palmar or plantar skin eruptions (eg, swelling, pain, redness, shedding or scaling of skin on hands or feet); hair loss; rash; itching; shortness of breath; difficulty breathing; pneumonia; facial swelling; back pain; tightness in chest or throat; abnormal blood counts; joint pain; oral fungal infection; opportunistic viral or bacterial infection; headache; chills; fever; dizziness; drowsiness; low blood pressure; chest pain; fast heartbeat; abnormal heart rhythm; diarrhea; nausea; stomach pain; vomiting; mouth ulcer; inflammation or redness of the tongue; constipation; appetite loss; difficulty swallowing; herpes simplex; weight loss; infection; inflammation of the retina; watery eyes; emotional instability.

Guidelines for Use:

- This medicine will be prepared and administered intravenously (IV; into a vein) by your health care provider in a medical setting.
- Dosage is individualized.
- Nausea and vomiting associated with therapy may be severe. Antiemetic medications may be necessary.
- You will almost certainly experience hair loss.
- Notify your doctor if you experience bloody stools.
- Your urine may turn reddish-colored for 1 to 2 days following therapy. This is not cause for concern.
- *Doxorubicin, liposome* — Notify your doctor if you experience an acute infusion-related reaction (eg, flushing, shortness of breath, facial swelling, headache, chills, back pain, tightness in the chest or throat, low blood pressure). This effect is more common with the first infusion and usually resolves in about a day.
- Do not undergo any vaccinations with live vaccines during doxorubicin therapy.
- Lab tests will be required to monitor therapy. Be sure to keep appointments.

If you have any questions, consult your doctor, pharmacist, or health care provider.

Generic Name *Brand Name Example*	Supplied As	Generic Available
Rx **Epirubicin HCl**		
Ellence	**Injection**: 2 mg/mL	No

For more information on chemotherapy treatment, see the introduction to this chapter.

Type of Drug:

Antineoplastic; anticancer drug; antitumor drug.

How the Drug Works:

This drug interferes with a number of biochemical and biological cellular functions to slow or stop cancer cell growth.

Uses:

As a component of adjuvant therapy in patients with evidence of axillary node tumor involvement following resection of primary breast cancer.

Precautions:

Do not use in the following situations:

- allergy to epirubicin or any of its ingredients
- allergy to other anthracyclines or anthracenediones
- liver dysfunction, severe
- myocardial infarction, recent
- myocardial insufficiency, severe
- previous treatment with other anthracyclines up to the maximum cumulative dose
- severely reduced neutrophil count, preexisting

Use with caution in the following situations:

- bone marrow suppression, preexisting
- kidney disease
- liver disease
- radiation therapy, previous

Pregnancy: There are no adequate and well-controlled studies in pregnant women. Fetal harm can occur if used in a pregnant woman. Use only if clearly needed and the potential benefits to the mother outweigh the possible hazards to the fetus.

Breastfeeding: It is not known if epirubicin appears in breast milk. Mothers should, however, discontinue breastfeeding during therapy. Consult your doctor before resuming breastfeeding.

Children: Safety and effectiveness in children have not been established. Pediatric patients have a greater risk for anthracycline-induced acute manifestations of cardiotoxicity and for chronic congestive heart failure.

Elderly: Female patients 70 years of age and older are at an increased risk of drug accumulation and must be monitored closely.

Lab tests will be required to monitor therapy. Tests include blood counts and heart, liver, and kidney function tests.

Drug Interactions:

Tell your doctor or pharmacist if you are taking or planning to take any over-the-counter or prescription medicines or dietary supplements while taking epirubicin. Doses of one or both drugs may need to be modified or a different drug may need to be prescribed. Cimetidine (eg, *Tagamet*) interacts with epirubicin.

Side Effects:

Every drug is capable of producing side effects. Many epirubicin users experience side effects. The frequency and severity of side effects depend on many factors including dose, duration of therapy, and individual susceptibility. Possible side effects include:

Digestive Tract: Nausea; vomiting; diarrhea; appetite loss.

Skin: Injection site reaction (possibly severe); hair loss; rash; itching; skin changes.

Other: Secondary leukemia; myelosuppression; absence of menstrual bleeding; hot flashes; abnormal blood counts; infection; fever; lethargy; eye inflammation.

Guidelines for Use:

- This medicine will be administered intravenously (IV; into a vein) by your health care provider in a medical setting.
- Dosage is individualized.
- Epirubicin can cause nausea, vomiting, and diarrhea. Antiemetic medications administered before therapy may reduce these side effects.
- Notify your doctor if you experience vomiting, dehydration, fever, evidence of infection, symptoms of congestive heart failure (eg, difficult or labored breathing, swelling of lower legs, fast heartbeat), or injection site pain.
- You will almost certainly experience hair loss. Hair usually starts to regrow within 2 to 3 months after therapy has ended.
- Your urine may turn reddish-colored for 1 to 2 days following therapy. This is not cause for concern.
- There is a risk of irreversible heart damage associated with treatment, as well as treatment-related leukemia.
- Epirubicin may cause chromosomal damage in sperm. Men undergoing treatment should use effective contraceptive methods.
- Women treated with epirubicin may develop irreversible absence of menstruation or premature menopause.
- Lab tests will be required to monitor therapy. Be sure to keep appointments.

If you have any questions, consult your doctor, pharmacist, or health care provider.

	Generic Name *Brand Name Examples*	Supplied As	Generic Available
Rx	**Idarubicin HCl**		
	Idamycin	**Powder for injection (lyophilized)**: 20 mg	No
	Idamycin PFS	**Injection**: 5 mg, 10 mg, 20 mg	No

For more information on chemotherapy treatment, see the introduction to this chapter.

Type of Drug:

Antineoplastic; anticancer drug; antileukemic drug.

How the Drug Works:

Leukemia is a disease in which the body makes too many white blood cells. Idarubicin interferes with the reproduction (growth) of white blood cells as well as other cells formed in the bone marrow.

Uses:

Used in combination with other approved antileukemic drugs for the treatment of acute myeloid leukemia (AML) in adults.

Precautions:

Do not use in the following situations:

- allergy to idarubicin or any of its ingredients
- bone marrow suppression, preexisting

Use with caution in the following situations:

- heart disease
- kidney disease
- liver disease

Pregnancy: There are no adequate and well-controlled studies in pregnant women. Use only if clearly needed and the potential benefits outweigh the possible hazards to the fetus.

Breastfeeding: It is not known if idarubicin appears in breast milk. Consult your doctor before you begin breastfeeding.

Children: Safety and effectiveness in children have not been established.

Lab tests will be required to monitor therapy. Tests include blood cell counts and liver and kidney function.

Drug Interactions:

Tell your doctor or pharmacist if you are taking or planning to take any over-the-counter or prescription medicines or dietary supplements while taking idarubicin. Doses of one or both drugs may need to be modified or a different drug may need to be prescribed.

Side Effects:

Every drug is capable of producing side effects. Many idarubicin users experience side effects. The frequency and severity of side effects depend on many factors including dose, duration of therapy, and individual susceptibility. Possible side effects include:

Digestive Tract: Nausea; vomiting; stomach cramps or pain; diarrhea; inflammation of the lining of the mouth.

Circulatory System: Chest pain; irregular heart rhythm; congestive heart failure.

Skin: Hair loss; rash; hives.

Other: Infection; bleeding; abnormal lab tests; bone marrow suppression; fever; headache; seizure; nerve pain; difficulty breathing; psychological changes.

Guidelines for Use:

- This medicine will be prepared and administered intravenously (IV; into a vein) by your health care provider in a medical setting.
- Dosage is individualized.
- Notify your doctor if you experience sore throat, fever, irregular heartbeat, difficulty breathing, or unusual bleeding or bruising.
- Lab tests will be required to monitor therapy. Be sure to keep appointments.

If you have any questions, consult your doctor, pharmacist, or health care provider.

	Generic Name *Brand Name Example*	Supplied As	Generic Available
Rx	**Valrubicin**		
	Valstar	**Solution for intravesical instillation**: 40 mg/mL	No

For more information on chemotherapy treatment, see the introduction to this chapter.

Type of Drug:

Antineoplastic; anticancer drug.

How the Drug Works:

This drug penetrates rapidly-dividing cancer cells, interfering with nucleic acid metabolism, which leads to extensive chromosomal damage, DNA damage, and arrested cancer cell growth in a significant percentage of patients.

Uses:

For intravesical therapy of BCG-refractory carcinoma in situ (CIS) of the urinary bladder in patients for whom immediate cystectomy would be associated with morbidity or mortality.

Precautions:

Do not use in the following situations:

allergy to any anthracycline
allergy to valrubicin or any of its ingredients (eg, polyoxyethyleneglycol triricinoleate [*Cremophor EL*])
perforated bladder or compromised integrity of bladder mucosa
small bladder capacity (ie, unable to tolerate a 75 mL instillation)
urinary tract infection, concurrent

Use with caution in the following situations: Severe irritable bladder symptoms.

Pregnancy: There are no adequate and well-controlled studies in pregnant women. Fetal harm can occur if a pregnant woman is exposed to valrubicin systemically. Use only if clearly needed and the potential benefits to the mother outweigh the possible hazards to the fetus.

Breastfeeding: It is not known if valrubicin appears in breast milk. However, any exposure of infants to this drug could pose sevre health risks. Consult your doctor before you begin breastfeeding.

Children: Safety and effectiveness in children have not been established.

Lab tests will be required to monitor therapy. Tests include bladder function, cystoscopy, biopsy, and urine cytology.

Drug Interactions:

Tell your doctor or pharmacist if you are taking or planning to take any over-the-counter or prescription medicines or dietary supplements while taking valrubicin. Doses of one or both drugs may need to be modified or a different drug may need to be prescribed.

Side Effects:

Every drug is capable of producing side effects. Many valrubicin users experience side effects. The frequency and severity of side effects depend on many factors including dose, duration of therapy, and individual susceptibility. Possible side effects include:

Urinary and Reproductive Tract: Increased urination; painful or difficult urination; urinary urgency; bladder spasm; blood in the urine; bladder pain; urinary incontinence; excessive urination at night; procedure-related local burning symptoms; urethral pain; pelvic pain; urinary tract infection; urinary retention.

Digestive Tract: Stomach pain; nausea; diarrhea; vomiting; gas.

Other: High blood sugar; swelling of the arms or legs; weakness; headache; general body discomfort; back, muscle, or chest pain; dizziness; rash; abnormal blood counts; fever; pneumonia; flushing.

Guidelines for Use:

- This medicine will be prepared and administered by your health care provider in a medical setting.
- Dosage is individualized.
- Your urine may become reddish-colored for the first 24 hours after administration. This is not cause for concern.
- Notify your doctor if you experience prolonged reddish-colored urine or prolonged irritable bladder symptoms (eg, bladder spasm, spontaneous discharge of the drug).
- Women should not become pregnant and men should refrain from engaging in procreative activities during treatment. Use an effective contraception method during treatment.
- Lab tests will be required to monitor therapy. Be sure to keep appointments.

If you have any questions, consult your doctor, pharmacist, or health care provider.

Generic Name *Brand Name Example*	Supplied As	Generic Available
Rx **Testolactone**		
Teslac	**Tablets:** 50 mg	No

For more information on chemotherapy treatment, see the introduction to this chapter.

Type of Drug:

Chemotherapy agent; anticancer drug.

How the Drug Works:

Testolactone is produced synthetically; it is related to testosterone but does not have the masculine effects of testosterone. It blocks the production of estrogen and helps to prevent the growth of breast cancers that are activated by estrogens. It may also protect tumor cells from being activated by other steroid hormones.

Uses:

Used with other anticancer drugs to treat symptoms of breast cancer in women after menopause.

Precautions:

Do not use in the following situations:

allergy to testolactone or any if its ingredients
breast cancer in men

Pregnancy: Adequate studies have not been done in pregnant women, or animal studies may have shown a risk to the fetus. Use only if clearly needed and potential benefits outweight the possible hazards to the fetus.

Breastfeeding: It is not known if testolactone appears in breast milk. Consult your doctor before you begin breastfeeding.

Children: Safety and effectiveness in children have not been established.

Lab tests may be required to monitor therapy. Tests may include calcium blood levels.

Drug Interactions:

Tell your doctor or pharmacist if you are taking or if you are planning to take, any over-the-counter or prescription medications or dietary supplements while taking testolactone. Doses of one or both drugs may need to be modified or a different drug may need to be prescribed. Testolactone interacts with oral anticoagulants (eg, warfarin).

Side Effects:

Every drug is capable of producing side effects. Many testolactone users experience side effects. The frequency and severity of side effects depend on many factors including dose, duration of therapy, and individual susceptibility. Possible side effects include:

Digestive Tract: Inflammation of the tongue; nausea; vomiting; appetite loss.

Other: Abnormal skin sensations; aches and swelling of the hands or feet; high blood pressure; hair loss.

Guidelines for Use:

- Contraceptive (birth control) measures are recommended during treatment. Contact your doctor if pregnancy is suspected.
- If a dose is missed, take or inject as soon as possible. If several hours have passed or it is nearing time for the next dose, do not double the dose to catch up, unless advised to do so by your doctor. If more than one dose is missed, contact your doctor or pharmacist.
- The usual dose is five tablets 4 times daily.
- Notify your doctor if appetite loss, nausea, vomiting, hair loss or swelling of the hands or feet occur.
- Lab tests are required to monitor treatment. Be sure to keep appointments.
- Store at room temperature.

If you have any questions, consult your doctor, pharmacist, or health care provider.

	Generic Name *Brand Name Examples*	Supplied As	Generic Available
Rx	**Bicalutamide**		
	Casodex	**Tablets:** 50 mg	No
Rx	**Flutamide**		
	Eulexin	**Capsules:** 125 mg	No
Rx	**Nilutamide**		
	Nilandron	**Tablets:** 50 mg	No

For more information on chemotherapy treatment, see the introduction to this chapter.

Type of Drug:

Chemotherapy agents; anticancer drugs.

How the Drug Works:

Antiandrogens prevent androgens (eg, testosterone) from binding to and activating tumor cells of the prostate.

Uses:

Bicalutamide and flutamide are for use in combination with other anticancer drugs to treat prostate cancer. Nilutamide is for use with surgical castration for the treatment of prostate cancer.

Precautions:

Do not use in the following situations:

allergy to the antiandrogen or any of its ingredients
liver disease, severe (nilutamide only)
respiratory insufficiency, severe (nilutamide only)

Use with caution in the following situations: Liver disease.

Vision changes may occur. Report any changes to your doctor.

Flutamide and bicalutamide should always be administered with other drugs (eg, leuprolide acetate). Do not stop or interrupt dosing without first consulting your doctor.

Tumors: Nilutamide has been associated with the development of benign tumors and bicalutamide has been associated with the development of both benign and cancerous tumors in animals. Bicalutamide may lead to male infertility, although long-term studies have not been conducted. Discuss any concerns with your doctor.

Children: Safety and effectiveness in children have not been established.

Lab tests will be required frequently during treatment. Tests may include liver function tests, PSA levels, and blood clotting tests.

Drug Interactions:

Tell your doctor or pharmacist if you are taking or if you are planning to take any over-the-counter or prescription medications or dietary supplements while taking antiandrogens. Doses of one or both drugs may need to be modified or a different drug may need to be prescribed. The following drugs and drug classes interact with antiandrogens:

- anticoagulants, oral (eg, warfarin)
- phenytoin (eg, *Dilantin*) (nilutamide only)
- theophylline (eg, *Theo-Dur*) (nilutamide only)

Side Effects:

Every drug is capable of producing side effects. Many antiandrogen users experience side effects. The frequency and severity of side effects depend on many factors including dose, duration of therapy, and individual susceptibility. Possible side effects include:

Digestive Tract: Constipation; nausea; diarrhea; vomiting; black vomit; gas; weight changes; dry mouth; black, bloody stools; appetite loss; stomach pain or problem; indigestion.

Nervous System: Dizziness; abnormal skin sensations; sleeplessness; anxiety; depression; confusion; nervousness; drowsiness; headache; weakness; decreased sensitivity; disease of the nerves.

Circulatory System: High blood pressure; hot flashes; chest pain; heart failure.

Respiratory System: Difficulty breathing; cough; sore throat; upper respiratory infection; pneumonia; bronchitis; sinus infection; congestion.

Skin: Rash; itching; hair loss; sweating; dry skin; injection site reaction; body hair loss.

Urinary and Reproductive Tract: Urination problems; blood in the urine; discolored urine; urinary tract infection or disorder; excessive urination at night; bladder inflammation or problems; rectal bleeding; inflammation.

Other: Swelling of hands or lower legs; general body, back, neck, breast, bone, pelvic, stomach, muscle or joint pain; leg cramps; fever; chills; high blood sugar; dehydration; gout; weakness; infections; flu syndrome; impotence; breast growth in males; anemia; impaired visual adaptation to light or dark; atrophy of testicles; sensitivity to light; fainting; cataract; soreness or stiffness; diabetes; sweating; abnormal vision; changes in sex drive; abnormal coloring; bone fracture; loss of libido; abnormal blood counts; decreased blood platelets; arthritis; increased liver function tests; intolerance to alcohol.

Guidelines for Use:

- Use exactly as prescribed.
- If a dose is missed, take it as soon as possible. If several hours have passed or it is nearing time for the next dose, do not double the dose to catch up, unless advised to do so by your doctor. If more than one dose is missed or it is necessary to establish a new dosage schedule, contact your doctor or pharmacist.
- Do not stop or interrupt dosing without first consulting your doctor.
- Lab tests/exams are required to monitor treatment. Be sure to keep appointments.
- Store at room temperature in a tightly sealed container. Avoid moisture and light.

Bicalutamide:

- Usual dose is one tablet daily (morning or evening) with or without food. If possible, try to take the tablet at the same time each day.
- Medicine may cause hot flashes, breast growth or breast pain.

Flutamide:

- Usual dose is two capsules 3 times daily, 8 hours apart.
- Notify your doctor if any of the following occurs: Itching, dark urine, appetite loss, yellowing skin or eyes, stomach pain/tenderness or flu-like symptoms.

Bicalutamide and Flutamide:

- Be sure to take this medicine in combination with your LHRH agonist analog (eg, leuprolide acetate) for proper treatment.

Nilutamide:

- May cause a delay in visual adaptation to the dark, ranging from seconds to a few minutes. Exercise caution in night driving or driving through tunnels. Wear tinted glasses.
- Notify your doctor if any of the following occurs: Difficulty in breathing, nausea/vomiting, abdominal pain or yellowing of the skin or eyes.
- Avoid alcohol.

If you have any questions, consult your doctor, pharmacist, or health care provider.

Generic Name *Brand Name Example*	Supplied As	Generic Available
Rx **Megestrol Acetate**		
Megace	**Tablets:** 20 mg, 40 mg	Yes
Megace	**Suspension, oral:** 40 mg/mL	No

For more information on chemotherapy treatment, see the introduction to this chapter.

Type of Drug:

Chemotherapy agents; anticancer drugs.

How the Drug Works:

Progestins can interfere with the way that estrogen and other steroid hormones activate tumor cells of the breast and endometrium.

Uses:

Tablet: To treat the symptoms of breast and endometrial cancers.

Oral suspension: To treat loss of appetite, weight loss or an unexplained, significant weight loss in patients with a diagnosis of AIDS.

Precautions:

Do not use in the following situations:

allergy to megestrol or any of its ingredients
diagnostic test for pregnancy
neoplastic disease, other
pregnancy
pregnancy, first trimester

Use with caution in the following situations:

blood clotting disorders, history of
diabetes

HIV infected women (oral suspension only) have reported breakthrough bleeding with the use of megesterol acetate.

Diabetics should monitor glucose more frequently; insulin requirements may increase.

Pregnancy:

Tablet – Studies have shown a potential adverse effect on the fetus. Use only if clearly needed and potential benefits outweigh the possible risks. Megestrol is not recommended for use during the first four months of pregnancy.

Oral suspension – Do not use during pregnancy. The risk of use in a pregnant woman clearly outweights any possible benefit. Megestrol is not recommended for use during the first four months of pregnancy.

Breastfeeding: Because of the potential for adverse effects on newborns, nursing should be discontinued if the patient is taking megesterol acetate. Consult your doctor before you begin breastfeeding.

Children: Safety and effectiveness in children have not been established.

Drug Interactions:

Tell your doctor if you are taking or if you are planning to take any over-the-counter or prescription medications or dietary supplements with progestins. Doses of one or both drugs may need to be modified or a different drug may need to be prescribed.

Side Effects:

Every drug is capable of producing side effects. Many patients experience side effects. The frequency and severity of side effects depend on many factors including dose, duration of therapy and individual susceptibility. Possible side effects include:

Digestive Tract: Nausea; vomiting; diarrhea; indigestion; constipation; dry mouth; weight changes; increased salivation; mouth sores and infection; gas; stomach pain.

Nervous System: Weakness; sleeplessness; confusion; convulsions; depression; abnormal skin sensations; headache; chest or general body pain; mood changes; abnormal thinking; disease of the nerves.

Circulatory System: High blood pressure; pounding in the chest; heart failure; enlargement of the heart.

Respiratory System: Difficulty breathing; cough; sore throat; lung disorder.

Skin: Rash; itching; hair loss; sweating; decreased sensitivity to touch; skin disorder; herpes.

Other: Carpal tunnel syndrome; swelling; high blood sugar levels; fever; urinary changes; breast growth in males; breakthrough menstrual bleeding; hot flashes; glucose intolerance; impotence; anemia; infection; enlargement of the liver; abnormal blood counts; protein in the urine; urinary incontinence; urinary tract infection; decreased sex drive.

Guidelines for Use:

- Contraceptive (birth control) measures are recommended during treatment. Contact your doctor if pregnancy is suspected.
- If a dose is missed, take or inject it at soon as possible. If several hours have passed or it is nearing time for the next dose, do not double the dose to catch up, unless advised to do so by your doctor. If more than one dose is missed, contact your doctor or pharmacist.
- Shake suspension well before using.
- Contact your doctor if chest or stomach pain, headache, nausea, vomiting or other adverse reactions occur.
- Store suspension at 59° to 77°F in a tight container. Protect from heat.
- Lab tests/exams are required to monitor treatment. Be sure to keep appointments.
- Store tablets at room temperature away from heat.

If you have any questions, consult your doctor, pharmacist, or health care provider.

	Generic Name *Brand Name Example*	Supplied As	Generic Available
Rx	**Diethylstilbestrol Diphosphate**		
	Stilphostrol	**Tablets:** 50 mg	Yes
	Stilphostrol	**Injection:** 0.25 g (as sodium salt)	No

For more information on chemotherapy treatment, see the introduction to this chapter.

Type of Drug:

Chemotherapy agents; anticancer drugs.

How the Drug Works:

Diethylstilbestrol diphosphate increases estrogen levels in the body that prevent the formation of androgens that stimulate tumor cells of the prostate.

Uses:

To treat symptoms of progressing prostate cancer where surgery is not possible.

Precautions:

Do not use in the following situations:

blood clotting disorders
breast cancer (except for metastatic disease)
estrogen-dependent tumors
women

Use with caution in the following situations:

asthma
bone diseases
depression
diabetes
epilepsy
gallbladder disease
heart problems
kidney disease
liver disease, history of
migraines
surgery, prior to

Estrogen use in men: Diethylstilbestrol should not be used in men with breast cancer (unless advised by a doctor), estrogen-dependent tumors or blood clots.

Diabetes: Diethylstilbestrol may decrease glucose (sugar) tolerance. Test blood sugar often.

High blood pressure: Diethylstilbestrol may increase blood pressure. Blood pressure should be checked frequently.

Vision changes may occur. Report any changes to your doctor.

Children: Use diethylstilbestrol with extreme caution in young patients who are still growing, because it may interfere with normal bone development.

Lab tests may be required to monitor therapy. Tests may include eye exams, complete blood counts, liver and kidney function tests, calcium blood levels, cholesterol and triglyceride blood levels, prostate specific antigen (PSA) levels, glucose (sugar) blood levels (diabetics), blood clotting tests, folic acid levels, blood pressure and heart rate.

Drug Interactions:

Tell your doctor or pharmacist if you are taking or planning to take any over-the-counter or prescription medications or dietary supplements while taking an estrogen. Doses of one or both drugs may need to be modified or a different drug may need to be prescribed.

Side Effects:

Every drug is capable of producing side effects. Many estrogen users experience side effects. The frequency and severity of side effects depend on many factors including dose, duration of therapy, and individual susceptibility. Possible side effects include:

Digestive Tract: Nausea; vomiting; stomach cramps; appetite loss; weight changes; bloating.

Nervous System: Headache; migraine; nervousness; dizziness; mood changes; depression; fatigue; involuntary movements; numbness/tingling around nose or mouth.

Skin: Unusual hair growth or loss; itching or burning in the rectal area; rash; skin discoloration; yellowing of eyes or skin.

Other: Intolerance to contact lenses; backache; breast tenderness or enlargement; changes in sex drive; vision problems; swelling of hands or feet; shortness of breath; chest pain; painful, difficult and frequent urination.

Guidelines for Use:

- If a dose is missed, take or inject it as soon as possible. If several more hours have passed or it is nearing time for the next dose, do not double the dose to catch up, unless advised to do so by your doctor. If more than one dose is missed, contact your doctor or pharmacist.
- Diabetic patients should be prepared to monitor their blood sugar levels more frequently. Loss of glucose control may occur.
- Promptly report any of the following symptoms to your doctor: Bloating, nausea, vomiting, stomach cramps, loss of appetite, fluid retention, swelling/tenderness of breasts, rash, mood changes, depression, nervousness, dizziness, chest pain, shortness of breath, numbness or tingling around nose or mouth, vision changes, swelling, painful or frequent urination, yellowing of skin or eyes.
- Those who wear contact lenses may notice a change in their eyes or vision. Lens wear may not be possible.
- Lab tests and exams are required to monitor treatment. Be sure to keep appointments.
- Store tablets and injection at room temperature (59° to 86°F). Protect from light.

If you have any questions, consult your doctor, pharmacist, or health care provider.

	Generic Name *Brand Name Examples*	Supplied As	Generic Available
Rx	**Tamoxifen Citrate**		
	Nolvadex	**Tablets**: 10 mg, 20 mg	Yes
Rx	**Toremifene Citrate**		
	Fareston	**Tablets**: 60 mg	No

Type of Drug:

Antiestrogen; anticancer drug.

How the Drug Works:

Estrogens may cause the growth of some types of breast tumors. Antiestrogens block the effects of estrogen on certain tissues in the body, including breast tissue. Antiestrogens may block the growth of breast tumors that are activated by estrogens.

Uses:

Tamoxifen: For the treatment of metastatic breast cancer in men and women.

For the treatment of breast cancer in postmenopausal women following surgery and breast irradiation.

To reduce the rick of invasive breast cancer in women with ductal carcinoma in situ (DCIS) following breast surgery and radiation.

To reduce the incidence of breast cancer in women at high risk for developing breast cancer.

Toremifene: For the treatment of metastatic breast cancer in postmenopausal women with estrogen-receptor (ER) positive or ER-unknown tumors.

Unlabeled Use(s): Occasionally doctors may prescribe tamoxifen for treatment of breast pain and enlargement.

Precautions:

Do not use in the following situations:

- allergy to the antiestrogen or any of its ingredients
- deep-vein thrombosis, history of (tamoxifen only when used to reduce the incidence of breast cancer)
- oral anticoagulant therapy, concomitant (tamoxifen only when used to reduce the incidence of breast cancer)
- pulmonary embolus, history of (tamoxifen only when used to reduce the incidence of breast cancer)
- thromboembolic disease (toremifene only)

Use with caution in the following situations:

- calcium blood levels, increased
- cataracts (tamoxifen only)
- cholesterol or triglyceride levels, increased (tamoxifen only)

deep-vein thrombosis (following surgery for breast cancer) (tamoxifen only when used to treat metastatic breast cancer or breast cancer following surgery and breast irradiation)
liver disease (tamoxifen only)
platelet count decreased (tamoxifen only)
pulmonary embolus (tamoxifen only when used to treat metastatic breast cancer or breast cancer following surgery and breast irradiation)
white blood cells decreased (tamoxifen only)

Vision changes may occur. Report any changes to your doctor.

Pregnancy: There are no adequate and well-controlled studies in pregnant women. Antiestrogens may cause fetal harm when administered to a pregnant woman. Use only if clearly needed and potential benefits to the mother outweigh the possible hazards to the fetus.

Breastfeeding: It is not known if antiestrogens appear in breast milk. A decision must be made whether to discontinue nursing or discontinue the drug, taking into account the importance of the drug to the mother. Consult your doctor before you begin breastfeeding.

Children: Safety and effectiveness in children have not been established Antiestrogens are not indicated for use in children.

Lab tests will be required to monitor therapy. Tests may include complete blood counts, calcium levels, white blood cell counts, liver function tests, platelet counts, breast examinations, mammograms, gynecological exams, and cholesterol and triglyceride blood levels.

Drug Interactions:

Tell your doctor or pharmacist if you are taking or if you are planning to take any over-the-counter or prescription medications or dietary supplements while taking an antiestrogen. Doses of one or both drugs may need to be modified or a different drug may need to be prescribed. The following drugs and drug classes interact with antiestrogens:

anticoagulants, oral (eg, warfarin)
bromocriptine (*Parlodel*)
chemotherapeutic agents (eg, methotrexate)
cytochrome P450 3A4 enzyme inducers (eg, phenobarbital, phenytoin, carbamazepine)
rifamycins (eg, rifampin)

Side Effects:

Every drug is capable of producing side effects. Many antiestrogen users experience side effects. The frequency and severity of side effects depend on many factors including dose, duration of therapy, and individual susceptibility. Possible side effects include:

Eyes or Ocular: Corneal changes; cataracts; need for cataract surgery; decline in color vision perception; retinal vein thrombosis; retinopathy; dry eyes; abnormal visual fields.

Digestive Tract: Nausea; vomiting; appetite loss; weight loss; stomach cramps; constipation.

Nervous System: Fatigue; depression; dizziness; light-headedness; headache.

Skin: Rash; skin changes; hair thinning or partial hair loss; flushing; sweating.

Urinary and Reproductive Tract: Abnormal vaginal bleeding and discharge; menstrual irregularities; ovarian cysts; vaginal itching; vaginal dryness; pelvic pain or pressure.

Other: Hot flashes; difficulty breathing; cough; pain; bone, tumor, or muscle pain; local disease flare; lesion size increase in soft tissue disease; new lesions; flushing or redness around the lesion; high blood calcium levels; elevated liver enzymes; decreased white blood cell counts; decreased platelet count; changes in triglyceride blood levels; changes in cholesterol levels; swelling of the arms or legs; distaste for food; fluid retention; increased creatinine; loss of sex drive; impotence; blood clot in lungs; blood clot in legs; endometrial cancer; heart failure.

Guidelines for Use:

- Dosage is individualized. Take exactly as prescribed.
- Do not change the dose or stop taking, unless advised by your doctor.
- Swallow tablets whole with a glass of water.
- May be taken without regard to meals.
- Do not become pregnant during therapy. If you are sexually active, barrier or nonhormonal contraceptive (birth control) measures are recommended during treatment and for 2 months following the discontinuation of treatment. Contact your doctor if pregnancy is suspected.
- Notify your doctor immediately if you experience marked weakness, sleepiness, mental confusion, difficulty talking, numbness, pain or swelling of legs, unexplained shortness of breath, coughing up blood, sudden chest pain, changes in vision, new breast lumps, vaginal bleeding, gynecological symptoms (eg, menstrual irregularities, changes in vaginal discharge, pelvic pain or pressure), bone pain, hot flashes, nausea, vomiting, weight gain, dizziness, headache, or loss of appetite.
- If a dose is missed, take it as soon as possible. If several hours have passed or it is nearing time for the next dose, do not double the dose to catch up, unless advised to do so by your doctor. If more than one dose is missed, contact your doctor or pharmacist.
- Bone or tumor pain may occur shortly after starting tamoxifen and usually subsides rapidly.
- Lab tests and exams will be required to monitor therapy. Be sure to keep appointments. Women who receive long-term tamoxifen therapy should have regular gynecological and vision exams.
- Store at room temperature (68° to 77°F) in a tightly closed container. Protect from heat and light. Do not use after the expiration date.

If you have any questions, consult your doctor, pharmacist, or health care provider.

	Generic Name *Brand Name Example*	Supplied As	Generic Available
	Estramustine Phosphate Sodium		
Rx	*Emcyt*	**Capsules:** Equivalent to 140 mg estramustine phosphate	No

For more information on chemotherapy treatment, see the introduction to this chapter.

Type of Drug:

Chemotherapy agents; anticancer drugs.

How the Drug Works:

Estramustine increases estrogen levels in the body that prevent the formation of androgens that stimulate tumor cells of the prostate.

Uses:

To treat the symptoms of prostate cancer.

Precautions:

Do not use in the following situations:

allergy to estradiol or nitrogen mustard
blood clotting disorder, active

Use with caution in the following situations:

blood clotting disorders, history
calcium blood levels, increased
cerebrovascular disease
congestive heart disease
coronary artery disease
diabetes
edema (fluid retention)
epilepsy
high blood pressure
kidney disease
liver disease
migraines
stroke

Estrogen use in men: Estramustine should not be used in men with blood clots.

Diabetes: Estramustine may decrease glucose (sugar) tolerance. Test blood sugar often.

High blood pressure: Estramustine may increase blood pressure. Blood pressure should be checked frequently.

Lab tests may be required to monitor therapy. Be sure to keep appointments. Tests may include: Liver function tests, calcium blood levels, total bilirubin.

Drug Interactions:

Tell your doctor or pharmacist if you are taking or planning to take any over-the-counter or prescription medications or dietary supplements while taking these medicines. Doses of one or both drugs may need to be modified or a different drug may need to be prescribed. The following drugs, drug classes and foods interact with this medicine:

- calcium-containing antacids
- milk, dairy products and calcium-rich foods

Side Effects:

Every drug is capable of producing side effects. Many patients experience side effects. The frequency and severity of side effects depend on many factors including dose, duration of therapy, and individual susceptibility. Possible side effects include:

Digestive Tract: Nausea; vomiting; diarrhea; appetite loss; gas; burning throat; thirst; bleeding; stomach ache.

Nervous System: Headache; anxiety; sleeplessness; mood changes; drowsiness; depression.

Circulatory System: Chest pain; heart failure; stroke; heart attack; difficulty breathing; hoarseness; upper respiratory discharge; swelling.

Skin: Rash; itching; dry skin; peeling skin at fingertips; easy bruising; flushing; hair loss; thinning hair; skin color changes.

Other: Watery eyes; breast tenderness or enlargement; hot flashes; pain in eyes; ringing in the ears; abnormal blood counts; leg cramps; night sweats.

Guidelines for Use:

- Contraceptive (birth control) measures are recommended during treatment. Contact your doctor if pregnancy is suspected.
- If a dose is missed, take it as soon as possible. If several hours have passed or it is nearing time for the next dose, do not double the dose to catch up, unless advised to do so by your doctor. If more than one dose is missed, contact your doctor or pharmacist.
- Take 3 to 4 times daily with water and at least 1 hour before or 2 hours after meals.
- Do not take milk, dairy products and calcium-rich foods or drugs (such as antacids) at the same time as estramustine.
- Prepare diabetic patients to monitor their blood sugar levels more frequently. Loss of glucose control may occur.
- Lab tests/exams are required to monitor treatment. Be sure to keep appointments.
- Store at 36° to 46°F.

If you have any questions, consult your doctor, pharmacist, or health care provider.

Generic Name *Brand Name Example*	Supplied As	Generic Available
Rx **Anastrozole**		
Arimidex	**Tablets:** 1 mg	No

Type of Drug:

Anticancer drug; antihormone; aromatase inhibitor.

How the Drug Works:

Anastrozole lowers estradiol (female sex hormones) levels and thus reduces or delays the growth of tumors in breast cancer patients.

Uses:

To treat advanced breast cancer in postmenopausal women whose disease continues to grow after tamoxifen therapy.

Precautions:

Use with caution in the following situations:

high cholesterol
pregnancy

Pregnancy: Studies have shown a potential adverse effect on the fetus. Use only if clearly needed and potential benefits outweigh the possible risks to the fetus.

Breastfeeding: It is not known if anastrozole appears in breast milk. Consult your doctor before you begin breastfeeding.

Children: Safety and effectiveness in children have not been established.

Lab tests may be required to monitor therapy. Be sure to keep appointments.

Drug Interactions:

Tell your doctor or pharmacist if you are taking or planning to take any over-the-counter or prescription medications or dietary supplements while taking this medicine. Doses of one or both drugs may need to be modified or another drug may need to be prescribed. Drugs metabolized by the cytochrome P450 oxidase enzyme system (eg, carbamazepine) may interact with this medicine.

Side Effects:

Every drug is capable of producing side effects. Many patients experience no, or minor, side effects. The frequency and severity of side effects depend on many factors including dose, duration of therapy, and individual susceptibility. Possible side effects include:

Digestive Tract: Nausea; vomiting; diarrhea; constipation; stomach pain; appetite changes.

Nervous System: Headache; weakness; dizziness; depression; abnormal skin sensations; drowsiness; sleeplessness; confusion; anxiety; nervousness.

Respiratory System: Difficulty breathing; increased cough; sore throat; sinus infection; bronchitis; congestion.

Skin: Rash; itching; thinning hair.

Other: Hot flushes; pain; muscle, joint, back, bone, pelvic, neck, breast or chest pain; general body discomfort; dry mouth; swelling of hands and feet; vaginal bleeding; weight gain; sweating; flu syndrome; fever; injury; infection; urinary tract infection; abnormal blood counts; anemia; abnormal lab tests; weight loss; fracture; high blood pressure; vein inflammation.

Guidelines for Use:

- Use exactly as prescribed.
- The usual dose is 1 tablet once daily.
- Take on an empty stomach.
- If a dose is missed, take it as soon as possible. If several hours have passed or it is nearing time for the next dose, do not double the dose to catch up, unless advised to do so by your doctor. If more than one dose is missed or it is necessary to establish a new dosage schedule, contact your doctor or pharmacist.
- May cause dizziness or drowsiness. Use caution while driving or performing other tasks requiring mental alertness, coordination, or physical dexterity.
- Inform your doctor if your are pregnant, become pregnant, are planning to become pregnant or if you are breastfeeding.
- Store at room temperature (68° to 77°F).

If you have any questions, consult your doctor, pharmacist, or health care provider.

	Generic Name *Brand Name Example*	Supplied As	Generic Available
Rx	**Letrozole**		
	Femara	**Tablets:** 2.5 mg	No

Type of Drug:

Anticancer drug.

How the Drug Works:

Letrozole lowers estrogen levels resulting in a reduction or a delay in the growth of estrogen-dependent breast tumors.

Uses:

To treat advanced breast cancer in postmenopausal women whose disease continues to progress after antiestrogen therapy.

Precautions:

Do not use in the following situations: Allergy to letrozole or any of its ingredients.

Use with caution in the following situations:

- liver impairment, severe
- liver tests, abnormal
- pregnancy

Pregnancy: Studies have shown a potential adverse effect to the fetus. Use only if clearly needed and potential benefits outweigh the possible risks.

Breastfeeding: It is not known if letrozole appears in breast milk. Consult your doctor before you begin breastfeeding.

Children: Safety and effectiveness in children have not been established.

Lab tests may be required to monitor treatment. Be sure to keep appointments.

Drug Interactions:

Tell your doctor or pharmacist if you are taking or planning to take any over-the-counter or prescription medications or dietary supplements with letrozole. Doses of one or both drugs may need to be modified or a different drug may need to be prescribed.

Side Effects:

Every drug is capable of producing side effects. Many letrozole users experience no, or minor, side effects. The frequency and severity of side effects depend on many factors including dose, duration of therapy, and individual susceptibility. Possible side effects include:

Digestive Tract: Nausea; vomiting; constipation; diarrhea; stomach pain; loss of appetite; indigestion.

Nervous System: Headache; drowsiness; dizziness; depression; anxiety.

Skin: Hot flushes; rash; itching.

Other: High blood pressure; difficulty breathing; coughing; fatigue; chest pain; swelling of the arms and legs; weakness; weight increase; viral infection; elevated cholesterol; muscle pain; skeletal pain; back pain; arm pain; leg pain; pain in the joints; excessive calcium in the blood; fracture; hair loss; increased sweating.

Guidelines for Use:

- The recommended dose of letrozole is one 2.5 mg tablet a day.
- May be taken with or without food.
- Inform your doctor if you are pregnant, become pregnant, are planning to become pregnant or if you are breastfeeding.
- This medicine may cause drowsiness or dizziness. Use caution while driving or performing other tasks requiring mental alertness, coordination or physical dexterity.
- Lab tests or exams may be required to monitor treatment. Be sure to keep appointments.
- Store at room temperature (59° to 86°F).

If you have any questions, consult your doctor, pharmacist, or health care provider.

	Generic Name *Brand Name Example*	Supplied As	Generic Available
Rx	**Goserelin Acetate**		
	Zoladex	**Implant:** 3.6 mg, 10.8 mg	No

Type of Drug:

Synthetic hormone; luteinizing hormone-releasing hormone (LHRH); gonadotropin-releasing hormone (GnRH) agonist analogue.

How the Drug Works:

Goserelin acetate inhibits the release of certain hormones responsible for causing the release of sex hormones, thereby decreasing sex hormone levels in men (testosterone) and women (estradiol). Decreased levels of sex hormones lead to a reduction in size and function of sex organs as well as regression of some tumors stimulated by sex hormones.

Uses:

To treat the symptoms of advanced prostate cancer when orchiectomy (castration) or estrogen administration is either not indicated or unacceptable to the patient. Used in combination with flutamide to manage locally confined stage T2b-T4 (Stage B2-C) prostate cancer. Treatment should begin 8 weeks prior to initiating radiation therapy and should be continued during radiation therapy.

To manage endometriosis including pain relief and lesion reduction (3.6 mg).

To treat symptoms of advanced breast cancer in pre– and perimenopausal women (3.6 mg).

To thin the endometrium prior to ablation procedures for dysfunctional uterine bleeding (3.6 mg).

Precautions:

Do not use in the following situations:

- allergy to LHRH, LHRH agonist analogues, or any ingredient of this drug
- pregnancy
- vaginal bleeding, abnormal
- women, breastfeeding
- women, childbearing potential
- women (10.8 mg implant only)

Use with caution in the following situations:

- anticonvulsant use
- bone cancer, metastatic
- corticosteroid use
- female chronic alcohol abuse
- high calcium levels
- males with the risk of ureteral obstruction or spinal cord compression
- osteoporosis, family history
- tobacco use

Contraception: Effective non–hormonal contraception must be used by all women of childbearing potential while using this drug and for 12 weeks following discontinuation of therapy.

Diagnostic test interference: Goserelin acetate therapy will interfere with diagnostic tests of pituitary–gonadotropic and gonadal function.

Pregnancy: Do not use during pregnancy. The risk of use in a pregnant woman clearly outweighs any possible benefit. Goserelin acetate can cause fetal harm when administered to a pregnant woman. There is a risk for pregnancy termination (miscarriage) due to possible hormonal imbalances as a result of goserelin acetate.

Breastfeeding: It is not known if goserelin acetate appears in human milk. There is a potential for serious adverse reactions in nursing infants of mothers receiving goserelin acetate. Consult your doctor before you begin breastfeeding.

Children: Safety and effectiveness in children have not been established.

Lab tests will be required to monitor therapy. Tests may include testosterone or estradiol blood levels, PSA levels, and pregnancy test.

Drug Interactions:

Tell your doctor or pharmacist if you are taking or planning to take any over-the-counter or prescription medications or dietary supplements while taking goserelin acetate. Doses of one or both drugs may need to be modified or a different drug may need to be prescribed.

Side Effects:

Every drug is capable of producing side effects. Many goserelin acetate users experience no, or minor, side effects. The frequency and severity of side effects depend on many factors including dose, duration of therapy, and individual susceptibility. Possible side effects include:

Digestive Tract: Diarrhea; vomiting of blood; nausea; constipation; gas; indigestion; appetite changes; ulcer; vomiting; dry mouth.

Nervous System: Headache; spinal cord compression; irritability; emotional instability; anxiety; depression; lethargy; dizziness; sleeplessness.

Circulatory System: Anemia; blood or tissue infection; chest pain; reduced blood flow to brain; stroke; blood clot in the lungs; varicose veins; bleeding; high blood pressure; fast or irregular heartbeat; congestive heart failure.

Urinary and Reproductive Tract: Sexual dysfunction; change in sex drive; decreased erections; ureteral or bladder obstruction; enlarged breasts; pelvic pain; breast pain; blood in urine; impotence; changes in urinary frequency; incontinence; urinary tract infection; difficult urination or inability to urinate; bladder inflammation; rectal bleeding; vaginal dryness; urinary urgency; pain or burning upon urination; vaginal inflammation; vaginitis; pain during intercourse; painful menstruation; heavy menstruation.

Skin: Herpes simplex; hives; itching; rash; sweating; acne; excessively oily skin; bruising.

Other: Hot flashes; weakness; abdominal pain; back, joint, or muscle pain; flu-like syndrome; diabetes mellitus; anemia; loss of bone mineral density; upper respiratory tract infection; implant site reaction; voice alterations; hair disorders; increased hair growth; weight gain; leg cramps; migraine; swelling; muscle tightness; sore throat; sinus infection; chronic obstructive lung disease; general pain; severe allergic reaction.

Guidelines for Use:

- *3.6 mg Implant:* Administer subcutaneously (just under the skin) every 28 days into the upper abdominal wall. It is also used in conjunction with the 10.8 mg dose for treatment of stage B2–C prostatic cancer.
- *10.8 mg Implant:* Administer subcutaneously (just under the skin) every 28 days into the upper abdominal wall.
- Every effort should be made to adhere to the 28–day schedule. A missed dose may cause breakthrough bleeding and pregnancy (females).
- *Stage B2–C Prostatic Carcinoma* – When goserelin acetate is given in combination with flutamide, start treatment at least 8 weeks prior to initiating radiation therapy and continue treatment during radiation therapy. Administer 1 goserelin acetate 3.6 mg depot followed in 28 days by 1 goserelin acetate 10.8 mg depot.
- *Prostate and Breast Cancer* – Intended for long-term administration unless clinically inappropriate. Transient worsening of symptoms or the occurrence of additional signs and symptoms of prostate or breast cancer may occasionally develop during the first few weeks of goserelin acetate treatment.
- *Endometriosis* – Recommended dosage is 3.6 mg every 28 days for 6 months. Retreatment cannot be recommended because safety data for periods longer than 6 months are not available. Pregnancy is contraindicated in women being treated for endometriosis or endometrial thinning. Therefore, a nonhormonal method of contraception should be used during treatment. If pregnancy occurs during treatment, discontinue goserelin acetate and advise the patient of the possible risks to the fetus.
- *Females* – Menstruation should stop with goserelin acetate. If regular menstruation persists, notify your doctor.
- Goserelin acetate may result in decrease or loss of bone mineral density or bone mineral loss in patients with major risk factors such as chronic alcohol abuse, tobacco abuse, significant family history of osteoporosis, or chronic use of bone density reducing drugs (eg, anticonvulsants, corticosteroids). Benefits must be weighed carefully before therapy with goserelin acetate is instituted.
- No dosage adjustment is necessary for patients with kidney or liver disease.
- This medication will usually be administered by a health care provider in a clinical setting. It is possible that it could be prescribed for home use in certain circumstances. In that event, follow the proper method of administration of goserelin acetate as described in the following instructions (or by your health care provider).

Guidelines for Use (cont.):

Administration Technique:

1. Inspect the package for damage prior to opening. If damaged, do not use.
2. Clean an area of the upper abdominal wall with an alcohol swab. A local anesthetic may be used.
3. Using aseptic technique, stretch or pinch the abdominal skin with one hand and grip the syringe barrel. Insert needle into the subcutaneous tissue. If a vessel is penetrated, blood will be seen instantly in the syringe chamber. Withdraw the needle, discard the unit, and inject with a new syringe elsewhere.
4. Change the direction of the needle so it parallels the abdominal wall. Push the needle in until the barrel hub touches the skin. Withdraw the needle 1 cm to create a space to discharge the goserelin acetate implant. Fully depress the plunger to discharge the implant.
5. Withdraw the needle. Bandage the site. Confirm discharge of goserelin acetate by ensuring tip of the plunger is visible within the tip of the needle. Dispose of the used needle and syringe in a safe manner. In the unlikely event of the need to surgically remove goserelin acetate, it may be localized by ultrasound.

- Store at room temperature.

If you have any questions, consult your doctor, pharmacist, or health care provider.

	Generic Name *Brand Name Example*	Supplied As	Generic Available
Rx	**Levamisole HCl**		
	Ergamisol	**Tablets:** 50 mg	No

Type of Drug:

Anticancer drug; immunomodulator.

How the Drug Works:

The exact mechanism of action of levamisole is unknown. It is believed the drug stimulates the body's natural immune system to produce the substances needed to fight infection and destroy tumors.

Uses:

Used in combination with fluorouracil after surgery in patients with Duke stage C colon cancer.

Precautions:

Do not use in the following situations: Allergy to levamisole or any of its ingredients.

Use with caution in the following situations: Liver impairment.

Mental impairment: Cases of an encephalopathy-like syndrome have been reported in patients treated with levamisole HCl. Symptoms may include confusion, coma, lethargy, weakness, seizures, speech disturbances, tingling in the hands or feet, and brain inflammation.

Blood disorders: Chronic use of levamisole may result in decreased white blood cell counts. Development of flu-like symptoms may be a sign of a serious blood disorder. Immediately report any flu-like symptoms (eg, fever, chills) to your doctor.

Pregnancy: Adequate studies have not been done in pregnant women. Use only if clearly needed and potential benefits to the mother outweigh the possible hazards to the fetus.

Breastfeeding: It is not known if levamisole appears in breast milk. Consult your doctor before you begin breastfeeding.

Children: Safety and effectiveness have not been established.

Lab tests will be required frequently during treatment with levamisole. Tests may include complete blood counts, electrolytes, and liver function tests.

Drug Interactions:

Tell your doctor or pharmacist if you are taking or planning to take any over-the-counter or prescription medications or dietary supplements with levamisole. Doses of one or both drugs may need to be modified or a different drug may need to be prescribed. The following drugs and drug classes interact with levamisole:

alcohol
anticoagulants (eg, warfarin)
phenytoin (eg, *Dilantin*)

Side Effects:

Every drug is capable of producing side effects. Many levamisole users experience side effects. The frequency and severity of side effects depend on many factors including dose, duration of therapy, and individual susceptibility. Possible side effects include:

Digestive Tract: Nausea; vomiting; diarrhea; appetite loss; stomach ache; constipation.

Nervous System: Dizziness; drowsiness; depression; confusion; anxiety; memory loss; weakness; difficulty concentrating; headache; nervousness; fatigue; sleeplessness.

Skin: Rash; itching; hair loss; skin inflammation; abnormal skin sensations.

Other: Abnormal blood cell and platelet counts; flu-like symptoms (eg, fatigue, fever, chills); infection; fluid retention; changes in taste or smell; inflammation of the mouth and gums; irritated eyes with watering; muscle and joint pain; blurred vision.

Guidelines for Use:

- Usual initial therapy is 50 mg levamisole HCl every 8 hours for 3 days (starting 7 to 30 days after surgery) with 450 mg/m^2/day flourouracil IV for 5 days (starting 21 to 34 days after surgery).
- Usual maintenance dosage is 50 mg levamisole HCl every 8 hours for 3 days every 2 weeks with 450 mg/m^2/day flourouracil IV once a week beginning 28 days after initiation of the 5-day course.
- Do not exceed recommended dose or frequency. The risk of serious side effects may be increased.
- Do not drink alcohol while taking this medication. A serious reaction (nausea, vomiting, flushing) may occur.
- If you miss a dose of this drug, wait until your next scheduled dose and resume taking it as before. Do not take an extra dose in an effort to catch up.
- Discontinue the drug immediately and contact your doctor if you experience any of the following symptoms: Confusion, lethargy, memory loss, muscle weakness, abnormal skin sensations, seizures, speech disturbances. These symptoms may be a sign of a serious condition.
- Notify your doctor immediately if you experience flu-like symptoms (eg, fatigue, fever, chills).
- Inform your doctor if you are pregnant, become pregnant, are planning to become pregnant, or are breastfeeding.
- Lab tests will be required during treatment. Be sure to keep appointments.
- Store at controlled room temperature (58° to 77°F). Protect from moisture.

If you have any questions, consult your doctor, pharmacist, or health care provider.

	Generic Name *Brand Name Examples*	Supplied As	Generic Available
Rx	**Carmustine**		
	BiCNU	**Powder for Injection:** 100 mg	No
	Gliadel	**Wafer:** 7.7 mg	No

For more information on chemotherapy treatment, see the introduction to this chapter.

Type of Drug:

Anticancer agent; alkylating agent; nitrosourea.

How the Drug Works:

Carmustine stops or slows the growth of cancerous cells by interfering with their reproduction.

Uses:

Injection: To treat brain tumors, cancer of the bone marrow, Hodgkin disease and non-Hodgkin lymphoma (as a secondary therapy in combination with other drugs in failure of response to primary therapy).

Wafer: Used as an adjunct to surgery or used after surgery to prolong survival after removal of certain brain tumors.

Precautions:

Do not use in the following situations: Allergy to carmustine or any of its ingredients.

Use with caution in the following situations:

bone marrow suppression (injection only)
complications of brain surgery (eg, seizures, abnormal wound healing) (wafer only)
lung disease (injection only)

Long-term use may cause secondary cancer.

Pregnancy: Studies have shown a potential effect to the fetus. Use only if clearly needed and potential benefits outweigh the possible risks.

Breastfeeding: It is not known if carmustine appears in breast milk. Either breastfeeding or drug therapy should be stopped, taking into account the importance of the drug to the mother. Consult your doctor before you begin breastfeeding.

Children: Safety and effectiveness in children have not been established.

Lab tests will be required frequently during treatment with carmustine. Be sure to keep appointments. Tests may include kidney, liver and lung function tests and blood counts.

Drug Interactions:

Tell your doctor or pharmacist if you are taking or if you are planning to take any over-the-counter or prescription medications or dietary supplements with carmustine. Doses of one or both drugs may need to be modified or a different drug may need to be prescribed. The following drugs interact with injectable carmustine:

cimetidine (eg, *Tagamet*)
phenytoin (eg, *Dilantin*)
mitomycin (*Mutamycin*)

Side Effects:

Every drug is capable of producing side effects. Many carmustine users experience no, or minor, side effects. The frequency and severity of side effects depend on many factors including dose, duration of therapy, and individual susceptibility. Possible side effects include:

Injection —

Circulatory System: Decreased blood platelets; abnormal blood counts; anemia.

Skin: Burning; excessive pigmentation; flushing; injection site burning.

Other: Nausea; vomiting; lowered ability to fight infection; liver toxicity; kidney abnormalities and damage; swelling of the retina and optic nerve (of the eye); watery eyes; lung toxicity.

Wafer —

Digestive Tract: Nausea; vomiting; diarrhea; constipation; bleeding.

Nervous System: Brain damage; brain or spinal cord swelling; brain infection; confusion; seizures; headache; one-sided paralysis; elevated brain pressure; drowsiness; acting unsensible; depression; abnormal thinking; clumsiness; dizziness; sleeplessness; coma; amnesia; paranoid reaction.

Circulatory System: Anemia; blood clots; high blood pressure; low blood pressure; decreased blood platelets; abnormal blood count; high blood sugar; low potassium count; salt depletion in blood.

Respiratory System: Pneumonia; lung clot; infection.

Other: Rash; fever; pain; abnormal healing; urinary tract infection; mouth infection; neck pain; accidental injury; back pain; allergic reaction; swelling of the arms and legs; weakness; chest pain; infection; eye pain; vision problems; double vision; difficulty in swallowing.

Guidelines for Use:

- This medicine will be prepared and administered by your health care provider.
- Carmustine injection is administered every 6 weeks and should be monitored weekly for at least 6 weeks after a dose.
- Carmustine injection contains no preservatives.
- *Injection* — Nausea and vomiting may occur. Use of drugs for nausea before dosing may help reduce and sometimes prevent these side effects.
- *Infections* — This drug may lower your body's ability to fight infection. Notify your doctor of any signs of infection, including fever, sore throat, rashes or chills.
- Contraceptive measures should be used during therapy.
- Lab tests or exams will be required to monitor treatment. Be sure to keep appointments.
- Store dry powder for injection in refrigerator (36° to 46°F).
- Store wafers at or below −4°F.

If you have any questions, consult your doctor, pharmacist, or health care provider.

	Generic Name *Brand Name Example*	Supplied As	Generic Available
Rx	**Lomustine (CCNU)**		
	CeeNu	**Capsules:** 10 mg, 40 mg, 100 mg	No
	CeeNu	**Dose pack:** Two 10 mg capsules, two 40 mg capsules, two 100 mg capsules	No

For more information on chemotherapy treatment, see the introduction of this chapter.

Type of Drug:

Chemotherapy drug; anticancer drug; alkylating agent; CCNU; nitrosourea.

How the Drug Works:

Lomustine stops the spread or growth of cancerous cells by interfering with their reproduction. This drug is often used with other anticancer drugs.

Uses:

To treat brain tumors in patients who have had surgery and/or radiation treatment.

To treat Hodgkin disease when other drugs have failed.

Precautions:

Do not use in the following situations: Allergy to lomustine or any of its ingredients.

Breathing: Lomustine can affect the lungs. Report any breathing difficulty to your doctor immediately.

Long-term use may cause secondary cancer.

Pregnancy: Studies have shown a potential adverse effect on the fetus. Use only if clearly needed and potential benefits outweigh the possible risks.

Breastfeeding: It is not known if lomustine appears in breast milk. Either breastfeeding or drug therapy should be stopped, taking into account the importance of the drug to the mother. Consult your doctor before you begin breastfeeding.

Lab tests will be required during treatment with lomustine. Blood counts should be monitored weekly for at least 6 weeks following a dose. Liver, kidney and lung function tests must be done periodically. Dosage adjustments may be necessary.

Drug Interactions:

Tell your doctor or pharmacist if you are taking or planning to take any over-the-counter or prescription medications or dietary supplements while taking this medicine. Doses of one or both drugs may need to be modified or a different drug may need to be prescribed.

Side Effects:

Most lomustine users experience side effects. The frequency and severity of side effects depend on many factors including dose, duration of therapy, and individual susceptibility. Possible side effects include:

Digestive Tract: Nausea; vomiting; appetite loss; sore throat.

Nervous System: Unusual tiredness; disorientation; clumsiness; slurred speech.

Respiratory System: Shortness of breath; dry cough; lung fibrosis.

Skin: Yellowing of the skin or eyes; unusual bleeding or bruising; hair loss.

Other: Fever; chills; sore throat; swelling of the lower legs or feet; sores on mouth or lips; kidney damage; abnormal liver and kidney function tests; abnormal blood counts; inflammation of the mouth; lowered ability to fight infection; anemia; visual disturbances; acute leukemia; bone marrow dysplasia.

Guidelines for Use:

- Take on an empty stomach to reduce nausea. Nausea and vomiting may occur 3 to 6 hours after an oral dose and usually lasts less than 24 hours, although loss of appetite may last for several days. Use of drugs for nausea before dosing may help reduce and sometimes prevent these side effects.
- Lomustine is given as a single oral dose and will not be repeated for at least 6 weeks.
- *Infections* — These drugs may lower your body's ability to fight infection. Notify your doctor of any signs of infection, including fever, sore throat, rashes or chills.
- Notify your doctor if unusual bleeding or bruising, shortness of breath, dry cough, swelling of feet or lower legs, yellowing of eyes and skin, confusion, inflammation of the mouth or unusual tiredness occurs.
- May cause appetite loss, nausea and vomiting and, less frequently, hair loss. Notify your doctor if these reactions become pronounced.
- Avoid alcohol for short periods after taking a dose of lomustine.
- Contraceptive (birth control) measures are recommended during therapy.
- Patients should be aware that lomustine is an anticancer drug and belongs to the group of medicines known as alkylating agents.
- Patients should be aware that there may be 2 or more different types and colors of capsules in the container in order to provide the proper dose.
- Lab tests/exams will be required to monitor treatment. Be sure to keep appointments.
- Store at room temperature (68° to 77°F) in a tightly sealed container.

If you have any questions, consult your doctor, pharmacist, or health care provider.

	Generic Name *Brand Name Example*	Supplied As	Generic Available
Rx	**Streptozocin**		
	Zanosar	**Powder for Injection:** 1 g	No

For more information on chemotherapy treatment, see the introduction to this chapter.

Type of Drug:

Anticancer agent.

How the Drug Works:

Streptozocin stops or slows the spread of cancerous cells by disrupting the growth of DNA.

Uses:

To treat cancer of the pancreas.

Precautions:

Do not use in the following situations: Allergy to streptozocin or any of its ingredients.

Use with caution in the following situations:

development of tumors at the injection site
kidney disease
use with other kidney toxic drugs

Pregnancy: Adequate studies have not been done in pregnant women. Use only if clearly needed and potential benefits outweigh the possible hazards to the fetus.

Breastfeeding: It is not known if streptozocin appears in breast milk. Consult your doctor before you begin breastfeeding.

Lab tests will be required frequently during treatment with streptozocin. Tests may include kidney and liver function tests, blood counts and urinalysis.

Drug Interactions:

Tell your doctor or pharmacist if you are taking or planning to take any over-the-counter or prescription medications or dietary supplements with streptozocin. Doses of one or both drugs may need to be modified or a different drug may need to be prescribed. The use of other drugs toxic to the kidney should be used with caution or not at all with this drug.

Side Effects:

Every drug is capable of producing side effects. Many streptozocin users experience no, or minor, side effects. The frequency and severity of side effects depend on many factors including the dose, duration of therapy, and individual susceptibility. Possible side effects include:

Digestive Tract: Nausea; vomiting; diarrhea; liver toxicity; elevated liver enzyme levels; low amounts of albumin in the blood.

Circulatory System: Blood toxicity; reduction in red and white blood cells; reduction in platelet count; abnormal glucose (sugar) tolerance.

Other: Kidney toxicity; excess urea in the blood; low amounts of phosphate in the blood; glucose in the urine.

Guidelines for Use:

- This medicine will be prepared and administered by your healthcare provider.
- Streptozocin injection contains no preservatives.
- Use gloves during preparation and administration.
- If streptozocin powder or solution contacts the skin, wash with soap and water.
- Inform your doctor if you are pregnant, become pregnant, are planning to become pregnant or if you are breastfeeding.
- Lab tests or exams will be required to monitor treatment. Be sure to keep appointments.
- Store in refrigerator (35° to 46°F) and protect from light.

If you have any questions, consult your doctor, pharmacist, or health care provider.

	Generic Name *Brand Name Example*	Supplied As	Generic Available
	Estramustine Phosphate Sodium		
Rx	*Emcyt*	**Capsules:** Equivalent to 140 mg estramustine phosphate	No

For more information on chemotherapy treatment, see the introduction to this chapter.

Type of Drug:

Chemotherapy agents; anticancer drugs.

How the Drug Works:

Estramustine increases estrogen levels in the body that prevent the formation of androgens that stimulate tumor cells of the prostate.

Uses:

To treat the symptoms of prostate cancer.

Precautions:

Do not use in the following situations:

allergy to estradiol or nitrogen mustard
blood clotting disorder, active

Use with caution in the following situations:

blood clotting disorders, history
calcium blood levels, increased
cerebrovascular disease
congestive heart disease
coronary artery disease
diabetes
edema (fluid retention)
epilepsy
high blood pressure
kidney disease
liver disease
migraines
stroke

Estrogen use in men: Estramustine should not be used in men with blood clots.

Diabetes: Estramustine may decrease glucose (sugar) tolerance. Test blood sugar often.

High blood pressure: Estramustine may increase blood pressure. Blood pressure should be checked frequently.

Lab tests may be required to monitor therapy. Be sure to keep appointments. Tests may include: Liver function tests, calcium blood levels, total bilirubin.

Drug Interactions:

Tell your doctor or pharmacist if you are taking or planning to take any over-the-counter or prescription medications or dietary supplements while taking these medicines. Doses of one or both drugs may need to be modified or a different drug may need to be prescribed. The following drugs, drug classes and foods interact with this medicine:

calcium-containing antacids

milk, dairy products and calcium-rich foods

Side Effects:

Every drug is capable of producing side effects. Many patients experience side effects. The frequency and severity of side effects depend on many factors including dose, duration of therapy, and individual susceptibility. Possible side effects include:

Digestive Tract: Nausea; vomiting; diarrhea; appetite loss; gas; burning throat; thirst; bleeding; stomach ache.

Nervous System: Headache; anxiety; sleeplessness; mood changes; drowsiness; depression.

Circulatory System: Chest pain; heart failure; stroke; heart attack; difficulty breathing; hoarseness; upper respiratory discharge; swelling.

Skin: Rash; itching; dry skin; peeling skin at fingertips; easy bruising; flushing; hair loss; thinning hair; skin color changes.

Other: Watery eyes; breast tenderness or enlargement; hot flashes; pain in eyes; ringing in the ears; abnormal blood counts; leg cramps; night sweats.

Guidelines for Use:

- Contraceptive (birth control) measures are recommended during treatment. Contact your doctor if pregnancy is suspected.
- If a dose is missed, take it as soon as possible. If several hours have passed or it is nearing time for the next dose, do not double the dose to catch up, unless advised to do so by your doctor. If more than one dose is missed, contact your doctor or pharmacist.
- Take 3 to 4 times daily with water and at least 1 hour before or 2 hours after meals.
- Do not take milk, dairy products and calcium-rich foods or drugs (such as antacids) at the same time as estramustine.
- Prepare diabetic patients to monitor their blood sugar levels more frequently. Loss of glucose control may occur.
- Lab tests/exams are required to monitor treatment. Be sure to keep appointments.
- Store at 36° to 46°F.

If you have any questions, consult your doctor, pharmacist, or health care provider.

ALKYLATING AGENTS — NITROGEN MUSTARDS

	Generic Name *Brand Name Examples*	Supplied As	Generic Available
Rx	**Chlorambucil**		
	Leukeran	**Tablets:** 2 mg	No
Rx	**Cyclophosphamide**		
	Cytoxan	**Tablets:** 25 mg, 50 mg	No
	Cytoxan	**Powder for Injection:** 75 mg mannitol/100 mg cyclophosphamide	No
Rx	**Ifosfamide**		
	Ifex	**Powder for injection:** 1 g, 3 g	No
Rx	**Mechlorethamine HCl**		
	Mustargen	**Powder for injection:** 10 mg	No
Rx	**Melphalan**[1]		
	Alkeran	**Tablets:** 2 mg	No

[1] Some of these products are available as an injection.

For more information on chemotherapy treatment, see the introduction to this chapter.

Type of Drug:

Anticancer drugs.

How the Drug Works:

Nitrogen mustard anticancer drugs interfere with the function of DNA, disrupting the reproduction of the cancer cells. They are often used in combination with other drugs.

Uses:

Chlorambucil: To treat malignant lymphomas, a certain type of leukemia and Hodgkin disease.

Cyclophosphamide: To treat cancer of the breast and ovaries, lymphomas, certain leukemias, multiple myeloma and Hodgkin disease. Also used for advanced mycosis fungoides (cancer of skin and lymph nodes), neuroblastoma (malignant tumor of embryonic ganglion cells), adenocarcinoma (malignant tumor originating from glandular cells) and retinoblastoma (malignant tumor of the retina). To treat nephrotic syndrome in children when other treatment regimens have failed.

Ifosfamide: To treat testicular cancer in combination with other approved anticancer drugs.

Mechlorethamine: To treat Hodgkin's disease (Stages III and IV), lymphosarcoma, chronic myelocytic or chronic lymphocytic leukemia, polycythemia vera, mycosis fungoides, bronchogenic cancer and metastatic cancer causing effusions.

Melphalan: To treat cancer of the ovaries and multiple myeloma.

Unlabeled Use(s): Occasionally doctors may prescribe chlorambucil for uveitis, inflammation of the brain caused by Behcet disease, and for treating certain types of nephropathy and rheumatoid arthritis. Cyclophosphamide has been prescribed for rheumatoid conditions (eg, arthritis, systemic lupus erythematous), Wegener granulomatosis, other steroid-resistant vasculidites, multiple sclerosis, polyarteritis nodosa and polymyositis.

Precautions:

Do not use in the following situations:

- allergy to the drug or to other nitrogen mustard drugs
- bone marrow depression, severe (cyclophosphamide and ifosfamide only)
- infectious diseases (mechlorethamine only)
- prior resistance to the drug

Use with caution in the following situations:

- abnormal blood counts
- abnormal uric acid levels (mechlorethamine)
- adrenal surgery
- anemia
- anesthesia use
- blood disorders (eg, decreased blood counts)
- bone marrow depression
- chemotherapy
- decreased blood platelets
- development of bleeding cysts, urinary (cyclophosphamide)
- infection, recent
- kidney disease
- liver disease
- pregnancy
- radiation
- tumor of the bone marrow
- tumors of the bone and nervous tissues (mechlorethamine)
- wounds

Fertility impairment: Nitrogen mustard agents may cause temporary or permanent infertility. These drugs can cause chromosome damage and can interfere with formation of sperm in males and eggs in females. They may also cause menstruation to stop.

Infections: These drugs may impair your body's ability to fight infection. Notify your doctor of any signs of infection including fever, sore throat, rashes or chills.

Long term use may cause secondary cancer.

Pregnancy: Studies have shown a potential adverse effect to the fetus. Use only if clearly needed and potential benefits outweigh the possible risks. Women should avoid becoming pregnant and proper birth control should be used. Contact your doctor immediately if pregnancy is suspected.

Breastfeeding: Cyclophosphamide and ifosfamide appear in breast milk. It is not known if the other nitrogen mustards appear in breast milk. Use during breastfeeding is not recommended. Consult your doctor before you begin breastfeeding.

Children: Safety and effectiveness in children have not been established.

Lab tests will be required during treatment.

Drug Interactions:

Tell your doctor or pharmacist if you are taking or planning to take any over-the-counter or prescription medications or dietary supplements with cyclophosphamide. Doses of one or both drugs may need to be modified or a different drug may need to be prescribed. The following drugs and drug classes interact with cyclophosphamide:

allopurinol (eg, *Zyloprim*)
anticoagulants (eg, warfarin)
chloramphenicol (eg, *Chloromycetin)*
corticosteroids (eg, *Prednisone*)
digoxin (eg, *Lanoxin)*
doxorubicin (eg, *Adriamycin)*
methotrexate (eg, *Folex*)
phenobarbital (eg, *Solfoton)*
quinolone antibiotics (eg, *Cipro*)
succinylcholine (eg, *Anectine)*
sulfonamides (eg, sulfisoxazole)
thiazide diuretics (eg, hydrochlorothiazide)

Side Effects:

Most nitrogen mustard users experience side effects. The frequency and severity of side effects depend on many factors including dose, duration of therapy, and individual susceptibility. Possible side effects include:

Blood: Bone marrow depression; decreased blood cell and platelet counts; anemias; abnormal red and white blood cell counts.

Skin: Unusual skin sensitivity; hair loss; discoloration (eg, yellowing of skin); rash.

Digestive Tract: Nausea; vomiting; diarrhea; mouth sores.

Urinary and Reproductive Tract: Prolonged or permanent infertility; cessation of menstruation; decreased sperm count; lesions.

Other: Allergic reaction; lung fibrosis; inflammation of the lungs.

Other:

Chlorambucil – Tremors; confusion; agitation; incoordination; seizures; inflammation of the corneas; inflammation of the bladder; fever; twitching; hallucinations; liver toxicity; pneumonia; leukemia; secondary cancer.

Cyclophosphamide – Stomach ache; appetite loss; colitis; new tumor growth; inflammation of the bladder; pigmentation of the skin; changes in nails.

Ifosfamide – Blood in the urine; infection; kidney impairment; liver dysfunction; pain at injection site.

Mechlorethamine – Blood clot; vein clot; allergic reaction; dizziness; ringing in the ears; diminished hearing; herpes zoster.

Melphalan – Allergy symptoms; inflamed blood vessels.

Guidelines for Use:

- Notify your doctor of unusual bleeding or bruising, black tarry stools, nausea, vomiting, weight loss, fever, chills, sore throat, cough, shortness of breath, seizures, lack of menstrual flow, unusual lumps or masses, flank or stomach pain, joint pain, sores in the mouth or on the lips, yellow discoloration of the skin or eyes, skin rash or pain of unknown origin.
- Contraceptive (birth control) measures are recommended during therapy for both men and women.
- *Cyclophosphamide* — May cause darkening of skin and changes in fingernails. Contact your doctor if these become pronounced. Take tablets on an empty stomach. If stomach upset is severe, take with food. Oral solution may be made from injectable cyclophosphamide and Aromatic Elixir. Store in refrigerator and use within 14 days.
- *Mechlorethamine* — May cause potential risk to reproductive capacity.
- *Melphalan* — Take under close medical supervision.
  Response may be gradual over many months; repeated courses or continuous therapy are important. The maximum benefit may be missed if treatment is ended too soon.
  Long term use may produce secondary cancers and infertility.
  Protect tablets from light. Dispense in glass container.
- These medicines may cause drowsiness and/or dizziness. Use caution while driving or performing other tasks requiring mental alertness, coordination or physical dexterity.
- Inform your doctor if you are pregnant, become pregnant, are planning to become pregnant or if you are breastfeeding.
- *Infections*—These drugs may lower your body's ability to fight infection. Notify your doctor of any signs of infection, including fever, sore throat, rashes or chills.
- Lab tests will be required during treatment with these medications. Be sure to keep appointments.
- Store at controlled room temperature (59° to 77°F).

If you have any questions, consult your doctor, pharmacist, or health care provider.

	Generic Name *Brand Name Example*	Supplied As	Generic Available
Rx	**Plicamycin**		
	Mithracin	**Powder for injection:** 2500 mcg/vial with 100 mg mannitol	No

For more information on chemotherapy treatment, see the introduction to this chapter.

Type of Drug:

Chemotherapy agent; anticancer drug.

How the Drug Works:

Plicamycin stops the growth of cancer cells by binding to the RNA material in the cancer cell and inhibiting it, interfering with cell reproduction. It also exhibits a calcium lowering effect.

Uses:

To treat tumors of the testicles when surgery or radiation therapy is not possible.

To lower abnormal amounts of calcium in the blood and urine caused by certain other types of cancer.

Precautions:

Do not use in the following situations:

- blood clotting disorders (eg, low platelet count)
- bone marrow function impairment
- bone marrow impairment
- nonhospitalized patients
- pregnancy

Use with caution in the following situations:

- electrolyte imbalance (eg, calcium, potassium, phosphorus)
- kidney disease
- liver disease

Pregnancy: Do not use during pregnancy. The risk of use in a pregnant woman clearly outweighs any possible benefit.

Breastfeeding: It is not known if plicamycin appears in breast milk. Consult your doctor before you begin breastfeeding.

Lab tests will be required during treatment. Tests may include: Liver and kidney function, complete blood counts and platelet counts, blood clotting tests (eg, protime) and electrolyte levels (eg, calcium).

Drug Interactions:

Tell your doctor or pharmacist if you are taking or planning to take any over-the-counter or prescription medications or dietary supplements while taking plicamycin. Doses of one or both drugs may need to be modified or a different drug may need to be prescribed.

Side Effects:

Most plicamycin users experience side effects. The frequency and severity of side effects depend on many factors including dose, duration of therapy, and individual susceptibility. Possible side effects include:

Digestive Tract: Nausea; vomiting; diarrhea; appetite loss; inflammation of the mouth.

Nervous System: Drowsiness; weakness; depression; headache; lethargy.

Circulatory System: Abnormal blood count; abnormal clotting.

Skin: Rash; facial flushing; unusual bruising.

Other: Sudden or prolonged bleeding; nosebleed; vomiting of blood; black or tarry stools; blood in urine; fever; general body discomfort; vein inflammation; pain or irritation at injection site; abnormal lab tests.

Guidelines for Use:

- This medicine will be prepared and administered by your health-care provider.
- Requires close monitoring of effects with lab tests. This medicine is usually limited to use in the hospital.
- *Infections* — These drugs may lower your body's ability to fight infection. Notify your doctor of any signs of infection including fever, sore throat, rashes or chills.
- Some of the most common side effects are nausea, vomiting and stomach upset. If these symptoms persist, your doctor may prescribe antinausea drugs.
- May cause lowered blood counts. Report any symptoms of unusual bleeding or bruising, bloody nose, black tarry stools or dark urine to your doctor.
- Inform your doctor if you are pregnant, become pregnant, are planning to become pregnant or if you are breastfeeding.
- Contraceptive measures (birth control) are recommended during treatment.
- Calcium supplements are sometimes needed during plicamycin therapy.
- Avoid sweet, fried, or fatty foods. Eat smaller light meals several times a day. Dry foods (eg, toast, crackers) and liquids (eg, soups, unsweetened apple juice) may be more easily digested.
- Lab tests will be required to monitor therapy. Be sure to keep appointments. Tests may include: Liver and kidney function tests and blood counts.
- Discard any unused solution. Fresh solutions must be prepared daily.
- Store in the refrigerator between 36° to 46°F.

If you have any questions, consult your doctor, pharmacist, or health care provider.

	Generic Name *Brand Name Examples*	Supplied As	Generic Available
Rx	**Interferon Alfa-2a**		
	Roferon-A	**Solution for Injection:** 3 million IU/vial, 9 million IU/vial, 18 million IU/vial, 36 million IU/vial	No
	Roferon-A	**Powder for Injection:** 18 million IU/vial (3 million IU/0.5 ml when reconstituted)	No
Rx	**Interferon Alfa-2b**		
	Intron A	**Solution for Injection:** 3 million IU/vial, 5 million IU/vial, 10 million IU/vial, 18 million IU/vial, 25 million IU/vial	No
	Intron A	**Powder for Injection:** 3 million IU/vial, 5 million IU/vial, 10 million IU/vial, 18 million IU/vial, 25 million IU/vial, 50 miliion IU/vial	No

Type of Drug:

Chemotherapy agents; anticancer drugs.

How the Drug Works:

This group of cancer drugs prevents cancer cell growth by unknown mechanisms or by directly destroying cancer cells. These agents are often used with other cancer drugs.

Uses:

Interferon Alfa-2a: To treat hairy-cell leukemia and AIDS-related Kaposi sarcoma in selected patients.

Interferon Alfa-2b: To treat hairy-cell leukemia, condylomata acuminata (venereal warts) and AIDS-related Kaposi sarcoma in selected patients, skin cancer and chronic hepatitis C.

Unlabeled Use(s): Occasionally doctors may prescribe alpha interferons for a wide range of cancer types and viral infections.

Precautions:

Do not use in the following situations:

allergy to the drug or any of its components
allergy to human interferon alpha
allergy to mouse immunoglobulin (IgG) (interferon alfa-2a only)
bone marrow depression (decreased blood cell counts and platelets)

Use with caution in the following situations:

- AIDS-related Kaposi sarcoma, rapidly progressive or life-threatening
- blood clotting disorders
- bone marrow disorders
- diabetes mellitus
- heart disease or conditions, history of
- kidney disease
- liver disease
- lung disease (eg, chronic obstructive pulmonary disease)
- neurologic disorders
- psoriasis (skin dryness, flaking)
- psychiatric disorders (eg, depression)
- seizure disorders (epilepsy)
- thyroid disease

Sensitivity to sunlight: Interferon Alfa-n3 may cause sensitivity to light. Avoid prolonged exposure to the sun. Use sunscreens and wear protective clothing until tolerance is determined.

Infections: These drugs may lower your body's ability to fight infection. Notify your doctor immediately of any signs of infection (fever, sore throat, rash or chills).

Pregnancy: Adequate studies have not been done in pregnant women, or animal studies may have shown a risk to the fetus. Use only if clearly needed and potential benefits outweigh the possible hazards to the fetus.

Breastfeeding: It is not known if these drugs appear in breast milk. Use is not recommended. A decision should be made whether to discontinue nursing or the drug, taking into account the importance of the drug to the mother. Consult your doctor.

Children: Safety and effectiveness in persons under 18 years of age have not been established.

Lab tests will be required to monitor treatment. Tests may include: Complete blood counts and platelet counts, liver function tests, bone marrow aspirations and electrocardiograms (EKG).

Drug Interactions:

Tell your doctor or pharmacist if you are taking or planning to take any over-the-counter or prescription medications or dietary supplements while taking this medicine. Doses of one or both drugs may need to be modified or a different drug may need to be prescribed.The following drugs and drug classes interact with this medicine:

myelosupressives (eg, zidovudine)
theophylline (eg,*Theo-Dur)*

Side Effects:

Every drug is capable of producing side effects. Most patients experience side effects. The frequency and severity of side effects depend on many factors including dose, duration of therapy, and individual susceptibility. Possible side effects include:

Interferon Alfa-n3 only: Impaired concentration; sensitivity to sunlight; increased salivation; hot feet; heat intolerance.

Interferon Alfa-2b only: Decreased sex drive; menstrual changes; leg cramps.

Flu-like Symptoms (common): Fever; drowsiness; chills; tiredness; sore throat; joint and muscle aches/pain; headache.

Digestive Tract: Appetite loss; diarrhea; constipation; stomach pain; indigestion; nausea; vomiting; gas; heartburn; inflammation of or dry/swollen mouth; taste changes; tongue sensitivity; thirst.

Nervous System: Dizziness; confusion; forgetfulness; incoordination; nervousness; drowsiness; sleep problems; anxiety; fatigue; mood disorders; emotional instability; depression; abnormal thinking; abnormal skin sensations; general body discomfort; rigidity; vertigo (feeling of whirling motion); numbness or tingling of hands or feet.

Circulatory System: Chest pain; abnormal heart rhythm; changes in blood pressure; abnormal blood counts; palpitations (pounding in the chest).

Respiratory System: Painful or difficult breathing; pneumonia; coughing; sinusitis; runny nose; chest congestion; nasal congestion; sore throat.

Skin: Hair loss; itching; rash; hives; flushing; dry skin; sweating; pain at injection site; yellowing of skin or eyes.

Other: Allergic reaction; swelling of hands or feet; back pain; night sweats; weight loss; inflammation of mucous membranes; hot flashes; cold sores; nosebleed; abnormal lab tests; lymph node swelling; abnormal vision; ear and eye pain; painful or difficult urination; temporary impotence.

Guidelines for Use:

- Therapy should begin in the hospital where you can be closely observed.
- Use exactly as prescribed.
- Read patient information sheet carefully. Follow the administration and preparation instructions (of injections) as outlined by your doctor.
- Drink plenty of fluids, especially during the initial stages of treatment.
- Do not change brands of interferon. Changes in dosage may be necessary when changing from one brand to another.
- If a dose is missed, inject it as soon as possible. If several hours have passed or it is nearing time for the next dose, do not double the dose to catch up, unless advised to do so by your doctor. If more than one dose is missed or it is necessary to establish a new dosage schedule, contact your doctor or pharmacist.
- The most common side effects are "flu-like" symptoms, such as fever, chills, drowsiness, fatigue, headache, sore throat, appetite loss, nausea, vomiting, muscle aches and joint pain. These appear to lessen over time. Some symptoms may be minimized by bedtime doses. Use acetaminophen (eg, *Tylenol*) to prevent or lessen fever and headache. Notify your doctor if these symptoms become pronounced during therapy.
- May cause drowsiness or dizziness. Use caution while driving or performing other tasks requiring alertness, coordination or physical dexterity.
- Notify your doctor if hives, itching, tightness in the chest, cough, difficulty breathing, visual problems, wheezing, low blood pressure or lightheadedness occurs.
- Contraceptive measures (birth control) are recommended during therapy with these drugs. Notify your doctor immediately if you suspect pregnancy.
- *Infections* — These drugs may lower your body's ability to fight infection. Notify your doctor immediately of any signs of infection (fever, sore throat, rash or chills).
- Avoid prolonged exposure to sunlight. Photosensitivity (sensitivity to sunlight) may occur. Wear protective clothing and use sunscreens until tolerance is determined (interferon alfa-n3 only).
- Lab tests will be required to monitor treatment. Be sure to keep appointments.
- Store in the refrigerator (36° to 46°F). Do not freeze or shake.

If you have any questions, consult your doctor, pharmacist, or health care provider.

	Generic Name *Brand Name Example*	Supplied As	Generic Available
Rx	**Tretinoin**		
	Vesanoid	**Capsules:** 10 mg	No

Type of Drug:

Antineoplastic; anticancer drug; chemotherapy agent.

How the Drug Works:

The exact mechanism of action is not known, but it appears that tretinoin decreases the growth (reproduction) of leukemia cells (acute promyelocytic leukemia cells) and promotes the growth of normal cells.

Uses:

To induce remission of acute promyelocytic leukemia (APL). Further therapy with other medications usually will be necessary.

Precautions:

Do not use in the following situations: Allergy to retinoids, its components or parabens.

Use with caution in the following situations:

high cholesterol or triglycerides
leukocytosis (high white blood cell count)
pregnancy

Retinoic acid-APL syndrome: A potentially serious drug reaction has occurred in patients given tretinoin to treat APL. Symptoms include: Fever, difficulty breathing or weight gain. Report these symptoms to your doctor immediately.

Pseudotumor cerebri (pressure in brain/head): High doses of tretinoin could produce symptoms such as: Headaches, nausea, vomiting or visual problems. Report these symptoms to your doctor immediately.

Pregnancy: Studies have shown a potential adverse effect on the fetus. Use only if clearly needed and potential benefits outweigh the possible risks.

Breastfeeding: It is not known if tretinoin appears in breast milk. Consult your doctor before you begin breastfeeding.

Children: Safety and effectiveness in children under 1 year of age have not been established.

Lab tests will be required to monitor therapy. Tests may include complete blood counts, coagulation profiles, liver function tests, triglyceride levels and cholesterol levels.

Drug Interactions:

Tell your doctor or pharmacist if you are taking or planning to take any over-the-counter or prescription medications or dietary supplements while taking this medicine. Doses of one or both drugs may need to be modified or a different drug may need to be prescribed.The following drugs and drug classes interact with this medicine:

cytochrome P-450 inducers or inhibitors (eg, phenobarbital, cimetidine)
ketoconazole (eg, *Nizoral*)

Side Effects:

Every drug is capable of producing side effects. Most patients experience side effects. The frequency and severity of side effects depend on many factors including dose, duration of therapy and individual susceptibility. Possible side effects include:

Typical Retinoid Toxicity: Headache; fever; skin/mucous membrane dryness; bone pain/inflammation; nausea; vomiting; rash; irritation of mucous membranes (eg, eye, nose); itching; increased sweating; abnormal vision/eye disorders; hair loss; skin changes; fatigue; weakness.

Digestive Tract: Appetite loss; bleeding; stomach pain/bloating; diarrhea; constipation; indigestion; enlargement of liver and spleen; ulcers; liver disorders.

Nervous System: Dizziness; abnormal skin sensations; anxiety; sleep changes; depression; confusion; agitation; hallucinations; difficulty walking (unsteady); tremors; convulsions; slow/slurred speech; facial paralysis; paralysis of one side of the body; weak reflexes; visual sensitivity to light; leg weakness; forgetfulness; drowsiness; unconsciousness.

Circulatory System: Abnormal heart rate; flushing; changes in blood pressure; vein inflammation/redness; blood clotting disorders; pressure in head; heart attack/failure; stroke.

Respiratory System: Breathing difficulties; pneumonia; bronchial asthma; swelling of the lungs/larynx; lung disease.

Other: Earache or feeling of fullness in the ears; hearing loss/disorders; general body discomfort; shivering; bleeding; infections; swelling of arms and legs; pain; chest discomfort; swelling; weight changes; muscle pain; facial swelling; pale skin; low body temperature; difficult or frequent urination; enlarged prostate; abnormal lab tests.

Guidelines for Use:

- Use exactly as prescribed.
- Take each dose with fluids (6 to 8 oz) at evenly spaced intervals throughout the day, preferably every 12 hours.
- May be taken with food. Drug absorption is enhanced when taken with food.
- If a dose is missed, take it as soon as possible. If several hours have passed or it is nearing time for the next dose, do not double the dose to catch up, unless advised to do so by your doctor. If more than one dose is missed or it is necessary to establish a new dosage schedule, contact your doctor or pharmacist.
- Notify your doctor immediately if you experience fever, difficulty breathing or weight gain. These can be signs of a serious medical condition.
- Notify your doctor if you experience eye pain, headache, nausea, vomiting, dizziness or abnormal vision. This especially applies to children.
- Notify your doctor if you are pregnant, become pregnant, are planning to become pregnant or if you are breastfeeding.
- Contraceptive measures (birth control) are recommended during therapy with this medicine and for 1 month after therapy.
- May cause sensitivity to bright light. Protect eyes and wear sunglasses.
- Lab tests will be required to monitor therapy. Be sure to keep appointments.
- Store at room temperature (59° to 86°F) in a tightly sealed container.

If you have any questions, consult your doctor, pharmacist, or health care provider.

	Generic Name *Brand Name Examples*	Supplied As	Generic Available
Rx	**Altretamine**		
	Hexalen	**Capsules:** 50 mg	No
Rx	**Hydroxyurea**		
	Hydrea	**Capsules:** 500 mg	No
Rx	**Mitotane**		
	Lysodren	**Tablets:** 500 mg	No
Rx	**Paclitaxel**		
	Taxol	**Injection:** 30 mg/5 mL single-dose vial	No
Rx	**Pentostatin**		
	Nipent	**Powder for injection:** 10 mg/vial	No
Rx	**Procarbazine**		
	Matulane	**Capsules:** 50 mg	No

Type of Drug:

Chemotherapy agents; anticancer drugs.

How the Drug Works:

This miscellaneous group of cancer drugs prevents cancer cell growth by stopping the adrenal gland from working or directly destroying cancer cells. These agents are often used with other cancer drugs.

Uses:

Altretamine: To treat ovarian cancer.

Hydroxyurea: To treat certain types of skin cancer (melanoma, primary squamous cell carcinoma), resistant chronic myelocytic leukemia and inoperable cancer of the ovary.

Mitotane: To treat inoperable cancer of the adrenal gland.

Paclitaxel: To treat ovarian cancer after failure of first-line or subsequent chemotherapy and to treat breast cancer after failure of combination chemotherapy or relapse within 6 months of adjuvant chemotherapy.

Pentostatin: To treat hairy cell leukemia.

Procarbazine: To treat Stage III and IV Hodgkin disease in combination with other anti-cancer drugs.

Unlabeled Use(s): Occasionally doctors may prescribe paclitaxel for a wide range of cancer types.

Precautions:

Do not use in the following situations:

allergy to the drug or any of its components
allergy to polyoxyethylated castor oil (paclitaxel only)
bone marrow depression (decreased blood cell counts and platelets)
CNS toxicity, severe (altretamine only)
severe neutropenia/low white blood cell count (paclitaxel only)

Use with caution in the following situations:

altretamine —
pregnancy

hydroxyurea —
anemia, severe
bone marrow depressant agents, use
kidney disease
pregnancy
radiation, recent

mitotane —
liver disease
long-term use
shock
trauma, severe

paclitaxel —
heart disease
liver disease
low blood pressure
peripheral neuropathy (burning or numbness in hands or feet)
pregnancy

pentostatin —
infections
nervous system, kidney, liver or lung toxicity
pregnancy
rash, severe

procarbazine —
bone marrow depressant agents, use
kidney disease
liver disease
pregnancy
radiation, recent

Infections: These drugs may lower your body's ability to fight infection. Notify your doctor immediately of any signs of infection (eg, fever, sore throat, rash, chills).

Mitotane long-term use: Continuous use of high doses may lead to brain or nervous system damage.

Paclitaxel allergy: All patients should be premedicated with corticosteroids, diphenhydramine and H_2 antagonists to avoid the occurrence of severe hypersensitivity reactions. Severe reactions such as low blood pressure, labored breathing requiring bronchodilators, edema (swelling) or severe hives require immediate discontinuation of the drug and aggressive symptomatic therapy.

Pregnancy: There are no adequate studies and well-controlled studies of mittane in pregnant women. Studies have shown all others agents have a potential adverse effect on the fetus. Use only if clearly needed and the potential benefits to the mother outweigh the possible hazards to the fetus.

Breastfeeding: It is not known if these drugs appear in breast milk. Use is not recommended. A decision should be made whether to discontinue nursing or the drug, taking into account the importance of the drug to the mother. Consult your doctor.

Children: Safety and effectiveness in children have not been established.

Elderly: Elderly patients may be more sensitive to the effects of hydroxyurea and may require a lower dose.

Lab tests will be required to monitor treatment. Be sure to keep appointments. Tests may include: Complete blood and platelet counts, liver and kidney function tests, or bone marrow aspirations. Neurologic exams should be performed regularly with altretamine use.

Drug Interactions:

Tell your doctor or pharmacist if you are taking or planning to take any over-the-counter or prescription medications or dietary supplements while taking one of these preparations Doses of one or both drugs may need to be modified or a different drug may need to be prescribed.The foliowing drugs and drug classes interact with these preparations:

altretamine —

antidepressants, MAO inhibitor class (eg, phenelzine)
cisplatin (eg, *Platinol)*
histamine H_2 antagonists (eg, cimetidine)
pyridoxine (eg, *Nestrex)*

mitotane —

cytochrome P-450 inducers or inhibitors (eg, phenobarbital, cimetidine)
warfarin (eg, *Coumadin)*
spironolactone (eg, *Aldactone)*

paclitaxel —

cisplatin (eg, *Platinol)*
ketoconazole *(Nizoral)*

pentostatin —

fludarabine *(Fludara)*
vidarabine *(Vira-A)*

procarbazine —

antihistamines (eg, diphenhydramine)
barbiturates (eg, phenobarbital)
digoxin (eg, *Lanoxin)*
ethyl alcohol
foods containing tyramine
hypotensive agents
levodopa (eg, *Larodopa)*
narcotics (eg, codeine)
phenothiazines (eg, chlorpromazine)
sympathomimetics (eg, pseudoephedrine)
tricyclic antidepressants (eg, amitriptyline)

Side Effects:

Every drug is capable of producing side effects. Most patients experience side effects. The frequency and severity of side effects depend on many factors including dose, duration of therapy, and individual susceptibility. Possible side effects include:

Flu-like Symptoms (common): Fever; chills; joint and muscle aches/pain; headache.

Digestive Tract: Appetite loss; diarrhea; constipation; stomach pain; indigestion; nausea; vomiting; gas; inflammation of mouth.

Nervous System: Dizziness; confusion; incoordination; mood disorders; disorders of consciousness; nervousness; drowsiness; anxiety; fatigue; weakness; abnormal skin sensations; sleepiness; depression; vertigo (feeling of whirling motion); numbness or tingling of hands or feet; seizures (altretamine only); CNS toxicity (pentostatin only).

Circulatory System: Chest pain; rapid heart rate; abnormal heart rhythm; changes in blood pressure; abnormal blood counts; anemia; bleeding; blood clots; slowed heart rate (paclitaxel only).

Respiratory System: Difficult breathing, upper respiratory infection; pneumonia; coughing; bronchitis; sinusitis; runny nose; sore throat; asthma (pentostatin only).

Skin: Hair loss; itching; redness; rash; hives; fiushing; dry skin; skin disorders; sweating; skin discoloration or swelling at injection site (paciitaxel only); boils (pentostatin only).

Other: Allergic reaction; swelling of hands or feet; inflammation of mucous membranes; bone marrow suppression; pain; infections; abnormal lab tests; painful or difficult urination; blood in urine; bone pain; blood poisoning; fainting; facial swelling; blurred or double vision; discoloration of nails (paclitaxel oniy); herpes zosterlshingles (pentostatin only); urinary tract infection (pentostatin oniy); eye irritation (pentostatin only); dental abnormalities (pentostatin only); swollen gums (pentostatin only); over-development of mammary glands in prepubertal and early pubertal boys (procarbazine only).

Guidelines for Use:

- Use exactly as prescribed.
- If a dose is missed, take or inject it as soon as possible. If several hours have passed or it is nearing time for the next dose, do not double the dose to catch up, unless advised to do so by your doctor. If more than one dose is missed or it is necessary to establish a new dosage schedule, contact your doctor or pharmacist.
- Flu-like symptoms (fever, drowsiness, chills, tiredness, sore throat, muscle aches, headache, joint pain) are common with these drugs. Notify your doctor if these become pronounced during therapy.
- Contraceptive measures (birth control) are recommended during therapy with these drugs. Notify your doctor immediately if you suspect pregnancy.
- May cause drowsiness or dizziness. Use caution while driving or performing other tasks requiring alertness, coordination or physical dexterity.
- *Infections* — These drugs may lower your body's ability to fight infection. Notify your doctor immediately of any signs of infection (fever, sore throat, rash or chills).
- *Altretamine* —
  Avoid taking altretamine at the same time as antidepressants such as phenelzine and tranylcypromine (MAO inhibitors), as this may result in severe orthostatic hypotension (dizziness, lightheadedness or fainting when rising quickly from a sitting or lying position).
  May cause nausea, vomiting, incoordination, dizziness, vertigo (feeling of whirling motion) or fatigue. Notify your doctor if these become pronounced.
  Store at room temperature (59° to 86°F).
- *Hydroxyurea* —
  Notify your doctor if fever, chills, sore throat, nausea, vomiting, appetite loss, diarrhea, sores in the mouth and on the lips, unusual bleeding or bruising occurs.
  Contents of the capsule may be emptied into a glass of water and taken immediately. Some material from the capsule contents may not dissolve and may float on the surface of the water. This is a potent medication and should be handled with care. Do not allow powder to come in contact with the skin, eyes or mucous membranes.
  May cause drowsiness, constipation, redness of the face, rash, itching, nausea, vomiting, appetite loss, pain or inflammation at irradiation site or hair loss.
  Notify your doctor if these become pronounced.
  Drink plenty of fluids.
  Store at room temperature (59° to 86°F) in a tightly closed container. Avoid excessive heat.

Guidelines for Use (cont.):

- *Mitotane* —
  Notify your doctor if nausea, vomiting, appetite loss, diarrhea, depression, rash or darkening of the skin occurs.
  Notify your doctor if difficulty breathing, dizziness, lightheadedness, swelling or hives occur.
  May cause muscle aches, fever, flushing or muscle twitching. Notify your doctor if these become pronounced.
  Store at room temperature (59° to 86°F).
- *Paclitaxel* —
  Read patient information sheet carefully. Follow the administration and preparation instructions (of injections) as outlined by your doctor.
  Before treatment with paclitaxel, you must be pretreated with medication to prevent serious allergic reactions.
  Notify your doctor if difficult breathing, dizziness, lightheadedness, edema (swelling) or severe hives occur.
  Store in the refrigerator (36° to 46°F). Freezing does not harm the drug. Keep in original package to protect from light. Reconstituted solution will keep for 27 hours at room temperature (77°F).
- *Pentostatin* —
  Read patient information sheet carefully. Follow the administration and preparation instructions (of injections) as outlined by your doctor.
  Notify your doctor if severe rash or signs of nervous system toxicity (eg, drowsiness, weakness) occur.
  Store viais in the refrigerator (36° to 46°F). Reconstituted solution will only keep for 8 hours since it does not contain any preservatives.
- *Procarbazine* —
  Avoid the following: Tyramine-containing foods, alcohol, antihistamines and sympathomimetics (eg, stimulant drugs or decongestants).
  Consult your doctor before using any prescription medications.
  Notify your doctor if cough, shortness of breath, thickened bronchial secretions, fever, chills, sore throat, unusual bleeding or bruising, vomiting of blood or black tarry stools occur.
  May cause muscle or joint pain, nausea, vomiting, sweating, tiredness, weakness, constipation, headache, difficulty swallowing, appetite loss, hair loss, or depression. Notify your doctor if these become pronounced.
  Store below 104°F, preferably between 59° to 86°F. Protect from light and moisture.

If you have any questions, consult your doctor, pharmacist, or health care provider.

Generic Name *Brand Name Example*	Supplied As	Generic Available
Rx **Pegaspargase**		
Oncaspar	**Injection:** 750 IU/ml	No

Type of Drug:

Chemotherapy agent; anticancer drug.

How the Drug Works:

Pegaspargase reduces asparagine levels in the body. Leukemic cells need asparagine to survive. Without it in the body, the leukemic cells die.

Uses:

To treat acute lymphoblastic leukemia (ALL). Is usually used in combination with other cancer drugs.

Precautions:

Do not use in the following situations:
- allergy to this medicine
- bleeding problems after taking this medicine
- pancreatitis, history of

Use with caution in the following situations:
- hepatotoxic drugs
- liver disease

Bleeding: Patients taking this medicine are at higher than usual risk for bleeding problems, especially if used in combination with other anticoagulant medications (eg, warfarin).

Infections: Pegaspargase may lower your body's ability to fight infection. Notify your doctor immediately of any signs of infections (eg, fever, sore throat, rash, chills).

Pregnancy: Adequate studies have not been done in pregnant women, or animal studies may have shown a risk to the fetus. Use only if clearly needed and potential benefits outweigh the possible hazards to the fetus.

Breastfeeding: It is not known if pegaspargase appears in breast milk. Use is not recommended. A decision should be made whether to discontinue nursing or the drug, taking into account the importance of the drug to the mother. Consult your doctor.

Lab tests will be required to monitor treatment. Be sure to keep appointments. Tests may include complete blood counts (CBC) and platelet counts, blood sugar, bone marrow aspirations, and liver function tests.

Drug Interactions:

Tell your doctor or pharmacist if you are taking or planning to take any over-the-counter or prescription medications or dietary supplements while taking this medicine. Doses of one or both drugs may need to be modified or a different drug may need to be prescribed. The following drugs and drug classes interact with this medicine:

anticoagulannts (eg, warfarin)
aspirin
methotrexate (eg, *Folex PFS)*
NSAIDs (eg, ibuprofen)

Side Effects:

Every drug is capable of producing side effects. Most patients experience side effects. The frequency and severity of side effects depend on many factors including dose, duration of therapy, and individual susceptibility. Possible side effects include:

Digestive Tract: Nausea; vomiting; diarrhea; cramps; constipation; gas; indigestion; lip numbness or sweliing; stomach pain; mouth or lip sores; appetite changes; difficulty swallowing.

Nervous System: Headache; abnormal skin sensations; convulsions.

Circulatory System: Low blood pressure; rapid heartbeat; chest pain; stroke; blood clots.

Skin: Rash; redness; swelling, hardness or pain at injection site; hives; itching.

Other: Swelling or pain in the hands or feet; cough; difficulty breathing; yellowing of skin or eyes; swelling; changes in blood sugar levels; unusual bleeding or bruising; night sweats; muscle/joint pain or stiffness; chills; fever; general body discomfort; anemia; abnormal blood or lab values.

Guidelines for Use:

- Use exactly as prescribed.
- Follow the injection procedure taught to you by your health care provider.
- Inject this medicine every 14 days.
- If a dose is missed, inject it as soon as possible. If several hours have passed or it is nearing time for the next dose, do not double the dose to catch up, unless advised to do so by your doctor. If more than one dose is missed or it is necessary to establish a new dosage schedule, contact your doctor or pharmacist.
- If rash, redness, swelling, pain, hives or difficulty breathing occurs, contact your doctor immediately.
- This medicine may lower your body's ability to fight infection. Notify your doctor of any signs of infection, including fever, sore throat, rashes or chills.
- This medicine raises the risks of bleeding problems. Avoid the use of aspirin or nonsteroidal anti-inflammatory agents (NSAIDs) while taking this medicine.
- This medicine may affect the ability of the liver to function normally in some patients. Therapy with this medicine may increase the toxicity of other medications. Contact your doctor if there is any yellowing of the skin or eyes.
- Diabetic patients may experience loss of glucose control. Be prepared to monitor blood sugar more often.
- Lab tests will be required to monitor treatment. Be sure to keep appointments.
- Visually inspect solution for particles and discoloration before use.
- Store refrigerated (36° to 46°F). Do not store at room temperature for more than 48 hours. Do not shake. Do not freeze or use if solution has been frozen.
- Discard any unused solution.

If you have any questions, consult your doctor, pharmacist, or health care provider.

	Generic Name *Brand Name Example*	Supplied As	Generic Available
Rx	**Porfimer Sodium**		
	Photofrin	**Cake or powder for injection:** 75 mg	No

Type of Drug:

Chemotherapy agent; anticancer drug.

How the Drug Works:

Porfimer is a photosensitizing agent used in laser therapy or photodynamic therapy (PDT) of tumors.

Uses:

To treat esophageal (food pipe) cancers in adults.

Precautions:

Do not use in the following situations:

allergy to porfimer sodium or related medications
esophageal fistula (hole in the throat; food pipe)
porphyria
tumors eroding into a major blood vessel

Light Sensitivity: Will cause sensitivity to the sun, bright indoor lights or car headlights. For 30 days, avoid exposure of skin and eyes to direct sunlight or bright indoor light (eg, examination lights, including dental lamps, operating room lamps, unshaded light bulbs at close proximity). Wear dark sunglasses and cover exposed skin with clothing when outside.

Chest Pain: Some patients may experience chest pain because of inflammation of the area being treated. This pain may be strong enough to warrant treatment. Contact your doctor if severe chest pain occurs.

Pregnancy: Adequate studies have not been done in pregnant women, or animal studies may have shown a risk to the fetus. Use only if clearly needed and potential benefits outweigh the possible hazards to the fetus.

Breastfeeding: It is not known if porfimer appears in breast milk. Mothers taking porfimer should not breastfeed. Consult your doctor.

Children: Safety and effectiveness in children have not been established.

Lab tests may be required to monitor therapy. Be sure to keep appointments.

Drug Interactions:

Tell your doctor or pharmacist if you are taking or planning to take any over-the-counter or prescription medications or dietary supplements while taking this medicine. Doses of one or both drugs may need to be modified or a different drug may need to be prescribed. The following drugs and drug classes interact with this medicine:

- alcohol
- allopurinol (eg, *Zyloprim)*
- beta-carotene (eg, *Max-Caro)*
- calcium channel blockers (eg, nifedipine)
- dimethyl sulfoxide *(Rimso-50)*
- glucocorticoid hormones (eg, hydrocortisone)
- griseofulvin (eg, *Fulvicin)*
- hypoglycemic agents (eg, sulfonylureas)
- mannitol (eg, *Osmitrol)*
- phenothiazines (eg, chlorpromazine)
- prostaglandin synthesis inhibitors (eg, NSAIDs)
- sulfonamides (eg, sulfisoxazole)
- tetracyclines (eg, doxycycline)
- thiazide diuretics (eg, hydrochlorothiazide)
- thromboxane A_2 inhibitors (eg, aspirin)

Side Effects:

Every drug is capable of producing side effects. Most patients experience side effects. The frequency and severity of side effects depend on many factors including dose, duration of therapy, and individual susceptibility. Possible side effects include:

Digestive Tract: Nausea; vomiting; constipation; diarrhea; indigestion; belching; appetite loss; weight loss; dark, bloody stools; vomiting of blood; stomach pain; difficulty swallowing; mouth sores.

Other: Dehydration; fever; cough; sore throat; general or back pain; difficulty breathing; pneumonia; unusual bleeding or bruising; difficult or painful urination; anemia; sensitivity to light; swelling of the hands or feet; swelling; weakness; tiredness; anxiety; confusion; sleeplessness; chest pain; rapid or unusual heartbeat; changes in blood pressure.

Guidelines for Use:

- Use exactly as prescribed.
- This medicine will be prepared and administered by your health care provider in a medical setting.
- Contact your doctor if severe chest pain occurs.
- *Light sensitivity* — Will cause sensitivity to the sun, bright lights or car headlights. For 30 days, avoid exposure of skin and eyes to direct sunlight or bright indoor light (eg, examination lights, including dental lamps, unshaded light bulbs at close proximity). Do not stay in a darkened room during this period, because exposure to indoor light is helpful in inactivating this medicine. Before exposing skin to bright indoor light or direct sunlight, test it for sensitivity. Expose a small skin area to sunlight for 10 minutes. If no sensitivity reactions (eg, rash, swelling, blistering) occurs within 24 hours, gradually resume normal outdoor activities. If a sensitivity reaction occurs with the skin test, continue precautions for another 2 weeks before retesting. The skin around the eyes may be most sensitive, so do not use the face for testing. UV (ultraviolet) sunscreens are not a protection against sensitivity reactions. Wear dark sunglasses and cover exposed skin with clothing when outside.
- Contraceptive measures (birth control) are recommended during treatment to avoid birth defects. Inform your doctor if you are pregnant, become pregnant, are planning to become pregnant or if you are breastfeeding.
- Lab tests may be required to monitor treatment. Be sure to keep appointments.
- Wipe up spills with a damp cloth. Avoid contact with skin and eyes. Use rubber gloves and eye protection. Dispose of all contaminated materials in a polyethylene bag.
- Store at room temperature (68° to 77°F). Reconstituted solution should be protected from bright light and used immediately.

If you have any questions, consult your doctor, pharmacist, or health care provider.

Generic Name *Brand Name Example*	Supplied As	Generic Available
Rx **Rituximab**		
Rituxan[1]	**Injection:** 10 mg/mL	No

[1] Preservative free.

Type of Drug:

Monoclonal antibody.

How the Drug Works:

Rituximab is a genetically engineered monoclonal antibody directed against the CD20 antigen found on the surface of malignant B lymphocytes associated with non-Hodgkin lymphoma.

Uses:

For recurring or untreatable low-grade or follicular, CD20–positive, B-cell non-Hodgkin lymphoma.

Precautions:

Do not use in the following situations:

allergy to murine (rats, mice) proteins or any rituximab ingredients
life-threatening heartbeat irregularities

Use with caution in the following situations:

coronary artery disease
difficulty breathing
heart rhythm disturbance, history
hives
low blood pressure
throat/tongue swelling

Pregnancy: Adequate studies have not been done in pregnant women or animal studies may have shown a risk to the fetus. Use only if clearly needed and potential benefits outweigh the possible hazards to the fetus.

Breastfeeding: It is not known if rituximab appears in breast milk. Consult your doctor before you begin breastfeeding or discontinue nursing until circulating rituximab serum levels are no longer detectable.

Children: The safety and effectiveness of rituximab in children have not been established.

Lab tests may be required to monitor treatment. Tests may include complete blood and platelet counts.

Drug Interactions:

Tell your doctor or pharmacist if you are taking or planning to take any over-the-counter or prescription medications or dietary supplements with rituximab. Doses of one or both drugs may need to be modified or a different drug may need to be prescribed. Blood pressure medicine (eg, valsartan) interacts with rituximab.

Side Effects:

Every drug is capable of producing side effects. Many patients experience no, or minor, side effects. The frequency and severity of side effects depend on many factors including dose, duration of therapy, and individual susceptibility. Possible side effects include:

Digestive Tract: Nausea; sensation of tongue or throat swelling; vomiting; throat irritation; stomach pain; diarrhea; indigestion; appetite loss; swelling of stomach.

Nervous System: Tiredness; headache; dizziness; anxiety; nervousness; agitation; sleeplessness.

Circulatory System: Low blood pressure; chest pain; fast or irregular heartbeat; abnormal blood cell counts; high blood pressure; agitation; sleeplessness; dizziness when rising to standing position; slow heartbeat.

Respiratory System: Difficulty breathing; nasal congestion; runny nose; sinus infection; bronchitis; respiratory disorder; increased cough.

Skin: Hives; rash; itching; abnormal skin sensations.

Senses: Eye infection; taste perversion; watery eyes.

Other: Pain at disease sites; weakness; back, muscle or joint pain; pain; high blood sugar; fluid retention; swelling of arms and legs; general body discomfort; tumor pain; pain at injection site; tight muscles; fever; chills; flushing; night sweats.

Guidelines for Use:

- This medicine will be prepared and administered by a health care provider in an outpatient setting.
- This medicine will be given as an intravenous (IV; into a vein) infusion once weekly for 4 doses (days 1, 8, 15, and 22).
- Premedication with acetaminophen (eg, *Tylenol*) and diphenhydramine (eg, *Benadryl*) are recommended before each infusion to reduce infusion-related side effects.
- Withhold high blood pressure medications 12 hours before therapy because short-lived low blood pressure may occur.
- Lab tests may be required to monitor treatment. Be sure to keep appointments.

If you have any questions, consult your doctor, pharmacist, or health care provider.

	Generic Name *Brand Name Example*	Supplied As	Generic Available
Rx	**Trastuzumab**		
	Herceptin	**Powder for injection**: 440 mg/vial	No

Type of Drug:

Antineoplastic; anticancer drug.

How the Drug Works:

Trastuzumab is a DNA-derived antibody that inhibits the growth of tumor cells that over-produce a specific protein (HER2 protein).

Uses:

Trastuzumab is indicated for the treatment of patients with metastatic breast cancer whose tumors over-produce the HER2 protein. Trastuzumab is used as a single agent for patients who have received one or more chemotherapy treatments or in combination with paclitaxel for patients who have not received chemotherapy for their metastatic disease.

Precautions:

Do not use in the following situations:

allergy to trastuzumab, Chinese hamster ovary cell proteins, or any ingredient of this product
radiation therapy to chest, history

Use with caution in the following situations:

anthracyclines, concurrent use
cardiac disease, history
cardiac dysfunction, preexisting
cardiac therapy, history
heart failure, congestive

Congestive heart failure associated with trastuzumab may be severe and has been associated with disabling cardiac failure, death, and stroke. Candidates for treatment should undergo thorough baseline cardiac assessment including history and physical exam and one or more of the following: EKG, echocardiogram, and MUGA scan. Monitoring may not identify all patients who will develop cardiac dysfunction.

Pregnancy: Adequate studies have not been done in pregnant women. Use only if clearly needed and potential benefits to the mother outweigh the possible hazards to the fetus.

Breastfeeding: It is not known if trastuzumab appears in breast milk. Consult your doctor before you begin breastfeeding. Because the potential for absorption and harm is unknown, women should be advised to discontinue nursing during trastuzumab therapy and for 6 months after the last dose of trastuzumab.

Children: Safety and effectiveness in children have not been established.

Elderly: Advanced age may increase the risk of heart problems. Because clinical experience is limited, it is not known if older patients respond differently than younger patients.

Lab tests may be required. Tests may include cardiac (heart) function tests and blood counts.

Drug Interactions:

Tell your doctor or pharmacist if you are taking or planning to take any over-the-counter or prescription medications or dietary supplements while taking trastuzumab. Dose of one or both drugs may need to be modified or a different drug may need to be prescribed. The following drugs and drug classes interact with trastuzumab:

anthracyclines (eg, doxorubicin)

cyclophosphamide (eg, *Cytoxan)*

Side Effects:

Every drug is capable of producing side effects. Many or most trastuzumab users experience side effects. The frequency and severity of side effects depend on many factors including dose, duration of therapy, and individual susceptibility. Possible side effects include:

Circulatory System: Heart failure (eg, shortness of breath, increased cough, sudden nighttime shortness of breath, ankle and leg swelling); low blood pressure; fast heartbeat.

Digestive Tract: Diarrhea; nausea; vomiting; stomach pain; loss of appetite.

Nervous System: Sleeplessness; dizziness; abnormal skin sensations; depression; inflammation of nerves; nerve pain; numbness.

Respiratory System: Increased cough; sinus infection or inflammation; congested or runny nose; sore throat; difficulty breathing.

Skin: Rash; itching; hives; acne; herpes simplex.

Other: Infection; body, back, bone, or joint pain; pain at tumor sites; weakness; fever; chills; headache; flu syndrome; accidental injury; allergic reaction; urinary tract infection; swelling of hands or feet; anemia; low white blood cell count.

Guidelines for Use:

- This medication will be prepared and administered by your health care provider in a medical setting.
- Chills and fever frequently occur with the first dose, but are infrequent with subsequent doses.
- Notify your doctor if you notice difficulty breathing, increased cough, shortness of breath while lying down, or swelling in the ankles or feet.
- Lab tests will be required to monitor therapy. Be sure to keep appointments.

If you have any questions, consult your doctor, pharmacist, or health care provider.

Antidotes
- Charcoal, Activated, 1633
- Flumazenil, 1635
- Ipecac, 1637
- Dexrazoxane, 1639
- Nalmefene HCl, 1641
- Naloxone, 1643

Chelating Agents
- Succimer, 1645

Anticholinesterase Muscle Stimulants, 1647

Urinary Tract Products
- Acetohydroxamic Acid, 1650
- Acidifiers, 1652
- Alkalinizers, 1655
- Bethanechol Chloride, 1658
- Cellulose Sodium Phosphate, 1660
- Cysteamine Bitartrate, 1662
- Dimethyl Sulfoxide, 1664
- Flavoxate, 1666
- Oxybutynin Chloride, 1668
- Tolterodine Tartrate, 1670
- Phenazopyridine HCl, 1672

Immunosuppressives
- Azathioprine, 1674
- Cyclosporine, 1676
- Mycophenolate Mofetil, 1680
- Muromonab-CD3, 1683
- Tacrolimus, 1686

Retinoids
- Isotretinoin, 1689

Miscellaneous Agents
- Bromocriptine Mesylate, 1693
- Cabergoline, 1696
- Chymopapain, 1698
- Cromolyn Sodium, Oral, 1700
- Disulfiram, 1702
- Naltrexone HCl, 1705
- Levomethadyl Acetate HCl, 1708
- Penicillamine, 1710
- Phosphate Binders, 1713
- Smoking Deterrents, 1715
  - Bupropion HCl, 1719
- Alprostadil, 1722
- Agents for Impotence
  - Sildenafil Citrate, 1724
- Yohimbine, 1727
- Interferon Beta, 1729
- Riluzole, 1732
- Glatiramer Acetate, 1734
- Thalidomide, 1736
- Etanercept, 1740
- Leflunomide, 1743

	Generic Name *Brand Name Examples*	Supplied As	Generic Available
otc	**Charcoal, Activated**	**Powder**	Yes
	Actidose-Aqua, Actidose with Sorbitol, Charcoaid, Liqui-Char, Superchar	**Liquid**	Yes

Type of Drug:

Poisoning antidote.

How the Drug Works:

Charcoal adsorbs (attaches to) toxic substances (eg, drugs, chemicals, poisons), forming a barrier between the particles and the stomach lining, thus preventing absorption of the toxic substance into the body.

Sorbitol may be added to some activated charcoal products because it improves the taste and does not leave a gritty residue.

Uses:

To treat poisonings and drug overdoses caused by swallowing.

Precautions:

Do not use when there is an overdose of cyanide, mineral acids and alkalies. Although not contraindicated, it is not effective for use in poisonings of alcohol or iron.

Drug Interactions:

Tell your doctor or pharmacist if you are taking or if you are planning to take any over-the-counter or prescription medications or dietary supplements with activated charcoal. Doses of one or both drugs may need to be modified or a different drug may need to be prescribed. Ipecac interacts with activated charcoal. Do not take concomitantly. Charcoal will decrease the effectiveness of any medication taken at the same time.

Side Effects:

Every drug is capable of producing side effects. Many activated charcoal users experience no, or minor, side effects. The frequency and severity of side effects depend on many factors including dose, duration of therapy and individual susceptibility. Possible side effects include constipation, diarrhea, black stools and vomiting.

Guidelines for Use:

- Use exactly as prescribed.
- Contact your doctor or poison control center for all poisonings or suspected poisonings.
- Give only to conscious (alert) persons.
- If ipecac syrup is also given, give the ipecac first; give activated charcoal after vomiting occurs.
- Do not mix charcoal with milk, ice cream or sherbet since they will decrease the effectiveness of the activated charcoal.
- Keep in a closed container.

If you have any questions, consult your doctor, pharmacist, or health care provider.

Generic Name *Brand Name Example*	Supplied As	Generic Available
Rx **Flumazenil**		
Romazicon	**Injection:** 0.1 mg/mL[1]	No

[1] Contains EDTA and parabens.

Type of Drug:

Antidote for benzodiazepine (eg, diazepam)-induced sedation.

How the Drug Works:

Flumazenil reverses the effects of benzodiazepines by inhibiting their activity. It counteracts sedation, memory loss and impaired movement.

Uses:

To reverse the sedative effects of benzodiazepines in cases of general anesthesia, diagnostic or therapeutic sedation, and overdose.

Precautions:

Do not use in the following situations:

allergy to benzodiazepines
allergy to flumazenil
benzodiazepine use to control a potentially life-threatening condition
cyclic antidepressant (eg, amitriptyline) overdose, serious

Use with caution in the following situations:

alcoholism
drug dependency
head injury
intensive care unit use
liver disease
mixed drug overdose
panic disorder, history
neuromuscular blocker use

Seizures: The reversal of benzodiazepine effects may be associated with seizures in certain individuals. Risk factors include: withdrawal from sedative-hypnotics (eg, triazolam); recent therapy with repeated doses of injectable benzodiazepines, jerking or seizure activity prior to flumazenil use in overdose; cyclic antidepressant poisoning.

Amnesia: Flumazenil does not consistently reverse amnesia. Patients cannot be expected to remember information told to them following administration. Therefore, instructions should be written down or given to a responsible family member.

Hypoventilation: Monitor patients who have received flumazenil for reversal of benzodiazepine effects (after conscious sedation or general anesthesia) for resedation, respiratory depression or other residual benzodiazepine effects for up to 120 minutes.

Pregnancy: Adequate studies have not been done in pregnant women. Use only if clearly needed and potential benefits outweigh the possibie hazards to the fetus.

Breastfeeding: It is not known if flumazenil appears in breast milk. Consult your doctor before you begin breastfeeding.

Children: Safety and effectiveness in children have not been established. Use is not recommended.

Drug Interactions:

Tell your doctor or pharmacist if you are taking or if you are planning to take any over-the-counter or prescription medications or dietary supplements with flumazenil. Doses of one or both drugs may need to be modified or a different drug may need to be prescribed.

Side Effects:

Every drug is capable of producing side effects. Many flumazenil users experience no, or minor, side effects. The frequency and severity of side effects depend on many factors including dose, duration of therapy and individual susceptibility. Possible side effects include:

Digestive Tract: Nausea; vomiting.

Nervous System: Seizures; dizziness; headache, fatigue; weakness; agitation; anxiety; nervousness; tremor; sleeplessness; vertigo (feeling of whirling motion); incoordination; emotional changes (eg, depression); abnormal sensations.

Other: Pain at injection site; reaction at injection site (eg, rash); sweating; abnormal or blurred vision; general body discomfort; flushing; hot flushes; dry mouth; palpitations (pounding in the chest); difficulty breathing.

Guidelines for Use:

- The reversal of benzodiazepine effects may be associated with seizures in certain individuals. Consult your doctor regarding sedative-hypnotic drug withdrawal, recent therapy with repeated doses of injectable benzodiazepines, jerking or seizures prior to flumazenil use, and cyclic antidepressant poisoning.
- Inform your doctor of any benzodiazepine, alcohol or sedative use prior to flumazenil therapy.
- Benzodiazepine effects may recur despite alertness at the time of discharge. Memory and judgment may be impaired.
- *Do not* drive or perform other tasks requiring alertness until at least 18 to 24 hours after discharge.
- *Do not* take any alcohol or nonprescription drugs for 18 to 24 hours after flumazenil use or if sedation persists.

If you have any questions, consult your doctor, pharmacist, or health care provider.

Generic Name	Supplied As	Generic Available
otc/ Rx **Ipecac**[1]	**Syrup**	Yes

[1] Contains alcohol.

Type of Drug:

Emetic; an agent that induces vomiting.

How the Drug Works:

Ipecac irritates the stomach lining and stimulates the vomiting center (chemoreceptor trigger zone, CTZ) in the brain.

Uses:

To treat drug overdoses and certain poisonings caused by swallowing.

Precautions:

Do not use in the following situations:

- breastfeeding
- corrosives (eg, alkalies, strong acids)
- poisoning by petroleum distillates
- pregnancy
- semiconscious or unconscious patients
- strychnine poisoning

Ipecac syrup abuse: Ipecac syrup may be abused by bulimic and anorexic patients. It has been implicated as the cause of severe heart problems and even death in several persons with eating disorders who used it regularly to cause vomiting.

Pregnancy: Not recommended for use during pregnancy. Adequate studies have not been done in pregnant women. Use only if clearly needed and potential benefits outweigh the possible hazards to the fetus.

Breastfeeding: It is not known if ipecac appears in breast milk. Use is not recommended. Contact your doctor.

Drug Interactions:

Tell your doctor or pharmacist if you are taking or if you are planning to take any over-the-counter or prescription medications or dietary supplements with ipecac. Doses of one or both drugs may need to be modified or a different drug may need to be prescribed. The following drugs and drug classes interact with ipecac.

- carbonated beverages
- charcoal, activated
- milk

Side Effects:

Every drug is capable of producing side effects. Many ipecac syrup users experience no, or minor, side effects. The frequency and severity of side effects depend on many factors including dose, duration of therapy and individual susceptibility. Possible side effects include diarrhea, drowsiness, stomach ache and vomiting.

When ipecac syrup does not cause vomiting, absorption may occur and may cause heart conduction disturbances, or even fatal inflammations of the heart muscle (see Precautions).

Guidelines for Use:

- Do not give to semiconscious or unconscious individuals. Have patient sit upright with head forward before administering dose.
- Always consult your doctor or poison control center in cases of accidental ingestion of toxic substances.
- Ipecac syrup may not work on an empty stomach. Give with plenty of water. Do not exceed recommended dosage.
- Do not take with milk or carbonated drinks (eg, soda).
- Do not confuse ipecac syrup with ipecac fluid extract, which is 14 times stronger and has caused some deaths.
- *Children (6 months to 1 year)* — 5 to 10 mL (1 to 2 tsp) followed by one-half to one glass of water. Syrup of ipecac should probably be given only with a doctor's advice or supervision. It is not recommended that ipecac be given to children less than 6 months of age.
- *Children (1 to 12 years)* — 15 mL (1 tbsp) followed by 1 to 2 glasses of water.
- *Adults* — 15 to 30 mL (1 to 2 tbsp) followed by 3 to 4 glasses of water.
- Repeat the dosage once if vomiting does not occur within 30 minutes.
- If vomiting does not occur within 30 minutes after the second dose, contact your doctor or poison control center.
- If vomiting does not occur after taking ipecac syrup, or if excessive doses are used, it may be absorbed into the body and cause problems with the heart. Contact your doctor.

If you have any questions, consult your doctor, pharmacist, or health care provider.

Generic Name *Brand Name Examples*	Supplied As	Generic Available
Rx **Dexrazoxane** *Zinecard*	**Injection:** 10 mg/mL	No

Type of Drug:

Cardioprotective (heart protective) agent.

How the Drug Works:

Dexrazoxane heaps protect women from heart problems caused by doxorubicin (chemotherapy) treatment of breast cancer.

Uses:

To reduce the chances and severity of heart problems caused by doxorubicin(chemotherapy) treatment of breast cancer. This medicine should not be used at the beginning of doxorubicin therapy. It is added after a certain amount of doxorubicin has been given.

Precautions:

Do not use in the following situations:

allergy to dexrazoxanle or to any of its components
chemotherapy that does not contain an anthracyclinle drug

Use with caution in the following situations:

FAC therapy (fluorouracil, doxorubicin, cyclophosphamide), initiation
myelosuppression (bone marrow suppression)

Pregnancy: Adequate studies have not been done in pregnant women, or animal studies may have shown a risk to the fetus. Use only if clearly needed and potential benefits outweigh the possible hazards to the fetus.

Breastfeeding: It is not known if dexrazoxane appears in breast milk. Consult your doctor before you begin breastfeeding.

Children: Safety and effectiveness for use have not been established.

Lab tests will be required durinlg treatment with dexrazoxane. Tests will include frequent blood counts.

Side Effects:

Every drug is capable of producing side effects. Many patients experience no, or minor, side effects. The frequency or severity of side effects depend on many factors including dose, duration of therapy and individual susceptibility. Possible side effects include:

Digestive Tract: Nausea, vomiting; diarrhea; appetite loss; difficulty swallowing; stomach ache; inflammation of mouth and throat.

Skin: Pain on injection; pain at injection site; redess/streaking; flushing; bruising; hives; rash; numbness.

Other: Fatigue; general body discomfort; fever; infection; blood clots; hair loss; bleeding.

Guidelines for Use:

- This medicine will be prepared and administered by a healthcare provider.
- *Infections* — This medicine, along with chemotherapy medicines, may lower your body's ability to fight infection. Notify your doctor of any signs of infection, including: fever, sore throat, rashes or chills.
- Lab tests and exams will be required to monitor therapy. Be sure to keep appointments.

If you have any questions, consult your doctor, pharmacist, or health care provider.

	Generic Name *Brand Name Examples*	Supplied As	Generic Available
Rx	**Nalmefene HCl** *Revex*	**Injection:** 1 mg/mL	No

Type of Drug:

Anti-opioid; antinarcotic; narcotic antagonist.

How the Drug Works:

Nalmefene prevents or reverses the effects of narcotics (opioids), including respiratory depression, sedation and hypotension (low blood pressure). Nalmefene can cause acute withdrawal symptoms in individuals who are narcotic addicts/abusers. Nalmefene does not produce tolerance, nor cause physical or psychological dependence.

Uses:

To completely or partially reverse narcotic effects, including respiratory depression. To manage known or suspected narcotic overdose.

Precautions:

Do not use in the following situations:
allergy to nalmefene

Use with caution in the following situations:
heart disease, preexisting
kidney disease
liver disease
patients who have received potentially cardiotoxic drugs
physical dependence on narcotics
surgery involving high use of narcotics

Pregnancy: Studies in pregnant women or in animals have been judged not to show a risk to the fetus. However, no drug should be used during pregnancy unless clearly needed.

Breastfeeding: Nalmefene appears in breast milk. Consult your doctor before you begin breastfeeding.

Children: Safety and effectiveness for use have not been established.

Drug Interactions:

Tell your doctor or pharmacist if you are taking or if you are planning to take any over-the-counter or prescription medications or dietary supplements while taking this medicine. Doses of one or both drugs may need to be modified or a different drug may need to be prescribed. Nalmefene may interact with flumazenil (*Romazicon*).

Side Effects:

Every drug is capable of producing side effects. Many patients experience no, or minor, side effects. The frequency or severity of side effects depend on many factors including dose, duration of therapy and individual susceptibility. Possible side effects include:

Digestive Tract: Nausea; vomiting.

Circulatory System: Rapid heartbeat; changes in blood pressure.

Other: Fever; dizziness; headache; chills; flushing; pain.

Guidelines for Use:

- This medicine will be administered by a healthcare provider.
- Difficulty breathing may occur even after using this medicine. Contact your doctor if you are experiencing difficulties.
- Patients using this medicine require careful monitoring by their healthcare providers.
- This medicine should be used with caution in patients with previous heart problems or who are taking drugs which affect the heart.
- This medicine can cause severe withdrawal symptoms and should be used with extreme caution in patients with a known physical dependence on or tolerance to narcotics, or following surgery involving high doses of narcotics.
- This medicine has no demonstrated abuse potential, is not addictive and is not a controlled substance, nor will it relieve pain.
- This medicine is not effective in cases where narcotics were not responsible for sedation and shortness of breath.
- Dosage adjustments may be necessary in patients with kidney failure.

If you have any questions, consult your doctor, pharmacist, or health care provider.

	Generic Name *Brand Name Examples*	Supplied As	Generic Available
Rx	**Naloxone HCl** *Narcan*[1]	**Injection:** 0.02 mg/mL, 0.4 mg/mL,[2] 1 mg/mL[2]	Yes

[1] Contains sodium chloride.
[2] Available with or without methyl and propylparabens.

Type of Drug:

Anti-opioid; antinarcotic; narcotic antagonist.

How the Drug Works:

Naloxone prevents or reverses the effects of narcotics (opioids) and certain narcotic analgesics (eg, codeine). The exact mechanism of action is not fully understood. Evidence suggests that narcotic effects are blocked by competition for the same receptor sites.

Naloxone does not produce tolerance, nor cause dependence. Naloxone will produce withdrawal symptoms in individuals who are narcotic addicts/abusers.

Uses:

To completely or partially reverse narcotic effects, including respiratory depression induced by narcotics (opioids). To diagnose suspected acute narcotic overdosage.

Unlabeled Use(s): Occasionally doctors may prescribe naloxone for improved circulation in refractory shock, reversal of alcoholic coma, dementia of the Alzheimer type and schizophrenia.

Precautions:

Do not use in the following situations:
- allergy to naloxone

Use with caution in the following situations:
- heart disease, preexisting
- patients who have received potentially cardiotoxic drugs
- physical dependence on narcotics, known or suspected (including newborns of dependent mothers)

Pregnancy: Studies in pregnant women or in animals have been judged not to show a risk to the fetus. However, no drug should be used during pregnancy unless clearly needed.

Breastfeeding: It is not known if naloxone appears in breast milk. Consult your doctor before you begin breastfeeding.

Side Effects:

Every drug is capable of producing side effects. Many patients experience no, or minor, side effects. The frequency and severity of side effects depend on many factors including dose, duration of therapy and individual susceptibility. Possible side effects include:

Digestive Tract: Nausea; vomiting.

Circulatory System: Increased heart rate; changes in blood pressure; heart attack.

Other: Sweating; seizures; excitement; tremors; fluid in the lungs.

Guidelines for Use:

- Naloxone does not produce tolerance or cause physical or psychological dependence.
- In the presence of physical dependence on narcotics, naloxone will produce withdrawal symptoms.
- Since the duration of action of some narcotics may exceed that of naloxone, patients should be kept under continued supervision and given repeated doses of naloxone if necessary.

If you have any questions, consult your doctor, pharmacist, or health care provider.

	Generic Name *Brand Name Example*	Supplied As	Generic Available
Rx	**Succimer**		
	Chemet	**Capsules:** 100 mg	No

Type of Drug:

Chelating agent.

How the Drug Works:

Succimer binds to lead in the body and then is excreted in the urine. This results in a reduction in the total amount of lead (which is poisonous) in the body.

Uses:

To treat lead poisoning in children with blood lead levels greater than 45 μg/dL. When using this drug, the source of the lead poisoning should always be identified and removed.

Precautions:

Do not use in the following situations: Allergy to succimer or any of its ingredients.

Use with caution in the following situations:

kidney disease
liver disease, history of

Pregnancy: Adequate studies have not been done in pregnant women. Use only when clearly needed and potential benefits to the mother outweigh the possible hazards to the fetus.

Breastfeeding: It is not known if succimer appears in breast milk. Consult your doctor before you begin breastfeeding.

Children: Safety and effectiveness for use in children under 1 year of age have not been established.

Lab tests will be required during treatment with succimer. Tests may include bloodcounts, blood lead levels, and liver function tests.

Side Effects:

Every drug is capable of producing side effects. Many succimer users experience no, or minor, side effects. The frequency and severity of side effects depend on many factors including dose, duration of therapy, and individual susceptibility. Possible side effects include:

Digestive Tract: Nausea; vomiting; diarrhea; appetite loss; stomach ache or cramps; loose stools.

Nervous System: Headache; dizziness; drowsiness.

Circulatory System: Irregular heartbeat.

Respiratory System: Cough; runny nose; nasal congestion.

Skin: Rash; itching; eruptions of skin and mucous membranes; abnormal skin sensations (burning, prickling, tingling).

Other: Fever; chills; head or body aches or pain; heavy head feeling; cloudy film in eyes; watery eyes; ear infection; plugged ears; cold or flu-like symptoms; sore throat; metallic taste in mouth; hemorrhoidal symptoms; fungal infections; decreased or difficult urination; protein in urine; abnormal blood counts; abnormal blood tests.

Guidelines for Use:

- Dosage is individualized.
- Do not stop taking or change the dose of the drug unless advised to do so by your doctor.
- Drink plenty of fluids.
- If dose is missed, take it as soon as possible. If several hours have passed or if it is nearing time for the next dose, do not double the dose to catch up, unless advised to do so by your doctor. If more than one dose is missed, contact your doctor or pharmacist.
- Identification of the source of the lead poisoning and its removal are critical to successful therapy. Succimer should not be used prophylactically to prevent further exposure to lead.
- In young children who are unable to swallow capsules, the contents of the capsule may be sprinkled on a small amount of food or on a spoon and followed with fruit drink.
- Contact your doctor immediately if you experience a rash.
- Uninterrupted therapy for greater than 3 weeks is generally not recommended.
- Patients should promptly report any indication of infection (eg, sore throat, fever), which may be a sign of low white blood cell count.
- Experience with this drug is limited; therefore, close observation by a doctor is required.
- Lab tests will be required to monitor therapy. Be sure to keep appointments.
- Store between 59° and 77°F and avoid excessive heat.

If you have any questions, consult your doctor, pharmacist, or health care provider.

	Generic Name *Brand Name Examples*	Supplied As	Generic Available
Rx	**Ambenonium Chloride**		
	Mytelase Caplets	**Tablets:** 10 mg	No
Rx	**Edrophonium Chloride**		
	Enlon,[1] Reversol,[1] Tensilon[1]	**Injection**: 10 mg/mL	No
Rx	**Edrophonium Chloride and Atropine Sulfate**		
	Enlon-Plus[1]	**Injection**: 10 mg edrophonium chloride and 0.14 mg atropine sulfate/ml	No
Rx	**Neostigmine Bromide**		
	Prostigmin	**Tablets:** 15 mg	No
Rx	**Neostigmine Methylsulfate**		
	Prostigmin	**Injection**: 0.25 mg/mL, 0.5 mg/mL, 1 mg/mL	Yes
Rx	**Pyridostigmine Bromide**		
	Mestinon	**Tablets:** 60 mg	No
	Mestinon Timespan	**Tablets, sustained-release:** 180 mg	No
	Mestinon	**Syrup:** 60 mg/5 mL	No
	Regonol	**Injection**: 5 mg/mL	No

[1] Contains sodium sulfite.

Type of Drug:

Muscle stimulants; anticholinesterase; cholinesterase inhibitor.

How the Drug Works:

Anticholinesterase muscle stimulants improve the transmission of nerve impulses in muscles so that the muscles are better able to work.

Uses:

To diagnose and treat myasthenia gravis (a disease which causes muscle weakness).

Used as an antidote for certain muscle relaxant drugs used during surgery.

To prevent and treat distention and urinary retention following surgery (neostigmine methylsulfate only).

Precautions:

Do not use in the following situations:

allergy to anticholinesterase muscle stimulants or any of their ingredients
allergy to bromides (neostigmine bromide and pyridostigmine only)
intestinal obstruction
peritonitis (inflammation of the lining of abdomen) (neostigmine methylsulfate only)
urinary obstruction

Use with caution in the following situations:

abnormal heart rhythm
asthma
epilepsy
kidney disease (pyridostigmine only)
obstruction of coronary artery, recent
overactive thyroid
peptic ulcer
slow heartbeat

Overdosage: Overdosage may result in cholinergic crisis which causes increased muscle weakness. Muscle weakness involving the respiratory muscles may lead to death.

Pregnancy: Safety for use during pregnancy has not been established. Although cholinesterase inhibitors are apparently safe for the fetus, they may ultimately affect the condition of the infant. Temporary muscular weakness has occurred in infants whose mothers used these drugs during pregnancy. Use only if clearly needed and the potential benefits outweigh the possible hazards to the fetus.

Breastfeeding: It is not known if anticholinesterase muscle stimulants appear in breast milk. Consult your doctor before you begin breastfeeding.

Children: Safety and effectiveness for use in children have not been established.

Sulfites: Some of these products may contain sulfite preservatives, which can cause allergic reactions in some individuals (eg, patients with asthma). Check package label when available or consult your doctor or pharmacist.

Drug Interactions:

Tell your doctor or pharmacist if you are taking or if you are planning to take any over-the-counter or prescription medications or dietary supplements with anticholinesterase muscle stimulants. Doses of one or both drugs may need to be modified or a different drug may need to be prescribed. The following drugs and drug classes interact with anticholinesterase muscle stimulants:

aminoglycosides (eg, gentamicin)
atropine
corticosteroids (eg, prednisone)
mecamylamine (*Inversine*)
succinylcholine (eg, *Anectine)*

Side Effects:

Every drug is capable of producing side effects. Many anticholinesterase muscle stimulant users experience no, or minor, side effects. The frequency and severity of side effects depend on many factors including dose, duration of therapy, and individual susceptibility. Possible side effects include:

Muscular System: Muscle cramps or spasms; muscle twitching; joint pain; weakness.

Eyes or Ocular: Increased tearing; blurred vision; double vision; redness; visual changes; decreased pupil size.

Digestive Tract: Nausea; vomiting; diarrhea; stomach pain or cramping; gas.

Nervous System: Convulsions; loss of consciousness; dizziness; drowsiness; headache.

Circulatory System: Changes in heart rate; abnormal heart rhythm; decreased blood pressure.

Skin: Rash; itching; sweating; flushing; hives.

Other: Vocal problems or difficulty speaking; difficulty swallowing; uncontrolled urination; increased urination; increased salivation; difficult or painful breathing; fainting.

Guidelines for Use:

- Dosage is individualized.
- Close supervision by your doctor is required during treatment to avoid overdosage.
- Do not crush or chew sustained-release tablets.
- Do not change the dose or stop taking unless advised to do so by your doctor. Frequently, therapy is required day and night (except ambenonium).
- *Oral products* — If a dose is missed, take it as soon as possible. If several hours have passed or if it is nearing time for the next dose, do not double the dose to catch up, unless advised to do so by your doctor. If more than one dose is missed or it is necessary to establish a new dosage schedule, contact your doctor or pharmacist.
- *Pyridostigmine* — Sustained-release tablets may develop some patchy discoloration over time. This does not change the effectiveness of the medicine and is no cause for concern.
- Keep a daily record of doses and note times of greatest fatigue or weakness.
- Contact your doctor immediately if you experience periods of extreme muscle weakness, diarrhea, vomiting, stomach cramps, increased salivation, decreased pupil size, or difficulty speaking or swallowing.
- Store at controlled room temperature (59° to 86°F).

If you have any questions, consult your doctor, pharmacist, or health care provider.

Generic Name *Brand Name Example*	Supplied As	Generic Available
Rx **Acetohydroxamic Acid**		
Lithostat	**Tablets:** 250 mg	No

Type of Drug:

Urinary enzyme inhibitor.

How the Drug Works:

Acetohydroxamic acid (AHA) inhibits the bacterial enzyme urease, thereby inhibiting ammonia production and urea decomposition in the urine. These two effects enable antibiotics to be more effective in treating chronic urinary tract infections.

Uses:

To aid antibiotic treatment of chronic urinary tract infections due to urea-splitting bacteria.

Precautions:

Do not use in the following situations:

allergy to acetohydroxamic acid or any of its ingredients
female patients who do not use adequate contraception
infection treatable with antibiotics alone
kidney disease, moderate to severe infection treatable with surgery and antibiotics
pregnancy
urinary infection with nonurease-producing bacteria

Use with caution in the following situations:

hemolytic anemia (Coombs negative)
kidney disease, mild

Pregnancy: Do not use during pregnancy. May cause fetal harm when given to a pregnant woman. The risk of use in a pregnant woman clearly outweighs any possible benefit. If you become pregnant while taking this medicine or plan to become pregnant, consult your doctor.

Breastfeeding: It is not known if acetohydroxamic acid appears in breast milk. Consult your doctor before you begin breastfeeding.

Children: Children with chronic recalcitrant urinary tract infections caused by urea-splitting bacteria may benefit from this drug. However, detailed studies involving dosage and dose intervals in children have not been established. If used in children, close monitoring will be required.

Lab tests may be required during treatment with acetohydroxamic acid. Tests may include complete blood counts, kidney function tests, urine cultures, and liver function tests.

Drug Interactions:

Tell your doctor or pharmacist if you are taking or planning to take any over-the-counter or prescription medications or dietary supplements with acetohydroxamic acid. Doses of one or both drugs may need to be modified or a different drug may need to be prescribed. The following drugs and drug classes interact with acetohydroxamic acid:

alcohol
heavy metals (eg, iron)

Side Effects:

Every drug is capable of producing side effects. Many acetohydroxamic acid users experience no, or minor, side effects. The frequency and severity of side effects depend on many factors including dose, duration of therapy, and individual susceptibility. Possible side effects include:

Digestive Tract: Nausea; vomiting; appetite loss.

Nervous System: Mild headache; shakiness; depression; anxiety; nervousness; fatigue.

Skin: Rash (especially after ingesting alcohol); hair loss.

Other: Vein inflammation of the lower extremities; palpitations (pounding in the chest); leg pain; abnormal blood counts; abnormal lab tests; general body discomfort.

Guidelines for Use:

- Read the patient package insert before using.
- Dosage is individualized.
- Do not stop taking or change the dose unless advised to do so by your doctor.
- Take on an empty stomach at least 1 hour before or 2 hours after a meal or snack.
- If dose is missed, take it as soon as possible. If several hours have passed or if it is nearing time for the next dose, do not double the dose to catch up, unless advised to do so by your doctor. If more than one dose is missed, contact your doctor or pharmacist.
- Do not take iron tablets or multivitamins with minerals at the same time. Take between dose of *Lithostat*.
- Avoid alcoholic beverages. A rash commonly appears 30 to 45 minutes after drinking alcohol. It is associated with a general feeling of warmth and spontaneously disappears within 30 to 60 minutes.
- Contact your doctor if you experience tiredness, nausea, vomiting, rash, lower extremity pain, appetite loss, or fatigue.
- Lab tests may be required to monitor therapy. Be sure to keep appointments.
- Store at room temperature (59° to 86°F) in a dry place.

If you have any questions, consult your doctor, pharmacist, or health care provider.

	Generic Name *Brand Name Examples*	Supplied As	Generic Available
Rx	**Potassium Acid Phosphate**		
	K-Phos Original	**Tablets:** 500 mg	No
Rx	**Potassium Acid Phosphate and Sodium Acid Phosphate**		
	K-Phos M.F.	**Tablets:** 155 mg potassium acid bphosphate and 350 mg sodium acid phosphate	No
	K-Phos No. 2	**Tablets:** 305 mg potassium acid phosphate and 700 mg sodium acid phosphate	No

Although controversy exists regarding the effectiveness of ascorbic acid as a urinary acidifier, it is often used for this purpose. For more information on ascorbic acid, see the Vitamin C (Ascorbic Acid) monograph in the Nutritionals chapter.

Type of Drug:

Urinary tract acidifiers.

How the Drug Works:

Urinary tract acidifiers increase the amount of acid in the urine. This lowers the pH of the urine.

Uses:

Makes the urine more acid and therefore less likely to support the growth of some bacteria. Also helps calcium dissolve in the urine, thereby reducing the risk of calcium stone formation. Increases the effect of the urinary tract anti-infective methenamine. Reduces odor and skin irritation caused by urine with high ammonia concentrations.

Precautions:

Do not use in the following situations:

increased blood phosphate levels
increased blood potassium levels
infected phosphate stones
kidney disease, severe

Use with caution in the following situations:

Addison's disease
dehydration
edema (fluid retention), body or lungs (sodium acid phosphate only)
heart disease (eg, heart failure)
high blood pressure (sodium acid phosphate only)
hypoparathyroidism (decreased function)
kidney disease, mild-to-moderate
liver disease (eg, cirrhosis)
pancreas, inflamed
rickets (vitamin D deficiency)
sodium in the blood, increased (sodium acid phosphate only)

sodium-restricted diet (sodium acid phosphate only)
tissue breakdown, extensive (eg, burns)
toxemia of pregnancy (sodium acid phosphate only)

Kidney stones: Patients with kidney stones may pass old stones when therapy is started.

Antacids: Avoid antacids which contain aluminum, calcium, or magnesium. These ingredients may prevent phosphate absorption.

Potassium supplements: Consider the potassium content of urinary acidifiers if potassium supplements, salt substitutes, or potassium sparing diuretics are being used. Potassium levels should be monitored in these situations.

Pregnancy: Adequate studies have not been done in pregnant women. Use only if clearly needed and potential benefits outweigh the possible hazards to the fetus.

Breastfeeding: It is not known if urinary acidifiers appear in breast milk. Consult your doctor before you begin breastfeeding.

Lab tests may be required during treatment with urinary acidifiers. Tests may include: Liver and kidney function tests; blood electrolyte (sodium, potassium, phosphorus, calcium) levels.

Drug Interactions:

Tell your doctor or pharmacist if you are taking or if you are planning to take any over-the-counter or prescription medications or dietary supplements with urinary acidifiers. Doses of one or both drugs may need to be modified or a different drug may need to be prescribed. The following drugs and drug classes interact with urinary acidifiers:

aluminum-, calcium-, or magnesium-containing antacids (eg, *Maalox*)
amiloride *(Midamor)*
corticosteroids (eg, prednisone)
corticotropin (eg, *Acthar*)
diazoxide (eg, *Proglycem*)
guanethidine (eg, *Ismelin*)
hydralazine (eg, *Apresoline*)
methyldopa (eg, *Aldomet*)
potassium supplements
reserpine (eg, *Serpasil*)
salicylates (eg, aspirin)
salt substitutes (eg, *Morton Salt Substitute*)
spironolactone (eg, *Aldactone*)
triamterene (*Dyrenium*)

Side Effects:

Every drug is capable of producing side effects. Many urinary acidifier users experience no, or minor, side effects. The frequency and severity of side effects depend on many factors including dose, duration of therapy, and individual susceptibility. Possible side effects include:

Digestive Tract: Stomach pain; nausea; vomiting; diarrhea.

Nervous System: Confusion; seizures; unusual tiredness; dizziness; headache.

Circulatory System: Fast or irregular heartbeat.

Respiratory System: Shortness of breath; difficulty breathing.

Other: Weakness or heaviness of legs; muscle cramps; numbness, tingling, pain or weakness in hands or feet; numbness or tingling around lips; swelling of feet or legs; low urine output; unusual thirst; bone or joint pain; weight gain; edema (fluid retention).

Guidelines for Use:

- Do not change the dose or stop taking this medicine unless advised to do so by your doctor.
- If a dose is missed, take it as soon as possible. If several hours have passed or if it is nearing time for the next dose, do not double the dose in order to catch up, unless advised to do so by your doctor. If more than one dose is missed or it is necessary to establish a new dosage schedule, contact your doctor or pharmacist.
- *Potassium Acid Phosphate and Sodium Acid Phosphate Tablets* — Take each dose with a full glass of water.
- *Potassium Acid Phosphate Tablets* — Dissolve prescribed number of tablets in a full glass of water before taking. Let tablets soak for 2 to 5 minutes. You may crush and stir the tablets to speed the dissolving time.
- Notify your doctor if stomach pain, nausea or vomiting, heart irregularities, or edema (fluid retention) occurs.
- Avoid antacids containing aluminum, calcium, or magnesium.
- Some patients experience a mild laxative effect. If this effect persists, contact your doctor.
- Inform your doctor if you are pregnant, become pregnant, are planning to become pregnant, or are breastfeeding.
- Lab tests may be required during therapy. Be sure to keep appointments.
- Store at controlled room temperature (59° to 86°F).

If you have any questions, consult your doctor, pharmacist, or health care provider.

	Generic Name *Brand Name Examples*	Supplied As	Generic Available
Rx	**Potassium Citrate**		
	Urocit-K	**Tablets:** 5 mEq, 10 mEq	No
Rx	**Potassium Citrate Combinations**		
	Polycitra-LC	**Solution:** 550 mg potassium citrate, 500 mg sodium citrate and 334 mg citric acid/5 mL	No
	Polycitra-K	**Solution:** 1100 mg potassium citrate and 334 mg citric acid/ 5 mL	No
otc	**Sodium Bicarbonate**	**Tablets:** 650 mg	Yes
		Powder	Yes
Rx	**Sodium Citrate and Citric Acid (Shohl's Solution, Modified)**		
	Bicitra	**Solution:** 500 mg sodium citrate and 334 mg citric acid/ 5 mL	No
	Oracit	**Solution**: 490 mg sodium citrate and 640 mg citric acid/ 5 mL	No

Type of Drug:

Urinary alkalinizer.

How the Drug Works:

Urinary alkalinizers make the urine less acidic (alkaline). This may help dissolve certain types of kidney stones and enhance the elimination of certain acidic drugs and other substances in the urine.

Uses:

To correct acid urine and systemic acidosis (excessive acid in the blood) due to disorders of the kidney tubules (renal tubular acidosis).

To limit the formation of uric acid crystals in the urine during the treatment of gout.

To help dissolve some types of kidney stones.

To alter the kidneys' elimination of certain medications.

Precautions:

Do not use in the following situations:

Addison's disease, untreated adrenal insufficiency
allergy to urinary alkalinizers or any of their ingredients
anticholinergic drug therapy, concurrent
dehydration, acute

- delayed stomach emptying (potassium citrate tablets only)
- diabetes mellitus, uncontrolled
- diuretic therapy, concurrent
- esophageal compression (potassium citrate tablets only)
- heart damage, severe
- heat cramps
- hyperkalemia (high blood potassium levels)
- intestinal obstruction or stricture (potassium citrate tablets only)
- kidney disease, severe
- kidney failure, chronic (potassium products only)
- peptic ulcer (potassium citrate tablets only)
- strenuous physical exercise in unconditioned patients
- tissue breakdown, extensive (eg, severe trauma)
- urinary tract infection

Use with caution in the following situations:

- congestive heart failure (sodium products only)
- disorders which cause swelling (sodium products only)
- high blood pressure (sodium products only)
- kidney disease
- low urine output
- sodium-restricted diet (sodium products only)
- toxemia of pregnancy (sodium products only)

Pregnancy: There are no adequate and well-controlled studies in pregnant women. Use only if clearly needed and the potential benefits to the mother outweigh the possible risks to the fetus.

Breastfeeding: It is not known if urinary alkalinizers appear in breast milk. Consult your doctor before you begin breastfeeding.

Children: Safety and effectiveness of potassium citrate tablets in children have not been established.

Lab tests may be required to monitor therapy. Tests may include serum potassium determinations and acid-base determinations.

Drug Interactions:

Tell your doctor or pharmacist if you are taking or if you are planning to take any over-the-counter or prescription medications or dietary supplements with urinary alkalinizers. Doses of one or both drugs may need to be modified or a different drug may need to be prescribed. The following drugs and drug classes interact with urinary alkalinizers:

- ACE inhibitors (eg, captopril)
- aluminum-based antacids (eg, *Amphojel*)
- anorexiants (eg, amphetamine)
- anticholinergic drugs (eg, atropine) (potassium citrate tablets only)
- chlorpropamide (eg, diabenese)
- lithium (eg, *Eskalith*)
- potassium-sparing diuretics (eg, amiloride, triamterene)
- salicylates (eg, aspirin)
- sympathomimetics (eg, pseudoephedrine)
- tetracyclines (eg, doxycycline)

Side Effects:

Every drug is capable of producing side effects. Many urinary alkalinizer users experience no, or minor, side effects. The frequency and severity of side effects depend on many factors including dose, duration of therapy, and individual susceptibility. Possible side effects include:

Digestive Tract: Stomach discomfort; vomiting; diarrhea; loose stools; nausea.

Other: Edema (fluid retention) (sodium products); gas; sour taste (citrate products); high blood pressure (sodium products).

Guidelines for Use:

- Dosage will be individualized.
- Do not change the dose or stop taking unless advised to do so by your doctor.
- Take with or after meals or a snack to avoid stomach discomfort.
- If a dose is missed, take it as soon as possible. If several hours have passed or if it is nearing time for the next dose, do not double the dose in order to catch up, unless advised to do so by your doctor. If several doses are missed, or it is necessary to establish a new dosage schedule, contact your doctor or pharmacist.
- *Potassium citrate tablets* — Stop taking and notify your doctor if you experience severe vomiting, severe stomach pain, vomiting of blood, or dark, tarry stools.
  Do not crush, chew, or suck on the tablet. Swallow whole.
  Following the release of the potassium citrate, the wax matrix of the tablet, which is not absorbable, is excreted in the stool. This is normal and no cause for concern.
- *Solutions* — Dilute with water; follow with more water, if desired. Refrigerate to mask taste.
- *Tablets* — Talk to you doctor if you have trouble swallowing the tablets or they seem to stick in your throat.
- *Sodium bicarbonate* — Dissolve each dose in a glass of water. Do not take until completely dissolved in water. Do not take if you are overly full from food or drink.
- Lab tests may be required to monitor therapy. Be sure to keep appointments.
- Store at controlled room temperature (59° to 86°F).

If you have any questions, consult your doctor, pharmacist, or health care provider.

Generic Name *Brand Name Examples*	Supplied As	Generic Available
Rx **Bethanechol Chloride**		
Urecholine	**Tablets:** 5 mg, 10 mg, 25 mg, 50 mg	Yes
Urecholine	**Injection**: 5 mg/mL	No

Type of Drug:

Cholinergic stimulant; bladder stimulant.

How the Drug Works:

Bethanechol chloride stimulates the muscles in the bladder to contract, which causes urination. It also stimlates digestive tract movement.

Uses:

To treat urinary retention (incomplete emptying of the bladder) after surgery or childbirth or due to neurogenic atony (nerve damage).

Unlabeled Use(s): Occasionally doctors may prescribe bethanechol for reflux esophagitis in adults and for gastroesophageal reflux in infants and children.

Precautions:

Do not use in the following situations:

- allergy to bethanechol chloride or any of its ingredients
- bladder obstruction
- bladder surgery, recent
- bronchial asthma, latent or active
- coronary artery disease
- digestive tract obstruction
- digestive tract lesions, acute
- epilepsy
- intestinal surgery, recent
- low blood pressure
- overactive thyroid
- Parkinson's disease
- peptic ulcer
- peritonitis
- slow heart rate
- spastic digestive tract disorders
- vagotonia, marked
- vasomotor instability

Use with caution in the following situations: Bladder infection.

Pregnancy: There are no adequate and well-controlled studies in pregnant women. Use only if clearly needed and potential benefits to the mother outweigh the possible hazards to the fetus.

Breastfeeding: It is not known if bethanechol appears in breast milk. Consult your doctor before you begin breastfeeding.

Children: Safety and effectiveness in children have not been established.

Drug Interactions:

Tell your doctor or pharmacist if you are taking or if you are planning to take any over-the-counter or prescription medications or dietary supplements with bethanechol. Doses of one or both drugs may need to be modified or a different drug may need to be prescribed. The following drugs and drug classes interact with bethanechol:

cholinergic drugs (eg, ambenonium)
ganglion-blocking compounds
procainamide (eg, *Pronestyl*)
quinidine (eg, *Cin-Quin*)

Side Effects:

Every drug is capable of producing side effects. Many bethanechol users experience no, or minor, side effects. The frequency and severity of side effects depend on many factors including dose, duration of therapy, and individual susceptibility. Possible side effects include:

Digestive Tract: Belching; diarrhea; stomach pain, cramps, or discomfort; rumbling stomach; nausea; abnormal salivation.

Respiratory System: Asthma attack; difficulty breathing.

Other: General body discomfort; urinary urgency; headache; fall in blood pressure with fast heart rate; sweating; flushing producing a feeling of warmth; facial warmth; visual disturbances; tearing of eyes; change in pupil size.

Guidelines for Use:

- Dosage is individualized.
- Do not stop taking or change the dose unless advised to do so by your doctor.
- Take tablets on an empty stomach at least 1 hour before or 2 hours after meals to avoid nausea or vomiting.
- If a dose is missed, take it as soon as possible. If several hours have passed or if it is nearing time for the next dose, do not double the dose in order to catch up, unless advised to do so by your doctor. If several doses are missed, or it is necessary to establish a new dosage schedule, contact your doctor or pharmacist.
- Injection is for subcutaneous (SC) (beneath the skin) administration only. It will be prepared and administered by your health care provider in a medical setting.
- May cause increased salivation, sweating, flushing, or stomach ache. Notify your doctor if these symptoms persist or become severe.
- May cause dizziness, lightheadedness, or fainting, especially when rising from a seated or lying position.
- Store tablets at controlled room temperature (59° to 86°F).

If you have any questions, consult your doctor, pharmacist, or health care provider.

Generic Name *Brand Name Example*	Supplied As	Generic Available
Rx **Cellulose Sodium Phosphate**		
Calcibind	**Powder**	No

Type of Drug:

Urinary tract product.

How the Drug Works:

Cellulose sodium phosphate alters the levels of calcium, magnesium, phosphate, and oxalate in the urine. Urine phosphate and oxalate levels increase. Urine calcium and magnesium levels decrease. Lowering of calcium in the urine leads to decreased formation of calcium-containing kidney stones.

Uses:

To reduce the formation of calcium containing kidney stones in absorptive hypercalciuria Type I (excess calcium levels in the urine).

Precautions:

Do not use in the following situations:

- allergy to cellulose sodium phosphate or any of its ingredients
- calcium levels in blood or urine, decreased
- hyperparathyroidism (overactive parathyroid)
- increased urine calcium levels other than absorptive hyper calciuria Type I
- magnesium levels, decreased in blood
- osteomalacia (softening of bone)
- osteitis (inflammation of bone)
- osteoporosis (brittle bones)
- oxalic acid or oxalates, increased in urine
- phosphate levels, decreased in blood

Use with caution in the following situations:

- ascites (fluid in the abdominal cavity)
- congestive heart failure

Pregnancy: Adequate studies have not been done in pregnant women. Because of the increased dietary calcium requirement in pregnant women, use only when clearly needed and potential benefits to the mother outweigh possible hazards to the fetus.

Breastfeeding: It is not known if cellulose sodium appears in breast milk. Consult your doctor before you begin breastfeeding.

Children: Because of the increased requirement for dietary calcium in growing children, use in children under 16 years of age is not recommended.

Lab tests will be required to monitor therapy. Tests may include blood levels of calcium, magnesium, copper, zinc, iron and parathyroid hormone, and complete blood counts.

Side Effects:

Every drug is capable of producing side effects. Many cellulose sodium phosphate users experience no, or minor, side effects. The frequency and severity of side effects depend on many factors including dose, duration of therapy, and individual susceptibility.

Digestive Tract: Diarrhea; indigestion; loose bowel movements; poor taste of the drug.

Circulatory System: Calcium and magnesium depletion; depletion of trace metals (ie, copper, zinc, iron).

Guidelines for Use:

- Dosage is individualized and may be adjusted over time.
- Do not stop taking or change the dose of the drug unless advised to do so by your doctor.
- Dietary changes are recommended, including:
  Avoid dairy products and reduce intake of calcium from other sources.
  Restrict oxalate in the diet by avoiding spinach and other dark greens, rhubarb, chocolate, and brewed tea.
  Avoid vitamin C supplements.
  Reduce your sodium intake.
  Drink plenty of fluids.
- Dissolve prescribed amount of the powder for each dose in water, soft drinks, or fruit juices. Take within 30 minutes of a meal, but do not take at the same time as magnesium supplements (eg, magnesium gluconate).
- Lab tests will be required to monitor therapy. Be sure to keep appointments.
- Store in a dry place at room temperature (59° to 86°F).

If you have any questions, consult your doctor, pharmacist, or health care provider.

Generic Name *Brand Name Example*	Supplied As	Generic Available
Rx **Cysteamine Bitartrate**		
Cystagon	**Capsules:** 50 mg, 150 mg	No

Type of Drug:

Urinary tract product.

How the Drug Works:

Cysteamine lowers the cystine content of cells in patients with cystinosis.

Uses:

To manage nephropathic cystinosis (a rare, serious kidney disease) in children and adults. This disease may cause kidney failure, other organ damage or growth reduction in children.

Precautions:

Do not use in the following situations:
allergy to cysteamine or penicillamine (eg, *Cuprimine)*

Use with caution in the following situations:

depression
drowsiness
lethargy
liver, digestive or blood disorders
neurologic problems
rash
seizures

Rash: Do not begin or continue use if a skin rash is present.

Lab tests: Cysteamine may cause abnormal blood counts (low white blood cells) and abnormal liver function tests. Lab tests will be required to monitor therapy.

Pregnancy: Adequate studies have not been done in pregnant women. Use only if clearly needed and potential benefits outweigh the possible hazards to the fetus.

Breastfeeding: It is not known if cysteamine appears in breast milk. Consult your doctor before you begin breastfeeding.

Children: Cysteamine is a safe and effective drug for use in children once nephropathic cystinosis is diagnosed.

Side Effects:

Every drug is capable of producing side effects. Many cysteamine users experience no, or minor, side effects. The frequency and severity of side effects depend on many factors including dose, duration of therapy and individual susceptibility. Possible side effects include:

Digestive Tract: Vomiting; diarrhea; constipation; appetite loss; nausea; bad breath; stomach ache; indigestion.

Nervous System: Fever; tiredness; weakness; drowsiness; headache; convulsions; seizures; incoordination; confusion; tremor; impaired hearing;

dizziness; jitteriness; abnormal dreams; lightheadedness; nervousness; abnormal thinking; depression; emotional instability; hallucinations.

Skin: Rash; hives.

Other: Dehydration; flushing; abnormal blood counts; abnormal liver function tests.

Guidelines for Use:

- Take in 4 divided doses about 6 hours apart, or as directed by your doctor.
- Young children may not be able to swallow the capsules. Contents of the capsules should be sprinkled over food or mixed in formula for children under 6 years of age. Other patients should follow their doctor's instructions with regard to food.
- Do not increase or decrease this medication without your doctor's approval.
- Upset stomach and indigestion are common side effects. If these are severe or become a nuisance, contact your doctor.
- If a dose is missed, take it as soon as possible. If several hours have passed or if it is nearing time for the next dose, do not double the dose to "catch up" (unless advised to do so by your doctor). If more than one dose is missed or if it is necessary to establish a new dosage schedule, contact your doctor or pharmacist. Use exactly as prescribed.
- If a skin rash develops, discontinue use of this medicine and contact your doctor immediately.
- Notify your doctor if any of the following occurs: fever; seizures; weakness; tiredness; drowsiness; incoordination; difficulty breathing; strange behavior; unusual thinking or emotions, depression; nausea; diarrhea; vomiting; appetite loss; abdominal pain.
- May cause drowsiness, dizziness or confusion. Avoid driving or performing other tasks requiring alertness or coordination until effects are known, then use caution.
- Lab tests will be required every 3 months. Tests will include: liver function tests and complete blood counts. Be sure to keep appointments.
- Store in a dry, safe place away from light and the reach of children.

If you have any questions, consult your doctor, pharmacist, or health care provider.

	Generic Name *Brand Name Example*	Supplied As	Generic Available
Rx	**Dimethyl Sulfoxide (DMSO)**		
	Rimso-50	**Solution, aqueous:** 50%	No

Dimethyl sulfoxide (DMSO) is available in a variety of forms not intended for human use (eg, veterinary and industrial solvents). Human use of such products should be discouraged because of their unknown purity. Because of its skin transport characteristics, impurities and contaminants may be systemically absorbed from topical use.

Type of Drug:

Local anti-inflammatory agent.

How the Drug Works:

DMSO has a broad range of pharmacological properties that include: Anti-inflammatory action, nerve blockade, diuresis, cholinesterase inhibition, vasodilation and muscle relaxation.

Uses:

For symptomatic relief of bladder inflammation.

There is no clinical evidence of effectiveness for treatment of bacterial urinary tract infections.

Unlabeled Use(s): DMSO has been used in the topical treatment of a wide variety of musculoskeletal disorders and collagen diseases and to enhance the absorption of other drugs through the skin. Such unlabeled uses, as well as many others, have not been approved by the FDA.

Precautions:

Allergic reaction: DMSO can cause an allergic reaction. Consult your doctor.

Pregnancy: Adequate studies have not been done in pregnant women. Use only if clearly needed and potential benefits outweigh the possible hazards to the fetus.

Breastfeeding: It is not known if DMSO appears in breast milk, but presence is likely. Consult your doctor before you begin breastfeeding.

Children: Safety and effectiveness have not been established.

Lab tests will be required at least every 6 months during treatment with DMSO. Tests may include: Liver and kidney function tests, full eye exams and complete blood counts.

Drug Interactions:

Tell your doctor or pharmacist if you are taking or if you are planning to take any over-the-counter or prescription medications or dietary supplements with DMSO. Doses of one or both drugs may need to be modified or a different drug may need to be prescribed.

Sulindac *(Clinoril)* interacts with DMSO.

Side Effects:

Every drug is capable of producing side effects. Many DMSO users experience no, or minor, side effects. The frequency and severity of side effects depend on many factors including dose, duration of therapy and individual susceptibility. Possible side effects include:

Topical Use: Garlic-like taste and odor on breath and skin; dermatitis; sedation; nausea; vomiting; headache; burning or aching eyes.

Other: Inflamed bladder.

Guidelines for Use:

- Caution — Use of veterinary and industrial forms of this drug is not recommended because of unknown purity.
- A garlic-like taste, breath and odor on skin may develop within a few minutes of use. The taste may linger for several hours. Odor on the breath and skin may be present for up to 72 hours.
- Obtain a complete eye exam before and during treatment with this drug.
- Lab tests will be required every 6 months. Tests will include: Liver and kidney function tests and complete blood counts.

If you have any questions, consult your doctor, pharmacist, or health care provider.

	Generic Name *Brand Name Example*	Supplied As	Generic Available
Rx	**Flavoxate HCl**		
	Urispas	**Tablets:** 100 mg	No

Type of Drug:

Urinary tract antispasmodic.

How the Drug Works:

Flavoxate relieves smooth muscle spasm of the urinary tract. It aids in the retention of urine and has local anesthetic and pain-relieving properties.

Uses:

For relief of painful urination, frequency, urgency, nighttime urination, incontinence and pain associated with urinary tract disorders. It is not a definitive treatment, but is compatible with other urinary tract drugs.

Precautions:

Do not use in the following situations:
achalasia (failure of certain sphincter muscles to relax)
bleeding of digestive tract
intestinal obstruction
stomach obstruction
urinary tract obstruction

Use with caution in the following situations: glaucoma

Pregnancy: Adequate studies have not been done in pregnant women. Use only if clearly needed and potential benefits outweigh the possible hazards to the fetus.

Breastfeeding: It is not known if flavoxate appears in breast milk. Consult your doctor before you begin breastfeeding.

Children: Safety and effectiveness in children under 12 have not been established.

Side Effects:

Every drug is capable of producing side effects. Many flavoxate users experience no, or minor, side effects. The frequency and severity of side effects depend on many factors including dose, duration of therapy and individual susceptibility. Possible side effects include:

Digestive Tract: Nausea; vomiting.

Nervous System: Nervousness; vertigo (feeling of whirling motion); headache; drowsiness; confusion.

Other: Dry mouth; high fever; painful or difficult urination; increased heart rate; palpitations (pounding in the chest); vision problems (eg, blurred vision); hives; skin disorders; abnormal blood counts.

Guidelines for Use:

- May cause drowsiness or blurred vision. Use caution while driving or performing other tasks requiring alertness, coordination or physical dexterity.
- May cause dry mouth, hives and rash. If these or other side effects persist or worsen, contact your doctor.

If you have any questions, consult your doctor, pharmacist, or health care provider.

	Generic Name *Brand Name Examples*	Supplied As	Generic Available
Rx	**Oxybutynin Chloride**		
	Ditropan	**Tablets:** 5 mg	Yes
	Ditropan	**Syrup:** 5 mg/5 mL	Yes

Type of Drug:

Urinary tract antispasmodic.

How the Drug Works:

Oxybutynin chloride reduces muscle spasms of the bladder by exerting direct relaxing effects on the muscle around the bladder and inhibiting the effect of chemicals which can cause bladder spasm.

Uses:

For symptomatic relief of certain bladder conditions, such as frequent or painful urination, urge, incontinence, and urinary leakage.

Precautions:

Do not use in the following situations:

glaucoma, angle-closure
intestinal weakness, elderly or debilitated
intestinal tract problems, paralyzed, obstructed, or inflammed
megacolon (dilated or enlarged colon)
myasthenia gravis
urinary tract obstruction
unstable blood pressure from blood loss

Use with caution in the following situations:

autonomic nervous system disorders
congestive heart failure
coronary artery disease
diarrhea
elderly
hiatal hernia
high blood pressure
hot weather
hyperthyroidism
ileostomy or colostomy
increased heart rate
irregular heartbeat
kidney disease
liver disease
prostate, enlarged
sweating, decreased
ulcerative colitis

Hot weather: Oxbutynin can cause heat prostration (fever and heatstroke) due to decreased sweating.

Diarrhea: Diarrhea may be a sign of partial intestinal obstruction especially in ileostomy or colostomy patients. If diarrhea is severe, discontinue use and contact your doctor.

Pregnancy: Adequate studies have not been done in pregnant women. Use only if clearly needed and potential benefits outweigh the possible hazards to the fetus.

Breastfeeding: It is not known if oxybutynin appears in breast milk. Consult your doctor before you begin breastfeeding.

Children: Safety and effectiveness in children under 5 years old have not been established.

Drug Interactions:

Tell your doctor or pharmacist if you are taking or if you are planning to take any over-the-counter or prescription medications or dietary supplements with oxybutynin. Doses of one or both drugs may need to be modified or a different drug may need to be prescribed. The following drugs and drug classes interact with oxybutynin.

digoxin (eg, *Lanoxin)*
haloperidol (eg, *Haldol)*
phenothiazines (eg, promethazine)
atenolol (eg, *Tenormin*)
acetaminophen (eg, *Tylenol)*
levodopa (eg, *Larodopa)*
nitrofurantoin (eg, *Macrodantin)*
amantadine (eg, *Symmetrel)*

Side Effects:

Every drug is capable of producing side effects. Many oxybutynin users experience no, or minor, side effects. The frequency and severity of side effects depend on many factors including dose, duration of therapy and individual susceptibility. Possible side effects include:

Digestive Tract: Nausea; vomiting; constipation.

Nervous System: Dizziness; sleeplessness; weakness; restlessness; drowsiness; hallucinations.

Circulatory System: Palpitations (pounding in the chest); rapid heart rate; flushing.

Other: Difficulty or inability to urinate; impotence; decreased tearing of eyes; vision problems; suppression of breast milk production; decreased sweating; dry mouth; rash; dilated pupils; fever; vision problems.

Guidelines for Use:

- Usual adult dose is 1 tablet 2 or 3 times per day. Adjust dosage to control symptoms.
- If a dose is missed, take it as soon as possible. If several hours have passed or if it is nearing time for the next dose, do not double the dose to catch up (unless advised by your doctor). If more than 1 dose is missed, contact your doctor or pharmacist.
- May cause drowsiness or blurred vision. Alcohol or sedatives may enhance these effects. Use caution when driving or performing other tasks requiring alertness, coordination, or physical dexterity until tolerance is determined.
- May cause dry mouth. If this or other side effects, especially diarrhea, persist or worsen, contact your doctor.
- Use caution in hot weather.
- Store at room temperature.

If you have any questions, consult your doctor, pharmacist, or health care provider.

Generic Name *Brand Name Examples*	Supplied As	Generic Available
Rx **Tolterodine Tartrate**		
Detrol	**Tablets:** 1 mg, 2 mg	No

Type of Drug:

Bladder muscle relaxant.

How the Drug Works:

Tolterodine acts on the muscles of the bladder, decreasing the pressures and urge to empty the bladder.

Uses:

For the treatment of patients with an overactive bladder with the symptoms of urinary frequency, urgency, and urinary incontinence.

Precautions:

Do not use in the following situations:

allergy to tolterodine
digestive tract obstruction
narrow-angle glaucoma, uncontrolled
urinary retention

Use with caution in the following situations:

bladder outflow obstruction
gastrointestinal obstructive disorders (pyloric stenosis)
kidney function, reduced
liver function, reduced
narrow-angle glaucoma, controlled

Pregnancy: There are no studies of tolterodine in pregnant women. Use only if the potential benefit justifies the potential risk to the fetus.

Breastfeeding: It is not known if tolterodine appears in breast milk. Therefore, tolterodine should be discontinued during breastfeeding.

Children: Safety and effectiveness in children have not been established.

Drug Interactions:

Tell your doctor or pharmacist if you are taking or if you are planning to take any over-the-counter or prescription medications or dietary supplements with tolterodine. Doses of one or both drugs may need to be modified or a different drug may need to be prescribed. The following drugs and drug classes interact with tolterodine.

azole antifungal agents (eg, ketoconazole, itraconazole, miconazole)
fluoxetine
macrolide antibiotics (eg, erythromycin, clarithromycin)

Side Effects:

Nervous System: Abnormal skin sensations; dizziness; drowsiness; feeling of whirling motion; nervousness; headache.

Digestive Tract: Abdominal pain; constipation; diarrhea; gas; indigestion; nausea; vomiting.

Respiratory System: Bronchitis; coughing; sore throat; upper respiratory tract infection; runny nose.

Urinary and Reproductive Tract: Painful, difficult, or frequent urination; urine retention; urination disorders; urinary tract infection.

Other: Dry mouth; dry skin; back, chest, and joint pain; fatigue; flu-like symptoms; falling; itching; rash; skin flushing or redness; abnormal vision; dry eyes; night blindness; weight gain; high blood pressure; infection; blurred vision.

Guidelines for Use:

- The recommended dose is 2 mg twice daily but it can be lowered to 1 mg twice daily based on individual need.
- For patients with reduced liver function or for those taking macrolide antibiotics or azole antifungal agents, the recommended dose is 1 mg twice daily.
- May cause dry mouth. If this or other side effects persist or worsen, contact your doctor.
- May cause drowsiness or blurred vision. Use caution while driving or performing other tasks that require alertness until tolerance is determined.
- Store at controlled room temperature (68° to 77°F).

If you have any questions, consult your doctor, pharmacist, or health care provider.

	Generic Name *Brand Name Examples*	Supplied As	Generic Available
	Phenazopyridine HCl		
otc	*Azo-Standard, Azo-Gesic, Uristat*	**Tablets:** 95 mg	No
otc	*Baridium, ReAzo*	**Tablets:** 97 mg	No
Rx	*Pyridium, Urogesic*	**Tablets:** 100 mg, 200 mg	Yes

For more information on urinary tract combinations containing phenazopyridine, see Urinary Anti-Infective Combinations in the Anti-Infectives chapter.

Type of Drug:

Urinary tract pain reliever.

How the Drug Works:

Phenazopyridine exerts a local analgesic (pain-relieving) action on the inner lining of the urinary tract. It relieves symptoms of pain, burning, urgency, and frequency only. It does not treat the cause of the pain (eg, infection).

Uses:

For symptomatic relief of pain, burning, urgency, frequent urination, and other discomforts due to irritation of the lower urinary tract.

Precautions:

Do not use in the following situations:

allergy to phenazopyridine
kidney function, reduced
liver disease

Urinary tract infection: Treatment of the discomforting symptoms of a lower urinary tract infection with phenazopyridine should not exceed 2 days.

Kidney/liver dysfunction: Yellowing of skin or eyes may indicate accumulation of the drug due to impaired kidney or liver function. The drug may need to be discontinued. Consult your doctor.

Pregnancy: Adequate studies have not been done in pregnant women. Use only if clearly needed and potential benefits outweigh the possible hazards to the fetus.

Breastfeeding: It is not known if phenazopyridine appears in breast milk. Consult your doctor before you begin breastfeeding.

Children: Phenazopyridine should not be given to children under 12 years of age unless prescribed by your doctor.

Lab tests: Phenazopyridine may interfere with some urine tests for sugar and ketones.

Side Effects:

Every drug is capable of producing side effects. Many phenazopyridine users experience no, or minor, side effects. The frequency and severity of side effects depend on many factors including dose, duration of therapy, and individual susceptibility. Possible side effects include: Stomach upset; headache; rash; itching; blue lips and fingertips; anemia; liver and kidney damage; fever; staining of contact lenses.

Guidelines for Use:

- Take exactly as prescribed or as the package labeling directs (OTC products).
- May cause stomach upset. Take with or after meals to decrease irritation.
- May cause urine to turn reddish orange. This is not harmful but may stain bedding or undergarments. Staining of contact lenses may occur.
- Treatment of urinary tract pain associated with a urinary tract infection should not exceed 2 days.
- Notify your doctor if any of the following occurs: Symptoms persist for more than 2 days or get worse; fever; chills; back pain; bloody urine.
- This medicine can interfere with lab tests including urine tests for sugar and ketones.
- Provides symptom (eg, pain, burning, urgency, frequency) relief only; it does not treat the cause of the symptoms (eg, infection).
- Store at room temperature.

OTC drugs —

- If symptoms persist for more than 5 days, contact your doctor.
- Do not give OTC drugs to children under 12 years of age unless instructed by your doctor.
- Do not use if you have liver or kidney problems unless instructed by your doctor.

If you have any questions, consult your doctor, pharmacist, or health care provider.

	Generic Name *Brand Name Example*	Supplied As	Generic Available
Rx	**Azathioprine**[1]		
	Imuran	**Tablets:** 50 mg	No

[1] This product is also available as an injection.

Type of Drug:

Drug used to suppress the immune system.

How the Drug Works:

The exact mechanism is not known. Azathioprine alters the immune response in the body, alters the production of antibodies and, in some instances, reduces inflammation.

Uses:

To prevent rejection of kidney transplants.

To treat severe rheumatoid arthritis that does not respond to other therapies.

Unlabeled Use(s): Occasionally doctors may prescribe azathioprine for treatment of chronic ulcerative colitis and generalized myasthenia gravis. However, serious side effects may offset any benefits the drug may offer. It also may be prescribed for controlling Behcet's syndrome, especially eye disease. It may be effective in treating Crohn's disease.

Precautions:

Do not use in the following situations:
- allergy to azathioprine
- pregnant rheumatoid arthritis patients

Serious infections are a constant hazard for patients on chronic immunosuppression, especially transplant recipients. Fungal, viral, bacterial and protozoal infections may be fatal and should be treated vigorously. Infection may occur as a result of bone marrow suppression or decreased white-cell counts. Azathioprine dose may have to be reduced or other drugs used.

Chronic use: Long-term use of azathioprine may increase the risk of developing tumors. Consult your doctor.

Pregnancy: Studies have shown a potential effect to the fetus. Use only if clearly needed and potential benefits outweigh the possible risks. Do not give to pregnant rheumatoid arthritis patients.

Breastfeeding: Azathioprine or its metabolites appear in breast milk. Use of azathioprine in nursing mothers is not recommended. Consult your doctor before you begin breastfeeding.

Children: Safety and efficacy in children have not been established. However, it has been used in children.

Lab tests will be required during treatment with azathioprine. Tests may include: Complete blood and platelet counts to monitor for blood disorders; liver function tests; and cultures to check for infections.

Drug Interactions:

Tell your doctor or pharmacist if you are taking or if you are planning to take any over-the-counter or prescription medications or dietary supplements while taking this medicine. Doses of one or both drugs may need to be modified or a different drug may need to be prescribed.The following drugs and drug classes interact with azathioprine.

ACE inhibitors (eg, captopril)
allopurinol (eg, *Zyloprim)*
anticoagulants (eg, warfarin)
sulfamethoxazole/trimethoprim (eg, *Bactrim)*
cyclosporine (eg, *Sandimmune)*
nondepolarizing neuromuscular blockers (eg, rocuronium bromide)
methotrexate (eg, *Folex PFS)*

Side Effects:

Every drug is capable of producing side effects. Most patients experience side effects. The frequency and severity of side effects depend on many factors including dose, duration of therapy and individual susceptibility. Possible side effects include:

Digestive Tract: Nausea; vomiting; diarrhea.

Other: Rash; fever; general body discomfort; muscle pain; infection; tumors; abnormal blood counts.

Guidelines for Use:

- Take exactly as prescribed.
- If stomach upset occurs, take in divided doses or with food.
- If a dose is missed, take it as soon as possible. If several hours have passed or if it is nearing time for the next dose, do not double the dose in order to "catch up" (unless advised to do so by your doctor). If more than one dose is missed or it is necessary to establish a new dosage schedule, contact your doctor or pharmacist.
- Notify your doctor if any of the following occurs: Unusual bleeding or bruising, fever, sore throat, mouth sores, signs of infection, stomach pain, pale stools or darkened urine.
- May cause nausea, vomiting, rash, fever, muscle pain and diarrhea. Notify your doctor if these persist or become bothersome.
- Contraceptive measures (birth control) are recommended during treatment to avoid birth defects. Inform your doctor if you are pregnant, become pregnant, are planning to become pregnant or if you are breastfeeding.
- Lab tests will be required to monitor therapy. Be sure to keep appointments.
- Visually inspect injection solution for particles or discoloration before use.
- Store at room temperature (59° to 77°F), away from moisture and light.

If you have any questions, consult your doctor, pharmacist, or health care provider.

	Generic Name *Brand Name Example*	Supplied As	Generic Available
Rx	**Cyclosporine**		
	Sandimmune	**Capsules, soft gelatin:** 25 mg, 50 mg, 100 mg	No
	Neoral	**Capsules, soft gelatin for microemulsion:** 25 mg, 100 mg	No
	Sandimmune[1]	**Oral solution:** 100 mg/mL	No
	Neoral	**Oral solution for microemulsion:** 100 mg/mL	No
	Sandimmune	**IV solution:** 50 mg/mL	No

[1] Contains alcohol.

Type of Drug:

Immunosuppressive; drug used to suppress the immune system in organ transplants.

How the Drug Works:

Cyclosporine is a potent immunosuppressive agent which increases the survival of transplants involving skin, kidney, liver, heart, pancreas, bone marrow, small intestine and lung. It is not known how cyclosporine suppresses the immune system.

Uses:

To prevent rejection of organ (eg, kidney, liver, heart) transplants. May be used with corticosteroids.

To treat chronic rejection in patients previously treated with other immunosuppressive agents (*Sandimmune* only).

Unlabeled Use(s): Occasionally doctors may prescribe cyclosporine for Crohn's disease, Graves ophthalmopathy, severe psoriasis, aplastic anemia, multiple sclerosis, alopecia areata, pemphigus and pemphigoid, dermatomyositis, polymyositis, lichen planus, Behcet's disease, uveitis, pulmonary sarcoidosis, biliary cirrhosis, myasthenia gravis, atopic dermatitis, insulin-dependent diabetes mellitus, lupus nephritis, nephrotic syndrome, psoriatic arthritis, pyoderma gangrenosum, rheumatoid arthritis, ulcerative colitis and corneal transplantation or other diseases of the eye which have an autoimmune component; pancreas, bone marrow and heart/lung transplants.

Precautions:

Do not use in the following situations: An allergy to cyclosporine or polyoxyethylated castor oil or coadministration of potassium-sparing diuretics.

Use with caution in the following situations:

- high blood levels of aluminum, potassium and uric acid (eg, gout)
- high blood pressure
- high dose methylprednisolone therapy
- kidney disease (other than transplant)

liver disease (other than transplant)
low blood levels of cholesterol or magnesium
malabsorption problems
seizures

Nervous system toxicity: Symptoms including headache, flushing, confusion, seizures, incoordination, hallucinations, mania, depression, sleep problems and blurred vision have been observed. Various studies have associated the symptoms with low cholesterol and magnesium levels, high levels of aluminum, kidney problems, high dose methylprednisolone and high blood pressure.

Diabetes: Kidney transplant patients have developed insulin-dependent diabetes meltitus after treatment with cyclosporine and prednisolone.

Immunosuppression: Increases susceptibility to infection and the possible development of lymphoma and other tumors may result from the degree of immunosuppression.

Pregnancy: Adequate studies have not been done in pregnant women, or studies in animals may have shown a risk to the fetus. Use only if clearly needed and potential benefits outweigh the possible hazards to the fetus.

Breastfeeding: Cyclosporine appears in breast milk. Avoid breastfeeding while taking this drug.

Children: Safety and effectiveness have not been established. Patients as young as 6 months have received the drug with no unusual side effects.

Lab tests may be required to monitor therapy. Be sure to keep appointments. Liver and kidney problems have occurred during therapy; therefore, close monitoring is needed.

Drug Interactions:

Tell your doctor or pharmacist if you are taking or if you are planning to take any over-the-counter or prescription medications or dietary supplements while taking this medicine. Doses of one or both drugs may need to be modified or a different drug may need to be prescribed. The following drugs and drug classes interact with this medicine.

allopurinol (eg, *Zyloprim*)
aminoglycosides (eg, gentamicin)
amiodarone (*Cordarone*)
amphotericin B
azathioprine (*Imuran*)
azole antifungals (eg, fluconazole)
bromocriptine (*Parlodel*)
calcium channel blockers (eg, nifedipine)
carbamazepine (eg, *Tegretol*)
clarithromycin (*Biaxin*)
colchicine
contraceptives, oral (eg, *Ortho-Novum*)
corticosteroids (eg, prednisolone)
cyclophosphamide (eg, *Cytoxan*)
danazol (*Danocrine*)
digoxin (eg, *Lanoxin*)
erythromycin (eg, *EES*)
histamine H_2 antagonists (eg, cimetidine)
imipenem-cilastatin (*Primaxin*)
lovastatin (*Mevacor*)
melphalan (*Alkeran*)

methyltestosterone (eg, *Testred*)
metoclopramide (eg, *Reglan*)
nafcillin (eg, *Nafcil*)
nondepolarizing muscle relaxants (eg, rocuronium bromide)
NSAIDs (eg, indomethacin)
octreotide (*Sandostatin*)
phenobarbital
phenytoin (eg, *Dilantin*)
potassium-sparing diuretics (eg, spironolactone)
quinolones (eg, ciprofloxacin)
rifabutin (*Mycobutin*)
rifampin (eg, *Rifadin*)
sulfamethoxazole/trimethoprim (eg, *Septra*)
tacrolimus (*Prograf*)
ticlopidine (*Ticlid*)
vaccines
vancomycin (eg, *Vancocin*)

Side Effects:

Every drug is capable of producing side effects. Many patients experience no, or minor, side effects. The frequency and severity of side effects depend on many factors including dose, duration of therapy and individual susceptibility. Possible side effects include:

Digestive Tract: Nausea; vomiting; stomach pain or discomfort; appetite loss; diarrhea; hiccups; peptic ulcer.

Nervous System: Confusion; seizures; tremors; headache; abnormal skin sensations.

Skin: Acne; unusual hair growth; brittle fingernails; flushing.

Other: Unusual growth of the gums; swelling of the breast (male or female); swelling; fever; hearing loss; ringing in the ears; signs of infection; muscle pain; sinus inflammation; weight loss; anemia; high blood sugar; cramps; blood clots; high blood pressure.

Guidelines for Use:

- Take exactly as directed by your doctor.
- Do not take with food or grapefruit juice.
- To improve the flavor of the oral solution, dilute with milk, chocolate milk, apple juice or orange juice (preferably at room temperature). Try to be consistent with the mixture you use. The combination of milk and *Neoral* may be unpalatable.
- If a dose is missed, take it as soon as possible. If several hours have passed or if it is nearing time for the next dose, do not double the dose in order to "catch up" (unless advised to do so by your doctor). If more than one dose is missed or it is necessary to establish a new dosage schedule, contact your doctor or pharmacist.
- Do not change from one brand of this drug to another without consulting your doctor or pharmacist. These products are not equivalent to each other.
- Do not stop taking this medication unless advised to do so by your doctor.
- See your doctor regularly to assure that the drug is working properly and that no serious side effects are developing.
- Use a glass container when mixing this medication. Stir well and drink at once. Rinse glass and drink again to assure that the entire dose was taken. Do not allow it to stand before drinking.
- *Oral solution* — Do not rinse the syringe used for measuring dosages before or after use. Getting water or chemicals in the medicine can cause variation in the dose. After use, replace the syringe in its protective cover.
- Injection should only be used in patients who cannot take the capsules or oral suspension.
- Contact your doctor if fever, sore throat, tiredness, urinary problems or unusual bleeding or bruising occurs.
- Discontinue use at first first appearance of signs of allergic reaction. Symptoms may include: Flushing of the face or upper chest, difficulty breathing, wheezing, changes in blood pressure and rapid heartbeat.
- Use mechanical contraceptive measures (eg, diaphragm, condom) during cyclosporine treatment. Do not use oral contraceptives. Contact your doctor if pregnancy is suspected.
- Diabetic patients may experience loss of glucose control. Be prepared to monitor blood sugar more often.
- Lab tests will be required to monitor therapy. Be sure to keep appointments.
- Visually inspect solutions for particles or discoloration.
- Store at room temperature (below 86°F). Protect from light.
- *Oral solution* — Store at room temperature (68° to 77°F). Do not refrigerate. If Neoral solution gets too cold, it may gel. If this happens, allow to warm to room temperature (77°F) before use. Once opened, contents must be used within 2 months.

If you have any questions, consult your doctor, pharmacist, or health care provider.

	Generic Name *Brand Name Examples*	Supplied As	Generic Available
Rx	**Mycophenolate Mofetil**		
	CellCept	**Capsules:** 250 mg	No
		Tablets: 500 mg	No
	Mycophenolate Mofetil HCl		
	CellCept Intravenous	**Powder for injection:** 500 mg	No

Type of Drug:

Immunosuppressant used to prevent rejection of transplanted organs.

How the Drug Works:

Inhibits an enzyme needed by T-cells and B-cells to produce an immune response to foreign proteins in the body.

Uses:

To prevent organ rejection in patients receiving allogenic kidney or heart transplants. Mycophenolate is used in combination with cyclosporine and corticosteroids.

Precautions:

Do not use in the following situations:

allergy to mycophenolate, mycophenolic acid (active metabolite), or any ingredient of this medicine

Use with caution in the following situations:

digestive system disease, active, serious
kidney disease, severe, chronic
women of childbearing potential

Pregnancy: Adequate studies have not been done in pregnant women. Use only if clearly needed and potential benefits outweigh the possible hazards to the fetus.

Breastfeeding: It is not known if mycophenolate or mycophenolic acid appears in breast milk. Because of the potential for serious adverse reactions in nursing infants, a decision should be made whether to discontinue nursing or discontinue the drug, taking into account the importance of the drug to the mother. Consult your doctor before you begin breastfeeding.

Children: Safety and effectiveness for use in children have not been established.

Lab tests will be required to monitor therapy. Tests will include complete blood counts and pregnancy tests.

Drug Interactions:

Tell your doctor or pharmacist if you are taking or if you are planning to take any over-the-counter or prescription medications or dietary supplements while taking mycophenolate mofetil. Doses of one or both drugs may need to be modified or a different drug may need to be prescribed. The following drugs and drug classes interact with mycophenolate mofetil:

acyclovir (eg, *Zovirax*)
antacids with magnesium and aluminum (eg, *Maalox*)
azathioprine (*Imuran*)
cholestyramine (eg, *Questran*)
contraceptives, oral (eg, *Ortho-Novum*)
cyclosporine (eg, *Sandimmune*)
ganciclovir (*Cytovene*)
phenytoin (eg, *Dilantin*)
probenecid (eg, *Benemid*)
salicylates (eg, aspirin)
theophylline (eg, *Theo-Dur*)
trimethoprim/sulfamethoxazole (eg, *Bactrim*)

Side Effects:

Every drug is capable of producing side effects. Many mycophenolate mofetil users experience no, or minor, side effects. The frequency and severity of side effects depend on many factors including dose, duration of therapy, and individual susceptibility. Possible side effects include:

Digestive Tract: Diarrhea; constipation; nausea; indigestion; stomach pain; vomiting; mouth sores; inflammation of the gums; appetite loss; gas; enlarged abdomen; inflammation of the esophagus.

Urinary and Reproductive Tract: Urinary tract infection; blood in urine; painful or difficult urination; infrequent urination; impotence.

Pulmonary: Difficulty breathing; cough; sore throat; bronchitis; pneumonia; asthma; sinus infection; sinus congestion.

Circulatory System: Chest pain; irregular heartbeat; rapid or slow heartbeat; pounding in the chest (palpitations); changes in blood pressure; blood clots; heart problems; heart failure.

Nervous System: Tremors; dizziness; headache; weakness; sleeplessness; anxiety; depression; drowsiness; abnormal skin sensations; agitation; confusion; nervousness.

Skin: Acne; rash; hair loss; excessive hairiness; itching; sweating; skin ulcers; skin infection; skin growth; bruising; skin disorder.

Muscular System: Pelvic, back, joint, and muscle pain; muscle weakness; leg cramps; muscle tightness.

Eyes or Ocular: Changes in vision; infection.

Other: Pain; chills; fever; infection; edema (fluid retention); swelling of the arms and legs; high blood sugar levels; general body discomfort; bleeding; weight gain; change in potassium levels; elevated cholesterol; low blood phosphorus levels; anemia; decreased blood platelets; change in white blood counts.

Guidelines for Use:

- Use exactly as prescribed.
- Injectable form is only used when patients cannot take medicines by mouth. The injectable form will be prepared and administered by your health care provider.
- Usual dosage for kidney transplant is 1 g taken orally twice daily on an empty stomach in combination with corticosteroids and cyclosporine. Usual dosage for heart transplant is 1.5 g taken orally twice daily.
- Take each dose 1 hour before or 2 hours after meals.
- Do not open or crush capsules. Do not crush tablets. Avoid inhalation or direct contact of the powder contained in the tablets or capsules with skin or mucous membranes. If contact occurs, wash skin thoroughly with soap and water; rinse eyes with plain water.
- Stagger doses of antacids and mycophenolate by at least 1 hour.
- This medicine is used in conjunction with corticosteroids (eg, prednisone) and cyclosporine.
- Use caution when rising from a sitting or lying position. Sit or lie down if you feel lightheaded. If dizziness or lightheadedness become bothersome, notify your doctor.
- If a dose is missed, take it as soon as possible. If several hours have passed or if it is nearing time for the next dose, do not double the dose in order to catch up (unless advised to do so by your doctor). If more than one dose is missed or it is necessary to establish a new dosage schedule, contact your doctor or pharmacist.
- Increased susceptibility to infection and the possible development of lymphoma may result from immunosuppression. Contact your doctor if you develop fever, fatigue, unusual bruising or bleeding, swollen lymph nodes, or skin growths.
- This medicine increases the chances of infections, lymphomas, and other malignancies, particularly of the skin. Tell your doctor is any of the following occur: Fever; chills; tiredness; bruising or bleeding; sore throat; mouth sores.
- For patients at increased risk of skin cancer, limit exposure to sunlight and UV light (eg, tanning beds) by wearing protective clothing and using a sunscreen with a high protection factor.
- Inform your doctor if you are pregnant, become pregnant, are planning to become pregnant, or if you are breastfeeding. Effective contraception must be used before beginning therapy, during therapy, and for 6 weeks following discontinuation of therapy. Use 2 reliable forms of contraception. Women of childbearing potential must have a negative pregnancy test result 1 week before beginning mycophenolate therapy.
- Lab tests will be required. Be sure to keep appointments.
- Store at room temperature (59° to 86°F).

If you have any questions, consult your doctor, pharmacist, or health care provider.

Generic Name *Brand Name Example*	Supplied As	Generic Available
Rx **Muromonab-CD3**		
Orthoclone OKT3	**Injection:** 5 mg/5 mL	No

Type of Drug:

Drug used to suppress the immune system; immunosuppressant.

How the Drug Works:

Muromonab-CD3 blocks the function of blood cells (T-cells) which play a major role in heart, kidney and liver transplant (organ) rejection.

Uses:

To treat heart, kidney or liver transplant rejection.

Precautions:

Do not use in the following situations:

- allergy to this medicine or any of its relatives
- breastfeeding
- fluid retention problems
- heart failure
- pregnancy
- seizures, history of

Use with caution in the following situations:

- angina, unstable
- calcium levels, low
- cardiac or respiratory arrest
- cardiovascular collapse
- cerebrovascular disease
- chronic obstructive pulmonary disease (COPD) (eg, breathing difficulties)
- coma
- dehydration, severe
- electrolyte imbalances, history of fever
- fluid in the lungs
- head trauma, history of
- heart attack, recent
- heart disease
- high blood pressure
- infection
- low blood sugar
- medications affecting the central nervous system
- septic shock
- shock
- uremia (eg, kidney disease)
- vascular disease

Immunosuppression: As a result of immunosuppression, organ transplant patients have an increased risk of developing serious infections and various types of cancer.

First Dose Effect: Fever (up to 107° F), chills, rigidity, headache, tremors, nausea, vomiting, diarrhea, stomach pain, general body discomfort, muscle/joint aches and pains, generalized weakness, fluid in the lungs or difficulty breathing can occur within 30 to 60 minutes of the first few doses.

Pregnancy: Adequate studies have not been done in pregnant women, or animal studies may have shown a risk to the fetus. Use only if clearly needed and potential benefits outweigh the possible hazards to the fetus.

Breastfeeding: It is not known if muromonab-CD3 appears in breast milk. Consult your doctor before you begin breastfeeding.

Children: Safety and effectiveness have not been established. Careful and frequent monitoring is required for children more than for adults. It is not known whether there may be significant long-term effects from the high fever, seizures, infections or meningitis from this treatment, especially in children under 1 year of age.

Lab tests and chest x-rays will be required before and during treatment with this medicine. Be sure to keep appointments.

Drug Interactions:

Tell your doctor or pharmacist if you are taking or if you are planning to take any over-the-counter or prescription medications or dietary supplements while taking this medicine. Doses of one of both drugs may need to be modified or a different drug may need to be prescribed. The following drug and drug classes interact with this medicine.

azathioprine (*Imuran*)
corticosteroids (eg, prednisolone)
cyclosporine (eg, *Sandimmune*)
indomethacin (eg, *Indocin*)

Side Effects:

Every drug is capable of producing side effects. Many patients experience no, or minor, side effects. The frequency and severity of side effects depend on many factors including dose, duration of therapy and individual susceptibility. Possible side effects include:

Digestive Tract: Nausea; vomiting; diarrhea; appetite loss; stomach pain; stomach bleeding.

Circulatory System: Chest pain or tightness; changes in heart rhythm; blood pressure changes; shock; heart attack.

Respiratory System: Shortness of breath; wheezing; difficult or painful breathing; hyperventilation; pneumonia; bronchospasm.

Skin: Rash; hives; itching; redness; flushing; excessive sweating.

Senses: Blindness; blurred vision; double vision; eye irritation; light sensitivity; hearing loss; ringing in the ears; ear infection.

Other: Infections (some severe); tremors; headache; fever; rigidity; chills; general body discomfort; flu-like syndrome; tiredness; weakness; muscle and joint pain/stiffness; vertigo (feeling of whirling motion); nasal/ear stuffiness; neck stiffness; meningitis; seizures.

Guidelines for Use:

- Use exactly as prescribed.
- If a dose is missed, inject it as soon as possible. If several hours have passed or it is nearing time for the next dose, do not double the dose in order to "catch up," unless advised by your doctor. If more than one dose is missed, contact your doctor or pharmacist.
- *First Dose Effect:* Fever, chills, rigidity, headache, tremors, nausea, vomiting, diarrhea, stomach or muscle/joint aches/pains, general body discomfort, weakness or difficulty breathing can occur within 30 to 60 minutes of the first few doses. Contact your doctor immediately if any of these occur.
- Notify your doctor immediately if any of the following occurs: Rash, hives, rapid heartbeat, chest pain, difficulty breathing or swallowing.
- Patients should know how they might react before driving or performing other tasks requiring alertness, coordination or physical dexterity.
- Lab tests will be required to monitor treatment. Be sure to keep appointments.
- Visually inspect solution for particles or discoloration before use.
- Store in the refrigerator between 36° and 46°F. Do not freeze or shake. After use, discard any unused solution.

If you have any questions, consult your doctor, pharmacist, or health care provider.

	Generic Name *Brand Name Example*	Supplied As	Generic Available
Rx	**Tacrolimus**		
	Prograf[1]	**Capsules:** 1 mg, 5 mg	No

[1] Some of these products are also available as an injection.

Type of Drug:

Drug used to suppress the immune system after organ (liver) transplants.

How the Drug Works:

Although the exact mechanism of action is not known, it appears tacrolimus suppresses organ graft rejection by inhibiting the activation of T-lymphocyte cells.

Uses:

To prevent organ (liver) transplant rejection. It is recommended that tacrolimus be used in conjunction with adrenal corticosteroids.

Unlabeled Use(s): Tacrolimus is being investigated for the treatment of kidney, bone marrow, heart, pancreas, pancreatic island cell and small bowel transplantation. It has also been used for the treatment of autoimmune disease and severe recalcitrant psoriasis.

Precautions:

Do not use in the following situations:

allergy to tacrolimus
allergy to HCO-60 polyoxyl 60 hydrogenated castor oil (injection only)
cyclosporine use within 24 hours
potassium-sparing diuretic use
other immunosuppressive use (except adrenal corticosteroids)

Use with caution in the following situations:

diabetes
Epstein-Barr virus
high blood pressure
high potassium levels
kidney disease
liver disease
long-term immunosuppressive use
lymphomas or skin cancer

Liver and kidney function: Due to the possibility of kidney damage, patients with kidney or liver disease should receive the lowest recommended dose. Further reductions in dosage may be required.

Diabetes: Transplant patients have developed insulin-dependent diabetes mellitus after treatment with tacrolimus.

Infection: Patients using immunosuppressants are at a higher risk of developing lymphomas and other malignancies (tumors), especially of the skin.

Nerve damage: Over half of liver transplant recipients experience nerve damage including tremors, headaches, changes in muscle coordination, mental status and sensory function. Seizures, coma and delirium have also been observed.

Pregnancy: Adequate studies have not been done in pregnant women. Use only if clearly needed and potential benefits outweigh the possible hazards to the fetus.

Breastfeeding: Tacrolimus appears in breast milk. Avoid breastfeeding while taking this drug. Consult your doctor before you begin breastfeeding.

Children: Tacrolimus has been used successfully in liver transplants in children less than 12 years of age. Younger patients usually require higher doses than adults.

Lab tests will be required during treatment with tacrolimus. Tests may include routine monitoring of kidney, blood and metabolic systems.

Drug Interactions:

Tell your doctor or pharmacist if you are taking or if you are planning to take any over-the-counter or prescription medications or dietary supplements while taking tacrolimus. Doses of one or both drugs may need to be modified or a different drug may need to be prescribed. The following drugs and drug classes interact with tacrolimus.

aminoglycosides (eg, kanamycin sulfate)
antifungals (Amphotericin B)
bromocriptine (*Parlodel*)
calcium channel blockers (eg, nifedipine)
carbamazepine (eg, *Tegretol*)
cimetidine (*Tagamet*)
cisplatin (eg, *Platinol*)
clarithromycin (*Biaxin*)
clotrimazole (eg, *Lotrimin*)
cyclosporine (*Sandimmune*)
danazol (*Danocrine*)
diltiazem (eg, *Cardizem*)
erythromycin (eg, *E-Mycin*)
fluconazole (*Diflucan*)
immunosuppressive agents (except adrenal corticosteroids)
itraconazole (*Sporanox*)
ketoconazole (*Nizoral*)
methylprednisolone (*Medrol*)
metoclopramide (eg, *Reglan*)
phenobarbital (eg, *Solfoton*)
phenytoin (eg, *Dilantin Infatab*)
potassium-sparing diuretics (eg, amiloride HCl)
rifabutin (*Mycobutin*)
rifampin (eg, *Rifadin*)
vaccines

Side Effects:

Every drug is capable of producing side effects. Many tacrolimus users experience no, or minor, side effects. The frequency and severity of side effects depend on many factors including dose, duration of therapy and individual susceptibility. Possible side effects include:

Digestive Tract: Diarrhea; enlarged abdomen; nausea; constipation; appetite changes; vomiting; stomach pain; bloating; indigestion; gas; liver damage or disease; hepatitis; intestinal bleeding or other problems.

Nervous System: Mood swings; stiffness; tremor; headache; sleeplessness; abnormal skin sensations; abnormal dreams; anxiety; confusion; depression; dizziness; hallucinations; incoordination; drowsiness; seizures; coma.

Circulatory System: High blood pressure; abnormal blood counts; chest pain; low blood pressure; fast heartbeat; abnormal heart rhythms; abnormal blood clotting; bleeding.

Respiratory System: Difficulty breathing; cough; asthma; sore throat; pneumonia; bronchitis; voice alteration; sinus infection.

Skin: Skin cancer; itching; hives; rash; bruising; hair loss; abnormai hair growth; sweating.

Urinary and Reproductive Tract: Urinary tract infection; infrequent urination; blood in the urine.

Other: Yellowing of the skin and eyes; weight loss; non-Hodgkin's lymphoma; infections related to Epstein-Barr virus; elevated blood sugar levels; fever; weakness; back pain; mouth infections; swelling of the arms and legs; vision changes; ringing in the ears; speech impairment; kidney failure; abnormal healing; abscesses; chills; hernia; sensitivity to sunlight; joint, muscle, back and general body pain; leg cramps; herpes; tumors; oral thrush; abnormal sensations.

Guidelines for Use:

- Take exactly as prescribed.
- The possibility of serious infection, nerve or kidney damage, diabetes and some cancers is increased with the use of this medicine.
- *Capsules* — Take in two divided doses every 12 hours on an empty stomach, or as directed by your doctor.
- Administer injectable form only in facilities that can handle emergency situations.
- If a dose is missed, take it as soon as possible. If several hours have passed or if it is nearing time for the next dose, do not double the dose in order to "catch up" (unless advised to do so by your doctor). If more than one dose is missed or it is necessary to establish a new dosage schedule, contact your doctor or pharmacist.
- Lab tests will be required to monitor therapy. Be sure to keep appointments.
- Notify your doctor immediately if you have any of the following: tremors, headache, dizziness, incoordination, abnormal sensations, suspected infections, changes in mental status, or decreased urination.
- *Injection patients* — Notify your doctor immediately if any of the following signs of an allergic reaction occurs: hives, itching, fluid retention or difficulty breathing.
- May cause drowsiness, dizziness or visual problems. Use caution while driving or performing other tasks requiring alertness, coordination or physical dexterity.
- Store at room temperature.

If you have any questions, consult your doctor, pharmacist, or health care provider.

Generic Name *Brand Name Example*	Supplied As	Generic Available
Rx **Isotretinoin**		
Accutane[1]	**Capsules**: 10 mg, 20 mg, 40 mg	No

[1] Contains edetate disodium, methyl- and propylparabens.

Type of Drug:

Agent for severe, disfiguring nodular acne resistant to standard therapies.

How the Drug Works:

The exact mechanism by which isotretinoin exerts its beneficial effect is not known. The drug reduces sebum (oil) secreted by specialized glands in the skin (sebaceous glands), changes some of the characteristics of the sebum, and may prevent abnormal hardening of skin cells (keratinization).

Uses:

To treat severe disfiguring nodular (red, swollen, tender lumps in the skin) acne unresponsive to conventional therapy including antibiotics.

Unlabeled Use(s): Occasionally doctors may prescribe isotretinoin for Darier-White disease, pityriasis rubra pilaris, lamellar ichthyosis, congenital ichthyosiform erythroderma, hyperkeratosis palmaris and plantaris, cutaneous T-cell lymphoma and leukoplakia, rosacea, lichen planus, psoriasis, or for prevention of second primary tumors in skin cancer of the head and neck.

Precautions:

Do not use in the following situations:

- allergy to isotretinoin or any of its ingredients (eg, parabens)
- breastfeeding
- depression
- pregnancy or likelihood of becoming pregnant
- psychosis
- sexually active women of child-bearing age not using 1 or more methods of effective contraception
- suicidal thoughts
- tetracycline therapy, concurrent
- vitamin A use, concurrent

Use with caution in the following situations:

- alcohol use
- blood donors
- diabetes
- high cholesterol or triglyceride levels
- liver disease

Depression: Depression and mood swings, including suicidal ideation, suicide attempts and suicide have been associated with isotretinoin use. Discontinuation of the drug may be insufficient; further testing may be necessary.

Pseudotumor cerebri: Pseudotumor cerebri (benign intracranial hypertension) has occurred with isotretinoin. Early signs and symptoms include headache, swelling of optic disk, nausea, vomiting, and visual disturbances. If present, discontinue drug immediately and consult your doctor or a neurologist.

Inflammatory bowel disease: Inflammatory bowel disease (including regional ileitis) has been temporally associated with isotretinoin in patients with no history of intestinal disorders. Discontinue treatment immediately if abdominal pain, rectal bleeding or severe diarrhea occur.

Visual disturbances: Visual disturbances such as decreased night vision and clouding in the eye have occurred during therapy with isotretinoin. Because the onset may be sudden, use caution when driving or operating any vehicle, especially at night. Stop using the drug and see your eye doctor if any visual problems occur.

Hearing impairment: Hearing impairment has been reported in patients taking isotretinoin and, in some cases, has persisted after discontinuing treatment. Discontinue drug immediately and consult your doctor if ringing in the ears or impared hearing occurs.

Pregnancy: Women who are pregnant or who may become pregnant must not use isotretinoin. There is an extremely high risk that serious birth defects will result if pregnancy occurs while taking this drug in any amount, even for short periods. Potentially, all exposed fetuses can be adversely affected.

Breastfeeding: It is not known if isotretinoin appears in breast milk. Because of the potential for side effects, do not take while breastfeeding.

Children: Safety and effectiveness in children have not been established.

Lab tests and eye exams may be required before and during treatment with isotretinoin. Tests may include: liver function tests, blood lipid tests (cholesterol, triglycerides, and lipoproteins), glucose tests, CPK tests, and pregnancy tests.

Drug Interactions:

Tell your doctor or pharmacist if you are taking or planning to take any over-the-counter or prescription medications or dietary supplements with isotretinoin. Doses of one or both drugs may need to be modified or a different drug may need to be prescribed. The following drugs and drug classes interact with isotretinoin:

vitamin A
tetracyclines (eg, minocycline)

Side Effects:

Every drug is capable of producing side effects. Many isotretinoin users experience side effects. The frequency and severity of side effects depend on many factors including dose, duration of therapy, and individual susceptibility. Possible side effects include:

Nervous System: Headache; depression; mood swings, suicidal thoughts; psychosis; pseudotumor cerebri; fatigue; dizziness; drowsiness; sleeplessness; lethargy; nervousness; seizures; suicidal thoughts.

Skin: Dry skin; rash; sloughing of skin; thinning of hair; sensitivity to sunlight; hives; crusty or oily skin; redness; fragile skin; itching; brittle nails;

cracking around corners of mouth; bruising; chapped or swollen lips; drying of mucous membranes; peeling of palms and soles; nosebleed, bleeding gums.

Senses: Visual disturbances; corneal clouding; cataracts; eye infection; dry eyes; decreased night vision; sensitivity to light.

Other: Dry nose or mouth; inflammatory bowel disease (see Precautions); blood or protein in urine; abnormal menstrual flow; bone, joint, or muscle pain or stiffness; chest pain; nausea; vomiting; stomachache; appetite loss; change in blood lipids; increase in liver enzymes; hepatitis; changes in blood counts; delayed wound healing; pus-filled swollen sores; increased blood sugar; swelling; rapid heart rate; weight loss; nausea; anemia; low platelet counts.

Guidelines for Use:

- Dosage is individualized. Take exactly as prescribed.
- Usually taken in 2 divided daily doses with meals for 15 to 20 weeks.
- Read the patient information leaflet available with the product and complete patient consent form prior to use.
- Do not crush or chew the capsules. Swallow whole.
- Take with food.
- If a dose is missed, take it as soon as possible. If several hours have passed or it is nearing time for the next dose, do not double the dose to catch up unless advised to do so by your doctor. If more than one dose is missed or it is necessary to establish a new dosage schedule, contact your doctor or pharmacist.
- Avoid drinking alcohol.
- Do not take vitamin supplements containing vitamin A while taking isotretinoin.
- A prescription will not be issued until a report of a negative pregnancy test has been received by your doctor and pregnancy testing will be repeated on a monthly basis. For your health and well-being, be sure to keep appointments.
- Sexually active women of childbearing potential should practice contraception 1 month before starting therapy, during therapy, and for 1 month after therapy is stopped.

Guidelines for Use (cont.):

- Two separate, reliable forms of contraception should be used at the same time unless abstinence is the chosen method.
- Contact the doctor immediately if pregnancy is suspected during therapy. Major birth defects have been associated with isotretinoin use. Discuss continuation of the pregnancy with your doctor.
- Worsening of acne may occur during the initial period of therapy. This does not suggest a therapeutic failure or a need to stop therapy.
- Isotretinoin may cause photosensitivity (sensitivity to sunlight). Avoid prolonged exposure to the sun or other forms of ultraviolet (UV) light (eg, tanning beds). Use sunscreens and wear protective clothing until tolerance is determined.
- Discontinue the drug and contact your doctor immediately if depression, visual disturbances, abdominal pain, rectal bleeding, severe diarrhea, or difficulty in controlling blood sugar occur.
- Do not donate blood for transfusion during therapy and for 30 days after stopping therapy.
- Patients may experience decreased tolerance to contact lenses during and after therapy.
- Avoid skin smoothing procedures, including waxing, dermabrasion, or laser procedures, during therapy and for 6 months after stopping therapy. There is an increased possibility of scarring.
- If the total nodule count has been reduced by 70% or more before completing 15 to 20 weeks of treatment, therapy may be stopped. After 2 months or more of therapy and if the acne returns, a second course of therapy may be started. Contraceptive measures must be followed for any following course of therapy.
- Lab tests will be required before and during therapy. Be sure to keep appointments.
- Store at 59° to 86°F. Protect from light.

If you have any questions, consult your doctor, pharmacist, or health care provider.

Generic Name *Brand Name Examples*	Supplied As	Generic Available
Rx **Bromocriptine Mesylate**		
Parlodel	**Capsules:** 5 mg	No
Parlodel	**Tablets:** 2.5 mg	No

Type of Drug:

Ergot alkaloid derivative; antiparkinson drug; fertility drug.

How the Drug Works:

Bromocriptine suppresses prolactin secretion from the pituitary gland in the brain. Excessive prolactin activity can be responsible for galactorrhea (excessive milk flow), amenorrhea (absence of menstruation) and infertility. By inhibiting prolactin release, bromocriptine can suppress galactorrhea and reinstate normal menstrual cycles.

Bromocriptine also reduces the secretion of growth hormones from the pituitary gland. This can help in the treatment of acromegaly (abnormal enlargement of the bones of the hands, feet or face).

It also acts on the chemicals in the brain to relieve some of the symptoms of Parkinson's disease.

Uses:

To treat female infertility and other disorders (eg, menstrual irregularities, reduced sex gland activities) caused by the secretion of too much prolactin, acromegaly and Parkinson's disease; also to reduce the size of some pituitary gland tumors before surgery.

Unlabeled Use(s): Occasionally doctors may prescribe bromocriptine mesylate to treat neuroleptic malignant syndrome, hyperprolactinemia associated with pituitary gland tumors, cocaine addiction and cyclical mastalgia.

Bromocriptine mesylate was previously used to reduce or prevent breast milk production in mothers who do not want to breastfeed following delivery. It is not used for this condition anymore.

Precautions:

Do not use in the following situations:

allergy to ergot alkaloids
high blood pressure, uncontrolled
heart or vascular disease, severe
pregnancy in patients with hyperprolactinemia

Use with caution in the following situations:

kidney disease
liver disease
peptic ulcers

Pregnancy: Studies in pregnant women or in animals have been judged not to show a risk to the fetus. However, no drug should be used during pregnancy unless clearly needed.

Breastfeeding: Since bromocriptine prevents lactation, mothers who wish to breastfeed should not use this drug.

Children: Safety and effectiveness in children under 15 years of age have not been established.

Lab tests or exams may be required to monitor treatment. Be sure to keep appointments.

Drug Interactions:

Tell your doctor or pharmacist if you are taking or if you are planning to take any over-the-counter or prescription medications or dietary supplements while taking this medicine. Doses of one or both drugs may need to be modified or a different drug may need to be prescribed. The following drugs and drug classes interact with this medicine.

erythromycin (eg, *E-Mycin*)
blood-pressure-lowering agents (eg, clonidine)
phenothiazines (eg, chlorpromazine)
sympathomimetics (eg, phenylpropanolamine)

Side Effects:

Every drug is capable of producing side effects. Many patients experience no, or minor, side effects. The frequency and severity of side effects depend on many factors including dose, duration of therapy and individual susceptibility. Possible side effects include:

Digestive Tract: Nausea; vomiting; diarrhea; constipation; stomach cramps; indigestion; appetite loss; dry mouth.

Nervous System: Psychological disturbances; headache; dizziness; tiredness; lightheadedness; fainting; drowsiness.

Other: Low blood pressure; orthostatic hypotension (dizziness or lightheadedness when rising from a seated or lying position); coldness or numbness in hands or feet; nasal congestion.

Guidelines for Use:

- Take with meals or food.
- Take the first dose while lying down. May cause drowsiness, dizziness or fainting, especially following the first dose. Avoid sudden changes in posture, such as rising from a sitting or lying position. Use caution when driving or performing other tasks requiring alertness, coordination or physical dexterity.
- Do not stop taking or change the dose unless advised to do so by your doctor.
- If a dose is missed, take it as soon as possible. If several hours have passed or it is nearing time for the next dose, do not double the dose in order to "catch up" (unless advised to do so by your doctor). If more than one dose is missed or it is necessary to establish a new dosage schedule, contact your doctor or pharmacist. Use exactly as prescribed.
- Contact your doctor immediately if you experience a persistent runny nose.
- Use mechanical contraceptive measures (eg, diaphragm, condom) during treatment. Do not use oral contraceptives. Perform a pregnancy test every 4 weeks during the amenorrheal (non-menstrual) period or if menstruation does not occur within 3 days of the expected date.
- Inform your doctor if you are pregnant, become pregnant, are planning to become pregnant or if you are breastfeeding.
- *Medical exams* may be required to monitor treatment. Be sure to keep appointments.
- Store below 77°F. Protect from light.

If you have any questions, consult your doctor, pharmacist, or health care provider.

	Generic Name *Brand Name Examples*	Supplied As	Generic Available
Rx	**Cabergoline**		
	Dostinex	**Tablets:** 0.5 mg	No

Type of Drug:

Dopamine receptor agonist.

How the Drug Works:

Inhibits secretion of prolactin from the pituitary gland; reduces prolactin levels in blood.

Uses:

For hyperprolactinemic disorders, either from an unknown cause or caused by pituitary adenomas (tumors).

Unlabeled Use(s): To shrink pituitary tumors; to treat Parkinson's disease; normalize androgen levels and improve menstrual cyclicity in polycystic ovary syndrome.

Precautions:

Do not use in the following situations:

uncontrolled high blood pressure

allergy to ergot derivatives

Use with caution in the following situations:

pregnancy-induced high blood pressure
liver impairment
use in conjuction with other medicines used to lower blood pressure
suppression of physiologic lactation

Pregnancy: Studies in pregnanct women or in animals have been judged not to show a risk to the fetus. However, no drug should be used during pregnancy unless clearly needed.

Breastfeeding: It is not known if cabergoline appears in breast milk. Consult your doctor before you begin breastfeeding.

Children: Safety and effectiveness have not been established.

Lab tests are required to monitor treatment. Be sure to keep appointments.

Drug Interactions:

Tell your doctor or pharmacist if you are taking or planning to take any over-the-counter or prescription medications or dietary supplements while taking this medicine. Doses of one or both drugs may need to be modified or a different drug may need to be prescribed. The following drugs and drug classes interact with cabergoline: Dopamine (D_2)-antagonists (eg, phenothiazines); antihypertensive drugs (eg, methyldopa).

Side Effects:

Digestive Tract: Nausea; constipation; abdominal pain; indigestion; vomiting; diarrhea; gas.

Nervous System: Headache; dizziness; drowsiness; depression; nervousness; feeling of whirling motion; abnormal skin sensations; abnormal movements; confusion; hallucinations.

Circulatory System: Low blood pressure.

Urinary and Reproductive Tract: Breast pain; painful menstruation.

Other: Weakness; fatigue; dry mouth; pain; hot flashes; abnormal vision; itching; swelling of feet or ankles.

Guidelines for Use:

- May take with or without food. Take with food if GI upset occurs.
- Take this medicine twice a week as directed by your doctor. Increases in dosage of medication should occur no less often than every 4 weeks after physician assessment of response.
- If response is not noted after increase in dose, the lowest dose that achieves benefit should be used and other therapies considered.
- After normal serum prolactin levels are maintained for 6 months, therapy may be discontinued.
- This medicine may cause drowsiness or dizziness. Use caution while driving or performing other tasks requiring mental alertness, coordination or dexterity.
- Inform your doctor if you are pregnant, become pregnant or are planning to become pregnant.
- Lab tests or exams will be required to monitor treatment. Be sure to keep appointments. Tests will include serum prolactin levels.
- Store at controlled room temperature (68° to 77°F).

If you have any questions, consult your doctor, pharmacist, or health care provider.

	Generic Name *Brand Name Examples*	Supplied As	Generic Available
Rx	**Chymopapain** *Chymodiactin*[1]	**Powder for injection, lyophilized:** 4000 pKat units chymopapain	No

[1] Preservative free.

Type of Drug:

Enzyme that breaks down proteins.

How the Drug Works:

When injected into the cushioning disc between the bones in the lower spine (lumbar), chymopapain breaks down the proteins in the disc. This reduces pressure in the disc and relieves symptoms of disc compression.

Uses:

To treat documented herniated (protruding) intervertebral discs in the lumbar (lower) spine which have not responded to conservative therapy.

Precautions:

Do not use in the following situations:

- allergy to chymopapain, papaya, or papaya derivatives
- circulating chymopapain-specific IgE antibodies
- displaced vertebrae
- injection of chymopapain, history
- lesions producing spinal motor or sensory dysfunction (eg, cauda equina lesion)
- paralysis, severe and progressing as indicated by rapidly progressing neurological dysfunction
- spinal cord tumor
- spinal stenosis, significant
- use in any other region of the spinal cord other than the lumbar area

Use with caution in the following situations:

- beta blocker therapy, current use
- cerebrovascular disorders (eg, stroke), history or family history
- females (particularly black females)
- general anesthesia use
- high blood pressure, history
- injections at 2 or more disc sites
- iodine allergy
- surgery of lumbar spine, history

Allergic reactions (mild to severe) have occurred rarely with chymopapain use. The reactions have occurred more frequently in females (particularly black females) and patients receiving general anesthesia.

Symptoms can be immediate or delayed up to 2 hours. They can last for a few minutes to several hours or longer. Symptoms may include decreased blood pressure, dizziness, difficulty breathing, and irregular heartbeat. A delayed reaction (rash, hives, itching) may occur for up to 15 days after injection.

Pregnancy: Adequate studies have not been done in pregnant women. Use only if clearly needed and potential benefits outweigh the possible hazards to the fetus.

Children: Safety and effectiveness have not been established; do not use chymopapain in children.

Lab tests and exams may be required before therapy. Tests include preoperative screening test for chymopapain-specific IgE antibody.

Side Effects:

Every drug is capable of producing side effects. Chymopapain may cause no, or minor, side effects. The frequency and severity of side effects depend on many factors including dose, duration of therapy, and individual susceptibility. Possible side effects include:

Symptoms of Anaphylaxis: Difficulty breathing; palpitations (pounding in the chest); redness; flushing; rash; goosebumps; itching; stomach problems; skin inflammation; low blood pressure; bronchospasm; irregular heartbeat; cardiac arrest; hives; redness or discharge around the eye; runny nose; coma.

Other: Back pain, stiffness, or soreness; tingling, weakness, or pain in the legs; foot drop; cramping in calves; paraplegia or paraparesis (eg, cauda equina syndrome); back spasm; subarachnoid or cerebral hemorrhage; seizures; burning sensation in the lower back; decreased sensitivity to pain; abnormal skin sensations; numbness in the legs or toes; disc inflammation.

Guidelines for Use:

- This medication will be prepared and administered by your health care provider.
- Chymopapain is *only* used in a hospital setting by doctors experienced and trained in the diagnosis of lumbar disc disease and all standard treatment methods, including surgery. Doctors and their support personnel are to be competent in the diagnosis and management of all potential complications from chymopapain use.
- *Postinjection pain* — You may experience pain or involuntary muscle spasm in the lower back for several days. A lingering stiffness or soreness may persist for several months. This is not uncommon.
- Notify your doctor immediately if you experience a rash of any type, hives, or itching as late as 15 days after the procedure. These symptoms may be signs of an allergic reaction.
- Lab tests may be required to monitor therapy. Be sure to keep appointments.

If you have any questions, consult your doctor, pharmacist, or health care provider.

Generic Name *Brand Name Example*	Supplied As	Generic Available
Rx **Cromolyn Sodium**		
Gastrocrom	**Oral concentrate:** 100 mg/5 mL	No

Cromolyn sodium is also available as a respiratory inhalant and antiallergy agent for the eyes. See the corresponding monographs.

Type of Drug:

Mast cell stabilizer; antiallergy.

How the Drug Works:

Cromolyn sodium is a mast cell stabilizer. Mast cells, which are distributed throughout the body, contain storage granules containing potent inflammatory materials (eg, histamine) that are released by a variety of stimuli. Patients with mastocytosis have a greater than normal accumulation of mast cells. Oral cromolyn sodium reduces histamine release from these cells and decreases symptoms caused by histamine.

Uses:

To prevent attacks and relieve the symptoms of mastocytosis. These symptoms include diarrhea, flushing, headaches, vomiting, hives, stomach pain, nausea, and itching.

Precautions:

Do not use in the following situations: Allergy to cromolyn sodium or any of its ingredients.

Use with caution in the following situations:
kidney disease
liver disease

Pregnancy: There are no adequate and well-controlled studies in pregnant women. Use only if clearly needed and the potential benefits to the mother outweigh the possible risks to the fetus.

Breastfeeding: It is not known if cromolyn sodium appears in breast milk. Consult your doctor before you begin breastfeeding.

Children: Use in children under 2 years of age is not recommended and should be used only in those patients with severe diseases where the benefits clearly outweigh the risks.

Drug Interactions:

Tell your doctor or pharmacist if you are taking or if you are planning to take any over-the-counter or prescription medications or dietary supplements with cromolyn sodium. Doses of one or both drugs may need to be modified or a different drug may need to be prescribed.

Side Effects:

Every drug is capable of producing side effects. Many oral cromolyn sodium users experience no, or minor, side effects. The frequency and severity of side effects depend on many factors including dose, duration of therapy, and individual susceptibility. Possible side effects include:

Digestive Tract: Diarrhea; nausea; stomach pain.

Nervous System: Headache; irritability; anxiety.

Other: Rash; itching; general body discomfort; muscle or joint pain; sensitivity to light; pounding in the chest; rapid heart rate; fluid retention.

Guidelines for Use:

- Dosage will be individualized. Your doctor may increase or decrease your dose depending on your response to the medication.
- For maximum effectiveness, take at regular intervals as directed by your doctor. To prevent relapses, maintain the dosage regimen prescribed by your doctor.
- Break open ampule(s) and squeeze liquid contents into a glass of water. Stir solution and drink all of the liquid. Discard the empty ampule.
- Mix with water only. Do not mix with milk, fruit juice, or foods.
- Take at least one-half hour before meals and at bedtime.
- Do not use if ampule contains particles or becomes discolored.
- Store between 59° and 86°F. Protect from light. Leave ampules in foil pouch until ready for use.

If you have any questions, consult your doctor, pharmacist, or health care provider.

Generic Name *Brand Name Example*	Supplied As	Generic Available
Rx **Disulfiram**		
Antabuse	**Tablets:** 250 mg, 500 mg	Yes

Type of Drug:

Anti-alcoholic.

How the Drug Works:

Disulfiram blocks the normal breakdown of alcohol and allows an unpleasant by-product (acetaldehyde) to accumulate. This by-product produces numerous side effects, including flushing, throbbing in the head and neck, throbbing headache, nausea, vomiting, painful and difficult breathing, sweating, thirst, chest pain, heart pounding, increased heart rate, low blood pressure, feeling of whirling motion, weakness, blurred vision, marked uneasiness, fainting, hyperventilation, and confusion.

Uses:

To aid in the management of selected chronic alcoholic patients who wish to remain in a state of enforced sobriety so that supportive and psychotherapeutic treatment may be applied to best advantage.

Disulfiram is not a cure for alcoholism. When used alone, without proper motivation and support therapy, it is unlikely that it will have any substantive effect on the drinking pattern of the chronic alcoholic patient.

Precautions:

Do not use in the following situations:

alcohol or alcohol-containing products (eg, some cough syrups, sauces, aftershave lotions), use of
allergy to disulfiram or any of its ingredients
allergy to rubber
allergy to thiuram derivatives used in pesticides
heart disease, severe
metronidazole use, current or recent
paraldehyde use, current or recent
psychosis

Use with caution in the following situations:

brain damage
diabetes mellitus
epilepsy
kidney disease
liver disease
rubber contact dermatitis
underactive thyroid

Disulfiram-alcohol reaction: Disulfiram plus alcohol, even small amounts, produces flushing, throbbing in the head and neck, throbbing headaches, fainting, nausea, vomiting, sweating, thirst, chest pain, heart pounding, painful and difficult breathing, increased heart rate, weakness, feeling of whirling motion, blurred vision, low blood pressure, hyperventilation, marked uneasiness, and confusion. In severe reactions, there may be collapse, irregular heart rhythm, heart attack, acute congestive heart failure, unconsciousness, convulsions, and death. The intensity of the reaction is generally proportional to the amounts of disulfiram and alcohol ingested. Mild reactions may occur in the sensitive individual when the blood-alcohol level is low. The reaction may last from 30 to 60 minutes to several hours, or as long as there is alcohol in the blood.

Ethylene dibromide (a fumigant also found in antiknock gasolines) and its vapors may be harmful to patients receiving disulfiram. Avoid exposure.

Pregnancy: Safety for use during pregnancy has not been established. Use only if clearly needed and the potential benefits to the mother outweigh the potential risks to the fetus.

Breastfeeding: It is not known if disulfiram appears in breast milk. Consult your doctor before you begin breastfeeding.

Lab tests will be required during treatment with disulfiram. Tests may include: Liver function tests and complete blood counts. Patients with a history of rubber contact dermatitis should be tested for allergy to disulfiram before administration.

Drug Interactions:

Tell your doctor or pharmacist if you are taking or if you are planning to take any over-the-counter or prescription medications or dietary supplements with disulfiram. Doses of one or both drugs may need to be modified or a different drug may need to be prescribed. The following drugs and drug classes interact with disulfiram.

alcohol
anticoagulants, oral (eg, warfarin)
benzodiazepines (eg, diazepam)
chlorzoxazone (eg, *Paraflex*)
hydantoins (eg, phenytoin)
isoniazid (eg, *Laniazid*)
metronidazole (eg, *Flagyl*)
theophyllines (eg, aminophylline)

Side Effects:

Every drug is capable of producing side effects. Many disulfiram users experience no, or minor, side effects. The frequency and severity of side effects depend on many factors including dose, duration of therapy, and individual susceptibility. Possible side effects include:

Nervous System: Drowsiness; fatigue; headache; psychotic reaction.

Other: Rash; acne; metallic or garlic-like aftertaste; impotence; abnormal liver function; optic neuritis; peripheral neuritis; polyneuritis; peripheral neuropathy.

Guidelines for Use:

- Dosage will be individualized. Use exactly as prescribed.
- Tablets may be crushed and mixed with liquid to insure ingestion.
- Depending on the individual patient, maintenance dosage may be required for months or even years.
- Never use in intoxicated individuals or without an individual's knowledge. Patient's relatives should be instructed accordingly.
- Do not take for at least 12 hours after drinking alcohol. A reaction may occur for up to 2 weeks after disulfiram has been stopped.
- If a dose is missed, take it as soon as possible. If several hours have passed or if it is nearing time for the next dose, do not double the dose to catch up, unless advised to do so by your doctor. If more than one dose is missed, or it is necessary to establish a new dosage schedule, contact your doctor or pharmacist.
- Avoid alcohol in all forms. This includes: Alcoholic beverages including beer and wine, vinegars, many liquid medications (including prescription and nonprescription products), some sauces, aftershave lotions, colognes, liniments, backrubs, etc.
- Always read product labels or ask your pharmacist about alcohol content of all liquid medications before choosing one.
- May cause drowsiness. Use caution while driving or performing other tasks requiring alertness, coordination, or physical dexterity.
- The alcohol-disulfiram reaction can have serious adverse effects on the heart and respiratory systems.
- When taking disulfiram, always carry identification that describes the symptoms most likely to occur as a result of the disulfiram-alcohol reaction. Include the phone numbers of your doctor or the medical facility that should be contacted in case of an emergency.
- Lab tests will be required during therapy. Be sure to keep appointments.
- Store at room temperature.

If you have any questions, consult your doctor, pharmacist, or health care provider.

Generic Name *Brand Name Examples*	Supplied As	Generic Available
Rx **Naltrexone HCl**		
ReVia	**Tablets:** 50 mg	No

Type of Drug:

Pure opioid antagonist; anti-opioid; antinarcotic.

How the Drug Works:

Naltrexone blocks the effects of alcohol and intravenous (IV) opioids (eg, narcotic pain relievers, heroin). The exact mechanism of action is unknown. It is believed that naltrexone blocks the effects of opioids by competitive binding at opioid receptors. Therefore, if patients self-administer alcohol, heroin or any other opiate they will not feel the effects ("high") of the drug.

Uses:

To aid in the treatment of alcohol dependence and narcotic addiction by blocking the drug's effects. It has not been shown to provide any benefit except as part of a full plan of management for the addictions.

Unlabeled Use(s): Occasionally doctors may prescribe naltrexone for the treatment of postconcussional syndrome unresponsive to other treatments. It has also been used in eating disorders.

Precautions:

Do not use in the following situations:

- acute opioid withdrawal
- allergy to naltrexone
- failure of NARCAN challenge test
- hepatitis, acute
- liver failure
- opioid dependency
- opioid use (within 7 to 10 days)
- opioid analgesic use

Use with caution in the following situations:

- liver disease, active or history of

Drug-free condition should be maintained for at least 7 to 10 days before starting naltrexone.

Severe opioid withdrawal syndromes have been reported in addicts currently using narcotics who have ingested naltrexone. Symptoms usually appear within 5 minutes and last up to 48 hours. Symptoms may include confusion, severe drowsiness and hallucinations. Fluid loss due to vomiting and diarrhea may require IV fluid replacement.

Self-administering large amounts of opioids in an attempt to overcome the blockade is very dangerous and may lead to a fatal overdose.

Pregnancy: Adequate studies have not been done in pregnant women. Use only if clearly needed and potential benefits outweigh the possible hazards to the fetus.

Breastfeeding: It is not known if naltrexone appears in breast milk. Consult your doctor before you begin breastfeeding.

Children: Safety and effectiveness have not been established in children under 18.

Drug Interactions:

Tell your doctor or pharmacist if you are taking or if you are planning to take any over-the-counter or prescription medications or dietary supplements while taking naltrexone. Doses of one or both drugs may need to be modified or a different drug may need to be prescribed. The following drugs and drug classes may interact with naltrexone:

- disulfiram (eg, *Antabuse*)
- opioid containing medicines (eg, opioid analgesics, narcotic pain relievers)
- thioridazine (eg, *Mellaril*)

Side Effects:

Every drug is capable of producing side effects. Many naltrexone users experience no, or minor, side effects. The frequency and severity of side effects depend on many factors including dose, duration of therapy and individual susceptibility. Possible side effects include:

Digestive Tract: Nausea; vomiting; stomach cramps/pain; appetite loss; diarrhea; constipation.

Nervous System: Sleeplessness; anxiety; headache; changes in energy level; irritability; dizziness; fatigue; depression; drowsiness; suicidal thoughts.

Other: Bone, joint or muscle pain; skin rash; chills; increased thirst; delayed ejaculation; impotence; abnormal blood counts and liver function tests; liver problems; tearfulness; nasal symptoms; yawning.

Guidelines for Use:

- Always carry identification indicating that you are taking naltrexone.
- Take without regard to food.
- If a dose is missed, take it as soon as possible. If several hours have passed or if it is nearing time for the next dose, do not double the dose in order to "catch up" (unless advised to do so by your doctor). If more than one dose is missed or it is necessary to establish a new dosage schedule, contact your doctor or pharmacist.
- Do not share your medication with anyone else.
- Do not take this medicine until you are opioid-free for at least 7 to 10 days, and after successful completion of the NARCAN challenge test.
- Take only as directed by your doctor. Attempts to self-administer heroin or any other opiate in small doses will result in no perceived effect. However, self-administration of large doses may result in serious injury, coma or death.
- Patients taking naltrexone may not benefit from opioid-containing medicines, such as cough and cold preparations, antidiarrheals and some pain relievers. Use a nonopioid-containing alternative, if available.
- Naltrexone may cause liver injury when taken in large doses, or in people who develop liver disease from other causes. If you develop abdominal pain lasting more than a few days, white bowel movements, dark urine or yellowing of the eyes, stop taking naltrexone and contact your doctor immediately.
- Lab tests will need to be done often to detect early liver damage. Be sure to keep appointments.
- Naltrexone should be used only as part of a comprehensive alcohol or drug treatment program.
- Store in a dry, dark place at room temperature.

If you have any questions, consult your doctor, pharmacist, or health care provider.

	Generic Name *Brand Name Example*	Supplied As	Generic Available
C-II	**Levomethadyl Acetate Hydrochloride (LAAM)**		
	ORLAAM	**Oral Solution:** 10 mg	No

Type of Drug:

Synthetic opioid analgesic used as an anti-opioid/antinarcotic.

How the Drug Works:

LAAM suppresses the symptoms of withdrawal in opiate-dependent individuals by acting as a substitute for morphine-like opiates. Chronic administration also can produce enough tolerance to block the "high" associated with injectable opiates.

Uses:

For the management of opiate (eg, heroin, morphine) dependence. LAAM is intended for use as part of a comprehensive treatment plan.

Precautions:

Do not use in the following situations: allergy to LAAM

Use with caution in the following situations:

- Addison's disease
- asthma and other respiratory conditions
- elderly or debilitated
- head injury
- heart conduction abnormality, existing or potential
- hypothyroidism (underactive thyroid)
- increased intracranial pressure
- kidney disease
- liver disease
- prostatic hypertrophy
- stomach conditions, acute
- urethral stricture

Pregnancy: Adequate studies have not been done in pregnant women. LAAM use is not recommended during pregnancy.

Breastfeeding: It is not known if LAAM appears in breast milk. Consult your doctor before you begin breastfeeding.

Children: LAAM is not recommended in children under 18 years of age.

Drug Interactions:

Tell your doctor or pharmacist if you are taking or if you are planning to take any over-the-counter or prescription medications or dietary supplements with levomethadyl acetate hydrochloride. Doses of one or both drugs may need to be modified or a different drug may need to be prescribed. The following drugs and drug classes interact with levomethadyl acetate hydrochloride.

- alcohol
- antidepressants
- antifungals (eg, ketoconazole)
- antihistamines
- benzodiazepines (eg, diazepam)
- carbamazepine (eg, *Tegretol)*
- cimetidine (eg, *Tagamet)*
- erythromycin (eg, *E-Mycin)*

meperidine (*Demerol)*
methadone (eg, *Dolophine)*
narcotic antagonists/agonists
opioids
phenobarbital (eg, *Barbita)*
phenytoin (eg, *Dilantin- 125)*
propoxyphene (eg, *Darvon)*
rifampin
sedatives (eg, benzodiazepines)
tranquilizers (eg, phenothiazines)

Side Effects:

Every drug is capable of producing side effects. Many LAAM users experience no, or minor, side effects. The frequency and severity of side effects depend on many factors including dose, duration of therapy and individual susceptibility. Possible side effects include:

Digestive Tract: Abdominal pain; constipation; diarrhea; dry mouth; nausea; vomiting.

Nervous System: Abnormal dreams; anxiety; decreased sex drive; depression; euphoria (exaggerated sense of well being); headache; decreased sensitivity to stimulation; sleeplessness; nervousness; sleepiness.

Circulatory System: Slow heart beat; light-headedness upon rising.

Respiratory System: Nasal congestion; cough; yawning.

Skin: Rash; sweating.

Other: Weakness; back pain; chilis; edema (fluid retention); hot flashes; flu-like symptoms;general body discomfort; blurred vision; tearing; difficult ejaculation; impotence; muscle and joint pain.

Guidelines for Use:

- Do not take more frequently than prescribed. These drugs can be addicting.
- Do not take daily. Daily use of the usual doses will lead to serious overdose.
- The full effects of LAAM will not be felt for several days.
- Use or abuse of other psychoactive drugs or alcohol may result in fatal overdose.
- If transferring from LAAM to methadone, wait 48 hours after the last dose of LAAM before taking the first dose of methadone or other narcotics.
- May impair mental and/or physical abilities. Use caution while driving or performing other tasks requiring alertness, coordination and/or physical dexterity.
- Current regulations mandate monthly pregnancy tests in female patients of childbearing potential.
- Patients should inform their adult family members that, in the event of overdose, the treating physician or emergency room staff should be told that the patient physically dependent on narcotics, is being treated with LAAM, a long-acting opioid that is likely to outlast naloxone-induced reversal and which requires prolonged observation and careful monitoring.

If you have any questions, consult your doctor, pharmacist, or health care provider.

	Generic Name *Brand Name Examples*	Supplied As	Generic Available
Rx	**Penicillamine**		
	Cuprimine	**Capsules:** 125 mg, 250 mg	No
	Depen	**Tablets:** 250 mg	No

Type of Drug:

Arthritis agent, chelating agent; antidote. Drug to decrease cystine kidney stone formation.

How the Drug Works:

The exact manner by which penicillamine works in arthritis is unknown. It may have anti-inflammatory activity or it may interfere with immune mechanisms which are responsible for arthritis-type problems.

Penicillamine is a chelating agent. Chelating agents combine with metal. Penicillamine removes excess copper from the systems of people with Wilson's disease. It may also be used in poisoning by binding with metals (iron, mercury, lead, arsenic).

Penicillamine reduces excessive excretion of amino acids in the urine, which leads to kidney stone formation, by chemically reacting with the stones, making them more soluble.

Uses:

To treat rheumatoid arthritis.

To treat Wilson's disease (disease characterized by copper deposits in the body due to faulty copper metabolism).

To treat kidney stone formation due to cystinuria.

Unlabeled Use(s): Occasionally doctors may prescribe penicillamine for treatment of primary biliary cirrhosis and scleroderma (thickening and hardening of the skin).

Precautions:

Do not use in the following situations:

breastfeeding
kidney disease
penicillamine-related aplastic anemia, history
penicillamine-related decrease in white blood cells
pregnancy

Use with caution in the following situations: myasthenic syndrome. Progression to myasthenia gravis has occurred. Symptoms usually disappear when the drug is stopped.

Pregnancy: Use only when clearly needed and when the potential benefits outweigh the possible hazards to the fetus. There are possible hazards of penicillamine to the developing fetus. Report promptly any missed menstrual periods or other indications of possible pregnancy to your doctor.

Breastfeeding: Safety of penicillamine use while breastfeeding is not established. Do not breastfeed while taking this drug.

Children: The safety and effectiveness of penicillamine in juvenile rheumatoid arthritis have not been established.

Lab tests will be required during treatment with penicillamine. Tests may include: Urine tests, liver function tests, x-rays, complete blood count and platelet count and an antinuclear antibody (ANA) test.

Drug Interactions:

Tell your doctor or pharmacist if you are taking or if you are planning to take any over-the-counter or prescription medications or dietary supplements with penicillamine. Doses of one or both durgs may need to be modified or a different drug may need to be prescribed. The following drugs and drug classes interact with penicillamine.

antacids
anticancer drugs (eg, methotrexate)
antimalarial drugs (eg, quinine sulfate)
digoxin (eg, *Lanoxin)*
gold therapy (eg, auranofin)
iron salts (eg, ferrous sulfate)
oxyphenbutazone
phenylbutazone (eg, *Butazolidin)*

Side Effects:

Every drug is capable of producing side effects. Many penicillamine users experience side effects. The frequency and severity of side effects depend on many factors including dose, duration of therapy and individual susceptibility. Possible side effects include:

Digestive Tract: Nausea; vomiting; stomach pain; appetite loss; diarrhea; reactivated peptic ulcer; colitis.

Respiratory System: Breathing difficulty; coughing or wheezing; shortness of breath.

Skin: Rash; itching; unusual bruising or bleeding; yellowing of skin or eyes; hot flashes.

Other: Fever; chills; joint pain; mouth sores; ringing in the ears; hair loss; muscle weakness; sore throat; breast enlargement; altered taste perception; abnormal liver function tests; protein and blood in urine; abnormal blood counts.

Guidelines for Use:

- Take on an empty stomach (1 hour before meals or 2 hours after meals). Take at least 1 hour apart from any other drugs, food or milk.
- Drink ample water while taking this drug.
- Notify your doctor promptly if fever, sore throat, chills, bruising or bleeding occurs.
- Periodically see your doctor to make certain that the drug is working properly and to insure that no serious side effects are developing.
- Do not stop taking this medication without first consulting your doctor. If therapy is interrupted, do not start taking the medication again without first consulting your doctor.
- May increase the dietary need for pyridoxine and iron. Daily supplements may be required.

If you have any questions, consult your doctor, pharmacist, or health care provider.

	Generic Name *Brand Name Example*	Supplied As	Generic Available
Rx	**Calcium Acetate**		
	PhosLo	**Tablets:** 667 mg (25.3% calcium)	No

Type of Drug:

Mineral.

How the Drug Works:

Patients with advanced kidney disease show signs of phosphate retention and some degree of hyperphosphatemia (excessive phosphates in the blood). Efforts to control hyperphosphatemia include reduction of dietary phosphate intake, interference of the absorption of phosphates in the stomach with phosphate binders, and removal of phosphates from the body by dialysis. Calcium acetate binds in the stomach to dietary phosphate, preventing its absorption and increasing its removal.

Uses:

To control excessive amounts of phosphates in the blood in patients with advanced kidney disease. It is not a calcium supplement and should not be used with other calcium supplements.

Precautions:

Do not use in the following situations:

digitalis use
high blood calcium levels

Pregnancy: Adequate studies have not been done in pregnant women. Use only if clearly needed and potential benefits outweigh the possible hazards to the fetus.

Breastfeeding: It is not known if calcium acetate appears in breast milk. Consult your doctor before you begin breastfeeding.

Children: Safety and effectiveness for use in children have not been estabiished.

Lab tests may be required during treatment with calcium acetate. Tests may inciude calcium biood levels.

Drug Interactions:

Tell your doctor or pharmacist if you are taking or if you are planning to take any over-the-counter or prescription medications or dietary supplements with caicium acetate. Doses of one or both drugs may need to be modified, or a different drug may need to be prescribed. The following drugs and drug classes interact with calcium acetate.

antacids, nonprescription
calcium supplements
digitalis
tetracyclines (eg, doxycycline)

Side Effects:

Every drug is capable of producing side effects. Many calcium acetate users experience no, or minor, side effects. The frequency and severity of side effects depend on many factors including dose, duration of therapy and individual susceptibility. Possible side effects inciude:

Mild hypercalcemia: Nausea; vomiting; constipation; appetite ioss.

Severe hypercalcemia: Confusion; delirium; stupor; coma.

Guidelines for Use:

- Do not take other calcium supplements or nonprescription antacids while taking this drug.
- Take with meals.
- If hypercalcemia develops, dosage should be reduced or treatment should be discontinued immediately, depending upon the severity of the condition.
- *Calcium toxicity* from calcium acetate may cause confusion, delirium, stupor and coma. Chronic use may cause calcification of blood vessels and tissue.
- Monitor calcium blood levels twice weekly during the early dose adjustment period.
- Store at room temperature.

If you have any questions, consult your doctor, pharmacist, or health care provider.

	Generic Name *Brand Name Examples*	Supplied As	Generic Available
	Nicotine		
Rx	*Habitrol*	**Transdermal System:** 7 mg/day, 14 mg/day, 21 mg/day	No
	Prostep	**Transdermal System:** 11 mg/day, 22 mg day	No
otc	*Nicoderm CQ*	**Transdermal System:** 7 mg/day, 14 mg/day, 21 mg/day	No
	Nicotrol	**Transdermal System:** 5 mg/day, 10 mg/day, 15 mg/day	No
	Nicotrol NS	**Nasal Spray:** 10 mg/mL	No
	Nicorette	**Chewing Gum:** 2 mg/square	No
	Nicorette DS	**Chewing Gum:** 4 mg/square	No

Type of Drug:

Smoking deterrents. Aids to stop smoking. Nicotine treatment should be used as part of a comprehensive behavioral smoking-cessation program.

How the Drug Works:

Nicotine has a variety of effects on the body. It is possible to become dependent on and abuse nicotine. As a smoking deterrent, nicotine is released and absorbed into the body. This lower level of nicotine may then help prevent physical signs of nicotine withdrawal after stopping smoking.

Uses:

To temporarily aid a cigarette smoker who is trying to quit smoking.

Precautions:

Do not use in the following situations:

allergy to any component of this medicine

Use with caution in the following situations:

angina, severe
asthma (nasal spray only)
cardiovascular disease
irregular heart rhythm, severe
diabetes, insulin dependent
endocrine diseases
heart attack, history
heartburn (gum only)
high blood pressure, severe
inflammation of mouth of throat (gum only)
kidney disease, severe
liver disease
nasal disorders, chronic (eg, allergy, congestion, polyps, sinus problems) (nasal spray only)
peptic ulcer
peripheral vascular disease
pheochromocytoma (tumor of the adrenal gland)
pregnancy
skin disorders (patch only)
temporomandibular disease (TMJ), active (gum only)
thyroid, overactive

Labor and delivery: The effects of smoking deterrents on the mother and fetus are unknown. Do not use during labor and delivery.

Pregnancy: Smoking and smoking deterrents are not recommended during pregnancy. Studies have shown a potential adverse effect on the fetus. Use only if clearly needed and potential benefits outweigh the possible risks.

Breastfeeding: Nicotine appears in breast milk. Do not use during breastfeeding. Consult your doctor.

Children: Safety and effectiveness have not been established. These products are not intended for use by children or adolescents. The amounts of nicotine that are tolerated by adult smokers can produce symptoms of poisoning and could prove fatal if applied or ingested by children. Therefore, keep these products out of the reach of children. Contact your doctor if a child chews or swallows a piece of nicotine gum.

Drug Interactions:

Tell your doctor or pharmacist if you are taking or if you are planning to take any over-the-counter or prescription medications or dietary supplements while taking this medicine. Doses of one or both drugs may need to be modified or a different drug may need to be prescribed. Stopping smoking, with or without nicotine substitutes, may change the response to the following drugs and drug classes.

acetaminophen (eg, *Tylenol)*
adrenergic agonists (eg, isoproterenol, phenylephrine)
adrenergic antagonists (eg, prazosin, labetalol)
caffeine
imipramine (eg, *Tofranil)*
insulin
oxazepam (*Serax)*
pentazocine (eg, *Talwin)*
propranolol (eg, *Inderal)*
theophylline (eg, *Theo-Dur)*

Side Effects:

Every drug is capable of producing side effects. Many smoking deterrent users experience no, or minor, side effects. The frequency and severity of side effects depend on many factors including dose, duration of therapy and individual susceptibility. Possible side effects include:

Skin (patches) – Burning; itching; redness; rash; swelling; hives; sweating.

Nasal spray – Nasal irritation, ulcers or blisters; congestion; runny nose; sore throat; hoarseness; watery eyes; sneezing; cough; smell or taste changes; numbness of burning of nose or mouth; earache; flushing; sinus problems; eye irritation or burning.

Gum – Mouth or tongue sores; injury to teeth or lining of the mouth; gum bleeding; jaw ache.

Digestive Tract: Belching; stomach pain; gas; diarrhea; nausea; excess saliva; constipation; vomiting; increased appetite; hiccups.

Nervous System: Drowsiness; dizziness; anxiety; moodiness; restlessness; cravings; irritability; headache; sleeplessness; abnormal dreams;

abnormal skin sensations; confusion; depression; apathy; tremors; weakness; fainting; clumsiness; difficulty concentrating; hearing loss; cold sweats.

Other: Dry mouth; sore throat; sinus infection; joint or muscle pain; back pain; pounding in the chest; acne; difficulty breathing; loss of menstruation; weight gain.

Guidelines for Use:

- Use exactly as prescribed. Read patient information sheet carefully.
- Stop smoking completely when starting these medicine. People who smoke while taking this medicine may experience side effects more profound than those experienced from smoking alone.
- Keep these products, including both used and unused patches, nasal spray and gum, out of the reach of children and pets.
- *Chewing Gum* — Most patients require approximately 9 to 12 pieces of gum per day during the first month of treatment. Do not exceed 20 pieces of 4 mg gum or 30 pieces of 2 mg gum per day.Avoid eating and drinking for 15 minutes before and during chewing nicotine gum.

  It may take a few days for you to adjust to the unpleasant taste of the gum.

  Slowly chew one piece of gum whenever you have an urge to smoke. Chew each piece slowly and intermittently for about 30 minutes. Chewing quickly can release the nicotine too quickly, leading to effects similar to oversmoking (eg, nausea, hiccups or throat irritation).

  Stop using the gum or initiate gradual withdrawal after 2 to 3 months of usage and complete use by 4 to 6 months. Do not use beyond 6 months.

  Stop using the gum immediately and contact your doctor if severe rash, itching or hives occurs. Stop using this gum if the gum sticks to dental work.

  Store below 86°F, away from heat and light (eg, not in parked cars in summer).

Guidelines for Use (cont.):

- *Patches* — Apply patch promptly upon removal from the protective pouch. Use only if pouch is intact. Apply patch once a day to non-hairy, clean, dry skin on the upper body or upper outer arm. After 24 hours, remove the used patch and apply a new patch to an alternate skin site. Skin sites should not be reused for at least a week. (Note: Remove *Nicotrol* at bedtime. It is for waking use only.) Do not use the same patch for more than 24 hours.
  Dosage may vary. Refer to patient package insert or consult your doctor for recommended dosing schedules. Once the appropriate dosage has been selected, continue therapy at that dosage for the prescribed time.
  If you are unable to stop smoking within 4 weeks, therapy should be discontinued. Therapy should not continue for longer than 3 months (5 months for *Nicotrol)* in patients who have stopped smoking because of the harmful and addictive effects of nicotine.
  Following application or removal, wash hands with water only. Do not use soap. Avoid contact with eyes.
  Discontinue use and consult your doctor if you experience severe or persistent skin reactions.
  Patch disposal — Fold patch over itself, place in pouch and discard.
  Patch storage — Store below 86°F. A slight discoloration of the patch is not significant. Do not store out of the pouch. Once out of the protective pouch, apply promptly since nicotine evaporates and the patch may lose its strength.
- *Nasal Spray* — Administer the spray with head tilted back slightly. Do not sniff, swallow or inhale through the nose as spray is administered.
  Avoid contact with eyes, mouth or ears. Contact your doctor immediately if such contact occurs.
  If solution is spilled, clean up immediately with an absorbent cloth or paper towel. Avoid contact with skin. Wash area of spill several times. If solution comes into contact with skin, lips, mouth, eyes or ears, rinse immediately with water only.
  This medicine may cause nasal irritation.
  Do not continue for longer than 6 months because of the harmful and addictive effects of nicotine.
  Discard bottle with the child-resistant cap in place.
  Store at room temperature below 86°F.

If you have any questions, consult your doctor, pharmacist, or health care provider.

Generic Name *Brand Name Example*	Supplied As	Generic Available
Rx **Bupropion HCl**		
Zyban	**Tablets, sustained-release**: 150 mg	No

Type of Drug:

Non-nicotine smoking deterrent; antidepressant.

How the Drug Works:

The exact mechanism by which bupropion helps patients stop smoking is unknown. It may alter chemicals in the brain (neurotransmitters) that suppress the urge to smoke.

Uses:

An aid to smoking cessation treatment.

Bupropion is also used as an antidepressant. See the Bupropion HCl monograph in the Central Nervous System Drugs chapter.

Precautions:

Do not use in the following situations:

allergy to bupropion or any of its ingredients
anorexia nervosa
bulimia
bupropion use for depression (eg, *Wellbutrin*), concurrent
monoamine oxidase inhibitor (MAOI) use, concurrent or within 14 days
seizure disorders

Use with caution in the following situations:

alcohol, excessive
attempted suicide, history of
brain tumor
diabetes treated with oral hypoglycemics or insulin
drug abuse
head injury, history of
heart attack, recent
heart disease
kidney disease
liver disease
manic depression (bipolar disorder)
seizure, history or risk of
therapy that lowers seizure threshold (eg, antipsychotics, antidepressants, theophylline, systemic steroids, benzodiazepine withdrawal)

Pregnancy: There are no adequate and well-controlled studies in pregnant women. Use during pregnancy only if clearly needed and the potential benefits to the mother outweigh the possible risks to the fetus.

Breastfeeding: Bupropion is excreted in human milk. Serious side effects could potentially occur in the nursing infant. Decide whether to discontinue the drug or discontinue breastfeeding, taking into account the importance of the drug to the mother. Consult your doctor before you begin breastfeeding.

Children: Safety and effectiveness have not been established in children under 18 years of age.

Elderly: Older patients are known to metabolize drugs more slowly and to be more sensitive to antidepressant drugs. Use the lowest effective dose.

Drug Interactions:

Tell your doctor or pharmacist if you are taking or if you are planning to take any over-the-counter or prescription medications or dietary supplements with bupropion. Doses of one or both drugs may need to be modified or a different drug may need to be prescribed. The following drugs and drug classes interact with bupropion:

- antiarrhythmics (eg, propafenone, flecainide)
- antidepressants (eg, fluoxetine, amitriptyline)
- antipsychotics (eg, phenothiazines)
- barbiturates (eg, phenobarbital)
- beta blockers (eg, metoprolol)
- carbamazepine (eg, *Tegretol*)
- cimetidine (eg, *Tagamet*)
- hydantoins (eg, phenytoin)
- levodopa (eg, *Sinemet*)
- monoamine oxidase inhibitors (eg, phenelzine)
- nicotine transdermal system (eg, *Nicoderm CQ*)
- ritonavir (*Norvir*)
- systemic corticosteroids (eg, prednisone)
- theophylline (eg, *Slo-Phyllin*)

Side Effects:

Every drug is capable of producing side effects. Many bupropion users experience no, or minor, side effects. The frequency and severity of side effects depend on many factors including dose, duration of therapy, and individual susceptibility. Possible side effects include:

Digestive Tract: Nausea; vomiting; constipation; indigestion; appetite changes; stomach pain; dry mouth; mouth sores; diarrhea; gas.

Nervous System: Seizures; tremor; dizziness; delusions; hallucinations; confusion; agitation; anxiety; sleep disturbances; headache; activation of psychosis or mania; sleeplessness; decreased memory; depression; nervousness; irritability; drowsiness; disturbed concentration.

Circulatory System: Changes in blood pressure; pounding in chest; chest pain.

Skin: Rash; itching; excessive sweating; flushing; dry skin; hives.

Other: Taste changes; blurred vision; ringing in the ears; frequent urination; fever; joint pain; weight changes; urinary urgency; muscle pain; allergic reaction; weakness; abnormal skin sensations; shortness of breath; hot flushes; sore throat.

Guidelines for Use:

- Usual adult dosage is 300 mg/day, given in 2 equally divided doses of 150 mg separated by at least 8 hours. Dosing should begin at 150 mg/day given as a single dose in the morning. Based on response, dose may be increased to 150 mg twice daily.
- Do not exceed 300 mg of bupropion sustained-release tablets daily for smoking cessation. Single doses should not exceed 150 mg because of the risk of seizures.
- Do not crush, chew, or divide tablets.
- Do not change the dose or stop taking, unless advised to do so by your doctor.
- May be taken without regard to meals. Take with food if stomach upset occurs.
- If a dose is missed, take it as soon as possible. If several hours have passed or if it is less than 8 hours before your next dose, do not double the dose to catch up. Never take more than 150 mg at one time. If several doses are missed or it is necessary to establish a new dosage schedule, contact your doctor or pharmacist. Usual duration of therapy is 7 to 12 weeks. Longer periods of therapy are acceptable under your doctor's guidance.
- To maximize your chance of quitting smoking, you should not stop smoking until you have been taking bupropion for 1 week. You should set a date to stop smoking during the second week you are taking bupropion.
- This medicine should not be used in combination with *Wellbutrin* or any other medication containing bupropion.
- It is not physically dangerous to smoke and use this medicine at the same time. However, continuing to smoke after the date you set to stop smoking will seriously reduce your chance of breaking your smoking habit.
- Using bupropion and nicotine patches (eg, *Nicoderm CQ*) at the same time can raise your blood pressure. Use both only under your doctor's supervision.
- Do not smoke if you are using bupropion and nicotine patches at the same time.
- Avoid alcohol to reduce the risk of seizures caused by bupropion.
- Do not take in combination with MAO inhibitors or within 14 days of discontinuing treatment with an MAOI.
- May cause drowsiness. Use caution while driving or performing other tasks requiring alertness, coordination, or physical dexterity.
- Bupropion has a characteristic odor. If present, this odor is normal.
- Do not share your medicine with anyone else.
- Counseling and support are an important component of smoking cessation.
- Store at 68° to 77°F. Protect from light and moisture.

If you have any questions, consult your doctor, pharmacist, or health care provider.

	Generic Name *Brand Name Examples*	Supplied As	Generic Available
Rx	**Alprostadil**		
	Caverject	**Injection:** 11.9 mcg, 23.2 mcg	No

Type of Drug:

Agent for impotence.

How the Drug Works:

Alprostadil induces penile erection by relaxing certain muscles of the penis and increasing arterial blood flow to the penis. When the effect of alprostadil wears off, the erection disappears and blood flow returns to normal.

Uses:

To treat erectile dysfunction (impotence) in adult males. It may also be used with other tests to diagnose erectile dysfunction.

Precautions:

Do not use in the following situations:

allergy to this medicine
children
deformity of penis
leukemia
men who are advised not to engage in sexual activity
newborns
penile implants
sickle cell anemia
tumors, bone marrow
women

Use with caution in the following situations:

anticoagulant (eg, warfarin) use
lung disease
prolonged or painful erections

Drug Interactions:

Tell your doctor or pharmacist if you are taking or if you are planning to take any over-the-counter or prescription medications or dietary supplements while taking this medicine. Doses of one or both drugs may need to be modified or a different drug may need to be prescribed. Anticoagulants (eg, warfarin) interact with this medicine (causing an increased risk of bleeding after injection).

Side Effects:

Every drug is capable of producing side effects. Many patients experience no, or minor, side effects. The frequency or severity of side effects depend on many factors including dose, duration of therapy and individual susceptibility. Possible side effects include:

Nervous System: Headache; dizziness.

Respiratory System: Respiratory infection; flu syndrome; sinus infection; nasal congestion; cough.

Other: Injection site bruising or bleeding; prolonged erection; prostate disorder or pain (possibly difficult urination); penile pain; itching, redness, rash, swelling, hardening (lumps) or discoloration of the skin; yeast infection; numbness; irritation; skin tearing; high blood pressure; back pain.

Guidelines for Use:

- Carefully follow the preparation and injection instructions included in each package. Many side effects can be reduced if the proper administration technique is used.
- Examine each vial for discoloration or particles. Discard such vials. Do not shake the contents of reconstituted (mixed) vials.
- The reconstituted vial is designed for one use only. Use it immediately. Discard any solution that remains after the proper dose has been withdrawn from the vial. Do not store or freeze.
- Do not change the dose without asking your doctor.
- Discard needle properly after each use. Do not re-use or share needles or syringes. Do not allow anybody else to access or use your medicine.
- Erections usually occur within 5 to 20 minutes after injection and last about 1 hour. If it lasts longer than 6 hours, contact your doctor immediately.
- Do not use this medicine more than 3 times per week. Wait at least 24 hours between each use.
- If penile redness, swelling, tenderness, pain, lumps, hardening of the skin or curving of the erect penis occurs, contact your doctor immediately.
- A small amount of bleeding at the injection site may occur. This is normal.
- This medicine offers no protection from the transmission of sexually transmitted diseases such as HIV (the virus that causes AIDS). A small amount of bleeding at the injection site can increase the risk of transmitting serious blood-born diseases between partners.
- Regular medical checkups are necessary to monitor treatment. Be sure to keep appointments.
- Store below 77°F for up to 3 months. Do not freeze, store in checked luggage during air travel or leave in a closed automobile.

If you have any questions, consult your doctor, pharmacist, or health care provider.

Generic Name *Brand Name Examples*	Supplied As	Generic Available
Rx **Sildenafil Citrate**		
Viagra	**Tablets:** 25 mg, 50 mg, 100 mg	No

Type of Drug:

Agent for impotence (erectile dysfunction).

How the Drug Works:

Sildenafil citrate produces smooth muscle relaxation in the penis, allowing blood to flow in and cause an erection.

Sildenafil citrate has no effect in the absence of sexual stimulation or arousal.

Uses:

To treat erectile dysfunction (eg, impotence) due to a variety of causes.

Precautions:

Do not use in the following situations:

allergy to sildenafil or any of its ingredients
children
women
organic nitrates, regular or intermittent use in any dose form (eg, nitroglycerin, isosorbide dinitrate as sublingual tablets, tablets, capsules, transdermal patches, ointments, nasal sprays)

Use with caution in the following situations:

abnormal heart rhythm, life-threatening (within the last 6 months)
bleeding disorders (eg, hemophilia)
cardiovascular disease, preexisting
elderly (65 years of age or older)
heart failure or coronary artery disease causing unstable angina
high blood pressure (BP greater than 170/110)
kidney function impairment, severe
leukemia
liver disease
low blood pressure, resting (BP less than 90/50)
multiple myeloma
myocardial infarction (within the last 6 months)
penile deformity (eg, Peyronie's disease)
penile implants or other erectile dysfunction treatments
priapism (eg, prolonged or painful erections)
retinitis pigmentosa
sickle cell anemia
stroke (within the last 6 months)
ulcers, active peptic

Pregnancy: There are no adequate and well-controlled studies in pregnant women. Sildenafil citrate is not indicated for use in women, children, or newborns.

Elderly: The elimination of sildenafil citrate is reduced in healthy patients over 65 years of age. The starting dose should not be over 25 mg.

Lab tests may be required before beginning treatment with sildenafil. A thorough medical history and physical exam must be done to determine erectile dysfunction, underlying causes, and appropriate treatment.

Drug Interactions:

Tell your doctor or pharmacist if you are taking or if you are planning to take any over-the-counter or prescription medications or dietary supplements with sildenafil. Doses of one or both drugs may need to be modified or a different drug may need to be prescribed. The following drugs interact with sildenafil.

amlodipine (eg, *Norvasc*)
beta blockers, non-specific (eg, atenolol, propranolol)
cytochrome P450 3A4 inducers (eg, rifampin)
cytochrome P450 3A4 inhibitors (eg, cimetidine, erythromycin, itraconazole)
high-fat meals may slow absorption with concurrent drug administration
loop diuretics (eg, furosemide)
organic nitrates (eg, nitroglycerin, all dose forms)
potassium-sparing diuretics (eg, spironolactone)

Side Effects:

Every drug is capable of producing side effects. Many sildenafil users experience no, or minor, side effects. The frequency and severity of side effects depend on many factors including dose, duration of therapy, and individual susceptibility. Possible side effects include:

Circulatory System: Chest pain; heart block; heart muscle damage; flushing; fast heartbeat; low blood pressure; heart failure; blood clots in brain; palpitations (pounding in chest); dizziness; fainting; low blood pressure when rising from a seated or lying position; abnormal heart rhythm; angina; cardiac arrest.

Digestive Tract: Vomiting; colon inflammation; difficulty swallowing; stomach pain; dry mouth; gum, stomach, tongue, or mouth inflammation; rectal bleeding; indigestion; diarrhea.

Nervous System: Dizziness; vertigo (feeling of a whirling motion); headache; migraine; tremors; depression; sleeplessness; drowsiness; decreased reflexes; abnormal dreams; abnormal skin sensations; nerve pain; nerve disease; incoordination; muscle stiffness or weakness; decreased sensitivity to touch.

Respiratory System: Asthma; difficulty breathing; laryngitis; increased cough; increased sputum; sinus inflammation; sore throat; nasal congestion; bronchitis; respiratory tract infections.

Skin: Sweating; skin ulcers; herpes simplex; hives; itching; skin inflammation; flushing; rash.

Senses: Eye pain; cataract; dry eyes; ear pain; ringing in ears; sensitivity to light; eye inflammation; pupil dilation; abnormal vision; color tinge to vision; blurred vision; double vision; deafness; eye bleeding.

Urinary and Reproductive Tract: Frequent urination; urinary tract infection; breast enlargement; inability to control bladder; abnormal ejaculation; genital swelling; bladder inflammation; excessive nighttime urination; inability to achieve orgasm; prolonged erection; priapism (painful erection longer than 6 hours in duration); blood in the urine.

Other: Back, muscle, joint, or bone pain; gout; thirst; high blood sugar; low blood sugar; shock; weakness; pain; chills; accidental injuries or falling; allergic reactions; facial swelling; flu-like syndrome; swelling; unstable diabetes; tendon rupture or inflammation; swelling of hands or feet; abnormal liver function tests; joint pain or inflammation; anemia; high blood uric acid levels; high blood sodium levels; decreased white blood cell counts.

Guidelines for Use:

- Sildenafil is not indicated for use in women, children, or newborns.
- A thorough physical exam and medical history assessing cardiovascular and general health status and confirming erectile dysfunction, including a determination of potential underlying causes, is necessary prior to beginning treatment.
- Recommended dosage is 50 mg taken approximately 1 hour before sexual activity. It may be taken 30 minutes to 4 hours before sexual activity. Dose may be increased to a maximum recommended dose of 100 mg or decreased to 25 mg based on effectiveness and patient tolerance. Maximum dosage frequency is once daily.
- Sildenafil has no effect in the absence of sexual stimulation or arousal.
- Do not use sildenafil citrate in combination with any nitrate medications (eg, nitroglycerin, isosorbide in any dose form) as it may cause a severe, possibly fatal drop in blood pressure.
- After therapy with sildenafil, it is not known when nitrates, if needed, can be safely administered.
- Patients who experience symptoms (eg, chest pain, dizziness, nausea) upon initiation of sexual activity should be advised to refrain from further activity and notify their doctor of the episode.
- Contact your doctor if you experience any unusual side effects.
- There is a potential for cardiac risk associated with sexual activity in patients with preexisting cardiovascular disease. Therefore, treatments for erectile dysfunction should not be generally used in men for whom sexual activity is inadvisable because of their underlying cardiovascular status.
- Prior to prescribing sildenafil, physicians should carefully consider whether their patients with underlying cardiovascular disease could be affected adversely by vasodilatory effects (transient decreases in supine blood pressure), especially in combination with sexual activity.
- Taking sildenafil citrate with a high-fat meal reduces the absorption rate which can result in a delay in onset of effect.
- Do not use sildenafil in combination with any other erectile dysfunction treatment.
- This medicine offers no protection from sexually transmitted diseases such as HIV (the virus that causes AIDS).
- Seek immediate medical assistance in the event of an erection that persists longer than 4 hours. If priapism (painful erection longer than 6 hours in duration) is not treated immediately, penile tissue damage and permanent loss of potency could result.
- Store at controlled room temperature (59° to 86°F).

If you have any questions, consult your doctor, pharmacist, or health care provider.

Generic Name *Brand Name Examples*	Supplied As	Generic Available
Rx **Yohimbine**		
Aphrodyne, Yocon, Yohimex	**Tablets:** 5.4 mg	No

Type of Drug:

Alpha adrenergic blocker. Drug for impotence (unlabeled).

How the Drug Works:

Yohimbine causes the release of the nervous system chemical norepinephrine. Norepinephrine affects the body in a variety of ways including: Increased blood flow to the penis, stimulation of mood, local anesthesia, mild decrease in urine output, and changes in blood pressure.

Uses:

Yohimbine has no FDA approved uses.

Unlabeled Use(s): Occasionally doctors may prescribe yohimbine for orthostatic hypotension and to dilate the pupil. Yohimbine may also be used as an aphrodisiac.

Precautions:

Do not use in the following situations:

allergy to yohimbine
kidney disease

Use with caution in the following situations:

duodenal ulcers
heart disease
psychiatric patients
stomach ulcers

Pregnancy: Do not use during pregnancy.

Children: Not intended for use in children.

Elderly: Not intended for use in elderly patients.

Drug Interactions:

Tell your doctor or pharmacist if you are taking or if you are planning to take any over-the-counter or prescription medications or dietary supplements with yohimbine. Doses of one or both drugs may need to be modified or a different drug may need to be prescribed. Antidepressants and other mood-modifying drugs interact with yohimbine.

Side Effects:

Every drug is capable of producing side effects. Many yohimbine users experience no, or minor, side effects. The frequency and severity of side effects depend on many factors including dose, duration of therapy and individual susceptibility. Possible side effects include:

Nervous System: Nervousness; irritability; tremors; dizziness; headache; increased motor activity; incoordination.

Circulatory System: Increased heart rate; heart pounding (palpitations); increased blood pressure.

Other: Runny nose; "goosebumps"; flushing; decreased urination.

Guidelines for Use:

- Yohimbine has no FDA approved use.
- If the inability to urinate, elevated blood pressure and heart rate, increased motor activity, nervousness, irritability or tremor occurs, reduce the dosage by half, followed by gradual increases to the original dose. Consult your doctor.
- Results of therapy for longer than 10 weeks are unknown.

If you have any questions, consult your doctor, pharmacist, or health care provider.

Generic Name *Brand Name Example*	Supplied As	Generic Available
Rx **Interferon Beta-1a**		
Avonex	**Powder for Injection (lyophilized):** 0.33 mg (6.6 mIU)	No
Rx **Interferon Beta-1b**		
Betaseron	**Powder for Injection (lyophilized):** 0.3 mg (9.6 mIU)	No

Type of Drug:

An antiviral and immunoregulatory.

How the Drug Works:

The mechanisms by which interferon beta works on multiple sclerosis are not clearly understood.

Uses:

For use in ambulatory patients with relapsing-remitting multiple sclerosis (MS) to slow the accumulation of physical disability or reduce the frequency and severity of attacks. Relapsing-remitting MS is characterized by recurrent attacks of neurologic dysfunction followed by complete or incomplete recovery.

Unlabeled Use(s): Occasionally, doctors may prescribe interferon beta to treat AIDS, AIDS-related Kaposi's sarcoma, herpes of the lips or genitals, certain cancers and acute non-A/non-B hepatitis.

Precautions:

Do not use in the following situations: Do not use if you are allergic to interferon beta, albumin human or any other component of the formulation.

Use with caution in the following situations:

- depression
- heart disease
- seizure disorder
- suicidal thoughts

Mental disorders/suicidal thoughts: Depression and thoughts of suicide can be a side effect of interferon beta. These symptoms should be reported immediately to your doctor.

Pregnancy: Adequate studies have not been done in pregnant women, or animal studies may have shown a risk to the fetus. Use only if clearly needed and potential benefits outweigh the possible hazards to the fetus. Spontaneous abortions have occurred during this therapy.

Breastfeeding: It is not known if interferon beta appears in breast milk. Consult your doctor before you begin breastfeeding.

Children: Safety and efficacy in children under 18 years of age have not been established.

Lab tests may be required before starting and during treatment with interferon beta. Be sure to keep appointments.

Drug Interactions:

Tell your doctor or pharmacist if you are taking or if you are planning to take any over-the-counter or prescription medications or dietary supplements while taking this medicine. Doses of one or both drugs may need to be modified or a different drug may need to be prescribed. Antidepressants and other mood-modifying drugs interact with this medicine.

Side Effects:

Every drug is capable of producing side effects. Many patients experience no, or minor, side effects. The frequency and severity of side effects depend on many factors including dose, duration of therapy and individual susceptibility. Possible side effects include:

Digestive Tract: Diarrhea; constipation; vomiting; nausea; appetite loss; indigestion; stomach pain; dry mouth.

Nervous System: Sleeplessness; depression; confusion; weakness; slurred speech; convulsions; dizziness; drowsiness; migraines; headache.

Circulatory System: Palpitations (pounding in the chest); rapid heartbeat; chest pain; flushing; fainting; high blood pressure; unusual bleeding/bruising; cold hands and feet.

Respiratory System: Sinus infection; difficulty breathing; laryngitis.

Skin: Sweating; hair loss; sunlight sensitivity; hives; herpes; shingles; splotchiness.

Urinary and Reproductive Tract: Painful menstruation; heavy menstrual bleeding; breast pain; fibrous cysts in the breast or ovaries; pelvic pain; frequent urination; vaginal infection; lumps in the breast.

Other: Pain and tenderness at the injection site; fever; flu-like symptoms; pain; chills; general body discomfort; joint and muscle pains or spasms; weight changes; eye irritation; vision problems; inner ear infections; hearing loss; infections; goiter; swelling; suicidal thoughts; abnormal lab values.

Guidelines for Use:

- Use exactly as prescribed.
- *Beta-1a* — usual dose is 1 vial once a week.
- *Beta-1b* — usual dose is 1 vial every other day.
- Follow the mixing process and injection procedure taught to you by your healthcare provider. Your first self-administered injection should be given under the supervision of a health care professional. A patient information sheet is provided.
- If a dose is missed, inject it as soon as possible. If it is nearing the next dose, do not double the dose in order to "catch-up" (unless advised to do so by your doctor). If more than one dose is missed or it is necessary to establish a new dosage schedule, contact your doctor or pharmacist.
- If you become pregnant or plan to become pregnant, discontinue using the medicine and talk to your doctor. Spontaneous abortions have occurred during use of interferon beta.
- May cause sunlight sensitivity. Avoid long exposure to the sun. Use sunscreens and protective clothing until tolerance is known.
- Flu-like symptoms are not uncommon following the beginning of therapy. Acetaminophen may be used to relieve fever and muscle pain.
- Contact your doctor immediately if depression or suicidal thoughts occur.
- Lab tests may be required to monitor therapy. Be sure to keep appointments.
- Store in the refrigerator (36°-46°F). If refrigerator is unavailable, interferon beta-1a may be stored at room temperature for up to 30 days. Use reconstituted solution within 3 hours (6 hours for Beta-1a). Discard any unused solution.

If you have any questions, consult your doctor, pharmacist, or health care provider.

Generic Name *Brand Name Example*	Supplied As	Generic Available
Rx **Riluzole**		
Rilutek	**Tablets:** 50 mg	No

Type of Drug:

Neuroprotective agent.

How the Drug Works:

Riluzole may prevent damage to certain brain cells (motor neurons) responsible for controlling muscle functions.

Uses:

To prolong survival in patients with amyotrophic lateral sclerosis (ALS, Lou Gehrig's disease).

Precautions:

Do not use in the following situations:
allergy to this medicine or its ingredients

Use with caution in the following situations:
kidney disease
liver disease

Pregnancy: Adequate studies have not been done in pregnant women, or animal studies may have shown a risk to the fetus. Use only if clearly needed and potential benefits outweigh the possible hazards to the fetus.

Breastfeeding: It is not known if riluzole appears in breast milk. Breastfeeding is not recommended. Contact your doctor before you begin breastfeeding.

Children: Safety and efficacy in children have not been established.

Elderly: Dosage may need to be adjusted due to reduced kidney or liver function in the elderly.

Lab tests will be required to monitor therapy. Be sure to keep appointments.

Drug Interactions:

Tell your doctor or pharmacist if you are taking or if you are planning to take any over-the-counter or prescription medications or dietary supplements with this medicine. Doses of one or both drugs may need to be modified or a different drug may need to be prescribed. The following drugs or drug classes interact with this medicine.

amitriptyline (eg, *Elavil)*
caffeine
cigarette smoke
food, charcoal broiled
omeprazole (*Prilosec)*
quinolones (eg, ciprofloxacin)
rifampin (eg, *Rifadin)*
tacrine (*Cognex)*
theophylline (eg, *Theo-Dur)*

Side Effects:

Every drug is capable of producing side effects. Many patients experience no, or minor, side effects. The frequency and severity of side effects depend on many factors including dose, duration of therapy and individual susceptibility. Possible side effects include:

Digestive Tract: Nausea; vomiting; diarrhea; appetite loss; indigestion; weight loss; stomach pain; gas; dry mouth; inflamed or sore mouth; teeth problems.

Skin: Rash; itching; eczema; hair loss.

Nervous System: Dizziness; vertigo (feeling of whirling motion); headache; weakness; drowsiness; abnormal skin sensations; depression; sleeplessness.

Other: General body discomfort; joint or back pain; difficulty breathing; pneumonia; nasal congestion; cough; swelling of hands and feet; high blood pressure; fast heartbeat; vein inflammation; postural hypotension (dizziness or lightheadedness when rising quickly from a sitting or lying position); difficult or painful urination; tight muscles; soreness; stiffness; inflexibility.

Guidelines for Use:

- Use exactly as prescribed.
- Usual dose is one tablet every 12 hours. Take at the same time of day (eg, in the morning and evening) each day.
- Take on an empty stomach, at least 1 hour before or 2 hours after a meal.
- Women and Japanese patients may require a lower dose.
- If a dose is missed, take the next tablet as originally planned. Do not try to "catch up" (unless advised to do so by your doctor).
- This medicine may cause drowsiness or dizziness, especially when rising or standing. If these symptoms should occur, sit or lie down and contact your doctor. Use caution while driving or performing other tasks requiring alertness, coordination or dexterity.
- To reduce the risk of liver damage, avoid drinking excessive alcohol while taking this medicine.
- Tell your doctor if you smoke. It may reduce the effectiveness of this medicine.
- Contact your doctor immediately if fever or any illness occurs.
- Lab tests will be required to monitor therapy. Be sure to keep appointments.
- Store at room temperature (68°-77°F), away from bright light.

If you have any questions, consult your doctor, pharmacist, or health care provider.

Generic Name *Brand Name Examples*	Supplied As	Generic Available
Rx **Glatiramer Acetate**		
Copaxone	**Powder for Injection, lyophilized:** 20 mg glatiramer acetate and 40 mg mannitol/ 2 mL vial	No

Type of Drug:

Agent to reduce frequency of relapses in relapsing-remitting multiple sclerosis (MS).

How the Drug Works:

The mechanism of action by which glatiramer acetate works on MS is unknown. Glatiramer is thought to possibly modify the immune process that may cause MS.

Uses:

Indicated in the reduction or frequency or relapses in patients with relapsing-remitting MS.

Precautions:

Do not use in the following situations:
allergy to glatiramer acetate or mannitol

Use with caution in the following situations:
immune disorders

Pregnancy: There are no adequate or well controlled studies in pregnant women. However, no drug should be used during pregnancy unless clearly needed.

Breastfeeding: It is not known if glatiramer acetate appears in breast milk. Consult your doctor before you begin breastfeeding.

Children: The safety and effectiveness of glatiramer acetate have not been established in individuals less than 18 years of age.

Side Effects:

Every drug is capable of producing side effects. Many patients experience side effects. The frequency and severity of side effects depend on many factors including dose, duration of therapy and individual susceptibility. Possible side effects include:

Digestive Tract: Nausea; appetite loss; diarrhea; stomach irritation; stomach disorder; vomiting; stomach pain; indigestion; gum disease; mouth sores.

Nervous System: Anxiety; depression; dizziness; tremor; agitation; confusion; foot drop; nervousness; rapid eye movement; speech disorder; feeling of whirling motion; migraine.

Circulatory System: Fast heartbeat; pounding in the chest; fainting; unusual bruising; lymph node disorder; high blood pressure.

Respiratory System: Difficulty breathing; bronchitis; difficulty swallowing; nasal congestion; laryngitis; rapid breathing.

Urinary and Reproductive Tract: Urinary urgency; painful menstruation; impotence; vaginal and yeast infections; menstrual disorder; blood in urine.

Skin: Hives; rash; flushing; itching; skin nodule; sweating; redness.

Senses: Ear pain; eye disorder.

Body as a Whole: Injection site reactions; chest pain; weakness; infection; pain; joint pain; muscle soreness or tightness; chills; cyst; facial swelling; fever; flu syndrome; neck pain or rigidity; general swelling; swelling of arms and legs; accidental injury; general body discomfort.

Guidelines for Use:

- The usual dose is 20 mg/day.
- Deliver by subcutaneous route only.
- Follow the injection procedure taught to you by your healthcare provider. Patient instructions for use are enclosed in each package; follow the instructions provided with the medicine exactly. Perform your first self-administered injection under the supervision of a healthcare professional.
- Do not stop taking this medicine or change the dose without checking with your doctor.
- Inform your physician if you are pregnant, if you are planning to become pregnant or if you become pregnant while taking this medication.
- Inform your physician if you are nursing.
- The reconstituted product contains no preservative; it should be used immediately. Before reconstitution with diluent, store in freezer at -4° to 14°F. Store diluent at room temperature.

If you have any questions, consult your doctor, pharmacist, or health care provider.

	Generic Name *Brand Name Examples*	Supplied As	Generic Available
Rx	**Thalidomide** *Thalomid*	**Capsules:** 50 mg	No

Type of Drug:

Immune system modulator.

How the Drug Works:

The exact mechanism of action is unknown. It appears that thalidomide modifies some immune system effects which are responsible for the skin changes seen in erythema nodosum leprosum (ENL).

Uses:

For the acute treatment of the cutaneous (skin) manifestations of moderate to severe erythema nodosum leprosum (ENL).

Also for maintenance therapy for prevention and suppression of the cutaneous (skin) manifestations of ENL recurrence.

This drug is not indicated as monotherapy for ENL treatment in the presence of moderate to severe neuritis (nerve inflammation).

Thalidomide is approved for marketing only under a special restricted distribution program called "System for Thalidomide Education and Prescribing Safety (S.T.E.P.S.)." Only prescribers and pharmacists registered under the program are allowed to prescribe and dispense the product. Patients must be advised of, agree to, and comply with the requirements of the S.T.E.P.S. program to receive the product.

Precautions:

Do not use in the following situations:

- allergy to thalidomide or any of its ingredients
- neuritis, moderate to severe
- pregnancy or the possibility of pregnancy

Use with caution in the following situations:

- HIV infection
- low blood pressure
- neuritis, preexisting

Pregnancy: Do not use during pregnancy. The risk of use in a pregnant woman clearly outweighs any possible benefit. If thalidomide is taken during pregnancy, it can cause severe birth defects or death to an unborn baby. Even a single dose (50 mg) taken by a pregnant woman can cause severe birth defects. When there is no alternative treatment, women of childbearing potential may be treated with thalidomide, provided adequate precautions are taken to avoid pregnancy. Women must commit either to abstain continuously from sexual intercourse or use 2 methods of reliable birth control, including at least 1 highly effective method (eg, IUD, hormonal contraception) and 1 additional effective method (eg, latex condom, diaphragm, cervical cap), beginning 4 weeks prior to initiating treatment with thalidomide, during therapy, and for 4 weeks following discontinuation of therapy. This should be done even when there has been a history of infertility, unless due to a hysterectomy or because the patient has been postmenopausal for at least 24 months.

Women of childbearing potential must have pregnancy testing (sensitivity of at least 50 mIU/mL). A written report of a negative pregnancy test must be obtained before the prescription is written. The test should be performed within the 24 hours before beginning thalidomide therapy and then weekly during the first month of therapy, then monthly thereafter in women with regular menstrual cycles or every 2 weeks in women with irregular menstrual cycles. Perform pregnancy testing and counseling if a patient misses her period or if there is any abnormality in menstrual bleeding. If pregnancy occurs during treatment, thalidomide must be discontinued immediately. Under these conditions, the patient should be referred to an OB/GYN experienced in reproductive toxicity for further evaluation and counseling.

Because it is not known whether thalidomide is present in the ejaculate of males receiving the drug, males receiving thalidomide must always use a latex condom when engaging in sexual activity with women of childbearing potential.

Breastfeeding: It is not known whether thalidomide appears in breast milk. A decision should be made whether to discontinue nursing or discontinue the drug, taking into account the importance of the drug to the mother. Consult your doctor before you begin breastfeeding.

Children: Safety and efficacy in children under 12 years of age have not been established.

Lab tests will be required before, during, and after treatment. Tests may include: Pregnancy tests, peripheral neuropathy detection, blood counts, and viral load in HIV patients.

Drug Interactions:

Tell your doctor or pharmacist if you are taking or planning to take any over-the-counter or prescription medications or dietary supplements with thalidomide. Doses of one or both drugs may need to be modified or a different drug may need to be prescribed. The following drugs may interact with thalidomide:

- alcohol
- barbiturates (eg, phenobarbital)
- chlorpromazine (eg, *Thorazine*)
- drugs associated with neuropathy (eg, isoniazid, amiodarone, clofibrate)
- reserpine

A variety of drugs (eg, protease inhibitors, phenytoin, carbamazepine, rifampin, rifabutin, griseofulvin, broad-spectrum antibiotics) may interact with oral contraceptives and render them less effective. This increases the risk of pregnancy.

Side Effects:

Every drug is capable of producing side effects. Many thalidomide users experience no, or minor, side effects. The frequency and severity of side effects depend on many factors including dose, duration of therapy, and individual susceptibility. Possible side effects include:

Nervous System: Agitation; dizziness; sleeplessness; nervousness; abnormal skin sensations; drowsiness; tremor; feeling of whirling motion; headache; dizziness when rising; numbness, tingling, or pain in hands or feet.

Skin: Acne; fungal skin inflammation; nail disorder; itching; rash; sweating.

Digestive Tract: Loss of appetite; stomach pain; constipation; diarrhea; dry mouth; gas; nausea; fungal infection (mouth); tooth pain.

Urinary and Reproductive Tract: Protein in urine; blood in urine; impotence.

Respiratory System: Sore throat; sinus infection; congested or runny nose.

Other: Anemia; swelling of feet or ankles; decreased white blood cell count; increased viral load (in HIV patients); low blood pressure; slow heart hate; accidental injury; weakness; back pain; infection; neck pain; neck stiffness; pain; liver function test abnormalities; chills; fever; general body discomfort; swollen glands.

Guidelines for Use:

- Thalidomide must only be administered in strict compliance with all of the terms outlined in the S.T.E.P.S. (System for Thalidomide Education and Prescribing Safety) program. Thalidomide may only be prescribed by prescribers registered with the S.T.E.P.S. program and only dispensed by pharmacists registered with the S.T.E.P.S. program.
- For an episode of cutaneous ENL, the recommended dose is 100 to 300 mg once daily with water, preferably at bedtime and at least 1 hour after the evening meal. Patients weighing less than 110 lbs. should be started at the low end of the dose range.
- In patients with a severe cutaneous ENL reaction, or in those who have previously required higher doses to control the reaction, thalidomide dosing may be initiated at higher doses, up to 400 mg once daily at bedtime or in divided doses with water, at least 1 hour after meals.
- Dosing with thalidomide should usually continue until signs and symptoms of active reaction have subsided, usually a period of at least 2 weeks. Patients may then be tapered off medication in 50 mg decrements every 2 to 4 weeks.
- Patients who have a documented history of requiring prolonged maintenance treatment to prevent the recurrence of cutaneous ENL or who flare during tapering off medication, should be maintained on the minimum dose necessary to control the reaction. Tapering off medication should be attempted every 3 to 6 months, in decrements of 50 mg every 2 to 4 weeks.

Guidelines for Use (cont.):

- Thalidomide should never be used by women who are pregnant or who could become pregnant while taking the drug.
- Women of childbearing potential must have pregnancy testing before and during therapy.
- Women must commit either to abstain continuously from sexual intercourse or use 2 methods of reliable birth control, including at least 1 highly effective method (eg, IUD, hormonal contraception) and 1 additional effective method (eg, latex condom, diaphragm, cervical cap), beginning 4 weeks prior to initiating treatment with thalidomide, during therapy, and continuing 4 weeks following discontinuation of therapy.
- Discontinue thalidomide immediately if pregnancy is suspected or identified.
- Males receiving thalidomide must always use a latex condom when engaging in sexual activity with women of childbearing potential.
- Women using oral contraceptives to prevent pregnancy should be aware that HIV-protease inhibitors, griseofulvin, rifampin, phenytoin, carbamazepine, and broad-spectrum antibiotic therapy can reduce the effectiveness of oral contraceptives.
- Thalidomide is known to cause nerve damage that may be permanent. Peripheral neuropathy is a common, potentially severe and irreversible, side effect of treatment. Symptoms (eg, numbness, tingling, or pain in the hands and feet) may occur after thalidomide treatment has been stopped and may resolve slowly or not at all. If symptoms develop, notify your physician immediately. If appropriate, your physician will discontinue thalidomide immediately to limit further damage. Testing at monthly intervals will be required for the first 3 months of therapy and periodically thereafter during treatment.
- Contact your doctor immediately if you experience a skin rash, fever, fast heartbeat, or low blood pressure. These may be signs of an allergic reaction and may necessitate therapy discontinuation.
- May cause drowsiness, dizziness, or blurred vision. Use caution while driving or performing other tasks requiring alertness, coordination, or physical dexterity until tolerance is determined. Patients should sit upright for a few minutes prior to standing up.
- May cause photosensitivity (sensitivity to sunlight). Avoid prolonged exposure to the sun or other forms of ultraviolet (UV) light (eg, tanning beds). Use sunscreens and wear protective clothing until tolerance is determined.
- In patients with moderate to severe neuritis associated with a severe ENL reaction, corticosteroids may be started along with thalidomide. Steroid usage may be tapered or discontinued when the neuritis has improved.
- Do NOT share this medication with anyone else.
- Patients taking thalidomide cannot donate blood. Male patients should not donate sperm.
- Lab tests will be required during therapy. Be sure to keep appointments.
- Store between 59° and 86°F. Protect from light.

If you have any questions, consult your doctor, pharmacist, or health care provider.

	Generic Name *Brand Name Example*	Supplied As	Generic Available
Rx	**Etanercept**		
	Enbrel	**Powder for injection:** 25 mg[1]	No

[1] Contains 0.9% benzyl alcohol.

Type of Drug:

Agent for rheumatoid arthritis.

How the Drug Works:

Etanercept binds to and inhibits one of the chemical mediators (tumor necrosis factor) that is responsible for the inflammation and joint destruction of rheumatoid arthritis.

Uses:

For reducing the signs and symptoms and delaying structural damage in patients with moderately to severely active rheumatoid arthritis. Etanercept can be used in combination with methotrexate in patients who do not respond adequately to methotrexate alone.

For reducing the signs and symptoms of moderately to severely active polyarticular-course juvenile rheumatoid arthritis in patients who have had an inadequate reponse to one or more disease-modifying antirheumatic drugs (DMARDs).

Unlabeled use(s): Occasionally doctors may prescribe entanercept for psoriatric arthritis or psoriasis.

Precautions:

Do not use in the following situations:

- allergy to etanercept or any of its ingredients
- infection, active
- sepsis (infection of blood)
- vaccines, live

Use with caution in the following situations:

- blood abnormalities, history of demylelinating disorders of the central nervous system (eg, multiple sclerosis)
- diabetes, poorly controlled
- immunosuppression

Immunosuppression: There is a possibility that etanercept may reduce the body's defense mechanism against infections and cancers. The safety and efficacy of etanercept in patients with immunosuppression or chronic infections have not been evaluated.

Pregnancy: There are no adequate and well-controlled studies in pregnant women. Use only if clearly needed and potential benefits to the mother outweigh the possible hazards to the fetus.

Breastfeeding: It is not known if etanercept appears in breast milk. A decision should be made whether to discontinue nursing or discontinue the drug, taking into account the importance of the drug to the mother. Consult your doctor before you begin breastfeeding.

Children: Safety and effectiveness have not been established in children under 4 years of age. Childhood immunizations should be up-to-date before starting etanercept therapy. Pediatric patients receiving etanercept who have a significant exposure to varicella virus (chickenpox) should temporarily stop etanercept therapy and be evaluated for treatment with varicella-zoster immune globulin.

Elderly: No overall differences in safety or effectiveness were observed in elderly patients compared with younger patients. Because there is a higher incidence of infections in the elderly population, caution should be used in treating the elderly.

Drug Interactions:

Tell your doctor or pharmacist if you are taking or are planning to take any over-the-counter or prescription medications or dietary supplements while taking etanercept. Doses of one or both drugs may need to be modified or a different drug may need to be prescribed. To date, there have been no drug interaction studies.

Side Effects:

Every drug is capable of producing side effects. Many etanercept users experience no, or minor, side effects. The frequency and severity of side effects depend on many factors including dose, duration of therapy, and individual susceptibility. Possible side effects include:

Injection Site Reaction: Mild to moderate redness; itching; pain; swelling.

Digestive Tract: Stomach pain; indigestion; vomiting; nausea.

Nervous System: Headache; dizziness.

Respiratory System: Upper respiratory tract infection; sinus infection; bronchitis; pneumonia; difficulty breathing; runny nose; cough.

Other: Kidney, joint, skin, bone, blood, or wound infection; foot abscess; leg ulcer; rash; sore throat; skin or mouth ulcer; hair loss; weakness; swelling of the feet or ankles.

Guidelines for Use:

- Dosage is individualized. Use exactly as prescribed.
- Etanercept is intended for use under the guidance and supervision of a physician. Patients may self-inject only if their physician determines that it is appropriate, and with medical follow-up as necessary after proper training in injection technique.
- Carefully follow the storage, preparation, administration, and disposal techniques taught to you by your health care provider.
- The usual dosage for adults is 25 mg subcutaneously (beneath the skin) twice weekly.
- The usual dosage for children is 0.4 mg/kg (maximum dose 25 mg) subcutaneously twice weekly for 3 months in patients 4 to 17 years of age.
- Doses should be separated by 72 to 96 hours and injection sites should be rotated. New injections should be given at least 1 inch from an old site and never into areas where the skin is tender, bruised, red, or hard.
- Visually inspect the solution for particles or discoloration before use. Do not use if the solution is discolored, cloudy, or has particles.
- Contact your doctor immediately if you experience persistent fever, bruising, bleeding, or pale skin while taking this medicine.
- Stop taking etanercept and contact your doctor immediately if an anaphylactic reaction or other serious allergic reaction occurs.
- If you are sensitive to latex, do not handle the needle cover of the syringe containing the diluent.
- Live vaccines should not be given concurrently with etanercept.
- Juvenile arthritis patients should be up-to-date with all immunizations prior to initiating therapy with etanercept.
- Methotrexate, corticosteroids (eg, prednisone), salicylates, nonsteroidal anti-inflammatory drugs (NSAIDs), or analgesics may be continued during treatment with etanercept.
- Injection-site reactions generally occur in the first month of use and subsequently decrease in frequency. The duration of reactions is typically 3 to 5 days.
- Improvement in symptoms may be noted within 1 to 2 weeks of starting therapy but, in some cases, may take up to 3 months.
- Arthritis symptoms will recur, usually within 1 month, following discontinuation of etanercept.
- Dose tray must be refrigerated at 36° to 46°F. Do not freeze. Reconstituted solution must be refrigerated and used within 6 hours of mixing. Do not use a dose tray beyond the date stamped on the carton.

If you have any questions, consult your doctor, pharmacist, or health care provider.

	Generic Name *Brand Name Examples*	Supplied As	Generic Available
Rx	**Leflunomide**		
	Arava	**Tablets:** 10 mg, 20 mg, 100 mg	No

Type of Drug:

Agent for treating active rheumatoid arthritis.

How the Drug Works:

Leflunomide appears to inhibit enzymes responsible for abnormal tissue development or growth. It may also have anti-inflammatory activity (reduces swelling, pain).

Uses:

For the treatment of active rheumatoid arthritis (RA) in adults to reduce signs and symptoms and to retard structural damage. May be used in conjunction with aspirin, nonsteroidal anti-inflammatory agents (NSAIDs), or low-dose corticosteroids (eg, prednisone).

Precautions:

Do not use in the following situations:

allergy to leflunomide or any of its ingredients
liver function impairment
positive hepatitis B or C serologies
pregnancy or the possibility of pregnancy

Use with caution in the following situations:

bone marrow dysplasia
immunodeficiency, severe
kidney disease
uncontrolled infections, severe

Pregnancy: Do not use during pregnancy or in women of childbearing potential who are not using reliable contraception. The risk of use in a pregnant woman clearly outweighs any possible benefit. Pregnancy must be excluded before the start of treatment, and patients must be fully counseled on the potential for serious risks, such as birth defects, to the fetus. Pregnancy must be avoided during treatment and prior to the completion of the drug elimination procedure after treatment. If there is any delay in the onset of menses or any other reason to suspect pregnancy, the physician must be notified immediately. In addition, to minimize any possible risk, men taking leflunomide who are considering fathering a child should discuss discontinuing use of leflunomide and completing the drug elimination procedure with their doctor.

Breastfeeding: It is not known if leflunomide appears in breast milk. Many drugs are excreted in breast milk and there is a potential for serious adverse reactions in nursing infants from leflunomide. The decision should be made whether to discontinue nursing or discontinue the drug, taking into account the importance of the drug to the mother. Consult your doctor before you begin breastfeeding.

Children: Safety and effectiveness in children have not been studied. Use of leflunomide in patients under 18 years of age is not recommended.

Lab tests may be required before, during, and after therapy. Tests may include liver enzymes and kidney function.

Drug Interactions:

Tell your doctor or pharmacist if you are taking or are planning to take any over-the-counter or prescription medications or dietary supplements while taking leflunomide. Doses of one or both drugs may need to be modified or a different drug may need to be prescribed. The following drugs and drug classes interact with leflunomide.

- charcoal
- cholestyramine (eg, *Questran*)
- hepatotoxic drugs (eg, methotrexate, isoniazid)
- immunosuppression medications (eg, systemic steroids, azathioprine, cyclosporine)
- NSAIDs (eg, ibuprofen, naproxen)
- rifampin (eg, *Rifadin*)
- tolbutamide (eg, *Orinase*)

Side Effects:

Every drug is capable or producing side effects. Many leflunomide users experience no, or minor, side effects. The frequency and severity of side effects depend on many factors including dose, duration of therapy, and individual susceptibility. Possible side effects include:

Digestive Tract: Stomach pain; appetite loss; diarrhea; indigestion; stomach or intestinal irritation; nausea; mouth ulcer; vomiting; gallstones; colitis; constipation; heartburn; gas; inflammation of gums; dark, bloody stools; mouth fungal infection; enlarged salivary gland; dry mouth; mouth inflammation; tooth disorder; taste changes.

Nervous System: Weakness; dizziness; headache; abnormal skin sensations; migraine; anxiety; depression; sleeplessness; nerve pain; sleep disorder; sweating; feeling of whirling motion.

Circulatory System: High blood pressure; chest pain; palpitations (pounding in the chest); fast heartbeat; blood vessel inflammation; varicose veins; anemia; flushing.

Respiratory System: Bronchitis; increased cough; respiratory tract infection; sore throat; pneumonia; runny nose; sinus infection; asthma; difficulty breathing; lung disorder.

Urinary and Reproductive Tract: Protein in urine; bladder inflammation; painful or difficult urination; blood in the urine; menstrual disorder; vaginal fungal infection; prostate disorder; urinary frequency; urinary tract infection.

Skin: Hair loss; rash; inflamed and itching skin; dry skin; acne; contact dermatitis; fungal skin infection; hair discoloration; skin nodule; subcutaneous nodule; rash; skin disorder; skin discoloration; skin ulcer; sweating; viral skin infection; nail disorder.

Eyes or Ocular: Blurred vision; cataract; eye inflammation; eye disorder.

Other: Abnormal liver enzymes, primarily ALT and AST; allergic reaction; flu-like syndrome; infection; accidental injury; muscle, back, neck, joint, pelvic, or bone pain; low blood potassium levels; weight loss; leg cramps; joint disorder; abscess; cyst; hernia; general body discomfort; hyperthyroidism; unusual bruising; swelling of arms and legs; hyperlipidemia; bursitis; muscle cramps; bone necrosis; tendon rupture; fever; high blood sugar levels; nosebleed; abnormal muscle enzymes.

Guidelines for Use:

- A loading dose is needed to provide a more rapid beneficial effect. The usual recommended starting dosage is one (1) 100 mg tablet per day for 3 days.
- Following the loading dose, the usual daily dosage is one (1) 20 mg tablet per day. Daily doses higher than 20 mg are not recommended due to increased risk of side effects.
- If dosing at 20 mg/day is not well tolerated, the dose may be decreased to 10 mg/day.
- Aspirin, nonsteroidal anti-inflammatory agents (eg, ibuprofen), or low-dose corticosteroids (eg, prednisone) may be continued during therapy with leflunomide.
- The combined use of leflunomide with antimalarials (eg, hydroxychloroquine), injectable or oral gold, D penicillamine, azathioprine, or methotrexate has not been adequately studied.
- Do not use if you are pregnant or may become pregnant. Pregnancy must be excluded before the start of treatment. Pregnancy must also be avoided prior to the completion of the drug elimination procedure after treatment. If there is any reason to suspect pregnancy, the physician must be notified immediately.
- To minimize any possible risk to the fetus, men taking leflunomide who are considering fathering a child should discuss discontinuing use of leflunomide with their doctor.
- There is a potential for immunosuppression with leflunomide.
- The risk of malignancy or lymphoproliferative disorders from the immunosuppression is not known.
- Vaccination with live vaccines during leflunomide therapy is not recommended.
- Beneficial effects should be noted within 1 month of starting therapy, but further improvement in symptoms may progress during the first 6 months of therapy.
- Leflunomide is converted in the body to a very long-acting byproduct (metabolite) which may remain in the body for up to 2 years following discontinuation of therapy. In situations in which the metabolite needs to be eliminated more rapidly (eg, planned pregnancy or toxicity), a drug elimination procedure using cholestyramine will need to be used.
- Lab tests will be required before, during, and after therapy. Be sure to keep appointments.
- Store at controlled room temperature (59° to 86°F). Protect from light.

If you have any questions, consult your doctor, pharmacist, or health care provider.

Glucose (Blood) Tests, 1749

Glucose (Urine) Tests, 1753

Ketone Tests, 1757

Occult Blood Tests, 1760

Ovulation Tests, 1763

Pregnancy Tests, 1765

Protein Tests, 1767

Urinary Tract Infection Tests, 1769

Miscellaneous (Urine) Tests, 1771

	Brand Name Examples	Supplied As	Test For
otc	*Accu-Chek Advantage*	**Test Strips:** For blood	Glucose meter (*Accu-Chek*)
otc	*Chemstrip bG*	**Test Strips:** For blood	Visual glucose and glucose meter (*Accu-Chek*)
otc	*Dextrostix, Glucostix*	**Test Strips:** For blood	Visual glucose and glucose meter (*Glucometer*)
otc	*Diascan*	**Test Strips:** For blood	Visual glucose and glucose meter (*Diascan*)
otc	*Glucofilm, Glucometer Elite, Glucometer Encore*	**Test Strips:** For blood	Glucose meter (*Glucometer*)
otc	*One Touch*	**Test Strips:** For blood	Glucose meter (*One Touch*)
otc	*First Choice*	**Test Strips:** For blood	Glucose meter (*Diascan, Glucometer, One Touch*)
otc	*Tracer bG*	**Test Strips:** For blood	Glucose meter (*Tracer*)

Diagnostic or therapeutic decisions should not be based on a single test result. If you have any questions regarding your test results, contact your doctor. For information on diabetes and diabetes medications, see insulin and sulfonylureas.

Type of Drug:

For detection of glucose (sugar) in blood.

How the Drug Works:

Specially treated test strips indicate the blood glucose concentration. Regular monitoring of glucose aids in the control of diabetes. It will help determine medication, dietary and exercise needs and help decrease the complications (eg, neuropathies, retinopathies) and problems during pregnancy.

Uses:

To monitor blood glucose levels in diabetics. To aid in control of the condition.

To aid in determining medication regimes, diet, and exercise programs for diabetics.

To help prevent development of complications during pregnancy.

Precautions:

Do not use in the following situations:
dehydration, severe
illness, severe
internal use
shock

Normal blood glucose levels — Approximate ranges:

Nondiabetic fasting adults – 60 to 110 mg/dL.

Nondiabetic adults (1 to 2 hours after eating) – 110 to 180 mg/dL.

Diabetics – Results will vary depending on diet, medication dose, exercise, etc. Consult your doctor to determine your target blood glucose level.

Newborns – Not all tests strips or glucose meters are intended for testing newborn blood samples. Read manufacturers' instructions carefully.

Specimen collection and handling: All blood glucose test strips require a finger or earlobe stick. An automatic lancet device punctures the skin to obtain a single drop of blood. A manual lancet is more painful and laceration size and puncture depth cannot be predicted. These are important because they control the volume of the drop of blood. The size of the test pad varies among manufacturers. It must be completely covered with blood.

A single drop of blood is placed on the test strip. Begin timing when the test pad is covered completely. In some tests, the blood drop is wiped from the test strip at the end of the timed period. Timing is critical. The wiping or blotting technique and the recommended tissue paper or cotton for blotting may vary by manufacturer. The test strip is placed in the glucose meter. The results are read from the meter display. The visual test is read against the color key.

Storage and handling: A bottle of test strips can be used for 4 months after being opened. Always write the date the bottle is first opened on the bottle label. Never use the test strips past the expiration date indicated on the bottle label or foil packet. Use of strips beyond the expiration date may yield inaccurate results.

Keep unused test strips in the original bottle with cap tightly closed. Always replace the cap immediately and tightly. Never transfer test strips to another bottle.

Leave the drying agent in the bottle. The drying agent absorbs moisture and keeps the strips dry. Never put cotton or other material in the bottle. Do not use discolored strips. Keep your fingers or other objects from touching the test pads before testing. Touching the pads could cause inaccurate test results.

Keep strip vial away from small children. A child could choke on the cap or drying agent, which could be harmful if swallowed.

Store at room temperature (59° to 86°F). Do not store bottle in direct sunlight. Do not freeze. Do not store in cabinets with bleach or products containing bleach.

Drug Interactions:

Tell your doctor or pharmacist if you are taking or planning to take any over-the-counter or prescription medications or dietary supplements while testing for blood glucose. The following drugs and drug classes may interact with the test to cause questionable results:

acetaminophen (eg, *Tylenol*)
aspirin (large amounts)
dopamine (large amounts)
fluoride
methyldopa (large amounts)
vitamin C

Guidelines for Use:

- Follow instructions on the label exactly.
- Monitor blood for glucose as prescribed. Monitor urine ketones if your blood glucose level has been greater than 300 mg/dL for 2 consecutive blood glucose determinations.
- Blood glucose monitoring is recommended to achieve normal blood sugar levels. Keep track of your blood glucose results so that adjustments in your treatment program can be made more easily.
- Participate in a thorough diabetes education program so that you understand diabetes and all aspects of its treatment, including diet, exercise, personal hygiene and how to self-monitor blood glucose.
- Apply the blood drop, time the reaction, blot the test pads and read the test results the same way each time you do the test.
- *Diabetics — Monitor glucose:*
  When you have a cold, the flu or any other kind of illness.
  When you "feel" the signs of low or high blood sugar (greater than 240 mg/dL) or when your blood sugar is well over the range your doctor has set for you (if you do blood glucose monitoring).
  When you are under unusual physical or emotional stress.
  During pregnancy or after a testing pattern has been established with your doctor or educator.
- Have all the materials you need before beginning the test: Test strips, timer (stop-watch or watch with a second hand), sterile lancet, cotton or rayon balls, alcohol wipes, and glucose meter.
- Color vision is needed to properly read visual, but not meter, test results. Have someone else confirm the visual test results if in doubt.
- Quality control and sample tests may be required before testing.
- If test results seem questionable, check expiration date on the label, repeat the test using a new test strip, run controls, check glucose meter and check procedure (timing).
- If you are unable to identify the cause of a low or high test result, contact your doctor or diabetes educator. Know the symptoms of hyperglycemia (high blood sugar), which include thirst, hunger and frequent and excessive urination and those of hypoglycemia (low blood sugar), which include trembling, sweating, blurred vision, rapid heartbeat, and tingling or numbness around mouth or fingertips.
- If you experience stomach pain, vomiting or difficulty breathing, contact your doctor immediately.
- Individuals with high uric acid, bilirubin cholesterol, triglyceride or hematocrit levels may have lowered glucose levels.
- Diabetes education may be obtained through your local chapter of the American Diabetes Association.

If you have any questions, consult your doctor, pharmacist, or health care provider.

	Brand Name Examples	Supplied As	Test For
otc	*Chemstrip uGK, Keto-Diastix*	**Test strips:** for urine	Glucose and ketones (acetoacetic acid)
otc	*Chemstrip 2GP*	**Test strips:** for urine	Glucose and protein
otc	*Chemstrip bG, Clinistix, Diastix*	**Test strips:** for urine	Glucose
otc	*Clinitest*	**Tablets:** for urine	Glucose, lactose, fructose, galactose and pentose

Diagnostic or therapeutic decisions should not be based on a single test result. If you have any questions regarding your test results, contact your doctor. For information on diabetes and diabetes medications see insulin and sulfonylureas.

Type of Drug:

For detection of glucose (sugar) in urine.

How the Drug Works:

Glucose does not normally appear in the urine, but when too much glucose builds up in the blood, the excess spills over from the kidney into the urine where it can be detected by specially designed plastic test strips and reagent tablets containing chemicals which detect glucose in urine. Color changes occur according to the amount of sugar present.

Regular monitoring of glucose levels aids in the control of diabetes. It will help determine medication, exercise and dietary needs and help decrease complications (eg, kidney and eye problems) and problems during pregnancy.

Ketones appear in the urine when the body breaks down body fats to use as a source of energy or food. This can occur in fasting individuals, out-of-control diabetics and individuals on starvation diets.

Proteins in the urine may be an early sign of kidney disease.

Uses:

To detect glucose in urine.

To aid diabetics in monitoring medication regimens, diet and exercise programs.

To help prevent the development of complications and problems during pregnancy.

Precautions:

Not for internal use.

Avoid contact with skin, mucous membranes or clothing. If contact occurs, flush the affected area with large amounts of water. If test strips, tape, or tablets are eaten or rubbed in the eyes, contact your doctor or local poison control center immediately. If eaten, do not induce vomiting; instead, drink large amounts of water or milk. If contact with the eyes occurs, flush with water for 15 minutes. Get prompt medical attention.

Specimen collection and handling: Collect fresh urine in a clean, dry container and test as soon as possible. (An alternate method is to pass the test strips directly through the urine stream). If testing cannot be done within an hour after collection, refrigerate. Let it return to room temperature before testing. Prolonged exposure of unpreserved urine to room temperature (59° to 86°F) may result in bacterial contamination and bacterial consumption of the glucose. Urine preservatives may also affect the accuracy of test results.

Storage and handling:

For bottled strips – Store at room temperature (59° to 86 F). Do not store the bottle in direct sunlight. Protect from light, heat, and moisture. Keep unused test strips in the original bottle with the cap tightly closed. Always replace the cap immediately and tightly. A new bottle of test strips can be used for 6 months after first being opened. Always write the date you first opened the bottle on the bottle label. Do not use the product after the expiration date. Use of strips beyond the expiration date may yield inaccurate test results. Never transfer strips to another bottle. Do not remove drying agent from the bottle. The agent absorbs moisture and keeps the strips dry. Never put cotton or other materials in the bottle. If test areas are discolored or darkened, throw the strip away and use a strip from a new bottle.

For tablets – Tablets have prolonged stability in the unopened container if stored at room temperature between 59° and 86°F. Do not refrigerate. Do not store in direct sunlight. Once the bottle is opened, protect from moisture. Excessive moisture may cause a chemical reaction and a bottle explosion may occur. Use tablets on a regular basis and do not store for extended periods of time after the bottle is opened. Recap the bottle tightly immediately after removing a tablet. Tablets in foil must be used immediately upon opening. Protect tablets from light, heat and moisture. Do not open the bottle in a steamy bathroom. Moisture causes tablets to turn a deeper shade of blue. If tablets darken or if test results seem questionable or inconsistent with expected findings:
Confirm that product is within expiration date shown on label or foil. Check performance with a positive control. If proper result is not obtained, discard and retest with a fresh tablet.

Tablets: Sugars other than glucose will cause a positive test result. These sugars include: Lactose, fructose, galactose, and pentose.

Ketones: High levels of ketones may cause false positive test results for urine containing small amounts of glucose.

Drug Interactions:

Tell your doctor or pharmacist if you are taking or planning to take any over-the-counter or prescription medication or dietary supplements while testing for urine glucose. The following drugs and drug classes may interact with the test to cause questionable results:

aspirin (large amounts)
nalidixic acid *(NegGram)*
nitrofurantoin (eg, *Furadantin)*
phenazopyridine (eg,*Pyridium)*
riboflavin
sulfa drugs (eg, sulfonamides)
vitamin C (ascorbic acid)

Clinitest only —

cephalosporins (eg, cephalexin)
penicillin
probenecid (eg, *Benemid)*
x-ray contrast media (IV)

Consider all drug interactions reported for protein test strips and ketone test strips when appropriate.

Guidelines for Use:

- Follow instructions on the label exactly.
- Glucose is not normally detected in urine.
- Monitor urine for glucose and ketones as prescribed. Monitor urine ketones if your biood glucose level has been greater than 300 mg/dL for 2 consecutive blood glucose determinations. Blood glucose monitoring is recommended to achieve normal blood sugar levels. Keep track of your blood glucose results so that adjustments in your treatment program can be made more easily.
- Participate in a thorough diabetes education program so that you understand diabetes and all aspects of its treatment, including diet, exercise, personal hygiene, and how to self-monitor blood or urine glucose.
- *Diabetics — Monitor glucose:*
  When you have a cold, the flu or any other kind of illness.
  When you "feel" the signs of high blood sugar (more than 240 mg/dL) or when your blood sugar is well over the range your doctor has set for you (if you do blood glucose monitoring).
  When you are under unusual physical or emotional stress.
  During pregnancy after a testing pattern has been established with your doctor or educator.
- Have all the materials you need before beginning the test: Test strips, timer (stopwatch or watch with a second hand), and a clean dry container.
- Color vision is needed to properly read test results. Have someone else confirm the test results if in doubt.
- If test results seem questionable, check expiration date on the label, repeat the test using a new test strip or tablet and a fresh urine specimen.
- If your are unable to identify the cause of a low or high test result, contact your doctor or diabetes educator. Know the symptoms of hyperglycemia (high blood sugar), which include thirst, hunger and frequent and excessive urination and those of hypoglycemia (low blood sugar), which include trembling, sweating, blurred vision, rapid heartbeat, and tingling or numbness around mouth or fingertips.
- Individuals with high uric acid, bilirubin cholesterol, triglyceride, or hematocrit levels may have lowered glucose levels.
- Diabetes education may be obtained through your local chapter of the American Diabetes Association.
- Some of these items can cause burns. Avoid contact with skin, eyes, mucous membranes, and clothing. Keep away from children.

If you have any questions, consult your doctor, pharmacist, or health care provider.

	Brand Name Examples	Supplied As	Test For
otc	*Acetest*	**Tablets:** For blood, serum, plasma, or urine	Acetoacetic acid and acetone
otc	*Chemstrip K*	**Test strips:** For urine	Acetoacetic acid and acetone
otc	*Ketostix*	**Test strips:** For urine	Acetoacetic acid

Diagnostic or therapeutic decisions should not be based on a single test result. If you have any questions regarding your test results, contact your doctor.

Type of Drug:

For detection of ketones (acetone, acetoacetate, or acetoacetic acid, also known as "ketone bodies" or "ketones").

How the Drug Works:

Specially treated tablets *(Acetest)* or plastic test strips *(Chemstrip K, Ketostix)* detect the presence of ketones in the urine and blood (*Acetest* only). Ketones are substances that are formed when the body breaks down fats and carbohydrates for energy or food. When there are too many ketones in the body, they spill over into the urine. Ketones may be found in the urine of people who are fasting, on starvation diets, or in diabetics who have a very high blood sugar level because of lack of insulin. Ketones are not present in normal urine.

Uses:

To detect ketones in urine.

To monitor for diabetic ketoacidosis, a complication of diabetes that may lead to diabetic coma. Ketoacidosis occurs in uncontrolled diabetes.

Acetest only — To detect ketones in urine and in blood.

Precautions:

Not for internal use. Do not chew or swallow.

Do not touch the testing patch of test strips with skin or mucous membranes. If contact occurs, flush the affected area with large amounts of water. If test pads are eaten or rubbed in the eyes, contact your doctor immediately.

Liver and kidney function tests requiring the administration of phthalein compounds such as bromsulfophthalein, phenolsulfonphthalein (PSP), or phenylketones (large quantities) may interfere with the ketone tests.

Specimen collection and preparations: Collect fresh urine in clean dry container and test as soon as possible. If testing cannot be done within an hour, refrigerate immediately. Let urine return to room temperature

(59° to 86°F) before testing. Mix urine thoroughly before testing. Urine that is not tested right away or use of urine preservatives may affect test results.

Storage and handling:

For Acetest tablets – These tablets are stable in the unopened container if stored at temperatures between 59° and 86°F. Protect from heat, moisture, and light. Once opened, stability is decreased with exposure to moisture, heat, and light. The bottle must be recapped promptly after removing a tablet. Tablets should be used on a regular basis and not stored for an extended period of time after the bottle is opened. Tan-to-brown discoloration or darkening of the tablet is an indication of deterioration.

For ChemStrip K – Avoid contact with skin and mucous membranes. Keep unused test strips in the original bottle with the cap tightly closed. *ChemStrip K* will remain stable in the original capped vial until the listed expiration date. To avoid moisture, replace the original stopper, which contains a drying agent, immediately after use. Store at room temperature (59° to 86°F). Protect from heat, moisure, and light. Do not freeze.

For Ketostix – Keep fingers or other objects from touching the reagent area before testing. Store at room temperatures between 59° and 86°F. Protect from heat, moisture, and light. Keep unused test strips in the original bottle with the cap tightly closed. Always replace the cap immediately and tightly. A new bottle can be used for 6 months. Always write the date you first opened the bottle on the bottle label. Do not use the strips after the expiration date has passed. Never transfer strips to another bottle. Do not remove the drying agent from bottle. It absorbs moisture and keeps the strips dry. Never put cotton or other materials in the bottle. If the reagent area becomes discolored or darkened, throw the strip away and use a strip from a new bottle. If using the individual foil-wrapped strips, do not remove strips until just prior to use.

Drug Interactions:

Tell your doctor or pharmacist if you are taking or if you are planning to take any over-the-counter or prescription medications or dietary supplements while testing for ketones. The following drugs and drug classes interact with the tests to cause questionable results.

8-hydroxyquinolone
levodopa (eg, *Larodopa)*
mesna *(Mesnex)*
nitrofurantoin (*Furadantin)*
phenazopyridine (eg, *Pyridium)*
phenylketone (see Precautions)
phthalein compounds (eg, bromsulfophthalein) (see Precautions)
sulfhydryls
sulfisoxazole and phenazopyridine (eg, *Azo-Sulfisoxazole)*
vitamin B_2 (riboflavin)

Guidelines for Use:

- Follow the instructions on the label EXACTLY.
- Monitor urine for glucose and ketones as prescribed. Monitor urine ketones especially if your blood glucose level has been more than 250 mg/dL for 2 consecutive blood glucose determinations. Blood glucose monitoring is essential to achieve normal blood sugar levels. Keep track of your blood glucose results so that adjustments in your treatment program can be made more easily.
- Ketones are not present in normal urine. Ketones in urine could be a sign of illness, stress, or poor diabetes control. Immediately report any positive test result to your doctor.
- Have all of the materials you need before beginning the test: Test strips or tablets, timer (stopwatch or watch with second hand), and a clean dry container. For *Acetest* you will need a dropper and a clean, white piece of paper.
- Color vision is needed to properly read test results. Have someone else confirm results if in doubt.
- If test results seem questionable, confirm that product is within the expiration date on the bottle. Repeat the test using a new test strip or tablet and fresh urine specimen.
- *Acetest* — When a drop of urine is put onto a tablet, the drop should be absorbed within 30 seconds. If absorption takes more than 30 seconds, the tablets have been exposed to moisture and may not give good results.
- As with all laboratory tests, definitive diagnostic or therapeutic decisions should not be based on any single result or method.
- Patients with diabetes should test for ketones:

  When you have a cold, the flu, or any other kind of illness.

  When your urine sugar test results show you are spilling large amounts of sugar (at least 2% for at least 2 tests in a row or several days).

  When you feel the signs of high blood sugar (more than 240 mg/dL) or when your blood sugar is well over the range your doctor or educator has set for you.

  When you are under unusual physical or emotional stress.

  Regularly during pregnancy.
- Participate in a diabetes education program so that you understand diabetes and all aspects of its treatment, including diet, exercise, personal hygiene, and how to self-monitor blood glucose.
- Diabetes education materials may be obtained through your local chapter of the American Diabetes Association.
- Do not use opened or unopened product after expiration date.
- For storage and stability see Precautions.

If you have any questions, consult your doctor, pharmacist, or health care provider.

	Brand Name Examples	Supplied As	Test For
otc	*ColoCare*[1]	**Pads:** For toilet bowl	Occult blood
otc	*ColoScreen*[2], *ColoScreen-ES*[2]	**Slides:** For stool	
otc	*EZ Detect*[1]	**Tissue:** For toilet bowl	
otc	*Heme-Chek*[2]	**Slides:** For stool	
otc	*Hemoccult*[2]	**Slides:** For stool	
otc	*Hemoccult SENSA*[2]	**Slides:** For stool	

[1] Flushable.
[2] Return test results to doctor's office.

Diagnostic or therapeutic decisions should not be based on a single test result. If you have any questions regarding your test results, contact your doctor.

Type of Drug:

For detection of occult blood ("hidden" blood or blood that is difficult to see) in the stool (feces).

How the Drug Works:

Tests for occult blood screen for unseen blood cells in the stool itself or in the toilet water around the stool. Specially treated pads turn a different color in the presence of blood.

Occult blood in the stool (feces) may be an indication of a disease in the digestive or gastrointestinal tract such as hemorrhoids, diverticulitis, fissures, ulcers, polyps, colitis, or colorectal cancer (cancer in colon or rectal area).

Uses:

To screen for early signs of digestive tract diseases, including ulcers, colitis, polyps, fissures, diverticulitis, hemorrhoids, and colorectal cancer.

Recommended for people older than 40 years of age and for those who have a personal or family history of lower intestinal disorders or colorectal cancers.

These tests *do not* replace regular physical and rectal examinations by your doctor. However, they may show the need for further examinations.

Precautions:

Not for internal use.

Diet: Eat a normal, well-balanced diet for 2 days before and throughout the testing period (eg, well-cooked poultry, raw beef, lamb), tuna fish, peanuts, high fiber foods such as bran cereal and popcorn, and plenty of raw or cooked lettuce, spinach, corn, prunes, grapes, plums, and apples.). Such a diet reduces the number of false positive results and at the same time the roughage helps to uncover "silent" lesions which may bleed only intermittently. Do not eat red or rare meat, horseradish, turnips, radishes, broccoli, cauliflower, cantaloupe, melons, or large amounts of citrus fruits. Consult your doctor before altering or discontinuing a special diet.

Do not use until 3 days after menstrual bleeding has ceased, or while you have bleeding hemorrhoids or constipation. Do not use any rectal ointments, suppositories, or certain medications (see Drug Interactions) for 2 days prior to or during the test period. Contact your doctor before stopping any drug therapy.

Kits containing a positive control package: Avoid contact with eyes, skin, clothing, heat, or open flame. In case of an accidental spill or direct contact, wash the affected area with large amounts of water. If ingested, administer large amounts of water. Do not induce vomiting. Call the poison control center.

Toilet cleaners, disinfectants, and deodorizers in the toilet bowl and tank can interfere with test results. Remove these items and flush repeatedly until water is clear.

Perform the test on 3 consecutive bowel movements. If the sequence is broken, continue the test until 3 bowel movements have been tested. Some digestive tract bleeding occurs intermittently. Checking 3 consecutive bowel movements will offer a better chance of finding lower intestinal bleeding.

Quality control tests or tests for toilet water quality may be required. Read individual test directions carefully.

Specimen collection and preparation of slides, collection papers, and filter papers returned to doctor's office:
1. Provide all information requested on outside of packet: Name, address, date, doctor, etc.
2. Collect sample from the toilet bowl.
3. Using the applicator provided, apply a thin smear to the slide or paper.
4. Close the cover. Place slide away from heat and light.
5. Mail or deliver to doctor's office.

Specimen collection and preparation of flushable tissue and pads: Carefully drop tissue or pad into toilet bowl. Wait the required length of time, then read the results as directed.

Drug Interactions:

Tell your doctor or pharmacist if you are taking or planning to take any over-the-counter or prescription medications or dietary supplements while testing for occult blood. The following drugs and drug classes may interact with the test, leading to questionable results.

anticoagulants (eg, warfarin)
antimetabolites (eg, methotrexate)
aspirin
cancer chemotherapeutic drugs
corticosteroids (eg, hydrocortisone)
dipyridamole (eg, *Persantine*)

iron
mineral oil
nonsteroidal anti-inflammatory drugs (eg, indomethacin)
phenylbutazone (eg, *Butazolidin)*
reserpine (eg, *Serpasil)*
vitamin C (ascorbic acid), largeamounts

Guidelines for Use:

- Read the product instructions carefully prior to testing. Follow the directions on the package label EXACTLY.
- A positive test indicates the presence of blood but does not necessarily mean that a serious condition exists. Discuss all positive test results with your doctor.
- *False negative results* (a false reading even though blood is actually present) can be caused by an improper sampling technique, ingestion of more than 250 mg a day of vitamin C (ascorbic acid), large amounts of citrus fruits, use of expired reagents or kits that have been improperly stored, or lesions not bleeding at the time of the test.
- *False positive results* (a positive reading even though no blood is actually present) can be caused by drugs causing gastrointestinal bleeding (see Drug Interactions), red or rare meat, foods such as horseradish, turnips, broccoli, cauliflower, or melons (eg, cantaloupe), toilet bowl cleaners, and sources of nongastrointestinal bleeding such as nosebleeds, menstruation, and hematuria (blood in the urine).
- The best results are achieved when 3 consecutive stool specimens are tested.
- Follow special diet for 2 days prior to testing (see Precautions). Do not change diet or prescription medications without first discussing it with your doctor.
- Have all the materials you need on hand before beginning the test: Testing package, pencil or pen, timer (stopwatch or watch with a second hand), and a clean, dry container.
- For some tests, color vision may be needed to properly read the test results. Have someone else confirm results if in doubt.
- Hema-Chek *slide test* — Use a clean container or toilet paper to collect sample. Do not collect from the toilet bowl.
- Store slide tests at room temperature in a dry place. Protect from heat and light. Keep bottle tightly closed.
- *Pad and tissue tests* —
  Remove all toilet cleaners and disinfectants from the toilet bowl and tank. Flush several times.
  Flush the toilet after urinating. Then have bowel movement.
  Do not throw toilet paper in toilet following bowel movement.
  Protect from heat, sunlight, or fluorescent light. Store at room temperature (59° to 86°F). Do not store in the bathroom or in an area where there is a high humidity or moisture level. Do not store in the refrigerator or in an area where the temperature will exceed 86°F. Keep out of the reach of children. Do not use after expiration date on pouch.

If you have any questions, consult your doctor, pharmacist, or health care provider.

	Brand Name Examples	Supplied As	Test For
otc	*Answer Quick & Simple*	**Test kit:** For urine (5 days)	Luteinizing hormone
otc	*ClearPlan Easy*	**Test kit:** For urine (5 days)	
otc	*First Response Ovulation Predictor*	**Test kit:** For urine (5 days)	
otc	*Healthcheck Ovulation Detector*	**Test kit:** For urine (6 days)	
otc	*OvuKIT Self-Test*	**Test kit:** For urine (9 days)	
otc	*OvuQUICK Self-Test*	**Test kit:** For urine (6 days)	
otc	*OvuSign*	**Test kit:** For urine (7 days)	
otc	*SureStep*	**Test kit:** For urine (5 days)	

Diagnostic or therapeutic decisions should not be based on a single test result. If you have any questions regarding your test results, contact your doctor.

Type of Drug:

Tests to predict time of ovulation and fertility.

How the Drug Works:

Ovulation predictor kits test for the presence of luteinizing hormone (LH) in the urine. The pituitary gland increases LH production 12 to 16 days before menstruation begins. This "LH surge" causes an ovarian follicle to rupture and releases a mature egg in 1 to 1.5 days (24 to 40 hours). The onset of the LH surge (and therefore ovulation) can be estimated by using the ovulation predictor tests for several days.

An egg survives for 12 to 24 hours after ovulation. If the egg and sperm are not united shortly after ovulation, conception will not occur.

It is possible the LH surge and ovulation will not occur during every menstrual cycle. Onset of menstrual bleeding does not always mean ovulation has occurred.

Uses:

To aid in planning pregnancy; to determine fertile time of menstrual cycle.

Precautions:

Not for internal use.

Menopause: Women entering menopause may have high LH levels during their entire menstrual cycle.

Day for beginning testing is determined by the approximate length of the menstrual cycle, the first day being the onset of bleeding (even spotting), the last being the day before bleeding onset. Test kits vary regarding the date to begin testing. Follow manufacturers' instructions carefully.

Specimen collection and handling: Collect urine in the urine cup from the kit or in a clean, dry container. If testing cannot be done in 3 to 4 hours after collecting the urine specimen, cover and refrigerate immediately. Let it return to room temperature before testing. Do not freeze specimen. For best results, do the test the same day as the urine was collected.

Time: Allow enough time to complete the test.

Drug Interactions:

Tell your doctor or pharmacist if you are taking or if you are planning to take any over-the-counter or prescription medications or dietary supplements while testing for LH surge (ovulation). The following drugs and drug classes may interact with the test to cause questionable results:

thyroid stimulating hormone (eg, *Thyrogen)*
hCG injection (eg, *A.P.L., Profasi HP)*
menopropins (*Pergonal)*
steroids (eg, prednisone)

Guidelines for Use:

- *Do not use as a contraceptive aid.* Results cannot guarantee that pregnancy will not occur.
- Follow the directions on the label EXACTLY.
- Results may not be accurate during menopause, pregnancy, in the presence of ovarian cysts, or after an abortion.
- Not all women ovulate during every menstrual cycle.
- Drinking large quantities of water before the test may dilute the urine and interfere with the results.
- Have all the materials you need on hand before beginning the test: Test kit, timer (second hand and 30-minute timer), clean dry container, and pen or pencil for dating test. Be near a cold water faucet.
- Do test at the same time in the same room with the same lighting each day, if possible. It is best to test in the mid-morning (10 a.m.).
- Color vision is needed to properly read the test results. Have someone else confirm results if in doubt.
- Look for the FIRST noticeable change in color, not the darkest.

If you have any questions, consult your doctor, pharmacist, or health care provider.

	Brand Name Examples	Supplied As	Test For
otc	*Answer Plus, Answer Quick & Simple, Conceive Pregnancy, Fact Plus, Fortel Plus, RapidVue*	**Test Kit**	Human chorionic gonadotropin
otc	*Advance, Clearblue Easy, e.p.t. Quick Stick, First Response, One Step Midstream, QTest*	**Test Stick**	Human chorionic gonadotropin
otc	*Nimbus Quick Strip*	**Test Strips**	Human chorionic gonadotropin
otc	*Pregnosis*	**Slide Tests**	Human chorionic gonadotropin

Type of Drug:
For detection of pregnancy.

How the Drug Works:
Pregnancy home tests detect the presence of human chorionic gonadotropin (HCG) in the urine. HCG is a hormone produced by the placenta during pregnancy. HCG will cause menstruation to stop. HCG slowly builds up in the body and appears in measurable levels in the urine 1 to 3 days after the first missed period.

Uses:
To detect pregnancy.

Precautions:
Not for internal use.

Use only once and discard.

False results: False positive results (test result is positive when no pregnancy actually exists) and false negative results (pregnancy is present, but test result is negative) may occur: during menopause; when protein, blood or excessive thyroid hormone are present in the urine; with cold urine; in the presence of an ovarian cyst or ectopic pregnancy (outside the uterus); with certain drugs (see Drug Interactions); performing the test too early; or when the test directions are not followed exactly.

Specimen collection and preparation: Collect fresh urine in a clean dry container or container provided. Do not use a wax cup. (Some products, however, may not require urine collection in a container.) For the best results, the sample should be the first morning urine. If testing cannot be done immediately, cover and refrigerate. Do not freeze. Let urine return to room temperature before testing. Do not mix or shake urine. Use the urine at the top of the container. Be sure to test the urine the same day.

Time: Depending on the test kit chosen, the time required for the test is often less than 5 minutes. Most test kits require 3 minutes or less to complete. Allow enough time to complete the test.

Drug Interactions:

Tell your doctor or pharmacist if you are taking or if you are planning to take any over-the-counter or prescription medications or dietary supplements while testing for pregnancy. The following drugs and drug classes may interact with the test to cause questionable results.

anticonvulsants (eg, carbamazepine)
antiparkinson agents (eg, biperiden)
HCG (eg, *A.P.L., Profasi HP)*
methadone (eg, *Dolophine)*
oral contraceptives (eg, *Ortho-Novum)*
phenothiazines (eg, chlorpromazine)
steroids (eg, prednisone)

Guidelines for Use:

- Follow the instructions EXACTLY.
- For best results, use the first urine of the day.
- Consult your doctor or pharmacist if you are taking any medication (eg, birth control pills) which could cause questionable tests results.
- If urine is cloudy, pink or red or has a strong odor, do not do the test. Wait 1 to 2 days and try the test then.
- Read instructions before beginning the test. Have all of the materials you need on hand: test kit, clean dry container, timer, and sink with cold running water.
- If test results seem questionable, check the expiration date on the test kit and repeat the test. Follow directions exactly.
- *Negative results* — Recount the number of days since your last period. Retest in 3 to 7 days. It is possible that not enough HCG has accumulated to cause a positive result. If you still do not have your period, contact your doctor. A health condition other than pregnancy may be causing your missed periods.
- *Positive results* — Contact your doctor to confirm the test results.
- Regardless of test results, contact your doctor if there are any signs of pregnancy (eg, delayed menstrual cycle, morning sickness).
- For some tests, color vision may be needed to properly read test results. Have someone else confirm results if in doubt.

If you have any questions, consult your doctor, pharmacist, or health care provider.

Brand Name Examples	Supplied As	Test For
otc *Albustix, Chemstrip Micral*	**Test strips:** For urine	Protein

Type of Drug:

For detection of protein in urine.

How the Drug Works:

Specially treated plastic test strips can detect protein in urine (proteinuria), which can be an early sign of kidney disease. Protein is not usually detected in urine. However, occasionally people with normal kidney function may have "trace" urine protein results. Contact your doctor if test results are positive.

Uses:

To detect protein in the urine. To screen for early signs of kidney disease, eclampsia (toxemia) in pregnant women.

Precautions:

Not for internal use.

Specimen collection and preparation: Collect urine in a clean container according to product instructions and test it as soon as possible. If testing cannot be done within an hour, refrigerate immediately. Let it return to room temperature before testing.

Storage/handling: Keep all unused strips in original bottle. Transfer to any other container may cause deterioration. Do not remove drying agent from bottle. Replace cap immediately and tightly after removing strip. Do not touch test area of the strip. Keep work area and containers free of detergents and other contaminants. Discoloration of the test area on the strip indicates deterioration.

Drug Interactions:

Tell your doctor or pharmacist if you are taking or if you are planning to take any over-the-counter or prescription medications or dietary supplements while testing for protein in the urine. The following drugs and drug classes may interact with the test results.

- antiseptics
- detergents
- nitrofurantoin (*Furadantin*)
- phenazopyridine (eg, *Pyridium*)
- skin cleansers (eg, chlorhexidine)
- sulfa drugs and phenazopyridine (eg, *Azo Gantanol*)
- urinary alkalinizers (antacids, sodium bicarbonate)
- vitamin B_2 (riboflavin)

Guidelines for Use:

- Follow the directions on the label EXACTLY.
- Proteins are not usually detected in urine. Contact your doctor to confirm test results.
- Have all of the materials you need on hand before beginning the test: test strips, timer (stopwatch or watch with a second hand), and clean dry container.
- If test results seem questionable, check the expiration date on the bottle and repeat the test using a new test strip and fresh urine specimen.
- Color vision is needed to properly read test results. Have someone else confirm results if in doubt.

If you have any questions, consult your doctor, pharmacist, or health care provider.

	Brand Name Examples	Supplied As	Test For
otc	*Chemstrip 2 LN*	**Test strips:** For urine	Leukocytes (white blood cells) and nitrites
otc	*Microstix-3*	**Test strips:**For urine	Nitrites and bacteria
otc	*UTI*	**Test strips:** For urine	Nitrites

Diagnostic or therapeutic decisions should not be based on a single test result. If you have any questions regarding your test results, contact your doctor.

Type of Drug:

Aid in the detection of urinary tract infections (UTIs).

How the Drug Works:

Nitrites can be detected in the first morning urine specimen in up to 90% of all people with UTIs (infections in kidneys or bladder). Urinary nitrate is often associated with UTIs. Specially treated plastic test strips are used to test for nitrites that are converted from nitrates by bacteria in the urine. Normally no nitrites are detectable in urine.

Leukocytes (white blood cells [WBCs]) are present in the urine of people with UTIs. Specially treated plastic strips detect enzymes from certain WBCs (neutrophils) in the urine. Red blood cells and cells from the urinary tract do not usually interfere with the test.

Bacteria may be detected in the urine specimens of people with UTIs. Specially treated plastic strips containing nutrients to support bacterial growth detect total bacterial and Gram-negative bacterial counts in the urine.

Uses:

To detect WBCs, bacteria, and nitrites. To aid in the detection of UTIs.

Precautions:

Not for internal use.

Caution: Nitrites are produced by some *(not all)* UTI causing bacteria. Therefore, a negative test result does not necessarily mean no infection exists.

White blood cell test strips: Avoid contact with skin and mucous membranes. If contact occurs, flush affected areas with large amounts of water. If test pads are eaten or rubbed in the eyes, contact your doctor or a poison control center immediately.

High urine protein (albumin) and vitamin C (ascorbic acid) levels will interfere with the test results for WBCs.

Drug Interactions:

Tell your doctor or pharmacist if you are taking or if you are planning to take any over-the-counter or prescription medications or dietary supplements while testing for UTIs. The following drugs and drug classes may interact with the tests to cause questionable results.

antibiotics (eg, cephalexin, gentamicin, nitrofurantoin)
phenazopyridine (eg, *Pyridium)*
vitamin C (ascorbic acid), large amounts

Guidelines for Use:

- A negative result with a test kit *does not* rule out the possibility that you may have a urinary tract infection (UTI).
- Consult your doctor if you experience symptoms of a UTI: Frequent urination, painful or burning urination, lower backache.
- Read the test instructions carefully before use. Follow the instructions on the label EXACTLY.
- Have all of the materials you need before beginning the test: Test strips, timer (stopwatch or watch with a second hand), and clean dry container.
- Do not open the vial in humid conditions, such as a steamy bathroom.
- Handle strips with clean, dry hands. Do not touch the test area of the strips.
- Do not use test strips if they are discolored or damaged.
- *Chemstrip 2 LN* — May be used on any fresh urine specimen or on urine collected under special conditions, such as first-morning specimens. Collect urine in a clean container and test as soon as possible after collection. If testing cannot be performed within one hour, refrigerate immediately. Return to room temperature before testing. Mix thoroughly before use. Do not use preservatives.
- Color vision is needed to properly read test results. Have someone else confirm results if in doubt.
- If test results seem questionable, check the expiration date on the bottle and repeat the test using a new test strip and a fresh urine specimen.
- Contact your doctor if the test results are positive or if you are unsure what your test results mean.
- Some medications may cause abnormal urine color and affect the readability of the test strip. Consult your doctor.
- *Vitamin C* (ascorbic acid) — Large doses of vitamin C (25 mg/dL or more) will give incorrect test results for nitrites.
- Store at room temperature (59° to 86°F) in a cool, dry place. Do not refrigerate. Keep out of direct sunlight. Close vial immediately after removing the test strip because prolonged exposure to air will cause the test strips to deteriorate.

If you have any questions, consult your doctor, pharmacist, or health care provider.

	Brand Name Examples	Glucose	Protein	pH	Blood	Ketones	Bilirubin	Urobilinogen	Nitrites	Leukocytes
otc	*Chemstrip uG*	x								
otc	*Nitrazine*			x						
otc	*Hemastix*				x					
otc	*Chemstrip K*					x				
otc	*Chemstrip 2 GP, Uristix*	x	x							
otc	*Chemstrip uGK*	x				x				
otc	*Combistix*	x	x	x						
otc	*Hema-Combistix*	x	x	x	x					
otc	*Uristix 4*	x	x						x	x
otc	*Chemstrip 4 the OB*	x	x		x					x
otc	*Chemstrip 6*	x	x	x	x	x				x
otc	*Labstix*	x	x	x	x	x				
otc	*Bili-Labstix, Bili-Labstix SG*[1]	x	x	x	x	x	x			
otc	*Chemstrip 7*	x	x	x	x	x	x			x
otc	*Multistix, Multistix SG*[1]	x	x	x	x	x	x	x		
otc	*Multistix 7, Multistix 8 SG*[1]	x	x	x	x	x			x	x
otc	*N-Multistix, N-Multistix SG*[1]	x	x	x	x	x	x	x	x	
otc	*Multistix 8, Multistix 9 SG*[1]	x	x	x	x	x			x	x
otc	*Chemstrip 9, Chemstrip 10 SG*[1], *Multistix 9, Multistix 10 SG*[1]	x	x	x	x	x	x	x	x	x

[1] Also tests specific gravity.

Do not base diagnostic or therapeutic decisions on a single test result. If you have any questions regarding your test results, contact your doctor.

Type of Drug:

Miscellaneous urine tests.

Uses:

Specialized test strips and test tapes detect:

Glucose — To detect glucose in urine. To aid diabetics in monitoring medication regimens and diet and exercise needs. To help reduce complications and problems during pregnancy.

Protein — To detect protein in the urine. To screen for early signs of kidney disease.

pH — To determine if urine is too acidic or too alkaline (basic). Normal pH range 4 to 8 (average pH is 6). Urine pH is influenced by diet and some disease states that affect the kidneys.

Blood — To detect occult (hidden/unseen) blood in urine. Blood may appear when there is disease or trauma in the urinary tract (kidney, bladder, etc.), with some drug therapy (eg, cyclophosphamide), or after extreme exertion (eg, running a marathon).

Ketones — To detect ketones in urine and blood. To monitor for diabetic ketoacidosis, a complication of diabetes, which may lead to diabetic coma.

Bilirubin — To detect bilirubin (a product of hemoglobin metabolism) in the urine. Used to diagnose and follow conditions such as hepatitis or gallbladder disease.

Urobilinogen — To detect urobilinogen (a product of bilirubin metabolism) in the urine. It is normally found in the urine. Increased levels of urobilinogen may occur when there is liver damage.

Nitrite — To detect nitrites in the urine. To aid in the detection of urinary tract infections (UTIs).

Leukocytes (white blood cells) — To detect white blood cells in the urine. To aid in the detection of UTIs.

Specific gravity — To detect the kidney's ability to concentrate urine. (Most accurate if patient is fluid-restricted).

Drug Interactions:

Tell your doctor or pharmacist if you are taking or if you are planning to take any over-the-counter or prescription medications or dietary supplements while using these tests. The following drugs and drug classes may interact with the tests to cause questionable results.

nitrofurantoin (eg, *Furadantin*)
phenazopyridine (eg, *Pyridium*)
sulfa drugs and phenazopyridine (eg, *Azo-Sulfisoxazole*)
vitamin B_2 (riboflavin)
vitamin C (ascorbic acid), large amounts

Consider all drug interactions reported for the individual test kits when using urine tests.

Guidelines for Use:

- Have all the materials you need before beginning the test: Testing packet, pencil or pen, timer (stopwatch or watch with a second hand), and clean, dry container.
- Follow instructions EXACTLY as provided.
- If test results seem questionable, check the expiration date on the packet and repeat the test.
- Color vision is needed to properly read test results. Have someone else confirm results if in doubt.

If you have any questions, consult your doctor, pharmacist, or health care provider.

APPENDIX

The Home Medicine Cabinet, A-3

Oral Dosage Forms That Should Not Be Crushed or Chewed, A-7

International System of Units, A-17

Normal Laboratory Values, A-19

FDA Pregnancy Categories, A-29

Poison Center Hotline, A-31

Drug Names That Look Alike and Sound Alike, A-33

The Home Medicine Cabinet

The cost associated with office visits to doctors for diagnosis and treatment of minor conditions due to an accidental injury or illness amounts to hundreds of millions of dollars annually. In many instances, the time and money spent visiting the doctor can be avoided if you have a properly stocked home medicine cabinet and a basic knowledge of first aid and self care.

A properly stocked home medicine cabinet must include, but not be limited to, typical first-aid items. Having key drugs and devices available and knowing how to use them may prevent delays in treating discomforting symptoms. However, if significant relief is not achieved or the condition worsens during the first 24 hours after the accident or onset of symptoms, do not hesitate to contact a pharmacist or doctor.

When we refer to the home medicine cabinet, the tendency is to think of a bathroom cabinet or drawer. However, the humidity and temperature fluctuations of the bathroom may accelerate the deterioration of certain drugs. The bathroom is a less than ideal place to store these health care items. Also, some items are bulky (eg, cool mist vaporizer, heating pad, ice pack) and it may not be practical to store them with other times. Think primarily of storing the items for the home medicine cabinet in a cool, dry area out of the reach of children. The upper portion of a hall or bedroom closet are good storage areas. Consolidation of many of the items in a locked fishing tackle box or plastic "tub" is a good idea.

Basic Inventory

The ideal inventory for a home medicine cabinet varies widely. Contents should reflect the nature, size, lifestyle, location, age, and health status of the individual or family. The basic inventory for a household that includes one or more children is included in the following table. These items may prevent costly and unnecessary trips to the emergency room or doctor's office, but must not be used as substitutes for appropriate medical attention.

First-aid items: First-aid items are most frequently employed to manage cuts, scrapes, bites, stings, sprains, and strains. Thoroughly clean all wounds involving broken skin. Mild soap and warm water are very effective. Hydrogen peroxide (3%) may be used if the wound is dirty and very sensitive. The bubbling action of the peroxide helps to physically remove debris. The antiseptic/antibacterial action of hydrogen peroxide is limited, however, and should not be overestimated. If the wound is painful, a local anesthetic spray may be applied. If no allergies to the drug exist, a thin layer of multiple antibiotic ointment or cream may be applied to a superficial wound each time the dressing is changed. Cover all wounds involving broken skin with a loose protective dressing for a few days and change the dressing at least once daily.

Hydrocortisone ointment or cream (0.5% or 1%) is useful in treating local pain, irritation, itching, and inflammation associated with bites, stings, sunburn, and contact dermatitis associated with poison ivy, oak, or sumac. If the allergic reaction is severe, oral diphenhydramine (eg, *Benadryl*) capsules or tablets may be required to provide relief. Oatmeal baths and calamine lotion may be useful if local inflammation is widespread, such as chickenpox. Isopropyl alcohol is included as an agent to rub on sprains and strains. If used as an antiseptic on a fresh wound, it will burn for several seconds.

An ice pack is recommended to control inflammation, pain, and swelling of bites, stings, sprains, and strains. Apply it as soon after the injury as possible. Heat should not generally be applied to a sprain or strain for 24 to 48 hours after the acute injury.

Cold and Allergy Items: Antihistamines, decongestants or both will provide symptomatic relief of seasonal allergic rhinitis and the common cold. Antihistamines work best in relieving allergic symptoms and are sometimes overvalued in treating the common cold.

Home Medicine Cabinet — Basic Inventory
First Aid Items
Assorted Adhesive Bandages (eg, *Band-Aids*) – 1 box
Sterile Gauze Pads (2″ x 2″) – 1 box
Waterproof Adhesive Tape (½″ x 5 yards) – 1 roll
Blunt Scissors
Elastic Bandage (2″ to 3″ wide)
Ice Pack (6″ to 9″ diameter)
Heating Pad (dry or moist heat)
Hydrogen Peroxide (3%) – 8 oz
Triple Antibiotic Ointment (eg, *Neosporin, Mycitracin*)
Local Anesthetic Spray (eg, *Bactine, Medi-Quick*) – 1 aerosol can
Isopropyl ("rubbing") alcohol (70%) – 16 oz
Hydrocortisone Ointment or Cream (0.5% or 1%) – ½ oz tube
Cold and Allergy Items
Diphenhydramine (eg, *Benadryl*) 25 mg capsule or tablet – 24 count
Chlorpheniramine maleate (eg, *Chlor-Trimeton*) 4 mg tablet – 24 count
Pseudoephedrine (30 or 60 mg) tablet – 24 count
Gastrointestinal Items
Antacid (eg, *Maalox, Mylanta*) – 12 oz
H_2 antagonist (eg, *Pepcid AC*)
Antidiarrheal (eg, *Kaopectate, Donnagel, Imodium A-D*) – 8 oz
Analgesic Items
Aspirin (325 mg) tablet – 50 count
Nonsteroidal anti-inflammatory drug (eg, *Advil, Motrin, Aleve*)
Acetaminophen (325 mg) tablet, capsule, or gelcap – 50 count
Sunscreen
Waterproof or water-resistant sunscreen with an SPF rating of ≥ 15
Miscellaneous Items
Oral fever thermometer
Rectal fever thermometer (for small children)
Pair of tweezers
Cool mist humidifier
Syrup of ipecac – 1 oz
Phone number of nearest poison control center

Gastrointestinal Products: Stomach upset, heartburn, and acid indigestion may be relieved with gastrointestinal products. Simple, uncomplicated diarrhea should respond to *Kaopectate, Donnagel,* or *Imodium A-D.*

Analgesic Items: Fever-reducing drugs and pain relievers are essential components of the home medicine cabinet. Standard fever-reducing drugs are aspirin and acetaminophen. Pain is the most common medical symptom. Over 30 million Americans suffer from headaches each week. Because of the suspected link between aspirin use and Reye's syndrome, do not give aspirin to children experiencing pain or fever. Acetaminophen is as effective as aspirin as an analgesic and fever-reducing drug. Therefore, treat children with symptoms of neuralgia, arthralgia, myalgia, headache, fever, or general discomfort associated with viral conditions such as chickenpox or influenza with acetaminophen. Liquid or chewable acetaminophen may be preferable for children. Nonsteroidal anti-inflammatory drugs (eg, ibuprofen, naproxen) are alternatives to aspirin or acetaminophen as analgesics and fever-reducing agents in a variety of clinical situations.

Sunscreens: The association of excessive exposure to ultraviolet (UV) light and skin cancers of various types is real. Sunscreens are stongly recommended, regardless of skin type, if exposure to sunlight is to be lengthy.

Tweezers are useful for removing splinters and other foreign objects embedded in the skin.

A cool mist humidifier, properly maintained and cleaned after use, helps to provide symptomatic relief from dry mucous membranes of the nasal passages and throat associated with colds and flu.

Finally, one ounce of ipecac syrup is an emergency drug that should be in every home in the event of childhood poisoning. Doses for children are smaller than adult doses. Call the nearest poison control center before administering ipecac to determine the proper dose or whether it should be used at all. Ipecac must not be used to treat some types of poisoning.

Conclusion

A host of other items may be appropriate additions to the home medicine cabinet. These often include foot powder; antifungal ointments, solutions, creams, or sprays; laxatives; vitamins; minerals; eye drops; lotions; and so forth. The core items recommended should serve most families well. Other items may be added as needed.

Do not neglect your home medicine cabinet. At times, medicine cabinets need first aid themselves. Remove and discard old, outdated, and deteriorated items periodically. Throw away any product that has changed its color, consistency, or odor, as they have probably "gone bad." Keep remaining items orderly so they may be found when needed. If symptoms do not respond to treatment or worsen rapidly after being treated with appropriate items in the home, do not hesitate to contact a pharmacist or doctor.

Oral Dosage Forms That Should Not Be Crushed or Chewed

Crushing, chewing, or breaking many drug formulations can affect their rate of absorption and could cause adverse or toxic side effects. Many of these products are intended to be released over a long period of time or at a specific time after administration.

Absence of a drug from this list should NOT imply that it is acceptable to chew or crush the drug. Consult your pharmacist or doctor if you have any questions.

Drug Product	Manufacturer	Dosage Form	Reason/Comments
Aciphex	Janssen	Tablet	Slow release
Accutane	Roche	Capsule	Mucous membrane irritant
Actifed 12 Hour	GlaxoSmithKline	Capsule	Slow release (b)
Acutrim	Novartis Consumer Health	Tablet	Slow release
Adalat CC	Bayer Corp.	Tablet	Slow release
Aerolate SR, JR, III	Fleming & Co.	Capsule	Slow release (a,b)
Afrinol Repetabs	Schering-Plough	Tablet	Slow release
Allegra-D	Hoechst-Marion Roussel	Tablet	Slow release
Allerest 12 Hour	Novartis Consumer Health	Caplet	Slow release
Artane Sequels	ESI Lederle	Capsule	Slow release (a,b)
Arthritis Bayer TR	Bayer Corp.	Capsule	Slow release
Arthrotec	Searle	Tablet	Enteric coated
ASA Enseals	Lilly	Tablet	Enteric coated
Asacol	Procter & Gamble	Tablet	Slow release
Ascriptin A/D	Rhone-Poulenc Rorer	Tablet	Enteric coated
Ascriptin Extra Strength	Rhone-Poulenc Rorer	Tablet	Enteric coated
Atrohist LA	Adams	Tablet	Slow release (b)
Atrohist Pediatric	Celltech	Capsule	Slow release (a,b)
Atrohist Plus	Adams	Tablet	Slow release (b)
Atrohist Sprinkle	Adams	Capsule	Slow release (a,b)
Azulfidine EN-tabs	Pharmacia & Upjohn	Tablet	Enteric-coated
Baros	Lafayette	Tablet	Effervescent tablet (f)
Bayer Enteric-coated	Bayer Corp.	Caplet	Enteric coated
Bayer Low Adult 81 mg	Bayer Corp.	Tablet	Enteric coated
Bayer Regular Strength 325 mg Caplets	Bayer Corp.	Caplet	Enteric coated
Betachron E-R	Inwood	Capsule	Slow release

Drug Product	Manufacturer	Dosage Form	Reason/Comments
Betapen-VK	Bristol-Myers Squibb	Tablet	Taste (e)
Biaxin-XL	Abbott	Tablet	Slow release
Biohist-LA	Wakefield	Tablet	Slow release (h)
Bisacodyl	(Various Mfr.)	Tablet	Enteric coated (c)
Bontril-SR	Carnrick	Capsule	Slow release
Breonesin	Sanofi Winthrop	Capsule	Slow release
Brexin LA	Savage	Capsule	Slow release
Calan SR	Searle	Tablet	Slow release (h)
Cama Arthritis Pain Reliever	Novartis	Tablet	Multiple compressed tablet
Carbatrol	Athena Neurosciences	Capsule	Slow release (a)
Carbiset-TR	Nutripharm	Tablet	Slow release
Cardene SR	Syntex	Capsule	Slow release
Cardizem	Marion-Merrell Dow	Tablet	Slow release
Cardizem CD	Marion-Merrell Dow	Capsule	Slow release (a)
Cardizem SR	Marion-Merrell Dow	Capsule	Slow release (a)
Carter's Little Pills	Carter	Tablet	Enteric coated
CartiaXT	Andrx	Capsule	Slow release
Ceclor CD	Lilly	Tablet	Slow release
Ceftin	GlaxoSmithKline	Tablet	Taste (b) Use suspension for children
CellCept	Roche	Capsule, Tablet	Teratogenic potential (i)
Charcoal Plus	Kramer	Tablet	Enteric coated
Chloral Hydrate	(Various Mfr.)	Capsule	Liquid in capsule (b)
Chlor-Trimeton 12-Hour	Schering-Plough	Tablet	Slow release (b)
Choledyl SA	Parke-Davis	Tablet	Slow release (b)
Cipro	Bayer Corp.	Tablet	Taste (e)
Claritin-D	Schering-Plough	Tablet	Slow release
Claritin-D 24 Hour	Schering-Plough	Tablet	Slow release
Codimal-LA	Schwarz Pharma	Capsule	Slow release
Codimal-LA Half	Schwarz Pharma	Capsule	Slow release
Colace	Bristol-Myers	Capsule	Taste (e)
Colestid	Pharmacia & Upjohn	Tablet	Slow release
Comhist LA	Roberts	Capsule	Slow release (a)
Compazine Spansule	SmithKline Beecham	Capsule	Slow release (b)
Congess SR, JR	Fleming & Co.	Capsule	Slow release
Contac 12-Hour	SmithKline Beecham	Capsule	Slow release (a,b)
Contac Maximum Strength	SmithKline Beecham	Capsule	Slow release (a,b)
Cotazym-S	Organon Teknita	Capsule	Enteric coated (a)
Covera-HS	Searle	Tablet	Slow release
Creon 10, 20, 25	Solvay	Capsule	Enteric coated (a)

Drug Product	Manufacturer	Dosage Form	Reason/Comments
Cystospaz-M	PolyMedica	Capsule	Slow release
Cytoxan	Mead Johnson Oncology	Tablet	May be crushed but maker recommends using injection.
Cytovene	Roche	Capsule	Skin irritant
D.A. II	Dura	Tablet	Slow release (h)
Dallergy	Laser	Capsule	Slow release
Dallergy-D	Laser	Capsule	Slow release
Dallergy-JR	Laser	Capsule	Slow release
Deconamine SR	Bradley	Capsule	Slow release (b)
Defen-LA	Horizon	Tablet	Slow release (h)
Depakene	Abbott	Capsule	Slow release, mucous membrane irritant (b)
Depakote	Abbott	Capsule	Enteric-coated
Desoxyn Gradumets	Abbott	Tablet	Slow release
Desyrel	Bristol-Myers Squibb	Tablet	Taste (e)
Dexatrim, Max. Strength	Thompson Medical	Tablet	Slow release
Dexedrine Spansule	SmithKline Beecham	Capsule	Slow release
Diamox Sequels	ESI Lederle	Capsule	Slow release
Dilacor XR	Rhone-Poulenc Rorer	Capsule	Slow release
Dilatrate SR	Schwarz Pharma	Capsule	Slow release
Disobrom	Geneva Pharm.	Tablet	Slow release
Disophrol Chronotab	Schering-Plough	Tablet	Slow release
Dital	UAD	Capsule	Slow release
Ditropan XL	Alza	Tablet	Slow release
Dolobid	Merck	Tablet	Irritant
Donnatal Extentab	Robins	Tablet	Slow release (b)
Donnazyme	Robins	Tablet	Enteric coated
Drisdol	Sanofi Winthrop	Capsule	Liquid filled (d)
Drixoral	Schering-Plough	Tablet	Slow release (b)
Drixoral Plus	Schering-Plough	Tablet	Slow release
Drixoral Sustained Action	Schering-Plough	Tablet	Slow release
Dulcolax	Novartis Consumer Health	Tablet	Enteric coated (c)
Duratuss	Whitby	Tablet	Slow release (h)
Dura-Vent A	Dura	Tablet	Slow release (h)
Dura-Vent/DA	Dura	Tablet	Slow release (h)
Dynabac	Sanofi Winthrop	Tablet	Enteric coated
DynaCirc CR	Novartis	Tablet	Slow release
Easprin	Parke-Davis	Tablet	Enteric coated
EC-Naprosyn	Syntex	Tablet	Enteric coated
Ecotrin Adult Low Strength	SmithKline Beecham	Tablet	Enteric coated

Drug Product	Manufacturer	Dosage Form	Reason/Comments
Ecotrin Maximum Strength	SmithKline Beecham	Tablet	Enteric coated
Ecotrin Regular Strength	SmithKline Beecham	Tablet	Enteric coated
E.E.S. 400	(Various Mfr.)	Tablet	Enteric coated (b)
Effexor XR	Wyeth-Ayerst	Capsule	Slow release
Efidac/24	Novartis	Tablet	Slow release
Efidac/24 Chlor-pheniramine	Novartis	Tablet	Slow release
E-Mycin	Pharmacia & Upjohn	Tablet	Enteric coated
Endafed	Forest	Capsule	Slow release
Entex LA	Procter & Gamble	Tablet	Slow release (b)
Entex PSE	Procter & Gamble	Tablet	Slow release
Equanil	Wyeth-Ayerst	Tablet	Taste (e)
Ergomar	Lotus	Tablet	Sublingual form (g)
Eryc	Warner-Chilcott	Capsule	Enteric-coated (a)
Ery-Tab	Abbott	Tablet	Enteric coated (b)
Erythrocin Stearate	Abbott	Tablet	Enteric coated
Erythromycin Base	(Various Mfr.)	Tablet	Enteric coated
Eskalith CR	SmithKline Beecham	Tablet	Slow release
Exgest LA	Schwarz Pharma	Tablet	Slow release
Extendryl JR	Fleming	Capsule	Slow release
Extendryl S-R	Fleming	Capsule	Slow release (b)
Fe 50	UCB	Tablet	Slow release
Fedahist Gyrocaps	Schwarz Pharma	Capsule	Slow release (b)
Fedahist Timecaps	Schwarz Pharma	Capsule	Slow release (b)
Feldene	Pfizer	Capsule	Mucous membrane irritant
Feocyte	Dunhall	Tablet	Slow release
Feosol	SmithKline Beecham	Tablet	Enteric coated (b)
Feosol Spansule	SmithKline Beecham	Capsule	Slow release (a,b)
Feratab	Upsher-Smith	Tablet	Enteric coated (b)
Fergon	Bayer Corp.	Capsule	Slow release (a)
Fero-Grad-500	Abbott	Tablet	Slow release
Ferro-Sequels	Self Care	Tablet	Slow release
Feverall Sprinkle	Upsher-Smith	Capsule	Taste (a) Place in water or soft food
Flomax	Boehringer Ingelheim	Capsule	Slow release
Fumatinic	Laser	Capsule	Slow release
Gastrocrom	Medeva	Capsule	May be dissolved in water
Geocillin	Roerig	Tablet	Taste
Glucotrol XL	Pfizer	Tablet	Slow release
Gris-PEG	Allergan	Tablet	Crushing may precipitate as larger particles
Guaifed	Muro	Capsule	Slow release

Drug Product	Manufacturer	Dosage Form	Reason/Comments
Guaifed-PD	Muro	Capsule	Slow release
Guaifenex LA	Ethex	Tablet	Slow release (h)
Guaifenex PSE	Ethex	Tablet	Slow release (h)
Humibid DM	Adams	Tablet	Slow release
Humibid DM Sprinkle	Adams	Capsule	Slow release (a)
Humibid LA	Adams	Tablet	Slow release
Humibid Sprinkle	Adams	Capsule	Slow release (a)
Hydergine LC	Sandoz	Capsule	Liquid in capsule (b)
Hydergine Sublingual	Sandoz	Tablet	Sublingual route (b)
Iberet	Abbott	Tablet	Slow release (b)
Iberet 500	Abbott	Tablet	Slow release (b)
ICaps Plus	Ciba Vision	Tablet	Slow release
ICaps Time Release	Ciba Vision	Tablet	Slow release
Ilotycin	Dista	Tablet	Enteric coated
Imdur	Key	Tablet	Slow release (h)
Inderal LA	Wyeth-Ayerst	Capsule	Slow release
Inderide LA	Wyeth-Ayerst	Capsule	Slow release
Indocin SR	Merck	Capsule	Slow release (a,b)
Ionamin	Medeva	Capsule	Slow release
Isoptin SR	Knoll Pharm.	Tablet	Slow release
Isordil Sublingual	Wyeth-Ayerst	Tablet	Sublingual form (g)
Isordil Tembid	Wyeth-Ayerst	Tablet	Slow release
Isosorbide Dinitrate Sublingual	(Various Mfr.)	Tablet	Sublingual form (g)
K + 8	Alra	Tablet	Slow release (b)
K + 10	Alra	Tablet	Slow release (b)
Kadian	Zeneca	Capsule	Slow release (a)
Kaon Cl	Pharmacia & Upjohn	Tablet	Slow release (b)
K-Dur	Key	Tablet	Slow release
K-Lease	Pharmacia & Upjohn	Capsule	Slow release (a,b)
Klor-Con	Upsher-Smith	Tablet	Slow release (b)
Klotrix	Bristol-Myers Squibb	Tablet	Slow release (h)
K-Lyte	Bristol-Myers Squibb	Tablet	Effervescent tablet (f)
K-Lyte/Cl	Bristol-Myers Squibb	Tablet	Effervescent tablet (f)
K-Lyte DS	Bristol-Myers Squibb	Tablet	Effervescent tablet (f)
K-Tab	Abbott	Tablet	Slow release (b)
Levbid	Schwarz Pharma	Tablet	Slow release (h)
Levsinex Timecaps	Schwarz Pharma	Capsule	Slow release
Lexxel	Merck	Tablet	Slow release
Lithobid	Solvay	Tablet	Slow release
Lodrane LD	ECR Pharmaceutical	Capsule	Slow release (a)
Lodine-XL	Wyeth-Ayerst	Tablet	Slow release

Drug Product	Manufacturer	Dosage Form	Reason/Comments
Mag-Tab SR	Niche	Tablet	Slow release
Mestinon Timespan	Zeneca	Tablet	Slow release (b)
Mi-Cebrin	Lilly	Tablet	Enteric coated
Mi-Cebrin T	Lilly	Tablet	Enteric coated
Micro K	Robins	Capsule	Slow release (a,b)
Monafed	Monarch	Tablet	Slow release
Monafed DM	Monarch	Tablet	Slow release
Motrin	Ortho-McNeil	Tablet	Taste (e)
MS Contin	Purdue Frederick	Tablet	Slow release (b)
Muco-Fen-DM	Wakefield	Tablet	Slow release (h)
Muco-Fen-LA	Wakefield	Tablet	Slow release (h)
Naldecon	Apothecon	Tablet	Slow release (b)
Naprelan	Wyeth-Ayerst	Tablet	Slow release
Nasatab LA	ECR Pharmaceutical	Tablet	Slow release (h)
Nexium	Astra Zeneca	Capsule	Slow release (a)
Nico-400	Jones Medical	Capsule	Slow release (j)
Nicotinic Acid	(Various Mfr.)	Capsule, Tablet	Slow release
Nitro Bid Plateau	Hoechst-Marion Roussel	Capsule	Slow release (a)
Nitroglyn	Key	Capsule	Slow release (a)
Nitrong	Wharton	Tablet	Sublingual route (g)
Nitrostat	Parke-Davis	Tablet	Sublingual route (g)
Nitro-Time	Time-Cap Labs	Capsule	Slow release
Nolamine	Carnrick	Tablet	Slow release
Nolex LA	Carnrick	Tablet	Slow release
Norflex	3M Pharmaceuticals	Tablet	Slow release
Norpace CR	Searle	Capsule	Slow release
Ondrox	Unimed	Tablet	Slow release
Optilets-500 Filmtab	Abbott	Tablet	Enteric coated
Optilets-M-500 Filmtab	Abbott	Tablet	Enteric coated
Oragrafin	Bristol-Myers Squibb	Capsule	Liquid in capsule
Oramorph SR	Roxane	Tablet	Slow release (b)
Ornade Spansule	SmithKline Beecham	Capsule	Slow release
OxyContin	Purdue Frederick	Tablet	Slow release
Pabalate	Robins	Tablet	Enteric coated
Pabalate SF	Robins	Tablet	Enteric coated
Pancrease	Ortho McNeil	Capsule	Enteric coated (a)
Pancrease MT	Ortho McNeil	Capsule	Enteric coated (a)
Panmist Jr, LA	Pan American Lab	Tablet	Slow release (h)
Panmycin	Pharmacia & Upjohn	Capsule	Taste
Pannaz	Pan American Lab	Tablet	Slow release (h)

Drug Product	Manufacturer	Dosage Form	Reason/Comments
Papaverine Sustained Action	(Various Mfr.)	Capsule	Slow release
Pathilon Sequels	ESI Lederle	Capsule	Slow release (a)
Pavabid Plateau	Hoechst-Marion Roussel	Capsule	Slow release (a)
PBZ-SR	Novartis Pharm	Tablet	Slow release (b)
Pentasa	Hoechst-Marion Roussel	Tablet	Slow release
Perdiem	Novartis Pharm	Granules	Wax coated
Peritrate SA	Parke-Davis	Tablet	Slow release (h)
Permitil Chronotab	Schering	Tablet	Slow release (b)
Phazyme	Schwarz Pharma	Tablet	Slow release
Phazyme 95, 125	Schwarz Pharma	Tablet	Slow release
Phenergan	Wyeth Ayerst	Tablet	Taste (c)
Phyllocontin	Purdue Frederick	Tablet	Slow release
Plendil	Astra Merck	Tablet	Slow release
Pneumomist	ECR Pharmaceutical	Tablet	Slow release (h)
Polaramine Repetabs	Schering-Plough	Tablet	Slow release (b)
Prelu-2	Boehringer Ingelheim	Capsule	Slow release
Prevacid	TAP Pharmaceutical	Capsule	Slow release
Prilosec	Astra Merck	Capsule	Slow release
Pro-Banthine	Schiapparelli Searle	Tablet	Taste
Procainamide HCL SR	(Various Mfr.)	Tablet	Slow release
Procanbid	Parke-Davis	Tablet	Slow release
Procardia	Pfizer	Capsule	Delays absorption (b,e)
Procardia XL	Pfizer	Tablet	Slow release, AUC is unaffected
Profen II	Wakefield	Tablet	Slow release (h)
Profen-LA	Wakefield	Tablet	Slow release (h)
Pronestyl SR	Bristol-Myers Squibb	Tablet	Slow release
Propecia	Merck	Tablet	Pregnant women should exercise caution in handling this product
Proscar	Merck	Tablet	Pregnant women should exercise caution in handling this product
Proventil Repetabs	Schering-Plough	Tablet	Slow release (b)
Prozac	Lilly	Capsule	Slow release (a)
Quibron-T/SR	Roberts	Tablet	Slow release (b)
Quinaglute Dura-Tabs	Berlex	Tablet	Slow release
Quinidex Extentabs	Robins	Tablet	Slow release
Quin-Release	Major	Tablet	Slow release

Drug Product	Manufacturer	Dosage Form	Reason/Comments
Respa-1st	Respa	Tablet	Slow release (h)
Respa-DM	Respa	Tablet	Slow release (h)
Respa-GF	Respa	Tablet	Slow release (h)
Respahist	Respa	Capsule	Slow release (a)
Respaire SR	Laser	Capsule	Slow release
Respbid	Boehringer Ingelheim	Tablet	Slow release
Ritalin-SR	Novartis	Tablet	Slow release
Robimycin	Robins	Tablet	Enteric coated
Rondec TR	Dura	Tablet	Slow release (b)
Ru-Tuss DE	Knoll	Tablet	Slow release
Sinemet CR	DuPont Pharm	Tablet	Slow release
Singlet for Adults	SmithKline Beecham	Tablet	Slow release
Slo-Bid Gyrocaps	Rhone-Poulenc Rorer	Capsule	Slow release (a)
Slo-Niacin	Upsher-Smith	Tablet	Slow release (h)
Slo-Phyllin GG	Rhone-Poulenc Rorer	Capsule	Slow release (b)
Slo-Phyllin Gyrocaps	Rhone-Poulenc Rorer	Capsule	Slow release (a,b)
Slow FE	Novartis Consumer Health	Tablet	Slow release (b)
Slow FE with Folic Acid	Novartis Consumer Health	Tablet	Slow release
Slow-K	Novartis	Tablet	Slow release (i)
Slow-Mag	Searle	Tablet	Slow release
Sorbitrate SA	Zeneca	Tablet	Slow release
Sorbitrate Sublingual	Zeneca	Tablet	Sublingual route
Sparine	Wyeth-Ayerst	Tablet	Taste (e)
S-P-T	Fleming	Capsule	Liquid gelatin thyroid suspension
Sudafed 12 hour	Warner Lambert Consumer Health Products	Capsule	Slow release (b)
Sudal 60/500	Atley	Tablet	Slow release
Sudal 120/600	Atley	Tablet	Slow release
Sudex	Atley	Tablet	Slow release (h)
Sular	Zeneca	Tablet	Slow release
Sustaire	Pfizer	Tablet	Slow release (b)
Syn-RX	Adams Lab	Tablet	Slow release
Syn-Rx DM	Adams Lab	Tablet	Slow release
Tavist-D	Novartis Consumer Health	Tablet	Multiple compressed tablet
Teczam	Hoechst-Marion Roussel	Tablet	Slow release
Tedral SA	Parke-Davis	Tablet	Slow release (b)
Tegretol-XR	Novartis	Tablet	Slow release
Teldrin Maximum Strength	SmithKline Beecham	Capsule	Slow release (a)

Drug Product	Manufacturer	Dosage Form	Reason/Comments
Tepanil Ten-Tab	3M Pharmaceuticals	Tablet	Slow release
Tessalon Perles	Forest	Capsule	Slow release
Theo-24	UCB Pharma	Tablet	Slow release (b)
Theobid Duracaps	Ross	Capsule	Slow release (a,b)
Theoclear LA	Schwarz Pharma	Capsule	Slow release (b)
Theochron	Inwood	Tablet	Slow release
Theo-Dur	Key	Tablet	Slow release (b)
Theo-Dur Sprinkle	Key	Capsule	Slow release (a,b)
Theolair SR	3M Pharmaceuticals	Tablet	Slow release (b)
Theo-Sav	Savage	Tablet	Slow release (h)
Theo-Span SR	Major	Tablet	Slow release
Theo-Time SR	Major	Tablet	Slow release
Theovent	Schering-Plough	Capsule	Slow release (b)
Theo-X	Schwarz Pharma	Tablet	Slow release
Thorazine Spansule	SmithKline Beecham	Capsule	Slow release
Tiamate	Hoechst-Marion Roussel	Tablet	Slow release
Tiazac	Forest	Capsule	Slow release
Toprol XL	Astra	Tablet	Slow release (h)
Touro A & D	Dartmouth	Capsule	Slow release
Touro EX	Dartmouth	Tablet	Slow release
Touro LA	Dartmouth	Tablet	Slow release
T-Phyl	Purdue Frederick	Tablet	Slow release
Trental	Hoechst Marion Roussel	Tablet	Slow release
Triaminic	Novartis	Tablet	Enteric coated (b)
Triaminic-12	Novartis	Tablet	Slow release (b)
Triaminic TR	Novartis	Tablet	Multiple compressed tablet (b)
Tri-Phen-Chlor Time Release	Rugby	Tablet	Slow release
Tri-Phen-Mine SR	Zenith Goldline	Tablet	Slow release
Triptono Caplets	Del Pharm	Tablet	Slow release
Tuss-LA	Hyrex	Tablet	Slow release
Tuss Ornade Spansule	SmithKline Beecham	Capsule	Slow release
Tylenol Extended Relief	McNeil Consumer Products	Capsule	Slow release
ULR-LA	Geneva Pharm.	Tablet	Slow release
Ultrase	Scandipharm	Capsule	Enteric coated (a)
Ultrase MT	Scandipharm	Capsule	Enteric coated (a)
Uni-Dur	Key	Tablet	Slow release
Uniphyl	Purdue Frederick	Tablet	Slow release
Urocit-K	Mission	Tablet	Wax coated
Verelan	ESI Lederle	Capsule	Slow release (a)

Drug Product	Manufacturer	Dosage Form	Reason/Comments
Volmax	Muro	Tablet	Slow release
Wellbutrin SR	GlaxoSmithKline	Tablet	Anesthetize mucous membrane
Wygesic	Wyeth-Ayerst	Tablet	Taste
ZORprin	Knoll Pharm.	Tablet	Slow release
Zyban	GlaxoSmithKline	Tablet	Slow release
Zymase	Organon Teknika	Capsule	Enteric coated

Revised by John F. Mitchell, PharmD, FASHP, from an article originally appearing in *Hosp Pharm 2000;* 35:553-567.

(a) Capsule may be opened and the contents taken without crushing or chewing; soft food such as applesauce or pudding may facilitate administration; contents may generally be administered via nasogastric tube using an appropriate fluid provided entire contents are washed down the tube.
(b) Liquid dosage forms of the product are available; however, dose, frequency of administration, and manufacturers may differ from that of the solid dosage form.
(c) Antacids and/or milk may prematurely dissolve the coating of the tablet.
(d) Capsule may be opened and the liquid contents removed for administration.
(e) The taste of this product in a liquid form would likely be unacceptable to the patient; administration via nasogastric tube should be acceptable.
(f) Effervescent tablets must be dissolved in the amount of diluent recommended by the manu- fac turer.
(g) Tablets are made to disintegrate under the tongue.
(h) Tablet is scored and may be broken in half without affecting release characteristics.
(i) Skin contact may enhance tumor production; avoid direct contact.

International System of Units

The *Système international d 'unités* (International System of Units) or *SI* is a modernized version of the metric system. The primary goal of the conversion to SI units is to revise the present confused measurement system and to improve test-result communications.

The SI has 7 basic units from which other units are derived:

Base Units of SI		
Physical quantity	Base unit	SI symbol
length	meter	m
mass	kilogram	kg
time	second	s
amount of substance	mole	mol
thermodynamic temperature	kelvin	K
electric current	ampere	A
luminous intensity	candela	cd

Combinations of these base units can express any property, although, for simplicity, special names are given to some of these derived units.

Representative Derived Units		
Derived unit	Name and symbol	Derivation from base units
area	square meter	m^2
volume	cubic meter	m^3
force	newton (N)	$kg{\bullet}m{\bullet}s^{-2}$
pressure	pascal (Pa)	$kg{\bullet}m^{-1}{\bullet}s^{-2}$ (N/m^2)
work, energy	joule (J)	$kg{\bullet}m^2{\bullet}s^{-2}(N{\bullet}m)$
mass density	kilogram per cubic meter	kg/m^3
frequency	hertz (Hz)	1 $cycle/s^{-1}$
temperature degree	Celsius (°C)	°C = °K −273.15
concentration		
mass	kilogram/liter	kg/L
substance	mole/liter	mol/L
molality	mole/kilogram	mol/kg
density	kilogram/liter	kg/L

Prefixes to the base unit are used in this system to form decimal multiples and submultiples. The preferred multiples and submultiples listed below change the quantity by increments of 10^3 or 10^{-3}. The exceptions to these recommended factors are within the middle rectangle.

Prefixes and Symbols for Decimal Multiples and Submultiples		
Factor	Prefix	Symbol
10^{18}	exa	E
10^{15}	peta	P
10^{12}	tera	T
10^{9}	giga	G
10^{6}	mega	M
10^{3}	kilo	k
10^{2}	hecto	h
10^{1}	deka	da
10^{-1}	deci	d
10^{-2}	centi	c
10^{-3}	milli	m
10^{-6}	micro	μ
10^{-9}	nano	n
10^{-12}	pico	p
10^{-15}	femto	f
10^{-18}	atto	a

To convert drug concentrations to or from SI units:

Conversion factor (CF) = 1000/mol wt

Conversion *to* SI units: μg/ml x CF = μmol/L

Conversion *from* SI units: μmol/L ÷ CF = μg/ml

Normal Laboratory Values

In the following tables, normal reference values for commonly requested laboratory tests are listed in traditional units and in SI units. The tables are a guideline only. Values are method dependent and "normal values" may vary between laboratories.

BLOOD, PLASMA, OR SERUM		
	Reference Value	
Determination	Conventional Units	SI Units
Ammonia (NH_3) – diffusion	20-120 mcg/dL	12-70 mcmol/L
Ammonia Nitrogen	15-45 µg/dL	11-32 µmol/L
Amylase	20-100 units/dL	37-185 U/L
Anion Gap ($Na^+-[Cl^-+HCO_3^-]$) (P)	7-16 mEq/L	7-16 mmol/L
Antinuclear antibodies	negative at 1:10 dilution of serum	negative at 1:10 dilution of serum
Antithrombin III (AT III)	80-120 U/dL	800-1200 U/L
Bicarbonate: Arterial Venous	21-28 mEq/L 22-29 mEq/L	21-28 mmol/L 22-29 mmol/L
Bilirubin: Conjugated (direct) Total	≤ 0.2 mg/dL 0.1-1 mg/dL	≤ 4 mcmol/L 2-18 mcmol/L
Calcitonin	Female: ≤ 20 pg/mL Male: ≤ 40 pg/mL	Female: ≤ 20 ng/L Male: ≤ 40 ng/L
Calcium: Total Ionized	8.6-10.3 mg/dL 4.4-5.1 mg/dL	2.2-2.74 mmol/L 1-1.3 mmol/L
Carbon dioxide content (plasma)	21-32 mmol/L	21-32 mmol/L
Carcinoembryonic antigen	< 3 ng/mL	< 3 mcg/L
Chloride	95-110 mEq/L	95-110 mmol/L
Coagulation screen: Bleeding time Prothrombin time Partial thromboplastin time (activated) Protein C Protein S	 3-9.5 min 10-13 sec 22-37 sec 0.7-1.4 µ/mL 0.7-1.4 µ/mL	 180-570 sec 10-13 sec 22-37 sec 700-1400 U/mL 700-1400 U/mL
Copper, total	70-160 mcg/dL	11-25 mcmol/L
Corticotropin (ACTH adrenocorticotropic hormone) – 0800 hr	< 60 pg/mL	< 13.2 pmol/L

BLOOD, PLASMA, OR SERUM				
	Reference Value			
Determination	**Conventional Units**		**SI Units**	
Cortisol: 0800 hr 1800 hr 2000 hr	5-30 mcg/dL 2-15 mcg/dL ≤ 50% of 0800 hr		138-810 nmol/L 50-410 nmol/L ≤ 50% of 0800 hr	
Creatine kinase: Female Male	20-170 IU/L 30-220 IU/L		0.33-2.83 mckat/L 0.5-3.67 mckat/L	
Creatine kinase isoenzymes, MB fraction	0-12 IU/L		0-0.2 mckat/L	
Creatinine	0.5-1.7 mg/dL		44-150 mcmol/L	
Fibrinogen (coagulation factor I)	150-360 mg/dL		1.5-3.6 g/L	
Follicle-stimulating hormone (FSH): Female Midcycle Male	 2-13 mIU/mL 5-22 mIU/mL 1-8 mIU/mL		 2-13 IU/L 5-22 IU/L 1-8 IU/L	
Glucose, fasting	65-115 mg/dL		3.6-6.3 mmol/L	
Glucose Tolerance Test (Oral)	mg/dL		mmol/L	
	Normal	Diabetic	Normal	Diabetic
Fasting	70-105	> 140	3.9-5.8	> 7.8
60 min	120-170	≥ 200	6.7-9.4	≥ 11.1
90 min	100-140	≥ 200	5.6-7.8	≥ 11.1
120 min	70-120	≥ 140	3.9-6.7	≥ 7.8
(γ) - Glutamyltransferase (GGT): Male Female	9-50 units/L 8-40 units/L		9-50 units/L 8-40 units/L	
Haptoglobin	44-303 mg/dL		0.44-3.03 g/L	
Hematologic tests:				
Fibrinogen	200-400 mg/dL		2-4 g/L	
Hematocrit (Hct), female	36%-44.6%		0.36-0.446 fraction of 1	
male	40.7%-50.3%		0.4-0.503 fraction of 1	
Hemoglobin A_{1C}	2.2%-5%		0.053-0.075	
Hemoglobin (Hb), female	12-16 g/dL		7.4-9.9 mmol/L	
male	14-18 g/dL		8.7-11.2 mmol/L	
Leukocyte count (WBC)	3800-9800/mcL		3.8-9.8 x 10^9/L	
Erythrocyte count (RBC), female	3.5-5 × 10^6/mcL		3.5-5 x 10^{12}/L	
male	4.3-5.9 × 10^6/mcL		4.3-5.9 x 10^{12}/L	
Mean corpuscular volume (MCV)	80-97.6 mcm^3		80-97.6 fl	
Mean corpuscular hemoglobin (MCH)	27-33 pg/cell		1.66-2.09 fmol/cell	
Mean corpuscular hemoglobin concentrate (MCHC)	33-36 g/dL		20.3-22 mmol/L	
Erythrocyte sedimentation rate (sedrate, ESR)	≤ 30 mm/hr		≤ 30 mm/hr	

BLOOD, PLASMA, OR SERUM		
	Reference Value	
Determination	**Conventional Units**	**SI Units**
Erythrocyte enzymes: Glucose-6-phosphate dehydrogenase (G-6-PD)	250-5000 units/10^6 cells	250-5000 mcunits/cell
Ferritin	10-300 ng/mL	10-300 mcg/L
Folic acid: normal	> 3.1-12.4 ng/mL	7-28.1 nmol/L
Platelet count	150-450 × 10^3/mcL	150-450 × 10^9/L
Reticulocytes	0.5%-1.5% of erythrocytes	0.005-0.015
Vitamin B_{12}	223-1132 pg/mL	165-835 pmol/L
Iron: Female	30-160 mcg/dL	5.4-31.3 mcmol/L
Male	45-160 mcg/dL	8.1-31.3 mcmol/L
Iron binding capacity	220-420 mcg/dL	39.4-75.2 mcmol/L
Isocitrate Dehydrogenase	1.2-7 units/L	1.2-7 units/L
Lactate dehydrogenase isoenzymes		
Fraction 1	14%-26% of total	0.14-0.26 fraction of total
Fraction 2	29%-39% of total	0.29-0.39 fraction of total
Fraction 3	20%-26% of total	0.20-0.26 fraction of total
Fraction 4	8%-16% of total	0.08-0.16 fraction of total
Fraction 5	6%-16% of total	0.06-0.16 fraction of total
Lactate dehydrogenase	100-250 IU/L	1.67-4.17 mckat/L
Lactic acid (lactate)	6-19 mg/dL	0.7-2.1 mmol/L
Lead	< 20 mcg/dL	≤ 2.41 mcmol/L
Lipase	10-150 IU/L	10-150 IU/L
Lipids:		
Total Cholesterol		
Desirable	< 200 mg/dL	< 5.2 mmol/L
Borderline-high	200-239 mg/dL	< 5.2-6.2 mmol/L
High	> 239 mg/dL	> 6.2 mmol/L
LDL		
Desirable	< 130 mg/dL	< 3.36 mmol/L
Borderline-high	130-159 mg/dL	3.36-4.11 mmol/L
High	> 159 mg/dL	> 4.11 mmol/L
HDL		< 0.91 mmol/L
Desirable	< 40 mg/dL	
High	≥ 60 mg/dL	
Triglycerides		
Desirable	< 200 mg/dL	< 2.26 mmol/L
Borderline-high	200-400 mg/dL	2.26-4.52 mmol/L
High	400-1000 mg/dL	4.52-11.3 mmol/L
Very high	> 1000 mg/dL	> 11.3 mmol/L
Magnesium	1.3-2.2 mEq/L	0.65-1.1 mmol/L
Osmolality	280-300 mOsm/kg	280-300 mmol/kg
Oxygen saturation (arterial)	94%-100%	0.94-1 fraction of 1
PCO_2, arterial	35-45 mm Hg	4.7-6 kPa

BLOOD, PLASMA, OR SERUM		
	Reference Value	
Determination	**Conventional Units**	**SI Units**
pH, arterial	7.35-7.45	7.35-7.45
PO_2, arterial: Breathing room air[1]	80-105 mm Hg	10.6-14 kPa
On 100% O_2	> 500 mm Hg	
Phosphatase (acid), total at 37°C	0.13-0.63 IU/L	2.2-10.5 IU/L or 2.2-10.5 mckat/L
Phosphatase alkaline[2]	20-130 IU/L	20-130 IU/L or 0.33-2.17 mckat/L
Phosphorus, inorganic,[3] (phosphate)	2.5-5 mg/dL	0.8-1.6 mmol/L
Potassium	3.5-5 mEq/L	3.5-5 mmol/L
Progesterone		
Female	0.1-1.5 ng/mL	0.32-4.8 nmol/L
Follicular phase	0.1-1.5 ng/mL	0.32-4.8 nmol/L
Luteal phase	2.5-28 ng/mL	8-89 nmol/L
Male	< 0.5 ng/mL	< 1.6 nmol/L
Prolactin	1.4-24.2 ng/mL	1.4-24.2 mcg/L
Prostate specific antigen	0-4 ng/mL	0-4 ng/mL
Protein: Total	6-8 g/dL	60-80 g/L
Albumin	3.6-5 g/dL	36-50 g/L
Globulin	2.3-3.5 g/dL	23-35 g/L
Rheumatoid factor	< 60 IU/mL	< 60 kIU/L
Sodium	135-147 mEq/L	135-147 mmol/L
Testosterone: Female	6-86 ng/dL	0.21-3 nmol/L
Male	270-1070 ng/dL	9.3-37 nmol/L
Thyroid Hormone Function Tests:		
Thyroid-stimulating hormone (TSH)	0.35-6.2 mcU/mL	0.35-6.2 mU/L
Thyroxine-binding globulin capacity	10-26 mcg/dL	100-260 mcg/L
Total triiodothyronine (T_3)	75-220 ng/dL	1.2-3.4 nmol/L
Total thyroxine by RIA (T_4)	4-11 mcg/dL	51-142 nmol/L
T_3 resin uptake	25%-38%	0.25-0.38 fraction of 1
Transaminase, AST (aspartate aminotransferase, SGOT)	11-47 IU/L	0.18-0.78 mckat/L
Transaminase, ALT (alanine aminotransferase, SGPT)	7-53 IU/L	0.12-0.88 mckat/L
Transferrin	220-400 mg/dL	2.20-4.00 g/L
Urea nitrogen (BUN)	8-25 mg/dL	2.9-8.9 mmol/L

BLOOD, PLASMA, OR SERUM		
	Reference Value	
Determination	**Conventional Units**	**SI Units**
Uric acid	3-8 mg/dL	179-476 mcmol/L
Vitamin A (retinol)	15-60 mcg/dL	0.52-2.09 mcmol/L
Zinc	50-150 mcg/mL	7.7-23 mcmol/L

[1] Age dependent
[2] Infants and adolescents up to 104 U/L
[3] Infants in the first year up to 6 mg/dL

URINE		
	Reference Value	
Determination	**Conventional Units**	**SI Units**
Calcium[1]	50-250 mg/day	1.25-6.25 mmol/day
Catecholamines: Epinephrine Norepinephrine	 < 20 mcg/day < 100 mcg/day	 < 109 nmol/day < 590 nmol/day
Catecholamines, 24-hr	< 110 μg	< 650 nmol
Copper[1]	15-60 mcg/day	0.24-0.95 mcmol/day
Creatinine: Child Adolescent Female Male	8-22 mg/kg/day 8-30 mg/kg/day 0.6-1.5 g/day 0.8-1.8 g/day	71-195 μmol/kg/day 71-265 μmol/kg/day 5.3-13.3 mmol/day 7.1-15.9 mmol/day
pH	4.5-8	4.5-8
Phosphate[1]	0.9-1.3 g/day	29-42 mmol/day
Potassium[1]	25-100 mEq/day	25-100 mmol/day
Protein Total At rest	 1-14 mg/dL 50-80 mg/day	 10-140 mg/L 50-80 mg/day
Protein, quantitative Sodium[1]	< 150 mg/day 100-250 mEq/day	< 0.15 g/day 100-250 mmol/day
Specific Gravity, random	1.002-1.030	1.002-1.030
Uric Acid, 24-hr	250-750 mg	1.48-4.43 mmol

[1] Diet dependent

DRUG LEVELS†			
		Reference Value	
Drug Determination		Conventional Units	SI Units
Aminoglycosides	Amikacin		
	(trough)	1-8 mcg/mL	1.7-13.7 mcmol/L
	(peak)	20-30 mcg/mL	34-51 mcmol/L
	Gentamicin		
	(trough)	0.5-2 mcg/mL	1-4.2 mcmol/L
	(peak)	6-10 mcg/mL	12.5-20.9 mcmol/L
	Kanamycin		
	(trough)	5-10 mcg/mL	nd
	(peak)	20-25 mcg/mL	nd
	Netilmicin		
	(trough)	0.5-2 mcg/mL	nd
	(peak)	6-10 mcg/mL	nd
	Streptomycin		
	(trough)	< 5 mcg/mL	nd
	(peak)	5-20 mcg/mL	nd
	Tobramycin		
	(trough)	0.5-2 mcg/mL	1.1-4.3 mcmol/L
	(peak)	5-20 mcg/mL	12.8-21.8 mcmol/L
Antiarrhythmics	Amiodarone	0.5-2.5 mcg/mL	1.5-4 mcmol/L
	Bretylium	0.5-1.5 mcg/mL	nd
	Digitoxin	9-25 mcg/L	11.8-32.8 nmol/L
	Digoxin	0.8-2 ng/mL	0.9-2.5 nmol/L
	Disopyramide	2-8 mcg/mL	6-18 mcmol/L
	Flecainide	0.2-1 mcg/mL	nd
	Lidocaine	1.5-6 mcg/mL	4.5-21.5 mcmol/L
	Mexiletine	0.5-2 mcg/mL	nd
	Procainamide	4-8 mcg/mL	17-34 mcmol/mL
	Propranolol	50-200 ng/mL	190-770 nmol/L
	Quinidine	2-6 mcg/mL	4.6-9.2 mcmol/L
	Tocainide	4-10 mcg/mL	nd
	Verapamil	0.08-0.3 mcg/mL	nd
Anticonvulsants	Carbamazepine	4-12 mcg/mL	17-51 mcmol/L
	Phenobarbital	10-40 mcg/mL	43-172 mcmol/L
	Phenytoin	10-20 mcg/mL	40-80 mcmol/L
	Primidone	4-12 mcg/mL	18-55 mcmol/L
	Valproic acid	40-100 mcg/mL	280-700 mcmol/L

DRUG LEVELS†			
		Reference Value	
Drug Determination		Conventional Units	SI Units
Antidepressants	Amitriptyline	110-250 ng/mL[3]	500-900 nmol/L
	Amoxapine	200-500 ng/mL	nd
	Bupropion	25-100 ng/mL	nd
	Clomipramine	80-100 ng/mL	nd
	Desipramine	115-300 ng/mL	281-1125 nmol/L
	Doxepin	30-250 ng/mL	107-537 nmol/L
	Imipramine	100-300 ng/mL	nd
	Maprotiline	200-300 ng/mL	nd
	Nortriptyline	50-150 ng/mL	nd
	Protriptyline	160-250 ng/mL	266-950 nmol/L
	Trazodone	800-1600 ng/mL	nd
Antipsychotics	Chlorpromazine	50-300 ng/mL	150-950 nmol/L
	Fluphenazine	0.13-2.8 ng/mL	nd
	Haloperidol	5-20 ng/mL	10-30 nmol/L
	Perphenazine	0.8-1.2 ng/mL	nd
	Thiothixene	2-57 ng/mL	nd
Miscellaneous	Amantadine	300 ng/mL	nd
	Amrinone	3.7 mcg/mL	nd
	Chloramphenicol	10-20 mcg/mL	31-62 mcmol/L
	Cyclosporine[1]	250-800 ng/mL (whole blood, RIA)	nd
		50-300 ng/mL (plasma, RIA)	nd
	Ethanol[2]	0 mg/dL	0 mmol/L
	Hydralazine	100 ng/mL	nd
	Lithium	0.6-1.2 mEq/L	0.6-1.2 mmol/L
	Salicylate	100-300 mg/L	724-2172 mcmol/L
	Sulfonamide	5-15 mg/dL	nd
	Theophylline	10-20 mcg/mL	55-110 mcmol/L
	Vancomycin		
	(trough)	5-15 ng/mL	nd
	(peak)	20-40 mcg/mL	nd

† The values given are generally accepted as desirable for treatment without toxicity for most patients. However, exceptions are not uncommon.

[1] 24 hour trough values [2] Toxic: 50-100 mg/dL (10.9-21.7 mmol/L) [3] Parent drug plus N-desmethyl metabolite

nd – No data available

Classification of Blood Pressure*			
	Reference Value		
Category	Systolic (mm Hg)		Diastolic (mm Hg)
Optimal†	< 120	and	< 80
Normal	< 130	and	< 85
High-normal	130-139	or	85-89
Hypertension‡			
Stage 1	140-159	or	90-99
Stage 2	160-179	or	100-109
Stage 3	≥ 180	or	≥ 110

Adopted from the Sixth Report of the Joint National Committee on Prevention, Detection, Evaluation, and Treatment of High Blood Pressure, National Institutes of Health

* For adults age 18 and older who are not taking antihypertensive drugs and not acutely ill. When systolic and diastolic blood pressures fall into different categories, the higher category should be selected to classify the individual's blood pressure status. In addition to classifying stages of hypertension on the basis of average blood pressure levels, clinicians should specify presence or absence of target organ disease and additional risk factors.

† Optimal blood pressure with respect to cardiovascular risk is below 120/88 mm Hg. However, unusually low readings should be evaluated for clinical significance.

‡ Based on the average of two or more readings taken at each of two or more visits after an initial screening.

FDA Pregnancy Categories

The rational use of any medication requires a risk versus benefit assessment. Among the myriad of risk factors which complicate this assessment, pregnancy is one of the most perplexing.

The FDA has established five categories to indicate the potential of a systemically absorbed drug for causing birth defects. The key differentiation among the categories rests upon the degree (reliability) of documentation and the risk vs benefit ratio. Pregnancy Category X is particularly notable in that if any data exists that may implicate a drug as a teratogen and the risk vs benefit ratio does not support use of the drug, the drug is contraindicated during pregnancy. These categories are summarized below:

FDA Pregnancy Categories	
Pregnancy Category	**Definition**
A	Controlled studies show no risk. Adequate, well-controlled studies in pregnant women have failed to demonstrate risk to the fetus.
B	No evidence of risk in humans. Either animal findings show risk, but human findings do not; or if no adequate human studies have been done, animal findings are negative.
C	Risk cannot be ruled out. Human studies are lacking, and animal studies are either positive for fetal risk or lacking. However, potential benefits may justify the potential risks.
D	Positive evidence of risk. Investigational or postmarketing data show risk to the fetus. Nevertheless, potential benefits may outweigh the potential risks. If needed in a life-threatening situation or a serious disease, the drug may be acceptable if safer drugs cannot be used or are ineffective.
X	Contraindicated in pregnancy. Studies in animals or human, or investigational or post-marketing reports have shown fetal risk which clearly outweighs any possible benefit to the patient.

Regardless of the designated Pregnancy Category or presumed safety, no drug should be administered during pregnancy unless it is clearly needed and potential benefits outweigh potential hazards to the fetus.

Poison Center Hotline

The American Association of Poison Control Centers (AAPCC) has established a national toll-free poison center hotline. Now everyone in the United States can call

1-800-222-1222

to reach the local poison center. Poison Center services are available 24 hours a day, seven days a week.

The phone number can be used for a poison emergency, or questions about poisons and poison prevention.

Regardless of where the call is placed, the hotline automatically connects callers to the closest poison control center. Existing local poison center numbers will still connect callers to their poison centers.

Callers who use a TTY/TDD and non-English speaking callers can also use this hotline.

Drug Names That Look Alike and Sound Alike

No drug name is without problems. Any name can be written or spoken poorly enough so that it can be mistaken for another. Listed in the accompanying table are drug names that can look and/or sound alike. Some are dangerously close, whereas others require incomplete prescribing information, poor communications skills, poor listening, and/or a lack of knowledge about the drugs for an error to result. To reduce errors, practitioners must share the common goal of drug name safety with pharmaceutical manufacturers, the Food and Drug Administration (FDA), the World Health Organization (WHO), the United States Adopted Name Council (USANC), and the United States Pharmacopeia (USP).

The potential for errors can be reduced by:

- Pretesting proposed names for error potential
- Careful selection of brand names and generic names by manufacturers, FDA, WHO, and USANC
- Legible handwriting
- Clear oral communications
- Writing complete drug orders
- Specifying the dosage form (eg, tablet)
- Specifying the drug strength (eg, 100 mg)
- Specifying directions (eg, take one daily with breakfast)
- Specifying the purpose/indication (eg, take one daily with breakfast to control blood pressure)
- Printing orders for new or rarely prescribed drugs
- Using computer-generated orders
- For those involved in drug dispensing and administration, being aware of the drugs that are available and paying careful attention to the work at hand
- Knowing the patient's condition/problems, to ascertain if the drug name that has been read or heard is indicated
- Double-checking completed prescriptions in the pharmacy
- Educating patients about their drug regimens (this serves as another final check that the prescription was properly read and dispensed)

If prescriptions are not computer generated, they should be formatted so that prescribers must print the name and strength in blocks like these:

The blocks should be preprinted in a 30% tint of black so that the lines appear as a light, but visible grey. This will prevent a T from looking like an I (if the top of the T falls across the block outline), an E from looking like an F, an L from looking like an I, a 7 from looking like a 1, and a 2 from looking like a 7.

The more identical attributes that drug products with similar names possess, the more likely it is that mix-ups will occur. These identical attributes are: having similar looking labels (eg, made by same manufacturer), being the same dosage form, being the same strength, having the same dosage schedule, requiring the same storage conditions (eg, refrigerated items or controlled substances) and being used for the same purpose. Also the more new drug names introduced, the more problems there will be; therefore, those companies that assign brand names to generic products worsen the problem.

*Note: Please e-mail suggestions for additions or deletions to this list to Neil M. Davis, MS, PharmD, FASHP, President, Safe Medication Practices Consulting, Inc., at: neilmdavis@neilmdavis.comBenjamin Teplitsky, retired Chief Pharmacist of Veterans Administration Hospitals in Albany, NY and Brooklyn, NY, originally developed "Look-Alike, Sound-Alike Drugs."

This list has been prepared to sensitize health professionals and their support personnel to the need for proper communication when writing, speaking, reading, and hearing drug names.

*Proprietary (brand) names are capitalized; other names are in lower case letters.

Accolate ....Accupril
Accolate ....Aclovate
Accupril ....Accolate
Accupril ....Accutane
Accupril ....Aciphex
Accurbron ....Accutane
Accutane ....Accupril
Accutane ....Accurbron
acetazolamide .....acetohexamide
acetohexamide ....acetazolamide
acetylcholine ....acetylcysteine
acetylcysteine .....acetylcholine
Aciphex ....Accupril
Aciphex ....Aricept
Aclovate ....Accolate
Acthar ....Acthrel
Acthar ....Acular
Acthrel ....Acthar
Acular ....Acthar
adapalene ....Adapin
Adapin ....adapalene
Adderall ....Inderal
Adeflor M ....Aldoclor
Adriamycin ....Idamycin
Afrin ....aspirin
Aggrastat ....Aggrenox
Aggrenox ....Aggrastat
Albutein ....albuterol
albuterol ....Albutein
albuterol ....atenolol
Alcaine ....Alcare
Alcare ....Alcaine
Aldactazide ....Aldactone
Aldactone ....Aldactazide
Aldoclor ....Adeflor M
Aldoclor ....Aldoril
Aldomet ....Aldoril
Aldomet ....Anzemet
Aldoril ....Aldoclor
Aldoril ....Aldomet
Aleve ....Alesse
Alfenta ....Sufenta
alfentanil ....Anafranil
alfentanil ....fentanyl
alfentanil ....sufentanil
Alkeran ....Leukeran
Alor 5/500 ....Alora
Alora ....Alor 5/500
alprazolam ....alprostadil
alprazolam ....lorazepam
alprostadil ....alprazolam
Altace ....alteplase
Altace ....Artane
alteplase ....Altace
alteplase ....anistreplase
Alupent ....Atrovent
Amaryl ....Amerge
Ambenyl ....Aventyl
Ambien ....Amen
Amen ....Ambien
Amerge ....Amaryl
Amicar ....amikacin
Amicar ....Amikin
amikacin ....Amicar
Amikin ....Amicar
amiloride ....amiodarone
amiloride ....amlodipine
aminophylline ......amitriptyline
aminophylline ......ampicillin
amiodarone ....amiloride
amitriptyline ....aminophylline
amitriptyline ....nortriptyline
amlodipine ....amiloride
amoxapine ....amoxicillin
amoxicillin ....amoxapine
ampicillin ....aminophylline
Anafranil ....alfentanil
Anafranil ....enalapril
Anafranil ....nafarelin
Anaprox ....Anaspaz
Anaspaz ....Anaprox
Ancobon ....Oncovin
anisindione ....anisotropine
anisotropine ....anisindione
anistreplase ....alteplase
Antabuse ....Anturane
Anturane ....Antabuse
Anturane ....Artane
Anusol ....Aplisol
Anusol ....Aquasol
Anzemet ....Aldomet
Aplisol ....Anusol
Aplisol ....Aplitest
Aplisol ....Atropisol
Aplitest ....Aplisol
Apresazide ....Apresoline
Apresoline ....Apresazide
Aquasol ....Anusol
Aricept ....Aciphex
Aricept ....Ascriptin
Artane ....Altace
Artane ....Anturane
Asacol ....Os-Cal
Ascriptin ....Aricept
Asendin ....aspirin
aspirin ....Afrin
aspirin ....Asendin
Atarax ....Ativan
Atarax ....Marax
atenolol ....albuterol
atenolol ....timolol
Atgam ....Ativan
Ativan ....Atarax
Ativan ....Atgam
Ativan ....Avitene
Atropisol ....Aplisol
Atropisol ....Aplisol
Atrovent ....Alupent
Aventyl ....Ambenyl
Aventyl ....Bentyl
Avitene ....Ativan
Avonex ....Avelox
azatadine ....azathioprine
azathioprine ....azatadine
azathioprine ....Azulfidine
azidothymidine ....azathioprine
azithromycin ....erythromycin
Azulfidine ....azathioprine
bacitracin ....Bactrim

bacitracin	Bactroban
baclofen	Bactroban
baclofen	Beclovent
Bactrim	bacitracin
Bactroban	bacitracin
Bactroban	baclofen
Banthine	Brethine
Beclovent	baclofen
Beminal	Benemid
Benadryl	benazepril
Benadryl	Bentyl
Benadryl	Benylin
benazepril	Benadryl
Benemid	Beminal
Benoxyl	Brevoxyl
Benoxyl	Peroxyl
Bentyl	Aventyl
Bentyl	Benadryl
Benylin	Benadryl
Benylin	Ventolin
benztropine	bromocriptine
bepridil	Prepidil
Betadine	betaine
Betagan	Betagen
Betagen	Betagan
betaine	Betadine
betaxolol	bethanechol
bethanechol	betaxolol
Betoptic	Betoptic S
Betoptic S	Betoptic
Bicillin	Wycillin
Brethine	Brethaire
Brevoxyl	Benoxyl
bromocriptine	benztropine
Bronkodyl	Bronkosol
Bronkosol	Bronkodyl
bupivacaine	mepivacaine
bupropion	buspirone
buspirone	bupropion
butabarbital	Butalbital
Butalbital	butabarbital
Cafergot	Carafate
Caladryl	calamine
calamine	Caladryl
calcifediol	calcitriol
calcitonin	calcitriol
calcitriol	calcifediol
calcitriol	calcitonin
calcium glubionate	calcium gluconate
calcium gluconate	calcium glubionate
Capastat	Cepastat
Capitrol	Captopril
Captopril	Capitrol
Carafate	Cafergot
Carbatrol	Cartrol
Carbex	Surbex
Carboplatin	Cisplatin
Cardene	Cardura
Cardene	codeine
Cardene SR	Cardizem SR
Cardizem SR	Cardene SR
Cardura	Cardene
Cardura	Cordarone
Cardura	Coumadin
Cardura	K-Dur
carteolol	carvedilol
Cartrol	Carbatrol
carvedilol	carteolol
Catapres	Cetapred
Catapres	Combipres
cefamandole	cefmetazole
cefazolin	cefprozil
cefmetazole	cefamandole
Cefobid	cefonicid
cefonicid	Cefobid
Cefotan	Ceftin
cefotaxime	cefoxitin
cefotaxime	ceftizoxime
cefotaxime	cefuroxime
cefotetan	cefoxitin
cefoxitin	cefotaxime
cefoxitin	Cefotetan
cefoxitin	Cytoxan
cefprozil	Cefazolin
ceftazidime	ceftizoxime
Ceftin	Cefotan
Ceftin	Cefzil
ceftizoxime	cefotaxime
ceftizoxime	ceftazidime
cefuroxime	cefotaxime
cefuroxime	deferoxamine
Cefzil	Ceftin
Cefzil	Kefzol
Celebrex	Cerebyx
Cepastat	Capastat
cephapirin	cephradine
cephradine	cephapirin
cephradine	cephapirin
Cerebyx	Celebrex
Cerebyx	Cerezyme
Ceredase	Cerezyme
Cerezyme	Cerebyx
Cerezyme	Ceredase
Cetaphil	Cetapred
Cetapred	Catapres
Cetapred	Cetaphil
Chenix	Cystex
chlorambucil	Chloromycetin
Chloromycetin	chlorambucil
chlorpromazine	chlorpropamide
chlorpromazine	clomipramine
chlorpromazine	prochlorperazine
chlorpropamide	chlorpromazine
Chorex	Chymex
Chymex	Chorex
Cidex	Lidex
Ciloxan	cinoxacin
Ciloxan	Cytoxan
cimetidine	simethicone
cinoxacin	Ciloxan
Cisplatin	Carboplatin
Citracal	Citrucel
Citrucel	Citracal
Clinoril	Clozaril
clofazimine	clozapine
clofibrate	clorazepate
clomiphene	clomipramine
clomiphene	clonidine
clomipramine	chlorpromazine
clomipramine	clomiphene
clonazepam	lorazepam
clonidine	clomiphene
clonidine	quinidine
clorazepate	clofibrate
clotrimazole	co-trimoxazole
Cloxapen	clozapine
clozapine	clofazimine
clozapine	Cloxapen
Clozaril	Clinoril
Clozaril	Colazal
codeine	Cardene
codeine	Lodine
Colazal	Clozaril
Combipres	Catapres
Combivent	Combivir
Combivir	Combivent
Compazine	Copaxone
Comvax	Recombivax
Copaxone	Compazine
Cordarone	Cardura
Cordran	Cordarone
Cort-Dome	Cortone
Cortone	Cort-Dome
Cortrosyn	Cotazym
Cotazym	Cortrosyn
co-trimoxazole	clotrimazole
Coumadin	Cardura
Coumadin	Kemadrin
Cozaar	Zocor
cyclobenzaprine	cycloserine
cyclobenzaprine	cyproheptadine
cyclophosphamide	cyclosporine
cycloserine	cyclobenzaprine
cycloserine	cyclosporine
cyclosporine	cyclophosphamide
cyclosporine	cycloserine

Drug name	Confused with
cyclosporine	Cyklokapron
Cyklokapron	cyclosporin
cyproheptadine	cyclobenzaprine
Cystex	Chenix
Cytadren	cytarabine
cytarabine	Cytadren
cytarabine	vidarabine
CytoGam	Cytoxan
Cytosar U	Cytovene
Cytosar U	Cytoxan
Cytotec	Cytoxan
Cytovene	Cytosar U
Cytoxan	cefoxitin
Cytoxan	Ciloxan
Cytoxan	CytoGam
Cytoxan	Cytosar U
Cytoxan	Cytotec
dacarbazine	Dicarbosil
dacarbazine	procarbazine
Dacriose	Danocrine
Dalmane	Demulen
Dalmane	Dialume
Danocrine	Dacriose
Dantrium	Daraprim
dapsone	Diprosone
Daranide	Daraprim
Daraprim	Dantrium
Daraprim	Daranide
Darvocet-N	Darvon-N
Darvon-N	Darvocet-N
daunorubicin	dactinomycin
daunorubicin	doxorubicin
deferoxamine	cefuroxime
Delsym	Desyrel
Demerol	Demulen
Demerol	Dymelor
Demulen	Dalmane
Demulen	Demerol
Depen	Endep
Depo-Estradiol	Depo-Testadiol
Depo-Medrol	Solu-Medrol
Depo-Testadiol	Depo-Estradiol
Dermatop	Dimetapp
Desferal	Disophrol
desipramine	disopyramide
desipramine	imipramine
desoximetasone	dexamethasone
Desoxyn	digoxin
Desyrel	Delsym
Desyrel	Zestril
dexamethasone	desoximetasone
Dexedrine	Dextran
Dexedrine	Excedrin
Dextran	Dexedrine
DiaBeta	Zebeta
Dialume	Dalmane
Diamox	Trimox
diazepam	diazoxide
diazepam	Ditropan
diazoxide	diazepam
diazoxide	Dyazide
Dicarbosil	dacarbazine
dichloroacetic acid	trichloracetic acid
diclofenac	Diflucan
diclofenac	Duphalac
dicyclomine	doxycycline
dicyclomine	dyclonine
Diflucan	diclofenac
Diflucan	disulfiram
digoxin	Desoxyn
digoxin	doxepin
Dilantin	Dilaudid
Dilaudid	Dilantin
dimenhydrinate	diphenhydramine
Dimetane	Dimetapp
Dimetapp	Dermatop
Dimetapp	Dimetane
diphenhydramine	dimenhydrinate
Diprosone	dapsone
dipyridamole	disopyramide
Disophrol	Desferal
disopyramide	desipramine
disopyramide	dipyridamole
disulfiram	Diflucan
dithranol	Ditropan
Ditropan	diazepam
Ditropan	dithranol
dobutamine	dopamine
Dolobid	Slo-bid
Donnagel	Donnatal
Donnatal	Donnagel
dopamine	dobutamine
dopamine	Dopram
Dopar	Dopram
Dopram	dopamine
Dopram	Dopar
doxacurium	doxapram
doxacurium	doxorubicin
doxapram	doxacurium
doxapram	doxazosin
doxapram	doxepin
doxapram	doxorubicin
doxazosin	doxapram
doxazosin	doxepin
doxazosin	doxorubicin
doxepin	digoxin
doxepin	doxapram
doxepin	doxazosin
doxepin	Doxidan
Doxidan	doxepin
Doxil	Doxy
Doxil	Paxil
Doxinate	doxapram
doxorubicin	dactinomycin
doxorubicin	daunorubicin
doxorubicin	doxacurium
doxorubicin	doxapram
doxorubicin	doxazosin
doxorubicin	idarubicin
Doxy	Doxil
doxycycline	dicyclomine
doxycycline	doxylamine
doxylamine	doxycycline
dronabinol	droperidol
droperidol	dronabinol
Duphalac	diclofenac
Dyazide	diazoxide
dyclonine	dicyclomine
Dymelor	Demerol
Dynabac	Dynacin
Dynabac	DynaCirc
Dynacin	Dynabac
Dynacin	DynaCirc
DynaCirc	Dynabac
DynaCirc	Dynacin
Ecotrin	Edecrin
Edecrin	Ecotrin
Efidac	Efudex
Efudex	Efidac
Elavil	Equanil
Elavil	Mellaril
Eldepryl	enalapril
Eldopaque Forte	Eldoquin Forte
Eldoquin Forte	Eldopaque Forte
Elmiron	Imuran
Emcyt	Eryc
enalapril	Anafranil
enalapril	Eldepryl
Enduronyl Forte	Inderal 40 mg
enflurane	isoflurane
Entex	Tenex
ephedrine	epinephrine
epinephrine	ephedrine
Epogen	Neupogen
Equagesic	EquiGesic (veterlnary)
Equanil	Elavil
EquiGesic (veterinary)	Equagesic
Eryc	Emcyt
Erythrocin	Ethmozine
erythromycin	azithromycin
erythromycin	Ethmozine
Esimil	Estinyl
Esimil	Ismelin
Estinyl	Esimil

Estraderm	Testoderm
Ethamolin	ethanol
ethanol	Ethamolin
ethanol	Ethyol
Ethmozine	Erythrocin
Ethmozine	erythromycin
ethosuximide	methsuximide
Ethyol	ethanol
etidocaine	etidronate
etidronate	etidocaine
etidronate	etomidate
etomidate	etidronate
Eurax	Evoxac
Eurax	Serax
Eurax	Urex
Evoxac	Eurax
Excedrin	Dexedrine
Factrel	Sectral
fentanyl	alfentanil
Feosol	Fer-In-Sol
Feridex	Fertinex
Fer-In-Sol	Feosol
Fertinex	Feridex
Fioricet	Fiorinal
Fiorinal	Fioricet
Fiorinal	Florinef
flecainide	fluconazole
Flexeril	Floxin
Flexon	Floxin
Flomax	Fosamax
Flomax	Volmax
Florinef	Fiorinal
Florvite	Folvite
Floxin	Flexeril
Floxin	Flexon
fluconazole	flecainide
Fludara	FUDR
Flumadine	flunisolide
Flumadine	flutamide
flunisolide	Flumadine
flunisolide	fluocinonide
fluocinolone	fluocinonide
fluocinonide	flunisolide
fluocinonide	fluocinolone
fluoxetine	fluvastatin
flutamide	Flumadine
fluvastatin	fluoxetine
folic acid	folinic acid
folinic acid	folic acid
Folvite	Florvite
Fosamax	Flomax
fosinopril	lisinopril
FUDR	Fludara
Fulvicin	Furacin
Furacin	Fulvicin
furosemide	Torsemide
Gantanol	Gantrisin
Gantrisin	Gantanol
Genpril	Genprin
Genprin	Genpril
Glaucon	glucagon
glimepiride	glipizide
glipizide	glimepiride
glipizide	glyburide
glucagon	Glaucon
Glucotrol	glyburide
glutethimide	guanethidine
glyburide	glipizide
glyburide	Glucotrol
GoLYTELY	NuLytely
gonadorelin	gonadotropin
gonadorelin	guanadrel
gonadotropin	gonadorelin
guaifenesin	guanfacine
guaifenesin	guanfacine
guanabenz	guanadrel
guanabenz	guanfacine
guanadrel	gonadorelin
guanadrel	guanabenz
guanethidine	glutethimide
guanethidine	guanidine
guanfacine	guaifenesin
guanfacine	guanabenz
guanfacine	guanidine
guanidine	guanethidine
guanidine	guanfacine
halcinonide	Halcion
Halcion	halcinonide
Halcion	Haldol
Halcion	Healon
Haldol	Halcion
Haldol	Halog
Halog	Haldol
Halotestin	Halotex
Halotestin	halothane
Halotex	Halotestin
halothane	Halotestin
Healon	Halcion
Heparin	Hespan
Hespan	Heparin
Humalog	Humulin
Humulin	Humalog
Hycodan	Hycomine
Hycodan	Vicodin
Hycomine	Hycodan
hydralazine	hydroxyzine
hydrochlorothiazide	hydroflumethiazide
hydrocortisone	hydroxychloroquine
hydroflumethiazide	hydrochlorothiazide
hydromorphone	morphine
hydroxychloroquine	hydrocortisone
hydroxyprogesterone	medroxyprogesterone
hydroxyurea	hydroxyzine
hydroxyzine	hydralazine
hydroxyzine	hydroxyurea
Hygroton	Regroton
Hytone	Vytone
Idamycin	Adriamycin
Idarubicin	doxorubicin
Iletin	Lente
imipenem	Omnipen
imipramine	desipramine
Imodium	Indocin
Imodium	Ionamin
Imuran	Elmiron
Imuran	Inderal
indapamide	iodamide
indapamide	iopamidol
indapamide	Iopidine
Inderal	Adderall
Inderal	Imuran
Inderal	Inderide
Inderal	Isordil
Inderal 40 mg	Enduronyl Forte
Inderide	Inderal
Indocin	Imodium
Indocin	Vicodin
interferon 2	interleukin 2
interferon alfa-2a	interferon alfa-2b
interferon alfa-2b	interferon alfa-2a
interleukin 2	interferon 2
interleukin 2	interleukin 11
Intropin	Isoptin
iodamide	indapamide
iodapamide	Iopidine
iodine	Iopidine
iodine	Lodine
Ionamin	Imodium
iopamidol	indapamide
Iopidine	indapamide
Iopidine	iodapamide
Iopidine	iodine
Iopidine	Lodine
Ismelin	Esimil
Ismelin	Isuprel
isoflurane	enflurane
Isoptin	Intropin
Isopto Carbachol	Isopto Carpine
Isopto Carpine	Isopto Carbachol
Isordil	Inderal
Isordil	Isuprel
Isuprel	Ismelin

Isuprel	Isordil
Kaochlor	K-Lor
K-Dur	Cardura
Kefzol	Cefzil
Kemadrin	Coumadin
Klaron	Klor-Con
K-Lor	Kaochlor
Klor-Con	Klaron
K-Phos Neutral	Neutra-Phos-K
lactose	lactulose
lactulose	lactose
Lamictal	Lamisil
Lamictal	Lomotil
Lamisil	Lamictal
lamivudine	lamotrigine
lamotrigine	lamivudine
Lanoxin	Levsinex
Lanoxin	Lonox
Lantus	Lente
Lasix	Lidex
Lasix	Luvox
Lasix	Luxiq
Lente	Iletin
Lente	Lantus
Leukeran	Alkeran
Leukeran	Leukine
Leukine	Leukeran
Leustatin	lovastatin
Levatol	Lipitor
Levbid	Lithobid
levothyroxine	liothyronine
Librax	Librium
Librium	Librax
Lidex	Cidex
Lidex	Lasix
Lioresal	lisinopril
liothyronine	levothyroxine
Lipitor	Levatol
lisinopril	fosinopril
lisinopril	Lioresal
Lithobid	Levbid
Lithobid	Lithostat
Lithobid	Lithotabs
Lithonate	Lithostat
Lithostat	Lithobid
Lithostat	Lithonate
Lithostat	Lithotabs
Lithotabs	Lithobid
Lithotabs	Lithostat
Livostin	lovastatin
Lodine	codeine
Lodine	iodine
Lodine	Iopidine
Lomotil	Lamictal
Loniten	Lotensin
Lonox	Lanoxin
Lonox	Loprox
Loprox	Lonox
Lopurin	Lopressor
Lopurin	Lupron
Lorabid	Lortab
lorazepam	alprazolam
lorazepam	clonazepam
Lortab	Lorabid
Lotensin	Loniten
Lotensin	lovastatin
Lotronex	Lovenox
Lotronex	Protonix
lovastatin	Leustatin
lovastatin	Livostin
lovastatin	Lotensin
Lovenox	Lotronex
Luminal	Tuinal
Lupron	Lopurin
Lupron	Nuprin
Luvox	Lasix
Luxiq	Lasix
Maalox	Maolate
Maalox	Marax
magnesium sulfate	manganese sulfate
manganese sulfate	magnesium sulfate
Maolate	Maalox
Maranox	Marax
Marax	Atarax
Marax	Maalox
Marax	Maranox
Maxidex	Maxzide
Maxzide	Maxidex
Mebaral	Medrol
Mebaral	Mellaril
mecamylamine	mesalamine
Medrol	Mebaral
medroxyprogesterone	hydroxyprogesterone
medroxyprogesterone	methylprednisolone
medroxyprogesterone	methyltestosterone
Mellaril	Elavil
Mellaril	Mebaral
melphalan	Mephyton
mephenytoin	Mephyton
mephenytoin	phenytoin
mephobarbital	methocarbamol
Mephyton	melphalan
Mephyton	mephenytoin
mepivacaine	bupivacaine
Mesantoin	Mestinon
Mestinon	Mesantoin
Mestinon	Metatensin
metaproterenol	metipranolol
metaproterenol	metoprolol
Metatensin	Mestinon
methazolamide	metolazone
methenamine	methionine
methicillin	mezlocillin
methionine	methenamine
methocarbamol	mephobarbital
methsuximide	ethosuximide
methylprednisolone	medroxyprogesterone
methyltestosterone	medroxyprogesterone
metipranolol	metaproterenol
metolazone	methazolamide
metolazone	metoprolol
metoprolol	metaproterenol
metoprolol	metolazone
metyrapone	metyrosine
metyrosine	metyrapone
Mevacor	Mivacron
mezlocillin	methicillin
miconazole	Micronase
miconazole	Micronor
Micro-K	Micronase
Micronase	miconazole
Micronase	Micro-K
Micronase	Micronor
Micronor	miconazole
Micronor	Micronase
Midrin	Mydfrin
Mifeprex	Mirapex
Milontin	Miltown
Milontin	Mylanta
Miltown	Milontin
Minocin	Mithracin
Minocin	niacin
MiraLax	Mirapex
Mirapex	Mifeprex
Mirapex	MiraLax
Mithracin	Minocin
mithramycin	mitomycin
mitomycin	mithramycin
Mivacron	Mevacor
Moban	Mobidin
Mobidin	Moban
Modane	Mudrane
Monopril	Monurol
Monurol	Monopril
morphine	hydromorphone
Mudrane	Modane
Myambutol	Nembutal
Mycelex	Myoflex
Myciguent	Mycitracin
Mycitracin	Myciguent
Mydfrin	Midrin
Mylanta	Milontin
Mylanta	Mynatal

Myleran	Mylicon
Mylicon	Myleran
Mynatal	Mylanta
Myoflex	Mycelex
nafarelin	Anafranil
Naldecon	Nalfon
Nalfon	Naldecon
naloxone	naltrexone
naltrexone	naloxone
Narcan	Norcuron
Nasarel	Nizoral
Navane	Norvasc
Navane	Nubain
Nembutal	Myambutol
Nephro-Calci	Nephrocaps
Nephrocaps	Nephro-Calci
Neumega	Neupogen
Neupogen	Epogen
Neupogen	Nutramigen
Neurontin	Noroxin
Neutra-Phos-K	K-Phos Neutral
niacin	Minocin
nicardipine	nifedipine
Nicobid	Nitro-Bid
Nicoderm	Nitroderm
Nicorette	Nordette
nifedipine	nicardipine
nifedipine	nimodipine
Nilstat	Nitrostat
Nilstat	Nystatin
nimodipine	nifedipine
Nitro-Bid	Nicobid
Nitroderm	Nicoderm
nitroglycerin	nitroprusside
Nitrol	Nizoral
nitroprusside	nitroglycerin
Nitrostat	Hyperstat
Nitrostat	Nilstat
Nitrostat	Nystatin
Nizoral	Nasarel
Nizoral	Nitrol
Norcuron	Narcan
Nordette	Nicorette
Norgesic #40	Norgesic Forte
Norgesic Forte	Norgesic #40
Noroxin	Neurontin
nortriptyline	amitriptyline
Norvasc	Navane
Norvasc	Vascor
Nubain	Navane
NuLytely	GoLYTELY
Nuprin	Lupron
Nutramigen	Neupogen
Nystatin	Nilstat
Nystatin	Nitrostat
OctreoScan	octreotide
OctreoScan	Oncoscint
octreotide	OctreoScan
Ocufen	Ocuflox
Ocuflox	Ocufen
olanzapine	olsalazine
olsalazine	olanzapine
Omnipen	Imipenem
Omnipen	Unipen
OncoScint	OctreoScan
Oncovin	Ancobon
Ophthaine	Ophthetic
Ophthetic	Ophthaine
Optiray	Optivar
Optivar	Optiray
Oretic	Oreton
Oreton	Oretic
Orinase	Ornade
Ornade	Orinase
Os-Cal	Asacol
oxaprozin	oxazepam
oxazepam	oxaprozin
oxybutynin	OxyContin
OxyContin	oxybutynin
oxymetazoline	oxymetholone
oxymetholone	oxymetazoline
oxymetholone	oxymorphone
oxymorphone	oxymetholone
paclitaxel	paroxetine
paclitaxel	Paxil
panadol	pindolol
pancuronium	pipecuronium
Paraplatin	Platinol
Paregoric	Percogesic
Parlodel	pindolol
paroxetine	paclitaxel
paroxetine	pyridoxine
Patanol	Platinol
Pathilon	Pathocil
Pathocil	Pathilon
Pathocil	Placidyl
Paxil	Doxil
Paxil	paclitaxel
Paxil	Plavix
Paxil	Taxol
Pediapred	Pediazole
Pediazole	Pediapred
Penetrex	Pentrax
penicillamine	penicillin
penicillin	penicillamine
penicillin G potassium	penicillin G procaine
penicillin G procaine	penicillin G potassium
pentobarbital	phenobarbital
pentosan	pentostatin
pentostatin	pentosan
Pentrax	Penetrex
Pentrax	Permax
Perative	Periactin
Percocet	Percodan
Percodan	Percocet
Percodan	Percogesic
Percodan	Periactin
Percogesic	Paregoric
Percogesic	Percodan
Periactin	Persantine
Peridex	Precedex
Permax	Pentrax
Permax	Pernox
Pernox	Permax
PerOxyl	Benoxyl
Persantine	Periactin
phenobarbital	pentobarbital
phentermine	phentolamine
phentolamine	phentermine
Phenytoin	mephenytoin
pHisoDerm	pHisoHex
pHisoHex	pHisoDerm
pHisoHex	Phos-Ex
PhosChol	PhosLo
PhosChol	Phosphocol P32
Phos-Flur	PhosLo
PhosLo	PhosChol
PhosLo	Phos-Flur
Phosphocol P32	PhosChol
physostigmine	Prostigmin
physostigmine	pyridostigmine
pindolol	Panadol
pindolol	Parlodel
pindolol	Plendil
pipecuronium	pancuronium
Pitocin	Pitressin
Pitressin	Pitocin
Placidyl	Pathocil
Platinol	Paraplatin
Platinol	Patanol
Plavix	Paxil
Plendil	pindolol
Plendil	Pletal
Pletal	Plendil
Polocaine	prilocaine
Ponstel	Pronestyl
Posicor	Proscar
Posicor	Psorcon
pralidoxime	Pramoxine
pralidoxime	pyridoxine
Pramoxine	pralidoxime
Pravachol	Prevacid
Pravachol	propranolol
PreCare	Precose
Precedex	Peridex
Precose	PreCare

Drug	Confused with
prednisolone	prednisone
prednisone	prednisolone
prednisone	Primidone
Premarin	Primaxin
Premarin	Remeron
Premphase	Prempro
Prempro	Premphase
Prepidil	bepridil
Prevacid	Pravachol
Prevacid	Prevpac
Preven	Prevnar
Prevnar	Preven
Prevpac	Prevacid
prilocaine	Polocaine
prilocaine	Prilosec
Prilosec	prilocaine
Prilosec	Prinivil
Prilosec	Prozac
Primaxin	Premarin
primidone	prednisone
Prinivil	Prilosec
Prinivil	Proventil
ProAmatine	protamine
Probenecid	Procanbid
probenecid	Procanbid
Procanbid	Probenecid
Procanbid	probenecid
procarbazine	dacarbazine
prochlorperazine	chlorpromazine
Prokine	procaine
Proloprim	Protropin
promazine	promethazine
promethazine	promazine
Pronestyl	Ponstel
propranolol	Pravachol
Proscar	Posicor
Proscar	ProSom
Proscar	Prozac
Proscar	Psorcon
ProSom	Proscar
ProSom	Prozac
ProSom	Psorcon
Prostigmin	physostigmine
protamine	ProAmatine
protamine	Protopam
protamine	Protropin
Protonix	Lotronex
Protopam	protamine
Protopam	Protropin
Protropin	Proloprim
Protropin	Protamine
Protropin	Protopam
Proventil	Prinivil
Prozac	Prilosec
Prozac	Proscar
Prozac	ProSom
Psorcon	Proscar
Psorcon	ProSom
Pyridium	pyridoxine
pyridostigmine	physostigmine
pyridoxine	paroxetine
pyridoxine	pralidoxime
pyridoxine	Pyridium
Quarzan	quazepam
Quarzan	Questran
quazepam	Quarzan
Questran	Quarzan
quinidine	clonidine
quinidine	quinine
quinidine	Quinora
quinine	quinidine
Quinora	quinidine
ranitidine	rimantadine
ranitidine	ritodrine
Reglan	Regonol
Reglan	Renagel
Regonol	Reglan
Regonol	Renagel
Regranex	Repronex
Remeron	Premarin
Renacidin	Remicade
Renagel	Reglan
Renagel	Regonol
Repronex	Regranex
reserpine	risperidone
Restasis	Retavase
Restoril	Vistaril
Restoril	Zestril
Retavase	Restasis
Retrovir	ritonavir
Revex	ReVia
ReVia	Revex
Ribavirin	riboflavin
riboflavin	Ribavirin
rifabutin	rifampin
Rifadin	Ritalin
Rifamate	rifampin
rifampin	rifabutin
rifampin	Rifamate
rifampin	rifapentine
rimantadine	ranitidine
risperidone	reserpine
Ritalin	Rifadin
ritodrine	ranitidine
ritonavir	Retrovir
Roxanol	Roxicet
Roxicet	Roxanol
Sandimmune	Sandoglobulin
Sandimmune	Sandostatin
Sandoglobulin	Sandimmune
Sandoglobulin	Sandostatin
Sandostatin	Sandimmune
Sandostatin	Sandoglobulin
saquinavir	Sinequan
Sarafem	Serophene
Sectral	Factrel
Sectral	Septra
selegiline	Stelazine
Septa	Septra
Septra	Sectral
Septra	Septa
Serax	Eurax
Serax	Xerac
Serentil	Serevent
Serentil	sertraline
Serevent	Serentil
Serophene	Sarafem
sertraline	Serentil
simethicone	cimetidine
Sinequan	saquinavir
Slo-bid	Dolobid
Slow FE	Slow-K
Slow-K	Slow FE
Solu-Medrol	Depo-Medrol
somatrem	somatropin
somatropin	somatrem
somatropin	sumatriptan
sotalol	Stadol
Sporanox	Suprax
Stadol	sotalol
Stelazine	selegiline
Sufenta	Alfenta
Sufenta	Survanta
sufentanil	alfentanil
sulfadiazine	sulfasalazine
sulfamethizole	sulfamethoxazole
sulfamethoxazole	sulfamethizole
sulfasalazine	sulfadiazine
sulfasalazine	sulfisoxazole
sulfisoxazole	sulfasalazine
sumatriptan	somatropin
Suprax	Sporanox
Surbex	Carbex
Surbex	Surfak
Surfak	Surbex
Survanta	Sufenta
Synagis	Synalgos-DC
Synalgos-DC	Synagis
Taxol	Paxil
Taxol	Taxotere
Taxotere	Taxol
Tazicef	Tazidime
Tazidime	Tazicef
Tegretol	Toradol
Tegretol	Trental
Tenex	Entex

Tenex ....Ten-K
Tenex ....Xanax
Ten-K ....Tenex
terbinafine ....terbutaline
terbutaline ....terbinafine
terbutaline ....tolbutamide
terconazole ....tioconazole
Testoderm ....Estraderm
testolactone ....testosterone
testosterone ....testolactone
Theolair ....Thyrolar
TheraFlu ....Thera-Flur
Thera-Flur ....TheraFlu
thiamine ....Thorazine
thioridazine ....thiothixene
thioridazine ....Thorazine
thiothixene ....thioridazine
Thorazine ....thiamine
Thorazine ....thioridazine
Thyrogen ....Thyrolar
Thyrolar ....Theolair
Thyrolar ....Thyrogen
timolol ....atenolol
Timoptic ....Viroptic
tioconazole ....terconazole
TobraDex ....Tobrex
tobramycin ....Trobicin
Tobrex ....TobraDex
tolazamide ....tolbutamide
tolbutamide ....terbutaline
tolbutamide ....tolazamide
tolnaftate ....Tornalate
Toradol ....Tegretol
Toradol ....Torecan
Torecan ....Toradol
Tornalate ....tolnaftate
Torsemide ....furosemide
tramadol ....Toradol
tramadol ....Trandate
Trandate ....tramadol
Trandate ....Trental
Travatan ....Xalatan
Trental ....Tegretol
Trental ....Trandate
tretinoin ....trientine
triamcinolone ......Triaminicin
triamcinolone ......Triaminicol
Triaminic ....Triaminicin
Triaminic ....TriHemic
Triaminicin ....triamcinolone
Triaminicin ....Triaminic
Triaminicol ....triamcinolone
triamterene ....trimipramine
trichloroacetic acid ....dichloroacetic acid

trientine ....tretinoin
trifluoperazine .....triflupromazine
Triaminic ....TriHemic
trimeprazine ....trimipramine
trimipramine ....triamterene
trimipramine ....trimeprazine
Trimox ....Diamox
Trimox ....Tylox
Trobicin ....tobramycin
Tronolane ....Tronothane
Tronothane ....Tronolane
Tuinal ....Luminal
Tuinal ....Tylenol
Tylenol ....Tuinal
Tylenol ....Tylox
Tylox ....Trimox
Tylox ....Tylenol
Ultane ....Ultram
Ultram ....Ultane
Unicap ....Unipen
Unipen ....Omnipen
Unipen ....Unicap
Urex ....Eurax
Urised ....Urispas
Urispas ....Urised
Valcyte ....Valium
Valium ....Valcyte
valsartan ....Valstar
Valstar ....valsartan
Vancenase ....Vanceril
Vanceril ....Vancenase
Vanceril ....Vansil
Vaniqa ....Viagra
Vansil ....Vanceril
Vantin ....Ventolin
Vascor ....Norvasc
Vasocidin ....Vasodilan
Vasodilan ....Vasocidin
Vasosulf ....Velosef
Velosef ....Vasosulf
Ventolin ....Benylin
Ventolin ....Vantin
VePesid ....Versed
Verelan ....Virilon
Verelan ....Vivarin
Verelan ....Voltaren
Versed ....VePesid
Vexol ....VoSol
Viagra ....Vaniqa
Vicodin ....Hycodan
Vicodin ....Indocin
vidarabine ....cytarabine
vinblastine ....vincristine
vinblastine ....vinorelbine
vincristine ....vinblastine

vinorelbine ....vinblastine
Vioxx ....Zyvox
Virilon ....Verelan
Viroptic ....Timoptic
Visine ....Visken
Visken ....Visine
Vistaril ....Restoril
Vivarin ....Verelan
Volmax ....Flomax
Voltaren ....Verelan
VoSol ....Vexol
Vytone ....Hytone
Wellbutrin ....Wellcovorin
Wellbutrin ....Wellferon
Wellcovorin ....Wellbutrin
Wellcovorin ....Wellferon
Wellferon ....Wellbutrin
Wellferon ....Wellcovorin
Wycillin ....Bicillin
Xalatan ....Travatan
Xanax ....Tenex
Xanax ....Xopenex
Xanax ....Zantac
Xerac ....Serax
Xopenex ....Xanax
Zagam ....Zyban
Zantac ....Xanax
Zantac ....Zofran
Zarontin ....Zaroxolyn
Zaroxolyn ....Zarontin
Zebeta ....DiaBeta
Zebeta ....DiaBeta
Zestril ....Desyrel
Zestril ....Restoril
Zestril ....Zostrix
Zocor ....Cozaar
Zofran ....Zantac
Zofran ....Zosyn
ZORprin ....Zyloprim
Zostrix ....Zestril
Zostrix ....Zovirax
Zosyn ....Zofran
Zosyn ....Zyvox
Zovirax ....Zostrix
Zyban ....Zagam
Zyloprim ....ZORprin
Zyprexa ....Zyrtec
Zyrtec ....Zyprexa
Zyvox ....Vioxx
Zyvox Zosyn

Patient Drug Facts

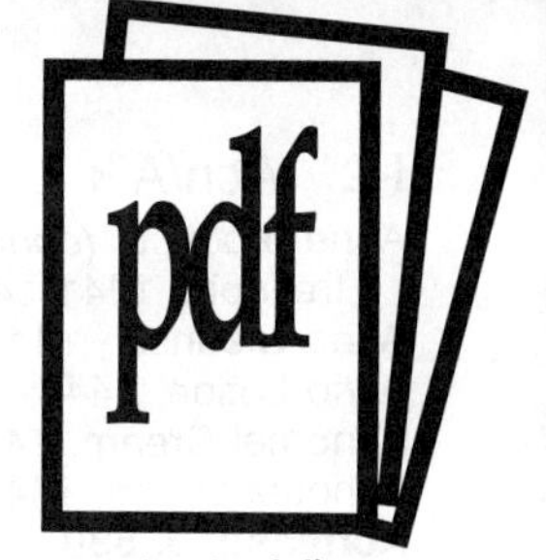

The *Patient Drug Facts* Annual Index lists all generic names (in bold), brand names, and drug group names included in *Patient Drug Facts.* Index entries may refer to more than one doseform of a product (ie, tablets, capsules, elixir, cream) when all forms are included on a single page. Separate index entries are included when multiple forms of a product appear on different pages or when products are listed in more than one therapeutic group.

GENERAL INDEX

.44 Magnum, 587
2-Ethylhexyl p-methoxycinnamate, 1521
2-Ethylhexyl salicylate, 1516, 1517, 1518, 1520, 1521
4-Way Long Lasting Nasal Spray, 517
5-Aminosalicylic acid agents, 1019-1021
5-ASA, 1019-1021
5-HT3 receptor antagonists, 696-698
6-MP, see Mercaptopurine
8-Hour Bayer Caplets, 601
8-Methoxypsoralen, 1460
20-20, 587
357 HR Magnum, 587
666 Cold Preparation Maximum Strength Liquid, 545

A-200, 1244
A and D, 1496
Abacavir, 1190
Abacavir sulfate/Lamivudine/Zidovudine, 1190
Absorbine Jr., 1131, 1514
Abuval Sport, 1519-1520
Acacia, 985
Acarbose, 272
Accolate, 468
Accu-Check, 1749
Accupril, 390
Accutane, 1689
Acebutolol HCl, 379
Acel-Imune, 1264
Aceon, 390
Acephen, 598
Aceta, 597
Aceta-Gesic Tablets, 529, 609
Acetaminophen, 597-600
  in antacid combinations, 929
  buffered, 598
  in migraine combinations, 668
  in narcotic pain relievers, 623-629
  in nonnarcotic pain relievers, 608-611
  in nonprescription sleep aids, 822
  in skeletal muscle relaxants, 889
  in upper respiratory combinations, 522-523, 529, 537-541, 545-547, 549-553, 557-561, 563-564
Acetaminophen and pentazocine, 633
Acetaminophen Uniserts, 598
Acetaminophen w/Codeine Elixir, 623
Acetaminophen w/Codeine Tablets, 623-624
Acetasol, 1400
Acetasol-HC, 1400
Acetazolamide
  as anticonvulsant, 825-827
Acetazolamide *(cont.)*
  as diuretic, 313
Acetest, 1757
Acetic acid
  in anorectal preparations, 1431
  in antifungal combinations, 1136
  in douche products, 1425
  in otic preparations, 1400
Acetohexamide, 278
Acetohydroxamic acid, 1650-1651
Acetone
  in acne products, 1444, 1447-1448
  in antifungal combinations, 1135-1136
Acetylcholine chloride intraocular, 1319
Acetylcysteine, 485
Achromycin, 1094
Acidifiers
  urinary tract, 1652-1654
Aciphex, 968
Acitretin, 1454-1456
Aclovate, 247
Acne products
  azelaic acid, 1438-1439
  benzoyl peroxide, 1435-1437
  combinations, 1444-1449
  sulfur, 1440
  tazarotene, 1464-1466

Acne products *(cont.)*
tretinoin, 1441-1443
Acno Cleanser, 1447
Acno Lotion, 1444
Acnomel Cream, 1444
Acnotex Lotion, 1444
Acrivastine, 530
ACT, 35
ACT for Kids, 35
ActHIB, 1268
Acticin, 1244
Actidose with Sorbitol, 1633
Actidose-Aqua, 1633
Actifed Cold & Allergy Tablets, 533
Actifed Cold & Sinus Maximum Strength Tablets, 538
Actigall, 973
Actimmune, 1242
Actinex, 1528
Actiq, 615
Actisite, 1412
Activase, 116
Active immunization agents, 1258-1261
Activella, 161
Actonel, 305
Actos, 275
ACU-dyne, 1505
Acular, 1356
Acyclovir, 1164
Adalat CC, 369
Adderall, 575
Adenine arabinoside, see Vidarabine
Adipex-P, 579
Adipost, 579
Adolph's Salt Substitute, 434
Adprin-B, 601
Adprin-B, Extra Strength, 601
Adprin-B Coated Tablets, 606
Adrenal cortical steroids
corticosteroid combinations topical, 254-257
corticosteroids topical, 247-253
corticotropin, 235-238
glucocorticoids, 239-246
mineralocorticoid, 258-261
Adrenal steroid inhibitors
aminoglutethimide, 262-263
Adrenalin Chloride, 455, 501
Adrenaline Chloride, 455
Adriamycin PFS, 1560
Adriamycin RDF, 1560
Adsorbocarpine, 1319
Advair Diskus, 471
Advance, 1765
Advanced Formula Di-Gel, 921
Advantage, 1749
Advil, 638
Advil, Junior Strength, 638
Advil Cold & Sinus Tablets, 523
Advil Flu & Body Ache Tablets, 523
Advil Liqui-Gels, 638
AeroBid, 471
AeroBid-M, 471
Aerocaine, 1485
Aerotherm, 1485
Aerozoin, 1498
Afrin, 501
Aftate for Athlete's Foot, 1131
Aftate for Jock Itch, 1131
A/G Pro, 56
Agenerase, 1182
Aggrenox, 95
Agoral, 1001
AH-chew D, 501
AH-chew Tablets, 542
Airet, 455
Akarpine, 1319
AK-Cide, 1372
AK-Cide Suspension, 1372
AK-Con, 1339
AK-Dex, 1348
AK-Dilate, 1339
AK-Homatropine, 1345
Akineton, 891
AK-Nefrin, 1339
Akne-mycin, 1098
AK-Neo-Dex Solution, 1370
AK-Pentolate, 1345
AK-Pred, 1348
AKPro, 1325
AK-Spore H.C., 1371
AK-Spore H.C. Ophthalmic Suspension, 1370
AK-Spore H.C. Otic, 1397
AK-Sulf, 1366
AK-Tob, 1366
AK-Tracin, 1366
AK-Trol, 1372
AK-Trol Suspension, 1371
Akwa Tears, 1383, 1386
Alacol DM Syrup, 547
Ala-Cort, 249
Alamag Plus Suspension, 924
Alamag Suspension, 924
Alamast, 1353
Ala-Quin Cream, 254
Ala-Scalp, 249
Alasulf, 1111
Albalon, 1339
Albendazole, 1199-1200
Albenza, 1199
Albustix, 1767
Albuterol sulfate, 455
Albuterol sulfate/Ipratropium bromide, 482-484
Alclometasone dipropionate, 247
Alcohol
in acne products, 1440, 1444, 1446-1448
in anorectal preparations, 1430, 1431
in antifungal combinations, 1135, 1136
in antiseborrheic combinations, 1479
in poison ivy treatment products, 1512
in topical antihistamines, 1502
Aldactazide, 327
Aldactone, 320
Aldocor-150 Tablets, 431
Aldocor-250 Tablets, 431
Aldomet, 421
Aldoril -15 Tablets, 431
Aldoril -25 Tablets, 431
Aldoril D30 Tablets, 431
Aldoril D50 Tablets, 431
Alendronate sodium, 305
Alesse, 177
Aleve, 639
Aleve Cold & Sinus Tablets, 523
Aleve Sinus & Headache Tablets, 523
Alferon N, 1237
Alginic acid, 922
Alkalinizers
urinary tract, 1655-1657
Alka-Mints, 30, 917

INDEX

Alka-Seltzer, 929
Alka-Seltzer, Extra Strength, 929
Alka-Seltzer Extra Strength Antacid and Pain Relief Effervescent Tablets, 606
Alka-Seltzer Flavored Antacid and Pain Relief Effervescent Tablets, 606
Alka-Seltzer Original Antacid and Pain Relief Effervescent Tablets, 606
Alka-Seltzer Plus Cold & Sinus Liqui-Gels, 522
Alka-Seltzer Plus Cold & Sinus Tablets, 522
Alka-Seltzer Plus Cold & Cough Liqui-Gels, 550
Alka-Seltzer Plus Cold & Cough Medicine Effervescent Tablets, 549
Alka-Seltzer Plus Cold Medicine Effervescent Tablets, 537
Alka-Seltzer Plus Cold Medicine Liqui-Gels, 538
Alka-Seltzer Plus Flu Medicine Effervescent Tablets, 549
Alka-Seltzer Plus Liqui-Gels Flu Medicine, 546
Alka-Seltzer Plus Night-Time Cold Liqui-Gels, 553
Alka-Seltzer Plus Night-Time Cold Medicine Effervescent Tablets, 552
Alkeran, 1602
Alkets, 917, 922
Alkets, Extra Strength, 917
Alkylating agents
  carmustine, 1593-1595
  estrogen/nitrogen mustard, 1581-1582, 1600-1601
  lomustine, 1596-1597
  nitrogen mustards, 1602-1605
  streptozocin, 1598-1599
Allantoin
  in mouth and throat products, 1420
  in skin cleansers, 1529
  in upper respiratory combinations, 572
  in vaginal anti-infectives, 1111
Allegra, 495
Allegra-D Tablets, 533
Aller-Chlor, 494
Allercreme Skin, 1498
Allercreme Ultra, 1498
Allerest Eye Drops, 1339
Allerest Maximum Strength Tablets, 532
Allerfrim Syrup, 533
Allerfrim Tablets, 533
Allergan Enzymatic, 1393
Allergen Ear Drops, 1400
Allergy, 494
Allergy Drops, 1339
Allergy Drops, Maximum Strength, 1339
AllerMax, 495, 689, 891
AllerMax Allergy and Cough Formula, 495
AlleRx Dose Pack Tablets, 543
AlleRx-D Tablets, 543
Allfen-DM Tablets, 569
All-Nite Children's Cold/Cough Relief Liquid, 560
All-Nite Liquid, 552
Allopurinol, 655-659
Almacone, 921, 924
Almacone II Double Strength Suspension, 925
Almora, 39
Almotriptan, 674-675
Almotriptan malate, 674
Alocril, 1353
Aloe vera
  in acne products, 1444, 1447-1448
  in anorectal preparations, 1431
  in diaper rash products, 1507
Alomide, 1353
Alophen Pills, 991
Alora, 155
Alpha-2 adrenergic agonist, 1311-1312
Alpha Keri, 1499
Alpha Keri Shower and Bath, 1525
Alpha Keri Therapeutic, 1499
Alpha-1-adrenergic blockers, 386-389
Alpha-adrenergic blocking agents, 1337-1338
Alphagan, 1311
Alpha-glucosidase inhibitors, 272-274
Alphatrex, 247
Alprazolam, 710
Alprostadil, 1722-1723
Alramucil, 978
Alrex, 1351
Altace, 390
Alteplase, recombinant, 116
ALternaGEL, 917
Altretamine, 1615
Alu-Cap, 917
Aludrox Suspension, 925
Alumina, Magnesia, and Simethicone Suspension, 924
Alumina-magnesia, 606
Aluminum acetate
  in astringents, 1526
  in otic preparations, 1400
Aluminum carbonate gel basic, 917
Aluminum chloride, 1531
Aluminum chloride hexahydrate, 1449, 1527
Aluminum hydroxide
  in analgesics, 921-923, 924-927
  in antacid combinations, 921-923, 924-927
  in modified iron products, 72
  in nonnarcotic analgesics, 610
Aluminum hydroxide gel, 917
Aluminum magnesium hydroxide sulfate, 917
Aluminum oxide, 1446
Aluminum Paste, 1528
Aluminum sulfate, 1529
Alupent, 456
Alu-Tab, 917
Amacodone Tablets, 625
Amantadine, 1167-1169
Amantadine HCl
  as antiparkinson agent, 895
  as antiviral agent, 1167
Amaphen w/Codeine No. 3 Capsules, 624
Amaryl, 278
Ambenonium chloride, 1647
Ambien, 817

Amcinonide, 247
Amen, 166
Amerge, 676
Americaine First Aid, 1485
Americaine Otic, 1400
Amigesic, 602
Amiloride and hydrochlorothiazide, 327
Amiloride HCl, 320
Aminacrine HCl, 1111
Amino acid combinations, 56-57
Amino acids, 55
Aminoglutethimide, 262-263
Aminoglycosides
oral, 1031-1033
Aminophylline, 462
Aminoquinolines, 1141-1143
Aminoxin, 18
Amiodarone, 343-345
Amitone, 30, 917
Amitriptyline HCl, 760
Amitriptyline HCl and chlordiazepoxide, 807
Amitriptyline HCl and perphenazine, 807
Amlexanox, 1414-1415
Amlodipine, 368, 432
Ammonium alum, 1425
Ammonium Cl, 328
Amobarbital sodium, 812
Amoxil, 1084
Amogel PG, 1016
Amosan, 1420
Amoxapine, 760
Amoxicillin, 1084
for Helicobacter pylori infections, 947-949
Amoxicillin and potassium clavulanate, 1084
Amoxil Pediatric Drops, 1084
Amphetamine aspartate, 575
Amphetamine mixtures, 575
Amphetamine sulfate, 575
Amphetamines, 575-578
Amphojel, 917
Amphotericin B, 1130, 1132
Ampicillin, 1084
Amprenavir, 1182
Amylase, 961-962, 971
Amytal Sodium, 812
Anbesol, 1481
Anabolic steroids, 142-145
Anacin Caplets and Tablets, 610
Anacin P.M. Caplets, 608
Anacin Tablets, Maximum Strength, 610
Anadrol-50, 142
Anafranil, 760
AnaGuard, 455
Analgesic Balm, 1514
Analgesics
acetaminophen, 597-600
and antihistamines, 529
aspirin and salicylates, 601-605
buffered aspirin, 606-607
butorphanol tartrate, 631-632
and decongestant and antihistamine combinations, 537-541, pediatric, 541
and decongestants, 522-523, pediatric, 523-524
diflunisal, 613-614
narcotic, 615-622
narcotic pain reliever combinations, 623-630
nonnarcotic combinations, 608-612
pentazocine, 633-635
topical capsaicin, 1500-1501
tramadol, 636-637
Analpram-HC Cream, 254
Analpram-HC Cream 2.5, 254
Anaplex HD Liquid, 554
Anaplex-DM Liquid, 548
Anaprox, 639
Anaprox DS, 639
Anaspaz, 931
Anastrozole, 1583-1584
Anbesol, 1420, 1481
Anbesol Cool Mint, 1420
Anbesol Maximum Strength, 1420, 1481
Ancef, 1037
Andehist DM Oral Drops, 559
Andehist-DM Syrup, 548
Andehist Drops, 536
Andehist Syrup, 531
Androderm, 149
Androgen inhibitors
finasteride, 153-154
Androgens, 149-152, 1569-1570
Android, 149
Anectine, 1648
Anestacon, 1481
Anesthetics
local in anorectal preparations, 1430
topical for mucous membranes, 1481-1484 for skin disorders, 1485-1488
Anexsia 5/500 Tablets, 625
Anexsia 7.5/650 Tablets, 626
Angiotensin converting enzyme inhibitors, 390-394
Angiotensin II receptor antagonists, 395-397
Anisindione, 111
Anistreplase, 116
Anitplatelet agents
dipyridamole and aspirin, 95-97
Anodynos DHC Tablets, 625
Anorectal preparations, 1430-1434
Ansaid, 638
Answer Plus, 1765
Answer Quick & Simple, 1763, 1765
Antabuse, 1702
Antacid Suspension, 924
Antacid Tablets, 917
Antacid Tablets, Extra Strength, 917
Antacids, 917-920
combinations capsules and tablets, 921-923
liquids, 924-928 powders and effervescent tablets, 929-930
Antazoline phosphate, 1343
Anthracyclines
daunorubicin, 1558-1559
doxorubicin, 1560-1562
epirubicin, 1563-1564
idarubicin, 1565-1566

INDEX

Anthracyclines *(cont.)*
valrubicin, 1567-1568
Anthra-Derm Drithocreme, 1450
Anthralin, 1450-1451
Antiandrogens, 1571-1573
Antianginals
nitrates, 337-342
Antianxiety agents
benzodiazepines, 710-715
buspirone, 716-718
hydroxyzine, 719-720
meprobamate, 721-723
Antiarrhythmics
amiodarone, 343-345
disopyramide, 346-348
dofetilide, 349-351
flecainide, 352-353
mexiletine, 354-355
moricizine, 356-358
procainamide, 359-360
propafenone, 361-362
quinidine, 363-365
tocainide, 366-367
Antibiotic and steroid combinations, 1370-1373
Antibiotic combinations, 1104-1107
Antibiotics
aminoglycosides, 1031-1033
aztreonam, 1034-1036
carbapenem, 1074-1075
cephalosporins, 1037-1044
chloramphenicol, 1045-1047
erythromycin, 1061-1062
fluoroquinolones, 1069-1073
imipenem-cilastatin, 1076-1078
lincosamides, 1048-1051
macrolides, 1052-1058
meropenem, 1074-1075
metronidazole, 1079-1081
multiple, 1098
mupirocin, 1082-1083
as ophthalmic anti-infectives, 1366-1369
otic, 1397-1399
Antibiotics *(cont.)*
oxalodinones, 1066-1068
penicillins, 1084-1088
plicamycin, 1606-1607
spectinomycin hydrochloride, 1059-1060
tetracyclines, 1089-1093 topical, 1094-1095
topical, 1098-1100
trimethoprim, 1096-1097
triple, 1099
vancomycin, 1063-1065
Anticholinergic and antispasmodic combinations, 931-935
Anticholinergic and decongestant and antihistamine combinations, 542-543
pediatric, 544
Anticholinergic combinations, 936-938
Anticholinergics, 689-692, 891-894
Anticholinesterase muscle stimulants, 1647-1649
Anticoagulants
tinzaparin sodium, 109-110
Anticonvulsants
acetazolamide, 825-827
carbamazepine, 828-831
clonazepam, 832-835
felbamate, 836-838
gabapentin, 839-841
hydantoins, 842-846
lamotrigine, 864-866
levetiracetam, 870-871
oxazolidinediones, 847-848
oxcarbazepine, 849-851
primidone, 855-857
succinimides, 861-863
tiagabine, 867-869
topiramate, 858-860
valproic acid, 872-875
zonisamide, 852-854
Antidepressants
bupropion, 724-726
citaprolam hydrobromide, 737-739
fluoxetine, 730-733
fluvoxamine, 734-736
Antidepressants *(cont.)*
monoamine oxidase inhibitors, 743-748
nefazodone, 727-729
paroxetine, 749-751
sertraline, 752-753
tetracyclic compounds, 740-742
trazodone, 754-756
tricyclic, 760-769
venlafaxine, 757-759
Antidiabetic agents
alpha-glucosidase inhibitors, 272-274
glyburide/metformin, 289-291
insulin, 264-271
meglitinides, 283-285
metformin, 286-288
sulfonylureas, 278-282
thiazolidinediones, 275-277
Antidiarrheals
bismuth subsalicylate, 1007-1009
combination products, 1016-1018
difenoxin, 1010-1012
diphenoxylate, 1010-1012
lactobacillus, 1013
loperamide, 1014-1015
Antidotes
charcoal activated, 1633-1634
dexrazoxane, 1639-1640
flumazenil, 1635-1636
ipecac, 1637-1638
nalmefene HCl, 1641-1642
naloxone, 1643-1644
Antiemetic/antivertigo agents
anticholinergics, 689-692
cannabinoids, 693-695
5-HT3 receptor antagonists, 696-698
phenothiazines, 699-704
phosphorated carbohydrate, 705-706
Antiestrogens, 1578-1580
Antiflatulents, 959-960
Antifungal combinations
topical, 1135-1137

Antifungals
clotrimazole, 1114-1115
fluconazole, 1116-1117
griseofulvin, 1118-1120
itraconazole, 1121-1123
ketoconazole, 1124-1127
nystatin, 1128-1129
topical preparations, 1130-1134
vaginal preparations, 1138-1140
Antiherpes virus agents, 1164-1166
Antihist-1, 494
Antihistamine and analgesic combinations, 529
Antihistamine and decongestant and analgesic combinations, 537-541
pediatric, 541
Antihistamine and decongestant and anticholingeric combinations, 542-543
pediatric, 544
Antihistamine and decongestant combinations, 530-534
pediatric, 535-537
Antihistamine and expectorant and decongestant combinations, 529
pediatric, 530
Antihistamines, 494-500
azelastine, 1360-1361
topical, 1502-1504
Antihyperlipidemics
bile acid sequestrants, 435-438
clofibrate, 439-441
fenofibrate, 442-444
gemfibrozil, 445-447
HMG-CoA reductase inhibitors, 448-451
Antihypertensive combinations, 430-433
Antihypertensives
alpha-1-adrenergic blockers, 386-389
angiotensin converting enzyme inhibitors, 390-394
angiotensin II receptor antagonists, 395-397
carvedilol, 413-415
clonidine, 398-400
Antihypertensives *(cont.)*
guanabenz acetate, 401-402
guanadrel sulfate, 403-404
guanethidine monosulfate, 405-407
guanfacine, 408-409
hydralazine, 410-412
labetalol, 416-418
mecamylamine, 419-420
methyldopa, 421-423
minoxidil, 424-426
miscellaneous, 432
reserpine, 427-429
Antihypotensive agents, see Vasopressor/antihypotensive agents
Anti-infectives
antituberculosis drugs, 1222-1232
atovaquone, 1232-1233
inferferon alfa-N3, 1237-1238
interferon alfacon-1, 1239-1241
interferon gamma-1B, 1242-1243
ophthalmic antibiotics, 1366-1369 antiviral agents, 1376-1377
natamycin, 1374-1375
steroid and antibiotic combinations, 1370-1373
pediculicides, 1244-1246
pentamidine isethionate, 1234-1236
scabicides, 1244-1246
urinary fosfomycin tromethamine, 1212-1213 methenamine, 1209-1211
nalidixic acid, 1214-1215 nitrofurantoin, 1216-1218
vaginal, 1111-1113 combinations, 1111
Anti-inflammatory agents
ophthalmic corticosteroids, 1348-1350
Antimalarials
aminoquinolines, 1141-1143
Antimalarials *(cont.)*
atovaquone and proguanil HCl, 1154-1155
halofantrine HCl, 1152-1153
mefloquine, 1144-1146
pyrimethamine, 1147-1148
quinine sulfate, 1156-1157
sulfadoxine and pyrimethamine, 1149-1151
Antimetabolites, 1541-1545
capecitabine, 1546-1548
Antiminth, 1203
Antineoplastic agents, 1537-1540
miscellaneous, 1615-1620
Anti-obesity agents
orlistat, 1025-1027
Antiparasitics
albendazole, 1199-1200
ivermectin, 1207-1208
mebendazole, 1201-1202
pyrantel, 1203-1204
thiabendazole, 1205-1206
Antiparkinson agents
anticholinergics, 891-894
dopaminergics, 895-899
entacapone, 912-913
pergolide mesylate, 906-908
pramipexole, 900-902
ropinirole, 903-905
selegiline, 909-911
Antipsychotics, 770-780
clozapine, 791-793
olanzapine, 787-790
quetiapine fumarate, 781-783
risperidone, 784-786
Antipyrine, 1400
Antiretroviral agents
non-nucleoside reverse transcriptase inhibitors, 1195-1198
nucleoside reverse transcriptase inhibitors, 1190-1194

INDEX

Antiretroviral agents *(cont.)*
  nucleotide analog
    reverse transcriptase
    inhibitors, 1187-1189
  protease inhibitors,
    1182-1186
Antirheumatic agents
  gold compounds, 646-
    648
  hydroxychloroquine,
    649-650
  methotrexate, 651-654
Antiseborrheic products
  combinations,
    1479-1480
  miscellaneous, 1475-
    1478
  selenium sulfide, 1473-
    1474
  shampoos, 1479
Antiseptics
  topical, 1505-1506
Antispasmodic and anti-
  cholinergic combina-
  tions, 931-935
Antithymocyte globulin (equine), 1251
Antithymocyte globulin (rabbit), 1249
Antithyroid agents, 294-
  296
Antituberculosis drugs,
  1222-1232
Anti-Tuss, 513
Antitussive and expecto-
  rant combinations,
  562-566
  pediatric, 567
Antitussive combinations,
  541-556
  pediatric, 556-561
Antitussives
  narcotic, 506-508
  nonnarcotic, 509-512
Antitussives with expecto-
  rants, 567-571
  pediatric, 571
Anti-ulcer agents
  misoprostol, 955-956
  sucralfate, 957-958
Antivert, 689
Antivert/25 Chewable, 689
Antivertigo agents, see
  Antiemetic/antivertigo
  agents
Antiviral agents, 1158-1160
  amantadine, 1167-1169
Antiviral agents *(cont.)*
  antiherpes virus agents,
    1164-1166
  cidofovir, 1170-1172
  ganciclovir, 1161-1163
  ophthalmic, 1376-1377
  oseltamivir phos-
    phate, 1180-1181
  ribavirin, 1173-1175
  rimantadine, 1176-1177
  zanamivir, 1178-1179
Antrizine, 689
Anturane, 666
Anucort-HC, 1430
Anumed-HC, 1430
Anusol, 1430, 1431
Anusol HC-1, 249, 1430
Anzomet, 696
AOSept, 1394
AOSept Disinfecting, 1394
Apacet, 597
APAP, see Acetamino-phen
APAP with chlorzoxa-zone, 889
Apatate Liquid, 48
Apatate Tablets, 48
Aphrodyne, 1727
Aphthasol, 1414
Aplisol, 1304
Aplitest, 1304
Appetite suppressants
  non-amphetamine, 579-
    583
  sibutramine, 584-586
Apple blossom oil, 1530
Apraclonidine HCl, 1328-1329
Apresazide 25/25 Cap-
  sules, 430
Apresazide 50/50 Cap-
  sules, 430
Apresazide 100/50 Cap-
  sules, 430
Apresoline, 410
Apri, 177
Aprodine Syrup, 533
Aprodine Tablets, 533
Aqua-Ban, 328
Aqua-Ban Plus, 328
Aquacare, 1496
Aquachloral Supprettes,
  817
Aquafresh Sensitive Teeth,
  1418
AquaMEPHYTON, 124
Aquanil, 1525
Aquasite, 1383
Aquatab C Tablets, 565
Aquatab DM Tablets, 570
AquatabD Dose Pack Tab-
  lets, 526
AquatabD Tablets, 527
Aquatensen, 323
Aquavit-E, 27
AR Eye Drops - Astringent,
  1339
Ara-A, see Vidarabine
Aralen, 1141
Aralen HCl, 1141
Arava, 1743
Arcobee with C Caplets,
  49
Ardeparin sodium, 107-108
Aredia, 305
Argesic Cream, 1515
Argesic-SA, 602
Aricept, 803
Arimidex, 1583
Aristocort, 241
Aristocort A, 250
Aristocort Forte, 241
Aristocort Intralesional, 241
Aristospan Intra-articular,
  241
Aristospan Intralesional,
  241
Armour Thyroid, 299
Arnica, 1527
Artane, 892
Artane Sequels, 892
Artha-G, 602
ArthriCare Lotion, 1515
ArthriCare Rub, 1514
ArthriCare Ultra Rub, 1515
Arthritis Foundation Pain
  Reliever, 601
Arthritis Foundation Pain
  Reliever Aspirin Free,
  597
Arthritis Pain Formula Aspi-
  rin Free, 597
Arthritis Pain Ascriptin
  Coated Caplets, 606
Arthritis Regular Strength
  Coated Tablets, 606
Arthropan, 601
Arthrotec Tablets, 611
ArthroTherapy Gel, 1515
Arth-Rx Lotion, 1515
Artificial Tears, 1386
Artificial Tears, 1383

Artificial tears, 1383-1385
inserts, 1383
solutions, 1383
Artificial Tears Plus, 1383
ASA with methocarbamol, 889
ASA with orphenadrine citrate, 889
Asacol, 1019
Ascorbic acid, 6, 20-22, 49-50
Ascorbic acid with iron, 75, 76
Ascriptin Coated Caplets, Maximum Strength, 606
Asendin, 760
Aspercreme, 1514
Aspercreme Rub, 1514
Aspergum, 601
Aspirin
in antacid combinations, 929
buffered, 606-607
Children's, 601
in migraine combinations, 668
in narcotic pain relievers, 623-629
in nonnarcotic pain relievers, 608-611
and salicylates, 601-605
in skeletal muscle relaxants, 889
in upper respiratory combinations, 549
Aspirin and dipyridamole, 95-97
Aspirin and pentazocine, 633
Aspirin Free Anacin Maximum Strength, 597
Aspirin Free Excedrin Caplets, 608
Aspirin Free Pain Relief, 597
Aspirin Regimen Bayer Adult Low Strength with Calcium Caplets, 606
Aspirin w/Codeine Tablets No. 2, 623
Aspirin w/Codeine Tablets No. 3, 623
Aspirin w/Codeine Tablets No. 4, 624
Asprimox Extra Protection for Arthritis Pain, 601
Astelin, 494
AsthmaHaler Mist, 455
Astramorph PF, 616
Astringents
aluminum acetate, 1526
Atacand, 395
Atarax, 495, 719
Atarax 100, 495, 719
Atenolol, 379, 432
ATG, see Antithymocyte globulin (equine)
ATG rabbit, see Antithymocyte globulin (rabbit)
Atgam, 1251
Ativan, 710
Atorvastatin calcium, 448
Atovaquone, 1232-1233
Atovaquone and proguanil HCl, 1154-1155
Atromid-S, 439
Atropine, 936
Atropine-1, 1345
Atropine Care, 1345
Atropine Sulfate, 1345
Atropine sulfate
in anticholinergic combinations, 936
in antidiarrheal combination products, 1016, 1017
in cycloplegic mydriatics, **1345**
in upper respiratory combinations, 543
in urinary anti-infective combinations, 1219, 1220
Atropine sulfate and edrophonium chloride, 1647
Atropine sulfate with difenoxin, 1010
Atropine sulfate with diphenoxylate, 1010
Atropisol, 1345
Atrosept, 1220
Atrovent, 479
A/T/S, 1061
Attapulgite
in acne products, 1445
in antidiarrheal combination products, 1017
Attenuvax, 1277
Atuss DM Syrup, 549
Atuss EX Syrup, 570
Atuss HD Liquid, 555
Atuss MS Liquid, 555
Atuss-G Syrup, 566
Augmentin, 1084
Auralgan Otic, 1400
Auranofin, 646
Auro Ear Drops, 1400
Aurocaine 2, 1400
Aurocaine Ear Drops, 1400
Auro-Dri, 1400
Aurolate, 646
Aurothioglucose, 646
Auroto Otic, 1400
Avandia, 275
Avapro, 395
AVC, 1111
Aveeno, 1498, 1512
Aveeno Acne Treatment, 1525
Aveeno Cleansing for Acne-Prone Skin, 1446
Aveeno Combination Skin, 1525
Aveeno Dry Skin, 1525
Aveeno Regular, 1499
AveenoOilated Bath, 1499
Avelox, 1069
Aventyl, 760
Aventyl Pulvules, 760
Avita, 1441
Avobenzone, 1517-1519
Avonex, 1729
Axert, 674
Axid AR, 950
Axid Pulvules, 950
Axocet Capsules, 608
Aygestin, 166
Ayr Baby Saline Nose Spray/Drops, 517
Ayr Saline Mist, 517
Ayr Saline Nasal Drops, 517
Azactam, 1034
Azatadine maleate, 494, 534
Azathioprine, 1674-1675
Azdone Tablets, 625
Azelaic acid, 1438-1439
Azelastine, 494, 1360-1361
Azelex, 1438
Azithromycin, 1052
Azmacort, 471
Azo-Gesic, 1672
Azopt, 1330
Azo-Standard, 1672
Azo-Sulfisoxazole, 1219

INDEX

Aztreonam, 1034-1036
Azulfidine, 1101
Azulfidine EN-tabs, 1101

B & O Supprettes No. 15A Suppositories, 626
B & O Supprettes No. 16A Suppositories, 627
B C w/Folic Acid Plus Tablets, 49
B-12 Tablets, 48
B-50 Caps Capsules, 51
B-50 Super B Complex Tablets, 51
B-100 Ultra B Complex Timed-Release Tablets, 51
Babee Teething, 1420
Baby Numz•it, 1420
Baby Orajel, 1420
Bacampicillin HCl, 1084
Bacid, 1013
Baciguent, 1098
Bacitracin
ophthalmic, 1366, 1371
topical, 1098
Backache Maximum Strength Relief, 602
Baclofen, 876-878
Bactine Antiseptic Anesthetic, 1485
Bactrim, 1108, 1219, 1458
Bactrim DS, 1108, 1219
Bactrim Pediatric, 1219
Bactroban, 1082
Bactroban Nasal, 1082
Bain de Soleil All Day Extended Protection, 1517, 1520
Bain de Soleil GentleBlock, 1517
Bain de Soleil Kids, 1517
Bain de Soleil Mademoiselle, 1520
Bain de Soleil Mega Tan, 1521
Bain de Soleil Orange Gelee, 1519-1520
Bain de Soleil Tanning Mist, 1521
Bain de Soleil Tropical Deluxe, 1521
Balamine DM Oral Drops, 559
Balamine DM Syrup, 548, 559
Balanced B-50 Capsules, 51
Balanced B-100 Capsules, 51
Balmex, 1497-1498
Balmex Diaper Rash, 1507
Balneol Perianal Cleansing, 1431
Balnetar, 1475
Balsalazide disodium, 1019
Balsam peru
in anorectal preparations, 1430
in diaper rash products, 1507
in skin cleansers, 1529
Banalg Hospital Strength Lotion, 1514
Banalg Muscle Pain Reliever, 1514
Banana Boat Action Sport, 1519
Banana Boat Baby, 1516
Banana Boat Dark Tanning, 1521
Banana Boat Faces Plus, 1519
Banana Boat Kids, 1517
Banana Boat Maximum, 1516
Banana Boat Sport, 1516, 1520
Banana Boat Ultra, 1517
Banatol Infantol Pink, 1016
Bancap HC Capsules, 625
Banophen, 495, 689, 891
Banophen Allergy, 495
Banophen Softgels, 495
Bar soaps
modified, 1525
Barbidonna, 936
Barbidonna No. 2, 936
Barbiturate combinations, 812
Barbiturates, 812-816
Baridium, 1672
Barley malt extract, 977
Basaljel, 917
Basic fuchsin, 1135
Basis All Clear, 1525
Basis Cleaner Clean Face Wash, 1525
Basis Comfortably Clean Face Wash, 1525
Basis Sensitive Skin, 1525
Bath oils, 1499
Bay Tet, 1252
Bayer Aspirin Tablets and Caplets, Maximum Strength, 601
Bayer Buffered, 601
Bayer Children's, 601
Bayer Enteric 500, Extra Strength, 601
Bayer Enteric Coated Caplets, Regular Strength, 601
Bayer Low Adult Strength, 601
Bayer Plus, Extra Strength, 601
Bayer PM Aspirin Plus Sleep Aid Caplets, Extra Strength, 610
Bayer Select Maximum Strength, 602
BayGam, 1249
BayHep B, 1249
BayRab, 1251
BayRho-D Full Dose, 1251
BayRho-D Mini Dose, 1252
BC Powder Original Formula, 610
B-Complex plus C High Potency Timed-Release Tablets, 49
B-Complex Tablets, 48
B-Complex with Vitamin B-12 Tablets, 51
Bebegyn, 1111
Becaplermin, 1467-1468
Beclomethasone dipropionate, 471, 490
Beconase AQ Nasal, 490
Beconase Inhalation, 490
Beepen-VK, 1085
Beeswax
in anorectal preparations, 1430-1431
in skin cleansers, 1530
Beldin, 509
Belix, 689, 891
Belladonna
in anticholinergic combinations, 936-937
in narcotic pain relievers, 626-627
Belladonna alkaloids
in migraine combinations, 668
in upper respiratory combinations, 543

Belladonna Alkaloids with Phenobarbital, 936
Bell/ans, 918
Bellergal-S, 936
Ben Gay, 1514
Ben Gay Ultra Strength Cream, 1514
Benadryl, 495, 689, 891, 1502
Benadryl, 2, Maximum Strength, 1502
Benadryl 25, 689, 891
Benadryl Allergy, 495, 891
Benadryl Allergy & Cold Tablets, 540
Benadryl Allergy & Sinus Fastmelt Dissolving Tablets, 533
Benadryl Allergy & Sinus Headache Tablets and Gelcaps, 540
Benadryl Allergy & Sinus Liquid, 533
Benadryl Allergy & Sinus Tablets, 533
Benadryl Allergy Kapseals, 891
Benadryl Allergy Ultratab, 495
Benadryl Children's Allergy & Cold Fastmelt Tablets, 537
Benadryl Children's Allergy & Sinus Liquid, 537
Benadryl Dye Free, 891
Benadryl Dye Free Allergy Liqui Gels, 891
Benadryl Dye Free Allergy Liqui-Gels, 495
Benadryl Dye-Free Allergy, 495
Benadryl Kapseals, 891
Benadryl Maximum Strength Severe Allergy & Sinus Headache Tablets, 540
Benazepril, 431-432
Benazepril HCl, 390
Benazepril HCl and hydrochlorothiazide, 390
Bendroflumethiazide, 323, 430, 431
Benoquin, 1528
Benoxyl 5, 1435
Benoxyl 10, 1435
Bensulfoid, 1440
Bensulfoid Cream, 1444
Bentonite, 1529
Bentonite magma, 1512
Bentyl, 931
Benylin, 509
Benylin Cough, 689, 891
Benylin Expectorant Liquid, 567
Benylin Pediatric, 509
Benza, 1505
Benzac 5 and 10, 1435
Benzac W 2.5, 5 and 10, 1435
Benzac W Wash 5 and 10, 1435
Benzagel, 1435
Benzalkonium chloride
in acne products, 1446-1447
in antiseborrheic combinations, 1479
in antiseptics/germicides, 1505
in douche products, 1425
in mouth and throat products, 1422
in poison ivy treatment products, 1512
in skin cleansers, 1529
in topical antihistamines, 1502
Benz-all, 1505
Benzamycin, 1061, 1435
Benzedrex, 517
Benzethonium chloride
in acne products, 1446-1447
in topical antihistamines, 1502
Benzocaine
in anorectal preparations, 1430
in antifungal combinations, 1135
in antitussives, 509
in lozenges, 1417-1418
in mouth and throat products, 1420-1422
for mucous membranes, 1481
in otic preparations, 1400
in poison ivy treatment products, 1512
in skin cleansers, 1528, 1530-1531
Benzocaine *(cont.)*
for skin disorders, 1485-1486
in topical antihistamines, 1502
Benzodent, 1420
Benzodiazepines, 710-715
Benzoic acid
in antifungal combinations, 1135-1136
in urinary anti-infective combinations, 1219-1220
Benzoin, 1499
Benzonatate, 509
Benzophenone-3, 1516-1520
Benzoyl peroxide
in acne products, 1435-1437
in antibiotics, 1061
cleansers, 1435
combinations, 1435
creams, 1435
gels, 1435
lotions, 1435
in topical corticosteroids, 254
Benzphetamine HCl, 579
Benzthiazide, 323
Benztropine mesylate, 891
Benzyl acetate, 1136
Benzyl alcohol
in acne products, 1444-1445, 1448
in anorectal preparations, 1430-1431
in antifungal combinations, 1135-1136
in mouth and throat products, 1416, 1421
in skin cleansers, 1531-1532
Benzyl benzoate, 1430
Bepridil HCl, 368
Berocca Tablets, 49
Beta-adrenergic blocking agents, 379-385
Beta-blockers, 1313-1315
Betadine, 1505
Betadine Medicated Disposable Douche, 1425
Betagan Liquifilm, 1313
Betalin S, 10
Betamethasone, 239

INDEX

Betamethasone acetate and betamethasone sodium phosphate, 239
Betamethasone dipropionate, 247
Betamethasone sodium phosphate, 239
Betamethasone sodium phosphate and betamethasone acetate, 239
Betamethasone valerate, 247
Betapace, 379
Betapace AF, 379
Betapentane tannate, 556
Betaseron, 1729
Betatrex, 247
Beta-Val, 247
Betaxolol HCl
ophthalmic, 1313
systemic, 379
Betaxon, 1313
Bethanechol chloride, 1658-1659
Bethaprim, 1108
Bethaprim DS, 1108
Bethaprim SS, 1108
Betopic S, 1313
Biavax II, 1277
Biaxin, 1052
Bicalutamide, 1571
Bicitra, 1655
BiCNU, 1593
Bicozene, 1485
Bile acid sequestrants, 435-438
Bili-Labstix, 1771
Bili-Labstix SG, 1771
Bimatoprost, 1322
Bioflavinoids, 58-59
Biohist-LA Tablets, 532
Biological response modifier
levamisole, 1591-1592
Biosun Faces, 1519
Biperiden, 891
Biphasic oral contraceptives, 177-178
Bisacodyl
in bowel evacuation kits, 1005
in laxatives, 991
Bismuth subcarbonate, 1016-1017
Bismuth subgallate
in anorectal preparations, 1431
Bismuth subgallate *(cont.)*
in antidiarrheal combination products, 1016-1017
Bismuth subnitrate, 1529
Bismuth subsalicylate
in antidiarrheal products, 1007-1009, 1016-1017
for Helicobacter pylori infections, 944-946
Bisoprolol fumarate
in antihypertensive combinations, 430
as beta-adrenergic blocking agent, 379
Bisphosphonates, 305-308
Bitolterol mesylate, 455
Black-Draught, 991, 1001
Blairex Sterile Saline, 1393
Bleph-10, 1366
Blephamide, 1372
Blephamide Suspension, 1372
BlisterGard, 1498
Blistex, 1522
Blistex DCt, 1521
Blistex Lip, 1420
Blistex Lip Medex, 1420
Blis-To-Sol, 1135
Blocadren, 379
Bluboro Powder, 1526
Boil-Ease, 1485, 1528
Biosun Professional Sun Protection, 1516
Bonine, 689
Bontril PDM, 579
Bontril Slow-Release, 579
Boric Acid, 1527
Boric acid
in antifungal combinations, 1135-1136
in otic preparations, 1400
in skin cleansers, 1530
Boric acid ointment, 1527
Borofair Otic, 1400
Borofax, 1527
Boropak, 1526
Boston Advance Cleaner, 1390
Boston Advance Comfort, 1390
Boston Advance Comfort Formula Convenience Pack, 1390
Boston Cleaner (original formula), 1390
Boston Conditioning, 1390
Boston One Step Liquid, 1390
Boston Reconditioning Drops, 1390
Boston Rewetting Drops, 1387, 1390
Boston Simplicity Multi-Action, 1390
Bowel evacuants
kits for, 1005-1006
polyethylene glycol, 1003-1004
B-Plex Tablets, 49
B.P.P.-Lemmon, 1016
Brasivol, 1446
Breathe Right Children's Colds Nasal Strips, 572
Breezee Mist, 1131
Breonesin, 513
Brethine, 456
Brevicon, 177
Brewers Yeast 500 Tablets, 48
Brexin-L.A. Capsules, 532
Brimonidine tartrate, 1311
Brinzolamide, 1330
Brofed Liquid, 530
Bromanate DM Cold & Cough Elixir, 558
Bromanate Elixir, 535
Bromatane DX Syrup, 547
Bromfed Capsules, 531
Bromfed DM Cough Syrup, 547
Bromfed Syrup, 530
Bromfed Tablets, 531
Bromfed-PD Capsules, 536
Bromfenex Capsules, 531
Bromfenex-PD Capsules, 536
Bromo Seltzer, 598, 929
Bromocriptine mesylate, 895, 1693-1695
Brompheniramine maleate, 530-531, 535-536, 538, 541, 547-548, 554, 558
Brompheniramine Maleate/Pseudoephedrine HCl Syrup, 531, 535
Bronchodilators
sympathomimetics, 455-461

Bronchodilators *(cont.)*
xanthine derivatives, 462-467
Broncholate Syrup, 524
Brondelate Elixir, 521
Bronkaid Dual Action Tablets, 524
Bucladin-S Softabs, 689
Buclizine HCl, 689
Budesonide, 471, 490
Buffered aspirin, 606-607
Buffered Aspirin Enteric Coated Tablets, 606
Bufferin Arthritis Strength Pain Reliever Caplets, 606
Bufferin Coated Tablets, 606
Bufferin Extra Strength Coated Caplets, 606
Buf-Puf Acne Cleansing, 1446
Bullfrog Body Gel, 1517
Bullfrog Body Lotion, 1517
Bullfrog for Babies, 1516
Bullfrog for Kids, 1517
Bullfrog Magic Block, 1517
Bullfrog Quick Gel, 1519
Bullfrog Quick Stick, 1517
Bullfrog Sport Lotion, 1516
Bullfrog SuperBlock, 1516
Bumetanide, 317
Bumex, 317
Bupap Tablets, 608
Buphenyl, 126
Bupropion, 724-726
Bupropion HCl, 1719-1721
Burn preparations
mafenide, 1469-1470
silver sulfadiazine, 1471-1472
Buro-Sol, 1526
Burow's Solution, 1526
Burow's Solution, Modified, 1400
BuSpar, 716
Buspirone, 716-718
Busulfan, 1552-1553
Butabarbital sodium
in anticholinergic combinations, 936-937
as sedative, 812
Butalbital
in narcotic analgesics, 624
Butalbital *(cont.)*
in nonnarcotic analgesics, 608-610
Butalbital, Acetaminophen and Caffeine Tablets, 609
Butalbital Compound Capsules and Tablets, 610
Butamben picrate, 1485
Butesin Picrate, 1485
Butibel, 936-937
Butisol, 812
Butoconazole nitrate, 1138
Butorphanol tartrate, 631-632
Butylene glycol, 1447
Bydramine Cough, 509

CFactors "1000" Plus, 58
Cabergoline, 1696-1697
Cafatine-PB, 668
Cafcit, 587
Cafergot, 668
Caffedrine, 587
Caffeine
as CNS stimulant, 587-589
in diuretics, 328
in migraine combinations, 668
in narcotic analgesics, 624, 626, 629
in nonnarcotic analgesics, 608-610
in skeletal muscle relaxants, 889
Caffeine and sodium benzoate, 587
Caffeine citrate, 538
Calaclear, 1512
Cala-gen, 1502, 1512
Calagesic, 1512
Calamine, 1512
Calamine
in poison ivy treatment products, 1512
in skin cleansers, 1528
in topical antihistamines, 1502
Calamycin, 1502
Calan, 369
Calan SR, 369
Calcarb 600 with Vitamin D Tablets, 53
Cal-Carb Forte, 29-30
Calcet Tablets, 53
Calcibind, 1660
CalciChew, 30
Calci-Chew, 917
Calcifediol, 23
Calciferol, 23
Calciferol Drops, 23
Calcijex, 23
Calcimar, 302
Calcionate, 29
Calcipotriene, 1452-1453
Calciquid, 29
Calcitonin, 302-304
Calcitonin-Salmon, 302
Cal-Citrate, 29
Calcitrol, 23
Calcium, 5, 29-32
Calcium 500 mg with D Tablets, 53
Calcium 600 mg with D Tablets, 53
Calcium 600 with Vitamin D Tablets, 53
Calcium acetate, 1526, 1713
Calcium and vitamin D, 53-54
Calcium ascorbate, 20
Calcium carbonate
in analgesics, 606
in antacids, 917, 921-927
in antidiarrheal combination products, 1016
in histamine H2 antagonists, 950
in laxatives, 978
nutritional, 29
Calcium caseinate, 1507
Calcium channel blocking agents, 368-374
Calcium citrate, 29
Calcium 600-D Tablets, 53
Calcium glubionate, 29
Calcium gluconate, 29
Calcium hydroxide, 1512
Calcium lactate, 29
Calcium pantothenate, 17
Calcium Rich Rolaids, 921
Calcium salts of sennosides A & B, 991
Caldecort, 249
Calderol, 23
Calglycine, 922
Calicylic Creme, 1493
Cal-Mint, 30
Calmol 4, 1431

INDEX

Calm-X, 689
Caltrate 600, 29
Caltrate 600 Plus, 29-30
Caltrate 600+D, 29
Caltrate 600+D Tablets, 53
Caltrate 600+Soy, 29
Cameo, 1499
Campho-Penique, 1528
Camphor
 in acne products, 1447
 in anorectal preparations, 1431
 in antifungal combinations, 1135
 in mouth and throat products, 1420, 1422
 in poison ivy treatment products, 1512
 in rubs and liniments, 1514
 in skin cleansers, 1528-1531
 in topical antihistamines, 1502
 in upper respiratory combinations, 572
Camptosar, 1549
Camptothecins, 1549-1551
Candesartan cilexetil, 395
Cankaid, 1405
Cannabinoids, 693-695
Cantharidin, 1489-1490
Cantil, 931
Cantri, 1111
Capastat Sulfate, 1222
Capecitabine, 1546-1548
Capital w/Codeine Suspension, 623
Capitrol, 1475
Capoten, 390
Capozide 25/15, 432
Capozide 25/25, 432
Capozide 50/15, 432
Capozide 50/25, 432
Capreomycin, 1222
Capsaicin, 1500-1501
Captopril, 390
 in antihypertensive combinations, 432
Carafate, 957
Carbachol
 intraocular, 1319
 topical, 1319
Carbamazepine, 828-831
Carbamide peroxide
 in mouth and throat products, 1405-1406
 in otic preparations, 1400
Carbapenem antibiotics
 meropenem, 1074-1075
Carbastat, 1319
Carbenicillin indanyl sodium, 1084
Carbetapentane citrate, 562
Carbetapentane tannate, 544
Carbex, 909
Carbidopa, 895
Carbinoxamine Compound Drops, 559
Carbinoxamine Compound Syrup, 548
Carbinoxamine maleate, 531, 536, 543, 548, 556, 558-559
Carbinoxamine Oral Drops, 536
Carbinoxamine Syrup, 536
Carbodex DM Drops, 559
Carbodex DM Syrup, 547
Carbofed DM Oral Drops, 558
Carbofed DM Syrup, 547
Carbohydrate, 977-978
Carbomer 940, 1530
Carbonic anhydrase inhibitors, 313-316
 brinzolamide, 1330-1331
 dorzolamide, 1330-1331
Carboptic, 1319
Cardec DM Syrup, 548
Cardec-S Liquid, 531
Cardene, 368
Cardene SR, 368
Cardiac glycosides, 329-332
Cardioquin, 363
Cardizem, 368
Cardizem CD, 368
Cardizem SR, 368
Cardura, 386
Carisoprodol, 885
Carisoprodol compound, 889
Carmol 10, 1496
Carmol 20, 1496
Carmol 40, 1496
Carmol HC, 1430
Carmol HC Cream, 254
Carmustine, 1593-1595
L-Carnitine, 63-64
Carnitor, 63
Carteolol HCl
 as beta-adrenergic blocking agent, 379
 for glaucoma, 1313
Cartia XT, 368
Cartrol, 379
Carvedilol, 413-415
Casanthranol, 998-999, 1001
Cascara sagrada, 991, 998-999
Cascara Sagrada Aromatic Fluid Extract, 991
Casodex, 1571
Caspin's Lotion, 1515
Castaderm, 1135
Castel Minus, 1135
Castel Plus, 1135
Castellani Paint, 1135
Castor oil
 in acne products, 1447
 in laxatives, 991
 in skin cleansers, 1529
Cataflam, 638
Catapres, 398
Catapres-TTS-1, 398
Catapres-TTS-2, 398
Catapres-TTS-3, 398
Catrix, 1498
Caverject, 1722
CCNU, see Lomustine
Ceclor, 1037
Ceclor CD, 1037
Cecon, 20
Cedax, 1038
CeeNu, 1596
Cefaclor, 1037
Cefadroxil, 1037
Cefadyl, 1039
Cefazolin sodium, 1037
Cefdinir, 1037
Cefepime hydrochloride, 1037
Cefixime, 1037
Cefizox, 1038
Cefmetazole sodium, 1037
Cefobid, 1037
Cefonicid sodium, 1037
Cefoperazone sodium, 1037
Cefotan, 1038

Cefotaxime sodium, 1038
Cefotetan disodium, 1038
Cefoxitin sodium, 1038
Cefprozil, 1038
Ceftazidime, 1038
Ceftibuten, 1038
Ceftin, 1039
Ceftizoxime sodium, 1038
Ceftriaxone sodium, 1038
Cefuroxime, 1039
Cefzil, 1038
Celebrex, 638
Celecoxib, 638
Celestone, 239
Celestone Phosphate, 239
Celestone Soluspan, 239
Celexa, 737
CellCept, 1680
CellCept Intravenous, 1680
Cellulase, 971
Cellulose sodium phosphate, 1660-1661
Celluvisc, 1383
Celontin Kapseals, 861
Cenafed Plus Tablets, 533
Cenestin, 156
Cenolate, 20
Centrax, 710
Cepacol, 1417-1418
Cepacol ColdCare, 1417
Cepacol Maximum Strength, 1417-1418
Cepacol Sore Throat Liquid, 522
Cepacol Sugar Free Maximum Strength, 1417
Cepastat Cherry, 1417
Cepastat Extra Strength, 1417
Cepastat Fast-Acting, 1417
Cephalexin HCl monohydrate, 1039
Cephalexin monohydrate, 1039
Cephalosporins, 1037-1044
Cephapirin sodium, 1039
Cephradine, 1039
Cephulac, 983
Ceptaz, 1038
Cerebyx, 842
Ceresin wax, 1529
Cerezyme, 309
Cerumenex Drops, 1400
Cervical cap, 170
Ceta Cleanser, 1525
Cetacaine, 1486
Cetacort, 249
Cetalkonium chloride, 1420
Cetaphil, 1525
Cetaphil Oily Skin, 1525
Cetapred, 1372
Cetearyl alcohol, 1445
Cetethyl morpholinium ethosulfate, 1431
Cetirizine HCl
- as antihistamine, 494
- in upper respiratory combinations, 532

Cetyl alcohol
- in acne products, 1444-1445
- in skin cleansers, 1532

Cetylpyridinum chloride
- in douche products, 1425
- in lozenges, 1417
- in mouth and throat products, 1421
- in mouthwash, 1418
- in throat spray, 1418

Cevi-Bid, 20
Chapstick Flava-Craze, 1522
Chapstick Ultra, 1521
Charcoal, 959
Charcoal, activated, 1633-1634
Charcocaps, 959
Chardonna-2, 936
Chatcoaid, 1633
Chelated magnesium, 39
Chelating agents
- succimer, 1645-1646

Chemet, 1645
Chemical disinfection systems
- for soft (hydrogel) contact lenses, 1394

Chemstrip 6, 1771
Chemstrip 7, 1771
Chemstrip 9, 1771
Chemstrip 2 GP, 1771
Chemstrip 2 LN, 1769
Chemstrip 10 SG, 1771
Chemstrip 4 the OB, 1771
Chemstrip bG, 1749, 1753
Chemstrip 2GP, 1753
Chemstrip K, 1757, 1771
Chemstrip Micral, 1767
Chemstrip uG, 1771
Chemstrip uGK, 1753, 1771
Cheracol Cough Syrup, 567
Cheracol D Cough Formula Syrup, 568
Cheracol Plus Liquid, 568
Chiggerex, 1485
Chigger-Tox, 1485
Children's Advil, 638
Children's Elixir DM Cough & Cold Elixir, 558
Children's Feverall, 598
Children's Genapap, 597
Children's Halenol, 598
Children's Mapap, 597
Children's Motrin, 638
Children's Nasalcrom, 476
Children's Panadol, 597, 598
Children's Silapap, 597
Children's Sudafed, 501
Children's Tylenol, 597, 598
Chlo-Amine, 494
Chlorpheniramine Maleate/ Pseudoephedrine HCl ER Capsules, 532
Chloral Hydrate, 817
Chloral hydrate, 817
Chloramphenicol
- in ophthalmic anti-infectives, 1366, 1370-1371
- in otic antibiotics, 1397
- systemic, 1045-1047
- topical, 1098

Chlorbutanol, 1529
Chlorcyclizine HCl, 254
Chlordiazepoxide
- as antianxiety agent, 710
- in anticholinergic combinations, 937

Chlordiazepoxide and amitriptyline HCl, 807
Chlordiazepoxide and Clidinium Bromide, 937
Chloresium, 1527
Chloresium, 1527
Chlorhexidine, 1407-1408
Chlorhexidine gluconate
- as antiseptic, 1505
- as mouth and throat product, 1407

Chloride, 33

Chlorambucil, 1602
Chloromycetin
ophthalmic, 1366
topical, 1098
Chloromycetin Otic, 1397
Chloromycetin Sodium Succinate, 1045
Chloromycetin/Hydrocortisone for Suspension, 1370
Chlorophyll derivatives, 1136, 1527
Chloroptic, 1366
Chloroquine hydrochloride, 1141
Chloroquine phosphate, 1141
Chlorostat, 1505
Chlorothiazide, 323
Chloroxine, 1475
Chloroxylenol
in antifungal combinations, 1135
in otic preparations, 1400
in topical antihistamines, 1502
Clorpactin, 1506
Chlorphenesin carbamate, 885
Chlorpheniramine maleate
systemic, 494
topical, 1502
in upper respiratory combinations, 529-530, 532, 534, 536-539, 541-543, 548-551, 554-555, 559-562, 566
Chlorpheniramine tannate, 530, 534-535, 537, 544, 556
Chlorpheniramine Tannate/Pseudoephedrine Tannate Suspension, 537
Chlorpropamide, 278
Chlorpromazine, 699
Chlorpromazine HCl, 770
Chlorthalidone, 323, 430, 432
Chlor-Trimeton, 494
Chlor-Trimeton Allergy 8-Hour, 494
Chlor-Trimeton Allergy 12-Hour, 494
Chlor-Trimeton Allergy-D 4 Hour Tablets, 534
Chlor-Trimeton Allergy-D 12 Hour Tablets, 534
Chlorzoxazone, 885
Chlorzoxazone with APAP, 889
Chlorthalidone, 432
Cholac, 983
Cholecalciferol, 23
Choledyl SA, 462
Cholestyramine, 435
Choline, 65
Choline bitartrate, 65
Choline salicylate, 601, 602
Choline theophyllinate, 462
Cholinesterase inhibitors
ophthalmic, 1316-1318
systemic, 803-806
Chooz, 30, 917
Choriogonadotropin alfa, 202-203
Chorionic gonadotropin, 204-206
Chromagen Capsules, 77, 78
Chromelin Complexion Blender, 1527
Chronulac, 983
Chymodiactin, 1698
Chymopapain, 1698-1699
Ciba Vision Daily Cleaner, 1393
Ciba Vision Saline, 1393
Ciclopirox, 1132
Ciclopirox olamine, 1130
Cidex, 1506
Cidex Formula-7, 1506
Cidex PA, 1506
Cidex Plus, 1506
Cidofovir, 1170-1172
Ciloxan, 1366
Cimetidine, 950
Cinoxate, 1519
Cipro, 1069
Ciprofloxacin, 1069
Ciprofloxacin HCl, 1366
Citaprolam hydrobromide, 737-739
Citra pH, 918
Citracal, 29
Citracal Caplets + D, 29
Citracal Liquitab, 29
Citrate, 33
Citrate of Magnesia, 988
Citric acid
in acne products, 1447-1448
in analgesics, 598, 606
in anorectal preparations, 1431
in antacid combinations, 929
in laxatives, 978
Citric acid and sodium citrate, 1655
Citrocarbonate, 929
Citrucel, 977
Citrucel Sugar Free, 977
Citrus Calcium+D Tablets, 53
Claforan, 1038
Clarithromycin
for Helicobacter pylori infections, 947-949
as macrolide, 1052
Claritin, 496
Claritin Reditabs, 496
Claritin-D 12 Hour Tablets, 534
Claritin-D 24 Hour Tablets, 534
Cleaning, soaking, and wetting solutions
for hard contact lenses, 1387
Cleaning and soaking solutions
for hard contact lenses, 1387
Cleaning solutions
for rigid gas permeable contact lenses, 1390
Cleaning solutions and gels
for hard contact lenses, 1387
Cleaning/soaking solutions
for rigid gas permeable contact lenses, 1390
Clean-N-Soak, 1387
Clear Eyes, 1339
Clear Eyes ACR, 1339, 1343
Clear Total Lice Elimination System, 1244
Clearasil 10, 1435
Clearasil Adult Care Cream, 1444
Clearasil Antibacterial Soap, 1446

Clearasil Clearstick Maximum Strength, 1444
Clearasil Clearstick Regular Strength, 1444
Clearasil Double Clear Maximum Strength Pads, 1444
Clearasil Double Clear Regular Strength Pads, 1444
Clearasil Double Textured Pads Maximum Strength, 1447
Clearasil Double Textured Pads Regular Strength, 1447
Clearasil Maximum Strength, 1435
Clearasil Medicated Deep Cleaner, 1447
Clearblue Easy, 1765
Clearly Cala-gel, 1502
ClearPlan Easy, 1763
Clemastine fumarate
as antihistamine, 494
in upper respiratory combinations, 539
Cleocin, 1111
Cleocin HCl, 1048
Cleocin Pediatric, 1048
Cleocin Phosphate, 1048
Cleocin T, 1048
Clerz 2, 1387
Clerz 2 Lubricating and Rewetting Drops, 1394
Clidinium bromide, 937
Climara, 155
Clinacort, 241
Clinalog, 241
Clinda-Derm, 1048
Clindamycin HCl, 1048
Clindamycin phosphate, 1111
Clinistix, 1753
Clinitest, 1753
Clinoril, 640
Clobetasol propionate, 247
Clocortolone pivalate, 247
Cloderm, 247
Clofibrate, 439-441
Clomid, 214
Clomiphene citrate, 214-216
Clomipramine HCl, 760
Clonazepam, 710, 832-835
Clonidine HCl, 398-400, 432
Clopidogrel bisulfate, 119-121
Clopra, 965
Clorazepate dipotassium, 710
Clotrimazole, 1114-1115, 1130, 1132, 1138
Clove, 1420
Cloxacillin sodium, 1085
Clozapine, 791-793
Clozaril, 791
CMV-IGIV, see Cytomegalovirus immune globulin intravenous (human)
CNS stimulants
amphetamines, 575-578
appetite suppressants non-amphetamine, 579-583 sibutramine, 584-586
caffeine, 587-589
methylphenidate, 590-593
pemoline, 594-596
Coal tar
in antifungal combinations, 1135
as antiseborrheic agent, 1475-1476, 1479
Cocaine HCl, 1481
Cocamidopropyl betaine, 1448
Cocoa butter
in anorectal preparations, 1430, 1431
in mouth and throat products, 1420
Cod liver oil, 1507
Cod Liver Oil USP, 47
Codal-DH Syrup, 556
Codal-DM Syrup, 553
Codeine, 615, 889
Codeine Phosphate, 615
Codeine phosphate
in antidiarrheal combination products, 1016
in antitussives, 506
in narcotic pain relievers, 623-624
in upper respiratory combinations, 544, 545, 562, 567
Codeine Phosphate and Guaifenesin Tablets, 567
Codeine Sulfate, 615
Codeine sulfate, 506
Codiclear DH Syrup, 570
Codimal DH Syrup, 556
Codimal DM Syrup, 553
Codimal PH Syrup, 545
Oxycodone terephthalate, 627
Cogentin, 891
Cognex, 803
Colace, 995
Colace-T, 995
Colax Tablets, 998
Colazal, 1019
Colchicine, 658-661
Colchicine and probenecid, 658, 662
Cold & Cough Tussin Softgels, 563
Cold Symptoms Relief Maximum Strength Tablets, 550
Coldec D Tablets, 531
Coldec DM Syrup, 548
Coldmist JR Tablets, 525
Coldmist LA Tablets, 527
Colesevelam HCl, 435
Colestid, 435
Colestipol HCl, 435
Colfed-A Capsules, 532
Colistin, 1397
Collagen, 1447
Colloidal alumina, 1136
Colloidal oatmeal
in acne products, 1446
in poison ivy treatment products, 1512
Colloidal sulfur, 1479
Collyrium Fresh, 1339
ColoCare, 1760
Colony-stimulating factor
filgrastim, 131-133
sargramostim, 134-136
ColoScreen, 1760
ColoScreen-ES, 1760
Col-Probenecid, 658, 662
Coly-Mycin S Otic, 1397
Colyte, 1003
Colyte Flavored, 1003
Combination oral contraceptives, 170
Combipatch, 162
Combipres 0.1 Tablets, 432
Combipres 0.2 Tablets, 432

INDEX

Combipres 0.3 Tablets, 432
Combistix, 1771
Combivent, 482
Combivir, 1190
Comfort Eye Drops, 1339
Compazine, 699, 771
Compazine Spansules, 699
Complete Allergy Relief, 495
Complex 15, 1498
Compound W, 1493
Compound W Wart Remover for Kids, 1493
Compoz Nighttime Sleep Aid, Maximum Strength, 822
Comtan, 912
Comtrex Acute Head Cold & Sinus Pressure Relief, Multi-Symptom Maximum Strength Tablets, 538
Comtrex Allergy-Sinus Treatment, Maximum Strength Tablets, 538
Comtrex Cough and Cold Relief, Multi-Symptom Maximum Strength Tablets, 550
Comtrex Day & Night Cold & Cough Relief, Multi-Symptom Maximum Strength Tablets, 550
Comtrex Flu Therapy & Fever Relief Day & Night, Multi-Symptom Maximum Strength Tablets, 539
Comtrex Multi-Symptom Deep Chest Cold & Congestion Relief Softgels, 563
Comtrex Multi-Symptom Maximum Strength Non-Drowsy Cold & Cough Relief Tablets, 546
Comtussin HC Syrup, 554
Conceive Pregnancy, 1765
Concentrated Phillips' Milk of Magnesia, 918
Conceptrol, 1428
Conceptrol Contraceptive Inserts, 1428
Concerta, 590
Condoms
  female, 170
Condoms *(cont.)*
  male, 170
Condylox, 1491
Congestac Tablets, 526
Conjugated estrogens, 155, 161
Constilac, 983
Constulose, 983
Contac Day & Night Allergy/Sinus Relief Tablets, 541
Contac Day & Night Cold & Flu Tablets, 552
Contac Severe Cold & Flu Maximum Strength Tablets, 550
Contact lenses
  hard products for, 1387-1389
  rigid gas permeable products for, 1390-1392
  soft (hydrogel) products for, 1393-1396
Contraceptive methods, 170-201
Contraceptive systems
  intrauterine progesterone, 189-191
  levonorgestrel implant, 192-194
  levonorgestrel-releasing intrauterine system, 195-198
Contraceptive transdermal system
  norelgestromin/ethinyl estradiol, 199-201
Contrin Capsules, 77
Contrin Capsules, 78
ConvaTec Aloe Vesta Perineal, 1431
Cool Hot Gel, 1514
Cool'n'Hot Gel, 1514
Copaxone, 1734
Cope Analgesic Tablets, 610
Coppertone All Day, 1516-1517, 1520
Coppertone Aloe and Vitamin E, 1522
Coppertone Bug & Sun, 1517, 1520
Coppertone Gold Dark Tanning, 1521
Coppertone Gold Tan Magnifier, 1521
Coppertone Kids, 1517-1518
Coppertone Kids Colorblock, 1517
Coppertone Kids Spray 'n Splash, 1518
Coppertone Kids Wacky Foam, 1516
Coppertone Moisturizing Suntan, 1521
Coppertone Natural Fruit Flavor, 1522
Coppertone Oil-Free, 1516-1517, 1520
Coppertone Shade, 1516-1518
Coppertone Shade UVA Guard, 1518
Coppertone Sport, 1516, 1518, 1520
Coppertone to Go, 1518, 1520
Coppertone Water Babies, 1516, 1518
Coppertone Water Babies Little Licks, 1521
Coppertone Water Babies Lotion, 1516
Cordarone, 343
Cordran, 248
Cordran SP, 248
Coreg, 413
Corgard, 379
Coricidin 'D' Cold, Flu, & Sinus Tablets, 541
Coricidin HBP Cold & Flu Tablets, 529
Coricidin HBP Cough & Cold Tablets, 548
Coricidin HBP Maximum Strength Flu Tablets, 549
Corn Huskers, 1498
Corn starch, 1507
Cornmint oil, 1447
Corrective Mixture with Paregoric, 1016
Correctol, 995
Correctol Extra Gentle, 995
Correctol Tablets, 998
CortaGel, 249
Cortaid Intensive Therapy, 249
Cortaid Maximum Strength, 249
Cortaid Sensitive Skin with Aloe, 249

Cortastat, 239
Cortastat 10, 239
Cortastat LA, 239
Cortef, 239, 240
Cortenema, 239
Cortic Ear Drops, 1400
Corticaine, 1430
CortiCool, 249
Corticosteroid combinations
topical, 254-257
Corticosteroids
inhalants, 471-475
as ophthalmic anti-inflammatory agents, 1348-1350
topical, 247-253
Corticotropin, 235-238
Cortifoam, 239
Cortisol, see Hydrocortisone
Cortisone acetate, 239
Cortisporin, 1371
Cortisporin Otic, 1397
Cortisporin Suspension, 1370
Cortisporin-TC, 1397
Cortizone-5, 249
Cortizone-10, 249
Cortizone-10 External Anal Itch Relief, 249
Cortizone for Kids, 249
Cortizone-10 Plus, 249
Cortizone-10 Quick Shot, 249
Cortrosyn, 235
Corzide Tablets 40/5, 431
Corzide Tablets 80/5, 430
Cosopt, 1332
Cosyntropin, 235
Cotazym Capsules, 961
Cotazym-S Capsules, 961
Cotrim, 1108, 1219
Cotrim DS, 1108
Cotrim D.S., 1219
Cotrim Pediatric, 1108, 1219
Cottonseed oil, 1530
Coumadin, 111
Coumarin derivatives, 111-115
Covera-HS, 369
Covicone, 1498
Cozaar, 395
C.P.-DM Drops, 558
C-PHED Tannate Suspension, 534
CPM 8/PSE 90/MSC 2.5 Tablets, 543
CP-TANNIC Suspension, 534
Creon 5 Capsules, 961
Creon 10 Capsules, 961
Creon 20 Capsules, 961
Crest Sensitivity Protection, 1418
m-cresyl acetate, 1400
Cresylate, 1400
Crinone, 166
Crixivan, 1182
Crolom, 1353
Cromolyn sodium
inhalant, 476-478
ophthalmic, 1353
oral, 1700-1701
Crotamiton, 1244
Cruex, 1114, 1130
Super DEC B-100 Tablets, 51
Cuprimine, 1710
Curel, 1498
Curel Moisturizing, 1498
Curretab, 166
Cutar Bath Oil, 1475
Cutemol, 1498
Cuticura Medicated Antibacterial, 1525
Cuticura Ointment, 1444
Cutivate, 248
Cyanocobalamin, 6
Cyclizine, 689
Cyclobenzaprine, 885
Cyclocort, 247
Cyclogyl, 1345
Cyclomydril, 1345
Cyclopentolate HCl, 1345
Cyclophosphamide, 1602
Cycloplegic mydriatics, 1345-1347
Cycloserine, 1222
Cyclosporine, 1676-1679
Cycofed Syrup, 544
Cycrin, 166
Cydec Oral Drops, 536
Cydec-DM Drops, 559
Cydec-DM Syrup, 548, 559
Cylert, 594
Cyproheptadine HCl, 494
Cystagon, 1662
Cysteamine bitartrate, 1662-1663
Cystex, 1220
Cystospaz, 931
Cystospaz-M, 931
Cytadren, 262
CytoGam, 1249
Cytomegalovirus immune globulin intravenous (human), 1249
Cytomel, 299
Cytotec, 955
Cytovene, 1161
Cytoxan, 1602
Cytuss HC Liquid, 554

D.A. Chewable Tablets, 542
D.A. II Tablets, 542
Daily Cleaner, 1393
Dakin's Solution Full Strength, 1506
Dakin's Solution Half Strength, 1506
Dalalone, 239
Dalalone D.P., 239
Dalalone L.A., 239
Dallergy Extended Release Tablets, 542
Dallergy Syrup, 542
Dallergy Tablets, 542
DALLERGY-JR Capsules, 536
Dalmane, 817
d'ALPHA E 400, 27
d'ALPHA E 1000, 27
Dalteparin sodium, 104-106
Damason-P Tablets, 625
Danaparoid sodium, 93-94
Danazol, 220-222
Danocrine, 220
Dantrium, 879
Dantrium Intravenous, 879
Dantrolene sodium, 879-881
Dapa, 597
Dapa Extra Strength, 597
Dapiprazole HCl, 1337
Daranide, 313
Daraprim, 1147
Darvocet-N 50 Tablets, 628
Darvocet-N 100 Tablets, 628
Darvon Compound-65 Pulvules, 629
Darvon Pulvules, 616
Darvon-N, 616
Daunorubicin, 1558-1559
Daunorubicin citrate liposome, 1558

INDEX

DaunoXome, 1558
Dayhist-1, 494
Daypro, 639
Dayto Sulf, 1111
DC Softgels, 995
DDAVP, 226
ddI, see Didanosine
Debrox Drops, 1400
Decadron, 239
Decadron Phosphate, 1348
Deca-Durabolin, 142
Decaject, 239
Decaject-L.A., 239
Declomycin, 1089
Decodult Tablets, 537
Decohistine DH Liquid, 544
Decolate Tablets, 529
Deconamine SR Capsules, 532
Deconamine Syrup, 532
Deconamine Tablets, 532
Decongestant(s), 501-505
Decongestant, antihistamine, and analgesic combinations, 537-541
  pediatric, 541
Decongestant, antihistamine, and anticholingeric combinations, 542-543
  pediatric, 544
Decongestant, antihistamine, and expectorant combinations, 529
  pediatric, 530
Decongestant and analgesic combinations, 522-523
  pediatric, 523-524
Decongestant and antihistamine combinations, 530-534
  pediatric, 535-537
Decongestant and expectorant combinations, 524-528
  pediatric, 528
Deconomed SR Capsules, 532
Deconsal II Tablets, 526
Deep-Down Rub, 1514
Defen-LA Tablets, 526
Degest 2, 1339
Dehistine Syrup, 542
Del Aqua-5, 1435
Del Aqua-10, 1435
Delatestryl, 149
Delavirdine mesylate, 1195
Delestrogen, 155
Delfen Contraceptive, 1428
Del-Mycin, 1061
Delsym, 509
Delta D3, 23
Delta-D2, 23
Deltasone, 240
Deltavac, 1111
Demadex, 317
Demecarium bromide, 1316
Demeclocycline, 1089
Demerol, 615
Demi-Regroton Tablets, 430
Demulon 1/35, 177
Demulen 1/50, 177
Denorex Extra Strength, 1475
Denorex Medicated, 1475
Depacon, 872
Depakene, 872
Depakote, 872
Depakote ER, 872
Depen, 1710
depMedalone 40, 240
depMedalone 80, 240
Depo-Estradiol, 155
Depogen, 155
Depoject-40, 240
Depoject-80, 240
Depo-Medrol, 240
Deponit, 338
Depopred, 240
Depo-Provera, 172
Depotest 100, 149
Depotest 200, 149
Depo-Testadiol, 161
Depotestogen, 161
Depo-Testosterone, 149
Dequasine, 56
Derma Viva, 1498
Dermacoat, 1485
Dermacort, 249
DermaFlex, 1485
Dermamycin, 1502
Derma-Pax, 1502
Dermarest, 1502
Dermarest Plus, 1502
Dermasept Antifungal, 1135
Dermoplast, 1485
Desenex, 1130
De-Sensitize Plus, 1418
Deserpidine, 430
Desipramine HCl, 760
Desitin, 1497, 1507
Desitin Creamy, 1507
Desitin with Zinc Oxide, 1507
Desmopressin acetate, 226-228
Desogen, 177
Desogestrel, 177-178
Desogestrel and Ethinyl Estradiol, 177
Desonide, 247
DesOwen, 247
Desoximetasone, 248
Desoxyn, 575
Desoxyn Gradumends, 575
Desquam-E, 1435
Desquam-X 5 and 10, 1435
Desquam-X Wash, 1435
Desyrel, 754
Desyrel Dividose, 754
Detane, 1485
Detrol, 1670
Detussin Tablets, 553
Devrom, 1017
Dex GG TR Tablets, 570
Dexacidin, 1372
Dexacidin Suspension, 1371
Dexameth, 239
Dexamethasone
  ophthalmic, 1348, 1370-1372
  systemic, 239
Dexamethasone Intensol, 239
Dexamethasone phosphate, 1370, 1371
Dexamethasone sodium phosphate
  ophthalmic, 1348
  systemic, 239
Dexasporin, 1372
Dexbrompheniramine maleate, 534
Dexchlorpheniramine maleate
  as antihistamine, 494
  in upper respiratory combinations, 529
Dexpanthenol, 1496
Dexrazoxane, 1639-1640
Dextroamphetamine saccharate, 575
Dextroamphetamine sulfate, 575

Dextromethorphan HBr
as antitussive, 509
in upper respiratory combinations, 545-553, 557-565, 567-571
Dextromethorphan HCl, 1417
Dextropropoxyphene, 616
Dextrose, 705
Dextrostix, 1749
DHS Tar, 1475
DHS Zinc, 1475
DHT, 23
DHT, see Dihydrotachysterol
DHT Intensol, 23
DiaBeta, 278
Diabetic Tussin DM Liquid, 568
Diabetic Tussin Maximum Strength DM Liquid, 569
Diabetic ulcer agent
becaplermin, 1467-1468
Diabinese, 278
Diabismul, 1016
Dia-Eze, 1017
Dialoce Plus Capsules and Tablets, 998
Dialose, 995
Dialose Plus Capsules, 998
Diamox, 313, 825
Diamox Sequels, 313, 825
Diaparene, 1507
Diaparene Medicated, 1507
Diaparene Peri-Anal Medicated, 1507
Diaper rash products, 1507-1508
Diaphragm, 170
Dia-Quel, 1016
Diar-Aid, 1017
Diascan, 1749
Diasorb, 1017
Diastix, 1753
Diazepam
as antianxiety agent, 710
as muscle relaxant, 885
Diazepam Intensol, 710, 885
Diazolidinyl urea
in acne products, 1447-1448
Diazolidinyl urea *(cont.)*
in douche products, 1425
Dibasic calcium phosphate dihydrate, 29
Dibucaine
in anorectal preparations, 1430
for skin disorders, 1485
Dical-D Tablets, 53
Dicarbosil, 30
Dichloralphenazone, 668
Dichlorphenamide, 313
Diclofenac potassium, 638
Diclofenac sodium
in nonnarcotic analgesics, 611
ophthalmic, 1356
oral, 638
Dicloxacillin sodium, 1085
Dicomal-DH Syrup, 556
Dicomal-DM Syrup, 553
Dicumarol, 111
Dicyclomine, 931
Didanosine, 1190
Di-Delamine, 1502
Didrex, 579
Didronel, 305
Dienestrol, 155
n,n-diethyl m-toluamide, 1517, 1520
Diethylpropion HCl, 579
Diethylstilbestrol diphosphate, 1576
Difenoxin, 1010-1012
Difenoxin with atropine sulfate, 1010
Diflorasone diacetate, 248
Diflucan, 1116
Diflunisal, 613-614
Di-Gel, 924
Digestive aids
digestive enzymes, 961-964
metoclopramide, 965-967
miscellaneous products, 971-972
Digestive enzymes, 961-964
Digitek, 329
Digoxin, 329
Dihistine DH Elixir, 544
Dihistine Expectorant Liquid, 562
Dihydrocodeine bitartrate, 626
Dihydrotachysterol, 23
Dihydroxyacetone, 1527
Dihydroxypropyl theophylline, 462
Dilacor XR, 368
Dilantin-125, 842
Dilantin Infatab, 842
Dilantin Kapseals, 842
Dilantin with Phenobarbital Kapseals, 842
Dilatrate-SR, 337
Dilaudid, 615
Dilaudid Cough Syrup, 571
Dilor, 462
Dilor-400, 462
Dilor-G Liquid, 521
Dilor-G Tablets, 521
Diltia XT, 368
Diltiazem HCl, 368
Dimaphen DM Cold & Cough Elixir, 558
Dimaphen Elixir, 535
Dimenhydrinate, 689
Dimetabs, 689
Dimetane-DX Cough Syrup, 547
Dimetapp Children's Nighttime Flu Syrup, 558
Dimetapp Children's Non-Drowsy Flu Syrup, 557
Dimetapp Cold & Allergy Elixir, 535
Dimetapp Decongestant Plus Cough Infant Drops, 557
Dimethicone, 1481
Dimethyl sulfoxide, 1664-1665
Diocto, 995
Diocto C, 1001
Diocto-K, 995
Diocto-K Plus Capsules, 998
Dioctolose Plus Capsules, 998
Dioeze, 995
Diovan, 395
Dipentum, 1019
Diphen, 495
Diphen AF, 495, 509
Diphen Cough, 495, 509, 689, 891
Diphenhist, 495, 891

INDEX

Diphenhist Captabs, 495, 891
Diphenhydramine
as antiemetic/antivertigo agent, 689
as antiparkinson agent, 891
Diphenhydramine citrate
in nonnarcotic analgesics, 608
in upper respiratory combinations, 533, 536
Diphenhydramine HCl
as antihistamine, 495
as antiparkinson agent, 891
as antitussive, 509
in nonnarcotic analgesics, 608, 610
as nonprescription sleep aids, 822
as topical antihistamine, 1502
in topical corticosteroids, 254
in upper respiratory combinations, 529, 533, 536, 540-541, 552
Diphenoxylate, 1010-1012
Diphenoxylate with atropine sulfate, 1010
Diphtheria, tetanus, pertussis, hemophilus b vaccine, 1271-1272
Diphtheria, tetanus, pertussis vaccine, 1258, 1264-1267
Diphtheria and tetanus toxoids, adsorbed combined, 1264
Diphtheria and tetanus toxoids and acellular pertussis vaccine adsorbed, 1264
Diphtheria and tetanus toxoids and pertussis vaccine, 1264
Diphtheria and tetanus toxoids and pertussis vaccine adsorbed and hemophilus b conjugate vaccine, 1271-1272
Dipivefrin, 1325
Diprolene, 247
Diprolene AF, 247
Diprosone, 247
Dipyridamole, 88-89
Dipyridamole and aspirin, 95-97
Direct-acting miotics, 1319-1321
Dirithromycin, 1052
Disalcid, 602
Disalcid Amigesic, 602
Disanthrol Capsules, 998
Disinfecting Solution, 1394
Disinfecting/wetting/soaking solutions
for rigid gas permeable contact lenses, 1390
Disodium, 1444
Disodium lauryl sulfosuccinate, 1448
Disodiumcocoamphodiacetate, 1431
Disolan Capsules, 998
Disolan Forte Capsules, 998
Disonate, 995
Disoplex Capsules, 998
Disopyramide, 346-348
Disulfiram, 1702-1704
D.I.T.1-2, 1111
Ditropan, 1668
Diucardin, 323
Diurese, 323
Diuretics
carbonic anhydrase inhibitors, 313-316
combinations, 327
loop diuretics, 317-319
nonprescription, 328
potassium-sparing diuretics, 320-322
thiazides and related diuretics, 323-326
Diurigen, 323
Diuril, 323
Diutensen-R Tablets, 430
Divalproex sodium, 872
Dizmiss, 689
DMDM hydantoin
in anorectal preparations, 1431
in skin cleansers, 1530
DML, 1498
DMSO, see Dimethyl sulfoxide
Doan's PM, Extra Strength, 602
Docucal-P Softgels, 998
Docusate, 998-999
Docusate potassium, 995
Docusate sodium
in bowel evacuation kits, 1005
in laxative combinations, 1001
in modified iron products, 72
as stool softener, 995
in vaginal anti-infectives, 1111
Dofetilide, 349-351
DOK, 995
Dolacet Capsules, 625
Dolanex, 597
Dolasetron mesylate, 696
Dolobid, 613
Dolophine HCl, 615
Dolsed, 1220
Domeboro Powder Packets, 1526
Dome-Paste, 1528
Domol Bath and Shower, 1499
Donatussin DC Syrup, 566
Donatussin Drops, 530
Donatussin Syrup, 562
Donepezil HCl, 803
Donnagel, 1017
Donnagel-PG, 1016
Donnamar, 931
Donnapectolin-PG, 1016
Donnatal, 936
Donnatal Extentabs, 936
Donnazyme Tablets, 961
Dopaminergics, 895-899
Doral, 817
Dormarex 2, 689, 891
Dornase Alfa, 485
Doryx, 1089
Dorzolamide HCl, 1330
Dorzolamide HCl/Timolol maleate, 1332-1334
DOS Softgel, 995
Dosalax, 991
Dostinex, 1696
Double Strength Gaviscon-2, 922
Douche products, 1425-1427
Dovonex, 1452
Doxazosin mesylate, 386
Doxepin HCl
in topical antihistamines, 1502

Doxepin HCl *(cont.)*
in tricyclic antidepressants, 760
Doxidan Capsules, 998
Doxidan LiquiGels, 998
Doxil, 1560
Doxinate, 995
Doxorubicin, 1560-1562
conventional, 1560
liposome, 1560
Doxycycline
as antibiotic, 1089
as mouth and throat product, 939-941
Doxylamine succinate
in nonprescription sleep aids, 822
in upper respiratory combinations, 541, 552-553
DPT, see Diphtheria and tetanus toxoids and pertussis vaccine
Dr. Caldwell Senna, 992
Dr. DermiHeal, 1529
Dr. Scholl's Cracked Heel Relief, 1485
Dr. Scholl's Fungi Solution, 1131
Dramamine, 689
Dri/Ear, 1400
Drisdol, 23
Dristan Cold Multi-Symptom Formula Tablets, 538
Dristan Cold Non-Drowsy Maximum Strength Tablets, 522
Dristan 12-hr, 501
Dristan Nasal Spray, 517
Dristan Sinus Tablets, 523
Drithocreme HP 1, 1450
Dritho-Scalp, 1450
Drixomed Tablets, 534
Drixoral, 502
Drixoral Allergy Sinus Tablets, 541
Drixoral Cold & Allergy Tablets, 534
Dronabinol, 693
Dry E 400, 27
Dry Eye Therapy, 1383
Dry Eyes, 1383, 1386
Dryphen Multi-Symptom Formula Tablets, 538
Drysol, 1527
Drytex Lotion, 1447
DSMC Plus Capsules, 998
D-S-S, 995
DTaP, see Diphtheria and tetanus toxoids and acellular pertussis vaccine adsorbed
DTP, see Diphtheria and tetanus toxoids and pertussis vaccine
DTwP, see Diphtheria and tetanus toxoids and pertussis vaccine
Dulcagen, 991
Dulcolax, 991
Dull-C, 20
Duofilm, 1493
Duonate-12 Suspension, 535
Duoplant Gel, 1493
Duphalac, 983
Duplex T, 1475
Duradrin, 668
Duradryl JR Capsules, 544
Duradryl Syrup, 542
Duragesic, 615
Duramist Plus 12 Hour, 501
Duramorph, 616
DuraScreen, 1518, 1520
Duratears Naturale, 1383, 1386
Duratuss DM Elixir, 569
Duratuss GP Tablets, 528
Duratuss HD Elixir, 566
Duratuss Tablets, 528
Dura-Vent/DA Tablets, 542
Durex, 1428
Duricef, 1037
Dyazide, 327
Dycil, 1085
Dyclone, 1481
Dyclonine HCl
in lozenges, 1417-1418
for mucous membranes, 1481
in throat spray, 1418
Dyflex-G Tablets, 521
Dy-G Liquid, 521
Dynabac, 1052
Dynacin, 1089
DynaCirc, 368
DynaCirc CR, 368
Dynafed Asthma Relief Tablets, 524
Dynapen, 1085
Dynex Tablets, 527
Dyphylline
as bronchodilator, 462
Dyphylline *(cont.)*
in upper respiratory combinations, 521
Dyphylline-GG Elixir, 521
Dyrenium, 320

E-400, 27
Ear-Dry, 1400
EarSol-HC, 1400
Eastprin, 601
E-base, 1052
Echothiophate iodide, 1316
EC-Naprosyn, 639
Econazole nitrate, 1130
Econopred, 1348
Econopred Plus, 1348
Ecotrin Maximum Strength Tablets and Caplets, 601
Ecotrin Tablets and Caplets, 601
Ed A-Hist Liquid, 530
Ed A-Hist Tablets, 530
ED Tuss HC Syrup, 555
Ed-DOXY Caps, 1089
Edecrin, 317
Ed-Flex Capsules, 529
Edrophonium chloride, 1647
Edrophonium chloride and atropine sulfate, 1647
EDTA
in acne products, 1444-1448
in antacid combinations, 926
in anorectal preparations, 1430
in antifungal combinations, 1136
ED-TLC Liquid, 554
E.E.S. 200, 1052
E.E.S. 400, 1052
E.E.S. Granules, 1052
Efavirenz, 1195
Effer-K, 41
Effer-syllium, 978
Effexor, 757
Effexor XR, 757
Efidac 24, 494, 501
Eflornithine HCl, 1533-1534
Efudex, 1541
Elavil, 760

INDEX

Eldepryl, 909
Electrolyte mixtures
  oral, 33-34
Elimite, 1244
Elixophyllin, 462
Elixophyllin-GG Liquid, 521
Elixophyllin-KI Elixir, 521
Ellence, 1563
Elocon, 250
E-LOR Tablets, 629
Elta Block, 1517
Eltroxin, 299
Emcyt, 1581, 1600
Emetrol, 705
Emgel, 1061
Eminase, 116
EMLA, 1486
Emollients, 1496-1499
Empirin, 601
Empirin w/Codeine No. 3 Tablets, 623
Empirin w/Codeine No. 4 Tablets, 624
Emulsoil, 991
E-Mycin, 1052
Enalapril maleate, 390, 432
Enbrel, 1740
Encare, 1428
Endagen-HD Liquid, 554
Endal Tablets, 524
Enduron, 323
Enduronyl Forte Tablets, 430
Enduronyl Tablets, 430
Enerjets, 587
Engerix-B, 1289
Enlon, 1647
Enlon-Plus, 1647
Enoxaparin sodium, 101-103
Entacapone, 912-913
Entertainer's Secret, 1409
Entex HC Liquid, 566
Entex LA Tablets, 525
Entex Liquid, 524
Entex PSE Tablets, 528
Enulose, 983
Enviro-Stress Tablets, 49
Enzymatic cleaners
  for hard contact lenses, 1388
  for rigid gas permeable contact lenses, 1390
  for soft (hydrogel) contact lenses, 1393
Enzymes
  pegaspargase, 1621-1623
EPA Capsules, 60
Ephedrine HCl, 521, 524
Ephedrine Sulfate, 455
Ephedrine sulfate
  in anorectal preparations, 1431
  as bronchodilator, 455
  as decongestant, 501
  in nasal products, 517
  in upper respiratory combinations, 524
Ephedrine tannate, 544, 556
E-Pherol, 27
Epifoam Aerosol Foam, 254
Epifrin, 1325
E-Pilo-1, 1335
E-Pilo-2, 1335
E-Pilo-3, 1335
E-Pilo-4, 1335
E-Pilo-6, 1335
Epilyt, 1498
Epinal, 1325
Epinephrine, 455
Epinephrine bitartrate, 1335
Epinephrine borate, 1325
Epinephrine HCl
  as decongestant, 501
  ophthalmic, 1325
Epirubicin HCl, 1563-1564
Epitol, 828
Epivir, 1190
Epivir-HBV, 1190
Epoetin alfa, 128-130
Epogen, 128
Eprosartan mesylate, 395
Epsom Salt, 988
e.p.t. Quick Stick, 1765
Equagesic Tablets, 610
Equalactin, 977
Equanil, 721
Ergamisol, 1591
Ergocalciferol, 23
Ergoloid mesylates, 797-798
Ergotamine tartrate, 668
E•R•O Ear Drops, 1400
Eryc, 1052
Erycette, 1061
Eryderm 2, 1061
Erygel, 1061
Erymax, 1061
Ery-Ped, 1052
Ery-Ped 200, 1052
Ery-Ped 400, 1052
Ery-Ped Drops, 1052
Ery-Tab, 1052
Erythra-Derm, 1061
Erythrocin Lactobionate, 1053
Erythrocin Stearate, 1053
Erythromycin
  in acne products, 1435
  ophthalmic, 1366
  topical, 1061-1062, 1098
Erythromycin base, 1052
Erythromycin estolate, 1052
Erythromycin ethylsuccinate, 1052
Erythromycin ethylsuccinate and sulfisoxazole, 1104-1107
Erythromycin gluceptate, 1053
Erythromycin lactobionate, 1053
Erythromycin stearate, 1053
Eryzole, 1104
Esclim, 155
Eserine Sulfate, 1316
Esgic Tablets, 609
Esgic-Plus Tablets, 608
Esidrix, 323
Esimil Tablets, 432
Eskalith, 799
Eskalith CR, 799
Esomeprazole magnesium, 968
Esoterica, 1498
Espotabs, 991
Estar, 1476
Estazolam, 817
Ester-C Plus, Extra Potency, 58
Ester-C Plus 500 mg Vegicaps, 58
Ester-C Plus Multi-Mineral Formula Vegicaps, 58
Esterified estrogens, 155, 161
Estinyl, 155
Estrace, 155
Estraderm, 155
Estradiol, 155, 161-162

Estradiol cypionate, 155, 161
Estradiol cypionate/ medroxyprogesterone acetate, 174-176
Estradiol hemihydrate, 155
Estradiol valerate in oil, 155
Estramustine phosphate sodium, 1581, 1600
Estratab, 155
Estratest, 161
Estratest H.S., 161
Estring, 155
Estrogen(s), 155-160, 1576-1577
Estrogen and nitrogen mustard, 1581-1582, 1600-1601
Estrogen combinations, 161-163
Estrone aqueous, 155
Estropipate, 155
Estrostep, 178
Estrostep Fe, 178
Etanercept, 1740-1742
Ethacrynic acid, 317
Ethambutol hydrochloride, 1222
Ethanol, 1135
Ethchlorvynol, 817
Ethinyl estradiol, 155, 161, 177-178
Ethinyl estradiol/levonorgestrel, 186
Ethinyl estradiol/norelgestromin, 199-201
Ethionamide, 1222
Ethmozine, 356
Ethopropazine, 891
Ethosuximide, 861
Ethotoin, 842
Ethyl alcohol, 1449
Ethylhexyl p-methoxycinnamate, 1516-1518, 1520-1522
Ethynodiol diacetate, 177
Etidronate disodium, 305
Etodolac, 638
Etoposide, 1554-1555
Etrafon 2-10, 807
Etrafon Forte, 807
Eucalyptamint, 1514
Eucalyptamint 2000 Gel, 1515
Eucalyptol
in douche products, 1425
in mouth and throat products, 1420, 1422
in mouthwash, 1418
in skin cleansers, 1530
in topical antihistamines, 1502
Eucalyptol acetate, 1136
Eucalyptus oil
in acne products, 1447
in douche products, 1425
in lozenges, 1417
in skin cleansers, 1528, 1531
in upper respiratory combinations, 572
Eucerin, 1498
Eulexin, 1571
Eurax, 1244
Evac-Q-Kwik, 1005
Evac-U-Gen, 991
Evac-U-Lax Tablets, 991
Everone 200, 149
Evista, 164
Exact, 1447
Excedrin Extra Strength Caplets, Geltabs, and Tablets, 609
Excedrin Migraine, 668
Excedrin PM Tablets, 608
Exelderm, 1131
Exelon, 803
Ex-Histine Syrup, 542
Ex-Lax Chocolated, 991
Ex-Lax Extra Gentle Pills, 998
Ex-Lax Gentle Nature, 991
Ex-Lax Maximum Relief, 991
Ex-Lax Unflavored, 991
Exna, 323
Exocaine Odor Free Creme, 1514
Exocaine Plus Rub, 1514
Econazole, 1132
Expectorants, 513-516
and antitussives, 562-571, pediatric, 567, 571
and decongestants, 524-528, pediatric, 528
and decongestants and antihistamines, 529, pediatric, 530
Extendryl Chewable Tablets, 542
Extendryl JR Capsules, 544
Extendryl SR Capsules, 542
Extendryl Syrup, 542
Extra Action Cough Syrup, 568
Extra Potency Ester-C Plus, 58
Extra Strength Adprin-B, 601
Extra Strength Alka-Seltzer, 929
Extra Strength Alkets, 917
Extra Strength Antacid Tablets, 917
Extra Strength Bayer Enteric 500, 601
Extra Strength Bayer Plus, 601
Extra Strength Bayer PM Aspirin Plus Sleep Aid Caplets, 610
Extra Strength Doan's PM, 602
Extra Strength Gas-X, 959
Extra Strength Genaton, 922
Extra Strength Goody's Tablets, 610
Extra Strength Maalox, 921
Extra Strength Maalox Plus, 921
Extra Strength Maalox Plus Suspension, 925
Extra Strength Maalox Suspension, 925
Extra Strength Mintox Plus, 925
Extra Strength Tylenol PM Geltabs, 822
Eye Drops, 1339
Eye Drops Extra, 1339
Eyesine, 1339
EZ Detect, 1760
Ezide, 323

Fact Plus, 1765
Famciclovir, 1164
Famotidine, 950
Famvir, 1164
Fansidar, 1149
Fareston, 1578
Fastin, 579

INDEX

Fastlene, 587
Fat, 978
Father John's Liquid Medicine Plus, 549
Fat-soluble vitamins, 6
Feen-a-mint, 991
Feen-a-mint Chocolated, 991
Feen-a-mint Pills, 998
Felbamate, 836-838
Felbatol, 836
Feldene, 640
Felodipine, 368
Fem-1 Tablets, 609
Femara, 1585
Femcare, 1138
femhrt, 161
Femilax Tablets, 998
Femiron, 71
FemPatch, 155
Femstat, 1138
Fenesin, 513
Fenesin DM Tablets, 569
Fen-gen-sol, 71
Fen-In-Sol, 71
Fenofibrate, 442-444
Fenoprofen calcium, 638
Fentanyl, 615
Fe-O.D. Tablets, 75
Feosol, 71
Feostat, 71
Ferancee Tablets, 75
Ferancee-HP Tablets, 75
Feratab, 71
Fergon, 71
Fer-In-Sol, 71
Fer-Iron, 71
Fermalox, 72
Ferocyl, 72
Fero-Folic-500 Filmtabs, 76
Fero-Grad-500 Filmtabs, 75
Fero-Gradumet Filmtab, 71
Ferospace, 71
Ferotrinsic Capsules, 77
Ferralet, 71
Ferralet Slow Release, 71
Ferralyn Lanacaps, 71
Ferra-TD, 71
Ferretts, 71
Ferro-Docusate T.R., 72
Ferro-Dok TR, 72
Ferro-DS S.R., 72
Ferromar Caplets, 75
Ferro-Sequels, 72
Ferrous fumarate, 71-72
Ferrous gluconate, 71
Ferrous sulfate, 71-72
Ferrous sulfate exsiccated, 71
Fertility agents, 202-203
  chorionic gonadotropin, 204-206
  clomiphene citrate, 214-216
  follitropin alfa, 209-211
  follitropin beta, 212-213
  menotropins, 217-219
  urofollitropin, 207-208
Fe-Tinic 150 Forte Capsules, 76
Feverall Sprinkle Caps, 597
Fexofenadine HCl, 495, 533
Fiberall, 977-978
Fiberall Natural Flavor, 977
Fiberall Orange Flavor, 977
FiberCon, 977
Fiber-Lax, 977
FiberNorm, 977
Filgrastim, 131-133
Finac Lotion, 1444
Finasteride, 153-154
Finevin, 1438
Fioricet w/Codeine Capsules, 624
Fiorinal Capsules, 610
Fiorinal w/Codeine No. 3 Capsules, 624
Fiortal Capsules, 609
First Choice, 1749
First Response, 1765
First Response Ovulation Predictor, 1763
Fish oils, 60-62
Fisher-Price Sensitive Skin Sunblock for Kids, 1519
Fisher-Price Spray Mist Sunscreen for Kids, 1519
Fisher-Price Sunscreen for Kids, 1517
Flagyl, 1079
Flagyl 375, 1079
Flanders Buttocks, 1507
Flarex, 1348
Flatulex, 959
Flavons, 58
Flavored Colestid, 435
Flavoxate HCl, 1666-1667
Flecainide acetate, 352-353
Fleet Babylax, 981
Fleet Bisacodyl Uniserts, 991
Fleet Flavored Castor Oil, 991
Fleet Phospho-soda, 988
Fleet-Prep Kit # 1, 1005
Fleet-Prep Kit # 2, 1005
Fleet-Prep Kit # 3, 1005
Fletcher's Castoria, 992
Flexaphen, 889
Flexeril, 885
Flextra-DS Tablets, 608
Flomax, 386
Flonase, 490
Florical, 29-30
Florinef Acetate, 258
Florone, 248
Florone E, 248
Flovent, 471
Flovent Rotadisk, 471
Floxin, 1069
Fluticasone propionate, 248
Fluconazole, 1116-1117
Fludrocortisone acetate, 258
Flumadine, 1176
Flumazenil, 1635-1636
Flunisolide
  inhalant, 471
  intranasal, 490
Fluocinolone acetonide, 248
Fluocinonide, 248
Fluogen, 1282
Fluonid, 248
Fluoride, 35-38
  oral, 35
  topical, 35
Fluorigard, 35
Fluorinse, 35
Fluoritab, 35
Fluorometholone
  in ophthalmic anti-infectives, 1372
  in ophthalmic anti-inflammatory agents, 1348
Fluor-Op, 1348
Fluoroplex, 1541
Fluoroquinolones, 1069-1073
Fluorouracil, 1541
Fluoxetine, 730-733

Fluoxymesterone, 149
Fluphenazine decanoate, 770
Fluphenazine enanthate, 770
Fluphenazine HCl, 770
Flura-Loz, 35
Flurandrenolide, 248
Flurazepam HCl, 817
Flurbiprofen, 638
Flurbiprofen sodium, 1356
FluShield, 1282
Flutamide, 1571
Fluticasone propionate, 471, 490
Fluticasone propionate/ salmeterol, 471
Fluvastatin sodium, 448
Fluvirin, 1282
Fluvoxamine maleate, 734-736
Fluzone, 1282
FML, 1348
FML Forte, 1348
FML S.O.P., 1348
FML-S Suspension, 1372
Foamicon, 922
Foille Medicated FirstAid, 1485
Foille Plus, 1485
Folate, 6
Folic acid, 51-52, 76, 77-78, 81-82
Follistim, 212
Follitropin alfa, 209-211
Follitropin beta, 212-213
Foltrin Capsules, 78
Folvite, 81, 1458
Fomivirsen sodium, 1378-1379
Formic acid, 1532
Formula 405 AHA, 1525
Formula 405 Moisturizing, 1525
Formula E-400, 27
Fortaz, 1038
Fortel Plus, 1765
Fortovase, 1182
Fosamax, 305
Foscarnet, 1158-1160
Foscarnet sodium, 1158
Foscavir, 1158
Fosfomycin tromethamine, 1212-1213
Fosinopril sodium, 390
Fosphenytoin, 842
Fostex, 1435
Fostex 10 Wash, 1435
Fostex Acne Cleansing Cream, 1444
Fostex Acne Medication Cleansing Bar, 1446
Fostex Medicated Cover-Up, 1440
Fostril Lotion, 1444
Fototar, 1476
Fragmin, 104
Fructose, 705
Fulvicin P/G, 1118
Fulvicin-U/F, 1118
Fumasorb, 71
Fumatinic Capsules, 76
Fumerin, 71
FungiCure, 1131
Fungi•Nail, 1135
Fungizone, 1130
Fungoid, 1114, 1130
Fungoid Tincture, 1130
Furadantin, 1216
Furosemide, 317

Gabapentin, 839-841
Gabitril Filmtab, 867
Galantamine HBr, 803
Gallstone dissolving agents
  infusion, 975-976
  oral, 973-974
Gamimune N, 1250
Gamma benzene hexachloride, see Lindane
Gamma globulin, see Immune globulin (human)
Gammagard S/D, 1250
Gammar-P I.V., 1250
Ganciclovir, 1161-1163
Ganciclovir sodium, 1161
Gani-Tuss NR Liquid, 567
Gani-Tuss-DM NR Liquid, 568
Gantanol, 1101
Gantanol DS, 1101
Gantrisin, 1101
Garamycin
  ophthalmic, 1366
  topical, 1098
Gas-Ban, 922
Gas-Ban DS, 925
Gastrocrom, 1700
Gastro-Relief, 917
Gas-X, 959
Gas-X, Extra Strength, 959
Gatifloxacin, 1069
Gaviscon, 922, 926
Gaviscon-2, Double Strength, 922
Gaviscon Extra Strength Relief Formula, 922, 926
Gee-Gee, 513
Gelatin, 1528
Gel-Kam, 35
Gel-Tin, 35
Gelusil, 921, 924
Gemfibrozil, 445-447
Genac Tablets, 533
Genacol Maximum Strength Cold & Flu Relief Tablets, 550
Genagesic Tablets, 629
Genahist
  as antiemetic/antivertigo agent, 891
  as antihistamine, 495
  as antiparkinson agent, 689
Genapap Extra Strength, 597
Genapap Infants' Drops, 598
Genapax, 1138
Genaphed, 501
Genasal, 501
Genasoft Plus Softgels, 998
Genaton, 922, 926
Genaton, Extra Strength, 922
Genatuss, 513
Genatuss DM Syrup, 568
Gen-D-phen, 689
Genebs, 597
Genebs Extra Strength, 597
Generet-500 Tablets, 76
Geneye, 1339
Geneye AC Allergy Formula, 1343
Geneye Extra, 1339
Genoptic, 1366
Genotropin, 231
Genpril, 638
Genprin, 601
Gentacidin, 1366
Gentak, 1366
Gentamicin
  ophthalmic, 1366
  topical, 1098
Gentamicin sulfate, 1370-1371

INDEX

GenTeal Multidose, 1383
Gentian violet
topical, 1130, 1132
vaginal, 1138
Gentlax, 991
Gentlax S Tablets, 998
Genuine Bayer Aspirin Tablets and Caplets, 601
Gen-Xene, 710
Geocillin, 1084
Gerber Pediatric Electrolyte Solution, 33
Germicides
topical, 1505-1506
Gets-It, 1493
Gevrabon Liquid, 48
GFN 1000/DM 60 Tablets, 570
GFN 1200/DM 60 Tablets, 570
GFN 1200/DM 60/PSE 120 Tablets, 565
GFN 600/Phenylephrine 20 Tablets, 524
GFN/PSE Tablets, 528
Gliadel, 1593
Glatiramer acetate, 1734-1735
Glaucoma agents
alpha-2 adrenergic agonist, 1311-1312
beta-blockers, 1313-1315
combinations, 1335-1336
miotics cholinesterase inhibitor, 1316-1318
direct-acting, 1319-1321
prostaglandin agonists, 1322-1324
sympathomimetics, 1325-1327
Glaucon, 1325
Glibenclamide, 278
Glimepiride, 278
Glipizide, 278
Glucagon, 292-293
Glucagon Diagnostic Kit, 292
Glucagon Emergency Kit, 292
Glucocorticoids, 239-246
Glucofilm, 1749
Glucometer Elite, 1749
Glucometer Encore, 1749
Glucophage, 286
Glucophage XR, 286
Glucose elevating agents
glucagon, 292-293
Glucose tests
blood, 1749-1752
urine, 1753-1756
Glucostix, 1749
Glucotrol, 278
Glucotrol XL, 278
Glucovance, 289
Glutaraldehyde, 1506
Glutethimide, 817
Glutofac Caplets, 49
Glyburide, 278
Glyburide/metformin, 289-291
Glycerin, 981-982
in acne products, 1446-1447
in anorectal preparations, 1430, 1431
in antiseborrheic combinations, 1479
in diaper rash products, 1507
in laxatives, 985
in otic preparations, 1400
in poison ivy treatment products, 1512
in skin cleansers, 1529, 1531
Glycerin, USP, 981
Glycerin rectal liquid, 981
Glyceryl cocoate, 1448
Glyceryl guaiacolate, 513
Glyceryl stearate
in anorectal preparations, 1431
in skin cleansers, 1530, 1532
Glycine, 922
Glycopyrrolate, 931
Glycosaminoglycan anticoagulants
danaparoid sodium, 93-94
Glynase PresTab, 278
Gly-Oxide Liquid, 1405
Glyset, 272
Glytuss, 513
Gold Alka-Seltzer, 929
Gold compounds, 646-648
Gold sodium thiomalate, 646
GoLYTELY, 1003
Gonal-F, 209
Good Sense Maximum Strength Dose Sinus Tablets, 538
Good Sense Maximum Strength Pain Relief Allergy Sinus Gelcaps, 539
Goody's Body Pain Powder, 609
Goody's Extra Strength Headache Powder, 609
Goody's Tablets, Extra Strength, 610
Gordochom, 1135
Gordofilm, 1493
Gordogesic Cream, 1514
Goserelin acetate, 1587-1590
Gout agents
allopurinol, 655-659
colchicine, 658-661
probenecid, 662-665
sulfinpyrazone, 666-667
G/P 1200/60 Tablets, 527
GP-500 Tablets, 527
Granisetron HCl, 696
Grifulvin V, 1118
Grisactin, 1118
Grisactin Ultra, 1118
Griseofulvin, 1118-1120
Griseofulvin microsize, 1118
Griseofulvin ultramicrosize, 1118
Gris-PEG, 1118
Growth hormones
somatrem, 229-230
somatropin, 231-234
Guaifed Capsules, 527
Guaifed Syrup, 525
Guaifed-PD Capsules, 526
Guaifenesin
as expectorant, 513
in upper respiratory combinations, 521, 524-530, 562-571
Guaifenesin 1000 mg and Dextromethorphan HBr 60 mg LA Tablets, 570
Guaifenesin DM Syrup, 568
Guaifenesin-DM NR Liquid, 568
Guaifenesin/Pseudoephedrine HCl Tablets, 526
Guaifenex DM Tablets, 569

Guaifenex GP Tablets, 528
Guaifenex PSE 60 Tablets, 526
Guaifenex PSE 120 Tablets, 528
Guaifenex-Rx DM Tablets, 565
Guaifenex-Rx Tablets, 526
GuaiMax-D Tablets, 528
Guaipax PSE Tablets, 528
Guai-Vent/PSE Tablets, 528
Guanabenz acetate, 401-402
Guanadrel sulfate, 403-404
Guanethidine monosulfate, 405-407, 432
Guanfacine HCl, 408-409
Guiadrine DM Tablets, 569
Guiatuss, 513
Guiatuss AC Syrup, 567
Guiatuss CF Syrup, 563
Guiatuss DAC Liquid, 562
Guiatuss PE Liquid, 525
Guiatuss-DM Syrup, 568
Gum benzoin, 1422
Gynecort 5, 249
Gynecort 10, 249
Gyne-Lotrimin, 1138
Gyne-Lotrimin Combination Pack, 1138
Gyne-Sulf, 1111
Gynodiol, 155
Gynol II Extra Strength, 1428
Gynol II Original Formula, 1428

H. pylori agents, see Helicobacter pylori agents
H 9600 SR Tablets, 527
Habitrol, 1715
Haemophilus influenzae type b vaccine, 1258
Hair dressings
medicated, 1479
Halazepam, 710
Halcinonide, 248
Halcion, 817
Haldol, 770
Haldol Decanoate, 770
Haley's M-O, 1001
Halfan, 1152
Halfprin, 601
Halfprin 81, 601
Hall's Mentho-Lyptus, 1417
Halobetasol propionate, 248
Halofantrine HCl, 1152-1153
Halog, 248
Halog-E, 248
Haloperidol, 770
Halotestin, 149
Halotussin AC Liquid, 567
Halotussin DAC Syrup, 562
Haltran, 638
Hamamelis water, 1527. see also Witch hazel
Hard contact lens products, 1387-1389
Hard fat, 1431
Havrix, 1286
Hawaiian Tropic 15 Plus, 1520
Hawaiian Tropic 30 Plus, 1518
Hawaiian Tropic 45 Plus, 1516
Hawaiian Tropic Baby Faces, 1516
Hawaiian Tropic Dark Tanning, 1521
Hawaiian Tropic Super Waterproof, 1518, 1520
HBIG, see Hepatitis B immune globulin (human)
HC Derma-Pax Liquid, 254
HCTZ, see Hydrochlorothiazide
Head and Shoulders Dandruff, 1475
Head and Shoulders Intensive Treatment, 1473
Healthcheck Ovulation Detector, 1763
Heet Spray, 1514
Helicobacter pylori agents, 942
bismuth subsalicylate, metronidazole and tetracycline HCl, 944-946
lansoprazole/amoxicillin/clarithromycin, 947-949
ranitidine bismuth citrate, 942-943
Helidac, 944
Hema-Combistix, 1771
Hemaspan Tablets, 75
Hemastix, 1771
Heme-Check, 1760
Hemoccult, 1760
Hemoccult SENSA, 1760
Hemocyte, 71
Hemocyte Plus Tablets, 76
Hemocyte-F Tablets, 76
Hemophilus b conjugate vaccine, 1268-1270
Hemorrhoidal HC, 1430
Hem-Prep, 1431
Heparin, 98-100
Heparin Sodium, Multiple Dose Vials, 98
Heparin Sodium, Single Dose Ampules and Vials, 98
Heparin Sodium, Unit Dose, 98
Hepatitis A, inactivated and Hepatitis B, recombinant vaccine, 1293-1295
Hepatitis A vaccine, 1258
Hepatitis A vaccine, inactivated, 1286-1288
Hepatitis B immune globulin (human), 1249
Hepatitis B vaccine, 1258, 1289-1292
Herbal Laxative Tablets, 998
Herceptin, 1629
Hexachlorophene, 1505
Hexalen, 1615
Hib TITER, 1268
Hibiclens Antiseptic/Antimicrobial Skin, 1505
Hibistat Germicidal Hand, 1505
Hiprex, 1209
Histade Capsules, 532
Histamine H_2 antagonists, 950-954
Histatab Plus Tablets, 530
Hista-Vent DA Tablets, 542
Histex Liquid, 532
Histex SR Capsules, 531
Histinex HC Syrup, 554
Histinex PV Syrup, 555
Histussin D Liquid, 553
Histussin HC Syrup, 554
Hi-Vegi-Lip Tablets, 961
Hivid, 1190

INDEX

HMG-CoA reductase inhibitors, 448-451
HMS, 1348
Hold DM, 509
Homatropine MBr, 553
Homatropine, 1016
Homatropine HBr, 1345
Homosalate, 1516-1521
Hormones
- anastrozole, 1583-1584
- androgens, 1569-1570
- antiandrogens, 1571-1573
- antiestrogens, 1578-1580
- estrogens, 1576-1577
- goserelin acetate, 1587-1590
- letrozole, 1585-1586
- progestins, 1574-1575

H.P. Acthar Gel, 235
Humalog, 265
Humalog Mix 50/50, 265
Humalog Mix 75/25, 265
Humatin, 1031
Humatrope, 231
Humegon, 217
Humibid DM Tablets, 569
Humibid L.A., 513
Humibid Sprinkle, 513
HuMist Moisturizing Nasal Mist, 517
Humorsol, 1316
Humulin 50/50, 265
Humulin 70/30, 265
Humulin L, 264
Humulin N, 264
Humulin R, 264
Humulin R Regular U-500 (Concentrated), 264
Humulin U Ultralente, 264
Hurricaine, 1481
Hycamtin, 1549
Hycodan Syrup, 553
Hycosin Expectorant, 570
Hycotuss Expectorant Syrup, 570
Hydantoins, 842-846
Hydergine, 797
Hydergine LC, 797
Hydralazine HCl, 410-412, 432
Hydramine, 689
Hydramine Cough, 495, 509
Hydramyn, 689, 891
Hydrap-ES Tablets, 430
Hydrea, 1615
Hydrisalic Gel, 1493
Hydrisinol, 1498
Hydrocarbon gel, 1421
Hydrocet Capsules, 625
Hydrochlorothiazide
- in antihypertensive combinations, 430-432
- as diuretic, 323

Hydrochlorothiazide and amiloride, 327
Hydrochlorothiazide and benazepril HCl, 390
Hydrochlorothiazide and spironolactone, 327
Hydrochlorothiazide and triamterene, 327
Hydrocil Instant, 977
Hydrocodone bitartrate
- in narcotic pain relievers, 624-626
- in upper respiratory combinations, 553-556, 566, 570-571

Hydrocodone Bitartrate and Acetaminophen Capsules and Tablets, 625
Hydrocodone Bitartrate and Guaifenesin Liquid, 570
Hydrocodone CP Syrup, 554
Hydrocodone GF Syrup, 570
Hydrocodone HD Liquid, 554
Hydrocortisone
- in acne products, 1435
- as adrenal cortical steroid, 239, 249, 254
- in ophthalmic anti-infectives, 1370
- in otic preparations, 1400

Hydrocortisone acetate
- as adrenal cortical steroid, 239, 249
- in anorectal preparations, 1430
- in ophthalmic anti-infectives, 1370-1371

Hydrocortisone cypionate, 240
Hydrocortisone probutate, 249
Hydrocortisone sodium phosphate, 240
Hydrocortisone sodium succinate, 240
Hydrocortisone valerate, 249
Hydrocortone, 239
Hydrocortone Phosphate, 240
HydroDIURIL, 323
Hydroflumethiazide
- in antihypertensive combinations, 430
- as diuretic, 323

Hydrogel contact lenses, see Soft (hydrogel) contact lens products
Hydrogen peroxide, 1422
Hydromet Syrup, 553
Hydromide Syrup, 553
Hydromorphone, 615
Hydromorphone HCl, 571
Hydromox, 323
Hydron KGS Liquid, 571
Hydropane Syrup, 553
Hydro-Par, 323
Hydro-PC II Liquid, 554
Hydro-PC Liquid, 554
Hydropel, 1498
Hydropres-50 Tablets, 430
Hydro-Serp Tablets, 430
Hydroserpine #1 Tablets, 430
Hydroserpine #2 Tablets, 430
Hydro-Tussin DM Liquid, 569
Hydro-Tussin HC Syrup, 555
Hydro-Tussin HD Liquid, 566
Hydroxyamphetamine HBr, 1345
Hydroxychloroquine, 649-650
Hydroxychloroquine sulfate, 1141
Hydroxyethylcellulose, 1135
Hydroxyprogesterone caproate, 166
Hydroxypropyl cellulose, 1383
Hydroxyurea, 1615
Hydroxyzine, 495
Hydroxyzine HCl, 719

Hydroxyzine pamoate, 719
Hygroton, 323
Hylorel, 403
Hylutin, 166
Hyoscine HBr, see Scopolamine HBr
L-Hyoscyamine, 937
Hyoscyamine HBr
in anticholinergic combinations, 936
in antidiarrheal combination products, 1016-1017
Hyoscyamine sulfate
in anticholinergic combinations, 936-937
as anticholinergic/antispasmodic agent, 931
in digestive aids, 971
in upper respiratory combinations, 543
in urinary anti-infective combinations, 1219-1220
Hyosophen, 936
Hyphed Liquid, 555
Hy-Phen Tablets, 625
Hypnotics, 817-821
HypoTears, 1383, 1386
HypoTears PF, 1383
Hyrexin-50, 495
Hytakerol, 23
Hytinic, 72
Hytone, 249
Hytrin, 386
Hytuss, 513
Hytuss 2X, 513
Hyzaar Tablets, 432
Hyzine 50, 719

Iberet Filmtabs, 76
Iberet-500 Filmtabs, 76
Iberet-Folic-500 Filmtabs, 76
Ibuprofen
as nonsteroidal anti-inflammatory agent, 638
in upper respiratory combinations, 523, 524
Ichthammol, 1528
Icy Hot, 1514
Idamycin, 1565
Idamycin PFS, 1565
Idarubicin HCl, 1565-1566
Ifex, 1602
Ifosfamide, 1602
IG, see Immune globulin (human)
IgG, see Immune globulin (human)
IGIM, see Immune globulin (human)
IGIV, see Immune globulin intravenous (human)
Ilosone Pulvules, 1052
Ilotycin gluceptate, 1053
Imdur, 337
Imiglucerase, 309-310
Imipenem-cilastatin, 1076-1078
Imipramine HCl, 760
Imipramine pamoate, 760
Imitrex, 683
Immune globulin (human), 1249-1250
Immune globulin intravenous (human), 1250-1251
Immune globulins, 1249-1255
Immunization
active agents, 1258-1261
Immunologic agents
interferons, 1608-1611
Immunomodulator
etanercept, 1740-1742
Immunosuppressives
azathioprine, 1674-1675
cyclosporine, 1676-1679
muromonab-CD3, 1683-1685
mycophenolate mofetil, 1680-1682
tacrolimus, 1686-1688
Imodium, 1014
Imodium A-D, 1014
Imodium A-D Caplets, 1014
Imogam Rabies-HT, 1251
Impotence agents
sildenafil citrate, 1724-1726
Imuran, 1674
Inactivated polio vaccine, 1258
Inamrinone lactate, 333-334
Indapamide, 323
Inderal, 379
Inderal LA, 379
Inderide LA 40/25 Capsules, 431
Inderide LA 80/25 Capsules, 431
Inderide LA 80/50 Capsules, 431
Inderide LA 120/50 Capsules, 431
Inderide LA 160/50 Capsules, 431
Indinavir sulfate, 1182
Indochron E-R, 639
Indocin, 639
Indocin SR, 639
Indomethacin, 639
Infalyte Oral Solution, 33
Infants' Feverall, 598
Infant's Motrin, 638
Inferferon alfa-N3, 1237-1238
Infergen, 1239
Inflamase Forte, 1348
Inflamase Mild, 1348
Infliximab, 1022-1024
Influenza virus vaccine, 1258, 1282-1285
Infumorph, 616
INH, see Isoniazid
Inhalants
corticosteroids, 471-475
cromolyn sodium, 476-478
ipratropium bromide, 479-481
ipratropium bromide/albuterol sulfate, 482-484
mucolytics, 485-487
nedocromil sodium, 488-489
Innohep, 109
Inositol, 65
Insulin, 264-271
Insulin Analog Injection, 265
Insulin Glargine Injection, 265
Insulin injection
concentrated, 264
regular insulin, 264
Insulin zinc suspension, 264
Insulin zinc suspension, extended, 264

INDEX

Intal Inhaler, 476
Intal Nebulizer Solution, 476
Interferon(s), 1608-1611
Interferon alfa-2a, 1608
Interferon alfa-2b, 1608
Interferon alfacon-1, 1239-1241
Interferon beta, 1729-1731
Interferon beta-1a, 1729
Interferon beta-1b, 1729
Interferon gamma-1B, 1242-1243
Intranasal steroids, 490-493
Intrauterine progesterone, 189-191
Intrinsic factor with iron, 77-80
Intron A, 1608
Inversine, 419, 1648
Invirase, 1182
Iobid DM Tablets, 569
Iodex, 1505
Iodex w/Menthyl Salicylate Ointment, 1515
Iodine
  as antiseptic, 1505
  nutritional, 5
Iodine products
  expectorants, 297-298
  thyroid drugs, 513
Iodochlorhydroxyquin, 254
Iodoquinol, 254
Iodotope, 294
Ionamin, 579
Ionax, 1446
Ionax Astringent Cleanser, 1447
Ionax Foam, 1447
Ionil, 1479
Ionil T, 1479
Iopidine, 1328
Iosal II Tablets, 526
Iosopan, 917
Ipecac, 1637-1638
IPOL, 1273
Ipratropium bromide, 479-481
Ipratropium bromide/ albuterol sulfate, 482-484
Irbesartan, 395
Ircon, 71
Irinotecan, 1549
Irish moss, 985
Iron, 5
  with vitamin B12 and intrinsic factor, 77-80
  with vitamin C, 75
  with vitamins, 76
Iron oxides, 1529
Iron-containing products, 71-74
Iron-FA Tablets, 76
Iron-Folic 500 Tablets, 76
Irospan Capsules, 75
Irospan Tablets, 75
Ismelin, 405
Ismo, 337
Isobutane, 1512
Isocarboxazid, 743
Isoetharine HCl, 455
Isometheptene mucate, 668
Isoniazid, 1222
Isoniazid with rifampin, 1222
Isoniazid with rifampin and pyrazinamide, 1222
Isophane Insulin Suspension, 264
Isophane Insulin Suspension (NPH) and Regular Insulin Injection Combined, 265
Isopropanol, 1448
Isopropyl alcohol
  in acne products, 1440, 1444, 1447
  in antifungal combinations, 1135-1136
  in antiseborrheic combinations, 1479
  in otic preparations, 1400
  in skin cleansers, 1529, 1531
Isopropyl myristate, 1512
Isoproterenol, 455
Isoptin SR, 369
Isopto Atropine, 1345
Isopto Carbachol, 1319
Isopto Carpine, 1319
Isopto Cetapred Suspension, 1372
Isopto Homatropine, 1345
Isopto Hyoscine, 1345
Isopto P-ES, 1335
Isopto Plain, 1383
Isopto Tears, 1383
Isordil, 337
Isordil Titradose, 337
Isosorbide dinitrate, 337
Isosorbide mononitrate, 337
Isotretinoin, 1689-1692
Isoxsuprine HCl, 375-376
Isradipine, 368
Isuprel, 455
Itch-X, 1485
Itraconazole, 1121-1123
IUD, 170
Iveegam, 1250
Ivermectin, 1207-1208
Ivy-Rid, 1512

Jenest, 177
Jets, 56
Junior Strength Advil, 638
Junior Strength Motrin, 638
Juniper tar, 1528
Just for Kids, 35
Just Tears, 1383

K-99, 41
K+ 8, 41
K+ 10, 41
Kadian, 616
Kaletra, 1182
Kanamycin sulfate, 1031
Kanka, 1421
Kantrex, 1031
Kaochlor, 41
Kaochlor-SF, 41
Kaodene Non-Narcotic, 1017
Kaodene with Codeine, 1016
Kaodene with Paregoric, 1017
Kaodonna-PG, 1016
Kaolin
  in antidiarrheal combination products, 1016-1017
  in diaper rash products, 1507
Kaolin with Pectin, 1017
Kaon Elixir, 41
Kaon-Cl, 41
Kaon-Cl 10, 41
Kaopectate, 1017
Kaopectate Concentrate, 1017
Kaopectate II Caplets, 1014

Kaopectolin Gel with Belladonna, 1017
Kao-tin, 1017
Kapectolin, 1017
Kapectolin PG, 1016
Kapectolin with Paregoric, 1016
Karigel, 35
Karigel Maintenance Neutral, 35
Kasof, 995
Kay Ciel, 41
KBP/O, 1016
K-C, 1017
K-Dur 10, 41
K-Dur 20, 41
Keep Alert, 587
Keep Going, 587
Keflex, 1039
Keftab, 1039
Kefurox, 1039
Kefzol, 1037
Kemadrin, 891
Kenaject, 241
Kenalog, 250
Kenalog-10, 241
Kenalog-40, 241
Kenalog in Orabase, 1421
Keppra, 870
Keratolytics
  cantharidin, 1489-1490
  podofilox, 1491-1492
  salicylic acid topical, 1493-1495
Keri, 1498
Keri Creme, 1498
KeriCort-10, 249
Keri-Light, 1498
Kerlone, 379
Kerodex, 1498
Kestrone 5, 155
Ketoconazole, 1124-1127
Keto-Diastix, 1753
Ketone tests, 1757-1759
Ketoprofen, 639
Ketorolac tromethamine
  ophthalmic, 1356
  systemic, 639
Ketostix, 1757
Ketotifen fumarate, 1364-1365
Key-Pred, 240
Kid Kare Children's Cough/Cold Liquid, 560
KIE Syrup, 524
Kiss My Face, 1517-1519
Klonopin, 710, 832
Klor-Con, 41
Klor-Con/25, 41
Klor-Con 8, 41
Klor-Con 10, 41
Klor-Con/EF, 41
Klotrix, 41
K-Lyte DS, 41
K-Lyte/Cl, 41
K-Lyte/Cl 50, 41
Kobee Tablets, 51
Kolephrin GG/DM Liquid, 568
Kolephrin Tablets, 538
Kolephrin/DM Tablets, 550
Kondremul Plain, 985
Kondremul with Phenolphthalein, 1001
Konsyl, 977
Konsyl Fiber, 977
Konsyl-Orange, 977
Koromex, 1428
Koromex Clear, 1428
K-P, 1017
KPAB, see Potassium Para-Amino-benzoate
K-Pek, 1017
K-Phos M.F., 1652
K-Phos No. 2, 1652
K-Phos Original, 1652
Kronofed-A Capsules, 532
Kronofed-A Jr. Capsules, 532
K-Tab, 41
Kudrox Double Strength Suspension, 925
Kutrase, 971
Ku-Zyme, 971
Kwelcof Liquid, 570
Kytril, 696

LAAM, see Levomethadyl acetate hydrochloride
Labetalol HCl, 416-418
Labstix, 1771
Lac-Hydrin, 1498
Lac-Hydrin Five, 1498
Lacri-Lube S.O.P., 1386
Lacrisert, 1383
Lactic acid, 1425
LactiCare, 1498
Lactinex, 1013
Lactobacillus, 1013
Lactulose, 983-984
Lamictal, 864
Lamisil AT, 1131
Lamivudine, 1190
Lamivudine/Abacavir Sulfate/Zidovudine, 1190
Lamivudine/Zidovudine, 1190
Lamotrigine, 864-866
Lanabiotic, 1099
Lanacane, 1485
LanaCort 5, 249
LanaCort 10, 249
LanaCort Cool, 249
Lanolin
  in acne products, 1435, 1445-1446
  in anorectal preparations, 1431
  in diaper rash products, 1507
  in mouth and throat products, 1420
  in skin cleansers, 1528-1530
Lanolin and petrolatum, 1496
Lanoxicaps, 329
Lanoxin, 329, 1458
Lanoxin Pediatric, 329
Lansoprazole
  for Helicobacter pylori infections, 947-949
  as proton pump inhibitor, 968
Lantus, 265
Lariam, 1144
Larodopa, 895
Lasix, 317
Latanoprost, 1322
Laureth-4, 1440
Lax Pills, 991
Laxative Pills, 991
Laxatives
  bulk-reducing, 977-980
  combinations capsules and tablets, 998-1000 liquids, 1001-1002
  glycerin, 981-982
  lactulose, 983-984
  mineral oil, 985-987
  saline, 988-990
  stimulant, 991-994
  stool softeners, 995-997
LC-65, 1387, 1393
LC-65 Daily Cleaner, 1390
Lecithin, 65
Leflunomide, 1743-1745

INDEX

Lens Drops, 1387, 1390, 1394
Lens Plus, 1393
Lens Plus Daily Cleaner, 1393
Lens Plus Rewetting Drops, 1394
Lente Iletin I, 264
Lente Iletin II, 264
Lente Insulin, 264
Lescol, 448
Lescol XL, 448
Letrozole, 1585-1586
Leucovorin, 83-84
Leukeran, 1602
Leukine, 134
Leukotriene receptor antagonists/formation inhibitors, 468-470
Leureth-4, 1440
Levalbuterol HCl, 455
Levall 5.0 Liquid, 566
Levall Liquid, 562
Levamisole, 1591-1592
Levaquin, 1069
Levatol, 379
Levetiracetam, 870-871
Levlen, 177
Levlite, 177
Levobetaxolol HCl, 1313
Levobunolol HCl, 1313
Levocabastine HCl, 1358-1359
Levocarnitine, 63-64
Levodopa, 895
Levo-Dromoran, 615
Levofloxacin
ophthalmic, 1366
systemic, 1069
Levomethadyl acetate HCl, 615
Levomethadyl acetate hydrochloride, 1708-1709
Levonorgestrel, 177-178, 186, 192, 195
Levonorgestrel implants, 170, 192-194
Levonorgestrel/ethinyl estradiol, 186
Levonorgestrel-releasing intrauterine system, 195-198
Levora, 177
Levorphanol tartrate, 615
Levo-T, 299
Levothroid, 299
Levothyroxine sodium, 299
Levoxine, 299
Levoxyl, 299
Levsin, 931
Levsin Drops, 931
Levsin with Phenobarbital, 937
Levsinex Timecaps, 931
Levsin-PB Drops, 937
Lextron Ferrous Pulvules, 77
Lextron Pulvules, 77
Librax, 937
Libritabs, 710
Librium, 710
Lidex, 248
Lidex-E, 248
Lidocaine
in skin cleansers, 1529
for skin disorders, 1486
Lidocaine HCl
for mucous membranes, 1481
for skin disorders, 1485
LIG, see Lymphocyte immune globulin
Limbitrol, 807
Limbitrol DS, 807
Lime water, 1530
Lincocin, 1048
Lincomycin, 1048
Lincorex, 1048
Lincosamides, 1048-1051
Lindane, 1244
Linezolid, 1066
Liniments, 1514-1515
Lioresal, 876
Lioresal Intrathecal, 876
Liothyronine sodium, 299
Liotrix, 299
Lipase, 961-962, 971
Lipitor, 448
Lipotropic combinations, 65
Lipotropic products, 65-66
Lipram 4500 Capsules, 961
Lipram-CR10 Capsules, 961
Lipram-CR20 Capsules, 961
Lipram-PN10 Capsules, 961
Lipram-PN16 Capsules, 961
Lipram-UL12 Capsules, 961
Lipram-UL20 Capsules, 961
Liquibid-D Tablets, 525
Liqui-Char, 1633
Liqui-Doss, 1001
Liquifilm Tears, 1383
Liquifilm Wetting, 1387
Liquimat, 1440
Liquiprin, 597
Liquiprin Infants' Drops, 598
Lisinopril, 390, 432
Listerex Scrub, 1446
Listerine, 1418
Lithium, 799-802
Lithium carbonate, 799
Lithium citrate, 799
Lithobid, 799
Lithostat, 1650
Live yeast cell derivative, 1431
Livitamin w/Intrinsic Factor Capsules, 77
Livitrinsic-f Capsules, 77
Livostin, 1358
Lobana Body, 1498
Lobana Derm-Ade, 1496
Lobana Peri-Garde, 1496
Local anesthetics
in anorectal preparations, 1430
Local vasoconstrictors
in anorectal preparations, 1431
LoCHOLEST, 435
LoCHOLEST Light, 435
Lodine, 638
Lodine XL, 638
Lodosyn, 895
Lodoxamide tromethamine, 1353
Lodrane LD Capsules, 531
Lodrane Liquid, 531
Loestrin 1/20, 177
Loestrin 1.5/30, 177
Loestrin Fe 1/20, 177
Loestrin Fe 1.5/30, 177
Lomefloxacin HCl, 1069
Lomotil, 1010
Lomustine, 1596-1597
Loniten, 424
Lonox, 1010
Loop diuretics, 317-319
Lo/Ovral, 177
Loperamide, 1014-1015

Lopid, 445
Lopinavir/Ritonavir, 1182
Lopressor, 379
Lopressor HCT 50/25 Tablets, 431
Lopressor HCT 100/25 Tablets, 431
Lopressor HCT 100/50 Tablets, 431
Loprox, 1130
Lorabid, 1039
Loracarbef, 1039
Loratadine
as antihistamine, 496
in upper respiratory combinations, 534
Lorazepam, 710
Lorazepam Intensol, 710
Lorcet 10/650 Tablets, 626
Lorcet Plus Tablets, 626
Lorcet Tablets, 625
Lorcet-HD Capsules, 625
Loroxide, 1435
Lortab 5/500 Tablets, 625
Lortab 7.5/500 Tablets, 626
Lortab Liquid, 624
Lortab SA Tablets, 625
Lortab Tablets, 624
Losartan potassium, 395, 432
Lowsium Plus Suspension, 926
Lotemax, 1351
Lotensin, 390
Lotensin HCT, 390
Lotensin HCT Tablets 5/6.25, 432
Lotensin HCT Tablets 10/12.5, 432
Lotensin HCT Tablets 20/12.5, 431
Lotensin HCT Tablets 20/25, 431
Loteprednol etabonate, 1351-1352
Lotrel Capsules, 432
Lotrimin, 1114
Lotrimin AF, 1114, 1130
Lovastatin, 448
Lovenox, 101
Lowila Cake, 1525
Low-Ogestrel, 177
Lowsium, 917
Loxapine, 770
Loxitane, 770
Loxitane C, 770
Loxitane IM, 770
Lozenges, 1417-1418
Lozol, 323
LubraSol, 1499
Lubricants
ocular, 1386
Lubriderm, 1498, 1499, 1525
Lufyllin, 462
Lufyllin-400, 462
Lufyllin-EPG Tablets, 521
Lufyllin-GG Tablets, 521
Lugol's Solution, 297
Lumigan, 1322
Lunelle, 174
Luride, 35
Luride Lozi-Tabs, 35
Luvox, 734
Lyme disease vaccine, 1299-1301
LYMErix, 1299
Lymphocyte immune globulin, 1251
L-Lysine, 55
Lysodren, 1615

Maalox, 921
Maalox, Extra Strength, 921
Maalox Anti-Diarrheal Caplets, 1014
Maalox Daily Fiber Therapy, 977
Maalox Heartburn Relief, 927
Maalox Plus, 921
Maalox Plus, Extra Strength, 921
Maalox Plus Suspension, Extra Strength, 925
Maalox Suspension, 924
Maalox Suspension, Extra Strength, 925
Maalox Therapeutic Concentrate Suspension, 925
Macrobid, 1216
Macrodantin, 1216
Macrolides, 1052-1058
Mafenide, 1469-1470
Magaldrate, 917, 923, 926-927
Magaldrate Plus Suspension, 926
Magan, 602
Mag-Carb, 39
Magnalox, 924
Magnaprin Film Coated Tablets, 606
Magnesia, 917-918
Magnesium, 5, 39-40
Magnesium AA, 39
Magnesium amino acid chelate, 39
Magnesium carbonate
in analgesics, 606
in antacid combinations, 922, 926, 927
nutritional, 39
Magnesium chloride hexahydrate, 39
Magnesium citrate, 39
in bowel evacuation kits, 1005
in laxatives, 988
Magnesium gluconate dihydrate, 39
Magnesium hydroxide
in analgesics, 606
as antacid, 917-918
in antacid combinations, 921-923, 924-927
in histamine H_2 antagonists, 950
in laxative combinations, 1001
in laxatives, 988
in modified iron products, 72
in nonnarcotic analgesics, 610
Magnesium lactate, 39
Magnesium oxide
in analgesics, 606
in antacids, 918
nutritional, 39
Magnesium salicylate
in analgesics, 602
in nonnarcotic analgesics, 609
Magnesium salicylate tetrahydrate, 611
Magnesium sulfate
in bowel evacuation kits, 1005
in laxatives, 988
Magnesium trisilicate, 922
Magnox Suspension, 924
Magonate, 39
Magonate Natal, 39
Mag-Ox 400, 39, 918
Magsal Tablets, 610
Mag-SR, 39

INDEX

Mag-Tab SR, 39
Magtrate, 39
Major-gesic Tablets, 529
Malarone, 1154
Malarone Pediatric, 1154
Malathion, 1244
Mallamint, 30, 917
Mallazine Eye Drops, 1339
Maltsuprex, 977
Mammol, 1529
Mandelamine, 1209
Mannitol, 1606, 1734
Mantadil Cream, 254
Maolate, 885
Mapap Cold Formula Tablets, 550
Mapap Extra Strength, 597
Mapap Regular Strength, 597
Mapap Sinus Maximum Strength Geltabs, 522
Maprotiline HCl, 740
Maranox, 597
Marblen, 922, 926
Marcof Expectorant Syrup, 571
Marezine, 689
Margesic Capsules, 609
Margesic H Capsules, 625
Margesic No. 3 Tablets, 623
Marine Lipid Concentrate Capsules, 60
Marinol, 693
Marmine, 689
Marplan, 743
Marpres Tablets, 430
Marthritic, 602
Masoprocol, 1528
Masse Breast, 1498
Massengill Baking Soda and Water Disposable Douche, 1425
Massengill Disposable Douche, 1425
Massengill Douche, 1425
Massengill Extra Cleansing Disposable Douche, 1425
Massengill Extra Mild Disposable Douche, 1425
Massengill Medicated Disposable Douche, 1425
Massengill "Scented" Disposable Douche, 1425
Mast cell stabilizers, 1353-1355
Matulane, 1615
Mavik, 390
Max EPA Capsules, 60
Maxair Autohaler, 456
Maxair Inhaler, 456
Maxalt, 679
Maxalt-MLT, 679
Maxaquin, 1069
Maxidex, 1348
Maxifed DM Tablets, 564
Maxifed-G Tablets, 526
Maxifed Tablets, 527
Maxiflor, 248
Maximum Bayer Aspirin Tablets and Caplets, 601
Maximum Cramp Relief Pamprin Caplets, 609
Maximum Strength Allergy Drops, 1339
Maximum Strength Anacin Tablets, 610
Maximum Strength Anbesol, 1481
Maximum Strength Ascriptin Coated Caplets, 606
Maximum Strength Benadryl, 2, 1502
Maximum Strength Compoz Nighttime Sleep Aid, 822
Maximum Strength Midol, 638
Maximum Strength Midol Menstrual Caplets and Gelcaps, 608
Maximum Strength Midol PMS Caplets and Gelcaps, 608
Maximum Strength Midol Teen Caplets, 609
Maximum Strength Multi-Symptom Pamprin Caplets and Tablets, 608
Maximum Strength NoDoz, 587
Maximum Strength Nytol QuickGels, 822
Maximum Strength Sleepinal Softgels, 822
Maximum Strength Sominex, 822
Maximum Strength Unisom SleepGels, 822
Maxipime, 1037
Maxitrol, 1372
Maxitrol Suspension, 1371
Maxi-Tuss DM Liquid, 569
Maxi-Tuss HC Liquid, 555
Maxivate, 247
Maxolon, 965
Maxzide, 327
Maxzide-25MG, 327
Mazanor, 579
Mazindol, 579
Measles, mumps, and rubella virus vaccine, 1258, 1277-1279
Measles, mumps, and rubella virus vaccine, live, 1277
Measles (rubeola) and rubella virus vaccine, live, 1277
Measles (rubeola) virus vaccine, live, attenuated, 1277
Mebaral, 812
Mebendazole, 1201-1202
Mecamylamine HCl, 419-420
Mechlorethamine HCl, 1602
Meclan, 1094
Meclizine, 689
Meclocycline sulfosalicylate, 1094
Meclofenamate sodium, 639
Meda Cap, 597
Meda Tab, 597
Medent-DM Tablets, 565
Medicated Acne Cleanser, 1444
Medicated hair dressings, 1479
Medicone, 1430, 1431
Medigesic Capsules, 609
Medilax, 991
Mediplast, 1493
Medi-Quik, 1485
Medotar, 1476
Medrol, 240
Medroxyprogesterone acetate, 161, 166, 172
Medroxyprogesterone acetate/estradiol cypionate, 174-176
Medroxyprogesterone injection, 170
MED-Rx DM Tablets, 565
Medrysone, 1348
Mefenamic acid, 639
Mefloquine, 1144-1146
Mefoxin, 1038
Mega-B Tablets, 51

Megace, 166, 1574
Mega-Max EPA Capsules, 60
Megestrol acetate, 166, 1574
Meglitinides, 283-285
Melfiat-105, 579
Mellaril, 771
Mellaril-S, 771
Melphalan, 1602
Menadol, 638
Meni-D, 689
Menotropins, 217-219
Menthol
in acne products, 1444-1445, 1447-1448
in antifungal combinations, 1135-1136
in douche products, 1425
in lozenges, 1417
in mouth and throat products, 1420-1422
in mouthwash, 1418
in poison ivy treatment products, 1512
in rubs and liniments, 1514
in skin cleansers, 1528, 1530-1531
in topical antihistamines, 1502
in upper respiratory combinations, 572
Mentholatum Cherry Chest Rub for Kids, 572
Mentholatum Ointment, 572
Menthyl anthranilate, 1516, 1519, 1521
Mepenzolate bromide, 931
Mepergan Fortis Capsules, 628
Meperidine, 628
Meperidine HCl, 615
Mephenytoin, 842
Mephobarbital, 812
Mephyton, 124
Meprobamate
as antianxiety agent, 610
in nonnarcotic analgesics, 721-723
Mepron, 1232
Mercaptopurine, 1541
Meridia, 584
Meropenem, 1074-1075
Merrem I.V., 1074
Meruvax II, 1277
Mesalamine, 1019
Mesantoin, 842
Mescolor Tablets, 543
Mesoridazine besylate, 770
Mestinon, 1647
Mestinon Timespan, 1647
Mestranol, 177
Metadate CD, 590
Metadate ER, 590
Metahydrin, 323
Metallic aluminum, 1528
Metamucil, 977, 978
Metamucil Lemon-Lime Flavor, 978
Metamucil Orange Flavor, 977-978
Metamucil Sugar Free, 977
Metaproterenol sulfate, 456
Metatensin #2 Tablets, 430
Metatensin #4 Tablets, 430
Metaxalone, 885
Meted, Maximum Strength, 1479
Metformin, 286-288
Metformin/glyburide, 289-291
Methacort 40, 240
Methacort 80, 240
Methadone HCl, 615
Methadone HCl Diskets, 615
Methadone HCl Intensol, 615
Methadose, 615
Methagual, 1515
Methamphetamine HCl, 575
Methazolamide, 313
Methenamine, 1209-1211
Methenamine combinations, 1219-1220
Methenamine hippurate, 1209
Methenamine mandelate, 1209, 1219
Methenamine salts, 1209-1211
Methimazole, 294
Methionine, 1507
Methocarbamol, 885
Methocarbamol with ASA, 889
Methotrexate
as antineoplastic, 1541
as antipsoriatic, 1457-1459
as antirheumatic, 651-654
Methotrexate LPF Sodium, 1457, 1541
Methotrexate Sodium For Injection, 1457
Methotrexate Sodium Injection, 1457
Methoxsalen, 1460
Methscopolamine bromide, 931
Methscopolamine nitrate, 542
Methsuximide, 861
Methyl nicotinate, 1514
Methyl salicylate
in douche products, 1425
in mouthwash, 1418
in rubs and liniments, 1514
Methylbenzethonium chloride, 1507
Methylbenzethonium HCl, 1135
Methylcellulose, 977
Methyclothiazide
in antihypertensive combinations, 430
as diuretic, 323
Methyldopa, 431
Methyldopa HCl, 421-423
Methylene blue, 1219-1220
Methylene chloride, 1512
Methylin, 590
Methylin ER, 590
Methylparaben
in acne products, 1445-1447
in anorectal preparations, 1430-1431
Methylphenidate HCl, 590-593
Methylprednisolone, 240
Methylprednisolone acetate, 240
Methylprednisolone sodium succinate, 240
Methyltestosterone, 149, 161
Methysergide, **671-673**

INDEX

Methysergide maleate, 671
Meticorten, 240
Metimyd, 1372
Metimyd Suspension, 1372
Metipranolol HCl, 1313
Metoclopramide, 965-967
Metoclopramide Intensol, 965
Metolazone, 323
Metoprolol, 379
Metoprolol tartrate, 431
Metrodin, 207
MetroGel, 1079, 1111
Metronidazole, 1079-1081
for Helicobacter pylori infections, 944-946
in vaginal anti-infectives, 1111
Mevacor, 448
Mexiletine, 354-355
Mexitil, 354
Mexsana Medicated, 1507
MG217, 1475
MG217 Medicated Intensive Strength, 1476
Miacalcin, 302
Miacalcin, 302
Mi-Acid, 924
Micardis, 395
Micatin, 1130
Miconazole, 1132
Miconazole nitrate
topical, 1130
vaginal, 1138
Micrainin Tablets, 610
MICRhoGAM, 1252
Microcrystalline sulfur, 1440
Micro-K 10 Extentabs, 41
Micro-K Extentabs, 41
Micronase, 278
microNefron, 455
Micronor, 178
Microstix-3, 1769
Midamor, 320
Midodrine, 707-709
Midol, Maximum Strength, 638
Midol Menstrual Caplets and Gelcaps, Maximum Strength, 608
Midol PMS Caplets and Gelcaps, Maximum Strength, 608
Midol Teen Caplets, Maximum Strength, 609
Midrin, 668
Mifeprex, 146
Mifepristone, 146-148
Miglitol, 272
Migraine agents
almotriptan, 674-675
combinations, 668-670
methysergide, 671-673
naratriptan, 676-678
rizatriptan, 679-682
sumatriptan succinate, 683-686
zolmitriptan, 687-688
Migratine, 668
Milex Shur-Seal, 1428
Milk of Magnesia, 917, 988
Milk of Magnesia, Concentrated, 988
Milkinol, 985
Miltown, 721
Milontin Kapseals, 861
Milophene, 214
Mitotane, 1615
Milrinone lactate, 335-336
Mineral oil
in acne products, 1435
in anorectal preparations, 1430-1431
in antacid combinations, 926
in antiseborrheic combinations, 1479
as laxative, 985-987
in laxative combinations, 1001
in skin cleansers, 1528
Mineralocorticoid, 258-261
Minerals, 3-6
Minerals and electrolytes
calcium, 29-32
fluoride, 35-38
magnesium, 39-40
oral electrolyte mixtures, 33-34
potassium, 41-44
zinc, 45-46
Mini Two-Way Action Tablets, 524
Minipress, 386
Minitran, 338
Minocin, 1089
Minocycline HCl, 1089
Minoxidil
systemic, 424-426
topical, 1509-1511
Mintezol, 1205
Mintox Plus, 921
Mintox Plus, Extra Strength, 925
Minizide 1 Capsules, 432
Minizide 2 Capsules, 432
Minizide 5 Capsules, 432
Miochol-E, 1319
Miostat, 1319
Miotics
cholinesterase inhibitor, 1316-1318
direct-acting, 1319-1321
Miradon, 111
MiraFlow Extra Strength, 1387, 1393
Mirapex, 900
Miraphen PSE Tablets, 528
Mircette, 178
Mirena, 195
Mirtazapine, 740
Miscellaneous nasal products, 517
Misoprostol
as anti-ulcer agent, 955-956
in nonnarcotic analgesics, 611
Mithracin, 1606
Mitotic inhibitors
vinorelbine tartrate, 1556-1557
Mitran, 710
Mitrolan, 977
Mixed E 400, 27
Mixed E 1000, 27
M-M-R II, 1277
Moban, 771
Mobidin, 602
Mobigesic Backache Pain Reliever Tablets, 611
Mobisyl Cream, 1514
Moctanin, 975
Modane, 991
Modane Plus Tablets, 998
Modane Soft, 995
Modicon, 177
Modified bar soaps, 1525
Modified Burow's Solution, 1400
Modified iron products, 72
Moduretic, 327
Moexipril HCl, 390
Moi-Stir, 1409
Moi-Stir 10, 1409
Moi-Stir Swabsticks, 1409

Moisture Eyes, 1383
Moisture Eyes PM, 1386
Moisturel, 1498
Molie, 587
Molindone HCl, 771
Mol-Iron, 71
Mol-Iron w/Vitamin C Tablets, 75
Mollifene Ear Wax Removal Aid, 1400
Momentum Muscular Backache Formula, 602
Mometasone furoate, 250, 490
Monistat 3, 1138
Monistat 7, 1138
Monistat 7 Combination Pack, 1138
Monistat Dual-Pak, 1138
Monistat-Derm, 1130, 1138
Monoamine oxidase inhibitors, 743-748
Monobenzone, 1528
Monocid, 1037
Monoclonal antibody
  palivizumab, 1256-1257
  rituximab, 1627-1628
  trastuzumab, 1629-1630
Monoctanoin, 975
Monodox, 1089
Mono-Gesic, 602
Monoket, 337
Monophasic oral contraceptives, 177
Monopril, 390
Mono-Vacc Test (O.T.), 1304
Montelukast sodium, 468
Monurol, 1212
More-Dophilus, 1013
Moricizine, 356-358
Morphine, 1017
Morphine sulfate, 616
Morton Salt Substitute, 434
Motofen, 1010
Motrin, 638
Motrin, Junior Strength, 638
Motrin Children's Cold Suspension, 524
Motrin IB, 638
Motrin Sinus Headache Tablets, 523
Mouth and throat products
  amlexanox, 1414-1415
  benzyl alcohol, 1416
Mouth and throat products *(cont.)*
  carbamide peroxide, 1405-1406
  chlorhexidine, 1407-1408
  doxycycline, 939-941
  lozenges, 1417-1418
  miscellaneous, 1420-1424
  saliva substitutes, 1409-1411
Mouthkote, 1409
Mouthwash, 1418
Moxifloxacin HCl, 1069
M-R-Vax II, 1277
MS Contin, 616
MSIR, 616
MTX, see Methotrexate
Muco-Fen-DM Tablets, 569
Mucolytics, 485-487
Mucomyst, 485
Mucosil-10, 485
Mucosil-20, 485
Mucous membranes
  topical anesthetics for, 1481-1484
Multiple antibiotics, 1098
Multiple sulfonamides, 1101
Multistix, 1771
Multistix 7, 1771
Multistix 8, 1771
Multistix 8 SG, 1771
Multistix 9, 1771
Multistix 9 SG, 1771
Multistix 10 SG, 1771
Multistix SG, 1771
Mumpsvex, 1277
Mupirocin, 1082-1083
Murine Ear Drops, 1400
Murine Ear Wax Removal System, 1400
Murine Plus, 1339
Muro 128 2, 1383
Muro 128 5, 1383
Murocel, 1383
Murocoll-2, 1345
Muromonab-CD3, 1683-1685
Muscle relaxants
  baclofen, 876-878
  dantrolene sodium, 879-881
  skeletal, 885-888 combinations, 889-890
  tizanidine, 882-884
Mustargen, 1602
Myambutol, 1222
Myapap Drops, 598
Mycelex, 1114
Mycelex Twin Pack, 1138
Mycelex-7, 1138
Mycelex-G, 1138
Myciguent, 1098
Mycinettes, 1417
Mycitracin Triple Antibiotic, 1099
Mycobutin, 1222
Mycolog-II, 1135
Mycophenolate mofetil, 1680-1682
Mycostatin, 1128, 1138
Mycostatin Pastilles, 1128
Mydfrin 2.5, 1339
Mydriacyl, 1345
Mydriatic combinations, 1345
Mygel II Suspension, 925
Mygel Suspension, 924
Mykrox, 323
Mylagen, 924
Mylagen Gelcaps, 922
Mylagen II, 925
Mylanta, 921, 924
Mylanta Double Strength, 921, 925
Mylanta Gelcaps, 922
Mylanta Natural Fiber Supplement, 977
Myleran, 1552
Mylicon, 959
Mylicon-125, 959
Myoflex Creme, 1515
Mysoline, 855
Mytelase Caplets, 1647
Mytussin, 513
Mytussin AC Cough Syrup, 567
Mytussin DAC Liquid, 562
Mytussin DM Syrup, 568

ND Clear Capsules, 532
Nabi-HB, 1249
Nabumetone, 639
Nadolol
  in antihypertensive combinations, 431-432
  as beta-adrenergic blocking agent, 379
Nafarelin acetate, 223-225

INDEX

Nafazair, 1339
Naftifine, 1132
Naftifine HCl, 1130
Naftin, 1130
Naldecon Senior EX, 513
Naldecon Senior DX Liquid, 569
Nalfon Pulvules, 638
Nalidixic acid, 1214-1215
Nalmefene HCl, 1641-1642
Naloxone, 1643-1644
Naloxone and pentazocine, 633
Naltrexone HCl, 1705-1707
Nandrolone decanoate, 142
Naphazoline HCl
as decongestant, 501
ophthalmic, 1343
Naphazoline Plus, 1343
Naphcon, 1339
Naphcon Forte, 1339
Naphcon-A, 1343
Naphoptic-A, 1343
Naprelan, 639
Naprosyn, 639
Naproxen, 639
Naproxen sodium
as nonsteroidal anti-inflammatory agent, 639
in upper respiratory combinations, 523
Naqua, 323
Naratriptan HCl, 676-678
Narcan, 1643
Narcotic pain reliever combinations, 623-630
Nardil, 743
Nasacort, 490
Nasacort AQ, 490
Nasal Decongestant Sinus Non-Drowsy Tablets, 522
Nasal products miscellaneous, 517
NaSal Saline, 517
Nasalcrom, 476
Nasalide, 490
Nasatab LA Tablets, 527
Nasonex, 490
Natacyn, 1374
Natamycin, 1374-1375
Nateglinide, 283
Natural Brewers Yeast 7 1/2 grs Tablets, 48
Nature's Remedy Tablets, 999
Naturetin, 323
Nausetrol, 705
Navane, 771
Navelbine, 1556
N.B.P., 1099
NebuPent, 1234
Necon 0.5/35, 177
Necon 1/35, 177
Necon 1/50, 177
Necon 10/11, 177
Nedocromil sodium
as inhalant, 488-489
ophthalmic, 1353
Nefazodone, 727-729
NegGram, 1214
Nelfinavir mesylate, 1182
Nelova 0.5/35E, 177
Nelova 1/35E, 177
Nelova 1/50M, 177
Nelova 7/14, 177
Nelova 10/11, 177
Nembutal Sodium, 812
Neo-Castaderm, 1135
Neo-Cultol, 985
NeoDecadron, 1371
Neodecadron Solution, 1370
Neo-Dexameth, 1370
Neo-fradin, 1031
Neoloid, 991
Neomac, 1099
Neomixin, 1099
Neomycin sulfate
in ophthalmic anti-infectives, 1370- 1372
in otic antibiotics, 1397
systemic, 1031
topical, 1098
Neopap, 598
Neoral, 1676
Neosporin, 1098-1099
Neostigmine bromide, 1647
Neostigmine methylsulfate, 1647
Neo-Synephrine, 1339
Neo-Synephrine 12-Hour, 501
Neo-Synephrine Extra Strength, 501
Neo-Synephrine Mild Formula, 501
Neo-Synephrine Regular Strength, 501
Neo-Synephrine Viscous, 1339
Neotricin HC, 1371
Nephro-Calci, 29
Nephrocaps Capsules, 49
Nephro-Fer, 71
Nephron FA Tablets, 76
Nephron S-2, 455
Nephro-Vite OTC Tablets, 49
Nephro-Vite Rx Tablets, 49
Nephrox, 926
Neptazane, 313
Nervine, 822
Nestrex, 18
Neupogen, 131
NeuRecover-DA, 56
NeuRecover-SA, 56
Neurodep-Caps Capsules, 48
Neurontin, 839
NeuroSlim, 56
NeutraCare, 35
Neutrogena, 1525
Neutrogena Acne-Prone Skin, 1525
Neutrogena Antiseptic Cleanser for Acne-Prone Skin, 1447, 1525
Neutrogena Body, 1498
Neutrogena Drying Gel, 1444
Neutrogena Kids, 1518
Neutrogena Moisture, 1520
Neutrogena Non-Drying, 1525
Neutrogena Norwegian Formula, 1498
Neutrogena Oil-Free, 1518-1519
Neutrogena Oil-Free Acne Wash, 1447, 1525
Neutrogena Sensitive Skin, 1519
Neutrogena Sunblock, 1516, 1518, 1520
Neutrogena T/Gel, 1475
Neutrogena T/Gel Extra Strength, 1475
Nevirapine, 1195
New-Skin, 1498
New-Skin Antiseptic, 1498
Nexium, 968
Niacin, 6
Niacinamide/Nicotinamide, 14

Niacin/Nicotinic acid, 14-16
Niacor, 14
Nicardipine HCl, 368
N'ice, 1417
N'ice Vitamin C Drops, 20
Nicoderm CQ, 1715
Nicorette, 1715
Nicorette DS, 1715
Nicotinamide/Niacinamide, 14
Nicotine, 1715
Nicotinex, 14
Nicotinic acid/Niacin, 14-16
Nicotrol, 1715
Nicotrol NS, 1715
Nico-Vert, 689
Nidryl, 689, 891
Nifedical, 369
Nifedipine, 369
Niferex, 72
Niferex-150, 72
Niferex-150 Forte Capsules, 76
Niferex w/Vitamin C Tablets, 75
Nil, 1111
Nilandron, 1571
Nilstat, 1128
Nilutamide, 1571
Nimbus Quick Strip, 1765
Nimodipine, 369
Nimotop, 369
Nipent, 1615
Nisoldipine, 369
Nite Time Children's Liquid, 560
Nite Time Cold Formula for Adults Liquid, 552
Nitrates, 337-342
Nitrazine, 1771
Nitrek, 338
Nitro-Bid, 337
Nitrodisc, 338
Nitro-Dur, 338
Nitrofurantoin, 1216-1218
Nitrofurantoin microcrystals, 1216
Nitrogard, 337
Nitrogen mustards, 1602-1605
Nitrogen mustards and estrogen, 1581-1582, 1600-1601
Nitroglycerin, 337
Nitroglycerin Transdermal, 338
Nitroglycerin transdermal systems, 338
Nitrolingual, 337
NitroQuick, 337
Nitrostat, 337
NitroTab, 337
Nitro-Time, 337
Nivea, 1498
Nivea Creme, 1525
Nivea Moisturizing, 1498
Nivea Skin, 1498
Nivea Visage, 1525
Nix, 1244
Nizatidine, 950
Nizoral, 1124
N-Multistix, 1771
N-Multistix SG, 1771
Noctec, 817
NoDoz, Maximum Strength, 587
Nolahist, 496
Nolvadex, 1578
Nonnarcotic analgesic combinations, 608-612
Nonnarcotic antitussive combinations, 509
Non-nucleoside reverse transcriptase inhibitors, 1195-1198
Nonoxynol-9, 1428
Nonprescription sleep aids, 822-824
Nonsteroidal anti-inflammatory agents
ophthalmic, 1356-1357
systemic, 638-645
Nordette, 177
Norditropin, 231
Nordryl, 689
Norelgestromin/ethinyl estradiol, 199-201
Norethindrone, 177-178
Norethindrone acetate, 161-162, 166, 177-178
Norethindrone and Ethinyl Estradiol, 177
Norethindrone and Ethinyl Estradiol (7/14), 177
Norethindrone and Ethinyl Estradiol (10/11), 177
Norflex, 885
Norfloxacin, 1069
Norgesic, 889
Norgesic Forte, 889
Norgestimate, 161, 177-178
Norgestrel, 177-178
Norinyl 1+35, 177
Norinyl 1+50, 177
Normiflo, 107
Normodyne, 416
Noroxin, 1069
Norpace, 346
Norpace CR, 346
Norplant System, 192
Norpramin, 760
Nor-QD, 178
Nortriptyline HCl, 760
Norvasc, 368
Norvir, 1182
Norwegian Cod Liver Oil, 47
Norwich, 601
Norwich Extra Strength, 601
NoSalt, 434
Nose Better Gel, 572
Nostrilla 12 Hour, 501
Novacet Lotion, 1444
Novagest Expectorant with Codeine Liquid, 562
Novolin 70/30, 265
Novolin 70/30 PenFill, 265
Novolin 70/30 Prefilled, 265
Novolin L, 264
Novolin N, 264
Novolin N PenFill, 264
Novolin N Prefilled, 264
Novolin R, 264
Novolin R PenFill, 264
Novolin R Prefilled, 264
NovoLog, 265
NP•27, 1131
NPH Iletin I, 264
NPH Iletin II, 264
NPH Insulin, 264
Nucleoside reverse transcriptase inhibitors, 1190-1194
Nucleotide analog reverse transcriptase inhibitors, 1187-1189
Nucofed Capsules, 544
Nucofed Expectorant Syrup, 562
Nucofed Pediatric Expectorant Syrup, 567
Nucofed Syrup, 544
Nucotuss Expectorant Syrup, 562

INDEX

Nucotuss Pediatric Expectorant Syrup, 567
Nu-Iron, 72
Nu-Iron 150, 72
Numorphan, 616
Nupercainal
  as adrenal cortical steroid, 249
  in anorectal preparations, 1430-1431
  as topical anesthetic, 1485
Nuprin, 638
Nu-Salt, 434
Nutracort, 249
Nutraderm, 1498-1499
Nutraplus, 1496
Nutra-Soothe, 1499
Nutritional supplements
  amino acid combinations, 56-57
  amino acids, 55
  bioflavinoids, 58-59
  fish oils, 60-62
  levocarnitine, 63-64
  lipotropic products, 65-66
  para-aminobenzoic acid, 67-68
Nutropin, 231
Nutropin AQ, 231
Nydrazid, 1222
Nystatin, 1128-1129
  in antifungal combinations, 1135
  in topical antifungals, 1130, 1132
  in vaginal antifungals, 1138
Nystex, 1128
Nytol QuickCaps, 822
Nytol QuickGels, Maximum Strength, 822

Obenix, 579
Oby-Cap, 579
Oby-Trim, 579
Occlusal-HP, 1493
Occult blood tests, 1760-1762
Ocean Nasal Mist, 517
OCL, 1003
Octamide, 965
Octocrylene, 1516-1518, 1520-1521
Octoxynol-9
  in douche products, 1425
  in spermicides, 1428
Octreotide acetate, 139-141
Octyl dimethyl PABA, 1520-1521
Octyl methoxycinnamate, 1516-1522
Octyl salicylate, 1516-1522
OcuClear, 1339
Ocufen, 1356
Ocuflox, 1366
Ocular lubricants, 1386
Ocupress, 1313
Ocusert Pilo, 1319
Ocusulf-10, 1366
Odor-Eaters, 1131
Off-Ezy Wart Remover, 1493
Ofloxacin, 1069, 1366
Ogen, 155
Oil of Olay Foaming Face Wash Liquid, 1447
Oilatum, 1525
Oilatum-AD, 1525
Olanzapine, 787-790
Old, 1304
Old tuberculin, multiple puncture devices, 1304
Oleostearine, 1531
Olive oil, 1530
Olopatadine, 1362-1363
Olsalazine sodium, 1019
Omega-3 700 Capsules, 60
Omega-3 fatty acids, 60
Omeprazole, 968
OMNI, 35
Omnicef, 1037
OmniHIB, 1268
OMNIhist L.A. Tablets, 542
OMS Concentrate, 616
Oncaspar, 1621
Ondansetron HCl, 696
One Step Midstream, 1765
One Touch, 1749
Opcon-A, 1343
Operand, 1505
Ophthalmic anti-infectives
  antibiotics, 1366-1369
  antiviral agents, 1376-1377
  natamycin, 1374-1375
Ophthalmic anti-infectives *(cont.)*
  steroid and antibiotic combinations, 1370-1373
Ophthalmic anti-inflammatory agents
  corticosteroids, 1348-1350
Ophthalmic drug therapy, 1309-1310
Ophthalmic phototherapy, 1380-1382
Ophthalmic vasoconstrictors
  decongestants, 1339-1342
  combinations, 1343-1344
Ophthocort, 1371
Opiates
  in antidiarrheal combination products, 1016-1017
Opium
  in antidiarrheal combination products, 1016
  in narcotic pain relievers, 626-627
Opium and Belladonna Suppositories, 626
Opti-Clean Daily Cleaner, 1387, 1390, 1393
Opti-Clean II, 1387, 1390, 1393
Opticyl, 1345
Opti-Free, 1394
Opti-Free Daily Cleaner, 1387, 1390
Opti-Free Enzymatic Cleaner, 1393
Opti-Free Enzymatic Cleaner Especially for Sensitive Eyes, 1388, 1393
Opti-Free Express, 1394
Opti-Free Rewetting Drops, 1394
Opti-Free Supra Clens Daily Protein Remover, 1390, 1393
Optigene 3, 1339
Optimal Omega Capsules, 60
Optimine, 494
Optimoist, 1409

Optimum Stress Formula Capsules, 49
OptiPranolol, 1313
Opti-Soft, 1393
Opti-Soft Disinfecting, 1394
Opti-Tears Soothing Drops, 1387, 1390, 1394
Optivar, 1360
Opti-Zyme Enzymatic Cleaner, 1390
Opti-Zyme Especially for Sensitive Eyes, 1390
OPV, see Poliovirus vaccine, live, oral, trivalent
Orabase-B, 1421
Orabase-B Gel, 1481
OrabaseGel, 1421
Orabase-Plain, 1421
Oracit, 1655
Orajel, 1421
Orajel, Maximum Strength, 1421
Orajel Denture, 1421
Orajel Mouth-Aid, 1422, 1481
Orajel Perioseptic, 1405
Oral contraceptives, 170, 177-185
Oral-B Sensitive with Fluoride, 1418
Oramorph SR, 616
Orap, 794
Oraphen-PD, 597
Orazinc 110, 45
Orazinc 220, 45
Oretic, 323
Orexin Chewable Tablets, 48
Orgaran, 93
Original Alka-Seltzer, 929
Original Doan's, 602
Orimune, 1273
Orinase, 278
ORLAAM, 615, 1708
Orlistat, 1025-1027
Ornex No Drowsiness Maximum Strength Tablets, 522
Ornex No Drowsiness Tablets, 522
Orphenadrine citrate, 885
Orphenadrine citrate with ASA, 889
Ortho Dienestrol, 155
Ortho Evra, 199
Ortho Tri-Cyclen, 178
Ortho-Cept, 177
Orthoclone OKT3, 1683
Ortho-Cyclen, 177
Ortho-Est, 155
Ortho-Gynol Contraceptive, 1428
Ortho-Novum 1/35, 177
Ortho-Novum 1/50, 177
Ortho-Novum 7/7/7, 178
Ortho-Novum 10/11, 177
Ortho-Prefest, 161
Orudis, 639
Orudis KT, 639
Oruvail, 639
OsCal, 30
OsCal 500, 29
OsCal 250+D, 29
OsCal 250+D Tablets, 53
OsCal 500+D Tablets, 53
Oseltamivir phosphate, 1180-1181
Osteocalcin, 302
Ostercal-D 500 Tablets, 53
Ostiderm, 1529
Otic antibiotics, 1397-1399
Otic preparations
miscellaneous, 1400-1402
Otobiotic Otic, 1397
Otocain, 1400
Otrivin, 502
Otrivin Pediatric, 502
Outgro, 1529
Ovcon 35, 177
Ovcon 50, 177
Overtime, 587
Ovide, 1244
Ovidrel, 202
Ovral, 177
Ovrette, 178
OvuKIT Self-Test, 1763
Ovulation tests, 1763-1764
OvuQUICK Self-Test, 1763
OvuSign, 1763
Oxacillin sodium, 1085
Oxalodinones, 1066-1068
Oxandrin, 142
Oxandrolone, 142
Oxaprozin, 639
Oxazepam, 710
Oxazolidinediones, 847-848
Oxcarbazepine, 849-851
Oxiconazole, 1132
Oxiconazole nitrate, 1130
Oxipor VHC, 1476
Oxistat, 1130
Oxsoralen, 1460
Oxsoralen-Ultra, 1460
Oxtriphylline, 462, 521
Oxy 10 Balance, 1435
Oxy Medicated Cleanser & Pads Regular Strength, 1447
Oxy Medicated Pads Maximum Strength, 1448
Oxy Medicated Pads Sensitive Skin, 1448
Oxy Medicated Soap, 1446
Oxy Night Watch Maximum Strength Lotion, 1445
Oxy Night Watch Sensitive Skin Lotion, 1445
Oxy ResiDON'T Medicated Face Wash, 1448
OxyBalance, 1435
Oxybenzone, 1516-1522
Oxybutynin chloride, 1668-1669
Oxycet Tablets, 627
Oxychlorosene sodium, 1506
Oxycodone, 627-628
Oxycodone 2 Aspirin Tablets, 627
Oxycodone HCl, 616
Oxycodone HCl and Acetaminophen Tablets, 627
Oxycodone with Acetaminophen Capsules, 627
Oxycontin, 616
OxyFast, 616
OxyIR, 616
Oxymetazoline HCl
as decongestant, 501
in nasal products, 517
ophthalmic, 1339
Oxymetholone, 142
Oxymorphone HCl, 616
Oxyquinoline, 1444
Oxyquinoline sulfate, 1529, 1531
Oxysept Disinfection System, 1394
Oxytetracycline
in ophthalmic anti-infectives, 1370
in urinary anti-infective combinations, 1219
in vaginal anti-infectives, 1111
Oxytetracycline HCl, 1089

INDEX

Oxyzal Wet Dressing, 1529
Oysco D Tablets, 53
Oysco 500+D Tablets, 53
Oyst-Cal 500, 29
Oyst-Cal-D, 29, 53
Oyst-Cal-D 500, 29
Oyst-Cal-D 500 Tablets, 53
Oystercal 500, 29
Oystercal-D 250, 29
Oystercal-D 250 Tablets, 53

P-1000, 58
P & S Sebex, 1479
PABA, see Para-aminobenzoic acid
P-A-C Analgesic Tablets, 610
Pacerone, 343
Paclitaxel, 1615
Padimate O, 1521-1522
Pain Relief Cream, 1515
Pain-Bust R II Cream, 1514
Palgic DS Syrup, 536
Palgic-D Tablets, 531
Palivizumab, 1256-1257
Palmitate-A 5000, 7
Pamabrom, 608-609
Pamelor, 760
Pamidronate disodium, 305
Pamine, 931
Pamprin, Maximum Cramp Relief, 609
Pamprin Caplets and Tablets, Maximum Strength Multi-Symptom, 608
Panadol, 597
Panadol Infants' Drops, 598
Panadol Junior Strength, 597
Panalgesic Gold Cream, 1514
Panama Jack, 1521
Panama Jack Dark Tanning, 1521
Pan-C 500, 58
Pancof-HC Liquid, 555
Pancof-XP Liquid, 566
Pancrease Capsules, 961
Pancrease MT 4 Capsules, 961
Pancrease MT 10 Capsules, 961
Pancrease MT 16 Capsules, 962
Pancrease MT 20 Capsules, 962
Pancreatin, 961
Pancreatin 4X Tablets, 961
Pancreatin 8X Tablets, 961
Pancrelipase, 961-962
Pancrezyme 4X Tablets, 961
Pandel, 249
Panex, 597
Panfil-G Capsules, 521
Panfil-G Syrup, 521
Panglobulin, 1250
PanMist JR Tablets, 525
PanMist LA Tablets, 527
PanMist-DM Syrup, 564
PanMist-DM Tablets, 564
PanMist-S Syrup, 525
Pannaz S Syrup, 543
Pannaz Tablets, 543
Panoxyl, 1435
PanOxyl 5 and 10, 1435
PanOxyl AQ 2.5, 5 and 10, 1435
Panthoderm, 1496
Pantoprazole sodium, 968
Pantothenic acid, 17
Papain, 971
Papaverine HCl, 377-378
Papaya Enzyme, 971
Para-aminobenzoic acid (PABA), 67-68
Parabens
- in acne products, 1435, 1444-1447
- in anorectal preparations, 1430-1431
- in skin cleansers, 1530

Paraffin, 1528
Paraflex Caplets, 885
Parafon Forte DSC Caplets, 885
Paral, 817
Paraldehyde, 817
Parapectolin, 1016
Paregoric, 1016
Paremyd, 1345
Paricalcitol, 23
Parlodel, 895, 1693
Parlodel SnapTabs, 895
Parnate, 743
Paromomycin sulfate, 1031
Paroxetine HCl, 749-751
Parsidol, 891
Parva-Cal 250 Tablets, 53
Parva-Cal 500 Tablets, 53
Parvlex Tablets, 51, 76
Patanol, 1362
Pavabid Plateau Caps, 377
Paxil, 749
Paxil CR, 749
Paxipam, 710
Pazo Hemorrhoid, 1431
PCE Dispertab, 1052
PDP Liquid Protein, 56
P1E1, 1335
P2E1, 1335
P3E1, 1335
P4E1, 1335
P6E1, 1335
Peanut oil, 1530
Pectin, 1016, 1017
Pedameth, 1507
Pedia Care Children's Cold & Allergy Liquid, 536
Pedia Care Children's Long-Lasting Cough Plus Cold Liquid, 558
Pedia Care Cough-Cold Liquid, 560
Pedia Care Infants' Decongestant & Cough Drops, 557
Pedia Care Multi-Symptom Cold Liquid, 560
Pedia Care Night-Rest Cough & Cold Liquid, 561
Pedia Relief Decongestant Plus Cough Infants' Drops, 557
PediaCare Fever, 638
PediaCare Infants' Decongestant, 501
Pediaflor, 35
Pedialyte Freezer Pops, 33
Pedialyte Solution, 33
Pediapred, 240
Pediatex-D Liquid, 536
Pediatex-DM Liquid, 559
Pediatric Advil, 638
Pediatric Electrolyte Solution, 33
Pediatrics
- antitussive combinations, 556-561
- decongestant, antihistamine, and expectorant combinations, 530

Pediatrics *(cont.)*
decongestant and analgesic combinations, 523-524
decongestant and expectorant combinations, 528
Pedi-Bath Salts, 1499
Pedi-Boro Soak Packs, 1526
Pediculicides, 1244-1246
Pedi-Dri, 1128, 1130
Pedi-Vit A, 1498
PedvaxHIB, 1268
PEG-8 stearate, 1530
PEG-100 stearate, 1530, 1532
Peganone, 842
Pegaspargase, 1621-1623
PemADD, 594
PemADD CT, 594
Pemirolast potassium, 1353
Pemoline, 594-596
Penbutolol sulfate, 379
Penecort, 249
Penicillamine, 1710-1712
Penicillin V potassium, 1085
Penicillins
oral, 1084-1088
Pen-Kera, 1498
Penlac Nail Lacquer, 1130
Pentamidine isethionate, 1234-1236
Pentazocine, 633-635
Pentazocine and acetaminophen, 633
Pentazocine and naloxone, 633
Pentobarbital, 812
Pentobarbital sodium
in migraine combinations, 668
as sedative, 812
Pentolair, 1345
Pentostatin, 1615
Pentoxifylline, 122-123
Pentrax, 1475
Pentrax Gold, 1475
Pepcid, 950
Pepcid AC, 950
Pepcid Complete, 950
Pepcid RPD, 950
Peppermint oil
in acne products, 1447
Peppermint oil *(cont.)*
in mouth and throat products, 1420, 1422
Pepto Diarrhea Control, 1014
Pepto-Bismol, 1007
Pepto-Bismol, Maximum Strength, 1007
Peracetic acid, 1506
Percocet Tablets, 627
Percodan Tablets, 627
Percodan-Demi Tablets, 628
Percogesic Extra Strength Tablets, 529
Percogesic Tablets, 529
Percolone, 616
Perdiem Fiber, 978
Pergolide mesylate, 906-908
Pergonal, 217
Periactin, 494
Perianal hygiene products, 1431
PeriColace, 1001
Peri-Colace Capsules, 998
Peridex, 1407
Peridin-C, 58
Peri-Dos Softgels, 998
Perindopril erbumine, 390
PerioMed, 35
Periostat, 939, 1089
Peripheral vasodilators
isoxsuprine, 375-376
papaverine, 377-378
Permax, 906
Permethrin, 1244
Permitil, 770
Pernox Lathering Abradant Scrub Lotion, 1446
Pernox Scrub for Oily Skin, 1446
Peroxyl, 1422
Perphenazine
as antiemetic/antivertigo agent, 699
as antipsychotic, 771
Perphenazine and amitriptyline HCl, 807
Persa-Gel W, 1435
Persantine, 88
Pertussin CS, 509
Pertussin DM, 509
Petrolatum
in anorectal preparations, 1430-1431
Petrolatum *(cont.)*
in diaper rash products, 1507
in mouth and throat products, 1420
in skin cleansers, 1528-1531
in sunscreens, 1519
Petrolatum and lanolin, 1496
PFA, see Foscarnet sodium
Pfeiffer's Cold Sore, 1422
Phanatuss DM Cough Syrup, 568
Pharmadine, 1505
Pharmaflur, 35
Pharmaflur 1.1, 35
Phazyme, 959
Phazyme 95, 959
Phazyme 125, 959
Phenapap Tablets, 522
Phenaphen w/Codeine No. 3 Capsules, 623
Phenaphen w/Codeine No. 4 Capsules, 624
Phenaphen-650 w/Codeine Tablets, 623
Phenazopyridine HCl
in urinary anti-infective combinations, 1219
in urinary tract products, 1672-1673
Phendimetrazine tartrate, 579
Phendry, 891
Phendry, 689
Phenelzine, 743
Phenergan
as antiemetic/antivertigo agent, 699
as antihistamine, 496
Phenergan Fortis
as antiemetic/antivertigo agent, 699
as antihistamine, 496
Phenergan Plain
as antiemetic/antivertigo agent, 699
as antihistamine, 496
Phenergan VC Syrup, 530
Phenindamine tartrate, 496
Pheniramine maleate
in nasal products, 517

INDEX

Pheniramine maleate *(cont.)*
in ophthalmic decongestant combinations, 1343
in topical antihistamines, 1502
in upper respiratory combinations, 533, 537-538, 562
Phenobarbital
in anticholinergic combinations, 936-937
as sedative, 812
in upper respiratory combinations, 521
Phenobarbital with phenytoin sodium, 842
Phenol
in acne products, 1444
in antifungal combinations, 1135
in antiseborrheic combinations, 1479
in douche products, 1425
in lozenges, 1417
in mouth and throat products, 1420, 1422
in poison ivy treatment products, 1512
in skin cleansers, 1528-1531
in topical antihistamines, 1502
Phenolated Calamine, 1512
Phenolphthalein
as laxative, 991
in laxative combinations, 998-999, 1001
Phenoptic, 1339
Phenothiazines, 699-704
Phensuxide, 861
Phentermine HCl, 579
Phentermine resin, 579
Phenyl salicylate
in antidiarrheal combination products, 1016
in urinary anti-infective combinations, 1219-1220
Phenylalanine
in antacid combinations, 929
in laxatives, 977
Phenylbenzimidazole sulfonic acid, 1518
Phenylcarbinol, 1512
Phenylephrine HCl
in anorectal preparations, 1431
in cycloplegic mydriatics, 1345
in decongestants, 501
in nasal products, 517
in ophthalmic decongestant combinations, 1339, 1343
in otic preparations, 1400
in upper respiratory combinations, 522, 524-525, 529-530, 537-538, 542-543, 545, 549, 552-556, 562-563, 566
Phenylephrine tannate, 535, 544, 556
Phenylephrine Tannate/Chlorpheniramine Tannate/Pyrilamine Tannate Solution, 535
Phenylgesic Tablets, 529
Phenylmerconic nitrate, 1431
Phenyltoloxamine citrate
in digestive aids, 971
in nonnarcotic analgesics, 608-609, 611
in upper respiratory combinations, 529, 533, 537
Phenyltoloxamine dihydrogen citrate, 610
Phenytoin, 842
Phenytoin Sodium, 842
Phenytoin sodium, extended, 842
Phenytoin sodium, prompt, 842
Phenytoin sodium with phenobarbital, 842
Phillip's Laxative Gelcaps, 998
Phillip's LaxCaps, 998
Phillips' Milk of Magnesia, 917, 988
Phillips' Milk of Magnesia, Concentrated, 988
pHisoDerm Acne, 1525
pHisoDerm Baby, 1525
pHisoDerm Normal to Dry, 1525
pHisoDerm Normal to Oily, 1525
pHisoDerm Sensitive Skin, 1525
pHisoHex, 1505
PhosChol, 65
Phos-Flur, 35
PhosLo, 1713
Phosphate, 239
Phosphate binders, 1713-1714
Phospholine Iodide, 1316
Phosphonoformic acid, see Foscarnet sodium
Phosphorated carbohydrate, 705-706
Phosphoric acid, 705
Phosphorus, 5
Phospho-soda, 1005
Photofrin, 1624
Phototherapy
ophthalmic, 1380-1382
Phrenilin Forte Capsules, 608
Phrenilin Tablets, 609
Physostigmine
for glaucoma, 1316 in combinations, 1335
Phytonadione, 124-125
Pilagan, 1319
Pilocar, 1319
Pilocarpine HCl, 1319, 1335
Pilocarpine nitrate, 1319
Pilopine HS, 1319
Piloptic, 1319
Pilopto-Carpine, 1319
Pilostat, 1319
Pima, 513
Pimozide, 794-796
Pindolol, 379
Pin-Rid, 1203
Pin-X, 1203
Pioglitazone HCl, 275
Piperazine estrone sulfate, see Estropipate
Pirbuterol acetate, 456
Piroxicam, 640
PIV, see Poliovirus vaccine, inactivated
Placidyl, 817
Plan B, 186
Plaquenil, 1141
Plaquenil Sulfate, 649
Plavix, 119

Plegine, 579
Plendil, 368
Pliagel, 1393
Plicamycin, 1606-1607
Pneumococcal vaccine, 1258, 1296-1298
Pneumococcal 7-valent conjugate vaccine, 1302-1303
Pneumotussin 2.5 Cough Syrup, 570
Pneumovax 23, 1296
Pnu-Imune 23, 1296
Podiacin Soak'n Massage Gel, 1514
Podofilox, 1491-1492
Poison ivy treatment products, 1512-1513
Polaramine, 494
Polaramine Expectorant Liquid, 529
Polaramine Repetabs, 494
Polio vaccine, 1273-1276
Polio vaccine, inactivated, 1258
Poliovax, 1273
Poliovirus vaccine, inactivated, 1273
Poliovirus vaccine, live, oral, trivalent, 1273
Polycarbophil, 977
Polycitra-K, 1655
Polycitra-LC, 1655
Polydine, 1505
Polyethylene glycol, 1003-1004
Polygam S/D, 1250
Polymyxin B sulfate
  in ophthalmic anti-infectives, 1370-1372
  in otic antibiotics, 1397
  in topical antibiotics, 1098-1099
  in vaginal anti-infectives, 1111
Polymyxin B sulfate sterile, 1366
Polyoxyethylene nonyl phenol, 1111
Poly-Pred Suspension, 1370
Polyquaternium-10, 1532
Polysaccharide-iron complex, 72
Polysorbate 80, 1448
Polysporin, 1098-1099
Polytar, 1475
Polythiazide
  in antihypertensive combinations, 430, 432
  as diuretic, 323
Polyvinyl alcohol, 1446
Ponstel, 639
Pontocaine, 1486
Pontocaine HCl, 1481
Porfimer sodium, 1624-1626
Posterior pituitary hormones
  desmopressin acetate, 226-228
Posture, 29
Posture D-Chewable Tablets, 53
Posture D-Tablets, 53
Posture-D, 29
Potassium
  in antihypertensive combinations, 432
  in combinations, 41
  in electrolyte mixtures, 33
  in laxatives, 977-978
  nutritional, 41-44
Potassium 99, 41
Potassium acid phosphate, 1652
Potassium acid phosphate and sodium acid phosphate, 1652
Potassium bicarbonate, 929
  in laxatives, 978
Potassium chloride, 41
Potassium citrate, 1655
Potassium citrate combinations, 1655
Potassium clavulanate and amoxicillin, 1084
Potassium cocoyl, 1447
Potassium gluconate, 41
Potassium guaiacolsulfonate, 566, 570-571
Potassium Iodide, 513
Potassium iodide
  in expectorants, 513
  as thyroid drug, 297
  in upper respiratory combinations, 521, 524
Potassium nitrate, 1418
Potassium Para-Aminobenzoate (KPAB), 67
Potassium-sparing diuretics, 320-322
Povidone-iodine
  in antiseptics, 1505
  in douche products, 1425
  in skin cleansers, 1529
PrameGel, 1485
Pramipexole, 900-902
Pramipexole dihydrochloride, 900
Pramosone Cream, 254
Pramosone Cream 2.5, 254
Pramoxine HCl
  in anorectal preparations, 1430
  in otic preparations, 1400
  in poison ivy treatment products, 1512
  for skin disorders, 1485
  in topical corticosteroids, 254
Prandin, 283
Pravachol, 448
Pravastatin sodium, 448
Prax, 1485
Prazepam, 710
Prazosin, 386, 432
Precose, 272
Pred Forte, 1348
Pred Mild, 1348
Predalone 50, 240
Pred-G S.O.P., 1371
Pred-G Suspension, 1370
Prednisolone, 240
Prednisolone acetate
  as adrenal cortical steroids, 240
  in ophthalmic anti-infectives, 1370-1372
  in ophthalmic antiinflammatory agents, 1348
Prednisolone sodium phosphate
  as adrenal cortical steroids, 240
  in ophthalmic anti-infectives, 1372
  in ophthalmic anti-inflammatory agents, 1348
Prednisone, 240
Prednisone Intensol Concentrate, 240
Prefrin, 1339

INDEX

Prefrin Liquifilm, 1339
Pregnancy tests, 1765-1766
Pregnosis, 1765
Pregnyl, 204
Pre-Hist-D Tablets, 542
Prelone, 240
Prelu-2, 579
Premarin, 155
Premarin Intravenous, 155
Premphase, 161
Prempro, 161
Premsyn PMS Caplets, 608
Preparation H, 1431
Preparation H Anti-Itch, 249
Preservative Free Moisture Eyes, 1383
Preservative free saline solutions
  for soft (hydrogel) contact lenses, 1393
Preserved saline solution
  for soft (hydrogel) contact lenses, 1393
PreSun Sensitive, 1519
PreSun Ultra, 1517, 1519
Pretz-D, 501, 517
Prevacid, 968
Prevalite, 435
Preven, 186
PreviDent, 35
PreviDent 5000 Plus, 35
Prevnar, 1302
Prevpac, 947
Priftin, 1222
Prilocaine, 1486
Prilosec, 968
Primacor, 335
Primaquine phosphate, 1141
Primatene Mist, 455
Primatene Tablets, 524
Primaxin I.M., 1076
Primaxin I.V., 1076
Primidone, 855-857
Principen, 1084
Prinivil, 390
Prinzide 12.5 Tablets, 432
Prinzide 25 Tablets, 432
Privine, 501
ProAmatine, 707
Pro-Banthine, 931
Probenecid, 662-665
Probenecid and colchicine, 658, 662
Procainamide, 359-360
Pro-Cal-Sof, 995
Procan SR, 359
Procarbazine, 1615
Procardia, 369
Procardia XL, 369
Prochlorperazine
  as antiemetic/antivertigo agent, 699
  as antipsychotic, 771
Procrit, 128
Proctocort, 1430
ProctoCream-HC 2.5, 249
ProctoFoam, 1430
ProctoFoam-HC, 1430
ProctoFoam-HC Aerosol Foam, 254
Pro-Cute, 1498
Procyclidine, 891
Proderm Topical, 1529
Profasi, 204
Profen Forte DM Tablets, 565
Profen Forte Tablets, 527
Profen II DM Liquid, 563
Profen II DM Tablets, 565
Profen II Tablets, 525
Profenal, 1356
Pro-Free/GP Weekly Enzymatic Cleaner Tablets, 1390
Progestasert, 189
Progesterone, 166
  intrauterine, 189-191
Progesterone in oil, 166
Progestin-only oral contraceptives, 170, 178
Progestins
  as antineoplastics, 1574-1575
  as sex hormones, 166-169
Prograf, 1686
Proguanil HCl and atovaquone, 1154-1155
ProHIBiT, 1268
Prolex DH Liquid, 570
Prolixin, 770
Prolixin Decanoate, 770
Prolixin Enanthate, 770
Proloprim, 1096
Promazine HCl, 771
Prometh VC Plain Syrup, 530
Prometh VC w/Codeine Cough Syrup, 545
Prometh w/Codeine Cough Syrup, 544
Prometh w/Dextromethorphan Syrup, 553
Promethazine
  as antiemetic/antivertigo agent, 699
  in upper respiratory combinations, 530, 553
Promethazine HCl
  as antihistamine, 496
  in narcotic pain reliever combinations, 628
  in upper respiratory combinations, 544, 545
Promethazine HCl and Phenylephrine HCl Syrup, 530
Promethazine HCl w/Codeine Syrup, 544
Promethazine w/Dextromethorphan Cough Syrup, 553
Promethazone VC w/Codeine Cough Syrup, 545
Prometrium, 166
Promise Sensitive, 1418
Pronestyl, 359
Pronestyl-SR, 359
Pronto, 1244
Propacet 100 Tablets, 628
Propafenone HCl, 361-362
Propantheline bromide, 931
PROPApH Acne Maximum Strength Cream, 1445
PROPApH Cleansing for Oily Skin Lotion, 1445
PROPApH Cleansing for Sensitive Skin Pads, 1448
PROPApH Cleansing Lotion for Normal/Combination Skin, 1445
PROPApH Cleansing Maximum Strength Pads, 1448
PROPApH Cleansing Pads, 1445
PROPApH Foaming Face Wash, 1448
PROPApH Peel-Off Acne Mask, 1446
Propecia, 153

Prophyllin, 1136
Propine, 1325
Propionic acid, 1136
Propoxyphene, 616
Propoxyphene HCl, 629
Propoxyphene HCl Compound Capsules, 629
Propranolol Intensol, 379
Propoxyphene HCl w/Acetaminophen Tablets, 629
Propoxyphene Napsylate and Acetaminophen Tablets, 628
Propoxyphene napsylate, 628
Propranolol HCl
- antihypertensive combinations, 431
- beta-adrenergic blocking agent, 379

Propylhexedrine, 517
Propylene glycol
- in acne products, 1435, 1444, 1447-1448
- in anorectal preparations, 1430-1431
- in antifungal combinations, 1136
- in douche products, 1425
- in skin cleansers, 1530

Propylene glycol alginate, 1529
Propylthiouracil, 294
Proscar, 153
Prosed/DS, 1219
Pro-Sof Capsules, 995
Pro-Sof Plus Capsules, 998
ProSom, 817
Prostaglandin agonists, 1322-1324
Prostep, 1715
Prostigmin, 1647
Protease, 961-962, 971
Protease inhibitors, 1182-1186
ProTech First-Aid Stick, 1485, 1529
Protein, 5-6
Protein tests, 1767-1768
Proton pump inhibitors, 968-970
Protonix, 968
Protostat, 1079
Protriptyline HCl, 760
Protropin, 229
Protuss DM Tablets, 565
Protuss Liquid, 571
Protuss-D Liquid, 566
Proventil, 455
Proventil HFA, 455
Proventil Repetabs, 455
Provera, 166
Proxigel, 1405
Prozac, 730
Prozac Weekly, 730
Prozine-50, 771
Prulet, 991
PSE 120/MSC 2.5 Tablets, 543
Pseudoephedrine HCl
- as decongestant, 501
- in upper respiratory combinations, 522-528, 531-533, 535-541, 543-567

Pseudoephedrine sulfate
- as decongestant, 502
- in upper respiratory combinations, 529, 534

Pseudoephedrine tannate, 537
Pseudovent Capsules, 527
Pseudovent-PED Capsules, 528
Psorcon, 248
Psorcon E, 248
Psoriasis agents, 1460-1463
- acitretin, 1454-1456
- anthralin, 1450-1451
- calcipotriene, 1452-1453
- methotrexate, 1457-1459
- tazarotene, 1464-1466

PsoriGel, 1476
Psychotherapeutic agents
- ergoloid mesylates, 797-798
- lithium, 799-802
- pimozide, 794-796

Psychotherapeutic combinations, 807-811
Psyllium, 977-978
PTU, see Propylthiouracil
Pulmicort Respules, 471
Pulmicort Turbuhaler, 471
Pulmozyme, 485
Puralube, 1383
Pure Eyes Cleaner/Rinse, 1393
Pure Eyes Disinfecting/Soaking, 1393
Purge, 991
Purified water, 1425
Purinethol, 1541
Purpose, 1525
Purpose DrySkin, 1498
P-V-Tussin Syrup, 555
P-V-Tussin Tablets, 553
Pyrantel, 1203-1204
Pyrazinamide, 1222
Pyrazinamide with rifampin and isoniazid, 1222
Pyrethrins, 1244
Pyridium, 1672
Pyridostigmine bromide, 1647
Pyridoxine
- in nonnarcotic analgesics, 608
- nutritional, 6, 18-19

Pyridoxine HCl, 18
Pyrilamine maleate
- in nonnarcotic analgesics, 608
- in skin cleansers, 1530
- in topical antihistamines, 1502
- in upper respiratory combinations, 533, 537, 545, 553, 555-556

Pyrilamine tannate, 535
Pyrimethamine, 1147-1148
Pyrimethamine and sulfadoxine, 1149-1151
Pyrinyl Plus, 1244
Pyrithione zinc, 1475

QTest, 1765
Quad Tann Tablets, 544
Quadra-Hist D Capsules, 533
Quadra-Hist D PED Capsules, 537
Quazepam, 817
Quercetin, 58
Questran, 435
Questran Light, 435
Quetiapine fumarate, 781-783
Quiagel, 1017
Quiagel PG, 1016

INDEX

Quibron Capsules, 521
Quibron-300 Capsules, 521
Quibron-T Accudose, 462
Quibron-T/SR Accudose, 462
Quick Care Starting Solution, 1394
Quin B Strong B-25 Tablets, 51
Quinaglute Dura-Tabs, 363
Quinalan, 363
Quinapril HCl, 390
Quinethazone, 323
Quinidex Extentabs, 363
Quinidine, 363-365
Quinidine gluconate, 363
Quinidine polygalacturonate, 363
Quinidine sulfate, 363
Quinine sulfate, 1156-1157
Quinora, 363
Quinsana Plus, 1131
Quixin, 1366
QVAR, 471

RA Lotion, 1445
RabAvert, 1262
Rabeprazole sodium, 968
Rabies immune globulin (human), 1251
Rabies vaccine, 1262-1263
Racepinephrine, 455
Raloxifene HCl, 164
Ramipril, 390
Ranitidine, 950
Ranitidine bismuth citrate, 942-943
RapidVue, 1765
Rauwolfia serpentina, 430
Rauzide Tablets, 430
Ray Block, 1520
R&C, 1244
Rea-Lo, 1496
ReAzo, 1672
Rebetol, 1173
Reclomide, 965
Recombivax HB, 1289
Rectagene Medicated Rectal Balm, 1431
Red petrolatum, see Petrolatum
Redness Reliever, 1339
Redutemp, 597
Reese's Pinworm, 1203
Refenesen Plus Severe Strength Cough & Cold Medicine Tablets, 526
Refresh, 1383
Refresh Plus, 1383
Refresh PM, 1386
Refresh Tears, 1383
Reglan, 965
Regonol, 1647
Regranex, 1467
Regroton Tablets, 430
Regulace Capsules, 998
Regular Iletin II, 264
Regular Strength Bayer Enteric Coated Caplets, 601
Regulax SS, 995
Rehydrate Solution, 33
Relafen, 639
Relenza, 1178
Relief, 1339
Remeron, 740
Remeron SolTab, 740
Remicade, 1022
Reminyl, 803
Remular-S, 885
Renese, 323
Renese-R Tablets, 430
ReNu 1 Step, 1393
ReNu Effervescent, 1393
ReNu Lubricating and Rewetting Drops, 1394
ReNu Multi-Plus, 1394
ReNu Multi-Purpose, 1394
Repaglinide, 283
Repan CF Tablets, 608
Repan Tablets, 609
Reposans, 710
Repository corticotropin, 235
Requip, 903
Rescon 12 Hour Capsules, 532
Rescon-DM Liquid, 549
Rescon-GG Liquid, 524
Rescon-Jr. Capsules, 537
Rescon-MX Tablets, 543
Rescriptor, 1195
Rescula, 1322
Reserpine, 427-429, 430
Resorcinol
- in acne products, 1444-1445
- in antifungal combinations, 1135

Resorcinol *(cont.)*
- in topical antihistamines, 1502

Respa A.R. Tablets, 543
Respa-DM Tablets, 569
Respahist Capsules, 531
Respaire-60 SR Capsules, 526
Respaire-120 SR Capsules, 527
Respa-1st Tablets, 526
Respbid, 462
RespiGam, 1251
Respiratory syncytial virus immune globulin intravenous (human), 1251
Restore, 977
Restoril, 817
Retavase, 116
Reteplase, recombinant, 116
Retin-A, 1441
Retinoids
- isotretinoin, 1689-1692
- tretinoin, 1612-1614

Retrovir, 1190
Rev-Eyes, 1337
Reversol, 1647
Revex, 1641
ReVia, 1705
Rewetting solutions
- for hard contact lenses, 1387
- for rigid gas permeable contact lenses, 1390
- for soft (hydrogel) contact lenses, 1394

Rezamid Lotion, 1445
Rheaban, 1017
Rheumatrex Dose Pack, 1457
- antineoplastic, 1541
- antirheumatic, 651
- antipsoriatic, 1457

Rhinall, 501
Rhinatate Pediatric Suspension, 535
Rhinatate-NF Pediatric Suspension, 535
Rhinocort, 490
Rho(D) immune globulin (human), 1251
Rho(D) immune globulin IV (human), 1252
Rho(D) immune globulin micro-dose, 1252

RhoGAM, 1251
RhuliAerosol, 1512
RhuliGel, 1512
RhuliSpray, 1512
Ribavirin, 1173-1175
Riboflavin, 6, 12-13
RID, 1244
Rid-A-Pain Cream, 1515
Rid-A-Pain Dental, 1422
Rid-A-Pain HP Cream, 1515
Ridaura, 646
Ridenol, 597
Rifabutin, 1222
Rifadin, 1222
Rifamate, 1222
Rifampin, 1222
Rifampin with isoniazid, 1222
Rifampin with isoniazid and pyrazinamide, 1222
Rifapentine, 1222
Rifater, 1222
RIG, see Rabies immune globulin (human)
Rigid gas permeable contact lens products, 1390-1392
Rilutek, 1732
Riluzole, 1732-1733
Rimactane, 1222
Rimantadine, 1176-1177
Rimantadine HCl, 1176
Rimexolone, 1348
Rimso-50, 1664
Rinade B.I.D. Capsules, 532
Riopan Plus, 923
Riopan Plus Double Strength, 923
Riopan Plus Double Strength Suspension, 927
Riopan Plus Suspension, 926
Risedronate, 305
Risperdal, 771, 784
Risperidone, 771, 784-786
Ritalin, 590
Ritalin-SR, 590
Ritonavir/lopinavir, 1182
Rituxan, 1627
Rituximab, 1627-1628
Rivastigmine tartrate, 803
Rizatriptan, 679-682
Rizatriptan benzoate, 679
RMS, 616
Robafen CF Syrup, 563
Robafen PE Liquid, 525
Robaxin, 885
Robaxin-750, 885
Robaxisal, 889
Robinul, 931
Robinul Forte, 931
Robitussin, 513
Robitussin Allergy & Cough Liquid, 547
Robitussin CF Syrup, 563
Robitussin Cold, Cold & Congestion Softgels and Tablets, 564
Robitussin Cold, Cold & Cough Softgels, 563
Robitussin Cold, Multi-Symptom Cold & Flu Softgels, 563
Robitussin Cold, Multi-Symptom Cold & Flu Tablets, 564
Robitussin Cold Sinus & Congestion Tablets, 525
Robitussin Cough & Cold Infant Drops, 567
Robitussin Cough & Congestion Formula Liquid, 569
Robitussin DM Infant Drops, 571
Robitussin Flu Liquid, 549
Robitussin Honey Cough & Cold Liquid, 545
Robitussin Honey Flu Multi-Symptom Liquid, 546
Robitussin Honey Flu Nighttime Syrup, 551
Robitussin Honey Flu Non-Drowsy Syrup, 547
Robitussin Maximum Strength Cough & Cold Syrup, 545
Robitussin Night Relief Liquid, 553
Robitussin PE Liquid, 525
Robitussin Pediatric Cough & Cold Formula Liquid, 558
Robitussin Pediatric Night Relief Cough & Cold Liquid, 561
Robitussin Severe Congestion Liqui-Gels, 525
Robitussin Sugar Free Cough Liquid, 568
Robitussin-DM Liquid, 568
Rocaltrol, 23
Rocephin, 1038
Rofecoxib, 640
Roferon-A, 1608
Rogaine Extra Strength for Men, 1509
Rogaine for Men, 1509
Rogaine for Women, 1509
Rolaids, 30
Romazicon, 1635
Romilar AC Liquid, 567
Rondamine DM Syrup, 548
Rondec Oral Drops, 536
Rondec Syrup, 531
Rondec Tablets, 531
Rondec-DM Oral Drops, 558
Rondec-DM Syrup, 547
Rondec-TR Tablets, 531
Ropinirole, 903-905
Rosiglitazone maleate, 275
Rosin, 1528
Rowasa, 1019
Roxanol, 616
Roxanol 100, 616
Roxanol T, 616
Roxicet 5/500 Caplets, 627
Roxicet Tablets and Solution, 627
Roxicodone, 616
Roxicodone Intensol, 616
Roxilox Capsules, 627
Roxiprin Tablets, 627
R/S Lotion, 1445
RSV-IGIV, see Respiratory syncytial virus immune globulin intravenous (human)
R-Tanna 12 Suspension, 535
R-Tannic-S A/D Suspension, 535
Rubella and mumps virus vaccine, live, 1277
Rubella virus vaccine, live, 1277
Rubex, 1560
Rubs, 1514-1515
RuLox, 921
Rulox #1, 921
Rulox #2, 921
Rulox Plus Suspension, 925

INDEX

Rulox Suspension, 924
Rutin, 58
Ru-Vert-M, 689
RVPaque, 1519
Ryna Liquid, 532
Ryna-12 S Suspension, 535
Ryna-C Liquid, 544
Rynatan Pediatric Suspension, 535
Rynatan Tablets, 530
Rynatuss Pediatric Suspension, 556
Rynatuss Tablets, 544
Rythmol, 361

Sabin vaccine, see Poliovirus vaccine, live, oral, trivalent
Saccharin, 977-978
Safe Tussin Liquid, 569
SalAc Cleanser, 1448
Salactic Film, 1493
Salicylic Acid and Sulfur Soap, 1446
Salicylic Acid Cleansing Bar, 1446
Salagen, 1410
Sal-Clens Acne Cleanser Gel, 1445
Saleto Tablets, 610
Salflex, 602
Salicylamide, 529
Salicylate combinations, 602
Salicylates
  aspirin and, 601-605
Salicylic acid
  in acne products, 1444-1449
  in antifungal combinations, 1135, 1136
  in antiseborrheic combinations, 1479
  in mouth and throat products, 1421
  topical, 1493-1495
Saline laxatives, 988-990
Saline Solution, 1393
Salinex Nasal Drops, 517
Salinex Nasal Mist, 517
Saliva Substitute, 1409
Saliva substitutes, 1409-1411
Salivart, 1409
Salix, 1409
Salk vaccine, see Poliovirus vaccine, inactivated
Salmeterol/fluticasone propionate, 471
Salsalate, 602
Salsitab, 602
Salt substitutes, 434
Saluron, 323
Salutensin Tablets, 430
Sam-EPA Capsules, 60
Sandimmune, 1676
Sandoglobulin, 1250
Sandostatin, 139
Sani-Supp, 981
Sanorex, 579
Sansert, 671
Saquinavir, 1182
Sarafem, 730
Saratoga, 1530
Sargramostim, 134-136
Sarna Anti-Itch, 1530
SAStid Soap, 1446
Scabicides, 1244-1246
Scarlet red, 1530
Scarlet Red Ointment Dressings, 1530
Schamberg's, 1530
Scope, 1418
Scopolamine
  anticholinergic combinations, 936
  antiemetic/antivertigo agent, 689
Scopolamine HBr
  antidiarrheal combination products, 1016-1017
  cycloplegic mydriatic, 1345
  upper respiratory combinations, 543
Scopolamine nitrate, 543
Scott's Emulsion, 47
Scot-tussin, 513
Scot-Tussin Allergy, 495, 891
Scot-Tussin DM Cough Chasers, 509
Scot-Tussin DM Liquid, 548
Scot-Tussin Hayfebrol Liquid, 532
Scot-Tussin Original 5-Action Cold and Allergy Formula Syrup, 538
Scot-Tussin Original Clear 5-Action Cold and Allergy Formula, 538
Scot-Tussin Senior Clear Liquid, 569
SD alcohol
  in acne products, 1445, 1448
  in poison ivy treatment products, 1512
SD alcohol 40
  in acne products, 1445-1448
  in antiseborrheic combinations, 1479
  in douche products, 1425
Seale's Lotion Modified, 1445
Sea-Omega 30 Capsules, 60
Sea-Omega 50 Capsules, 60
Seba-Nil Cleansing Mask, 1447
Seba-Nil Oily Skin Cleanser, 1448
Sebasorb Lotion, 1445
Sebizon, 1475
Sebucare, 1479
Sebulex, 1479
Sebulex with Conditioners, 1479
Sebulon, 1475
Secobarbital sodium, 812
Seconal Sodium, 812
Sectral, 379
Sedapap Tablets, 608
Sedatives
  barbiturates, 812-816
  hypnotics, 817-821
Selective estrogen receptor modulator, 164-165
Selegiline HCl, 909-911
Selenium, 5
Selenium sulfide, 1473-1474
Selsun, 1473
Selsun Blue, 1473
Semicid, 1428
Semprex-D Capsules, 530
Senexon, 991
Senna
  bowel evacuation kits, 1005
  laxative, 991-992

Senna *(cont.)*
in laxative combinations, 998-999, 1001
Senna-Gen, 991
Sennosides, 1005
Senokot, 991
Senokot-S Tablets, 998
Senokotxtra, 991
Senolax, 991
Sensitive Eyes Cleaner, 1393
Sensitive Eyes Daily Cleaner, 1393
Sensitive Eyes Drops, 1394
Sensitive Eyes Plus Saline, 1393
Sensitive Eyes Saline, 1393
Sensitive Eyes Saline/Cleaning Solution, 1393
Sensitive Eyes Sterile Saline Spray, 1393
Sensitive teeth preparations, 1418
Sensodyne Cool Gel for Sensitive Teeth and Cavity Prevention, 1418
Sensodyne Extra Whitening for Sensitive Teeth, 1418
Sensodyne w/Baking Soda for Sensitive Teeth and Cavity Prevention, 1418
Sensodyne-SC Original Formula for Sensitive Teeth, 1418
Septa, 1099
Septi-Soft, 1505
Septra, 1108, 1219
Septra DS, 1108, 1219
Ser-Ap-Es Tablets, 430
Serax, 710
Sereine, 1387
Serentil, 770
Serevent, 456
Seromycin Pulvules, 1222
Serophene, 214
Seroquel, 781
Serostim, 231
Sertraline HCl, 752-753
Serutan, 978
Serzone, 727
Severe Congestion Tussin Softgels, 525
Sex hormones
anabolic steroids, 142-145
Sex hormones *(cont.)*
androgens, 149-152
contraceptives, 172-173
emergency contraceptives, 186-188
estrogen combinations, 161-163
estrogens, 155-160
medroxyprogesterone acetate/estradiol cypionate, 174-176
mifepristone, 146-148
oral contraceptives, 177-185
progestins, 166-169
selective estrogen receptor modulator, 164-165
Sexadecyl alcohol, 1528
SF 1.1, 35
SF 5000 Plus, 35
SFC, 1525
Shark liver oil, 1431
Shepard's Skin, 1498
Shohl's Solution, Modified, 1655
Siblin, 978
Sibutramine, 584-586
Sibutramine HCl monohydrate, 584
Silace, 995
Silace-C, 1001
Siladryl, 891
Silafed Syrup, 533
Silapap Infants' Drops, 598
Sildec-DM Oral Drops, 559
Sildec-DM Syrup, 548
Sildenafil citrate, 1724-1726
Silica
in douche products, 1425
in skin cleansers, 1529
Silicone No. 2, 1498
Silphen-DM, 509
Siltussin DM Cough Syrup, 568
Silvadene, 1471
Silver sulfadiazine, 1471-1472
Simethicone
antacid combinations, 921-925, 927
antiflatulent, 959
skin cleansers, 1530
Simplet Tablets, 539
Simron, 71
Simvastatin, 448
Sinemet 10-100, 895
Sinemet 25-100, 895
Sinemet 25-250, 895
Sinemet CR, 895
Sine-Off Night Time Formula Sinus, Cold, & Flu Medicine, 540
Sine-Off No-Drowsiness Formula Tablets, 522
Sine-Off Sinus Medicine Tablets, 539
Sinequan, 760
Singlet for Adults Tablets, 539
Singulair, 468
Sinumist-SR, 513
Sinus-Relief Maximum Strength Tablets, 522
Sinustop, 501
Sinutab Non-Drying Liquid Tablets, 525
Sinutab Sinus Allergy, Maximum Strength, 539
Sinutab Sinus Without Drowsiness Maximum Strength Tablets, 522
Sinutab Sinus Without Drowsiness Regular Strength Tablets, 522
SkeeterStik, 1485
Skelaxin, 885
Skeletal muscle relaxants, 885-888
combinations, 889-890
Skelid, 305
Skin cleansers, 1525
astringents, 1526
topical agents, 1527-1532
Skin disorders
topical anesthetics for, 1485-1488
Skin protectants, 1498-1499
Sleep aids
nonprescription, 822-824
Sleepinal Sotfgels, Maximum Strength, 822
Sloan's Liniment, 1515
Slo-Niacin, 14
Slo-Phyllin, 462, 1458
Slo-Phyllin GG Syrup, 521
Slow FE, 71
Slow-K, 41
Slow-Mag, 39

SLT Lotion, 1479
Smoking deterrents, 1715-1718
  bupropion HCl, 1719-1721
Snaplets-FR, 597
Soac-Lens, 1387
Soap-free cleansers, 1525
Soaps
  modified bar, 1525
Sodium
  in antacid combinations, 929
  in electrolyte mixtures, 33
  in laxatives, 977, 978
Sodium acetate, 1431
Sodium acid phosphate and potassium acid phosphate, 1652
Sodium acid phosphate monohydrate, 1219
Sodium alginate, 926
Sodium ascorbate, 75
Sodium benzoate and caffeine, 587
Sodium bicarbonate
  in analgesics, 598, 606
  in antacid combinations, 922, 929
  in antacids, 918
  in douche products, 1425
  in laxatives, 978
  in urinary tract products, 1655
Sodium biphosphate, 1219
Sodium bisulfite
  in anorectal preparations, 1430-1431
  in antifungal combinations, 1135
Sodium C12-14 olefin sulfonate, 1431
Sodium carboxymethylcellulose
  in antidiarrheal combination products, 1016-1017
  in laxative combinations, 998-999
Sodium chloride
  in douche products, 1425
  in nasal products, 517
Sodium citrate, 538
  in antacid combinations, 929
  in antacids, 918
  in upper respiratory combinations, 562
Sodium citrate and citric acid, 1655
Sodium cocoyl isethionate, 1448
Sodium fluoride, 35, 1418
Sodium hypochlorite, 1506
Sodium iodide I 131, 294
Sodium lactate, 1425
Sodium laureth sulfate, 1448
Sodium lauryl sulfate, 1425
Sodium perborate monohydrate, 1425
Sodium peroxyborate monohydrate, 1420
Sodium phenylbutyrate, 126-127
Sodium phosphate
  in bowel evacuation kits, 1005
  in laxatives, 988
Sodium Phosphates, 988
Sodium propionate, 1136
Sodium salicylate, 538
  in analgesics, 602
  in upper respiratory combinations, 562
  in urinary anti-infective combinations, 1220
Sodium stearate, 1136
Sodium Sulamyd, 1366
Sodium sulfacetamide
  in acne products, 1444, 1445
  in ophthalmic anti-infectives, 1372
Sodium Sulfacetamide 10 and Sulfur 5, 1445
Sodium thiosulfate
  in acne products, 1444
  in antifungal combinations, 1136
Sodol Compound, 889
Soft (hydrogel) contact lens products, 1393-1396
Solarcaine, 1485
Solarcaine Aloe Extra Burn Relief, 1485
SolBar PF, 1516-1517
Solganal, 646
Salmeterol xinafoate, 456
Soltice Quick-Rub, 1515
Solu-Cortef, 240
Solu-Medrol, 240
Solurex, 239
Solurex-LA, 239
Soma, 885
Soma Compound, 889
Soma Compound w/Codeine, 889
Somatrem, 229-230
Somatropin, 231-234
Sominex, 822
Sominex, Maximum Strength, 822
Sominex Pain Relief, 822
Soothaderm, 1530
Sorbitol, 1431
Sorbitrate, 337
Soriatane, 1454
Sorine, 379
Sotalol HCl, 379
Span C, 58
Span-FF, 71
Sparfloxacin, 1069
Sparine, 771
Spec-T, 1417
Spec-T Cough Suppressant, 509
Spectazole, 1130
Spectinomycin HCl, 1059-1060
Spectrobid, 1084
Spectrocin, 1098
Spectro-Jel, 1525
Spermicide, 170
Spermicides, 1428-1429
Spironolactone, 320
Spironolactone and hydrochlorothiazide, 327
Spirozide, 327
Sporanox, 1121
Sportscreme, 1514
S-P-T, 299
SSD, 1471
SSD AF, 1471
SSKI, 513
St. Joseph Adult Chewable Aspirin, 601
St. Joseph Aspirin-Free Fever Reducer for Children, 598
St. Joseph Aspirin-Free for Children, 597

St. Joseph Aspirin-Free Infants' Drops, 598
S-T Forte 2 Liquid, 554
Stadol NS, 631
Stahist Tablets, 543
Stamoist E Tablets, 527
Stanozolol, 142
Star-Otic, 1400
Staticin, 1061
Statuss Green Liquid, 555
Stavudine, 1190
Stay Awake, 587
Stearyl alcohol, 1444-1445
Stelazine, 772
Step 2, 1532
Sterapred, 240
SteriNail, 1136
Steroids. see also Adrenal cortical steroids, Anabolic steroids
  in anorectal preparations, 1430
  intranasal, 490-493
  and ophthalmic antibiotic combinations, 1370-1373
Stilphostrol, 1576
Stimate, 226
Stimulant laxatives, 991-994
Sting-Eze, 1502
Sting-Kill, 1485
Stool softeners, 995-997
Stop, 35
Storzine 2, 1319
Streptase, 116
Streptokinase, 116
Streptozocin, 1598-1599
Stri-Dex Cleansing Bar, 1446
Stridex Clear Gel, 1445
Stri-Dex Pads Maximum Strength, 1448
Stri-Dex Pads Oil Fighting Formula, 1448
Stri-Dex Pads Regular Strength, 1448
Stri-Dex Pads Sensitive Skin, 1448
Stromectol, 1207
Strong's Iodine Solution, 297
Strovite Tablets, 49
Stypto-Caine, 1531
Succimer, 1645-1646
Succinimides, 861-863
Sucralfate, 957-958
Sucrets, 1417
Sucrets, Children's, 1417
Sucrets 4-Hour Cough Suppressant, 509
Sucrets Maximum Strength, 1418
Sucrose, 977-978
Sudafed, 501
Sudafed 12 Hour, 501
Sudafed Children's Non-Drowsy Cold & Cough Liquid, 557
Sudafed Cold & Allergy Maximum Strength Tablets, 532
Sudafed Cold & Sinus Non-Drowsy Liqui-Caps, 522
Sudafed Maximum Strength Sinus Nighttime Plus Pain Relief Tablets, 540
Sudafed Multi-Symptom Cold & Cough Liquid Caps, 563
Sudafed Non-Drowsy Non-Drying Sinus Liquid Caps, 525
Sudafed Non-Drowsy Severe Cold Formula Maximum Strength Tablets, 546
Sudafed Sinus Headache Non-Drowsy Tablets, 523
Sudafed Sinus Nighttime Maximum Strength Tablets, 533
Sudal 60/500 Tablets, 526
Sudal-DM Tablets, 569
SudoGest, 501
SudoGest Sinus Maximum Strength Tablets, 523
Sular, 369
Sulconazole, 1132
Sulconazole nitrate, 1131
Sulf-10, 1366
Sulfabenzamide, 1111
Sulfacetamide, 1111
Sulfacetamide sodium
  ophthalmic, 1366
  topical, 1475
Sulfacet-R Lotion, 1445
Sulfadiazine, 1101
Sulfadoxine and pyrimethamine, 1149-1151
Sulfalax Calcium, 995
Sulfamerazine, 1101
Sulfamethazine, 1101
Sulfamethizole
  as sulfonamide, 1101
  in urinary anti-infective combinations, 1219
Sulfamethoxazole
  as sulfonamide, 1101
  in urinary anti-infective combinations, 1219
Sulfamethoxazole and trimethoprim, 1108-1110
Sulfamylon, 1469
Sulfanilamide, 1111
Sulfasalazine, 1101
Sulfathiazole, 1111
Sulfatrim, 1108, 1219
Sulfatrim DS, 1108
Sulfa-Trip, 1111
Sulfinpyrazone, 666-667
Sulfisoxazole
  as sulfonamide, 1101
  in urinary anti-infective combinations, 1219
  in vaginal anti-infectives, 1111
Sulfisoxazole and erythromycin ethylsuccinate, 1104-1107
Sulfoil, 1525
Sulfonamides, 1101-1103
  combinations, 1219
  multiple, 1101
  trimethoprim and sulfamethoxazole, 1108-1110
Sulfonylureas, 278-282
Sulforcin Lotion, 1445
Sulfoxyl Regular, 1435
Sulfoxyl Strong, 1435
Sulfur
  in acne products, 1435, 1440, 1444-1449
  in antiseborrheic combinations, 1479
  in skin cleansers, 1528
Sulfur Soap, 1446
Sulindac, 640
Sulmeprim, 1108
Sulpho-Lac, 1440
Sultrin Triple Sulfa, 1111
Sumatriptan succinate, 683-686
Summer's Eve, 249
Summer's Eve Disposable Douche, 1425
Summer's Eve Medicated Disposable Douche, 1425

INDEX

Summer's Eve Post-Menstrual Disposable Douche, 1425
Summit Extra Strength Coated Tablets, 609
Sumycin 250, 1089
Sumycin 500, 1089
Sumycin Syrup, 1089
Sun Splash, 1518
Sunscreens, 1516-1524
Super B Complex Capsules, 48
Super Calcium 1200, 30
Super Quints B-50 Tablets, 51
Superchar, 1633
Suppap, 598
Suprax, 1037
Suprofen, 1356
Surbex with C Filmtabs, 49
Surbex-T Filmtabs, 49
SureStep, 1763
Surfactant cleaning solutions
  for soft (hydrogel) contact lenses, 1393
Surfak Liquigels, 995
Surmontil, 760
Sustiva, 1195
SU-TUSS DM Liquid, 569
SU-TUSS HD Elixir, 566
Sweet'n fresh clotrimazole-7, 1138
Swim Ear, 1400
Symmetrel, 895, 1167
Sympathomimetics
  as bronchodilators, 455-461
  for glaucoma, 1325-1327
  and xanthine, 521
Synagis, 1256
Synalar, 248
Synalgos-DC Capsules, 626
Synarel, 223
Synemol, 248
Synthetic Conjugated Estrogens, A, 156
Synthroid, 299

T3, 299
T4, 299
Tacrine HCl, 803
Tacrolimus, 1686-1688
Tagamet, 950
Tagamet HB 200, 950
Talacen Caplets, 633
Talc, 1507
Talwin Compound Caplets, 633
Talwin Nx, 633
Tambocor, 352
Tamiflu, 1180
Tamoxifen citrate, 1578
Tamsulosin HCl, 386
Tanac, 1422
Tanafed Suspension, 534
Tannic acid
  in antifungal combinations, 1135
  in mouth and throat products, 1421-1422
  in skin cleansers, 1529
Tannic-12 Suspension, 556
Tannic-12 Tablets, 544
TAO, 1053
Tapanol Extra Strength, 597
Tapazole, 294
Tar derivatives
  in bath products, 1475
  in emollients, 1475-1476
  in shampoos, 1475
Tarsum, 1479
Tartrazine, 1444-1447
Tavist Allergy, 494
Tavist Allergy/Sinus Headache Tablets, 540
Tavist Sinus Maximum Strength Tablets, 523
Taxol, 1615
Tazicef, 1038
Tazarotene, 1464-1466
Tazicef, 1038
Tazidime, 1038
Tazorac, 1464
T/Derm, 1476
Teargen, 1383
Teargen II, 1383
Tearisol, 1383
Tears Naturale, 1383
Tears Naturale Free, 1383
Tears Naturale II, 1383, 1386
Tears Plus, 1383
Tears Renewed, 1383
Tebamide, 690
Tega-Vert, 689
Tegretol, 828
Tegretol-XR, 828
Tegrin, 1475
Tegrin Medicated Advanced Formula, 1475
Telmisartan, 395
Temazepam, 817
Temovate, 247
Temovate E, 247
Tempo, 921
Tempra Drops, 598
Tenecteplase, 116
Tenex, 408
Tenofovir disoproxil fumarate, 1187
Tenoretic 50 Tablets, 430
Tenoretic 100 Tablets, 430
Tenormin, 379
Tensilon, 1647
Tenuate, 579
Tenuate Dospan, 579
Tequin, 1069
Teraseptic, 1525
Terazol 3, 1138
Terazol 7, 1138
Terazosin, 386
Terbinafine, 1132
Terbinafine HCl, 1131
Terbutaline sulfate, 456
Terconazole, 1138
Terra-Cortril Suspension, 1370
Terramycin, 1089
Terramycin with Polymyxin B Sulfate
  as antibiotic, 1098
  as sulfonamide, 1111
Teslac, 1569
Tessalon Perles, 509
Testoderm, 149
Testoderm TTS, 149
Testolactone, 1569
Testopel, 149
Testosterone aqueous, 149
Testosterone cypionate, 149, 161
Testosterone enanthate, 149
Testosterone pellets, 149
Testosterone propionate, 149
Testosterone transdermal, 149
Testred, 149
Tetanus immune globulin (human), 1252
Tetanus toxoid adsorbed, 1264

Tetracaine HCl
for mucous membranes, 1481
in skin cleansers, 1531
for skin disorders, 1486
Tetracyclic compounds, 740-742
Tetracycline HCl
as antibiotic, 1089
for Helicobacter pylori infections, 944-946
topical, 1412-1413
Tetracyclines
systemic, 1089-1093
topical, 1094-1095
Tetrahydrozoline HCl
as decongestant, 502
ophthalmic, 1339, 1343
Tetramune, 1271
Tetrasine, 1339
Tetrasine Extra, 1339
Teveten, 395
T-Gen, 690
Thalidomide, 1736-1739
Thalitone, 323
Thalomid, 1736
Theo-24, 462
Theochron, 462
Theo-Dur, 462
Theolair, 462
Theolair-SR, 462
Theolate Liquid, 521
Theophylline
as bronchodilator, 462
in upper respiratory combinations, 521
Theophylline ethylenediamine, 462
Theo-X, 462
Therac Lotion, 1445
TheraFlu Flu, Cold & Cough and Sore Throat, Maximum Strength Powder, 551
TheraFlu Flu, Cold & Cough Night Time, Maximum Strength Powder, 551
TheraFlu Flu, Cold & Cough Powder, 551
TheraFlu Flu & Cold Medicine for Sore Throat, Maximum Strength Powder, 539
TheraFlu Flu & Cough Night Time, Maximum Strength Powder, 551
TheraFlu Flu & Sore Throat, Maximum Strength Powder, 540
TheraFlu Flu & Sore Throat Night Time, Maximum Strength Powder, 540
TheraFlu Flu and Cold Medicine Original Formula Powder, 539
TheraFlu Maximum Strength Flu, Cold & Cough Powder, 564
TheraFlu Maximum Strength Flu & Congestion Non-Drowsy Powder, 564
TheraFlu Maximum Strength NightTime Formula Flu, Cold & Cough Medicine Tablets, 550
TheraFlu Non-Drowsy Flu, Cold & Cough Maximum Strength Powder, 547
TheraFlu Non-Drowsy Formula Maximum Strength Tablets, 546
Theraflu Severe Cold & Congestion Night Time Maximum Strength Powder, 551
Thera-Flur-N, 35
Thera-gesic, 1514
Thera-Hist Cold & Allergy Syrup, 536
Thera-Hist Cold & Cough Syrup, 560
Thera-Hist Expectorant Chest Congestion Liquid, 528
Theramycin Z, 1061
TheraPatch Vapor Patch for Kids Cough Suppressant, 572
Therapeutic B Complex with C Capsules, 49
Therapeutic Bath, 1499
ThexForte Caplets, 49
Thiabendazole, 1205-1206
Thiamilate, 10
Thiamine
with folic acid, 51-52
nutritional, 6, 10-11, 48-50
Thiazide diuretic and ACEIs, 431-432
Thiazide diuretic and beta-blockers, 430-431
Thiazide diuretic and clonidine, 432
Thiazide diuretic and hydralazine, 430
Thiazide diuretic and prazosin, 432
Thiazide diuretic, reserpine and hydralazine, 430
Thiazide diuretics, 323-326
Thiazide diuretics and methyldopa, 431
Thiazide diuretics and miscellaneous antihypertensives, 432
Thiazide diuretics and reserpine derivatives, 430
Thiazolidinediones, 275-277
Thiethylperazine, 699
Thimerosal, 1505
Thioguanine, 1541
Thioridazine HCl, 771
Thiosulfil Forte, 1101
Thiothixene HCl, 771
Thonzonium bromide, 1397
Thorazine
as antiemetic/antivertigo agent, 699
as antipsychotic, 770
Thorazine Spansules
as antiemetic/antivertigo agent, 699
as antipsychotic, 770
Throat and mouth products, see Mouth and throat products
Throat sprays, 1418
Thrombolytic agents, 116-118
Thyme oil, 1531
Thymoglobulin, 1249
Thymol
in douche products, 1425
in mouth and throat products, 1420, 1422
in mouthwash, 1418
in skin cleansers, 1528
Thyrar, 299
Thyro-Block, 297
Thyroid desiccated, 299
Thyroid drugs
antithyroid agents, 294-296

INDEX

Thyroid drugs *(cont.)*
iodine products, 297-298
Thyroid hormones, 299-301
Thyroid Strong, 299
Thyrolar, 299
L-Thyroxine, 299
Ti•Baby Natural, 1519
Ti•Screen, 1518-1520
Ti•Screen Natural, 1519
Ti•Screen Sports Gel, 1519
Tiagabine, 867-869
Tiamate, 368
Tiazac, 368
Ticlid, 90
Ticlopidine HCl, 90-92
TIG, see Tetanus immune globulin (human)
Tigan, 690
Tikosyn, 349
Tilade, 488
Tiludronate disodium, 305
Time-Hist Capsules, 532
Timolide 10-25 Tablets, 431
Timolol maleate
in antihypertensive combinations, 431
ophthalmic, 1313
systemic, 379
Timolol maleate and dorzolamide HCl, 1332-1334
Timolol maleate/dorzolamide HCl, 1332-1334
Timoptic, 1313
Timoptic in Ocudose, 1313
Timoptic-XE, 1313
Tinactin, 1131
Tinactin for Jock Itch, 1131
TinBen, 1498
TinCoBen, 1498
Tine Test, 1304
Tine Test PPD, 1304
Ting, 1130-1131, 1136
Tinver, 1136
Tinzaparin sodium, 109-110
Tioconazole, 1138
Tisit, 1244
Titanium dioxide
in acne products, 1446
in antifungal combinations, 1136
Titanium dioxide *(cont.)*
in sunscreens, 1516, 1518-1520
Titanium oxide, 1517
Titralac, 922
Titralac Extra Strength, 922
Titralac Plus, 922, 926
Tizanidine, 882-884
TMP-SMZ, see Trimethoprim and sulfamethoxazole
TNKase, 116
TobraDex Suspension, 1370-1371
Tobramycin, 1366, 1370-1371
Tobrex, 1366
Tocainide, 366-367
Tofranil, 760
Tofranil-PM, 760
Tolazamide, 278
Tolbutamide, 278
Tolectin 200, 640
Tolectin 600, 640
Tolectin DS, 640
Tolfrinic Tablets, 76
Tolinase, 278
Tolmetin sodium, 640
Tolnaftate
in antifungal combinations, 1135-1136
in antifungal preparations, 1131-1132
Tolterodine tartrate, 1670-1671
Tolu-Sed DM Liquid, 568
Tom's of Maine Natural Cough & Cold Rub Cough Suppressant, 572
Tonocard, 366
Toothpaste, 1418
Top Care Maximum Strength Flu, Cold & Cough Medicine Night Time Powder, 551
Top Care Maximum Strength Soothing Cough & Head Congestion Relief Liquid, 545
Top Care Multi-Symptom Pain Relief Cold Tablets, 546, 550
Topamax, 858
Topic, 1531
Topical analgesics
capsaicin, 1500-1501
Topical anesthetics
for mucous membranes, 1481-1484
for skin disorders, 1485-1488
Topical antihistamines, 1502-1504
Topical antiseptics, 1505-1506
Topical combinations, 572
Topical germicides, 1505-1506
Topical starch, 1431
Topicort, 248
Topicort LP, 248
Topicycline, 1094
Topiramate, 858-860
Topotecan, 1549
Toprol XL, 379
TOPV, see Poliovirus vaccine, live, oral, trivalent
Toradol, 639
Torecan, 699
Toremifene citrate, 1578
Tornalate, 455
Torsemide, 317
Totacillin, 1084
Total, 1387
Touro Allergy Capsules, 531
Touro CC Tablets, 564
Touro DM Tablets, 569
Touro LA Tablets, 527
T-Phyl, 462
Trac Tabs 2X, 1219
Tracer bG, 1749
Tramadol HCl, 636-637
Trandate, 416
Trandolapril, 390
Transact, 1440
Transderm-Nitro, 338
Transderm-Scop, 689
Trans-Ver-Sal, 1493, 1495
Tranxene, 710
Tranxene-SD, 710
Tranxene-SD Half-Strength, 710
Tranylcypromine sulfate, 743
Trastuzumab, 1629-1630
Travatan, 1322
Travoprost, 1322
Trazodone, 754-756
Trecator-SC, 1222
Trental, 122

Tretinoin
as acne product, 1441-1443
as antineoplastic, 1612-1614
Tri Levlen, 178
Tri Super Flavons, 58
Triacin-C Cough Syrup, 545
Triacting Cold & Allergy Liquid, 536
Tri-Acting Cold & Allergy Syrup, 536
Tri-Acting Cold & Cough Syrup, 560
Triacting Liquid, 528
Triad Capsules, 609
Triam Forte, 241
Triam-A, 241
Triamcin, 241
Triamcinolone, 241
Triamcinolone acetonide
in antifungal combinations, 1135
in glucocorticoids, 241
in inhaled corticosteroids, 471
in intranasal steroids, 490
in mouth and throat products, 1421
in topical corticosteroids, 250
Triamcinolone diacetate, 241
Triamcinolone hexacetonide, 241
Triaminic AM Decongestant, 501
Triaminic AM Non-Drowsy Cough & Decongestant Liquid, 558
Triaminic Chest Congestion Liquid, 528
Triaminic Cold, Cough & Fever Liquid, 561
Triaminic Cold & Allergy Liquid, 536
Triaminic Cold & Cough Liquid, 560
Triaminic Cold & Cough Softchews Tablets, 560
Triaminic Cold & Night Time Cough Liquid, 561
Triaminic Cough & Congestion Liquid, 558
Triaminic Cough & Sore Throat Liquid, 558
Triaminic Cough Softchews Tablets, 560
Triaminic Infant Decongestant, 501
Triaminic Softchews Allergy Sinus & Headache Tablets, 523
Triaminic Softchews Tablets, 536
Triaminic Throat Pain & Cough Softchews Tablets, 557
Triaminic Vapor Patch for Cough, 572
Triaminicin Cold, Allergy, Sinus Medicine Tablets, 539
Triamonide 40, 241
Triamterene, 320
Triamterene and hydrochlorothiazide, 327
Triazolam, 817
Tribasic calcium phosphate, 29
Trichlormethiazide
in antihypertensive combinations, 430
as diuretic, 323
Trichotine Douche, 1425
Trichotine Liquid Douche Concentrate, 1425
Triclosan, 1446, 1448
Tricodene Cough & Cold Liquid, 545
Tricodene Sugar Free Liquid, 548
Tricor, 442
Tricyclic antidepressants, 760-769
Triderm, 250
Tridesilon, 247
Tridione, 847
Tridrate Dry Bowel Cleansing System, 1005
Triethanolamine polypeptide oleate-condensate, 1400
Triethanolamine salicylate
in rubs and liniments, 1514
in sunscreens, 1521
Trifluoperazine HCl, 772
Trifluorothymidine, see Trifluridine
Triflupromazine HCl
as antiemetic/antivertigo agent, 699
as antineoplastic, 772
Trifluridine, 1376
TriHemic 600 Tablets, 77, 78
Trihexy-2, 892
Trihexy-4, 892
Trihexyphenidyl HCl, 892
Tri-Hydroserpine Tablets, 430
Tri-Immunol, 1264
Tri-K, 41
Trilafon, 699, 771
Trileptal, 849
Trilisate, 602
Trimazide, 690
Trimethadione, 847
Trimethobenzamide HCl, 690
Trimethoprim, 1096-1097, 1219
Trimethoprim and sulfamethoxazole, 1108-1110
Trimipramine maleate, 760
Trimox, 1084
Trimox Pediatric Drops, 1084
Trinalin Repetabs Tablets, 534
Tri-Norinyl, 178
Trinsicon Capsules, 77-78
Triostat, 299
Triotann Pediatric Suspension, 535
Triotann-S Pediatric Suspension, 535
Trioxsalen, 1460
Tripedia, 1264
Tripelennamine HCl, 1502
Triphase oral contraceptives, 178
Triphasil, 178
Triple antibiotics, 1099
Triple Sulfa, 1101
Triple sulfa, 1111
Triple Sulfa No. 2, 1101
Triprolidine HCl, 533, 545
Triprolidine HCl w/Pseudoephedrine HCl Syrup, 533
Triptone, 689
Tri-Screen, 1522
Trisodium EDTA, 1448
Trisoralen, 1460

INDEX

Tristoject, 241
Tritec, 942
Tri-Tinic Capsules, 77
Tri-Vi-Sol Drops, 47
Trivora, 178
Trizivir, 1190
Trobicin, 1059
Trocaine, 1418
Troleandomycin, 1053
Tronolane, 1430, 1431
Tronothane HCl, 1485
Tropicacyl, 1345
Tropicamide, 1345
Trovafloxacin mesylate, 1069
Trovan, 1069
Trusopt, 1330
Trysul, 1111
T-Stat, 1061
Tuberculin, 1304
Tuberculin PPD multiple puncture device, 1304
Tuberculin purified protein derivative, 1304
Tuberculin tests, 1304-1305
Tubersol, 1304
Tucks, 1431
Tucks Hemorrhoidal, 1527
Tucks Take-Alongs, 1431
Tuinal 100 mg Pulvules, 812
Tuinal 200 mg Pulvules, 812
Tums, 30, 917
Tums 500, 30
Tums 500 E-X, 30
Tums 500 E-X Sugar Free, 30
Tums E-X, 917
Tums Ultra, 30, 917
Tur-bi-kal, 501
Tussafed Ex Syrup, 563
Tussafed HC Syrup, 566
Tussafed Syrup, 548
Tussafed-LA Tablets, 565
Tuss-DM Tablets, 569
Tussend Syrup, 555
Tussend Tablets, 555
Tussex Cough Syrup, 563
Tussi-12 S Suspension, 556
Tussi-12 Tablets, 544
TUSSI-bid Tablets, 570
Tussigon Tablets, 553
Tussionex Pennkinetic Suspension, 555
Tussi-Organidin NR Liquid, 567
Tussi-Organidin-DM NR Liquid, 568
Tussi-Organidin-S-NR Liquid, 567
Tussirex Sugar Free Liquid, 562
Tussirex Syrup, 562
Tusstat, 509, 689, 891
T-Vites Tablets, 49
Twice-A-Day 12 Hour, 501
Twilite, 822
Twinrix, 1293
Tylenol Allergy Sinus, Maximum Strength, 539
Tylenol Allergy Sinus NightTime, Maximum Strength Tablets, 540
Tylenol Caplets, 597
Tylenol Children's Cold Chewable Tablets, 541
Tylenol Children's Cold Liquid, 541
Tylenol Children's Cold Plus Cough Chewable Tablets, 559
Tylenol Children's Cold Plus Cough Suspension, 560
Tylenol Children's Flu Suspension, 561
Tylenol Children's Sinus Suspension, 523
Tylenol Cold Complete Formula Tablets, 550
Tylenol Cold Non-Drowsy Formula, 546
Tylenol Extended Relief, 597
Tylenol Extra Strength, 597, 598
Tylenol Flu Maximum Strength Non-Drowsy Gelcaps, 546
Tylenol Flu NightTime, Maximum Strength Gelcaps, 540
Tylenol Flu NightTime, Maximum Strength Liquid, 552
Tylenol Infant's Cold Concentrated Drops, 523
Tylenol Infants' Cold Decongestant & Fever Reducer Plus Cough Concentrated Drops, 557
Tylenol Infants' Drops, 598
Tylenol Junior Strength, 597
Tylenol Multi-Symptom Cold Severe Congestion Tablets, 564
Tylenol PM Extra Strength, 529
Tylenol PM Geltabs, Extra Strength, 822
Tylenol Regular Strength, 597
Tylenol Severe Allergy Tablets, 529
Tylenol Sinus NightTime, Maximum Strength Tablets, 541
Tylenol Sinus Non-Drowsy Maximum Strength, 523
Tylenol w/Codeine Elixir, 623
Tylenol w/Codeine No. 2, 623
Tylenol w/Codeine No. 3, 623
Tylenol w/Codeine No. 4, 624
Tylox Capsules, 627
Tympagesic, 1400
Tyrosum Cleanser Liquid and Packets, 1448
Tyzine, 502
Tyzine Pediatric, 502

UAA, 1220
Ultra Derm, 1498-1499
Ultra Mide 25, 1496
Ultra Tears, 1383
ULTRAbrom Capsules, 531
ULTRAbrom PD Capsules, 536
Ultralente Insulin, 264
Ultram, 636
Ultrase Capsules, 961
Ultrase MT 18 Capsules, 961
Ultrase MT 20 Capsules, 961
Ultravate, 248
Ultrazyme, 1393
Undecylenic acid, 1132, 1135-1136
Undecylenic acid and derivatives, 1131
Unguentine, 1531
Unguentine Plus, 1485

Uni-Ace, 598
Uni-Dur, 462
Unifiber, 977
Unilax Capsules, 998
Uniphyl, 462
Unisol, 1393
Unisol 4, 1393
Unisom Nighttime Sleep Aid, 822
Unisom SleepGels, Maximum Strength, 822
Unisom with Pain Relief, 822
Univasc, 390
Unoprostone isopropyl, 1322
Upper respiratory combinations, 518-572
Uracid, 1507
Urea
  in anorectal preparations, 1430
  in emollients, 1496
  in mouth and throat products, 1420
  in topical corticosteroids, 254
Ureacin-10, 1496
Ureacin-20, 1496
Urecholine, 1658
Urex, 1209
Uridon Modified, 1220
Urimar-T, 1219
Urinary Abtiseptic No. 2, 1220
Urinary anti-infectives
  combinations, 1219-1221
  fosfomycin tromethamine, 1212-1213
  methenamine, 1209-1211
  methenamine salts, 1209-1211
  nalidixic acid, 1214-1215
  nitrofurantoin, 1216-1218
Urinary tract infection tests, 1769-1770
Urinary tract products
  acetohydroxamic acid, 1650-1651
  acidifiers, 1652-1654
  alkalinizers, 1655-1657
  bethanechol chloride, 1658-1659
Urinary tract products *(cont.)*
  cellulose sodium phosphate, 1660-1661
  cysteamine bitartrate, 1662-1663
  dimethyl sulfoxide, 1664-1665
  flavoxate, 1666-1667
  oxybutynin chloride, 1668-1669
  phenazopyridine HCl, 1672-1673
  tolterodine tartrate, 1670-1671
Urine tests, 1771-1773
Urised, 1220
Urisedamine, 1219
Urispas, 1666
Uristat, 1672
Uristix, 1771
Uristix 4, 1771
Uritin, 1220
Urobak, 1101
Urobiotic-250, 1219
Urocit-K, 1655
Urofollitropin, 207-208
Urogesic, 1672
Urogesic Blue, 1219
Uro-Mag, 39, 918
Uro-Phosphate, 1219
Uroplus DS, 1108
Uroplus SS, 1108
Uroquid-Acid No.2, 1219
Ursodeoxycholic acid, 973
Ursodiol, 973
UTI, 1769

Vaccines
  active agents, 1258-1261
  diphtheria, tetanus, pertussis, 1264-1267
  diphtheria, tetanus, pertussis, hemophilus b, 1271-1272
  hemophilus b, 1268-1270
  hepatitis A, 1286-1288
  hepatitis A/hepatitis B, 1293-1295
  hepatitis B, 1289-1292
  influenza, 1282-1285
  lyme disease, 1299-1301
Vaccines *(cont.)*
  measles, mumps and rubella virus, 1277-1279
  pneumococcal, 1296-1298
  pneumococcal 7-valent conjugate, 1302-1303
  polio, 1273-1276
  rabies, 1262-1263
  varicella, 1280-1281
Vagifem, 155
Vaginal antifungals, 1138-1140
Vaginal anti-infectives, 1111-1113
  combinations, 1111
Vaginal preparations
  douche products, 1425-1427
Vaginal sponge, 170
Vagisec Plus, 1111
Vagisil, Maximum Strength, 1481
Vagisil, New Improved, 1481
Vagistat-1, 1138
Valacyclovir, 1164
Valentine, 587
Valergen 20, 155
Valergen 40, 155
Valium
  as antianxiety agent, 710
  as muscle relaxant, 885
Valproic acid, 872-875
Valrelease, 710
Valrubicin, 1567-1568
Valsartan, 395
Valstar, 1567
Valtrex, 1164
Vancenase AQ 84 Nasal, 490
Vancenase AQ Nasal, 490
Vancenase Nasal Inhaler, 490
Vanceril, 471
Vanceril Double Strength, 471
Vancocin, 1063
Vancoled, 1063
Vancomycin, 1063-1065
Vanex HD Liquid, 554
Vaniqa, 1533
Vanoxide-HC, 1435
Vanoxide-HC Lotion, 254
Vanquish Caplets, 610

INDEX

Vantin, 1038
VAQTA, 1286
Varicella vaccine, 1258
Varicella virus vaccine, live, 1280-1281
Varicella-zoster immune globulin (human), 1252
Varivax, 1280
Vascor, 368
Vaseretic 10-25 Tablets, 432
Vasocidin, 1372
VasoClear, 1339
VasoClear A, 1343
Vasocon Regular, 1339
Vasocon-A, 1343
Vasoconstrictors
 local in anorectal preparations, 1431
Vasodilan, 375
Vasopressor/antihypotensive agents
 midodrine, 707-709
Vasotec, 390
Vasotec I.V., 390
V-Dec-M Tablets, 527
Vectrin, 1089
Veetids, 1085
Velosef, 1039
Velosulin BR, 264
Venlafaxine HCl, 757-759
Venoglobulin-S, 1250
Ventolin, 455
Ventolin Nebules, 455
Ventolin Rotocaps, 455
VePesid, 1554
Veracolate Tablets, 999
Verapamil HCl, 369
Verelan, 369
Verelan PM, 369
Vermox, 1201
Verr-Canth, 1489
Versacaps Capsules, 526
Verteporfin, 1380-1382
Vesanoid, 1612
Vesprin, 699, 772
Vexol, 1348
Viagra, 1724
Vibramycin, 1089
Vibra-Tabs, 1089
Vicks 44D Cough & Head Congestion Relief Liquid, 545
Vicks 44E Cough & Chest Congestion Relief Liquid, 568
Vicks 44M Cough, Cold, & Flu Relief Liquid, 549
Vicks Children's NyQuil Cold/Cough Relief Liquid, 560
Vicks Chloraseptic, 1417
Vicks DayQuil LiquiCaps Multi-Symptom Cold/ Flu Relief Capsules, 546
Vicks DayQuil Multi-Symptom Cold/Flu Relief Liquid, 545
Vicks NyQuil Cough Syrup, 552
Vicks NyQuil Multi-Symptom Cold & Flu Relief LiquiCaps Capsules, 552
Vicks NyQuil Multi-Symptom Cold/Flu Relief Capsules, 552
Vicks Pediatric 44E Cough & Chest Congestion Relief Liquid, 571
Vicks Pediatric 44M Cough & Cold Relief Liquid, 560
Vicks Sinex, 501
Vicks Sinex 12 Hour, 501
Vicks VapoRub, 1515
Vicks VapoRub Cream, 572
Vicodin ES Tablets, 626
Vicodin Tablets, 625
Vicodin Tuss Syrup, 570
Vicon-C Capsules, 49
Vidarabine, 1376
Vi-Daylin ADC Oral Solution, 47
Videx, 1190
Videx EC, 1190
Vinegar, 1425
Vinorelbine tartrate, 1556-1557
Viogen-C Capsules, 49
Vioxx, 640
Vira-A, 1376
Viracept, 1182
Viramune, 1195
Virazole, 1173
Viread, 1187
Virilon, 149
Viroptic, 1376
Visine, 1339
Visine Allergy Relief, 1343
Visine L.R., 1339
Visine Moisturizing, 1339
Visken, 379
Vistaril
 as antianxiety agent, 719
 as antihistamine, 495
Vistide, 1170
Visudyne, 1380
Vita-Bee w/C Captabs, 49
Vita-C, 20
Vitamin(s), 3-6
 combinations calcium and vitamin D, 53-54
  vitamin B, 48 vitamin B with folic acid, 51-52
  vitamins A and D, 47
  vitamins B and C, 49-50
 fat-soluble, 6
 iron with, 76
 water-soluble, 6
Vitamin A
 in emollients, 1496
 nutritional, 6-9, 47
Vitamin A & D Tablets, 47
Vitamin A and Beta Carotene, 7
Vitamin A Palmitate, 7
Vitamin B
 with folic acid, 51-52
 nutritional, 6, 10-11, 48-50
Vitamin B_1, 48-50, 77
Vitamin B_2, 6, 12-13, 48-49 50, 77
Vitamin B_3, 14-16, 48-50, 77
Vitamin B_5, 48-50
Vitamin B_6, 6, 18-19, 48-50
Vitamin B_{12}
 with iron, 77-80
 nutritional, 48-50, 76, 85-87
Vitamin B_{12} with Folic Acid Tablets, 51
Vitamin B-100 Complex Tablets, 51
Vitamin C
 with iron, 75
 nutritional, 6, 20-22, 48-50, 76-78
Vitamin D
 calcium and, 53-54
 in emollients, 1496
 nutritional, 6, 23-26, 47
Vitamin D_2, 23
Vitamin D_3, 23

Vitamin E
in emollients, 1496
nutritional, 6, 27-28
Vitamin E 400 I.U., 27
Vitamin E 1000 I.U., 27
Vitamin E acetate, 1446
Vitamin K
as antihemorrhagic, 124-125
nutritional, 6
Vita-Plus E, 27
Vite E, 1496
Vitec, 1496
Vitelle Lurline PMS Tablets, 608
Vitravene, 1378
Vitron-C Tablets, 75
Vitron-C-Plus Tablets, 75
Vivactil, 760
Vivarin, 587
Vivelle, 155
Vivelle-Dot, 155
Volmax, 455
Voltaren
ophthalmic, 1356
oral, 638
Voltaren-XR, 638
VoSol HC, 1400
VoSol HC Otic, 1400
VoSol Otic, 1400
V.V.S., 1111
Vytone Cream, 254
VZIG, see Varicella-zoster immune globulin (human)

Warfarin sodium, 111
Wart-Off Maximum Strength, 1493
Water-soluble vitamins, 6
WCS-90, 1506
Welchol, 435
Wellbutrin, 724
Wellbutrin SR, 724
Wellcovorin, 83
Westcort, 249
Wet-N-Soak, 1390
Wet-N-Soak Plus, 1387, 1390
Wetting & Soaking, 1387
Wetting solutions
for hard contact lenses, 1387
Wetting/soaking solutions
for hard contact lenses, 1387
Wheat bran, 977
White Cloverine Salve, 1498
White petrolatum, see Petrolatum
Whitfield's, 1136
Wigraine, 668
WinRho SDF, 1252
Winstrol, 142
Witch hazel, 1527
in acne products, 1444, 1447
in anorectal preparations, 1431
Women's Tylenol Multi-Symptom Menstrual Relief Caplets, 609
Wondra, 1498
Wygesic Tablets, 629
Wysteria oil, 1530
Wytensin, 401

Xalatan, 1322
Xanax, 710
Xanthine combinations, 521
Xanthine derivatives, 462-467
Xanthine-sympathomimetic combinations, 521
Xeloda, 1546
Xenical, 1025
Xerac, 1440
Xerac AC, 1449
Xiral Tablets, 543
Xopenex, 455
X-Prep Bowel Evacuant Kit-1, 1005
X-Prep Bowel Evacuant Kit-2, 1005
X-Prep Senna Liquid Bowel Evacuant, 1005
X-Seb T Pearl, 1479
X-Seb T Plus, 1479
Xylocaine
for mucous membranes, 1481
for skin disorders, 1485
Xylocaine 10 Oral, 1481
Xylocaine Viscous, 1481
Xylocaine-MPF, 1481
Xylometazoline HCl, 502

Yellow wax, 1528
Yocon, 1727
Yohimbine, 1727-1728
Yohimex, 1727

Zaditor, 1364
Zafirlukast, 468
Zagam, 1069
Zalcitabine, 1190
Zanaflex, 882
Zanamivir, 1178-1179
Zanosar, 1598
Zantac, 950
Zantac 75, 950
Zantac 150, 950
Zantac 150 EFFERdose, 950
Zantac 300, 950
Zantryl, 579
Zarontin, 861
Zaroxolyn, 323
Z-Cof DM Syrup, 564
Zeasorb-AF, 1130
Zebeta, 379
Zefazone, 1037
Zemplar, 23
Zephiran, 1505
Zerit, 1190
Zestoretic Tablets, 432
Zestril, 390
Zetar, 1475
Ziac Tablets, 431
Ziagen, 1190
Zidovudine, 1190
Zidovudine/Lamivudine, 1190
Zidovudine/Lamivudine/Abacavir Sulfate, 1190
Zilactin, 1416
Zilactin-L, 1485
Zileuton, 468
Zinacef, 1039
Zinc
in lozenges, 1417
nutritional, 5, 45-46
Zinc 15, 45
Zinc acetate
in poison ivy treatment products, 1512
in topical antihistamines, 1502
Zinc chloride
in antifungal combinations, 1135
in mouth and throat products, 1422
Zinc gluconate, 45
Zinc oxide, 1528
in acne products, 1444

INDEX

Zinc oxide *(cont.)*
- in anorectal preparations, 1430-1431
- in antifungal combinations, 1136
- in diaper rash products, 1507
- in emollients, 1497
- in poison ivy treatment products, 1512
- in skin cleansers, 1528-1531
- in sunscreens, 1517, 1519
- in topical antihistamines, 1502

Zinc phenolsulfonate, 1016
Zinc stearate, 1136
Zinc sulfate
- nutritional, 45
- in ophthalmic decongestant combinations, 1343

Zinc sulfocarbolate, 1016
Zinc-220, 45
Zincate, 45
Zincfrin, 1343
Zincon, 1475
Zinecard, 1639
Ziradryl, 1502
Zirconium oxide, 1502
Zithromax, 1052
Zocor, 448
Zofran, 696
Zofran ODT, 696
Zoladex, 1587
Zoledronic acid, 305
Zolmitriptan, 687-688
Zoloft, 752
Zolpidem tartrate, 817
Zometa, 305
Zomig, 687
Zonalon, 1502
Zone-A Forte Lotion, 254
Zonegran, 852
Zonisamide, 852-854
Zonite Douche, 1425
ZORprin, 601
Zostrix, 1500
Zostrix-HP, 1500
Zoto-HC Ear Drops, 1400
Zovia 1/35E, 177
Zovia 1/50E, 177
Zovirax, 1164
ZTuss Expectorant Liquid, 566
Zyban, 1719
Zydone Capsules, 625
Zyflo Filmtabs, 468
Zyloprim, 655
Zymase Capsules, 962
Zyprexa, 787
Zyprexa Zydis, 787
Zyrtec, 494
Zyrtec-D 12 Hour Tablets, 532
Zyvox, 1066